WILLARD AND SPACKMAN'S

Occupational Therapy

WILLARD AND SPACKMAN'S

Occupational Therapy

EIGHTH EDITION

HELEN L. HOPKINS
EdD, OTR/L, FAOTA

Professor Emeritus
Temple University
College of Allied Health Professions
Department of Occupational Therapy
Philadelphia, Pennsylvania

HELEN D. SMITH
MOT, OTR/L, FAOTA

Associate Professor
Tufts University–Boston School of Occupational Therapy
Medford, Massachusetts

65 CONTRIBUTORS

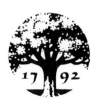

J. B. Lippincott Company
Philadelphia

Sponsoring Editor: Andrew Allen
Editorial Assistant: Miriam Benert
Project Editor: Mary Rose Muccie
Indexer: Alexandra Nickerson
Text Designer: Susan Hess Blaker
Cover Designer: Louis Fuiano

Art Director: Susan Hermansen
Production Manager: Helen Ewan
Production Coordinator: Kathryn Rule
Compositor: Circle Graphics
Printer/Binder: Courier Westford

8th Edition

3 5 6 4 2

Library of Congress Cataloging-in-Publication Data

Willard and Spackman's occupational therapy.—8th ed. / edited by
    Helen L. Hopkins, Helen D. Smith.
        p.   cm.
    Includes bibliographical references and index.
    ISBN 0-397-54877-X
    1. Occupational therapy.   I. Willard, Helen S.   II. Spackman,
Clare S.   III. Hopkins, Helen L.   IV. Smith, Helen D.   V. Title:
Occupational therapy.
RM735.W54   1993
615.8'515—dc20   92-32917
                                                                CIP

Any procedure or practice described in this book should be applied by the health-care practitioner
under appropriate supervision in accordance with professional standards of care used with regard to
the unique circumstances that apply in each practice situation. Care has been taken to confirm the
accuracy of information presented and to describe generally accepted practices. However, the authors,
editors, and publisher cannot accept any responsibility for errors or omissions or for any consequences
from application of the information in this book and make no warranty, express or implied, with
respect to the contents of the book.

Every effort has been made to ensure drug selections and dosages are in accordance with current
recommendations and practice. Because of ongoing research, changes in government regulations and
the constant flow of information on drug therapy, reactions and interactions, the reader is cautioned to
check the package insert for each drug for indications, dosages, warnings and precautions, particularly
if the drug is new or infrequently used.

To our families, friends, coworkers, and students,
with appreciation for their support and understanding,
and
to all past, present, and future occupational therapists.

Give a man a fish, and you feed him for a day. Teach a man to fish, and you feed him for a lifetime. —Chinese proverb

CONTRIBUTORS

Jane E. Johnston Allinder, BS, OTR/L
Occupational Therapist
Colerain School
Columbus, Ohio

Judith Atkins, BS, OTR
Supervisor, Occupational Therapy
Riley Hospital for Children
Indiana University Medical Center
Indianapolis, Indiana

Beverly K. Bain, EdD, OTR
Associate Adjunct Faculty and Coordinator
    of RSA Technology Grant
New York University, School of Education, Health, Nursing
    and Arts Professions
Department of Occupational Therapy
New York, New York

Olga Baloueff, MS, OTR/L
Associate Professor
Tufts University–Boston School of Occupational Therapy
Medford, Massachusetts

Nancy L. Beck, MA, OTR/L
Director of Rehabilitative Services
Belmont Center for Comprehensive Treatment
Philadelphia, Pennsylvania

David W. Beer, MA, PhD (candidate)
Adjunct Assistant Professor
University of Illinois at Chicago
College of Associated Health Professions
Department of Occupational Therapy
Chicago, Illinois

Florence Clark, PhD, OTR, FAOTA
Professor and Chair
University of Southern California
Department of Occupational Therapy
Los Angeles, California

Ellen S. Cohn, EdM, OTR/L
Academic Fieldwork Coordinator
Tufts University–Boston School of Occupational Therapy
Medford, Massachusetts

Mary A. Corcoran, PhD, OTR/L
Assistant Professor
Thomas Jefferson University
College of Allied Health Sciences
Department of Occupational Therapy
Philadelphia, Pennsylvania

Kathleen Hilko Culler, MS, OTR/L
Clinical Education Coordinator/Clinical Specialist
Rehabilitation Institute of Chicago
Department of Occupational Therapy
Chicago, Illinois

Mary Margaret Daub, EdM, OTR/L
Associate Professor
Temple University
College of Allied Health Professions
Department of Occupational Therapy
Philadelphia, Pennsylvania

Jean C. Deitz, PhD, OTR, FAOTA
Associate Professor
University of Washington
Department of Rehabilitation Medicine
Division of Occupational Therapy
Seattle, Washington

Rebecca Dutton, MA, OTR/L
Assistant Professor
Department of Occupational Therapy
Kean College of New Jersey
Union, New Jersey

Joyce M. Engel, PhD, OTR
Assistant Professor
University of Wisconsin, Madison
Department of Therapeutic Sciences
Occupational Therapy Program
Madison, Wisconsin

Cynthia F. Epstein, MA, OTR, FAOTA
Executive Director
Occupational Therapy Consultants, Inc.
Bridgewater, New Jersey

Rhoda P. Erhardt, MS, OTR/L, FAOTA
Consultant in Pediatric Occupational Therapy
Maplewood, Minnesota

Shereen D. Farber, PhD, OTR, FAOTA
Consultant in Private Practice
Neurorehabilitation Services and Sports Medicine Staff
World Skating Academy at PAN AM Plaza
Indianapolis, Indiana

Elaine Ewing Fess, MS, OTR, FAOTA, CHT
Director, Hand Research
Zionville, Indiana

Maureen Hayes Fleming, EdD, OTR/L, FAOTA
Associate Professor
Tufts University–Boston School of Occupational Therapy
Medford, Massachusetts

Linda L. Florey, MA, OTR, FAOTA
Chief, Rehabilitation Services
UCLA Neuropsychiatric Institute and Hospital
Los Angeles, California

Diane Gibson, MA, OTR/L
Former Director of Rehabilitation Services
Sheppard and Enoch Pratt Hospital
Baltimore, Maryland

Laura N. Gitlin, PhD
Associate Professor
Thomas Jefferson University
College of Allied Health Sciences
Philadelphia, Pennsylvania

Ruth Ann Hansen, PhD, OTR, FAOTA
Program Director and Associate Professor
Eastern Michigan University
Department of Associated Health Professions
Occupational Therapy Program
Ypsilanti, Michigan

Betty Risteen Hasselkus, PhD, OTR/L, FAOTA
Assistant Professor and Coordinator
University of Wisconsin, Madison
Department of Therapeutic Sciences
Occupational Therapy Program
Madison, Wisconsin

Judy Hill, BS, OTR
Clinical Manager, Occupational Therapy
Rehabilitation Institute of Chicago
Department of Occupational Therapy
Chicago, Illinois

Helen L. Hopkins, EdD, OTR/L, FAOTA
Professor Emeritus
Temple University
College of Allied Health Professions
Department of Occupational Therapy
Philadelphia, Pennsylvania

Ruth Humphry, PhD, OTR
Associate Professor
University of North Carolina
Medical School
Division of Occupational Therapy
Chapel Hill, North Carolina

Sharon Intagliata, MS, OTR/L
Former Director of Occupational Therapy
Rehabilitation Institute of Chicago
Department of Occupational Therapy
Chicago, Illinois
Independent Consultant, Private Practice
Riverside, Illinois

Karen Jacobs, MS, OTR/L, FAOTA
Assistant Professor
Boston University
Occupational Therapy Program
Boston, Massachusetts

Kaaren Jewell, MEd, OTR
Occupational Therapist
Carrboro Schools
Chapel Hill, North Carolina

Jerry A. Johnson, MBA, EdD, OTR/L, FAOTA
Professor and Graduate Coordinator
Thomas Jefferson University
College of Allied Health Sciences
Department of Occupational Therapy
Philadelphia, Pennsylvania

Nancy Allen Kauffman, EdM, OTR/L
Occupational Therapist
Private Practice
Newtown Square, Pennsylvania

Judith H. Kiel, MS, OTR
Associate Professor
Indiana University School of Medicine
Division of Allied Health Sciences
Occupational Therapy Program
Indianapolis, Indiana

Gary Kielhofner, DPH, OTR/L, FAOTA
Professor and Head
University of Illinois at Chicago
College of Associated Health Professions
Department of Occupational Therapy
Chicago, Illinois

Moya Kinnealey, PhD, OTR/L
Assistant Professor
Temple University
College of Allied Health Professions
Department of Occupational Therapy
Philadelphia, Pennsylvania

Susan H. Knox, MA, OTR, FAOTA
Doctoral Candidate
University of Southern California
Pediatric Occupational Therapist
Private Practice
Hollwood, California

Kirsten M. Kohlmeyer, MS, OTR
Acting Clinical Manager
Rehabilitation Institute of Chicago
Occupational Therapy Department
Chicago, Illinois

Lisa A. Kurtz, MEd, OTR/L
Director of Occupational Therapy
Children's Seashore House at Children's Hospital
    of Philadelphia
Philadelphia, Pennsylvania

Elizabeth A. Larson, MS, OTR
Doctoral Student
South Pasadena, California

Cheryl J. Leman, MA, OTR/L
Director, Burn Rehabilitation
Washington Hospital Center
Washington, District of Columbia

Ruth Ellen Levine, EdD, OTR/L, FAOTA
Professor and Chairman
Thomas Jefferson University
College of Allied Health Sciences
Department of Occupational Therapy
Philadelphia, Pennsylvania

Linda L. Levy, MA, OTR/L, FAOTA
Associate Professor
Temple University
College of Allied Health Professions
Department of Occupational Therapy
Philadelphia, Pennsylvania

Jeanne Ericsson Lewin, MS, OTR
Clinical Supervisor, Pediatric Team
Rehabilitation Institute of Chicago
Department of Occupational Therapy
Chicago, Illinois

Gladys Masagatani, MEd, OTR/L, FAOTA
Professor in Occupational Therapy
Eastern Kentucky University
Department of Occupational Therapy
Richmond, Kentucky

Cheryl Mattingly, PhD
Assistant Professor
University of Illinois at Chicago
College of Associated Health Professions
Department of Occupational Therapy
Chicago, Illinois

Lucy J. Miller, PhD, OTR
Executive Director
KID Foundation
Englewood, Colorado

Maureen E. Neistadt, ScD, OTR/L
Assistant Professor
University of New Hampshire
School of Health and Human Services
Department of Occupational Therapy
Durham, New Hampshire

Renee Okoye, MSHS, OTR/L
Occupational Therapist
Private Practice
Massapequa, New York

Lory P. Osorio, MPH, OTR
Executive Director
Stuart Circle Center, Inc.
Richmond, Virginia

Judith M. Perinchief, MS, OTR/L
Assistant Professor and Chairman
Temple University
College of Allied Health Professions
Department of Occupational Therapy
Philadelphia, Pennsylvania

Michael Pizzi, MS, OTR/L
Occupational Therapist
Private Practice
President, Positive Images and Wellness, Inc.
Consultant in Wellness and Health Promotion
Silver Spring, Maryland

Kathlyn L. Reed, PhD, LOTR, MLIS, FAOTA
Education/Information Services Librarian
Houston Academy of Medicine–Texas Medical Center Library
Houston, Texas

Gail Z. Richert, MS, OTR/L
Assistant Director, Rehabilitation Services
Sheppard and Enoch Pratt Hospital
Baltimore, Maryland

Joan C. Rogers, PhD, OTR/L, FAOTA
Professor of Occupational Therapy
Western Psychiatric Institute and Clinic
Pittsburgh, Pennsylvania

Sally E. Ryan, COTA, ROH
Faculty Assistant, Program in Occupational Therapy
College of St. Catherine
St. Paul, Minnesota

Jannette K. Schkade, PhD, OTR
Associate Professor
Texas Woman's University
School of Occupational Therapy
Dallas, Texas

Sally Schultz, PhD, OTR
Associate Professor
Texas Woman's University
School of Occupational Therapy
Denton, Texas

Sharan L. Schwartzberg, EdD, OTR/L, FAOTA
Professor and Chair
Tufts University–Boston School of Occupational Therapy
Medford, Massachusetts

Carole J. Simon, MS, OTR/L
Assistant Professor
Temple University
College of Allied Health Professions
Department of Occupational Therapy
Philadelphia, Pennsylvania

Helen D. Smith, MOT, OTR/L, FAOTA
Associate Professor
Tufts University–Boston School of Occupational Therapy
Medford, Massachusetts

Elinor Anne Spencer, MA, OTR/L, FAOTA
Director of Occupational Therapy Services
Blue Hill Memorial Hospital
Blue Hill, Maine

Ellen Dunleavey Taira, MPH, OTR/L
Director, Occupational Therapy
United Presbyterian Residence
Woodbury, New York

Sallie Elizabeth Taylor, MEd, OTR
Director, Evaluation and Rehabilitation Services
Health Line Corporate Health Services, Metro St. Louis, Inc.
St. Louis, Missouri

Marty Torrance, MS, OTR
Supervisor, Adult Service
Occupational Therapy Department
Indiana University Medical Center
Indianapolis, Indiana

Hilda P. Versluys, MEd, OTR/L
Assistant Professor
Tufts University–Boston School of Occupational Therapy
Medford, Massachusetts

PREFACE

Willard and Spackman's Occupational Therapy has, over the years, been a textbook written primarily for occupational therapy students. In preparation for this eighth edition and to evaluate the textbook's usefulness for students, questionnaires were sent during the summer of 1990 to all professional and technical educational programs in occupational therapy in the United States and to some educational programs in other countries. Detailed comments and constructive criticism were received from numerous programs and individual faculty members. As a result of the information received, changes and additions have been made to this edition.

This text uses a traditional approach to the dissemination of knowledge and assumes that students using this text will have had basic courses in the biologic and behavioral sciences. It is organized to cover major aspects of theory and practice in occupational therapy. This edition also reflects the growth of knowledge and new innovations in the field, including the beginning of the development of an academic discipline (Occupational Science) and the use of clinical reasoning for decision making in occupational therapy practice. Part I of the text deals with professional issues and Part II deals with practice issues. Ninety percent of the content is new and the remaining 10% has been revised and updated.

Part I, "Professional Issues," has five units. Unit I, "History and Philosophy," is an introduction to the field that considers the perspectives of both the occupational therapist and the occupational therapy assistant and includes chapters on the history of occupational therapy, developing an academic discipline, knowledge bases and specialized knowledge bases for occupational therapy, and the current basis for theory and philosophy in occupational therapy. Unit II, "Occupational Therapy Assessment and Treatment," includes chapters on occupational therapy assessment, performance areas, and tools of practice. Unit III includes information on the health care system. Unit IV covers the management aspects of occupational therapy and Unit V describes the various aspects of research in occupational therapy.

Part II, "Practice Issues: Occupational Therapy Intervention Across the Life Span," has five units. Unit VI discusses the implementation of occupational therapy in pediatrics. Unit VII contains chapters on the implementation of occupational therapy with adults and Unit VIII discusses the implementation of occupational therapy in geriatrics. Unit IX covers various environments for practice and Unit X discusses aspects of clinical reasoning in occupational therapy.

The appendices include selected official documents of the American Occupational Therapy Association to assist the reader in understanding the scope and practice of occupational therapy. These include the Code of Ethics, Standards of Practice, Uniform Terminology, Guidelines for Occupational Therapy Documentation, and Entry-Level Role Delineation. The appendices also include the Application of Uniform Terminology to Practice and the Hierarchy of Competencies Relating to the Use of Standardized Instruments and Evaluation Techniques by Occupational Therapists.

In our attempt to provide comprehensive coverage of occupational therapy, we have included work from 65 contributors, each with expertise in their area of practice. Fifty of these contributors are new and 15 have contributed to the previous edition. Of these contributors, 37 are educators, and 28 are clinicians, 8 of whom are in private practice. Two of the educators are anthropologists, one is a sociologist, one is a research librarian, and one is a graduate student. The contributors represent a wide geographic distribution, coming from 21 states and the District of Columbia. We thank them for their excellent contributions and for their assistance in providing a comprehensive overview of occupational therapy.

We thank Sarah D. Hertfelder and the Practice Division of the American Occupational Therapy Association for assisting us in identifying experts in specialized areas of practice. We also thank Andrew Allen of the J.B. Lippincott Company for his assistance and encouragement and Mary Rose Muccie and Miriam Benert for their editorial assistance. Thanks is also given to our families and friends, who provided moral support.

HELEN L. HOPKINS, EDD, OTR/L, FAOTA
HELEN D. SMITH, MOT, OTR/L, FAOTA

CONTENTS

WILLARD AND SPACKMAN'S

Occupational Therapy

PART I

Professional issues

UNIT I

History and philosophy

CHAPTER 1

An introduction to occupational therapy

SECTION 1A
Scope of occupational therapy

HELEN L. HOPKINS

KEY TERMS

Accreditation

Certification

Continuing Education

Essentials

Licensure

Occupational Science

Performance Areas

Performance Components

LEARNING OBJECTIVES

Upon completion of this section the reader will be able to:
1. *Define occupational therapy.*
2. *Describe the performance areas and performance components included within the parameters of occupational therapy.*
3. *Describe the varying locations for the practice of occupational therapy.*
4. *Describe the significance of the "Essentials."*
5. *Differentiate among accreditation, certification, licensure, and continuing education and describe the focus of each.*
6. *Describe the role of the American Occupational Therapy Association and the advantages of membership in the association.*

One of the American Occupational Therapy Association's founders, Dr. William Rush Dunton, Jr., stated, " . . . occupation is as necessary to life as food and drink" (Dunton, 1919). This was reiterated by Mary Reilly when she stated, "Man through the use of his hands as they are energized by mind and will can influence the state of his own health" (Reilly, 1962). When the National Society for the Promotion of Occupational Therapy (forerunner of the American Occupational Therapy Association) was established in 1917, the objectives of the association, as noted in the Constitution, were "the advancement of occupation as a therapeutic means, *the study of the effects of occupation upon the human being* and the dissemination of scientific knowledge of the subject" (Constitution of the National Society for the Promotion of Occupational Therapy, 1917). The objectives have remained the same throughout the history of the association. It is only now, with the development of a doctoral program in **occupational science** at the University of Southern California, that an effort is being made to develop an academic discipline. This discipline will study the effects of occupation on the human being and affirm the premises of both Dunton and Reilly, resulting in recognition of occupational therapy "as a vital area of inquiry" in which it will "achieve its potential as an integrated discipline" (Yerxa, 1991; Clark et al., 1991). (See also Chapter 3.)

Definition of occupational therapy

Over the course of the history of occupational therapy, the professional has been described and defined in many ways (see Chapter 2), but the earliest generally accepted definition was, "Occupational therapy is any activity, mental or physical, medically prescribed and professionally guided to aid a patient in recovery from disease or injury" (McNary, 1947).

As changes occurred in society and the demands for occupational therapy services grew, there was insufficient personnel to meet the needs. Thus, personnel from other disciplines, such as recreational therapy, art therapy, music therapy, and other therapies demanding specialized skills, assumed some of the activities of treatment that once fell within the parameters of occupational therapy,

Attempts were made over the years to modify the definition of occupational therapy to reflect changes that had occurred both in its practice and in its relations with the medical profession. Today, occupational therapists generally receive referrals from physicians and have the prerogative of determining the course of treatment on the basis of their own assessments rather than having treatment prescribed and directed by a physician (as in the early definition). In 1972, a new definition of occupational therapy was accepted by the Delegate Assembly of the American Occupational Therapy Association (AOTA). The current official definition is the following:

> Occupational therapy is the art and science of directing man's participation in selected tasks to restore, reinforce and enhance performance, facilitate learning of those skills and functions essential for adaptation and productivity, diminish or correct pathology, and to promote and maintain health. Its fundamental concern is the capacity, throughout the life span, to perform with satisfaction to self and others those tasks and roles essential to productive living and to the mastery of self and the environment. (Occupational Therapy: Its definition and functions, 1972, p. 204)

As the field of occupational therapy became better known and clarification of our practice was needed for the public, the following dictionary definition was adopted by the Representative Assembly in April 1986:

> Occupational Therapy: Therapeutic use of self-care, work and play activities to increase independent function, enhance development, and prevent disability. May include adaptation of task or environment to achieve maximum independence and to enhance quality of life. (Dictionary Definition, 1986, p. 852)

From these definitions, it can be seen that the major focus of occupational therapy intervention is the ***performance areas*** of self-care, work, and leisure, while consideration is given to the human and nonhuman environment and cultural and social environment within which the person is functioning. To assess and treat persons with performance deficits, the following ***performance components*** must be considered:

1. Sensory motor component: sensory integration (sensory awareness, sensory processing, and perceptual skills) neuromuscular (reflex, range of motion, muscle tone, strength, endurance, postural control, and soft tissue integrity), and motor (activity tolerance, gross motor coordination, crossing the midline, laterality, bilateral integration, praxis, fine motor coordination/dexterity, visual motor integration, and oral motor control)
2. Cognitive integration and cognitive components: level of arousal, orientation, recognition, attention span, memory, sequencing, categorization, concept formation, intellectual operations in space, problem solving, generalization of learning, integration of learning, and synthesis of learning
3. Psychosocial skills and psychological components: psychological (roles, values, interests, initiation of activity, termination of activity, and self-concept), social (social conduct, conversation, and self-expression), and self-management (coping skills, time management, and self-control). (See uniform terminology, Appendix C.)

Location of practice

Traditionally, most occupational therapists and occupational therapy assistants have practiced in institutional settings such as state hospitals, general hospitals, children's hospitals, rehabilitation centers, and schools for special children. With the passing of Public Law 94–142 (1975), which requires that all handicapped children receive free and "appropriate" education in the least restrictive setting and which includes occupational therapy as a "related service," many occupational therapists have been hired to work in the public school system with children with developmental disabilities; learning disabilities; speech, language, and hearing impairment; and physical, emotional, and mental impairment. Public Law 99–457 (1986) is based on the needs of children and families. It provides for early intervention services and includes occupational therapy (Dunn, 1989); thus, new positions have been created in neonatal units of hospitals and in community-based services, where therapists work with at-risk infants. Therefore, the number of therapists working with children has increased, with the result that about one third of all occupational therapists in the United States now work with children in public school systems, special schools, clinics, hospitals, and the community.

Just as both mental hospitals and hospitals for the mentally retarded began to move patients out into community settings, many occupational therapists moved from hospitals to mental health–mental retardation centers in the community. Occupational therapy services were provided in free-standing community centers, in sheltered workshops, in store-front walk-in units, in shelters for the homeless, and in various community living arrangements.

With the inception of the Prospective Payment System and the introduction of diagnostic-related groups (DRGs), which limit payment for a hospital stay according to a specified scale depending on the diagnosis, many patients were discharged sooner and "sicker," creating the need for more occupational therapy services in patients' homes or in long-term care facilities. Patients are admitted to rehabilitation centers before they are able to benefit from these services and are discharged before they are independent, thus requiring occupational therapy services in community agencies, in outpatient work-hardening units, or in patients' homes.

Currently, although occupational therapy services are available in more hospital settings than ever before, the greatest increase in services has been in the area of home care (Dataline, 1986; Devereaux, 1991). Many therapists work for corporations that provide occupational therapy services to hospitals, nursing homes, long-term care facilities, and home care. In addition, many therapists are working in private practice, not only in home care but also in physicians' offices and private practice agencies. Therapists are also working in industry, correctional institutions, hospice programs, and other nontraditional community settings.

Educational requirements for occupational therapists

Over the years, the educational requirements for the registered occupational therapist (OTR) have expanded from a 6- to 12-week course in 1918 to the current requirement of at least a baccalaureate degree, including study of biologic and behavioral sciences, pathologic conditions, and specific occupational therapy techniques. The educational programs must comply with the 1991 ***"Essentials and Guidelines for an Accredited Program for the Occupational Therapist"*** to be accredited by the American Medical Association Committee on Allied Health Education and Accreditation (CAHEA) and the AOTA. After completing a minimum of 6 months of full-time fieldwork, graduates of accredited programs are eligible to take the AOTA Certification Examination to become OTRs. All states that require licensure currently accept the AOTA's examination and educational requirements for state licensure. The required 6 months of full-time fieldwork is felt to provide the transition from the role of student to that of full-fledged professional practitioner. This is discussed further in Section 2 of this chapter.

The educational requirements for the occupational therapy assistant (COTA) are described in part B of this section.

Roles and functions of registered occupational therapists and certified occupational therapy assistants

As the number of COTAs increased and the tasks delegated to them expanded, role and relationship problems and conflicts arose (Hirama, 1986). Thus, in 1963, it became necessary to clarify roles and functions of OTRs and COTAs. In 1967, A Guide for the Supervision of the COTA was established, which stated that the COTA was to be supervised by "an OTR, an experienced COTA or an OTR designate" (Hirama, 1986). There was no further study until Ohio State University conducted a study of job descriptions through task analysis in 1972 (Schoen, 1972). In 1973, the AOTA received a grant to "Delineate Roles and Functions of Occupational Therapy Personnel" to serve as a basis for proficiency examinations (AOTA, 1973). However, it was not until 1981 that the first entry-level role delineation for OTRs and COTAs was approved by the Representative Assembly. In 1991, a new Entry-Level Role Delineation for Registered Occupational Therapists (OTRs) and Certified Occupational Therapy Assistants (COTAs) (AOTA, 1991) was approved by the Representative Assembly. (See Appendix F.) This role delineation should be used as a guideline for *entry-level practice* but should not be considered as a scope-of-practice statement.

Accountability

Because the demand for accountability is a driving force within the health care system today, the health care professions attempt to ensure the competence of practitioners in several ways. To ensure competence of entry-level practitioners, two processes are used to evaluate graduates of the educational programs: **accreditation** and **certification**. To maintain competence for practicing professionals, **continuing education** programs are perhaps the most widely used methods.

Accreditation

Accreditation is the process by which educational programs are evaluated against a set of standards that represent the knowledge, skills, and attitudes needed for competent practice in a specified field. Every occupational therapy program and every occupational therapy assistant program must be accredited every 5 to 8 years by demonstrating that its students are receiving an education that meets the standards specified in the "Essentials." Only those students who have graduated from an accredited occupational therapy program or an approved occupational

therapy assistant program are permitted to take the certification examination that allows them to practice in the field.

Certification

The certification process ensures that each practitioner has the knowledge, skills, and attitudes required for competent practice in the field. It is assumed that passing a written comprehensive examination that covers all aspects of the education of the OTR or COTA will verify that the practitioner has the entry-level knowledge and thus is competent to practice. For this reason, certification examinations have been developed for both levels of practice. To ensure that the practitioner has the skills and attitudes as well as the knowledge, all students are also required to have practical experience (fieldwork) under the supervision of an experienced practitioner. Students from all schools are evaluated using the Fieldwork Evaluation Reports approved by the AOTA in 1983 and 1987 (FWPR to FWE, 1986).

Successful completion of the required fieldwork assignments, along with completion of the didactic and laboratory portions of the educational program, determine eligibility to take the certification examination. This examination is developed by a qualified testing agency, but questions are written and checked for accuracy by practicing OTRs and COTAs. In 1988, an independent certification board, the American Occupational Therapy Certification Board (AOTCB), was established by the Association to reassure the public that the American Occupational Therapy Association is not a "closed shop" and is concerned with the public welfare. The AOTCB is responsible for screening examination questions and assessing the breadth and depth of the test to evaluate the competence of applicants for practice in occupational therapy. The board also can take disciplinary action against practitioners.

Licensure

For many years the American Occupational Therapy Association (AOTA) and most therapists believed that certification was sufficient to ensure competence of its practitioners. In 1974, however, the AOTA moved from a neutral stance to a positive position on **licensure** and encouraged occupational therapists to pursue licensure in their states. At this time, occupational therapy was not widely known by the public or other health care workers; this resulted in low status and prestige for the profession. It was felt that, with licensure, consumers of our services would be better protected and the status of the profession would be improved among third-party payors, thus providing increased coverage of occupational therapy services (Brayley, 1991).

In the late 1970s, several states (Florida, New York, Puerto Rico), feeling that nonqualified people were filling occupational therapy positions and thus putting the health and safety of the consumers at risk, pursued and obtained licensure for occupational therapists in their states. Since that time all but two states have attained some type of regulatory legislation, most having licensure laws. Most states license both OTRs and COTAs. Rules and regulations are developed by each State Licensure Board to clarify and enable enforcement of the law. Licensure allows consumers of OTR and COTA services as well as health care providers the option of filing complaints about the quality of care provided by OTRs and COTAs, and provides disciplinary procedures that can be enforced to protect the public. The AOTCB has developed an "information exchange," which is distributed to the regulatory boards of all states. The Board has also developed the Disciplinary Action Information Exchange Network (DAIEN) and has published a master list of disciplinary actions taken by AOTCB against OTRs, COTAs and occupational therapy students. State regulatory boards are invited to send disciplinary actions they have taken to the AOTCB for inclusion in the periodic DAIEN update so that all states will be informed regarding infringements of certification or licensure to further protect consumers of our services (Baum & Gray, 1991).

To retain competency in practice, practitioners need to update their knowledge and skills periodically. Most states have regulations requiring continued competency of its practitioners and require some method of determining this. One such method is to require practitioners to improve their practice through continuing education.

Continuing education

Since accountability to the public is demanded not only of the entry-level practitioner but of all therapists and assistants in active practice, it is mandatory that practitioners keep pace with changes in society, in medicine, and in the practice of occupational therapy. It is therefore important that all occupational therapists have a commitment to lifelong education.

The AOTA has recognized that opportunities for maintaining skills in traditional areas of practice as well as for gaining skills in new areas are often limited for practitioners because of the expense and availability of courses. For this reason, continuing education has been a high priority for the AOTA, and the Continuing Education Division was created in the national office to meet the needs of all practitioners. This division has provided resources for all members in many areas of practice through the development of "practice packets," which are updated constantly. In addition, the *Occupational Therapy News* publishes lists of continuing education programs conducted throughout the country that are sponsored by the AOTA, state and regional occupational therapy associations, individuals, and private educational agencies.

To provide education for members in developing or expanding areas of practice, the Continuing Education Division of the AOTA has developed courses and training programs in several areas, including "Training: Occupational Therapy Educational Management in Schools" (TOTEMS); "Planning and Implementing Vocational Readiness in Occupational Therapy" (PIVOT); "Role of Occupational Therapy with the Elderly" (ROTE); and "Strategies, Concepts and Opportunities for Program Development and Evaluation in Mental Health" (SCOPE). These courses have been given at numerous locations throughout the country in an attempt to make this information available and affordable to all members. Manuals for each training course are available for purchase by members who are unable to attend.

The Continuing Education Division of the AOTA has also developed a Self-Study Series, including "Assessing Function," "How to Work in the School System," and "Neurosciences Foundation of Human Performance." This division has also developed a workshop series in specialty areas and Re-entry Packets for therapists reentering practice after lengthy absence from practice.

Educational opportunities also are available through many colleges and universities. Some programs are given as continuing education courses, whereas others are given as advanced degrees in special areas of practice or as advanced work in education, administration, or research.

Many books in specialty areas of occupational therapy practice are now being published. These, along with articles in journals such as the *American Journal of Occupational Therapy*, the *Occupational Therapy Journal of Research*, the *Journal of Occupational Therapy in Health Care*, and special-interest newsletters, make information available to all members and help members stay informed of changes in occupational therapy and in society.

Licensure laws in many states require that each therapist acquire a specified number of continuing education units each year to retain a license. Some states have other requirements to ensure that therapists retain competence. Whether because of state licensure requirements or because of feelings of professional obligation, it is vital that all practitioners maintain their competence using any or all of the resources available and develop an attitude favoring lifelong learning.

Role of the professional organization

The AOTA is the official professional organization for occupational therapists and occupational therapy assistants. The Association was incorporated as the National Society for the Promotion of Occupational Therapy in March 1917. The present name was adopted in January 1923. The purposes of the Association, as indicated in the articles of incorporation as amended in 1976, are

> to advance the therapeutic value of occupation; to research the effects of occupation upon human beings and to disseminate that research; to promote the use of occupational therapy and to advance the standards of education and training in the field; to educate consumers about the effect of occupation upon their well-being; and to engage in such other activities as may be considered to be advantageous to the profession, its members and the consumer of occupational therapy services (Composite Articles, 1990).

The AOTA's national headquarters is in Rockville, Maryland, and has a paid staff to conduct Association business. The volunteer sector of the AOTA is made up of all members, including the officers and representatives who are elected to develop policies and procedures. The Representative Assembly is the policy-making body and is composed of elected representatives from each state, the elected officers of the Representative Assembly and the Association, the first alternate representative to the World Federation of Occupational Therapists, a COTA Representative, and the chair of the Student Committee. The Executive Board is the management body of the AOTA and directs its operations, with the national office staff conducting the day-to-day business.

There are three standing commissions of the Representative Assembly—Education, Practice, and Standards and Ethics. These recommend policies and procedures in their respective areas. The official bodies of the Association, composed of members from the volunteer sector, carry out business that enhances the education, research, and practice aspects of the profession. The standing committees of the Representative Assembly carry out the business of the Assembly. In addition, an independent Certification Board now conducts affairs related to certification of occupational therapists and occupational therapy assistants. Figure 1-1 shows the organizational chart of the AOTA.

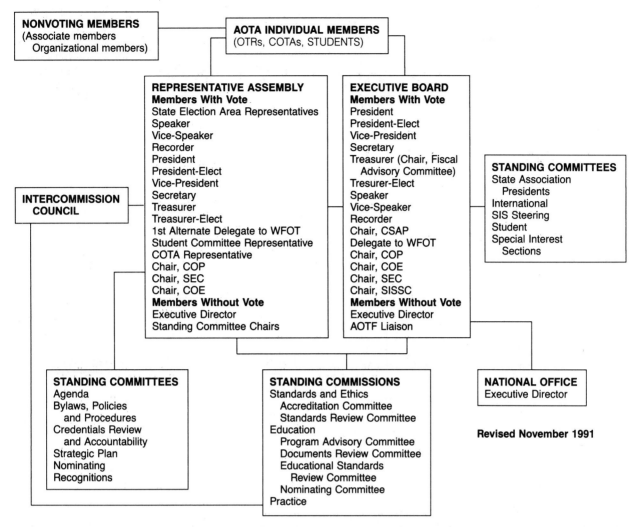

FIGURE 1-1. *Organizational chart of the American Occupational Therapy Association (AOTA). COP, Commission of Practice; SEC, Standards and Ethics Commission; COE, Commission on Education; CSAP, Committee of State Association Presidents; SISSC, Special Interest Section Steering Committee; AOTF, American Occupational Therapy Foundation.*

The national office of the AOTA is directed by an executive director, who has associate directors to administer the operations of five divisions: Professional Development, Professional Resource, Professional Relations, Finance and Operations, and Marketing. The national office staff provides services for membership through these divisions. Services provided include education, practice, continuing education, and legislative and political affairs.

Members of the AOTA receive numerous benefits. They receive a monthly journal; a news weekly; a quarterly specialty section newspaper; continuing education information and opportunities; national conferences; support for education, practice, and research; support for legislation at the national level; information on government and legal affairs; development and dissemination of information on standards of practice; position papers that define areas of practice to the public; dissemination of public information to enhance the public image of occupational therapy; and many others.

Professional responsibility

As a member of a health care profession, each OTR and COTA has professional responsibilities that must be met to enhance the public image of occupational therapy and to ensure the viability of the profession. Each person must take responsibility for his or her own competence as an OTR or a COTA and do whatever is needed to retain this competence. This can be done through reading of literature in the field; attendance at state, regional, and national meetings and conferences; and continuing or advanced education. Each OTR, COTA, and occupational therapy student also has an obligation to be involved in district, state, and national association affairs to the highest extent possible to be informed of changes in the field and other health care concerns. It is also an obligation for the therapist, assistant, and student to maintain membership in the state and national association and to support their activities so that these associations can continue to provide services that will benefit members and the general public.

Summary

The scope and location of practice in occupational therapy have been described. To differentiate between the roles and functions of OTR and COTA, the Representative Assembly of the American Occupational Therapy Association approved a role delineation in 1991, which can be used as a guideline for entry-level practice. (See Appendix F.) Each OTR and COTA has a professional responsibility to retain competence in his or her field. The professional organization assists practitioners in retaining competence by providing literature, seminars, self-study courses, and conferences. To ensure competence of practitioners in the field, several measures of accountability are used within the profession, including accreditation, certification, licensure, and continuing education.

References

American Occupational Therapy Association. (1991). Essentials and guidelines for an accredited program for the occupational therapist. *American Journal Of Occupational Therapy, 45*, 1077–1084.

American Occupational Therapy Association. (1990). Entry level role delineation for Registered Occupational Therapists (OTR's) and Certified Occupational Therapy Assistants (COTA's). *American Journal of Occupational Therapy, 44*, 1097–1102.

American Occupational Therapy Association. (1973). *Project to delineate the roles and functions of occupational therapy personnel in the detail needed to serve as a basis for the construction of proficiency examinations.* Washington, DC: Department of Health, Education, and Welfare, Public Health Services, National Institutes of Health, Bureau of Manpower Education, Division of Allied Health Manpower. Contract No. NO 1 AH 24172.

American Occupational Therapy Association. (1972). Occupational therapy: Its definition and functions. *American Journal of Occupational Therapy, 26*, 204.

Baum, C., & Gray, M. (January 1991). *Information exchange.* Rockville, MD: American Occupational Therapy Certification Board, Inc.

Brayley, C. (January 1991). What has licensure meant to occupational therapy in Pennsylvania. *Penn Point*, Pennsylvania Occupational Therapy Association.

Clark, F. A., Parham, D., Carlson, M. E., Frank, G., Jackson, J., Pierce, D., Wolfe, R. J., & Zemke, R. (1991). Occupational science: Academic innovation in the service of occupational therapy's future. *American Journal of Occupational Therapy, 45*, 300–310.

Composite Articles of Incorporation of the American Occupational Therapy Association as Amended. (1990). In *Reference manual of the official documents of the American Occupational Therapy Association, Inc.* Rockville, MD: AOTA.

Constitution of the National Society for the Promotion of Occupational Therapy. (1917). Baltimore: Sheppard Hospital Press.

Dataline: Occupational therapy services increase in the nation's hospitals. (1986). *Occupational Therapy News, 40*(4), 6.

Devereaux, E. B. (1991). Community based practice. *American Journal of Occupational Therapy, 45*, 944–946.

Dictionary definition of occupational therapy. (1986). Representative Assembly minutes. *American Journal of Occupational Therapy, 40*, 852.

Dunn, W. (1989). Occupational therapy in early intervention: New perspectives create better possibilities. *American Journal of Occupational Therapy, 43*, 717–721.

Dunton, W. R., Jr. (1919). *Reconstruction therapy.* Philadelphia: Saunders.

Education for All Handicapped Children Act. (Public Law 94–142). (1975). 20 USC:1401.

Education of the Handicapped Act. Amendments of 1986 (Public Law 99–457). (1986). 20 USC:1400.

From FWPR to FWE. (1986). *Occupational Therapy News, 40*(12), 9.

Hirama, H. (1986). A chronological review. In S. Ryan (Ed.), *The occupational therapy assistant: Roles and responsibilities* (pp. 23–34). Thorofare, NJ: Slack.

McNary H. (1947). The scope of occupational therapy. In H. Willard, & C. S. Spackman (Eds.), *Occupational therapy.* Philadelphia: Lippincott.

Reilly, M. (1962). Occupational therapy can be one of the great ideas of 20th century medicine. *American Journal of Occupational Therapy, 16*, 2.

Schoen, K.T. (1972). Development of occupational therapy job descriptions and curricula through task analysis. *Department of Health Education and Welfare Grant #D02 AH00964 01.2.* Columbus: Ohio State University.

Yerxa, E.J. (1991). Occupational therapy: An endangered species or an academic discipline. *American Journal Of Occupational Therapy, 45*, 680–685.

SECTION 1B
Scope of occupational therapy: the certified occupational therapy assistant

SALLY E. RYAN

KEY TERMS

Certification
Credentialing
Intraprofessional Team Building

Licensure
Role Delineation
Supervision

LEARNING OBJECTIVES

Upon completion of this section the reader will be able to:

1. *Discuss significant milestones in the history of certified occupational therapy assistants (COTAs).*
2. *Describe current educational and certification requirements for occupational therapy assistants.*
3. *Describe general COTA practice patterns.*
4. *Discuss basic principles of supervision as they relate to occupational therapy assistants.*
5. *Identify future roles and employment trends for COTAs.*

Celebration of the 30th anniversary of certified occupational therapy assistants (COTAs) in 1989 was an important milestone for the profession of occupational therapy. Throughout these years, as the number of COTAs increased markedly, tasks and responsibilities delegated to them expanded, and role and relationship issues and conflicts were identified. Although many of these issues have been successfully resolved, work continues on the development and implementation of policies, standards, and guidelines that will help to ensure effective registered occupational therapists (OTR) and COTA professional partnerships.

The purpose of this section is to provide the reader with basic information about the historical development, educational preparation, credentialing, and contemporary roles of the certified occupational therapy assistant. Principles and issues relative to patterns of **supervision**, **role delineation**, use, and **intra-professional team building** are an important focus. Future roles and employment trends will also be discussed with recommendations put forth to ensure continued growth and increased opportunities for technical personnel.

Historical perspectives

After World War II, the occupational therapy profession experienced a significant shortage of personnel, particularly in psychiatric facilities. In 1949, it was determined by the American Occupational Therapy Association (AOTA) Board of Management that a 1-year educational program to formally train occupational therapy assistants would help to alleviate this problem (Committee Reports, 1949). This initiative moved slowly; it wasn't until 1957 that the first standards for occupational therapy assistants were approved by the national association. Entitled "Requirements of an Acceptable Program and Curriculum Guide," the plan was implemented the following year (Crampton, 1958). The standards specified that the educational program be 12 weeks in length with a minimum of 460 clock hours devoted to training related to psychiatric technical practice. In 1959, the first occupational therapy assistant program was approved at Westborough State Hospital in Massachusetts (AOTA, undated). At the same time, it was recognized that a significant number of occupational therapy aides had received on-the-job training; thus, a grandfather clause was established allowing 336 of these persons to become certified for occupational therapy practice in psychiatry (Hirama, 1986).

In 1961, AOTA recognized the need for technical personnel in other practice settings. Therefore, programs were established to prepare occupational therapy assistants for work in general practice (Hirama, 1986). Shortly thereafter, programs were developed to train occupational therapy assistants in both general practice and psychiatry, the first being in Minnesota under the auspices of the Duluth Vocational–Technical School (1964). The first approved 2-year program was also in Minnesota at St. Mary's Junior College in Minneapolis (AOTA, 1965).

The addition of another level of personnel proved to be a challenge and a threat to some occupational therapists. COTAs were not always welcomed into the practice arena, particularly by those who had not worked with support personnel before or had not kept up to date in their knowledge and skills. Carr, a former occupational therapy assistant program director, addressed the problem in an article in the *American Journal of Occupational Therapy* in 1971. She stated, "Therapists away from current practice should be aware that what was taught fifteen years ago as functional treatment is taught to COTAs today as maintenance and supportive therapy" (Carr, 1971). Although this statement was made over 20 years ago, it continues to have relevance.

As the number of COTAs grew, legislation was enacted by the Delegate Assembly to grant them membership, voting rights, receipt of the professional journal, and eligibility for awards. More and more opportunities were made available for COTAs to serve on committees, councils, and other Association bodies, and they had a more active voice in AOTA. Through the establishment of the COTA Task Force and the COTA Advisory Committee in 1981 and 1984, respectively, more formalized mechanisms were developed, one of which was inclusion of specific COTA objectives in the Association's Strategic Plan (AOTA, 1990a).

Educational preparation

Standards for the education of occupational therapy assistants are referred to as *The Essentials and Guidelines of an Accredited Educational Program for the Occupational Therapy Assistant* (AOTA, 1991). Most of these programs last 2 years and grant the graduate an Associate in Science or an Associate in Arts degree. Some of the differences between technical and professional education are summarized in Table 1-1, prepared by the AOTA Entry-Level Study Committee (AOTA, 1985). Another document, developed by the AOTA Commission on Practice, entitled the "Entry-Level Role Delineation for Occupational Therapists, Registered (OTRs), and Certified Occupational Therapy Assistants (COTAs)," also serves as a guide for both education and beginning clinical practice (AOTA, 1990b.) See Appendix F for further information.

At this writing (1992) a total of 75 accredited occupational therapy assistant educational programs exist, located throughout the United States and in Puerto Rico.

Credentialing

Occupational therapy assistants are eligible for **certification** by the American Occupational Therapy Certification Board (AOTCB) once the following criteria are met (Gray, 1993):

Successful completion of an accredited educational program, including a minimal requirement of 12 weeks or 440 hours of level II fieldwork,
Submission of an application, and
Successful completion of the AOTCB certification examination for occupational therapy assistants.

This process is voluntary and currently the program offers only entry-level certification.

Many states have enacted regulatory legislation, such as **licensure**, registration, or statutory certification, which affects COTAs as well as OTRs. Specific information on the regulations may be obtained by contacting the individual state regulatory board or the AOTCB. Maintaining licensure, registration, or certification may mandate documentation of continuing education or other requirements. These vary from state to state.

Approximately 17,555 occupational therapy assistants are currently certified by the AOTCB and another 1100 join their ranks each year. This figure is current as of February 1992.

TABLE 1-1. *Knowledge and Skills to Be Developed at Various Levels of Education*

	Technical/Associate of Arts	Preprofessional/Bachelor's
Critical analysis	Analysis of standard problems	Develop skill in inquiry; abstract, logical thinking
Literacy	Communication Reading, reporting	Aware of the complexities of language; read aesthetically and critically
Understand numerical data	Gathering data Reporting Understanding some types of data	Basic concepts, ie, degree of risk, scatter, uncertainty, orders of magnitude, confidence levels, interpretation of graphs
History	General American and world history	Understanding history, its relationship to various social and environmental factors, and implications for the future
Science	The value of science, its role and limitations, and usefulness in addressing questions	Be intellectually at ease with science, understand its value and limitations, and the kinds of questions to be addressed
Values	Understand own values and value yourself; modify personal values, appreciate role of ethnic and other characteristics on values	Identify own values, critically analyze implications of actions and decisions for moral and ethical implications
Art	Appreciate and develop skill in arts and crafts as a means of expression	Appreciate fine and performing arts as a record and expression of human civilization
International multicultural understanding	Appreciate ethnic, religious cultural qualities	Access to a diversity of cultures; appreciate the language, customs, artifacts, and expressions of the culture
Study in depth	Begin study at introductory levels	Sequential learning, development of more sophisticated knowledge, imagination, synthesis
Communication	Clearly express self orally and in writing	Communicate ideas clearly; empathy, objectivity, ability to collaborate
Professional body of knowledge	Specific OT treatment techniques, basic science	Human development, biology and human science, statistics
Theory	Understand some concepts	Understand the nature and role of theories

(From AOTA: Entry Level Study Committee, June 1985.)

Practice patterns

Occupational therapy assistants work in a variety of health care settings. The 1990 AOTA Member Data Survey identified the following demographic and practice trends (AOTA, 1991b):

- 91%—female
- 90.2%—white
- 48.1%—between the ages of 30 and 39 years
- 70.7%—holding an associate degree
- 20%—currently pursuing additional educational degrees
- 72.2%—employed full time.

Skilled care nursing homes and intermediate care facilities employ the largest number of occupational therapy assistants (20%); school systems employ 17%; rehabilitation hospitals and centers, 10.9%; general hospitals, 9.4%; and psychiatric hospitals, 6.6%. The health problems most frequently seen by COTAs among patients and clients were the following (AOTA, 1991b)

- cerebrovascular accident/hemiplegia—30.3%
- mental retardation—11.4%
- developmental delay—8.9%
- schizophrenic disorders—6.6%
- cerebral palsy—6.0%

In addition to providing direct services to patients and clients, occupational therapy assistants are also serving in a number of administrative, consultative, supervisory, public relations, research, education, and fieldwork positions.

The Association's role delineation (AOTA, 1990b) provides more specific information on the entry-level roles and responsibilities of technical as well as professional personnel, which are organized around the general areas of the service provision process. Documentation, management, research, professional competence, promotion of the profession, and ethics are covered as well. (See Appendix F.)

Supervision guidelines

Throughout the history of the COTA, supervision has become an issue of frequent discussion and deliberation. For supervision to be successful, it must be a collaborative, ongoing effort between the supervisor and the supervisee, which is reciprocal and contributes to the professional growth of both parties (Ryan, 1992). It must be active and interactive. The document, "Supervision Guidelines for Certified Occupational Therapy Assistants," stresses the following points (AOTA, 1990c):

1. Implementation of treatment is the COTA's primary role.
2. A COTA may not conduct an evaluation independently or begin treatment before an OTR's evaluation.
3. The COTA contributes to the evaluation process by reporting observations, administering structured tests, and gathering pertinent data.
4. The OTR supervisor "is legally responsible for the outcomes of all occupational therapy services provided by the COTA."

5. "The frequency, amount and type of supervision indicated will vary with the service competence of the COTA and the setting and population characteristics."
6. If the COTA is not provided with adequate supervision, occupational therapy services must be discontinued.

Regulations such as those established by Medicare, Medicaid, and other third-party payors also have specific requirements relative to supervision. In addition, some state regulatory bodies have developed detailed supervisory regulations. More information on this subject may be found in the references cited in this section as well as in the bibliography.

Inherent in the topic of supervision is use. Technical personnel are frequently underused; this contributes to personnel shortages in a number of underserved areas. As Brooks succinctly stated (1982),

> With limited numbers of professionals available to meet the increase in demand for services, members must individually and collectively develop innovative strategies to deal with the constantly expanding role of occupational therapy. (p. 568)

She went on to challenge the profession to conduct research that would

> ... clearly demonstrate that OTRs working effectively with COTAs in a unified effort results in an expansion of occupational therapy services and is cost effective as well. (p. 568)

Overuse of COTAs is another area of concern. Every effort should be made by the supervisor to hire the appropriate level of personnel for the job that needs to be accomplished.

Another important consideration related to supervision is team building. Blechert and coworkers (1987) stress the importance of this for COTAs and OTRs. They state that team building has its foundation in satisfying three areas of needs (Blechert et al., 1987): "(a) administration, which leads to mutual respect; (b) mastery or effective performance; and (c) maturation or personal growth and professional socialization." They have developed a matrix that details stages of team development and is recommended as an outstanding tool for intraprofessional team building. Shannon (1988), a strong advocate of the team approach, reminds the profession and COTAs particularly that they "must become more assertive in expressing (their) beliefs and ideas, to the extent that a true partnership can evolve, characterized by mutual obligation, trust, and respect" (p. 198).

Future directions

The demand for occupational therapy services will continue to increase, as well as the demand and opportunities for occupational therapy assistants. A greater shift in roles and responsibilities may occur, provided that there is a more equitable geographic distribution of professional and technical personnel. OTRs will have increasingly more responsibilities for consultation, supervision, research, and program development, which will greatly influence the roles of occupational therapy assistants. In her discussion of future trends, Gilfoyle (1986) has stated,

> The upcoming years will see COTAs functioning more independently in the areas of evaluation, planning, and treatment. [More] Independent practice requires problem-solving abilities and skills to analyze and synthesize complex information. Thus, additional educational preparation will be necessary. (p. 405)

COTAs will see increasing opportunities to work with both the well and the frail elderly. The role of technical personnel will also increase in a number of other areas, including home health, substance abuse, independent living centers, work hardening, stress management, and hospice. It is recommended that educational preparation, including fieldwork, be modified to ensure that practitioners have the necessary knowledge, skills, and abilities. An additional recommendation is that technical and professional programs increase their emphasis on the collaborative and complimentary roles of the OTR and the COTA.

Summary

The role of the COTA has evolved for over 30 years. History chronicles significant changes in educational preparation, practice arenas, and specific roles and responsibilities. **Credentialing** (including accreditation, certification, and licensure), third-party reimbursement, and supervision standards all have had a direct influence on the use or underuse of the COTA. More effective collaboration and intraprofessional teamwork will result in the alleviation of personnel shortages and the provision of quality, cost-effective services in response to an ever-increasing demand for occupational therapy intervention.

References

American Occupational Therapy Association (undated). *Development of the certified occupational therapy assistant*. Rockville, MD: Author.

American Occupational Therapy Association. (1965). Board of Management report. *American Journal of Occupational Therapy, 19*, 100.

American Occupational Therapy Association. (1985). *Entry-Level Study Committee Report*. Rockville, MD: Author.

American Occupational Therapy Association. (1990a). *1991–1995 Strategic Plan*. Rockville, MD: Author.

American Occupational Therapy Association. (1990b). Entry-level role delineation for occupational therapists, registered (OTRs) and certified occupational therapy assistants (COTAs). *American Journal of Occupational Therapy, 12*, 1091–1103.

American Occupational Therapy Association. (1990c). Supervision guidelines for certified occupational therapy assistants. *American Journal of Occupational Therapy, 12*, 1089–1090.

American Occupational Therapy Association. (1991a). *Essentials and guidelines of an accredited educational program for the occupational therapy assistant*. Adopted by the Representative Assembly, June.

American Occupational Therapy Association. (1991b). Member data survey: Executive summary. *O. T. News*, June 6.

Blechert, T. F, Christiansen, M. F., & Kari, N. (1987). Intraprofessional team building. *American Journal of Occupational Therapy, 9*, 576–582.

Brooks, B. (1982). COTA issues: Yesterday, today, and tomorrow. *American Journal of Occupational Therapy, 9*, 567–568.

Carr, S. H. (1971). A modification of role for nursing home service. *American Journal of Occupational Therapy, 21*, 259–262.

Committee Reports: Education Committee. (1949). *American Journal of Occupational Therapy, 4*, 221.

Crampton, M. W. (1958). The recognition of occupational therapy assistants. *American Journal of Occupational Therapy, 12*, 269.

Gilfoyle, E. M. (1986). Epilogue. In S. E. Ryan (Ed.), *The certified occupational therapy assistant: Roles and responsibilities*. Thorofare, NJ: Slack.

Gray, M. (1993). Credentialing in occupational therapy. In S. E. Ryan (Ed.),

Practice issues in occupational therapy: Intraprofessional team building. Thorofare, NJ: Slack.

Hirama, H. (1986). The COTA: A chronological review. In S. E. Ryan (Ed.), *The occupational therapy assistant: Roles and responsibilities* (pp. 23–34). Thorofare, NJ: Slack.

Occupational therapy assistant education brochure. (1964). Duluth, MN: Duluth Vocational-Technical School.

Ryan, S. E. (1993). Supervision principles, patterns, and issues. In S. E. Ryan (Ed.), *Practice issues in occupational therapy: Intraprofessional team building.* Thorofare, NJ: Slack.

Shannon, P. H. (1988). Some messages for the COTA on image, imagery, and imagination. In J. A. Johnson (Ed.), *Certified occupational therapy assistants: Opportunities and challenges* (p. 198). New York: Haworth Press.

Bibliography

American Occupational Therapy Association (1991). *Executive summary on rules, regulations, and guidelines governing practice by and supervision of certified occupational therapy assistants.* Rockville, MD: Author.

Early, M. B. (1987). *Mental health concepts and techniques.* New York: Raven Press.

Hirama, H. (1990). *Occupational therapy assistant: A primer* (rev. ed.). Baltimore: Chess Publications.

Johnson, J. A. (Ed.). (1988). *Certified occupational therapy assistants: Opportunities and challenges.* New York: Haworth Press.

Punwar, A. (1988). *Occupational therapy: Principles and practice.* Baltimore: Williams & Wilkins.

Sabonis-Chafee, B. (1989). *Occupational therapy: Introductory concepts.* St. Louis: Mosby.

Schell, B. A. B. (1985). Guide to classification of occupational therapy personnel. *American Journal of Occupational Therapy, 12,* 803–810.

Wesley, S., & Bukatko, P. (1991). *A national study of the profession of occupational therapy.* Rockville, MD: American Occupational Therapy Certification Board.

SECTION 2

Fieldwork education: professional socialization

ELLEN S. COHN

KEY TERMS

Level I Fieldwork   *Fieldwork Educator*
Level II Fieldwork   *Supervision*
Learning Style   *Feedback*

LEARNING OBJECTIVES

Upon completion of this section the reader will be able to:

1. *Understand the role of fieldwork in developing professional competency.*
2. *Understand the roles and responsibilities of the key players in fieldwork education.*
3. *Be aware of the value of sharing one's learning style with the supervisor.*
4. *Understand the purpose of interviews for fieldwork placements.*
5. *Be aware of the impact of the transition from classroom to clinic.*
6. *Understand the process of supervision.*
7. *Understand the role of feedback and evaluation in the supervisory process.*

The consensus within the occupational therapy profession is that the fieldwork experience plays an integral role in professional development. In 1923, the first standards requiring fieldwork experiences were approved by American Occupational Therapy Association (AOTA). A survey of the literature reveals that fieldwork continues to function as the critical link between the academic world of theory and the clinical world of practice. This component of educational preparation functions as the gateway into our profession because all students must complete fieldwork requirements to become eligible to take the certification examination for occupational therapists and occupational therapy assistants.

The process and content of fieldwork experiences have been debated over the years. Yet the value of having an opportunity to integrate academic knowledge with application skills at progressively higher levels of performance and responsibility has always been acknowledged as important (Pressler, 1983). Christie, Joyce, and Moeller (1985) highlight that value by documenting the fieldwork experience as having the greatest impact on the development of a therapist's preference for a specific area of clinical practice. Of the 131 therapists surveyed, 55% indicated that clinical practice preferences were either formed or changed during the fieldwork experience, and another 24% noted that fieldwork experience expanded their interests to other areas of practice. Thus, the fieldwork experience can be rich and rewarding and is likely to have a tremendous impact on students' career choices.

Although it is understood that each student's fieldwork experience will be different, this section provides an overview of the fieldwork experience, a definition of the levels of fieldwork experiences recognized by the AOTA, and a description of the roles and responsibilities of the key players. The nature of the transition from the academic setting to the clinical world of practice, **learning styles**, and a description of the interview, supervisory, and evaluation processes are intended to familiarize students with the expectations and procedures of fieldwork settings.

Levels and purpose of fieldwork

Level I

The Essentials and Guidelines of an Accredited Educational Program for Occupational Therapists and Occupational Therapy Assistants outline the general fieldwork requirements for all students. The requirements are divided into two classifications, level I and level II fieldwork (AOTA, 1991). **Level I fieldwork** offers students practical experiences that are integrated throughout the academic program. The overall purpose of the level I fieldwork experience is to provide students with exposure to clinical practice through observation of clients and therapists. Through these observations students have the opportunity to examine their reactions to clients, themselves, other personnel, and the profession. Because the academic level, performance expectations, and specific purpose of the level I fieldwork experience vary throughout each occupational therapy curricula, the timing, length, requirements, and specific focus of the level I fieldwork experience are negotiated with each academic program on an individualized basis (AOTA, 1988).

Level II

The purpose of **level II fieldwork** is to "promote clinical reasoning and reflective practice; to transmit the values, beliefs, and ethical commitments of the field of occupational therapy; to communicate and model professional behaviors attending to the developmental nature of career growth and responsibility; and to develop and expand a repertoire of occupational therapy assessments and treatment interventions related to human performance" (COE, AOTA, 1991a, 1991b).

Students test firsthand the theories and facts learned in academic study and refine skills through interaction with patients under close supervision.

The requirements established by AOTA include a minimum of 6 months of level II fieldwork for occupational therapy students and a minimum of 2 months for occupational therapy assistant students (COE, AOTA, 1991a, 1991b). To offer students experience with a wide range of client ages and a variety of physical and mental health conditions, the 6 months are usually divided into two 3-month experiences in different clinical facilities. Some occupational therapy academic programs require an additional 3-month fieldwork experience to allow students to develop entry-level skills in a specialty area such as pediatrics, gerontology, hand therapy, and work hardening.

Occupational therapy students are expected to complete their fieldwork experience within 24 months after completion of academic preparation, whereas occupational therapy assistant students are expected to complete their level II requirement within 12 months after completion of academic preparation. Some academic programs include the level II fieldwork experiences in their degree requirements and offer corresponding academic credit, whereas other academic programs view the level II fieldwork experience as a professional requirement and do not offer academic credit for the experience. In either case, successful completion of level II fieldwork is an eligibility requirement for certification as a registered occupational therapist (OTR) or assistant (COTA). Fieldwork provides students with situations in which to practice interpersonal skills with patients

and staff and to develop characteristics essential to productive working relationships (COE, AOTA, 1988). For students, the overall purpose of the fieldwork experience is to gain mastery of occupational therapy reasoning and techniques to develop entry-level competency. Upon completion of the fieldwork experience, students are expected to demonstrate competence in the areas of assessment, planning, treatment, problem-solving, administration, and professionalism.

Although the goals and objectives specific to each fieldwork setting are initially delineated, occupational therapy students are expected to demonstrate competence in using the assessment tools and evaluation procedures routinely employed by occupational therapists. Occupational therapy assistant students are expected to collaborate in providing occupational therapy services with appropriate supervision to evaluate skills and plan programs, prevent deficits, and maintain or improve function in daily living skills and in underlying components. On the basis of the models and theories of occupational therapy practiced at the fieldwork centers, students should become proficient in implementing, justifying, and evaluating the effectiveness of treatment plans. Effective oral and written communication of ideas and objectives relevant to the roles and duties of an occupational therapist or occupational therapy assistant, including interaction with patients and staff in a professional manner, are expected of all students. Students are responsible for demonstrating a sensitivity to and respect for patient confidentiality. Finally, acquisition of professional characteristics that permit one to establish and sustain therapeutic relationships and to work collaboratively with others are expected in all fieldwork centers.

The aforementioned competencies require specific skill development and the ability to interact with others. Another expectation—more internal to the students' development of positive professional self-images—includes taking responsibility for maintaining, assessing, and improving self-competence.

Students are responsible for articulating their understanding of theoretical information and identifying their abilities to implement assessments or treatment techniques. Moreover, the ability to benefit from supervision as a resource for self-directed learning is critical for professional development. Thus, understanding and articulating one's individual learning style becomes essential to the supervisory process (Schwartz, 1980).

Roles and responsibilities

Upon completion of the prerequisite academic course work, occupational therapy and occupational therapy assistant students are eligible to begin their fieldwork experiences. Clearly defined objectives and guidelines provide students with the direction necessary for organizing their efforts toward achieving clinical competence. Considering the overall fieldwork objectives and the resources of the clinical facility, working toward mastery of the entry-level skills required for high-quality patient care is a mutual undertaking between the fieldwork educators and students. Both fieldwork educators and students are responsible for the process of evaluating student progress and modifying the learning experience within the environment. The roles and responsibilities of each of the participants in fieldwork education will be outlined.

Students

The responsibilities of the students are as follows:

1. Fulfilling all duties and responsibilities identified by the fieldwork educators and academic fieldwork coordinators within the designated times,
2. Complying with the professional standards identified by the fieldwork facility, the university, and the Principles of Occupational Therapy Ethics as approved by the Representative Assembly of the American Occupational Therapy Association in 1988 (see Appendix A),
3. Communicating with fieldwork educators to confirm the starting dates and other prerequisite information,
4. Securing documentation of adequate medical and professional insurance for the duration of the fieldwork experience,
5. Completing and presenting to the fieldwork educators one copy of the students' evaluation of the fieldwork experience (Cohn, 1991).

Fieldwork educators

The people responsible for the fieldwork education program must be registered occupational therapists with a minimum of 1 year of experience in direct client service. For occupational therapy assistant students, direct supervision can be provided by an OTR or COTA, also with a minimum of 1 year of experience.

Ultimate responsibility for the level II fieldwork experience must be assumed by an OTR. Although the minimum requirement is 1 year of experience, **fieldwork educators** should be competent clinicians who can serve as good role models or mentors for future practitioners. As stated in the Essentials and Guidelines of an Accredited Education Program for the Occupational Therapist, these people are formally titled "fieldwork educators," although "clinical educators," "fieldwork supervisors," and "student supervisors" are interchangeable titles (COE, AOTA, 1988).

Two areas of responsibility of fieldwork educators are administrative functions and direct day-to-day supervision. The administrative responsibilities of the fieldwork educator include, but are not limited to, the following:

1. Collaborating with the academic fieldwork coordinator in the development of a program that provides the best opportunity for the implementation of theoretical concepts offered as part of the academic educational program,
2. Creating an environment that facilitates learning, clinical inquiry, and reflection on one's practice,
3. Preparing, maintaining, and sending to the academic fieldwork coordinator current information about the fieldwork education center, including a statement of the conceptual models from which evaluation is derived and on which treatment is based,
4. Scheduling students in collaboration with the academic fieldwork coordinator,
5. Establishing objectives of the fieldwork experience and identifying the philosophy of the center,
6. Contributing to the evaluation of each student at midpoint and termination. One copy of the terminal document must be signed by both the fieldwork educator and the student

and sent to the fieldwork coordinator of the educational institution in which the student is enrolled,
7. Being familiar with the policy regarding the withdrawal of students from fieldwork experience of each educational institution from which students are accepted,
8. Notifying the academic fieldwork coordinator of any student for whom the fieldwork center is requesting withdrawal or of other problems that may arise,
9. Reviewing periodically the contractual agreement between the academic institution and the fieldwork center and ensuring that these agreements are signed,
10. Providing regular and periodic supervision of students.

The direct day-to-day supervisory responsibilities of the fieldwork educator include, but are not limited to, the following:

1. Providing an adequate orientation to the fieldwork education center and to specific department policies and procedures,
2. Assigning patients and clients to students and defining expectations clearly to students,
3. Supervising the provision of occupational therapy services and the documentation and oral reporting of students,
4. Assessing skills and knowledge of the students,
5. Meeting with students regularly to review performance and to provide guidance using behavioral language and observable data. As a result of supervisor's feedback, goals for change are developed collaboratively by students and supervisors.
6. Seeking out evaluation of own supervisory skills from appropriate people (COE AOTA, 1988).

Academic fieldwork coordinator

Each academic program has an academic fieldwork coordinator who functions as a liaison between the academic setting, the fieldwork educators, and the students. The responsibilities of the academic fieldwork coordinator are the following:

1. Assigning eligible students to fieldwork experience and confirming the assignment in writing to each fieldwork educator,
2. Ensuring that all written contracts or letters of agreement between the educational institution and the fieldwork education center are signed and periodically reviewed,
3. Making regular and periodic contacts with each fieldwork education center where students are placed,
4. Maintaining a current information file on each fieldwork education center where students are placed,
5. Identifying new sites for fieldwork education,
6. Developing and implementing a policy for withdrawal of students from a fieldwork education center,
7. Orienting students to the general purposes of fieldwork experience and providing them with necessary forms,
8. Reassigning students who do not complete their original fieldwork assignments in accordance with the educational institution's policies,
9. Developing fieldwork experience programs that provide the best opportunity for the implementation of theoretical concepts offered as part of the didactic curriculum,
10. Maintaining a collaborative relationship with fieldwork education centers,

11. Sending necessary information and forms for each student to the fieldwork educator (COE AOTA, 1988).

Knowledge of the fieldwork education programs is an important part of the academic fieldwork coordinator's job. Periodic visits are made to the fieldwork centers, or when on-site visits are unrealistic, telephone communication is maintained. The academic fieldwork coordinator is available for consultation to both students and fieldwork educators.

Transition from student to professional

The shift from the academic setting to the clinical fieldwork setting is an obvious, yet potentially underestimated life change. Occupational therapy students are making the environmental transition from the classroom to the clinic while simultaneously emerging from the role of students to the professional role of therapists. As with any transition, occupational therapy students leaving academia face a process of change from one structure, role, or sense of self to another. The struggle to assimilate into a new environment and to develop a new role may jolt students into disequilibrium, resulting in an inability to adjust. As is true of all life changes, the experience of disequilibrium can be an opportunity for growth, especially in the context of a supportive supervisory relationship. This time of transition results in changes in assumptions about oneself and the world and requires a corresponding change in behaviors and relationships.

As students move into fieldwork settings, they develop new relationships, learning styles, behaviors, and self-perceptions. Students may begin to reassess their suppositions about occupational therapy, the theories learned in school, and their views of themselves as therapists, learners, and individuals. Because individuals differ in their ability to adapt to change and because each

student will be placed in a different fieldwork setting, the transition will have a different impact on each student.

The nature of the clinical fieldwork environment is fundamentally different from that of the academic environment. Knowing and acknowledging some of the distinctions between the two settings may ease the transition and provide students with support to accept the challenges of fieldwork experiences (Table 1-2).

Within the fieldwork environment, the learning focus shifts to the application or implementation of therapy techniques in an applied interpersonal context. Techniques that were introduced in a simulated context now must be mastered and applied with attention to the patient's emotional needs. Abstract questions—appropriate in the academic environment—shift to pragmatic questions to reduce the possibility of error in one's thinking. For example, rather than thinking about the patient's function in the kitchen from an abstract perspective, the student has to think about the patient's function in the context of a specific kitchen in a small apartment and to attend to the patient's concerns about her family. Consequently, tolerance for ambiguity or uncertainty declines after students enter the fieldwork environment.

In the academic setting, students are accountable to themselves, and performance is evaluated on a summative basis through tests, assignments, and grades. Students choose whether to disclose grades to family or peers, and their performance does not affect others. In the fieldwork center, a student's performance is evaluated on a formative basis and may be observed by the entire health care term, especially at team meetings. Performance is no longer the private matter it was at school but is publicly observed, because it has a direct and critical impact on patients. Colleagues, patients, and their families then may offer meaningful feedback. Although all these opportunities may create disequilibrium or tension, they likewise constitute new ways in which students learn about themselves and their profession. The

TABLE 1-2. *Distinctions Between Academic and Clinical Settings*

	Academic Setting	Clinical Setting
Purpose	Facilitate dissemination of knowledge, development of creative thought and student growth, award degrees	Provide high-quality patient care
Faculty/supervisor accountability	1. To student 2. To university	1. To patient and family 2. To clinical center 3. To student
Student accountability	To self	To patients and families, supervisor, and clinical center
Pace	Dependent on curriculum; adaptable to student and faculty needs	Dependent on patient needs; less adaptable
Student/educator ratio	Many students to one faculty member	One student to one supervisor
Source of feedback	Summative at midterm or at the end of term; provided by faculty	Provided by patients and families, supervisor, and other staff; formative
Degree of faculty/supervisor control of educational experience	Able to plan, controlled	Limited control; various diagnoses and lengths of patient stay
Primary learning tools	Books, lectures, audiovisual aids, case studies, simulation	Situation of practice; patients, families, and staff
Conceptual learning	Abstract, theoretical	Pragmatic, applied in interpersonal context
Learning process	Teacher-directed	Patient-, self-, and supervisor-directed
Tolerance for ambiguity/uncertainty	High	Low
Lifestyle	Flexible to plan time around class schedule	Structured; flexible time limited to evenings and weekends

broad and diverse experience within the fieldwork setting challenges students to redefine their sense of self.

From an educational perspective, fieldwork education takes place in a situation in which fieldwork educators have little control. The organizational factors of the health care setting, combined with patient care factors such as the nature and complexity of the patient's problem, the length of stay, and fluctuation in patient load make it difficult to generalize for planning, especially in acute care settings. In settings that provide care for chronic patients, however, the fieldwork educators are able to plan ahead, since the patient population is more constant and the fieldwork educator knows which patients will be available during student placements. Conversely, in the academic setting, many of the factors that operate as fluctuating variables in the fieldwork setting are constant and inherently structured by the faculty.

The fieldwork educators' primary responsibility is patient care; they have an ethical imperative to ensure the welfare of patients. This appropriate professional ethic may constrain activities that may be desirable from the standpoint of education. A beneficial distinction between the academic environment and the clinic, which allows fieldwork educators to adapt to the constraints of the clinic, is the individualized supervisory relationship. This unique one-to-one relationship is a positive aspect of the fieldwork environment, since fieldwork educators have the luxury of adapting their styles to meet the needs of the learner.

Learning styles

Over two decades ago, Gail Fidler (1966), a prominent leader in our field, wrote, "Students bring to the learning experience a variety of attitudes, values, and previously learned responses. Some of these will need to undergo change, others to be enhanced and broadened" (p. 2). Kolb's research on learning styles addresses differences in how individuals learn and process information. He claims that each student has a preferred way of grasping and transforming information. Preference does not imply that these ways are the only or perhaps even the best ways for the student to learn. They are, however, the styles with which the student has the greatest experience and therefore represent the student's learning strengths.

A student's learning style is in fact not one style but many. Learning styles indicate the process by which a person most effectively and efficiently receives and arranges information. Some students process information in a step-by-step fashion versus first gaining a "big picture." Mentally categorizing ideas into a few large groupings rather than creating many smaller and more discrete groupings of the information is yet another example of how students might differ in the preferred learning style. Learning style is a dynamic process that can vary with subject matter and setting. For example, if listening to a lecture, viewing slides, and taking notes helps a student to organize the information being presented, he or she will have to adjust to a new way of organizing information during fieldwork where lecture and slides are not the primary teaching modalities (Kolb, 1984).

Although fieldwork educators ideally would like to match supervisor and learning styles, it is not feasible in most situations. Learning styles appear to be fluid as well as complex, making it unrealistic to match learners with supervisors Thus, learning style information is best used when learners take responsibility for sharing what they know about and how they learn with their supervisor. This notion is consistent with the shift from a teacher-directed learning situation to the self-directed, active, and ongoing professional role of occupational therapists and assistants. Sharing one's learning style can assist the fieldwork educator and student in determining effective strategies to help the student learn.

A number of learning style inventories have been developed to assist students in gaining insight into their learning style. Some fieldwork educators ask students to complete one of these inventories to facilitate the learning process (Crist, 1986; Geyer, 1988). These inventories are best used as a springboard to create awareness that learners differ. Other fieldwork educators may ask students to reflect on their past and present learning experiences as a way to understand their students' preferred learning style. In reflecting on past experiences, it is helpful for students to think about formal learning that took place in the classroom. In the context of fieldwork, it also becomes essential to reflect on informal or experiential learning situations (such as learning to sew at home), since fieldwork is experiential learning. By explicating their own learning strengths, weaknesses, and preferences, students can enhance their relationship with the fieldwork educator.

Fieldwork interviews

Many fieldwork educators require an interview to ensure that students understand the clinical expectations and the type of experience offered at their particular facility. Although these interviews are not a requirement for all fieldwork settings, the interview further serves to confirm the student's suitability for the particular fieldwork placement. Each academic program reserves fieldwork placements for a designated time, and students are then individually matched to the available placement. In most cases, only one student is scheduled to interview for a particular placement. Hence, the interview is usually noncompetitive and is designed for students and fieldwork educators to confirm assumptions. The fieldwork educators do have the right to decline acceptance of students based on the interview, however, just as students have the right to decline the particular fieldwork placement. The fieldwork educators notify either the students or the academic fieldwork coordinators of their intention to accept or deny the placement. In either case, the academic fieldwork coordinator serves as a liaison and consultant.

Because the interviews are designed to ensure a mutually agreeable match between students' career interests and fieldwork settings, a variety of professionally related questions may be generated by the fieldwork educators. For example, students may be asked to identify their clinical interests and long-term career goals, their expectations of the fieldwork experience, their frame of reference, or their experience in the academic setting. Additionally, some fieldwork educators ask questions to ascertain why students chose occupational therapy as a profession or why students desire to train in a particular fieldwork setting. Therefore, it is useful for students to learn about the facility and to consider their professional goals before the interview. It is important to note that each interviewer will ask his or her own set of questions and probe different aspects of students' backgrounds.

The process of becoming an occupational therapist involves developing a sense of professional identity and using the self as a therapeutic agent. Each student brings a unique composite of knowledge, skills, and personal style to the fieldwork experience. Therefore, depending on the type of facility, the role of occupational therapy, and the fieldwork educator's concept of supervision, the educator will ask different questions related to students' understanding of themselves. Students are commonly asked to identify experiences that may be relevant to fieldwork and to identify their strengths and weaknesses. Clarification of students' learning styles promotes an understanding of their preferred approach to learning and can assist both students and fieldwork educators in developing strategies to enhance the fieldwork experience. Since the fieldwork experience is a major life transition, the fieldwork educator may want to discuss a student's lifestyle, social supports, and perceived ability to enter a new system, to manage time, or to handle stress. These questions are intended to appraise the potential influences on a student's performance, and students should be prepared to discuss these important issues. Students, in turn, may use their fieldwork interview to clarify their assumptions about the fieldwork requirements, the structure of supervision, the types of patients treated, the frame of reference of the occupational therapy department, and the philosophy of the entire facility.

Supervisory relationship

In 1983, the AOTA defined supervision as a mutual understanding between supervisor and supervisee intended to promote growth and development while evaluating performance and maintaining standards (AOTA, 1983). **Supervision** is thus conceptualized as a dynamic teaching–learning relationship, an educational process that serves as a bridge between previously learned knowledge and clinical skill, and a mechanism that ensures an experiential learning environment. Because the goals and often the top priority in the clinical facility are directed toward providing high-quality care for patients, supervision will be structured to ensure such care for patients while simultaneously, and possibly secondarily, facilitating and managing the learning process for students. Within this framework, the fieldwork educator is a facilitator of learning who serves as a reflective model to be emulated as students progress toward greater responsibility in their role as occupational therapists (COE, AOTA, 1977).

The importance of the relationship between fieldwork educators and students is inherent within the supervisory context. Christie and coworkers (1985), in their study of 65 fieldwork centers, confirmed the longstanding belief that the relationship between students and fieldwork educators is the most significant aspect of the fieldwork experience. In the study, both students and educators perceived the supervisory process as the most critical element in distinguishing good from poor fieldwork experiences. Furthermore, communication and interpersonal skills were identified as distinguishing characteristics of effective supervision.

Each member in the supervisory relationship enters with his or her own assumptions and expectations. These expectations are based on the student's past experiences with other supervisors, parents, and other authority figures. These experiences, together with student's emerging paradigms of occupational therapy and professional goals, provide the foundation for the supervisory relationship. Supervisors in turn have a notion of the behaviors, skills, and attitudes necessary for effective entry-

level practice in their fieldwork settings. Initially, the delineation of expectations is a primary focus of supervision. After the expectations of both supervisors and students are defined, the focus shifts to providing feedback related to the stated expectations.

The feedback provided by the fieldwork educators is critical to a student's development. **Feedback,** defined as "knowledge of the results of individual's performance to the extent that individual's behavior is changed in a desirable direction," refers to a particular aspect of behavior, to a total behavioral sequence or performance, or to the nature of the message itself. For example, the message may convey information about the student's attitudes toward patients. This definition connotes an expectation that "some change will occur in the student's understanding, attitude, or behavior in response to feedback" (Freeman, 1985, p. 5). In a direct manner, feedback can help to identify the next step in the change process, to clarify steps that have taken place, to evaluate whether a particular step meets performance criteria for a specific task and whether it relates to or achieves the overall goals, and to clarify or modify those goals or expectations as needed. One of the key sources for feedback during the fieldwork experience is the fieldwork educator. It is important for students to recognize that fieldwork educators are not judging the student's worth or goodness but assessing how well the student is performing. Crist (1986) suggests that students "be willing to try new suggestions or ways, while evaluating their own biases and preferences." Feedback, given honestly and sincerely, is often the most valuable change agent for students (Freeman, 1985, p. 109).

Fieldwork evaluation

Frequently, students receive feedback informally during supervision meetings; however, formal mechanisms for providing feedback and evaluation of a student's performance, judgments, and attitudes are built into the fieldwork experience. There are two distinct purposes in fieldwork evaluation. One is the formative, ongoing process to direct student learning throughout the fieldwork experience, and the other is summative to document the level of skills attained at the completion of the fieldwork experience. Although these two processes are different, they are not mutually exclusive. The formative process occurs throughout the fieldwork experience so that students and fieldwork educators can compare perceptions, assess which student activities are important and which are less so, review objectives, plan new learning opportunities, and make necessary modifications in behaviors. As suggested by Yerxa (1988), counseling students is an important component of evaluation: "Counseling means to give students an objective, specific view of performance in such a way that students can be assured of their strengths and strengthened to improve their weaknesses" (p. 177). Counseling is a continuing process throughout the fieldwork experience and is usually specific to the setting.

The second process, which is cumulative, requires documentation of students' performance after completion of the fieldwork experience. The Fieldwork Evaluation (FWE) is the instrument adopted by the AOTA for evaluating performance of professional-level occupational therapy students in all fieldwork education centers (COE, AOTA, 1986). The FWE is designed to assess students' performance of specific professional tasks. It is an evaluation tool and is not intended to serve as a tool for the counseling process described by Yerxa.

The FWE consists of two sections. The first section has 51 behavioral statements depicting competent performance in five areas: assessment, planning, treatment, problem-solving, and administrative/professionalism. Each area is evaluated on the basis of performance, judgment, and attitude on a rating scale ranging from excellent to poor. The second section is a written summary of performance indicating particular strengths and weaknesses and any other information useful in documenting professional growth and learning. This form should serve as summary of what students already know of their performance. Completion, administration, and subsequent use of the FWE should be conducted with consideration of all legal and ethical implications regarding each student assessed. Such consideration includes the right to nonprejudicial evaluation, the right to privacy of information, and the right for students to appeal (AOTA, 1986).

The Guidelines for an Occupational Therapy Fieldwork Experience—Level II state that students should be evaluated at midterm and at completion of the fieldwork experience (AOTA, 1985). When used at midterm, the recommended ratings for each of the 51 tasks are satisfactory plus (S+), satisfactory (S), and unsatisfactory (U) (AOTA, 1986). Numerical scores are avoided at midterm to separate evaluation from any association with grades and to help students view the feedback as an aid to the development of professionalism. Furthermore, the avoidance of scores at midterm prevents inflated terminal scores, as evaluators have a tendency to expect greater scores at the end of the fieldwork experience. As the AOTA suggests,

> During the midterm review process, students and supervisors should collaboratively design a plan which would enable students to achieve entry level competence by the end of the fieldwork experience. This plan should include specific objectives and enabling activities to be used by students and supervisors in order to achieve the competence desired. (COE, AOTA, 1986, p. 8)

The Fieldwork Evaluation Form for the Occupational Therapy Assistant Student (FWE/OTA) is the instrument adopted by AOTA for evaluating performance of occupational therapy assistant students in all fieldwork centers. Developed in 1983, this instrument contains 24 competency items, subdivided into four sections: evaluation (five items); treatment (eight items); communication (four items); and professional behavior (seven items). Unlike the FWE, the FWE/OTA does not examine each evaluation item from three perspectives: performance, judgment, and attitude. Rather, it rates each item on a scale of 1 to 5 with criteria states for each level. In general, a score of 1 implies inability or severe difficulty in demonstrating the competency item; a score of 5 indicates exceptional ability in demonstrating the competency item. The 24 scored items, based on observable behaviors, were designed to reduce the subjectivity inherent in any evaluation. The "Comment Section" is provided for documenting observations of student performance and specific behaviors. Examples of specific examples are recorded in this section. These examples support the supervisors rationale for the given score.

The FWE/OTA is used in a formative manner at midterm to provide students with feedback and to develop strategies for improving performance. It is used in a summative manner after completion of the fieldwork experience, because the AOTA states that the FWE/OTA final scores be based on the last 2 weeks of the fieldwork experience (COE, AOTA, 1983).

There are no established guidelines to convert scores on the FWE or the FWE/OTA to academic letter grades. Performance in the clinical environment is not based on academic criteria; therefore, the official tools are designed to evaluate clinical competency. Some academic programs, however, have developed their own criteria to convert fieldwork performance scores to academic grades. This is not a standard practice across the country.

Finally, the intent of the fieldwork evaluation is not to differentiate between students, but to measure their achievement of specific competencies. Future employers will want assurance that students satisfy the entry-level requirements. The FWE data may be synthesized to provide the foundation for employment references.

Student evaluation of the fieldwork experience

Students also have the opportunity to provide the fieldwork educators and fieldwork facility with feedback. The Student Evaluation of Fieldwork Experiences form (SEFWE) is recommended for use by the Commission on Education (COE, AOTA, 1989). This form allows students to provide the facility with feedback about the orientation process, supervisor interaction, and the entire learning experience. The fieldwork facilities will then use this feedback to improve fieldwork programs, and the academic programs use this information to share with future students who are interested in training at the fieldwork facility.

Summary

A profession usually defines its boundaries by setting up criteria for entry. In occupational therapy, the fieldwork experience is an essential component of the entry criteria. The purpose of fieldwork is to provide learning experiences that foster professional competence and personal growth. It is the beginning of a lifelong process of connecting theory with practice. The depth of the experience is highly dependent on the degree to which students and fieldwork educators share the responsibility for teaching and learning.

References

American Occupational Therapy Association. (1983). *Reference manual of the official documents of the American Occupational Therapy Association*. Rockville, MD: American Occupational Therapy Association.

Christie, B. A., Joyce, P. C., & Moeller, P. L. (1985). Fieldwork experience 1: Impact on practice preference. *American Journal of Occupational Therapy*, *39*(10), 671–674.

Cohn, E. S. (1991). *Student fieldwork manual*. Medford, MA: Tufts University–Boston School of Occupational Therapy.

Commission on Education of the American Occupational Therapy Association. (1977). *Fieldwork experience manual for academic fieldwork coordinators, fieldwork supervisors and students*. Rockville, MD: American Occupational Therapy Association.

Commission on Education of the American Occupational Therapy Association. (1983). *Fieldwork evaluation for the occupational therapy assistant*. Rockville, MD: American Occupational Therapy Association.

Commission on Education of the American Occupational Therapy Association. (1985). *Guidelines for an occupational therapy fieldwork experience—level II*. Rockville, MD: American Occupational therapy Association.

Commission on Education of the American Occupational Therapy Association. (1986). *Fieldwork evaluation for the occupational therapist*. Rockville, MD: American Occupational Therapy Association.

Commission on Education of the American Occupational Therapy Association. (1988). *Guide to fieldwork education*. Rockville, MD: American Occupational Therapy Association.

Commission on Education of the American Occupational Therapy Association. (1991a). *Essentials and guidelines of an accredited educational program for the occupational therapist*. Rockville, MD: American Occupational Therapy Association.

Commission on Education of the American Occupational Therapy Association. (1991b). *Essentials and guidelines of an accredited educational program for the occupational therapy assistant*. Rockville, MD: American Occupational Therapy Association.

Crist, P. A. H. (1986). *Contemporary issues in clinical education*. Thorofare, NJ: Slack.

Fidler, G. (1966). Learning as a growth process. *American Journal of Occupational Therapy, 20*(1), 1–8.

Freeman, E. (1985). The importance of feedback in clinical supervision: Implications for direct practice. *Clinical Supervisor, 3*, 5–26.

Geyer, L. A. (1988). Affiliation supervision requires knowledge of learning styles. *Occupational Therapy Advance*, July 11, 1988, pp. 10–14.

Kolb, D. (1984). *Experiential learning: Experience as the source of learning and development*. Englewood Cliffs, NJ: Prentice-Hall.

Pressler, S. (1983). Fieldwork education: The proving ground of the profession. *American Journal of Occupational Therapy, 3*, 163–165.

Schwartz, K. B. (1980). *Fieldwork policies and procedures*. Medford, MA: Tufts University–Boston School of Occupational Therapy.

Yerxa, E. (1988). Problems of evaluating fieldwork students. In Commission on Education of the American Occupational Therapy Association (Eds.), *Guide to Fieldwork Education* (pp. 184–189). Rockville MD: American Occupational therapy Association.

Bibliography

Adelstein, L. A., Cohn, E. S., Baker, R. C., & Barnes, M. A. (1990). A part-time level 11 fieldwork program. *American Journal of Occupational Therapy, 44*, 60–65.

Cohn, E. S. (1989). Fieldwork education: Shaping a foundation for clinical reasoning. *American Journal of Occupational Therapy, 43*, 240–244.

Crepeau, B., & LaGarde, T. (Eds.). (1991). *Self-paced instruction for clinical education and supervision*. Rockville, MD: American Occupational Therapy Association.

Frum, D. C., & Opacich, K. J. (1987). *Supervision: The development of therapeutic competence*. Rockville, MD: American Occupational Therapy Association.

Jacobs, K., & Logigien, M. (Eds.). (1989). *Functions of a manager in occupational therapy*. Thorofare, NJ: Slack.

Kadushin, A. (1968). Games people play in supervision. *Social Work, 23*(62), 23–32.

Loganbill, C., Hardy, E., & Delworth, U. (1982). Supervision: A conceptual model. *Counseling Psychologist, 10*(1), 1–42.

SECTION 3

Ethics in occupational therapy

RUTH ANN HANSEN

KEY TERMS

Autonomy	Fidelity
Competency	Metaethics
Informed Consent	Normative Ethics
Beneficence	Justice
Equity	Distributive
Ethics	Nonmaleficence
	Paternalism

LEARNING OBJECTIVES

Upon completion of this section the reader will be able to:

1. *Understand and use key terms in discussions of ethical issues.*

2. *Identify utilitarian or teleologic reasoning and deontologic reasoning and distinguish between them.*

3. *Explain the uses and purposes of a professional code.*

4. *Discuss each principle of the Occupational Therapy Code of Ethics including the core ethical concepts described in each.*

5. *Know the ethical jurisdiction of the Standards and Ethics Commission of the American Occupational Therapy Association (AOTA), the American Occupational Therapy Certification Board (AOTCB), and the state regulatory boards (SRB).*

6. *Examine current ethical dilemmas in occupational therapy, discuss the issues and conflicts involved, and generate possible solutions to the dilemmas.*

Ethics is everybody's business. Thanks to the public media (newspapers, magazines, radio, and television), all of us are much more aware of the consequences of unethical conduct among stockbrokers, members of Congress, the judiciary, people in highly competitive businesses and, yes, health care professionals. You may have noticed that more and more people are using the word "ethics" in their everyday discussions of both personal and public issues.

Struggling with decisions about what is right or wrong in a given situation is an integral part of our lives. Decisions about what is right are based on personal, professional, and societal values. Ethical dilemmas occur when we encounter situations in which there is no clear right answer or when our values from different parts of our lives conflict. These dilemmas can cause us to feel uneasy or upset, and often create challenging differences of opinion with our professional colleagues.

The focus of this section is a discussion of the ethics of our profession—occupational therapy. To be comfortable discussing professional ethics, we need to understand several key terms and at least two major philosophical perspectives.

Definitions

Autonomy—the right of an individual to be self-determining; being self-sufficient in making and carrying out decisions about one's own life. Used when referring to patients' rights to make their own health care decisions; also used to describe health care professionals' rights to make decisions that are within their areas of professional expertise.

   Competency—having the cognitive and psychological abilities necessary to make decisions that are judged to be rational by other members of one's society. Can also include having the physical abilities to act on those decisions.

   Informed consent—the right of the individual to make choices about his or her own health care that are based on an understanding of the options available and the possible consequences of various alternatives. Connected to this idea is the notion that such choices should be made without coercion or external controlling influences.

Beneficence—holding the primary concern of doing good for others; the duty to try to bring about what is best for another person

Equity—the belief in the equality of all people. There is an accompanying duty to treat everyone equally that is an important consideration when deciding on the manner in which scarce resources will be allocated.

Ethics—the values and beliefs that are part of a particular group (social, cultural, professional); a guide for its members when determining right from wrong

   Metaethics—the branch of philosophy that examines the commonalities in the ways that human beings make decisions about what is right or moral

   Normative ethics—the examination of the day-to-day deliberations of members of a particular group about what is the "right thing to do."

Fidelity—the duty to be faithful to the patient and to the patient's best interests; includes the mandate to keep all patient information confidential

Justice—the concept of providing to an individual what is a "fair share" of resources (e.g., services, goods, money) or is that person's deserved or earned reward

   Distributive justice—the means of determining how resources will be apportioned or dispensed. This is a much-deliberated principle in health care today when determining how scarce resources (trained staff, equipment, or funding) will be allocated.

Nonmaleficence—the obligation to avoid doing harm to another or creating a circumstance in which harm could occur

Paternalism—acting or making decisions for another without that person's consent, usually done with the intent of doing what is best for that person

These terms are related to one another. Some, such as beneficence and nonmaleficence, are sometimes paired in discussions. Beneficence conveys the idea of doing good or what is best for an individual or group, whereas nonmaleficence implies an effort to avoid doing harm. For example, when an occupational therapist (OTR) works with a person who has been burned, the therapist may be playing out the principle of beneficence when working with the person to regain independence in activities of daily living. On the other hand, when the therapist applies a splint to prevent hand deformities, the major concern is that no further harm be done. Even though splinting may be painful over the short term, the person will have maximum hand function eventually. Here, the major concern is nonmaleficence.

Autonomy or self-determination, competency, and informed consent are concepts that are interdependent and intertwined. A person's ability to be self-directing and to make independent decisions is greatly valued in our society. At the same time, we all know that numerous people are not able to make autonomous decisions. These people may have temporary or permanent loss of cognitive or psychological functioning that interferes with their ability to reason and make sound judgments. As occupational therapists, we need to remind ourselves that persons who have physical, psychological, or cognitive disabilities, as well as young children and older adults, have the right to remain as autonomous as possible in their daily lives.

Determining whether a person is *competent* to make informed health care decisions is crucial when deciding whether the individual is *able* to make informed treatment choices. These decisions are not made easily and are often tied to legal decisions about whether or not a person requires a guardian. Again, we need to remind ourselves that we are obligated to inform those being served about the nature of the therapy provided, the goals of treatment, expected outcomes, and other treatment options.

Another critical principle is justice. Most people would agree that everyone should be treated fairly and receive the health care resources that they need and deserve. But how are those determinations to be made when money, time, equipment, and personnel are finite, limited resources? In most acute care settings, occupational therapy managers are deciding who gets treated, by whom, and for how long. Many of these decisions are based on the potential recipient's ability to pay for therapy, usually through some type of insurance coverage.

Understanding the terminology is important, but it is also necessary to have some familiarity with philosophy. Following is a description of two main theories in philosophy that help to explain the different ways that individuals perceive ethical situations and bring them to a personally satisfying resolution.

Two philosophical perspectives

"In the text *Medical Ethics*, edited by Monagle and Thomasma (1988), Glenn Graber presents an organization of basic philosophical theories used most frequently in medical ethics. He has divided theories regarding moral obligation into two major groups—teleological and deontological. At the risk of oversimplifying very complex material, I have developed the chart in Table 1-3 to give a few points of comparison between the two (Graber, 1988).

In my own research on ethical dilemmas in occupational therapy practice, many therapists explain that their major concern was assuring the best quality of life possible for their

TABLE 1-3. *Theories of Moral Obligation*

	Teleology	Deontology
How to determine right from wrong	By the consequences of an act	Identify what your duty is
Goal	To do good and avoid harm	To respect others
Principle for resolving conflict	Produce the greatest balance of good over evil	Weigh conflicting duties to determine which one is the primary or actual duty
	Produce the greatest good for the greatest number	

(From Graber, G.C. [1988]. Basic theories in medical ethics. In J.F. Monogle & D.C. Thomasma [Eds.], Medical ethics: A guide for health professionals [pp. 462–475]. Rockville, MD: Aspen.)

patients (Hansen, 1984). Quality of life for the patient as a fundamental issue is specifically mentioned by the deontologists Brody (1981) and Jonsen, Siegler, & Winslade (1982) but is not mentioned by any other major theorist which Graber cited.

When reading the literature on ethics it is important to determine the orientation of the author(s) because their philosophical base will influence what they consider to be the right course of action in a given situation. For example, an OTR is having difficulty deciding whether or not to share information with a patient about the use of the results of the functional assessment in making decisions about future placement. The agency for which the OTR works does not want this information shared with the patient since the management determines placement based on the census in various facilities and on a need to keep occupancy at the maximum to achieve the greatest profit margin. In other words, placement decisions are made for financial reasons over concerns about the least restrictive environment for the individual. The teleologist would weigh the decision based upon the consequences for the patient, the therapist, and the agency. Whereas, the deontologist would pay more attention to the duties of the various individuals to one another (patient, therapist, employer, family)." (Hansen, 1990, pp. 4–5).

It is important to remember that although these philosophical discussions may seem far removed from the everyday decisions that we make, they aren't. Differences of opinion among colleagues about the right answer or right solution to a problem may have their origins in a difference between deciding on the rank ordering of various duties or choosing the greatest good for the greatest number over a specific duty.

In addition to knowledge of some basic terminology and a brief overview of some philosophical perspectives, OTRs and certified occupational therapy assistants (COTAs) must understand the code of ethics of our profession.

Occupational therapy code of ethics

The Occupational Therapy Code of Ethics (AOTA, 1988) is a document that describes correct professional conduct for occupational therapy practitioners (OTRs and COTAs). These principles are also intended as a guide for students as future practitioners. What is the purpose of a professional code of ethics? Members of a profession write and publicly proclaim their codes to assure the general public that members of that particular profession are held to a higher standard of conduct than is expected of a lay person. Why does the profession of occupational therapy have a code of ethics? Because as occupational therapists, along with other health care professionals, we are

allowed special privileges that are not permitted to the general public. We have access to confidential information about patients and we are allowed to touch and manipulate the bodies of persons whom we serve.

The current Occupational Therapy Code of Ethics of AOTA outlines the general ethical principles and standards that we are expected to exemplify in our professional lives. It is important to remember from the outset that these principles are general in nature and will not provide the "right" answer to a particular ethical dilemma. (See Appendix A.)

Principle 1 centers around the ethical concepts of beneficence and autonomy. Occupational therapy practitioners are admonished to "demonstrate their concern for the welfare and dignity of the recipients of their services" (AOTA, 1988, p. 795). Under this principle, there are eight separate statements that provide clarification and specific examples of how these principles are "put into action." The practitioner must be sure that the following are carried out:

1. Services are provided with equity and without prejudice.
2. All potential recipients of services understand what therapy is planned and that they have the option of refusing.
3. All potential research subjects (patients, staff, students) are informed of the potential outcomes of the research and, in addition, students are informed of the expected outcomes of their educational experience.
4. Those receiving occupational therapy services are actively involved in setting treatment goals.
5. An objective relationship is maintained with all persons served.
6. All information gained in the practice, research, or educational arena remains confidential unless there is a threat of potential harm to another person.
7. No harm is done to the person receiving services nor to that person's property.
8. All fees for services are established in a fair and equitable manner and that the person is billed only for those services received.

Principle 2 emphasizes the need for occupational therapy practitioners to be competent in their practice. This means that the person must hold the necessary entry level credentials to practice (OTR or COTA) and includes additional credentials that may be state regulations or that are necessary for a particular specialization such as hand therapy or sensory integration. It requires that all practitioners involve themselves in an ongoing process of professional development to maintain and upgrade skills, and they must carry out their professional roles within their own levels of abilities and skills. In addition, if necessary services are outside the area of competence or expertise of an individual practitioner, he or she must either refer the potential client to someone more qualified or seek consultation with such an individual.

Principle 3 stresses the importance of adhering to the laws and regulations that govern the occupational therapy profession. This means that the individual must know and adhere to those local, state, and federal laws affecting occupational therapy, as well as all professional association policies and standards, and institutional or facilities protocols and guidelines. The practitioner is required to be sure that employers are informed of these regulations and that pertinent laws and regulations regarding documentation and billing are followed. Of course, abiding by and adhering to the Code itself as one type of professional policy is stressed.

Principle 4 highlights the need to avoid the use of false or exaggerated advertising or marketing strategies to attract prospective clients. The individual practitioner must be accurate in presenting the scope and limits of personal expertise and must avoid the use of "guarantees" or promises about cures or assured outcomes of treatment.

Principle 5 focuses on the need to maintain good relationships with fellow professionals. This implies the need to treat others with respect and courtesy, to provide appropriate supervision, and to appropriately recognize the contributions of others. Also included in this principle is the duty of "whistleblowing," that is, the obligation to report the illegal or unethical conduct of professional colleagues to appropriate authorities.

Principle 6 is a general statement that reminds practitioners to conduct themselves in a professional manner in all matters related to their roles as practitioners, educators, researchers, consultants, or managers. It also contains an admonition to avoid situations in which a conflict of interest may be present. This can happen when there is a perception of additional benefit to be gained beyond that which is readily apparent (e.g., urging a patient to buy a seating device from a particular company in which the therapist holds stock or from which the therapist will receive a commission).

As mentioned earlier, The Occupational Therapy Code of Ethics is an example of a document written by members of the occupational therapy profession to convey standards of ethical conduct. In fact, this Code was written by the American Occupational Therapy Association, Standards and Ethics Commission. It was subsequently reviewed by selected members of the Association and brought to the Representative Assembly of AOTA for final review and approval.

Ethical jurisdiction

When individuals have concerns about the misconduct of occupational therapy practitioners, they are often perplexed about where to go to seek guidance in determining what is ethically and legally permissible. General information about the three major organizations/groups that have jurisdiction over the profession of occupational therapy is provided in the following text. They are the American Occupational Therapy Association (AOTA), the American Occupational Therapy Certification Board (AOTCB), and state regulatory boards. Following the description of the purpose, scope, and regulatory power of each organiza-

tion are some guidelines for determining which of the three to contact in a given situation.

AOTA

The AOTA is a voluntary membership organization that represents and promotes the interest of persons who choose to become members. Because membership is voluntary, AOTA has no direct authority over practitioners (OTRs and COTAs) who are not members and no direct legal mechanism for preventing nonmembers who are incompetent, unethical, or unqualified from practicing. The Standards and Ethics Commission (SEC) is the component of AOTA that is responsible for the Code of Ethics (AOTA, 1988), the essentials for accreditation of educational programs (AOTA 1991a, 1991b), and the standards of practice (AOTA, 1983) of the profession. This group is responsible for informing and educating members about current ethical issues, upholding the practice and education standards of the profession, monitoring the behavior of members, and reviewing allegations of unethical conduct.

If a complaint is filed with the SEC, the Commission initiates an extensive, confidential review process. If a preliminary investigation review committee determines that there is sufficient evidence to warrant filing a complaint, a formal complaint is forwarded to a judicial council appointed by the president of AOTA to hear the case. If the person is found guilty of unethical conduct, several levels of sanction may be imposed depending on the severity of the infraction; these include (1) public censure, (2) temporary suspension of membership, and (3) revocation or permanent loss of membership.

AOTCB

The AOTCB is the national credentialing agency that certifies qualified persons as OTRs and COTAs through a written examination. That organization, by virtue of its purpose, has jurisdiction over all AOTCB certified occupational therapy practitioners as well as those eligible for AOTCB certification. AOTCB has developed "Grounds for Discipline" (AOTCB, 1991), used by that organization as a guide for considering possible disciplinary action. The three main categories of concern are incompetence, unethical behavior, and impairment. When AOTCB receives a complaint, they also initiate an intensive, confidential review process to determine whether the allegations are warranted. If so, depending on the seriousness of the misconduct, one of several sanctions are possible:

1. *Reprimand* (a formal expression of disapproval of conduct communicated privately and retained in the individual's certification file),
2. *Censure* (a formal expression of disapproval that is public),
3. *Ineligibility for certification* indefinitely or for a specified period of time,
4. *Probation* (a period of time in which the person is required to fulfill certain conditions such as education, supervision, counseling to remain certified),
5. *Suspension* or loss of certification for a specified period of time (often used when the person is required to complete a specific amount of public service or to participate in a rehabilitation program),
6. *Revocation* (permanent loss of certification).

State regulatory boards

State regulatory boards (SRBs) are public bodies created by state legislatures to ensure the health and safety of the citizens of that state. Their specific responsibility is to protect the public from potential harm that might be caused by incompetent or unqualified practitioners. State regulation may be in the form of licensure, registration, or certification. The legal guidelines of each state usually specify the scope of practice of the profession and the qualifications that must be met to practice. In addition, the board usually provides a description of ethical behavior. (In most instances, SRBs have adopted AOTA's Code of Ethics for this purpose.)

These state regulatory boards, by the very nature of their limited jurisdiction (ie, jurisdiction only over therapists practicing in their state) can monitor a profession closely. They have the authority by law to discipline members of a profession if the public is determined to be at risk. Boards can also intervene in situations in which the person has been convicted of an illegal act that is directly connected with professional practice. An example is fraud or misappropriation of funds through false billing practices.

Because each state board is primarily concerned with the protection of the public from harm, they will limit their review of complaints to those involving such a threat. In instances in which the state board determines that a person has violated the law, it can elect several different sanctions as a disciplinary measure. Examples are (1) public censure, (2) temporary suspension of practice privileges, and (3) permanent prohibition from practice in that state.

Where to go first

The AOTA, AOTCB, and state regulatory boards have specific jurisdictions over occupational therapy. Some areas of concern overlap, whereas others are distinct and unique. When deciding which of the three to contact for information and where to most effectively file a specific complaint, you need to answer the following three questions:

1. Did the alleged violation take place in a state that regulates occupational therapy?
2. Is the individual a member of AOTA?
3. What consequences would you consider appropriate if the complaint were determined to be justified?

If an alleged violation occurred in a state that has an occupational therapy regulatory law, both AOTA and AOTCB will recommend that you contact that state's regulatory board first. At the present time all states except Colorado, New Jersey, and Vermont have laws regulating the occupational therapy profession. Because each state has specific "local" jurisdiction and direct legal power, it is possible that the review will take place more quickly and any sanction that might be imposed will have an immediate and direct effect on the person.

If the incident occurred in a state without a regulatory law, you must determine whether the person is a member of AOTA. If so, you could contact AOTA or AOTCB. If not, your only recourse is to contact the AOTCB. If you must choose between the two organizations, you should determine what you would consider to be appropriate consequences if the person is judged to be in violation. AOTA actions can restrict or prohibit the person's ability to participate as a full member in the professional association, whereas AOTCB sanctions can suspend or revoke the violator's certification.

Within the past year, AOTA, AOTCB, and state regulatory boards have established a communication network, The Disciplinary Action Information Exchange Network (DAIEN), to notify the other organizations when any action is taken against an occupational therapy practitioner. The AOTCB's quarterly newsletter, *The Information Exchange*, publishes the DAIEN list, which is a master list of the names of persons who have been reported by the AOTCB, AOTA, and state regulatory boards as being subject to disciplinary action. Each group in turn decides whether to take additional action against the OTR or COTA who has been reprimanded for unethical or illegal conduct.

Summary

This section is intended to provide a background for readers about the various organizations that have ethical jurisdiction over occupational therapy. This information will be useful when determining where to seek guidance when ethical issues arise (Hansen, 1991).

Two ethical dilemmas

It is always difficult to translate abstract concepts into practical terms. You may be wondering what all this has to do with the everyday practice of occupational therapy. The two cases that are provided should help you to relate these ideas on a more pragmatic level. One is a discussion of a practice issue and the second is a management concern.

The cases are organized to provide you with the details of a situation and then a series of questions that should be considered when trying to resolve the ethical dilemma that is presented.

CASE 1

An occupational therapist is working for a for-profit, outpatient agency that provides rehabilitation services on a contractual basis. Mr. Alexander, who is 68 years old, had a stroke 3 months earlier. He was referred for occupational therapy services after his discharge from the hospital. His therapist, Ms. Kyle, has been working with Mr. Alexander on self-care activities for 1 hour, three times a week. He has made significant progress and Ms. Kyle decides to reduce his sessions to two ½-hour sessions each week.

When the administrator of the agency reads her report, he tells her not to reduce Mr. Alexander's time in treatment. The administrator explains that Mr. Alexander's insurance allows for up to 3 hours of occupational therapy a week and that is what should be provided in order to maximize the revenue of the agency.

Ms. Kyle is an experienced therapist and she knows that the 3 hours per week of therapy is not warranted. The administrator says that she must see him for the maximum amount of time that is "reimbursable." What should Ms. Kyle do?

The conflict in this situation is between the therapist's duty to her employer and her duty to the patient (and his insurance company). In thinking about this case you may want more information about the details. Often the reason why a situation is a dilemma is because all the facts are not available. If you take this case at face value, however, what are some of the questions/options that you might consider in bringing this issue to a satisfactory resolution?

The following are some possible points to think about:

1. What do Mr. Alexander and his family want? Does he feel that he needs more or less therapy to reach his goals?
2. Are there other types of therapy besides self-care training that should be provided for Mr. Alexander that are reimbursable? If not, can the 3 hours of treatment be justified to improve endurance and reduce the time needed to perform certain activities such as dressing?
3. What will happen if Ms. Kyle refuses to extend the amount of time that she sees the patient because in her best professional judgment, it is not needed? Is it worth taking the risk of getting fired?
4. What obligation does Ms. Kyle have to her employer and the agency? Is it part of her duty to make sure that the company remains viable?
5. What do the state and federal regulations and guidelines mandate in these situations? In other words, what is required to be practicing legally?

Of course, you will undoubtedly come up with other questions that should be taken into account when deliberating this case. Spend some time discussing them with your colleagues and try to reach a solution that all, or most, of you can agree is reasonable. After you have done this, role play the situation of providing this explanation to Mr. Alexander, his family, the agency administrator, and the third-party payor.

CASE 2

Ms. Scott is the director of an occupational therapy department in a large metropolitan hospital. The occupational therapy staff consists of six OTRs, two COTAs, and one aide. Recently the corporation that owns the hospital has been in serious financial difficulties and is attempting to implement all possible cost-saving measures to avoid bankruptcy. Mr. Wyatt, Ms. Scott's immediate supervisor and the administrator of all rehabilitation services, has asked her to find ways of cutting costs and increasing revenue.

The department implements several new procedures to achieve this goal but are told that more is needed. Two staff therapists (OTR) vacancies occur during this time and Mr. Wyatt tells Ms. Scott to convert them to three COTA positions. As he explains, "It will reduce our payroll budget and at the same time increase productivity."

Ms. Scott is concerned about providing the best possible treatment for the individuals that the department serves and in the most cost-effective manner possible.

In the previous situation it is possible for the two concerns of service and cost-effectiveness to come into conflict with one another. The following are some of the questions that arise when considering this dilemma:

1. What are the legal and ethical guidelines that describe the practice of OTRs and COTAs? What if any differences are there between the role of each? What type of supervision is required and by whom?
2. Would a change in staffing allow the department to maintain all services currently provided, including those in such specialty areas as neonatal intensive care and the traumatic brain injury acute care unit? If not, would essential services need to be cut or would the changes be in the form of shifts of emphasis and the provision of more services in areas that were previously underserved?
3. Are all the OTRs now on staff capable of providing the type of supervision necessary? Are they willing to reduce their direct patient contact and take on these supervisory responsibilities?
4. Is it realistic to expect that there are COTAs available in the community who would be interested in these new positions?
5. If the department is successful in making this transition, does it set a precedent for further shifts in staffing in the future?

Obviously, there are no clear answers to the questions posed. Again, it would be useful to discuss these and other issues that this dilemma generates with your professional peers. Try to look at this issue from the perspective of the OT manager, the administrator, the present and future staff, and the patients in the hospital. As in the previous case, test possible solutions by role playing an explanation of the "plan" to each of the involved parties.

Summary

Struggling with right and wrong in given situations is a part of everyday life. Ethical dilemmas are also found in the profession of occupational therapy, and it is necessary to get an overview of the professional ethics of occupational therapy. It is important to understand ethics terminology such as competence and informed consent. Two major philosophical perspectives—deontologic and teleontologic—can be applied to occupational therapy decisions. In addition, the purpose of professional codes and a discussion of each of the six principles contained in the AOTA code (AOTA, 1988) are important to understand. The ethical jurisdiction of the three major bodies—AOTA, AOTCB, and state regulatory boards—differ concerning the occupational therapy practice. The conflicts that exist between quality of service and cost-effectiveness in two cases illustrated herein can be used as a springboard for the clarification of the ethical issues that members of the profession encounter in their careers. You are urged to explore the literature on health care ethics more broadly and remain well versed about the issues involved in the emerging ethical challenges of our profession.

References

American Occupational Therapy Association. (1983). Standards of practice for occupational therapy. *American Journal of Occupational Therapy, 37,* 802–804.

American Occupational Therapy Association. (1988). Occupational therapy code of ethics. *American Journal of Occupational Therapy, 12,* 795–796.

American Occupational Therapy Association. (1991a). Essentials and guidelines of an accredited educational program for the occupational therapist. *American Journal of Occupational Therapy, 12,* 1077–1084.

American Occupational Therapy Association. (1991b). Essentials and guidelines of an accredited educational program for the occupational therapy assistant. *American Journal of Occupational Therapy, 12,* 1085–1092.

AOTCB (1991). Procedures for disciplinary action. Rockville, MD: AOTCB.

Brody, H. (1981). *Ethical decisions in medicine* (2nd ed.). Boston: Little, Brown.

Graber, G. C. (1988). Basic theories in medical ethics. In J. F. Monagle & D. C. Thomasma (Eds.), *Medical ethics: A guide for health professionals* (pp. 462–475). Rockville, MD: Aspen.

Hansen, R. A. (1984). Moral reasoning of occupational therapists: Implications for education and practice. (Doctoral dissertation, Wayne State University, 1984). *Dissertation Abstracts International, 45,* 761A.

Hansen, R. A. (1990). Lesson 10: Ethical considerations. In C. B. Royeen (Ed.), *AOTA self study series: Assessing function.* Rockville, MD: AOTA.

Hansen, R. A. (1991). Ethical jurisdiction of occupational therapy: The role of AOTA, AOTCB and State Regulatory Boards. *OT Week.*

Jonsen, A., Siegeler, M., & Winslade, W. (1982). *Clinical ethics: A practical approach to ethical decisions in clinical medicine.* New York: Macmillan.

CHAPTER 2

The beginnings of occupational therapy

KATHLYN L. REED

KEY TERMS

Addams, Jane

Archives of Occupational
   Therapy

Arts and Crafts Movement

Barton, George E.

Barton, Isabel Newton

British Journal of
   Occupational Therapy

Chicago School of Civics and
   Philanthropy

Dunton, William Rush, Jr.

Educational Standards

Henry B. Favill School of
   Occupations

Hull House

Humanism

Humanitarianism

Johnson, Susan C.

Kidner, Thomas B.

Maryland Psychiatric
   Quarterly

Mechanistic philosophy

Meyer, Adolf

Moral treatment

National Society for the
   Promotion of Occupational
   Therapy (NSPOT)

Occupational therapy and
   rehabilitation

Occupational Therapy Code of
   Ethics

Reconstruction aides

Rush, Benjamin

Slagle, Eleanor Clarke

Tracy, Susan E.

Vocational Rehabilitation Act
   and Amendments

LEARNING OBJECTIVES

Upon completion of this chapter the reader will be able to:

1. *Understand the social–cultural heritage of occupational therapy including humanism, humanitarianism, moral treatment, and the arts and crafts movements.*

2. *Become acquainted with the people who formulated the ideas and concepts on which occupational therapy is based and know where these people lived.*

3. *Learn the names and contributions of the founders of the National Society for the Promotion of Occupational Therapy/American Occupational Therapy Association.*

4. *Understand the world events that influenced the development of occupational therapy, including World War I and World War II.*

5. *Learn about federal legislation in the United States that has influenced the practice of occupational therapy.*

6. *Become acquainted with the concepts of educational standards, accreditation, registration, certification, and credentialing.*

7. *Understand the roles and functions of the American Occupational Therapy Association and the American Occupational Therapy Foundation.*

8. *Learn the concept of philosophy and the influence of different views of philosophy—organismic and mechanistic—on the development of occupational therapy practice and research.*

9. *Become acquainted with the development of occupational therapy worldwide and the formation of the World Federation of Occupational Therapists.*

To many people, history is boring, but the same people may spend hours tracing their family roots. A profession also has roots. The techniques, methods, modalities, and theories used in current occupational therapy practice all have historical roots. New ideas usually are based, at least in part, on concepts developed in earlier times. Knowledge of one's professional history is part of one's working life just as knowledge of one's family history is part of one's private life.

Development of a profession

Events that lead to the formation of a profession occur within a sociocultural context. Certain ideas and concepts develop and lead to action and doing. People, of course, do the thinking that develops the ideas, and the same or different people carry out the actions. The people happen to live in certain geographic areas in countries and cities. Common social backgrounds, cultural experiences, and land topography tend to facilitate or hinder communication among people who spread and share ideas. Out of the ideas develop concepts which, in the case of occupational therapy, can be used to develop models for viewing health and treating disease and dysfunction. Finally, ideas and concepts lead to conflict and change. Thus, the framework for this chapter includes a discussion of the sociocultural ideas and concepts that led to the creation of occupational therapy; the names of persons who contributed to the development and refinement of the profession; the places where these leaders of occupational therapy lived and interacted with other leaders; the role of the professional association in shaping the educational process for students and the practice of occupational therapy; the models of treatment that developed from the leaders of ideas; and, finally, the conflicts and changes that have resulted from ongoing refinement of ideas and concepts worldwide.

Social philosophy

The development of occupational therapy is woven into the fabric of human existence, but the tapestry became rich in the 19th and early 20th centuries. Occupation has been central to human existence, probably from the beginning of time. Many ideas have been presented throughout the centuries concerning who should work, what work should be performed, who should play, and when the playing should begin and end (Braude, 1983; Rodgers, 1974). Health and occupation became tied together because lack of health diminished the ability to engage in occupation.

English society and culture during the 19th century discussed the issues of occupation and health in numerous writings (Pressey & Rollins, 1904; Wagner, 1904). Many ideas and viewpoints appear but those that have influenced occupational therapy are related to the philosophy of humanism and the social values of humanitarianism that developed moral treatment and the arts and crafts movement. Thus, the roots of occupational therapy can be traced to English heritage as transmitted and altered by the American experience (Shi, 1985; Lears, 1981).

Moral treatment

Moral treatment evolved as a reaction to the prevailing approach to mental illness. Before the development of moral treatment, a person who was mentally ill was viewed as having lost all reason and therefore became animal-like, was considered a sinner or criminal, and possibly considered to be possessed by demons or supernatural spirits (Bynum, 1964). Such a person clearly was dangerous and could not be trusted in society, and therefore needed to be removed from it. Mental hospitals frequently whipped patients, chained them, and put them on exhibit for the curiosity of sightseers (Scull, 1979). Not everyone agreed that mental illness was a hopeless disorder. Some people suggested the cure was worse than the disease. Locking people in institutions almost guaranteed a deterioration of the mental processes. For example, what if a person were viewed as able to be responsible for his or her actions? What if an environment were set up that encouraged a person with mental problems to behave in a manner that was acceptable to society? What if a person who was mentally ill could be taught or retaught to behave according to the cultural norms? Would not such a person be considered morally sane? Thus, moral treatment stressed moral behavior.

The shift from pessimism to optimism about curing insanity occurred as thoughts about the causes of mental illness were shifting from somatic to psychological. Such thinking reflected the spirit of reform and **humanitarianism** that was sweeping both Western Europe and the United States. Dain (1964) suggests that the successes in astronomy and physics and the rapid strides in technology and political changes "were practical proofs of the Enlightenment's faith that man could control his environment and improve his life on earth" (p. 11). Thus, moral treatment evolved from both a humanitarian and a humanistic movement.

Arts and crafts movement

The **arts and crafts** movement was concerned more with general health than a specific area of disease (Eaton, 1949). Workers' general health was observed to be deteriorating in many large factories that were located in large cities. Knowledge of public health was meager in the 19th century, but a few people did understand the relationship of good physical health to physical exercise and clean air. Both were lacking in the factories and cities where people were required to work. They lived in situations that contributed to communicable diseases through lack of sanitation and occupational diseases because of poor ventilation and exposure to toxic agents (Naylor, 1971). As a reaction to the poor health and living conditions, the proponents of the arts and crafts movement suggested that people should return to the land (farming); live in small villages; make useful, functional products based on good designs; and become skilled craftspersons who could produce goods and services that promoted self-reliance (Marsh, 1982). Americans were not about to give up their factories or cities but were interested in the arts and crafts movement. Of specific interest was the concern for good design, good craftsmanship, self-reliance, and the role of craft work in promoting improved physical and mental health (Boris, 1986).

People and places—the pioneers

A French physician, **Philippe Pinel**, is usually credited with being the first to break the chains with which the mentally ill were bound. In 1793, he established practices that led to a more human approach to the treatment of persons with mental disorders (Pinel, 1962). His reforms were widely recognized and followed in Europe; however, American reformers did not choose to seek his counsel. Instead, they chose to visit reformers in England. The rationale was probably related to the Quaker religion rather than to specific disbelief in Pinel's ideas, since the English reformers were following a similar course toward humane treatment.

Among the most influential leaders in England was the Tuke family. **Samuel Tuke**, an English Quaker, was responsible for popularizing the treatment approach called moral treatment (Tuke, 1964). His grandfather, William Tuke, had founded the York Retreat in York, England, in 1796. William Tuke, like Pinel, did not believe that chains and punishment would help the mentally ill recover. Tuke believed most mental illness was curable. Instead of restraining the people, he released them as Pinel had done and clothed them. Tuke added the idea of encouraging patients to learn self-control and, with the use of attendants, engaged them in a variety of employment or amusements best adapted to different patients (Tuke, 1964).

American Quakers soon began to take note of moral treatment. *Thomas Scattergood*, a Quaker minister, visited the Retreat and returned with the concepts of "occupation and non-restraint." These concepts were used at the Friends Asylum for the Insane in Frankford, Pennsylvania, which opened in May, 1817 (Deutsch, 1949; Dain and Carlson, 1960). *Thomas Eddy*, a New York merchant and member of the Society of Friends, also visited the Retreat. He returned with the concept of "moral management"; this was later instituted at Bloomingdale Asylum, which was opened in New York City in 1821 (Deutsch, 1949.) The Asylum later moved to White Plains, in Westchester County, New York.

The first physician known to use the concepts of moral treatment and occupation in America was **Benjamin Rush**, also a Quaker. Rush is frequently considered the father of American psychiatry. He regarded insanity as a disease of the brain, in contrast to the prevailing theories in European medicine, which viewed insanity as a disorder of the body (Bynum, 1964). Rush (1962) also believed that "man was made to be active" (p. 117). He recommended exercise, labor, and music as part of the treatment for mental illness (Rush, 1962, pp. 224–226). Rush's ideas were actually ahead of their time. His book *Medical Inquiries and Observation Upon the Disease of the Mind* was published in 1812 (Rush, 1962). Moral treatment did not reach its full impact until about 1840.

Another early advocate of moral treatment was *Dr. Rufus Wyman*. He supervised the McLean Asylum near Boston, which opened in 1818. Wyman was specific about the use of moral treatment and occupation. He stated,

> But in mental disorders without symptoms of organic disease, a judicious moral management is more successful. It should afford agreeable occupation. It should engage the mind, and exercise the body: as swinging, riding, walking, sewing, embroidery, bowling, gardening, mechanic arts; to which may be added reading, writing, conversation, etc., the whole to be performed with order and regularity. (Wyman, 1830, p. 24)

Another physician, *Amariah Brigham*, superintendent of the Utica State Hospital in New York, outlined the benefits of moral treatment and occupation as follows: "employment of the mind . . . in fact, manual labor . . . proves more beneficial . . . by engaging the attention and direction of the mind to new subjects of thought than by its direct effect on the body" (Brigham, 1847, p. 11). In Rhode Island, Butler Hospital was opened in 1847 under Dr. Isaac Ray. In Connecticut, Dr. Eli Todd opened the Hartford Retreat now known as the Institute of Living (Jones, 1983). Finally, **Dr. Thomas Story Kirkbride** stressed the use of moral treatment and occupation throughout his term as superintendent of the Pennsylvania Hospital from 1840 to 1860. Kirkbride was involved in the organization of the Association of Asylum Medical Superintendents, which later became the American Psychiatric Association and thus was able to influence many other superintendents regarding the use and value of moral treatment and occupation (Tomes, 1964).

Moral treatment was practiced in America for many years and was successful (Bockoven, 1972b). However, the treatment required small numbers of patients, a high patient–staff ratio, and a homogeneous patient population (Kaplan et al., 1980). Moreover, moral treatment did not require drugs or other medical remedies that physicians saw as the true practice of medicine. Therefore, their support of moral treatment varied greatly from institution to institution. Finally, as the need for more psychiatric beds increased and the institutions for persons with mental disorders grew larger, the concepts of moral treatment could not

be continued and moral treatment was replaced with other forms of care until the 1960s, when many of the ideas reappeared as milieu therapy (Carlson & Dain, 1960).

The years between 1840 and 1860 became the golden years for the application of moral treatment and occupation in American mental hospitals (Bockoven, 1972b). After the Civil War, economic hard times beset the hospitals, the leading proponents died, the public lost interest, and the hospitals became overcrowded with new immigrants who were having difficulty adjusting to their new country (Bockoven, 1972a). As the use of moral treatment declined, so did the use of occupation (Bockoven, 1972c). However, occupation arose again in the early 1900s as occupational therapy (Bockoven, 1972c). Each of the institutions just mentioned was known to have an occupational therapist practicing in that hospital, as indicated by the first registry of occupational therapists published in 1932 (AOTA, 1932 National Directory).

The arts and crafts movement began when moral treatment ended, about 1860. **John Ruskin**, an English philosopher, is credited with popularizing the ideas; however, William Morris, an English artist, architect, and student of Ruskin, is better known in connection with movement (Ruskin, no date; Morris, 1901). Morris stressed the value of functional design and well-executed craftsmanship in all his work. This craftsmanship is seen most often in wallpaper and book printing, although Morris did many other types of artwork.

The arts and crafts movement, as it was translated into education and therapy, provided two approaches. One was known originally as ward occupations, invalid occupations, or amusements, and later as diversional therapy. The other was known by such names as manual training, vocational education, and occupational training. The two approaches had different objectives and competed for emphasis in occupational therapy. **Elizabeth Upham** summarized this conflict most succinctly,

> There are two theories upon which occupation from a therapeutic stand point has been based in the past. The first is the attitude . . . that the concrete value of occupation is its power to turn the patient's attention away from the disability, this in itself frequently constituting a real cure. This group of therapeutists makes occupation interesting, makes it approach normal activities, and makes the patient as little conscious of any abnormality as possible. There is, on the contrary, another smaller group of occupational therapeutists who believe the patient's disability should be uppermost in his mind. They related the occupation so closely to his disability that he is keenly conscious that occupation, as an interest or diversion, is not the primary concern, but as a part of his cure it is fundamental. He is taught to be faithful to that occupation as he would be in taking a drug and he develops a genuine interest in measuring his improvement by increased ability and length of periods of work. (Upham, 1918, pp. 18–19)

The first approach would become dominant in the practice of occupational therapy in psychiatry for persons with mental disorders. The second approach would become dominant in the practice of occupational therapy in physical disabilities, although some occupational therapists practicing in the area of mental health would revive the ideas as industrial therapy, work therapy, and finally psychiatric rehabilitation.

In 1904, **Dr. Herbert James Hall**, of Marblehead, Massachusetts, began seeking an alternative treatment to the "rest cure" for neurasthenia (Hall, 1905). Neurasthenia usually affected women, who experienced severe weakness when performing any work activity. Often neurasthenia was seen as the result of overwork (Beard, 1880). Today, the disorder probably would be classified as a stress disorder. Because the problem was originally attributed to overwork, the recommended treatment proposed by Silas Weir Mitchell, a neurologist, was total rest (Mitchell, 1891). Dr. Hall was not impressed by the recovery of persons put on rest cure and decided to try using occupations instead. He began by having the patient do a little needlework in bed, perhaps for only 10 minutes. Slowly he increased the time and later asked the patient to sit in a chair beside the bed while engaging in some simple craft activity. Later, patients "graduated" from Devereau Mansion, the boarding facility, to the Barn, a large building filled with weaving looms, ceramic molds, and various other crafts. He hired craftspersons to assist the patients in planning good designs and making commercially saleable products. He also recommended that his patients follow a schedule of work, rest, and relaxation. His ideas were drawn from the writings and ideas of the arts and crafts philosophers.

Hall's work was the first systematic study of the effects of occupation on mental health. He found that many of his patients improved when occupation and scheduled activity were used as a treatment approach (Hall, 1910). Hall was eclectic in his use of occupations and made use of both the ward occupation and manual training approaches. He later became president of the **National Society for the Promotion of Occupational Therapy (NSPOT)**. Hall was a prolific writer who authored several books that expanded his thoughts on arts and crafts as well as occupational therapy (Hall, 1913; Hall & Buck, 1915; Hall, 1923b).

Another person interested in arts and crafts was **Jane Addams**, a social service worker, who founded **Hull House** in Chicago, Illinois. In 1901, Addams decided to start a Labor Museum to show recent immigrants how making of craft items had changed over the years but the product was still basically the same (Addams, 1900). Her best example was spinning and weaving. Spinning initially was done on a variety of drop spindles, then on a spinning wheel, and finally on a machine. Weaving had followed a similar course. In the Labor Museum, the new immigrants could see how the craft used to be performed and listen to lectures about how manufacturing had changed the process but the purpose and product were the same. The Labor Museum was first developed by Jessie Luther, a crafts teacher, who 3 years later helped Herbert Hall set up the occupations at Devereau Mansion (Luther, 1902; Luther, 1918). In 1914, the Labor Museum served as a trial work rehabilitation program for immigrants who were having difficulty finding occupational skills that could lead to employment (Thomson, 1917; NSPOT, 1920). In 1917, the Labor Museum served as the site of an educational training program in cooperation with the Illinois Mental Hygiene Society for persons interested in becoming occupational therapists (Slagle, 1917). The Labor Museum emphasized primarily the manual training aspect of the arts and crafts movement.

A third application of arts and crafts developed in Jamaica Plain, Massachusetts in 1906, where **Susan Tracy**, a nurse, began a course to train nurses to use occupations in treatment of patients. Tracy wrote the first known book on occupational therapy, *Studies in Invalid Occupations*, in which she described the art or craft activity that she selected for each of her patients (Tracy, 1910). Tracy was a master clinician. Her analysis of the best occupations for each patient appears to be effortless. Therefore, the cognitive skills required to correctly assess a patient's

needs and interests are easily overlooked. Tracy also published some of the earliest known evaluation techniques for assessing patient's level of functional performance (Tracy, 1918). She was asked to be a founding member of the organization for occupational therapy, but she was busy setting up an occupational therapy department at Presbyterian Hospital in Chicago and thus declined the invitation to attend the meeting. Tracy also disagreed with the other founding members on the qualifications of therapists; she believed that trained nurses were the only persons who could learn to use occupations correctly with patients (Slagle, 1938). Nevertheless, Tracy did participate actively in the NSPOT as chair of the Committee on Teaching Methods and continued to maintain friendly relations with Slagle (Slagle, 1938). She was primarily interested in the use of ward occupations. Tracy died in 1928 (Portraits, 1928).

A fourth approach to using arts and crafts was developed by **Adolph Meyer**. Meyer immigrated from Switzerland in 1892, where he developed his early ideas about the causes and treatment of mental illness. He moved to Kankakee, Illinois to accept a position as a pathologist. There, he became acquainted with Julia Lathrop and the activities at Hull House. He was a frequent speaker in Illinois and was invited to give lectures at the courses on occupation offered at the **Chicago School of Civics and Philanthropy** from 1908 to 1911 even though he had moved to Worcester, Massachusetts and later to New York City. His next move was to Baltimore, where he started the Henry Phipps Clinic at Johns Hopkins Medical School (Mora, 1975).

Meyer saw mental disorders as resulting from disorganized habits or behavior that resulted in problems in living rather than any specific dysfunction of a given structure or function in the body or brain (Meyer, 1951). He reasoned that a person should organize his or her daily life into periods of work, play, rest, and sleep. The cycle of time and activity works to aid the person to achieve a balance and harmony with nature. Meyer presented the first organized model of occupational therapy in 1921 in his lecture entitled "The Philosophy of Occupation Therapy," which was the first article in the journal **Archives of Occupational Therapy** (Meyer, 1922).

Finally, another early proponent of occupational therapy was *Louis Haas*. Haas was a master craftsman who was hired by Bloomingdale Hospital in 1915, where he remained throughout his long professional career (Haas, 1924). Haas wrote extensively about the use of arts and crafts for therapeutic purposes and was especially influential in arguing for the role of men as occupational therapists (Haas, 1925a; Haas, 1925b). He wrote a textbook in 1925, *Occupational Therapy for the Nervous and Mentally Ill*, which was used for many years to teach occupational therapists about occupational therapy practices for persons with mental disorders (Haas, 1925c). Haas was active in NSPOT and served as its secretary in 1918; he was also a member of the **Board of Management** for several years.

People and places—the founders

In 1914, two people began a series of correspondences concerning the founding of an organization of persons interested in "occupation work," as occupational therapy was originally known. The initiating party was **George Edward Barton**, AIA (American Institute of Architecture), and the willing recipient was **Dr. William Rush Dunton, Jr.** (Dunton, 1926). Barton was an architect who had tuberculosis. During one of his recovery periods from an attack of tuberculosis, Barton began attending some lectures for nurses at the Clifton Springs Sanitarium in Clifton Springs, New York (Newton, 1917). He was interested in learning about the response of the human body to the therapeutics of occupation. In 1914, he began using the term "occupational therapy" rather than occupation work (Barton, 1915; Dunton, 1931). The term won rapid acceptance.

The correspondence of George Barton with Dr. Dunton did not go smoothly. Barton wanted the formation of the new organization to occur as he envisioned it and was afraid that Dr. Dunton's offer to help would lead to a physician takeover. Dr. Dunton tried to reassure Barton that no takeover was planned and finally the two men agreed on a date, place, and founding members of the organization, which was to be known as the National Society for the Promotion of Occupational Therapy (NSPOT or N-SPOT). Barton liked the name because he thought the initials implied a Johnny-be-ready attitude. The dates were to be March 15 to 17, 1917, in Clifton Springs, New York. The founding members were to be Barton, Dunton, Eleanor Clarke Slagle, Susan Johnson, Thomas Bissell Kidner, and *Isabel G. Newton*, who was Barton's secretary and later his wife (Dunton, 1946).

Barton continued his interest in occupations by starting Consolation House in Clifton Springs, where patients could continue their convalescence from chronic disorders and develop their vocational skills. Consolation House was an early example of the application of occupational therapy to manual training and vocational education in an outpatient setting (Newton, 1917; Barton, 1968). Barton's participation in the NSPOT was less active. Although he was elected president he was unable to attend the next meeting in September 1917 because of illness and did not participate thereafter (NSPOT, 1917a). Barton died in 1923 of recurring tuberculosis (Dunton, 1923b).

William Rush Dunton was a psychiatrist at the Shephard and Enoch Pratt Hospital in Towson, Maryland. He had been named for his uncle, Benjamin Rush, the well-known psychiatrist from Philadelphia who had used occupation in treating his patients and was a proponent of moral treatment (Licht, 1947a). Dr. Dunton himself had experimented with use of arts and craft activities in treating his patients and had started writing about his experiences in the *Maryland Psychiatric Quarterly* in 1912 in a column called Occupations and Amusements (Dunton, 1912). Dunton was editor of this *Quarterly*, and his editing skills would serve the new organization well when he became editor of the new journal on occupational therapy, *Archives of Occupational Therapy* (Dunton, 1946). Dunton also served the NSPOT as president and continued to actively support occupational therapy through his writings and correspondence. Among his many articles and books is a classic reference book, *Reconstruction Therapy* (Dunton, 1919). His long life, 99 years, certainly provided the young profession with a constant source of wisdom and counsel. Dunton's primary interest in using arts and crafts was as ward occupations. He stressed the diversional quality of occupational interests.

Dr. Dunton died in 1966 (Bing, 1967). His collection of letters, newspaper clippings, and other records form the basis of the occupational therapy archives collection now kept in Moody Medical Library in Galveston, Texas.

Eleanor Clarke Slagle was a social service worker student with Jane Addams at Hull House when she became inter-

ested in using arts and crafts at the suggestion of Addams and Julia Lathrop. Lathrop was instrumental in setting up a course on occupations and amusements at the Chicago School of Civics and Philanthropy, which conducted the classes under a state grant beginning in 1907 (Slagle, 1931). Slagle enrolled in the second class. After completion of the course she began helping to teach others about the use of arts and crafts and occupations. In 1912, Adolf Meyer, a psychiatrist, asked her to come to Johns Hopkins in Baltimore, Maryland to set up a department at the Henry Phipps Clinic, during which time she presented a paper on the history of the use of occupations as therapy (Slagle, 1914). Meyer knew Slagle from the time he worked at Kankakee State Hospital in Kankakee, Illinois. While in Baltimore, Slagle was introduced to Dr. Dunton at meetings of the American Medico-Psychological Association (Slagle, 1914).

In 1914, Slagle returned to Chicago to develop an Experimental Station run for several years by the Illinois Mental Hygiene Society at the *Labor Museum at Hull House*. In 1916, the program name was changed to the *Henry B. Favill School of Occupations* after a leading physician in the area (Favill, 1917). Slagle's activities led to an invitation from Barton and Dunton to attend the organization meeting of the NSPOT. Slagle served the NSPOT and the AOTA as president, vice president, and secretary/treasurer. In the latter capacity she organized and directed the activities of the national office headquarters throughout the 1920s until 1936 (Slagle, 1936). In addition, she was the Director of the Bureau of Occupational Therapy in the State of New York from 1920 until her death in 1942 (Slagle, 1934; Dunton, 1942). Her impact on occupational therapy has been acknowledged through the initiation of the Eleanor Clarke Slagle lectureship series, which recognizes therapists who also have made a substantial contribution to the profession (Meeting, House of Delegates, 1954, p. 24; Stattel, 1956).

In the practice of occupational therapy Slagle used both the ward occupation and manual training approaches by creating a series of steps through which a patient could progress from ward to workshop.

Susan Cox Johnson was an arts and crafts instructor originally from Texas. She had spent time in California and in the Philippines learning, teaching, and writing about textiles. After her return from the Philippines, she was hired by the state of New York to teach arts and crafts to the patients on Ward Island, a psychiatric facility (Johnson, 1917). Her activities were known to Barton, who invited her to attend the organization meeting. Johnson was deeply interested in the education of occupational therapists and in 1919 chaired a committee on education to develop standards (Johnson, 1919). Her report was not accepted for reasons not fully recorded in the minutes of the annual meeting. She apparently was not pleased by the lack of acceptance because she did not attend any meetings thereafter. Johnson used ward occupations in her approach to patients. She died in 1932 (Dunton, 1932a).

Thomas Bissell Kidner was an architect from England who was sent to Canada in 1900 to assist in the development of manual education in elementary schools. Such manual education frequently consisted of teaching arts and crafts as a means of developing hand skills, which were assumed by educators to lead to the development of occupational skills (Dunton, 1932b). Because many jobs still required considerable hand labor, manual skills were considered an essential part of the educational curriculum. In 1916, Kidner was asked to serve as the Vocational

Secretary to assist World War I Canadian soldiers to regain useful work skills after their war injuries healed. Barton heard of Kidner's appointment and invited Kidner to join the meeting at Clifton Springs to provide an international flavor (Dunton, 1926).

Shortly after the founding meeting, Kidner was invited to the United States to join the rehabilitation section of the Federal Board for Vocational Education, which was charged to provide vocational education and training to returning soldiers. After the war he became interested in designing institutions for persons with tuberculosis and was active in the National Tuberculosis Society (Kidner, 1922). He served as president of the AOTA for several years in the late 1920s when the process of registration was being developed and again briefly in 1930 when both the current president and vice president died within months of each other. Kidner was a capable leader and speaker for the cause of occupational therapy. He was committed to the manual training approach to occupational therapy. Kidner died in 1932 (Addresses, 1932).

Events

Legacy of World War I

No sooner had the National Society for the Promotion of Occupational Therapy completed its first annual meeting in September 1917 than the country was called to war by President Wilson in November. World War I had been ongoing in Europe since 1914. For 3 years the United States had resisted efforts to be drawn into the conflict but pressure had been mounting for some time. The pressure had not gone unnoticed by many physicians or the newly organized occupational therapists. Joel Goldthwait, an orthopedic surgeon from Boston and brother-in-law of Dr. Hall, had been studying the methods used by the Allies in Europe and Canada to aid wounded solders recover from war injuries (Goldthwait, 1917). He saw the use of curative workshops in which men were given occupations to maintain general physical and mental health or to regain the use of a particular body part such as the wrist or hand.

Based on recommendations from Goldthwait and others, several plans were submitted to the Secretary of War regarding the use of teachers and medical aides to assist in the reconstruction of the war wounded (Future of Disabled Soldiers, 1917). Initially, the plans called for men to fill the positions but not enough men could be found. Finally in March 1918, a call for women reconstruction aides in occupational therapy was issued (Sanderson, 1918; Haggerty, 1918). The purpose of the **reconstruction aides** was,

> . . . to hasten the recovery of the patients . . . promote contentment and make the atmosphere of these hospitals such that the time spent in convalescence will pass most pleasantly because the minds and hands of the patients are properly occupied in profitable pursuits. (Hospital Designated for Reconstruction, 1918, p. 8)

Reconstruction aides treated diagnoses including amputations, blindness, head and nerve injuries, osteomyelitis, tuberculosis, neurasthenia, hypochondriasis, hysteria, anxiety neurosis, anticipation neurosis, effort syndrome, exhaustion, timorousness and gas, and concussion syndrome (Hoppin, 1933). Some of the later diagnoses are no longer recognized but could be classified under a general diagnosis of stress disorders.

The war effort resulted in a number of positive gains for occupational therapy. Schools of occupational therapy were established, therapists were educated, public awareness was achieved, and many policies and procedures were developed as well as the definition and description of occupational therapy services. One early program was the occupational therapy service at Walter Reed General Hospital. The first reconstruction aides were employed in February 1918, and Bird T. Baldwin became the Director of Education in April of that year (Crane, 1927).

Baldwin immediately began developing the department of occupational therapy and the curative workshops. He was particularly interested in developing an individual prescription for each patient's problems and recording the progress that the patient was making in regaining the use of arms and legs by systematically measuring the increase in their range of motion and muscle strength. These efforts are recorded in the publication *Occupational Therapy Applied to Restoration of Function of Disabled Joints* (Baldwin, 1919). Although Baldwin's instruments were crude and cumbersome by today's standards, his objective of regularly recording each patient's progress cannot be faulted. The occupational therapy department at Walter Reed was a model department for many years, until the early 1930s, when severe cuts were made in funding because of the Great Depression.

One of the negative outcomes of the war was the decision to define occupational therapy by placing the discipline under medical authorities (The Vocational Rehabilitation Law, 1918; Federal Board of Vocational Education, 1920). The decision grew out of a dispute for power in the federal agencies concerned with medical and vocational education. The decision was made in favor of medical control, which meant that occupational therapy could not be offered by federal or state vocational rehabilitation programs that were funded with federal money.

Another loss was the failure to gain military status for the reconstruction aides. Their civilian status did not provide benefits that military personnel received (Ford, 1927). Most left the service after the war ended. Finally, along with the departure of the aides themselves went some of the skills developed during the war to treat physical disabilities. Occupational therapy practice returned to being primarily a service to persons with problems in mental health and psychiatry. As late as 1937, only 2% of occupational therapists were known to be working in orthopedics, whereas 59% were working in mental hospitals, 25% in general hospitals, 8% in tuberculosis hospitals, and 6% in other institutions (Hospital Service, 1937).

The practice of occupational therapy fared well during the 1920s. Hospitals were interested in expanding services and money was available to pay for the expansions. Expansion was particularly rapid along the Atlantic Coast, especially in New York, where Slagle provided a major influence; Maryland, where Dunton worked; and Pennsylvania, Massachusetts, and Washington, DC. The other expansion area was in the north central states including Michigan, Wisconsin, and Illinois. The southern states, midwestern states, except for Missouri, and west coast states had only sporadic contact with occupational therapy services (Roll call, 1922).

Many of the gains made during the 1920s were reversed during the 1930s. The Depression and the National Economy Act of 1933 resulted in deep cuts in occupational therapy budgets and personnel (McDaniel, 1968). Many clinics were closed or staffing was severely reduced. Schools of occupational therapy were also closed, including the school at Walter Reed Hospital (McDaniel, 1968).

World War II

The field of occupational therapy was ill prepared for the advent of World War II in 1941. In the U.S. Army only 12 people were working in occupational therapy, 8 of whom were registered therapists (Vogel et al., 1968a). Only five Army hospitals had occupational therapy services. This lack of preparedness was the legacy of World War I when occupational therapists failed to achieve military status. Civilian positions in the military had neither a reliable base of funding nor officers in Washington, DC to oversee their needs. The war years were spent trying to secure enough people to meet the need. Ultimately 899 people would be trained through the War Emergency training courses established at various schools of occupational therapy (Vogel et al., 1968a).

One of the most important outcomes of World War II was the development of departments of physical medicine (Vogel et al., 1968b). With the support of physical medicine, occupational therapy practice in physical disabilities was able to establish the foundation that had been lacking under the direction of orthopedics. For the first time many of the techniques were actually written and published through the government printing services (West, 1968; Occupational Therapy, 1944, 1951, 1962), the journal *Occupational Therapy and Rehabilitation*, and finally, through the first edition of a major textbook, Willard and Spackman's *Principles of Occupational Therapy* (Willard & Spackman, 1947).

Also in 1947, occupational therapists finally achieved military status (Messick, 1947). This recognition provided other opportunities to gain financial support from the federal government for the education of occupational therapy personnel and provided leadership training skills for members of the *American Occupational Therapy Association* (AOTA). Three presidents of the AOTA received at least some of their management skill training from the military, including Winifred Kahmann, Ruth Robinson, and Wilma West (In memoriam—Winifred Conrick Kahmann, 1982; Ruth Robinson, 1989; Ruben, 1990).

Finally, the numbers of therapists known to be employed increased dramatically as a result of the emphasis on education and training. At the beginning of the war in 1941, 2132 occupational therapists were employed, whereas in 1945, 3224 therapists were working (Arestad & Westmoreland, 1946). The maldistribution of manpower continued, however. Most therapists worked in the New England or north central states. The two exceptions were California and Texas. Practice areas continued to be dominated by mental health and psychiatry (54%), whereas general medicine and surgery had only 27% and tuberculosis, 10%. Practice in physical disabilities had only increased to 3% by 1953 (Arestad & Gordon, 1953). The shift to physical disabilities did not occur until the 1970s. Thereafter the number of occupational therapists practicing in psychiatry or mental health declined steadily and the number of therapists in mental health dropped steadily; now less than 10% of occupational therapists practice in the area of mental health (AOTA, Membership Survey, 1986).

The issue of work force continued to be a constant reminder of the occupational therapy's success and failure. The success was the recognition by health care providers that occupational therapy is a valuable health care service. The failure was in recruiting and training enough practitioners to meet the demand. The experience of World War II emphasized the need for more comprehensive planning for personnel development. Subsequently, planning led to the recognition that other levels of training could be used to augment the services of professional level personnel. In 1956, a report was adopted to recognize nonprofessional personnel in occupational therapy (Report, 1956). This report led to the creation of the *certified occupational therapy assistant* (COTA) level (Crampton et al., 1958). Today COTAs are working in positions alongside *registered occupational therapists* (OTRs), and their knowledge and talents have helped to expand the services of occupational therapy for many diverse health care needs.

Legislation

The first legislation that appears to have helped occupational therapy practice is the 1920 Civilian Industrial (Vocational) Rehabilitation Act (Public Law 236, 1920), which provided federal aid for vocational rehabilitation for persons disabled by accident or illness in industry. Facilities that were developed to rehabilitate injured workers could use the knowledge of occupational therapists about the therapeutic value of occupations. Unless the state paid for occupational therapy services, however, people employing occupational therapy techniques could not be paid as occupational therapists because of the original ruling in 1918 that made occupational therapy a medical, not an educational, service (Federal Board for Vocational Education, 1920). Thus, the services of occupational therapists were employed but the title of occupational therapist could not be used.

With the *Vocational Rehabilitation Act and amendments* in 1943 came a change to include payment for medical services (P. L. 133, 1943). Thus, occupational therapy could now be covered as a legitimate service. The 1954 amendments also included monies for training health professionals including occupational therapists (P. L. 565, 1954).

In 1965, *Medicare* (Title 18) became law under the amendments to the Social Security Act, 1933. Occupational therapy services were covered for inpatient services; however, limited coverage was available for outpatient services and none for private practitioners (P. L. 89–97, 1965). Again occupational therapists were not active in the legislative process and thus had no input into the original bill. Twenty-one years passed before efforts of occupational therapists would result in expanded coverage for occupational therapy services to include unrestricted coverage in outpatient centers and reimbursement for occupational therapists in private practice (Mallon, 1981).

The Education of the Handicapped Act was passed in 1975 (P. L. 94–142, 1975) and occupational therapy was included as a Related Service. This law was intended to ensure that children with handicaps received a "free and appropriate" education. In 1986, the act was amended (P. L. 99–457, 1986) to include infants and toddlers and handicapped preschoolers. The amendments called for the development of Early Intervention Programs for infants and toddlers and handicapped children ages 3 through 5. Occupational therapy was included as a primary service. The Education of the Handicapped Act and its amendments rapidly expanded the opportunities for occupational therapists practicing in the school system. Within a few years, the practice of occupational therapy in the school system became the fastest area of growth in the profession; this practice area now ranks second (AOTA, Membership Survey, 1986).

In 1988, the ***Technology-Related Assistance for Individuals with Disabilities Act*** was passed (P. L. 100–407, 1988). This act provides money to develop technologic aids designed to help persons with handicaps participate in society. The aids may assist in improving mobility and self-care, education, transportation, or communication. Occupational therapists along with rehabilitation engineers have an opportunity to develop technology that will improve the quality of life for persons with physical handicaps and other special needs.

In July 1990, the ***Americans with Disabilities Act (ADA)*** was passed (P. L. 101–336, 1990). This act extends many benefits to the handicapped as stated in the Rehabilitation Act of 1973, especially Section 504 (P. L. 93–112, 1973). The benefits of the 1973 legislation affected only institutions receiving federal funds. The ADA applies to all institutions, regardless of the source of funding. The ADA makes discrimination against persons with handicaps illegal in the workplace if the person has the skills necessary to perform the job but may require some modification of the environment to permit him or her to perform the job. Architectural barriers are addressed in detail with specifications that architects must follow when building new structures, which enable persons in wheelchairs to enter and make use of the facilities. Local public transportation and public buildings must also be accessible to persons in wheelchairs. Devices for persons with hearing impairments must be available in public places. Occupational therapists can be advocates for persons with handicaps to ensure that communities follow the requirements of the ADA.

The professional association and foundation

Formal organization is one of the means people use to notify the public that an idea is to be taken seriously and supported by interested parties. Thus, in 1917 a group of interested parties (mentioned previously) formed an organization originally called the National Society for the Promotion of Occupational Therapy, which was changed in 1921 to the American Occupational Therapy Association (AOTA; Hall, 1921). The association established guidelines for the development of an occupational therapy training program, recognition for qualified trainees, and publications of articles on subjects of interest to the practice of occupational therapy.

Educational standards—accreditation

The AOTA's first attempt to establish ***educational standards*** appeared in the *Maryland Psychiatric Quarterly* in 1919 (Emergency Course, 1918). Although prepared by the AOTA's Board of Management, the membership never voted to accept the Emergency Course of Training for Reconstruction Aides. The Surgeon General's Office decided it could not accredit programs for reconstruction aides in occupational therapy (Russell, 1918). Thus, the first attempt at educational standards was not supported. The second attempt was more successful; in 1923, the

Association adopted the Minimum Standards for Courses of Training in Occupational Therapy (Minimum Standards, 1924). The course was to take 12 months with at least 6 hours of work and lecture per day of classes. Subjects were to include psychology, anatomy, kinesiology, orthopedics, mental diseases, tuberculosis, general medical cases such as cardiac diseases, and practical work in arts and crafts.

In the late 1920s, members of the American Medical Association (AMA) were inspecting other training programs in medicine in addition to medical schools (Elwood, 1927). In 1931, the AOTA formally asked the AMA to examine schools of occupational therapy. These inspections led to a revision of the education standards, which were published in 1935 as the Essentials of an Acceptable School of Occupational Therapy (Essentials, 1935). Other major revisions occurred in 1943, 1949, 1965, 1972, and 1983. In 1958, the first standards were adopted for the education of occupational therapy assistants (Crampton et al., 1958). The current educational standards were adopted in 1991. The names of current documents are the Essentials and Guidelines of an Accredited Educational Program for the Occupational Therapist and Essentials and Guidelines of an Accredited Education Program for the Occupational Therapy Assistant (Essentials and Guidelines, 1991a; Essentials and Guidelines, 1991b).

The primary concerns in the standards have been the length of training, curriculum, selection of students, financial support, governance of the school, and facilities. Initially schools of occupational therapy could be offered in hospitals or private schools offering only an occupational therapy program, but by 1943 this requirement was changed to create stability in the occupational therapy program and support for the courses in the curriculum (Essentials, 1943). Professional level programs (OTR) are now offered only through universities or 4-year colleges. Technical level (COTA) programs for occupational therapy assistants were originally as short as 12 months and were offered in hospitals or state agencies (Crampton et al., 1958). COTA programs are now offered only in community or junior colleges and are 2-year programs.

The number of schools of occupational therapy fluctuated in the early years. During World War I, numerous schools were started but most did not survive after the war ended. The AMA inspectors visited 13 schools but ultimately only 5 were accredited in 1938: Boston School of Occupational Therapy, St. Louis School of Occupational and Recreational Therapy, Philadelphia School of Occupational Therapy, Milwaukee-Downer College, Department of Occupational Therapy, and the University of Toronto, Department of University Extension in Canada (Approved schools of occupational therapy, 1938). Kalamazoo State Hospital School of Occupational Therapy was given tentative approval, which was changed to accreditation the following year (1939). In 1990, 69 accredited programs existed at the professional level and 67 at the technical level. In addition, 28 programs offered master's level education and three offered doctoral programs in occupational therapy (Listing of education programs, 1990).

Credentialing

Standards to recognize competence to practice were requested almost from the beginning of the AOTA (Russell, 1918). Educational standards occupied the early years of the Association's energy. However, by 1925 the AOTA was ready to begin the process of establishing a registry of people who met basic qualifications as occupational therapists (Kidner, 1925). In 1932, the first registry of qualified therapists was published (AOTA National Directory, 1932). **Registration** could be achieved on the basis of successful graduation from an approved school of occupational therapy, 4 years of experience as an occupational therapist, or special work in occupational therapy such as an instructor. There were 318 persons who met the qualifications.

Beginning in 1941, registration and reregistration became contingent on membership in the AOTA (Reports of committees, 1941). Registration based on successful completion of an examination became a standard requirement in 1947 (Minutes, 1946). Canadian-trained occupational therapists had to pass the examination beginning in 1944 to be registered in the United States (Minutes, 1946). Before that time registration had been granted through reciprocity.

During the 1970s the government began revising the terminology associated with professional qualifications, as the guidelines for various health programs were introduced (U.S. Congress, 1976). Registration was defined as placing a person's name on a list. Certification was the process established by a voluntary organization to determine professional qualifications. A voluntary organization was defined as a nongovernment agency. **Licensure** was the process established by a governmental agency to determine professional qualification.

Thus, the correct term for the process begun by the AOTA became certification, although the designation of occupational therapist, registered (OTR) continues to be used because of its historical background. The term certified occupational therapy assistant is consistent with the accepted terminology. Technically, occupational therapy personnel are both certified and registered because they must complete a process of passing an examination established by a voluntary organization and then their names are placed on a list of qualified persons. In addition, most therapists must complete requirements to become licensed under the regulations established by a state licensing agency (AOTA, State Regulatory Information Packet, 1989).

The American Occupational Therapy Certification Board (AOTCB) was created in 1986 to separate the function of certification of practitioners from the setting of educational standards (AOTA certification, 1986). The government had established that conflict of interest and antitrust cases could be brought against an organization in which both the educational standards and the certification standards were approved by the same body. Before 1986, the Representative Assembly of the AOTA had approved both sets of standards. By creating a separate and autonomous certification board, the appearance of conflict was removed. Also, public members could be assigned to the AOTCB but could not serve on the Representative Assembly, whose members are elected by members of the AOTA. The AOTCB is now responsible for determining certification procedures, maintaining the examinations, and issuing documentation to those who qualify as registered occupational therapists or certified occupational therapy assistants (Baum & Gray, 1988).

Publication and public relations

Publication and public relations are the third major function of an association. During the first years of the AOTA, the *Maryland Psychiatric Quarterly* published articles about the AOTA meetings and subjects on occupational therapy. Dunton was the editor of *Maryland Psychiatric Quarterly*, so he controlled the content of the journal. In 1921, Dunton suggested that the Association establish a journal dedicated to occupational therapy (Fifth Annual Meeting, 1922). The following year the *Archives of Occupational Therapy* was launched under Dunton's editorship. The title was changed in 1925 to *Occupational Therapy and Rehabilitation* to broaden the appeal of the journal in hopes of increasing its circulation (Dunton, 1925). When Dunton decided to resign as editor in 1946, several problems regarding ownership arose and a decision was made by the publisher, Williams & Wilkins, to change the focus to physical medicine (Dunton, 1946). Meanwhile, the Association had been trying to establish a journal that it would own and control. The result was the launching of the **American Journal of Occupational Therapy** (AJOT; *American Journal of Occupation Therapy*, 1947).

For many years the official journals, *Archives of Occupational Therapy* and *Occupational Therapy and Rehabilitation*, conveyed personal notes and local events in addition to publishing full-length articles and recording the official Association records. In 1939, a newsletter was started to relieve the journal of personal notes and local events and to provide more timely correspondence than was possible with the journal publishing schedule (Cobb, 1939). The *Occupational Therapy Newsletter* continued until 1973 when it became the *Occupational Therapy Newspaper* and later the *O.T. News*. Beginning in 1990 the *O.T. News* was printed periodically and bound into *AJOT*. In addition, newsletters are published quarterly by the Special Interest Sections sponsored by the Association.

Originally want ads or job opportunities were printed on a green sheet and included with the *Occupational Therapy Newsletter*. Later they were printed in the back of the *American Journal of Occupational Therapy*. In 1987, *OT Week* was started as the a publication for listing job opportunities (*OT Week*, 1987). *OT Week* also serves as a source of information about a variety of health-related news items. Two other publications not owned by the AOTA serve a similar purpose of listing job opportunities and providing timely news articles about health issues and news items in occupational therapy practice. These newsletters are named *Occupational Therapy Forum* (*Occupational Therapy Forum*, 1986) and *Advance for Occupational Therapy* (*Advance for Occupational Therapy*, 1985).

Books published by the AOTA during the 1950s and 1960s were irregular. They included publications of the annual conference proceedings and government-sponsored institutes. In recent years the AOTA has become a publishing house for various literature of interest to occupational therapy personnel. The result has been a dramatic increase in availability of information on subjects of interest to the practitioners in occupational therapy.

Research

Research had been a concern of the AOTA since its inception. The founders were aware of the need to document the effects of occupational therapy intervention on the health of patients and clients; therefore, a Committee on Research and Efficiency was established (NSPOT, Constitution, 1917b). The difficulties were lack of trained researchers, lack of money to fund research activities, and lack of time to conduct the research projects. As master's level education became more available to therapists, there was a hope that the skills of research would begin to increase (Dunton, 1934; Editorial, *Clinical Research*, 1947). Other therapists learned skills at continuing education courses or inservice classes presented at their institutions.

Money was another matter. Few employers were willing to budget for research when the primary mission was service. Research activities could take time away from client services; this was not a popular idea with many employers. Thus, the AOTA again needed to provide leadership in funding research in occupational therapy. When the **American Occupational Therapy Foundation (AOTF)** was established in 1965, a workable solution was established (AOTF, 1975). Money donated to the Foundation was tax-deductible as a contribution. Therapists and companies could donate money to the Foundation and the Foundation would take the responsibility for evaluating research projects to be funded. The Foundation has become a major source of funds for budding researchers. Some therapists have been able to use their experience in writing grants for the Foundation to support their applications to larger funding agencies.

Organization of the association and foundation

The preceding sections have discussed some of the useful functions that a professional association can provide, but how the AOTA is organized to accomplish those functions has not been discussed.

When NSPOT began, the membership amounted to 40 people (NSPOT, List of Members, 1917c). In a small association, activities can be managed on a volunteer basis without the work becoming too burdensome. Eleanor Clarke Slagle is said to have run the AOTA from her kitchen for a few years, but the time came for a more suitable work environment and some paid help (Meetings, Board and House of Delegates, 1922; Sixth Annual Meeting, Office space, 1923). Now such an informal structure would be impossible. The AOTA has about 50,000 members and its headquarters is located in a three-story building in Rockville, Maryland. The National Office has an executive director and a staff of about 120 people (Bair, 1991). The vision, however, must continue to come from the members who volunteer their time to advance the cause of occupational therapy. Officers and chairpersons of committees are not paid.

The volunteer sector is composed of two groups; the **Executive Board** and the **Representative Assembly** (Incorporation Papers and Bylaws, 1989b). The AOTA has always had an Executive Board, although the original name was Board of Management. The purpose of the Executive Board is to manage the affairs of the Association. Although the early members of the Board had to both determine what was to be done and then do it, today the Board can direct the paid staff in the National Office through the Executive Director. During the early years Eleanor Clarke Slagle, as secretary/treasurer, organized the activities of the National Office. After her resignation, several Executive Secretaries were successively appointed by the Board. Not until the Association adopted the policy of hiring an Executive Director in 1947 did the issue of paying a person to manage the National Office become important (Meetings, Board of Management, 1948).

There were always plans for a Representative Assembly but reality forced a delay until 1939 (American Occupational Therapy Association, 1922). The purpose of the Representative Assembly is to make legislative and policy-making decisions. The Representative Assembly is composed of representatives elected from election areas composed of a state or class of people such as therapists living abroad. In the early years of the AOTA, people did not have enough money to permit representation from each state at each meeting. Therefore, the original idea of a Representative Assembly called the **House of Delegates** functioned only briefly in 1920. With the revision of the Constitution and Bylaws proposed in 1939, the House of Delegates was reestablished (Constitution, 1940). Delegates had to pay their own way to meetings or were supplemented by their state associations. Not until the early 1970s did the Association assume financial responsibility for getting its legislative and policy-making body to meetings. Representatives are now reimbursed for travel and *per diem* to attend the meetings of the Representative Assembly.

Under the direction of the Executive Board and the Representative Assembly, three major committees, called Commissions, carry out the major functions of the Association. The **Commission on Education** monitors the Essentials. When changes are needed to better prepare students to become practitioners, the Commission on Education makes recommendations for changes that are approved by the Representative Assembly. Changes in the Essentials of an Accredited Program for the Occupational Therapists must also be approved by the American Medical Association before they can be implemented because the collaborative arrangement established in 1933 continues today. As of 1991, changes in the Essentials of an Accredited Program for the Occupational Therapy Assistant are also jointly approved by the AMA and the AOTA. The Commission on Education also acts as a forum for the exchange of information and ideas on improving teaching methods or developing a better educational program. The Commission on Education is a continuation of the Committee on Education formed in 1920, chaired originally by Susan Johnson (Fifth Annual Meeting, p. 224).

The **Commission on Standards and Ethics** also evolved from early committee structure. Originally the concern was for determining the standards for membership in the Association. When the registration/certification process was added, the standards for determining who qualified as occupational therapy personnel had to be reviewed and approved. As the standards for educational programs (Essentials) were implemented, a committee was needed to review the qualifications of educational programs in collaboration with the American Medical Association. Ethical standards of conduct were also needed (**Occupational Therapy Code of Ethics**, 1989). The development, review, and enforcement of the standards became the responsibility of the Commission on Standards and Ethics. Since 1986, the Standards and Ethics Commission is responsible only for the accreditation or approval of educational programs and the ethical standards of conduct. The Occupational Therapy Certification Board is now responsible for certifying qualified occupational therapy personnel.

The third commission, the **Commission on Practice**, evolved more slowly and did not have a unique role until the changes in the Constitution in 1964. Originally the Committee on Teaching Methods was designed to examine the effectiveness of various techniques used to teach patients' activities. The Committee was chaired by Susan Tracy. Note that the focus was on patient treatment, not student training. Various other committees followed, often with a focus on one disease or technique.

The purpose of the Commission on Practice is to promote the quality of occupational therapy practice and practice standards. To meet this purpose, the Commission frequently writes position papers outlining model programs for the practice of occupational therapy with various patient/client groups or for persons with specific diseases or disorders (Standards of Practice, Position Papers, Roles and Function Papers, 1989).

Philosophy, concepts, and change

Models and theories

At the beginning of this chapter, the philosophy of humanism was mentioned briefly. Philosophy provides a value or belief system that influences or guides behavior and action (Gove, 1985). The value or belief system often functions without the person being aware of its existence. Behavior or actions occur but the person cannot always explain why he or she behaved in a certain way or did a particular action. Usually a value or belief system is present, which in turn is attributable to a recognized philosophy. Philosophy operates on several levels. At the top are philosophical beliefs called world views (Pepper, 1942). The *organismic* view is based on the idea that the person is active in determining and controlling his or her own behavior and can change that behavior when it is desired to do so. In contrast, the *mechanistic* world view is based on the belief that a person is passive and must be controlled by the society or environment in which he or she functions. In other words, the society or environment shapes the behavior and actions. The person simply conforms to the social environmental requirements. The organismic view also assumes holism. That is, a person is an integrated and organized entity and cannot be reduced to discrete parts. The mechanistic view assumes that a person is the sum of his or her discrete parts.

The history of occupational therapy has been influenced by both philosophies. *Humanism*, based on the organismic view, provided the initial framework for the development of ideas and concepts that the founders and early leaders used to describe what occupational therapy was and how it should be practiced (Abbognano, 1967). The individual was viewed as an active participant in treatment and was assumed to be functioning as an integrated whole who required assistance to reintegrate daily activities into a total living pattern. The ideas of humanism continued to guide occupational therapy until World War II. However, the apparent harmony of beliefs did not make all occupational therapists happy. At the beginning of this chapter a lengthy quote from Upham outlined the differing approaches of the arts and crafts movement as it was translated into therapeutic situations. The conflict between the two approaches—organismic and mechanistic—caused some serious differences of opinion and may have contributed to the decrease in the practice of occupational therapy with the physically disabled that used activities designed to direct the person's attention to the disabled part (Baldwin, 1919; Nell, 1923; Bowman, 1923).

In his classic work *The Structure of Scientific Revolutions*, Kuhn talks about the difficulty of the two radically different world views to communicate with each other (Kuhn, 1970). He does not explain the corollary that basically says that differing approaches or models within the same world view can argue, disagree, and denounce each other extensively because they inherently speak the same language but choose to look at a situation from a different vantage point. The vantage point or point of view makes a big difference in what is described. Dunton and Hall disagreed about the use of toy making as therapy. Dunton (1923a) saw toy making as diversional activity, whereas Hall (1923a) saw making toys as contributing to the person's return to society as a productive member. Both views were based on organismic and humanistic philosophy.

After World War II occupational therapists were increasingly pressured to adopt the biomedical model to become more scientific. The biomedical model, based on mechanistic world view, is organized around disease and pathology. Disease causes dysfunction in the cells of one or more body parts that are considered pathologic. Treatment is designed to repair the damaged parts. Under the biomedical model, occupational therapists viewed the individual as a passive recipient of treatment who needed to have therapy applied to specific body parts that had become dysfunctional. Function would be regained when the designated body parts were able to perform normally. The person was expected to cooperate in treatment—whether or not he or she thought the treatment would be beneficial—because the doctor, and therapist, knew what was the best treatment. Beginning in the 1960s, the trend began to reverse and occupational therapists began reexamining the original ideas that had guided the formation of occupational therapy as a practice discipline.

One of the early models of practice was *habit training*. Habit training was developed by Slagle, based on the idea of organizing the daily activities into cycles of work, play, rest, and sleep (Slagle, 1922). Both Meyer and Hall had advocated assisting patients to reestablish their habits into organized activities within an hourly schedule. For patients who had been hospitalized for many years or had lost many of the skills to perform daily skills, the schedule included performing simple work tasks and play activities. As the person's performance improved, the level of tasks and activities was increased until the person could perform work tasks at a competitive level of employment and perform self-care skills independently.

During the 1940s and 1950s, a marked trend toward organizing occupational therapy concepts under the mechanistic model existed. *Sidney Licht*, a physician, writer, and journal editor, suggested that occupational therapy should accept the scientific model and examine the component parts that permitted human movement. He divided occupational therapy into kinetic, metric, and tonic components (Licht, 1947b). Kinetic examined motion and was used to restore or improve muscle strength, joint mobilization, and coordination. Metric examined measurement and was used to increase work tolerance. Tonic looked at tone and was used to improve and maintain muscle and mental tone. The focus of the model is on the disease or trauma acting on the musculoskeletal parts that can be analyzed into individual muscles and joints with certain actions. Under this model, the concept of the person as a functioning, integrated whole who can act upon the environment is lost. Also under such a model, occupational therapy is a series of therapeutic exercises. If the person doing the exercises finds them useful or interesting, that is acceptable; however, the major objective is to regain the function of the parts, not the whole.

In the 1960s, occupational therapists rediscovered the original concepts of occupational therapy. Perhaps *Mary Reilly* best summarized the reaffirmation in her Eleanor Clarke Slagle lectureship in which she said, "Man, through the use of his hands as they are energized by mind and will, can influence the state of his own health" (Reilly, 1962, p. 2). This reaffirmation that a person is an active agent in promoting, maintaining, and regaining health and occupational performance is basic to the understanding of philosophy in occupational therapy.

The idea of a person as an active agent in health promotion and occupational performance is both simple to understand and complex to explain because a person can be active in so many areas covering a wide variety of subject knowledge. Thus, the knowledge base of occupational therapy includes humanities such as art and music; biologic sciences such as anatomy, physiology, and kinesiology; social sciences such as psychology, anthropology, and sociology; and aspects of applied sciences such as clinical medicine, ergonomics, child development, and business management. Developing practice models based on such an array of knowledge has proved to be a formidable task to occupational therapy. Which knowledge base should be considered primary? Is physiologic adaptation or psychosocial adaptation most important? How much does individual adaptation depend on interaction with the external physical environment? How much can the external physical environment be modified or adapted to meet the needs of a person with limited adaptive potential? How does adaptive ability change throughout the life cycle?

The variety of practice models developed during the past 30 years reflects the wide interpretation of human adaptation to and with the environment. **A. Jean Ayres**, for example, suggests that the primary adaptation occurs through the organization of the nervous system to information received from the vestibular, proprioceptive, and tactile senses, which are considered to be the oldest systems in the evolution of the brain. The practice model is called Sensory Integration (Ayres, 1972). **Gary Kielhofner** has looked at the organizational influence of time and occupation into cycles of activity following some the ideas proposed by Slagle and Reilly. The practice model is called Human Occupation (Kielhofner, 1980). Many other practice models or frames of reference are discussed more fully in Chapter 4.

Another problem in dealing with the complexity of concepts in occupational therapy is to find, understand, and perform research activities. Researchers traditionally have been trained in the scientific method, which is based on mechanistic philosophy. Research techniques based on **mechanistic philosophy** tended to stress the quantification of information into data using the research designs based on correlation between groups or an experimental group *versus* a control group. The data are collected in numeric form, which can be manipulated by statistical formulas based on normal variation of an attribute or characteristic. Such statistical formulas are therefore based on the concept of central tendency, that is, the tendency of an attribute or characteristic to cluster around the center called the *mean*. Persons whose findings do not cluster around the mean are considered to deviate from the mean by one or more standard deviations. Because occupational therapists often work with persons who deviate from the mean due to developmental differences, chronic diseases, social conditions, or other variables, the use of statistical procedures based on central tendency often are inappropriate. The individual may never be able to conform to the rules of central tendency. Deviation from the statistical mean may be translated by society with a label of a deviant (homosexual, crippled, deaf) from the social norm (mean). The person becomes an outcast for life.

Occupational therapists have had to recognize that research methods themselves are influenced by philosophy (Kielhofner, 1982). Research in occupational therapy needs to use research methods compatible with its organismic and humanistic philosophy. Such research methods must permit the individual to be described as a unique person, not as a datum among data or a deviant from the social norm. The individual must be viewed as the focus of the research. Comparisons with others may or may not be important. Among those research methods are a variety of qualitative research designs such as ethnography, case study, historical research, field studies, action research, interviewing techniques, evaluation research, and others that use qualitative design. Each method permits the person to be studied as a unique being, an "n" of one, with unique skills and talents. Use of qualitative design permits the person to be studied for what he or she can perform, not what he or she cannot perform. The focus is on studying who the person is and how he or she functions in the community and environment. The focus is on inclusion, not exclusion.

Scope of practice

The scope of occupational therapy knowledge and practice has at various times brought the profession into conflict with other professions including physical therapy, nursing, and education. Professional "turfdom" is a problem that develops as society changes its views about who is permitted to perform which health care and health education services. Physical therapists contend that some occupational therapists use modalities that rightfully belong to the domain of physical therapy practice such as paraffin baths, fluidotherapy, and ultrasound—heat modalities designed to increase circulation and decrease tightness of muscles and joints. Occupational therapists have countercharged that physical therapists should not be making hand splints. Nurses complain that occupational therapists perform activities of daily living (ADL), which nurses can perform equally as well, such as feeding, dressing, bathing, and grooming. Occupational therapists suggest that nurses are not trained to deal with difficult issues of ADL, which require adapted equipment and frequently do not have the time to spend helping severely disabled persons learn to perform the tasks with equipment aids. Educators complain that therapists do not have teaching certificates or teaching experience and that children lose time from the classroom to go to therapy. Occupational therapists countercharge that therapy enables the child to participate more actively in the educational process.

The issue of scope of practice has resurfaced again. A resolution was adopted by the Representative Assembly in 1989 to examine the use of physical agents by occupational therapists in various specialty areas of practice (Representative Assembly, 1989). The 1991 Representative Assembly adopted a new policy that stated,

> . . . physical agent modalities may be used by occupational therapy practitioners when used as an adjunct to/or in preparation for purposeful activity to enhance occupational performance and when applied by a practitioner who has documented evidence of possessing the theoretical background and technical skills for safe and competent integration of the modality into an occupational therapy intervention plan. (Association Policies, 1991, pp. 1112–1113)

Documentation in writing

Another problem in occupational therapy for many years was its apprentice approach to passing the art and science of occupational therapy from one generation of occupational therapists to the next. Generally inexperienced therapists learned directly from more experienced therapists. Little was actually published about the techniques, modalities, and media used by the practitioners of occupational therapy. Much of what was published provided superficial descriptions of clinical programs. The lack of publication on the "meat" of occupational therapy became a problem in two areas: public relations and reimbursement. In public relations the problem appears to have been most acute in communication with physicians. Physicians learned about occupational therapy from occupational therapists but very little published literature supported the contentions of occupational therapists that occupational therapy actually benefited patients in their recovery from chronic disorders, disabilities, or handicaps, or that occupational therapy might contribute to the prevention of certain health problems before they occurred.

The lack of publication about the effectiveness of occupational therapy continues to be a problem in getting reimbursement. Insurance carriers are reluctant to provide coverage for occupational therapy until they are convinced that the insurance dollar will result in some tangible benefit to the patient or client. Although some recent studies have shown the potential benefit of occupational therapy services, more research is needed to provide data to insurance carriers that occupational therapy is a necessary and useful service, not just a diversional or luxury service (Ostrow et al., 1985; Ostrow et al., 1987).

In both cases, better information to physicians and the results of studies of the effectiveness of occupational therapy services must be published. Occupational therapists have been improving their publication record. More journals are providing literature on occupational therapy to occupational therapists. Examples are *Occupational Therapy in Mental Health, Occupational Therapy Journal of Research, Physical and Occupational Therapy in Geriatrics, Physical and Occupational Therapy in Pediatrics, Occupational Therapy in Health Care, Journal of Hand Therapy, Occupational Therapy Practice,* and *Work.* However, there is a continuing need for occupational therapists to communicate the results of research in journals read by physicians and health care administrators (Reed, 1988).

Publication and retrieval of occupational therapy literature

For many years the primary source of occupational therapy literature was the official journal of the AOTA. That journal, whatever its title, was indexed in the primary indexing source of medical literature, **Index Medicus**. In 1966, *Index Medicus* became part of a computer database called **Medline**. The official journal, *American Journal of Occupational Therapy,* is indexed in Medline. However, no other journal devoted in part or in whole to occupational therapy is indexed in Medline. Thus, a large portion of occupational therapy literature is not seen by physicians. The other journals are seen by nurses and other allied health professionals who use the **Cumulative Index to Nursing and Allied Health Literature (CINAHL)** and *Psychological Abstracts.* Whereas CINAHL and *Psychological Ab-*

stracts provide excellent sources for recording journal literature, neither is very helpful in informing physicians. That communication must be done by learning which journal titles are indexed in *Index Medicus* and by making attempts to get articles, especially research articles published in those journals.

Occupational therapists are also fortunate to have a library organized and maintained jointly by the American Occupational Therapy Association and the American Occupational Therapy Foundation. The **Wilma L. West Library** is housed in the American Occupational Therapy Foundation. It contains over 3600 volumes on occupational therapy and related subjects and is available for use by members of the AOTA. The library contains monographs, textbooks, master's theses, doctoral dissertations, journals, and newsletters (AOTF, Silver celebration, 1990). Based on the library's collection, a database of occupational therapy literature also has been developed and maintained jointly by the AOTA and the AOTF. The database contains many articles and resources not available on other commercial databases such as articles from the newsletters of the Special Interest Sections and articles from the *Archives of Occupational Therapy* and *Occupational Therapy and Rehabilitation.* The database is available through O.T. Source, a communication software program that can be purchased from the Association (AOTA/F, O.T. Source, 1990).

In addition, the archives of the Association and the Foundation are available for use in research projects on the history of the profession. The archives are kept at the Moody Library in Galveston, Texas and include many of the original letters and documents of the founders. Several presidents of the Association and Foundation have contributed their working papers. Records of many committees and special projects are also included. In addition, a large collection of photographs and some films, slides, and videotapes are available. Archival materials need special care to preserve their usefulness. Heat, humidity, and an acid-free environment are essential to preserving historical documents. The occupational therapy archives are therefore kept with the Truman Bocker History of Medicine archive collection. A list of materials is available, but special arrangements must be made with the archivist at the Moody Library to use the materials (Bowman, 1985).

Occupational therapy worldwide

Occupational therapy has flourished in the United States owing to cultural acceptance of its basic concepts and a supportive system of government and private agencies. Other countries have found somewhat less acceptance and support, which has held back the development of occupational therapy as a recognized discipline in health care delivery services. Nevertheless, occupational therapy has enlarged its sphere of influence throughout the world.

Canada

In Canada, occupational therapy became known in 1917 when ward occupations were introduced in the Canadian military hospitals. Ward occupations were given to men confined to a hospital ward. Occupations included basketry, weaving, and other arts and crafts. The purpose of ward occupations was to provide mental stimulus and to bridge the gap between chronic invalidism and idleness and the work in the curative workshops (Sedgworth, 1920).

The first training class was organized in 1918 by Professor Haultain at the University of Toronto (Sedgworth, 1920). This school continued to train occupational therapists and was accredited under the Essentials of an Accredited School of Occupational Therapy by the AMA in 1938. In spite of this early history, the Canadian occupational therapists did not become formally organized until 1934 (Driver, 1968). In the same year the *Canadian Association of Occupational Therapists* began publishing a journal, the *Canadian Journal of Occupational Therapy* (*Canadian Journal*, 1933).

American occupational therapists specializing in physical disabilities owe much credit to the early work of physicians and occupational therapy aides in Canada. Canada was engaged in World War I for several years before the United States entered the conflict. Therefore, they already had experience in treating returning soldiers and sailors injured in battle or other mishaps. Of particular interest is the work on mechanotherapy at Hart House in Toronto under the direction of McKenzie and Bott (McKenzie, 1918; Bott, 1918). Bott designed much of the basic equipment used for measuring and exercising various limbs under Dr. McKenzie's direction.

Great Britain

Occupational therapy probably began in England and Scotland during World War I. Reports of American physicians studying the methods of caring for the wounded soldiers and sailors indicate that the curative workshops were using the ideas and activities of occupational therapy, although the label was not applied (Allaben, 1918; Scheme, 1921). Recognition of occupational therapy did not occur until the first school, Dorset House School of Occupational Therapy, was opened in 1930 by Dr. Elizabeth Casson (Obituary, 1955). The school was originally started in Bristol but later moved to Oxford. The Scottish Association of Occupational Therapists was formed in 1932 and the English Association of Occupational Therapists in 1936. In 1973, the Scottish and English associations joined together and are now one association. Their journals were combined to form the *British Journal of Occupational Therapy* (Jay, 1974).

Australia

Occupational therapy became known in Australia during World War II. The Australian Association of Occupational Therapists was begun in 1945. Sylvia Docker was most instrumental in developing occupational therapy in Australia, and a lecture series has been named in her honor (Sims, 1967). A journal was started shortly thereafter, which is known today as the *Australian Occupational Therapy Journal*.

World federation of occupational therapists

After World War II several countries formed an international organization to provide rehabilitation services to all countries affected by the war. Members of the World Congress on the Welfare of Cripples (now the International Society for the Rehabilitation of the Disabled) suggested that occupational therapists form an international organization to promote the development and use of occupational therapy. In 1951, a meeting was held in Liverpool, England to organize the *World Federation of Occupational Therapists* (*WFOT*). The founding members were Australia, Canada, Denmark, India, Israel, New Zealand, South Africa, Sweden, the United Kingdom, and the United States (Spackman, 1967). The WFOT holds conferences every 4 years in a different country to promote occupational therapy. Other activities include promoting standards for occupational therapy education, maintaining the ethics of the profession, advancing the practice and standards of occupational therapy, facilitating international exchange and placement of therapists and students, facilitating the exchange of information, seeking publication to promote research, and promoting international cooperation between occupational therapists and other allied professional groups (Constitution, 1952). Current membership in the WFOT includes 36 countries.

Summary

Occupational therapy is a product of and is dependent on a social environment that values the individual and believes that each person has the capacity to act on his or her own behalf to achieve through occupation a better state of health. Individual performance and self-initiated action are encouraged, especially when they lead toward a purpose or goal that the person wants to achieve. Occupational therapy has its foundations in the ideas and beliefs expressed in humanistic philosophy and the social values of humanitarianism. Occupational therapy has a rich and varied history because its fundamental principles can be expressed through many occupational endeavors and performed at many levels of skill. This rich heritage is a constant challenge to its practitioners to keep the fundamental founding principles of occupational performance and purposeful activity in mind while providing the diversity of options to which each patient or client is capable of achieving in his or her quest to obtain, maintain, or attain the maximum degree of health and well-being to which the person can reach.

Many challenges still need to be met as occupational therapists move away from the protective walls of the institutions and into the community in which the problems of living in today's world are ever present. As always, leaders and thinkers have been preparing the way for today and tomorrow. Two examples are the articles by Wiemer and West (1970) and by Bockoven (1971).

This chapter is a glimpse of the rich and varied heritage of occupational therapy. The curious reader can find many avenues left untouched and many tales to be told about the contribution of occupational therapy to the health and care of our patients and clients.

References

The 1989 Representative Assembly summary of minutes. (1989). *American Journal of Occupation Therapy, 43*(12), 845–846.

Abbognano, N. (1967). Humanism. In P. Edwards (Ed.), *The encyclopedia of philosophy* (Vol. 4, pp. 69–72). New York: Macmillan.

Addams, J. (1900). Labor Museum at Hull House. *The Commons, 5*(47), 1–4.

Addresses made at the memorial meeting for Thomas Bessell Kidner. (1932). *Occupational Therapy and Rehabilitation, 11*(6), 435–445.

Advance for Occupational Therapy. (1985, September). *1*(1).

Allaben, C. M. (1918). An English orthopedic hospital—for the treatment of chronic diseased soldiers and sailors. *Military Surgeon, 43,* 200–206.

American Journal of Occupational Therapy. (1947, February). *1*(1), 1–68.

American Occupational Therapy Association has enthusiastic annual session. (1922). *Modern Hospital, 14*(4), 340–342.

American Occupational Therapy Association [AOTA]. (1932). The *1932 National Directory of Qualified Occupational Therapists Enrolled in 1931 in the National Register.* New York: The Association.

American Occupational Therapy Association. (1986). *Membership survey.* Rockville, MD: The Association.

American Occupational Therapy Association. (1989). *State regulatory information packet.* Rockville, MD: The Association.

American Occupational Therapy Association and Foundation. (1990). *OT Source.* Rockville, MD: The Association.

American Occupational Therapy Foundation [AOTF]. (1975). The first decade: 1965–1975. *American Journal of Occupational Therapy, 29*(10), 636–40.

American Occupational Therapy Foundation. (1990). Silver celebration: Golden future. *OT Week, 4*(13), 18–19.

AOTA certification structure changed. (1986). *Occupational Therapy News, 40*(6), 1.

Approved schools of occupational therapy. (1938). *JAMA, 110*(13), 979–980.

Arestad, F. H., & Gordon, M. A. (1953). Hospital service in the United States. *JAMA, 152,* 160.

Arestad, F. H., & Westmoreland, M. G. (1946). Hospital service in the United States. *JAMA, 130,* 1085.

Association Policies (1991). *American Journal of Occupational Therapy, 45*(12), 1112–1113.

Ayres, A. J. (1972). The sensory modalities. In A. J. Ayres (Ed.), *Sensory integration and learning disorders* (pp. 55–74). Los Angeles: Western Psychological Services.

Bair, J. (1991). From my office. *OT Week, 5*(42), 2.

Baldwin, B. T. (1919). *Occupational therapy applied to restoration of function of disabled joints.* Takoma Park: Walter Reed General Hospital.

Barton, G. E. (1915). Occupational therapy. *Trained Nurse and Hospital Review, 54,* 138–140.

Barton, I. G. (1968). Consolation House, fifty years ago. *American Journal of Occupational Therapy, 22,* 344–345.

Baum C. M., & Gray, M. S. (1988). Certification: Serving the public interest. *American Journal of Occupational Therapy, 42*(2), 77–79.

Beard, G. M. (1880). *A practical treatice* on nervous exhaustion (neurasthenia). New York: Wm. Wood.

Bing, R. K. (1967). William Rush Dunton, Jr.: American psychiatrist and occupational therapist, 1986–1966. *American Journal of Occupational Therapy, 21*(3), 172–175.

Bockoven, J. S. (1971). Legacy of moral treatment—1800's to 1910. *American Journal of Occupational Therapy, 25*(5), 223–225.

Bockoven, J. S. (1972a). The breakdown of moral treatment (pp. 20–31). In J. S. Bockoven (Ed.), *Moral treatment in community mental health.* New York: Springer.

Bockoven, J. S. (1972b). Moral treatment defined. In J. S. Bockoven (Ed.), *Moral treatment in community mental health* (pp. 69–80). New York: Springer.

Bockoven, J. S. (1972c). Occupational therapy: A neglected source of community rehumanism. In J. S. Bockoven (Ed.), *Moral treatment in community mental health* (pp. 217–227). New York: Springer.

Boris, E. (1986). *Art and labor: Ruskin, Morris, and the craftsman ideal in America.* Philadelphia: Temple University Press.

Bott, E. A. (1918). Mechanotherapy. *American Journal of Orthopedic Surgery, 16,* 441–446.

Bowman, E. (1923). Report of the round table on crafts for the physically disabled. *Archives of Occupational Therapy, 2*(6), 467.

Bowman, I. (1985). *Guide to the archives of the American Occupational Therapy Association.* Rockville, MD: American Occupational Therapy Association.

Braude, L. (1983). *Work and workers: A sociological analysis* (2nd ed.). Malabar: Robert E. Krieger.

Brigham, A. (1847). Moral treatment of insanity. *American Journal of Insanity, 4*(1), 1–15.

Bynum, W. F. (1964). Rationales for therapy in British psychiatry: 1780–1835. *Medical History, 18*(4), 317–334.

Canadian Journal of Occupational Therapy, (1933, September), *1*(1).

Carlson, E.T, & Dain, N. (1960). The psychotherapy that was moral treatment. *American Journal of Psychiatry, 117,* 519–524.

Cobb M. R. (1939). News Letter. *1*(1),1–4.

Constitution. (1940). *Occupational Therapy and Rehabilitation, 19*(1), 67–70.

Constitution for a World Organization of Occupational Therapists. (1952). *American Journal of Occupational Therapy, 6,* 274–278.

Crampton, M. W., et al. (1958). Recognition of occupational therapy assistants. *American Journal of Occupational Therapy, 12*(5), 269–275.

Crane, A. G. (1927). Physical reconstruction and vocational education. Part 1. In A. G. Crane (Ed.), *Medical Department of the United States Army in the World War* (Vol. XIII, p. 58). Washington, DC: U.S. Government Printing Office.

Dain, N. (1964). *Concepts of insanity in the United States, 1789–1865* (p. 11). New Brunswick: Rutgers University Press.

Dain, N., & Carlson, E. T. (1960). Milieu therapy in the nineteenth century: Patient care at the Friend's asylum, Frankford, Pennsylvania, 1817–1861. *Journal of Nervous and Mental Disease, 131*(4), 277–290.

Deutsch, A. (1949). The rise of moral treatment. In A. Deutsch (Ed.), *The mentally ill in America: A history of their care and treatment from colonial times* (2nd ed. rev., pp. 88–113). New York: Columbia University Press.

Driver, M. F. (1968). A philosophic view of the history of occupational therapy in Canada. *Canadian Journal of Occupational Therapy, 35,* 53–60.

Dunton, W. R. (1912). Occupations and amusements. *Maryland Psychiatric Quarterly, 2*(1), 19–20.

Dunton, W. R. (1919). *Reconstruction therapy.* Philadelphia: W. B. Saunders.

Dunton, W. R. (1923a) A debate upon toy-making as a therapeutic occupation. *Archives of Occupational Therapy, 2*(1), 39–42.

Dunton, W. R. (1923b). Editorial: George Edward Barton. *Archives of Occupational Therapy, 2*(6), 409–410.

Dunton, W. R. (1925). Editorial. *Occupational Therapy and Rehabilitation, 4*(3), 227–228.

Dunton, W. R. (1926). An historical note. *Occupational Therapy and Rehabilitation, 5*(6), 427–439.

Dunton, W. R. (1931). Occupational therapy. *Occupational Therapy and Rehabilitation, 10*(2), 113–121.

Dunton, W. R. (1932a). Obituary—Susan C. Johnson. *Occupational Therapy and Rehabilitation, 11*(2), 153.

Dunton, W. R. (1932b). Obituary. *Occupational Therapy and Rehabilitation, 11*(5), 321–323.

Dunton, W. R. (1934). The need and value of research in occupational therapy. *Archives of Occupational Therapy, 13*(6), 325.

Dunton, W. R. (1942). Editorial: Eleanor Clarke Slagle. *Occupational Therapy and Rehabilitation, 21*(6), 373–374.

Dunton, W. R. (1946). Editorial. *Occupational Therapy and Rehabilitation, 25*(6), 267–268.

Eaton, A. H. (1949). *Handicrafts of New England* (p. xvii). New York: Harper & Brothers.

Editorial: Clinical research. (1947). *Occupational Therapy and Rehabilitation, 26*(1), 53–54.

Elwood, E. S. (1927). The National Board of Medical Examiners and Medical Education, and the possible effect of the Board's program on the spread of occupational therapy. *Occupational Therapy and Rehabilitation, 6*(5), 341–347.

Emergency Course of training for reconstruction aides. (1918). *Maryland Psychiatric Quarterly, 8*(2), 48–49.

Essentials of an acceptable school of occupational therapy. (1935). *JAMA, 104*(18), 1632–1633.

Essentials of an acceptable school of occupational therapy. (1943). *JAMA, 122*(8), 541–543.

Essentials and guidelines of an accredited educational program for the occupational therapist. (1991a). *American Journal of Occupational Therapy, 45*(12), 1077–1084.

Essentials and guidelines of an approved education program for the occupational therapy assistant. (1991b). *American Journal of Occupational Therapy, 45*(12), 1085–1092.

Favill, J. (1917). *Henry Baird Favill* (p. 87). Chicago: Rand McNally.

Federal Board for Vocational Education. (1920). *Industrial rehabilitation: A statement of policies to be observed in the administration of the Industrial Rehabilitation Act.* Bulletin 57 (p. 31). Washington, DC: U.S. Government Printing Office.

The Fifth Annual Meeting of the National Society for the Promotion of Occupational Therapy. (1922). *Archives of Occupational Therapy, 1,* 65.

The Fifth Annual Meeting of the National Society for the Promotion of Occupational Therapy. (1922). *Archives of Occupational Therapy, 1,* 224.

Ford, J. H. (1927). Administration American Expeditionary Forces, Vol. II, Circular No. 56. In J. H. Ford (Ed.), *Medical department of the United States Army* (Vol. II, p. 994). Administration: American Expeditionary Forces. Washington, DC: U.S. Government Printing Office.

The future of disabled soldiers: Recommendations of the conference called by the General Medical Board of the Advisory Commission of the Council of National Defense. (1917). *Modern Hospital, 9,* 124–125.

Goldthwait, J. E. (1917). The place of orthopedic surgery in war. *American Journal of Orthopedic Surgery, 15*(10), 679–686.

Gove, P. B. (1985). *Webster's third new international dictionary of the English language unabridged* (p. 1698). Springfield: Merriam-Webster.

Haas, L. J. (1924). One hundred years of occupational therapy, a local history. *Archives of Occupational Therapy, 3*(2), 83–100.

Haas, L. J. (1925a). The masculine side of occupational therapy. *Mental Hygiene, 9,* 743–752.

Haas, L. J. (1925b). The male occupational therapist. *Occupational Therapy and Rehabilitation, 4*(1), 53–56.

Haas, L. J. (1925c). *Occupational therapy for the nervously and mentally ill.* Milwaukee: Bruce.

Haggerty, M. E. (1918). Where can a woman serve? *Carry On, 1*(3), 26–29.

Hall, H. J. (1905). The systematic use of work as a remedy in neurasthenia and allied conditions. *Boston Medical and Surgical Journal, 152*(2), 29–32.

Hall, H. J. (1910). Work cure, a report of five years' experience at an institution devoted to the therapeutic application of manual work. *JAMA, 54*(1), 12–14.

Hall, H. J. (1913). Out-patient workshops—a new hospital department. *Modern Hospital, 1*(1), 101–103.

Hall, H. J. (1921). American Occupational Therapy Association is new name. *Modern Hospital, 17*(6), 554.

Hall, H. J. (1923a). In defense of toys. *Archives of Occupational Therapy, 1*(1), 43.

Hall, H. J. (1923b). *O.T. A New Profession.* Concord: Rumford Press.

Hall, H. J., & Buck, M. M. C. (1915). *The work of our hands.* New York: Moffat, Yard & Co.

Hoppin, L. B. (1933). *History of the World War reconstruction aides.* Millbrook: William Tyldsley.

Hospital Service in the United States. (1937). *JAMA, 108,* 1046.

Hospitals designated for reconstruction of disabled American soldiers

and policy to be pursued outlined by Surgeon General. (1918). *Official Bulletin, 2*(273), 8.

Incorporation papers and bylaws (1989). In American Occupational Therapy Association (pp. I.1–I.39). *Reference manual of official documents of the American Occupational Therapy Association,* Rockville, MD: The Association.

In memoriam—Winfred Conrick Kahmann. (1982). *American Journal of Occupational Therapy, 36*(7), 472–475.

Jay, P. (1974). From Chairman of Council Association of Occupational Therapists. *British Journal of Occupational Therapy, 37*(5), 70.

Johnson, S. C. (1917). Occupational therapy in New York City institution. *Modern Hospital, 8,* 414–415.

Johnson, S. C. (1919). Report of Committee on Admissions & Positions. *Proceedings of the Third Annual Meeting of the National Society for the Promotion of Occupational Therapy* (pp. 16–25). Towson, MD: Sheppard and Enoch Pratt Hospital.

Jones, R. E. F. (1983). Moral treatment: The basis of private mental hospital care. *Psychiatric Hospital, 14*(1), 5–9.

Kaplan, H. I., Freedman, A. M., & Sadock, B. J. (1980). Historical and theoretical trends in psychiatry. In H. I. Kaplan, et al. (Eds.), *Comprehensive textbook of psychiatry/III* (Vol. 1, pp. 63–64). Baltimore: Williams & Wilkins.

Kidner, T. B. (1922). Accommodation for occupational therapy in federal tuberculosis sanatoriums. *Modern Hospital, 18,* 292, 294.

Kidner, T. B. (1925). President's address. *Occupational Therapy and Rehabilitation, 4*(6), 407–416.

Kielhofner, G. (1980). A model of human occupation, Part two. Ontogenesis from the perspective of temporal adaptation. *American Journal of Occupational Therapy, 34*(10), 657–663.

Kielhofner, G. (1982). Qualitative research: Part one. Paradigmatic grounds and issues of reliability and validity. *Occupational Therapy of Journal Research, 2*(2), 67–79.

Kuhn, T. (1970). *The structure of scientific revolutions* (2nd ed.). Chicago: University of Chicago Press.

Lears, T. J. J. (1981). *No place of grace: Antimodernism and the transformation of American culture: 1880–1920.* New York: Pantheon Books.

Licht, S. (1947a). William Rush Dunton, Jr. *Occupational Therapy and Rehabilitation, 26*(2), 47–52.

Licht, S. (1947b). The objectives of occupational therapy. *Occupational Therapy and Rehabilitation, 26*(1), 17–22.

Listing of education programs in occupational therapy. (1990). *American Journal of Occupational Therapy, 44*(12), 1104–1116.

Luther, J. (1902). The Labor Museum at Hull House. *The Commons, 7*(70), 1–12.

Luther, J. (1918). Occupational treatment in nervous disorders. *Modern Hospital, 11*(1), 11–15.

Mallon, F. J. (1981). History of the occupational therapy medicare amendments. *American Journal of Occupational Therapy, 35*(4), 231–235.

Marsh, J. (1982). *Back to the land: The pastoral impulse in Victorian England from 1880 to 1914.* London: Quartet Books.

McDaniel, M. L. (1968). Occupational therapists before World War II (1917–1940). In R. S. Anderson (Ed.), *Army Medical Specialist Corps* (pp. 92–3). Washington, DC: U.S. Government Printing Office.

McKenzie, R. T. (1918). *Reclaiming the maimed: A handbook of physical therapy.* New York: Macmillan.

Meetings of the Board of Management. (1947). *American Journal of Occupational Therapy, 2*(1), 50–58.

Meetings of the Board and Members of the House of Delegates of the American Occupational Therapy Association. (1922). *Archives of Occupational Therapy, 1*(4), 317–355.

Meetings of the House of Delegates. (1954). *American Journal of Occupational Therapy, 8*(1), 24–35.

Messick, H. E. (1947). The new Women's Medical Specialist Corps. *American Journal of Occupational Therapy, 1*(5), 298–300.

Meyer, A. (1951). Remarks on habit disorganizations in the essential deteriorations, and their relation to deterioration of the psychasthenic, neurasthenic, hysterical and other constitutions. In E. Winters (Ed), *The collected papers of Adolf Meyer* (Vol. II, pp. 421–431). Baltimore: Johns Hopkins Press.

Meyer, A. (1922). The philosophy of occupational therapy. *Archives of Occupational Therapy, 1*(1), 1–10.

Minimum standards for courses of training in occupational therapy. (1924). *Archives of Occupational Therapy, 3*(4), 295–298.

Minutes of the Meeting of the Board of Management, May 10, 1946, and Committee Reports. (1946). *Occupational Therapy and Rehabilitation, 25*(3), 80–82.

Mitchell, S. W. (1891). *Fat and blood, an essay on the treatment of certain forms of neurasthenia and hysteria.* Philadelphia: J. B. Lippincott.

Mora, G. (1975). Adolf Meyer. In A. M. Freedman, et al. (Eds.), *Comprehensive textbook of psychiatry—II* (Vol. 1, pp. 6266–632). Baltimore: Williams & Wilkins.

Morris, W. (1901). *Hopes and fears for art.* London: Longmans Green & Co.

National Society for the Promotion of Occupational Therapy [NSPOT]. (1917a). *First Annual Meeting of the National Society for the Promotion of Occupational Therapy* (p. 9). Towson, MD: Sheppard Hospital Press.

National Society for the Promotion of Occupational Therapy. (1917b). *Constitution of the National Society for the Promotion of Occupational Therapy.* Towson, MD: Sheppard Hospital Press.

National Society for the Promotion of Occupational Therapy. (1917c). List of Members. In *First Annual Meeting of the National Society for the Promotion of Occupational Therapy* (pp. 6–7). Towson, MD: Sheppard Hospital Press.

National Society for the Promotion of Occupational Therapy. (1920). *Proceedings of the Fourth Annual Meeting of the National Society for the Promotion of Occupational Therapy* (pp. 35–37). Towson, MD: Sheppard Hospital Press.

Naylor, G. (1971). *The arts and crafts movement: A study of its sources, ideals and influences on design theory.* Cambridge, MA: MIT Press.

Nell, G. (1922). Occupational therapy for orthopedic cases. *Archives of Occupational Therapy, 1*(4), 269–278.

Newton, I. G. (1917). Consolation House. *Trained Nurse and Hospital Review, 59,* 321–326.

Obituary: Elizabeth Casson, OBE, MD, DPM. (1955). *British Medical Journal, 1*(Jan. 1), 48–49.

Occupational Therapy. (1944). War Department Training Manual TM8-291. Washington, DC: U.S. Government Printing Office.

Occupational Therapy. (1951, rev. 1962). Department of the Army Technical Manual TM8-291. Washington, DC: U.S. Government Printing Office.

Occupational Therapy Code of Ethics. In American Occupational Therapy Association. (1989). *Reference manual of the office documents of the American Occupational Therapy Association* (pp. III.1–III.2). Rockville, MD: The Association.

Occupational Therapy Forum. (1986, September). *1*(1).

Ostrow, P. C., Lieberman, P., & Merrill, C. S. (1985). *Outcomes of stroke rehabilitation.* Rockville, MD: American Occupational Therapy Association.

Ostrow, P. C., Spencer, F. M., & Johnson, M. (1987). *The cost-effectiveness of rehabilitation: A guide to research relevant to occupational therapy.* Rockville, MD: American Occupational Therapy Association.

OT Week. (1987, January). *1*(1).

Pepper, S. C. (1942). *World hypotheses.* Berkeley: University of California Press.

Pinel, P. (1962). *A treatise on insanity.* New York: Hafner (Facsimile of the London 1806 edition).

Portraits from the past: Susan E. Tracy. (1928). *Trained Nurse and Hospital Review, 75*(11), Cover Portrait.

Position papers. In American Occupational Therapy Association. (1989.) *Reference manual of the official documents of the American Occupational Therapy Association* (pp. V.1–V.16). Rockville, MD: The Association.

Pressey, E. P., & Rollins, C. P. (1904). *The arts and crafts and the individual.* Montague: New Clairvaux Press.

Public Law 236 (66th Congress, June 2, 1920, Industrial Rehabilitation Act, Smith-Fess Act).

Public Law 113 (78th Congress, June 6, 1943, Vocational Rehabilitation Amendments).

Public Law 565 (83rd Congress, August 3, 1954, Vocational Rehabilitation Amendments).

Public Law 89–97 (Social Security Act Amendments, Medicare, Title 18, Insurance for the Aged, July 30, 1965).

Public Law 93–112 (Rehabilitation Act, 1973).

Public Law 94–142 (Education of the Handicapped Act, 1975).

Public Law 99–457 (Education of the Handicapped Act Amendments, 1986).

Public Law 100–407 (Technology-Related Assistance for Individuals with Disabilities Act, August, 19, 1988).

Public Law 101–336 (Americans with Disabilities Act, July 26, 1990).

Reed, K. L. (1988). Serial publications in occupational therapy. *Bulletin of the Medical Library Association, 76*(2), 125–130.

Reilly, M. (1962). Occupational therapy can be one of the great ideas of 20th century medicine. *American Journal of Occupational Therapy, 16*(1), 1–9.

Report of the committee to plan implementation of recognition on non-professional personnel in the field of occupational therapy (1956). *American Journal of Occupational Therapy, 10*(1), 27–38.

Reports of committees. (1941). *Occupational Therapy and Rehabilitation, 20*(6), 409–421.

Rodgers, D. T. (1974). *The work ethic in industrial America: 1850–1920.* Chicago: University of Chicago Press.

Roles and Function papers. In American Occupational Therapy Association. (1989). *Reference manual of official documents of the American Occupational Therapy Association* (pp. VI.1–VI.69). Rockville, MD: The Association.

The roll call. (1922). *Modern Hospital, 19*(4), 370–1.

Ruth Robinson enjoyed a long and distinguished career. (1989). *Occupational Therapy News, 43*(5), 2.

Ruben, B. (1990). A lifetime of achievement: AOTA and AOTF present commendation to Wilma L. West. *OT Week, 4*(17), 4–5, 42.

Rush, B. (1962). *Medical inquiries and observations upon the diseases of the mind* (pp. 224–226). New York: Hafner (Facsimile of the Philadelphia 1812 edition).

Ruskin, J. (no date). *The stones of Venice* (Vol. II, p. 166). Boston: Dana Estes & Co.

Russell, J. E. (1918). Occupational therapy in military hospitals. *American Journal of Care for Cripples, 7,* 112–16.

Sanderson, M. (1918). *Circular of information concerning the employment of reconstruction aides* (2). [Washington], Medical Department, United States Army, March 27, Occupational Therapy Archives, Galveston, TX.

Scheme and organization of curative workshops. (1921). In R. Jones (Ed.), *Orthopaedic surgery of injuries* (Vol. 2, pp. 631–643). London: Oxford University Press.

Scull, A. T. (1979). Moral treatment reconsidered: Some sociological comments on an episode in the history of British psychiatry. *Psychological Medicine, 9,* 421–428.

Sedgworth, W. E. (1920). *Retraining Canada's disabled soldiers* (p. 37). Ottawa, Canada: J. de Labroquerie Tache.

Sedgworth, W. E. (1920). *Retraining Canada's disabled soldiers* (p. 24). Ottawa, Canada: J. de Labroquerie Tache.

Shi, D. E. (1985). *The simple life: Plain living and high thinking in American Culture.* New York: Oxford University Press.

Sims, G. E. (1967). Sylvia Docker lecture: Occupational therapy in Australia—the formative years. *Australian Occupational Therapy Journal, 14,* 29–44.

The Sixth Annual Meeting of the American Occupational Therapy Association. (1923). Office space. *Archives of Occupational Therapy, 2*(1), 49–82.

Slagle, E. C. (1914). History of the development of occupation for the insane. *Maryland Psychiatric Quarterly, 4*(1), 14–20.

Slagle, E. C. (1917). The Department of Occupational Therapy. *Institutional Quarterly, 10,* 29–32.

Slagle, E. C. (1922). Training aides for mental patients. *Archives of Occupational Therapy, 1*(1), 11–18.

Slagle, E. C. (1931). The training of occupational therapists. *Psychiatric Quarterly, 31*(5), 12–20.

Slagle, E. C. (1934). The occupational therapy programme in the state of New York. *Journal of Mental Science, 80,* 639–649.

Slagle, E. C. (1936). Editorial: From the heart. *Occupational Therapy and Rehabilitation, 16*(6), 343–345.

Slagle, E. C. (1938). Occupational therapy. *Trained Nurse and Hospital Review, 100,* 375–382.

Spackman, C. S. (1967). The World Federation of Occupational Therapists. *American Journal of Occupational Therapy, 21,* 301–309.

Standards of practice. In American Occupational Therapy Association. (1989). *Reference manual of the official documents of the American Occupational Therapy Association* (pp. IV.1–IV.24). Rockville, MD: The Association.

Stattel, F. (1956). Equipment design for occupational therapy. 1955 Eleanor Clarke Slagle lecture. *American Journal of Occupational Therapy, 10*(4, Pt. II), 194–99.

Thomson, E. E. (1917). Occupation and its relation to mental hygiene. *Modern Hospital, 8*(6), 397–8.

Tomes, N. (1964). *A generous confidence: Thomas Story Kirkbride and the art of asylum-keeping, 1840–1883.* London: Cambridge University Press.

Tracy, S. E. (1910). *Studies in invalid occupation: A manual for nurses and attendants.* Boston: Whitcomb & Barrows.

Tracy, S. E. (1918). Twenty-five suggested mental tests derived from invalid occupations. *Maryland Psychiatric Quarterly, 8*(1), 15–18.

Tuke, S. (1964). *Description of the Retreat, an institution near York, for insane persons of the Society of Friends.* London: Dowsons of Pall. (Original work published 1813).

Upham, E. G. (1918). *Ward occupations in hospitals* (pp. 18–19). Bulletin No. 25. Washington, DC: Federal Board for Vocational Education.

U.S. Congress. House Committee on Interstate and Foreign Commerce. (1976). *A discursive dictionary of health care.* Washington, DC: U.S. Government Printing Office.

The vocational rehabilitation law establishes national program. (1918). *Official Bulletin, 2* (July 13), 8.

Vogel, E. E., et al. (1968a). Training in World War II. In R. S. Anderson (Ed.), *Army Medical Specialist Corps* (p. 179). Washington, DC: U.S. Government Printing Office.

Vogel, E. E., et al. (1968b). Wartime organization and administration. In R. S. Anderson (Ed.), *Army Medical Specialist Corps* (p. 135). Washington, DC: U.S. Government Printing Office.

Wagner, C. (1904). *The simple life.* New York: Grosset & Dunlap.

West, W. L. (1968). Professional services of occupational therapists, World War II. In R. S. Anderson (Ed.), *Army Medical Specialist Corps* (pp. 287–338). Washington, DC: U.S. Government Printing Office.

Wiemer, R. B., & West, W. L. (1970). Occupational therapy in community health care. *American Journal of Occupational Therapy, 24*(5), 323–328.

Willard, H. S., & Spackman, C. S. (1947). *Principles of occupational therapy* (1st ed.). Philadelphia: J. B. Lippincott.

Wyman, R. (1830). *A discourse on mental philosophy as connected with mental disease.* Boston: Boston Daily Advertiser.

CHAPTER 3

Developing an academic discipline: the science of occupation

FLORENCE CLARK and ELIZABETH A. LARSON

"Occupation is the very life of life."

HAROLD BELL WRIGHT (1915)

The emergence of occupational science is both timely and timeless in its development as an academic discipline. Neither by a random course nor as a sudden unpredictable happening was occupational science formed at this time. The demands of a rapidly expanding practice, the need to have a unified perspective to guide intervention, and the recognition that only after the centrality of occupation to health is made clear to the public will the profession be sufficiently valued, created the context from which occupational science has sprung. The discipline addresses the form, function, and meaning of human endeavors. Its emergence seems timeless and gradual in that human beings have sought for centuries to comprehend the meaning and essence of existence—how to best lead a happy and productive life and how to form a sense of self not by dramatic events, but by our everyday understandings of and reactions to the many activities in which we engage.

This chapter begins by tracing the historical roots of occupational science. Next, the discipline's focus on the concept of occupation is discussed, and a method of organizing interdisciplinary knowledge using general systems theory is presented. Research and scholarship in occupational science are discussed in relation to the ethics and values of occupational therapy. The chapter concludes with a projection of how occupational science is apt to influence practice.

Roots in occupational therapy

The founders of the profession

Occupational science grew out of the profession of occupational therapy. In turn, the conceptual springboard for the establishment of occupational therapy was the Moral Treatment Movement (Bockoven, 1963). In the 1800s, proponents of moral treatment believed in,

> . . . the wholesome discipline of the well-regulated household, regular hours for food and for sleep, manual employment, reading, lectures, and other intellectual exercises and entertainments and various recreations and amusements . . . to procure a healthful exercise of the body, to abstract the mind from its delusions, to win back the patient to the regular and useful habits and practices of his former life. (Butler, 1843, as quoted by Harms, 1964, p. 287)

Clearly, this group recognized the health-promoting benefits of engagement in a broad spectrum of what we currently call ***"occupations."***

Consistent with this line of thinking, the founders of the occupational therapy profession, in the early 1900s, paid homage to the commonplace activities in which people engaged, as central to the living of a balanced and contented life. Adolph Meyer (1922), an early pioneer in occupational therapy, conceptualized the human being as "an organism that maintains and balances itself in the world of reality and actuality by being in active life and active use, i.e., using and living and acting its time in harmony with its own nature and the nature about it" (p. 641). Similarly, Dunton, an early president of the Occupational Therapy Association, extolled the virtues of occupation. He wrote,

> That occupation is as necessary to life as food and drink. That every human being should have both physical and mental occupation. That all should have occupations which they enjoy. These are more necessary when the vocation is dull or distasteful. . . . That sick minds, sick bodies, sick souls, may be healed through occupation. (Dunton, 1919, p. 17)

Clearly the belief that the full spectrum of human activity, that is, a customary round of occupations, was crucial to health and finding meaning in one's life took a central position in both the moral treatment movement and in the founding of the profession of occupational therapy. Note that early occupational therapists were concerned with helping patients enjoy a rich and productive menu of daily activities; they did not seem to regard occupations as treatment modalities to be inserted artificially into the day of patients to attain a discrete therapeutic goal.

The arts and crafts movement: a reaction to industrialization and scientifism

Unfortunately, the view described above, which emphasized the fundamental role that occupation plays in the natural framework of life, was powerfully struck down as the industrial revolution and scientific community began a trend of reductionism in examining the person and his or her world. Serret (1985) claims that the "mechanization of work caused people to be treated as machines and fitted as parts into greater wholes defined primarily by technology and business needs" (p. 10). Likewise ***science***, through advancements in technology, tended to an-

alyze problems into parts to find solutions. Bockoven noted that in psychiatry,

> The observation by pathologists of microscopic lesions in the central nervous system of patients who had been mentally ill made a profound impression on many psychiatrists. Psychiatry . . . accepted the then current notion of science that all phenomena were reducible to simple material units. (Bockoven, 1963, p. 189)

The impact of this trend was the fractionated view that people can be understood by the examination of the smallest units, a perspective that is identified with reductionism.

As reductionism and scientism were changing the thinking in the developing social sciences and professions, early occupational therapists continued to embrace a holistic view, advancing the arts and crafts movement in reaction to the industrial age. Gradually, the use of arts and crafts media became increasingly enfolded into the profession as a means of developing a sense of purposefulness and self-efficacy in patients who were not experiencing these feelings in the workplace.

Soon the complexion of occupational therapy began to be colored more and more by the prevailing influences associated with the industrial revolution, however. In the 1930s, as therapists began to widen their scope of practice to include those with orthopedic problems and industrial accident patients, in addition to patients who were mentally ill or had tuberculosis (Gritzer & Arluke, 1985), exercise was incorporated, "dovetailing, and supplementing, and extending, treatments by means of crafts" (*Physiotherapy Review*, 1932, p. 12). This revision of practice was viewed as trespassing on the turf of physiotherapy at a time when the demarcation between the two professions was not defined. As both fields continued to broaden their scope of patients and treatment methods, the distinctions between the two became increasingly blurred (Gritzer & Arluke, 1985).

The reductionistic period

By the 1940s, the holistic emphasis on the customary round of activity of patients and on their blend of ***work***, ***rest***, ***play***, and leisure no longer had the central position it had had in the founding years. As it began to recede into the periphery, the use of arts and crafts had come to be seen as the identifying medium of the profession. Now patients would experience occupational therapy as a segment of time, inserted here and there, in their daily routine, during which they would do an art or craft project of presumed therapeutic value; no longer was it the full spectrum of work, rest, and leisure with which it was identified in the founding years. Even this latter development was vulnerable to the further impact of reductionism in the next two decades, however.

The synergistic effects of world history in a context of continued reductionism furthered the transmutation of the profession. During World War II, occupational therapy was transferred from the "Trades and Industries" to the "Medical Division" in civil service classification (Gritzer & Arluke, 1985). This reclassification more closely aligned occupational therapy with the medical profession. Physicians, particularly those in physical medicine, were interested in broadening the role of occupational therapy and attributed its lack of growth to its " 'sterile preoccupation' with 'arty' pursuits such as basketry and weaving" (Gritzer & Arluke, 1985, p. 107). They further maintained that "occupational therapy has been covering only a limited portion of its proper field ... and that it should have more contact with medicine ... where it rightfully belonged" (*Report of the Baruch Committee on Physical Medicine*, April 1944, pp. 53, 77).

The intertwining of occupational therapy with the medical field inextricably changed the face of occupational therapy services. By becoming aligned with physicians, occupational therapists were increasingly more vulnerable to the reductionist tendencies with which medicine had become entrenched. The holism of the founders—their belief that the core of occupational therapy was to assist patients to be engaged daily in a customary round of satisfying and productive activity—appeared to be slowly vanishing from occupational therapy.

Against this background, in the 1950s there was a call for an "exact science" in occupational therapy (Hopkins, 1988). Clinical experience during and after the war had stressed precise measurement of physical dysfunction and carefully structured treatment protocols. Much of the intervention at this time had focused on the application of technology for treatment or for promotion of compensatory adaptation. The technologic skill needed by the therapist increased, and the traditional emphasis on occupation in the broad sense, although still verbalized, became increasingly less visible.

Movement toward a broader view

Also in the 1950s, leaders in the profession began to be concerned that the field had become so dominated by reductionist ideas that it was losing its identity. In an article published in 1958, Reilly described the "great scientific, social, and economic change ... of the day" and urged the profession to address "the disruptive influences of the 20th century rush of scientific advances" (p. 293). She claimed that, although the profession had tripled in size by World War II, it was "still troubled in the fifties by its own undigested growth" (Reilly, 1958, p. 293). What she meant was that the field of occupational therapy had expanded in the absence of a coherent philosophy. She went on to propose that its continued growth should be guided by a commitment to the ideas "that occupational therapy is any activity, physical or mental" and "occupational therapy treats the whole man" (p. 296). Reilly further asserted that "we would have to search out its [work's] central nature in human behavior.... The roles of concern to us might be those that man assumes in the spheres of occupation and recreation" (p. 297). Thus, her position was to invoke the profession to embrace its roots, its traditional emphasis on occupation.

Given the confusion that had resulted from the unbridled expansion of the profession, it is no surprise that in the 1960s leaders attempted to identify threads of philosophical coherence and organize the extant knowledge base. Lela Llorens (1970), for example, compiled the following list of theoretical orientations that were being applied in practice in the 1960s:

1. The emphasis on purposeful activity as delineated by A. J. Ayres
2. The focus on the communication process within the context of therapy as described by Gail Fidler
3. The construction of a holistic theory grounded in cognitive–perceptual–motor constructs, psychosocial theory, human development, and central nervous system functioning by Llorens and others

4. The highlighting of recapitulation of ontogenesis as it applied to the development of psychosocial, cognitive, and perceptual–motor theory by Ann Cronin Mosey
5. The emphasis on life space, mastery, and life tasks as specified by Sandra Watanabe
6. The focus on intrinsic motivation as described by Linda Florey

Although the compilation of this list made a significant contribution because it assembled in one paper many of the multiple orientations that were influencing treatment at the time, it also demonstrated to the astute reader that the various perspectives only vaguely demonstrated a sense of commonality. No perspective, in fact, even used the word occupation as a key term in its conceptualization, although each one did, in its own way, reflect remnants of the thinking of the original founders of occupational therapy, recast in new frameworks that were derived from the burgeoning availability of knowledge from scientific studies. In this period, Reilly (1966b) warned that "the fragmented disorganized knowledge which supports practice needs the consistency and unity which theory would demand" (p. 224). She was concerned that leaders in the field were importing knowledge from diverse disciplines into the occupational therapy literature, and instead of being directed toward enhancing our understanding of the concept of occupation, in some instances, it was displacing it.

As the decade of the 1970s began, Reilly and her students (Reilly, 1971; Matsutsuyu, 1971) argued for a reembracing of the concept of occupation in theory development in the field. To comprehend occupational behavior, Reilly (1971) urged the profession to include knowledge of human achievement, life space, lifestyle, role models, aspirations, occupational choice, and job satisfaction. Numerous papers were subsequently published by Reilly's students, which addressed these topics as a way of enhancing our understanding of occupation (Heard, 1977; Matsutsuyu, 1969, 1971; Robinson, 1977).

The paradigm quandary

Toward the end of this period Kielhofner and Burke (1977), using Kuhn's (1970) description of science, examined the nature and status of the theories that were being used in occupational therapy. Kuhn had defined a paradigm as a definition of a phenomenon, determined by consensus, which guides the purpose, nature, and scope of practice and research in a discipline. In Kielhofner and Burke's analysis, the occupation concept was seen as the founding paradigm of occupational therapy, which was eventually replaced by scientific reductionism. The result was a crisis, defined in the Kuhnian sense as a period in which there is a rise of competing schools of thought and a rejection of the old paradigm.

Perhaps in response to Kielhofner and Burke's analysis, in 1978, King suggested that "the very universality of the filling or occupying of time with purposeful behavior has made it difficult to form concepts that would help us to construct a theory or science of occupation" (p. 430). She identified that the profession needed a science of occupational therapy that would provide the following:

1. A unifying concept that will apply to all areas of specialization

2. A framework that will clearly distinguish occupational therapy theory and techniques from those of other disciplines
3. A model that is readily explainable to other professionals and to consumers
4. A theory that is adequate for scientific elaboration and refinement

A number of authors proposed ways of creating a paradigm that would meet the above requirements as well as encompass the rich history of the profession from the early years through the reductionist period. Although King (1978) suggested construction of a science of adaptive responses, reflecting the strain imposed by increasing technology on the human being's ability to adjust in society, Kielhofner and Burke (1980) introduced a model using a **general systems theory** called the "Model of Human Occupation." In this model, the human being was viewed as an "open system and his occupational behavior is the output of that open system" (p. 573).

Finally, Clark (1979) published a paper on human development through occupation in which she attempted to connect diverse theoretical approaches to view the human being as an adaptive creator. Although different in their emphases, each of these perspectives emphasized occupation, viewed the human being as interacting in the environment, was concerned with adaptation, and was directed toward unifying the field around a single theoretical orientation.

Not all theorists agreed on the need for a single paradigm. Mosey (1985), for example, suggested that only a continuing pluralistic identity would allow the profession of occupational therapy to grow; limiting the field to one element, she argued, would be stifling. Similarly, Labovitz and Miller (1986) did not view the development of a paradigmatic-level model as necessary or useful for practice.

Finally, although Christiansen (1981) advised that the theoretical core of occupational therapy be centered around the concept of occupation, a premise "that humankind has a natural drive toward activity, growth, productivity and creativity" (p. 120), he found flaws in Kielhofner and Burke's analysis. His criticism centered on the notion that since occupational therapy did not meet the criteria for a mature science, it could not have a paradigm in the Kuhnian sense.

The need for occupational science

Against this backdrop of conflicting perspectives, in 1981, Elizabeth J. Yerxa recommended that occupational therapy develop a basic science of human occupation. Yerxa's position was in concert with many of those already cited in its emphasis on the need for a unifying perspective centered on the concept of occupation. It is critical to note, however, that it departed from all others in its specification that the science be **basic** rather than applied. A basic science of occupation would have as its primary focus the explanation of occupation, whereas an applied science would advance knowledge on the use of occupation in treatment. In Yerxa's view, however, the science of occupation would ultimately be in the service of occupational therapy. As comprehensive and substantive knowledge about occupation was generated, she foresaw that therapists would draw on it to ascertain "the attributes of purposeful and self-directed activity designed for the disabled person to adapt to specific daily life challenges and endeavors within community, medical and institutional environ-

ments" (Yerxa, 1980, p. 534). In this way, while maintaining the importance of a basic science, Yerxa also made it clear that she intended the knowledge base to be relevant to the practitioners of occupational therapy.

Six years after Yerxa's recommendation, Kielhofner and Barris (1986a) echoed the sentiment that "the field" had "no readily identified structure of knowledge" (p. 68). They suggested, in contrast to Mosey (1985), that occupational therapy would need to be defined by consensus regarding its purpose and mission and the necessary perspective for knowledge in the field. In addition to the criteria listed by King (1978), these authors suggested that a paradigm in occupational therapy was needed: (a) to filter relevant knowledge into the field and determine how that knowledge would be interpreted and integrated; (b) to define the nature and scope of problems with which practitioners deal; and (c) to establish the goals, values, philosophical base, and ethics of the profession.

Timing is crucial in the formation of landmark events. If Yerxa's vision of a new basic science of occupation was to materialize, occupational therapists would need to be ready to embrace it. That is, they would need to see the value of having the proposed access to basic knowledge addressing occupation. Although the proposed discipline would be concerned with disability, it would also address occupation more broadly and thus be relevant to society at large, to general issues of wellness and life satisfaction. Kielhofner and Burke (1977) had maintained that the crisis in occupational therapy was felt not only by academics generating theory, but also by its practitioners.

Some perceived the advancing of a science as a potentially powerful way of resolving the profession's identity problems, its conflicts on the appropriate use of technology, its dilemmas on the degree of emphasis that should be placed on occupation, and the tendency for the public to undervalue it. Christiansen (1981), in advocating the need for a science, conveyed a sense of urgency when he wrote,

> ... the challenge of advancing our science may appear to be simply a matter of generating more research of higher caliber. A closer examination, however, reveals that the challenge is far greater than this; it involves the critical need to focus research efforts within the context of a unified theoretical structure. ... It is worth noting here that our failure to meet the challenge of research may ultimately lead to our demise as a viable discipline. (p. 116)

Meanwhile, in the broader culture, serious concern was developing about the impact of technology and reductionism on people's lives. The technology phase of the 50s had continued to grow into an increasingly sophisticated technology in the 1980s. Some became ill at ease with this technology. The products and uses of technology had bettered people's positions but also threatened them through destruction of environmental resources, creation of weapons for warfare of greater deadliness, and perhaps most critically, the devaluation of the individual (Beer, 1975). Beer (1975) goes so far as to say "that evolution may well have taken a wrong turning" (p. 23).

Examining things at their smallest levels to understand the whole "caused people to be treated as machines and fitted as parts into greater wholes defined primarily by technology and business needs" (Serret, 1985, p. 10). Human beings, in this sense, lost individual identity and value, being only a part or fraction of a greater whole. Much as the arts and crafts movement was a backlash against industrialism, the increasing technology continued to alienate us from a purposeful balanced lifestyle. In 1975, Beer suggested,

> Homo Faber sees the world in terms of the things he makes: then this is why our society is preoccupied with material wealth as its primary measure or achievement. . . . Homo Faber who invented work regards work as the "ethical" occupation: everything else is "play"—which is vaguely immoral, and is certainly not allowed to count as anything but a re-creation for work. Then this is why society is prepared to sustain men and their families only on the basis of the work that they do: it will in no circumstances reward them for playing. (p. 25)

The human being is more than just a component of the technology machine, but is a living active being who requires a purposeful, meaningful lifestyle that includes work, rest, and play. The devaluation of the human being throughout the industrial age is one social current that supported the need for the new science.

The emergence of occupational science

Amidst this confusion and hesitation to commit to one particular model of practice for the profession and in a social climate of concern about the impact of technology and reductionism on the people's lives, the faculty at the University of Southern California, led by Yerxa began to prepare a proposal for a doctoral degree in a new discipline, *"occupational science."* Although the proposal's primary aim was the delineation of a doctoral course of study, concurrently it successfully made the claim that a new scientific discipline was needed. Beyond its role in advancing knowledge for knowledge sake, the faculty made the case that the new discipline would benefit society in practical ways by increasing public knowledge about occupation and illuminating ways in which human lives could become more productive, satisfying, meaningful, and healthy (University of Southern California, 1989). A reading of this proposal reveals its strong conceptual ties with the thoughts of Mary Reilly. Its themes of recognizing the need for a scientifically sound knowledge base, the focus of which is on occupation, embracing a general systems theory and the traditional values of the profession, and viewing the human being as an occupational being can be traced to Reilly's publications (Reilly, 1958, 1962, 1966a).

In 1980, at the American Occupational Therapy Association Annual Conference, Yerxa for the first time publicly advocated the development of a science of occupation. In 1981, in her Foundation Report, she further advised that this science should be a basic science (as opposed to applied) and suggested several components, such as the focus of study (understanding of the nature of engagement in meaningful, purposeful, self-directed activity), the framework (general systems theory), and the methods (including phenomenology and ethnography). In 1982, an early model of the human subsystems (formed using a general systems approach) was developed by the faculty of the Department of Occupational Therapy, University of Southern California (USC, 1982). Under Yerxa's leadership, this faculty continued to mold and develop these ideas throughout the 80s.

Several grants facilitated the development of the doctoral proposal in occupational science (Department of Health and Human Services, Division of Maternal and Child Health Bureau, Grant #MCJ009048). Beginning in 1986, yearly symposia sponsored by the Division of Maternal and Child Health of the Department of Health and Human Services, were conducted with scholars from other disciplines to gain and share knowledge that is essential to the construction of this unique discipline (USC, 1989). The doctoral program in occupational science was approved in March 1989, and the first students were admitted in fall, 1989.

By 1991, Yerxa (1991c) had pinpointed that the new science needed to be true to the heritage of the occupational therapy founders, who viewed the person as active, capable, and free, and the agent of purposeful activity. This optimistic view identified all persons as capable beings, with resources and ability to adapt to change in complex societies. As described initially, the establishment of occupational science is both timely and timeless in its advent. Given the current social trends, it appears that occupational science is one of the great ideas of the 21st century (Yerxa et al., 1990).

This review has shown that occupational science had its roots in the conceptual themes that historically identified the practice of occupational therapy. Clearly, the focus that the science would give to the occupation concept represents a legacy from the founding period of the profession. Furthermore, the issues with which occupational science would grapple would be those that had plagued the profession: the reconciliation of technology with a broad view of occupation, the desirability of having a unified paradigm, and the survival of the occupation theme with encroaching reductionism. One thing was certain— that just as the profession's pioneers had celebrated the crucial role that occupation played in human existence, so too would the new science.

Definition of the science of occupation

Occupational science is a new social science, which grew out of occupational therapy. Its primary focus is the study of the human being as an occupational being, of how human beings realize their sense of life's meaning through purposeful activity (Yerxa et al., 1990; Clark et al., 1991). You may think of occupational science as addressing what anthropologists call the activity spectrum or stream of a species, that is, the range of activities that fill the day for a given species (White, 1991). The usefulness of occupational science is that it nurtures the practice of occupational therapy. This does not mean that occupational science is a single theory, a model, or a frame of reference. It is a basic social science, similar in form to academic disciplines such as anthropology, sociology, and psychology (Yerxa et al., 1990). Yerxa et al. (1990) state, "Occupational science is conceived as a basic science . . . as it deals with universal issues about occupation without concern for their immediate application in occupational therapy" (p. 4). Furthermore, Yerxa et al. propose that the applications of knowledge generated in occupational science to practice will be determined by practitioners.

Occupational science is classified as falling within the sciences (rather than the humanities) because its methods of data collection are systematic, disciplined, and subject to public scrutiny (Carlson & Clark, 1991). Carlson and Clark (1991) define science "as a systematic (rule-bound) and empirically based form of human inquiry undertaken by a community of scholars" (p. 236). Occupational science is considered to be more closely aligned to the social sciences than the physical sciences because its subject matter deals with human behavior (Homans, 1967).

Although the idea of a basic science of occupation is a recent innovation, we have shown that it is grounded in the beliefs of the founders of occupational therapy (Meyer, 1922), it evolved out of the occupational behavior perspective articulated by Reilly (1962, 1966, 1969), and it was seen as a partial solution to the problems that have historically plagued the rapidly expanding profession of occupational therapy. According to Mosey (1985), theories falling under the aegis of specific scientific disciplines constitute the corpus of knowledge that is applied in practice by professionals. Each theory on which therapists rely may provide a set of explanations about different phenomena. Occupational therapists typically draw from theories in psychology, anatomy, and physiology to construct their treatment approaches. Mosey (1985) defines frames of reference as "linking structures" that "answer the questions of how theories should be applied and when they should be applied" (p. 505). Finally, models may be defined as graphic or visual depictions of the relationships between variables.

In contrast to sensory integration theory as described by Ayres (1972), which is a frame of reference drawing from neuroanatomy, neurobiology, psychology, and other fields, the model of human occupation depicts relationships among variables for application in practice. It is expected that numerous theories about the nature, form, function, and meaning of occupation will be developed and coexist within the discipline of occupational science. These theories are likely to be differentially applied to practice in concert with others that therapists find useful in the construction of frames of reference. Occupational science's unique contribution to occupational therapy will be that of providing a corpus of knowledge sharply focused on the occupation concept. As an academic discipline, occupational science can potentially build professional unity by giving therapists a more explicit and expansive sense of the complexity and power of human occupation, but it is not likely to do so by claiming that only one frame of reference or theory should be used in practice.

Focus on occupation

If occupation is the point of focus of occupational science, how is it defined in the discipline? Because the science is new, we expect its definition to undergo revision. Yerxa et al. (1990) have provisionally defined occupation as the "specific 'chunks' of activity within the ongoing stream of human behavior which are named in the lexicon of the culture" (p. 5). Examples are skiing, grooming, dining, and making love (Figures 3-1 and 3-2). Engagement in occupation is assumed to influence health, either positively or negatively. For example, spending time taking illegal drugs is self-destructive, whereas daily aerobic activity is almost categorically health promoting. In their book, *Healthy pleasures*, Ornstein and Sobel (1989) describe a multitude of occupations that not only are enjoyable but also have been shown in studies to have a positive effect on health. The authors point out that certain occupations that we think of as ordinary or that we take for granted can have enormous health benefit. Examples are gazing at a crackling fire or sitting mesmerized by the illuminated movement of fish in a fishtank. While engaging in these ordinary activities, not only do we experience soothing effects, but our bodies are simultaneously being altered in positive ways physiologically.

The renowned linguist, anthropologist, and writer, Mary Catherine Bateson, at the Fourth Annual Occupational Science

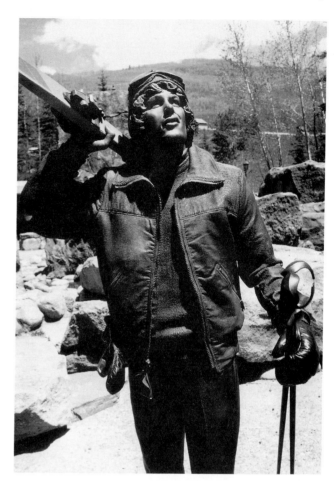

FIGURE 3-1. *J. Seward Johnson's sculpture, "Anticipation," conveys the feeling that one experiences in preparing for satisfying occupations. (Life-sized bronze sculpture, "Anticipation" by J. Seward Johnson, Jr. Photo, courtesy of Sculpture Placement, Ltd, Washington, DC.)*

Symposium (1991) in Philadelphia, presented her thoughts on the "chunking" aspect of the definition of occupation proposed by Yerxa et al. Bateson believes that only men typically have had the luxury of progressing from one chunk of activity to the next during the day. In contrast, according to Bateson's anthropologic work, women's occupations are enfolded onto one other. In other words, women do not enjoy the luxury of being able to think about one thing at a time. Bateson describes the activity spectrum of a village woman in Iran as follows,

> [She is] in a household with several children, probably at least one other woman, and one or two elderly people. In the course of a day's work, she prepares food; she keeps track of the children; she keeps track of the elderly people, including looking after them if they are sick; and if she has an hour here or there she sits down at the carpet loom, which is right in the center of the household. She can be interrupted at any moment, and yet after a few months she has a valuable carpet which is a unified work of art. (Bateson, in press, p. 9)

Bateson points out that when the day ends an observer might say that this woman didn't get much done, because the many things the woman did were "enfolded in these interlocking patterns" (Bateson, in press, p. 9). The centrality, therefore, of the notion of "chunks," in the definition of occupation concerns

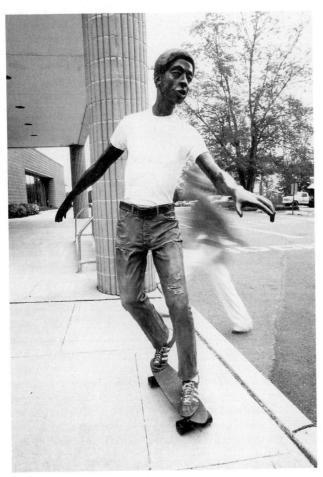

FIGURE 3-2. *In this sculpture, the concentration, coordination, and pleasure of engaging in a challenging physical task are communicated. (Life-sized bronze sculpture by J. Seward Johnson, Jr. Photo, courtesy of Sculpture Placement, Ltd, Washington, DC.)*

her, because it is considerably easier to categorize men's activities in this way in contrast to women's.

The philosopher Aaron Ben-Ze'ev was also invited to reflect on the definition of occupation as proposed in the science. In his paper entitled, "What is an Occupational Activity?" (in press), he proposes the following definition, "a repeated, complex, pattern of actions whose value is not limited to the value of its external results" (p. 2). This definition emphasizes the complexity and frequency of the activity and its intrinsic value. For Ben-Ze'ev, an occupational activity is a "complex pattern of actions of the whole system" (p. 3). A hand movement could not constitute an occupational activity, but when such a movement is used in a grooming situation, the "structured whole" could be called an occupational activity—if and only if it has intrinsic value, that is, experienced as satisfying in its own right. Thus, for Ben-Ze'ev, an occupational activity cannot be performed simply to achieve a functional outcome (dining for the purpose of food intake). Eating, according to Ben-Ze'ev, is not sufficiently complex to be categorized as an occupational activity; however, dining is an occupational activity because, in addition to satisfying hunger, it has an intrinsic value manifested in the pleasure it produces.

Ben-Ze'ev's work is notable in that it proposes a sharp distinction between an occupational and a nonoccupational activity. If his definition is accepted, the question arises as to how often therapists are actually employing occupation in clinics. If they are instead using nonoccupational activities, Ben-Ze'ev's prediction is that patients would want to finish the activity as soon as possible and would not be eager to repeat it. Thus, Ben-Ze'ev's work provokes us to think deeply about the requirements of occupational activity and the extent to which we have explored its full therapeutic valence. Ben-Ze'ev believes that the definition of occupation that he proposes will be useful in distinguishing occupational science from other social sciences.

In occupational science, occupation is seen as the means through which human beings realize their sense of life's meaning. Bateson (in press, p. 5) warns occupational scientists not to view occupation as something peripheral that is done here and there, but as the "web and woof" of the human being. Having studied the complex weave that constituted the lives of five women (Bateson, 1989) and now having read selected literature in occupational science, Bateson concludes,

> Now that I've looked at some of your materials and seen the titles of some of your papers, it is very clear to me that when I talk about composing a life, about how individuals weave together and combine many different kinds of activities, I am very precisely talking about occupations, particularly about how occupations fit together in the framework of a life. (Bateson, in press, p. 5)

Each day people make decisions about what they will and will not do, and they develop a daily itinerary of the things they may want to do, offset by the things they must do. For example, in our review of the diaries of over 75 female college students, we found tremendous variation in their patterns of occupation. Some spent the bulk of their time in occupations related to career or academic goals; others seemed to be consumed by activities related to grooming, dating, and the social scene.

Holland and Eisenhart (1990) published the findings of an ethnographic account that revealed that many women enter college with strong academic preparation and aspirations, but by the time they graduate these aspirations have been scaled down. While in college these same women invested exorbitant amounts of time and energy in finding and keeping their romantic partners. In occupational science, we are concerned with the reasons people choose one set of occupations over another, how investment in particular occupational patterns relates to life satisfaction, the effects of occupation on health, the ontogeny of occupational patterns, and how individuals experience joy in the world of activity and express their sense of life's meaning through their choices.

Complexity of occupation and organization of knowledge

Occupational scientists recognize that although occupation often appears ordinary and commonplace, it is infinitely complex. At the University of Southern California, The Model of the Human Subsystems that Influence Occupation (Clark et al., 1991) was developed to organize the interdisciplinary knowledge that is needed to construct comprehensive theories about occupation (Figure 3-3). It is crucial for the reader to recognize that this model is not conceived of as a final solution, however, but as a tentative heuristic for organizing knowledge.

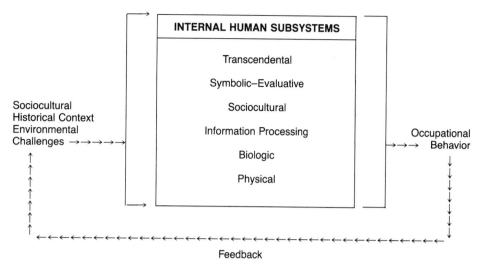

FIGURE 3-3. *Model of the human as an occupational being.* (*From* American Journal of Occupational Therapy.)

The model, using a general systems theory perspective, presents the person as a hierarchically arranged set of subsystems interacting as an open system in the environment over the lifespan from birth to old age. Occupations are seen as the output of the system through which the person negotiates and meets environmental challenges.

The six subsystems can be thought of as representing the knowledge areas that need to be addressed in developing multidisciplinary theories about occupation. Although provisional, the choice of the six subsystems was guided by the seminal works of Boulding (1956), Reilly (1974), and von Bertalanffy (1968). The following description introduces the reader to the conceptual underpinnings of each level and how the levels are being used to organize knowledge.

Physical subsystem

The physical subsystem "encompasses phenomenon that can be appropriately described by physiochemical processes" (Clark et al., 1991, p. 302). Included are physical matter, muscles, skin, and neural synapses. Occupational science does not address these phenomena in and of themselves, but only in relation to the role they play in the enactment of occupations. We have offered as an example (Clark et al., 1991) explanations of the physical requirements of hand use during purposeful activity as falling within this level.

More recently, an occupational scientist (Zemke, in press) presented a paper at the Fourth Annual Occupational Science Symposium, in which she urged the discipline to examine Edelman's (1987, 1989) theory of neural Darwinism to gain an understanding of the ways in which physical structures (in this case neuronal groups) seem to govern much of how reality is constructed and, therefore, by extension, how occupation is experienced. Even more interesting is the implication in Edelman's theory that the actual neuronal networks that will be used are sorted and selected through the person's experience of activity in the physiocospatial and social world. These networks, so determined, shape consciousness, and with it the interpretations we bring to our experiences. If Edelman's theory is correct (he cites much research to support it), the everyday occupations of children are key in determining how they will perceive and experience the world as adults. Furthermore, this theory can lead to conceptions of innovative rehabilitation techniques such as those proposed by Bach-y-Rita (1990), in which the mind is seen as a powerful moderator of rehabilitation outcomes.

Biologic subsystem

In a past publication cited by Clark et al. (1991), the physical subsystem was separated from the biologic system on the basis of being concerned with living systems involved in biologic adaptation (von Bertalanffy, 1968). At this level we described the phenomena of concern as the biologic urge for competence, the role that sensory integration plays in the execution of occupations, and the exploratory behaviors that result from the coupling of the two. Continued theory development at this level, we believe, will assist us in separating the biologic from the social influences on occupation, in appreciating the role that occupation has played in evolution, and in identifying the biologic foundations of occupation.

To understand the evolutionary roots of occupation and to get a glimpse at the activity spectrum of another closely related species, occupational scientists are now studying chimpanzee occupation and drawing on literature in ethology and primatology (Wood, in press). It is expected that work of this kind will identify the survival advantages of occupations, answer questions about the meaning and cause of particular occupations in nonhuman primate groups, shed light on what happens when particular species experience occupation-deprivation, and allow us to trace the evolutionary advantages of various occupational patterns.

Jane Goodall's (1986) work on the chimpanzees living in Gombe has been found to be particularly useful in demonstrating the crucial role that occupations such as sexual behavior and grooming play in chimpanzee communities, not only by enabling survival, but also by becoming the contexts within which position in the dominance hierarchy is jockeyed, negotiated, and regulated. For example, grooming, in addition to being performed for the functional purpose of insect removal, is just as significantly engaged in, particularly by males, as a display of deference to males of higher status. Through attention to this work, occupational scientists have at hand an ethologic model of inquiry that may be used to study human activity spectra and through which occupations can begin to be viewed in more complex ways. Occupational scientists have vast literature at their disposal that documents typical days of the chimpanzees of Gombe; they need now to build just as rich a repository on human occupation.

Information processing subsystem

At this level the focus is on the cognitive processes that are employed by human beings to successfully enact occupations. Theoretically, phenomena such as "perceptual and conceptual functions, learning, memory and planning" (Clark et al., p. 303) are addressed here. We have included Reilly's (1974) work on rules in relation to the development of skill at this level of the system.

Several theorists from the discipline of psychology have done work that is particularly relevant in understanding information processing at this level. Neisser (1976), for example, describes specifically how schemata, attention, imagination, and perceptual anticipation are needed to execute everyday activities, such as playing a game of chess (Figure 3-4). He maintains that the cognitive maps that people use while engaged in such activity are not confined simply to the rules of the game but include an overlay of social meaning and know-how on the part of the player on what to perceive. A person's decision to execute the next move in a certain way depends on choices about what to see, his or her perception of an opponent's demeanor and the anticipation of that opponent's next move, as well as on the person's own knowledge of the goals of and moves that are possible in the game. According to Neisser (1976),

> The rules of chess do not control the master's perception; they make it possible by giving him something to perceive . . . the chess player is neither totally free to look and move where he chooses nor entirely at the mercy of his environment. The control of eye movements and all adaptive behavior is only comprehensible as an

interaction. . . . One of the characteristics of a good chess player is his skill in picking up relevant information from the board. (pp. 180–181)

Equally fascinating is Bruner's (1990) account of how children enter into the world of meaning through everyday activity. Before they can speak, he maintains, they already grasp, in what he calls a "prelinguistic" (p. 71) way, the significance and meaning of situations. Such practical understanding is demonstrated as the child begins to regulate social interactions. For example, he cites a study published by Chandler et al. (1989), in which it was found that during a hide-and-seek game, children as young as age 2 years would withhold information when it was in their self-interest to do so. Later, as the child matures, he or she makes sense out of everyday experience by constructing progressively more complex narratives or stories about his or her experiences.

Sociocultural system

Clark et al. (1991) described the sociocultural subsystem as focusing on perceived social and cultural expectations. Just as occupational and gender roles influence sense of identity, so, too, do they, to a certain extent, determine choices of and commitment to specific occupations. Belenky et al. (1986) cite numerous studies that indicate that girls and women find it more difficult than men and boys to assert their authority, express themselves in public so that the attention of others is commanded, and maximally use their abilities in the working world. These same girls and women would be likely then to refrain from entering political arenas, assuming leadership positions in team meetings, and choosing high status professions that allegedly require stretching to the outer limits of their capabilities. The authors state, "All women grow up having to deal with historically and culturally engrained definitions of femininity and womanhood—one common theme being that women, like children, should be seen and not heard" (Belenky et al., 1986, p. 5).

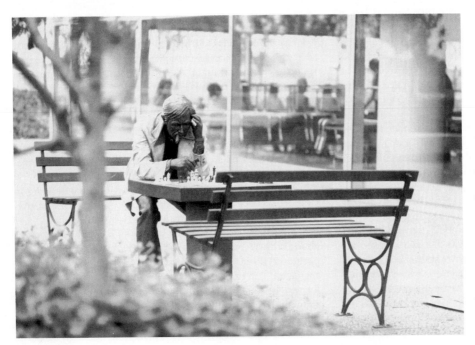

FIGURE 3-4. *During the game of chess, master players are able to pick up relevant information from the board. (Life-sized bronze sculpture by J. Seward Johnson, Jr. Photo, courtesy of Sculpture Placement, Ltd, Washington, DC.)*

Thus, a comprehensive understanding of occupation requires careful analysis of the sociocultural context in which it occurs. Consistent with Vygotsky's theory (see Wertsch, 1979, 1985), occupational science at this level recognizes the powerful impact that sociocultural context and history have on the developing child. The study of human occupation then involves examining its social origins. Also, particular occupations need to be viewed as possessing a physical form as well as a social dimension. Take, for example, the occupation of making music together. Schutz (1976) elucidates the social nature of playing chamber music when he states that the musicians become disturbed if the arrangement prevents the co-performers from seeing one another. While playing their instruments, musicians must attend to their own part and simultaneously tune in to the timing and emotional expression of those with whom they are playing.

Symbolic evaluative subsystem

The symbolic evaluative level is concerned with the symbolic systems that are used to appraise the individual's valuing of occupations. As already mentioned, for Ben Ze'ev, activities must possess some intrinsic value for them to be deemed occupational. Aesthetic, moral, emotional, and economic value systems can be employed to appraise the significance of particular activities. For example, one may find a particular job boring and demoralizing, but stay employed for reasons of economic gain. In this case, Ben Ze'ev would classify the activity as nonoccupational. In contrast, a person may want to walk on the beach because of its aesthetic appeal or because the billowing breezes simply feel good. Finally, a person may choose to become invested in a "food for the homeless project" sponsored by the church because of a blend of moral conviction, that is, the activity is seen as a good thing to do, and emotion—feeling loved by God for being charitable. All of this means that to understand how individuals piece their lives together through occupation, we must probe to understand the symbolic systems that reside in their consciousness and through which they evaluate the significance and meaning of occupation.

Moore (1991), for example, describes how the image of self as honorable, in contrast to economic utility, governs the Big Man's choice to hold a competitive feast. In these rituals, the defeated rivals of the Big Man are invited to join him at a huge party at which they will be showered with gifts. In this context, gifts are not a token of winning but of losing. Participation in the feast allows the Big Man to see himself as honorable, but in the process, he depletes his people of needed resources. A vision of honor, in this instance, preempts economic utility. Moore concludes that "individuals strive to live interactive and coupled lives in accordance with cultural models of honor" (p. 1).

Just as images of honor can govern commitment to specific occupations, so do emotions play a crucial role in how we live our daily lives. Zajonc (1980) differentiates feeling from thinking, concluding that each is governed by independent systems, although one can influence the other. He sees the affective system as primary, tending to be irrevocable, implicating the self and difficult to describe in words. He would take the position that our choices of occupation are influenced by feelings as much as they are by our thoughts. Harré et al. (1985) similarly highlight emotion as central to human choices to act in particular ways.

Finally, in their stunning body of research using the experiential sampling method, Mihalyi Csikszentmihalyi et al. (Csikszentmihalyi, 1975; Csikszentmihalyi et al., 1977) have shown how emotions are actually modified by the degree of match between a person's skill level and the challenge embedded in the occupation before him or her. People are happy, he maintains, when they feel in control of their lives, when their bodies and minds are being challenged but not to the point of stress, when they are gradually mastering new skills. It would seem that the knowledge produced about this state, which Csikszentmihalyi calls "flow," could be applied widely to the practice of occupational therapy. Choices of occupation seem to be emotionally laden, but reciprocally, occupation can modify emotional state.

Transcendental subsystem

This subsystem is concerned with the sense of meaning the person ascribes to his or her everyday experiences over the course of a lifetime (Clark et al., 1991). Mary Catherine Bateson (1989, in press) has addressed this aspect of occupation when she speaks of life as an improvisational art form, analogous to a still life painting in which a mandolin, one or two apples, and drafting tools are arranged in a composition. Although each element seems unrelated, they nevertheless form a unity. Similarly, in life, according to Bateson, the diverse occupations in which we engage ultimately are unified by themes that define our personhood. At this level, the explanation of occupation is similar to viewing a still life or listening to a symphony, in which new movements that have different tempos but are united by certain themes emerge in time. Yerxa et al. (1990) suggest that human beings are authors of their life experience and must adapt to each successive chapter. As David Polinghorne (1988) suggests:

> We achieve our personal identities and self-concept through the use of narrative configuration, and make our existence into a whole by understanding it as an expression of a single unfolding and developing story. We are in the middle of our stories and cannot be sure how they will end; we are constantly having to reverse the plot as new events are added to our lives (p. 150).

Summary

Through reference to the Model of the Human as an Occupational Being, we have provided a glimpse at the vast interdisciplinary intellectual territory that needs to be traversed for an explanation of human occupation. When we think about our patients as occupational beings, we must address all these levels, but in doing so, we must guard against losing our sense of the essence of the person. People, after all, are individuals with hopes, dreams, ambitions, loves, and disappointments, not conglomerations of subsystems. The hierarchical systems approach used here allows us to coherently import into the science interdisciplinary knowledge that sheds light on the complexity of occupation, but systems thinking requires us to first and foremost view people as actors negotiating in a world of meaning.

The research and scholarship program in occupational science

Assumptions and ethics

How will we guide decisions about the proper research methodologies for occupational science and for the selection of knowledge to be assimilated into the discipline? Yerxa (1991b) believes that the assumptions and ethics that have always guided occupational therapy should also be relied on in the development of occupational science. She accords centrality to the following assumptions:

> Occupational therapy provides therapeutic intervention to human beings, not to muscles or synapses or superegos.
> Human beings are complex, multileveled systems who act on and interact with their environments.
> Unique human qualities include language, history, culture, and the endowment of life experiences with spiritual meaning.
> Occupational therapy is designed to enable people to adapt to the challenges of their environments through the use of their hands, mind, and will (Reilly, 1962).
> Occupational therapy, grounded in humanistic values, has an ethical responsibility to persons with chronic conditions.
> Human beings have interests, goals, aspirations, and plans that, when achieved, provide a valued sense of efficacy.
> Occupational therapy is concerned with how occupation enables persons to achieve competence and economic self-sufficiency and to contribute to themselves and others.
> Although it may be provided in a medical milieu, occupational therapy is different from and complementary to medicine in its thought process, view of the human being, and scientific foundation.
> Occupational therapy's knowledge is based on a synthesis of evolutionary biology, the social sciences, and the humanities; medicine's foundation rests in the physical and natural sciences.
> Occupational therapy views the individual as embedded in the stream of time (evolutionary, developmental, and learning) (Reilly, 1974, p. 200)

These assumptions, according to Yerxa, imply that research in occupational science should be neither reductionist nor tied to traditional methods of scientific inquiry. For although she views experimental methods as acceptable for the study of physical matter, she regards them as inadequate for developing theory about human occupation. The reasons are convincing.

First, traditional scientific method usually requires artificial environments in which to do experiments. But human occupation is context-bound and therefore study occurs with the most credulity in natural settings. Second, traditional methodologies are not designed to apprehend a sense of how the person is experiencing and interpreting life events. Rather, the emphasis on objectivity discourages taking into account the person's point of view. Finally, traditional research methodology, because of its reductionist focus, does not lend itself to the study of complex systems changing over time. Adopting Gergen's (1982) view, Yerxa believes the research methodologies for occupational science and the studies we deem as most relevant to it should emphasize context embeddedness, change through time, and voluntary action.

Yerxa (1991b) judges the traditional experimental approach to advancing science to be in violation of the ethics of occupation

therapy. She claims that "its treatment of subjects as objects and its use of statistical tools, reduces persons to less than human beings, for example, to muscles, synapses, or homeostatic mechanisms" (p. 201). Autonomy, choice, and even individuality are lost in this approach. Yerxa (1991c) goes on to suggest that occupation scientists invent new methods of scientific inquiry that are particularly well suited to the study of the interpretive dimension of occupation. The qualitative approaches she lists as having the potential for advancing occupational science are the life history method (Langness & Frank, 1981), naturalistic inquiry (Lincoln & Guba, 1985), systems theory (Sameroff, 1982), ethnography (Geertz, 1973), and historical methods (Stone, 1979), and others.

Currently, graduate students in the occupational science program at the University of Southern California are exploring the use of the methods just mentioned for furthering occupational science. Using ethnographic methods, Krishnigiri (in press) studied mate selection in a sample of Indian college-age students; Pierce (in press), the occupations of scholars; and Jackson (in press), the meaning with which a group of senior citizens had imbued their occupations over a lifetime. Currently, Clark and her students are using naturalistic inquiry to study the person-oriented adaptive systems of former high school students with disability who are living in the community. As an extension of this line of research, the University of Southern California Department of Occupational Therapy was just awarded a grant from the American Occupational Therapy Foundation to study the person-centered adaptive systems used by adolescents with disability making the transition to independent living, people with spinal cord injury, and a group of well elderly. A mix of qualitative and quantitative approaches (ideally) adapted to be in accord with the ethics and assumptions of occupational therapy will be used in the implementation of this project.

Finally, Mihalyi Csikszentmihalyi (1991) believes that the research program on occupation will become bona fide as a new science only after it has discovered "a set of laws specific to occupations that are not reducible to the symbolic systems of already existing disciplines" (Csikszentmihalyi, 1990, p. xvi). The primary goal of occupational science is to disseminate knowledge about the form, function, and meaning as well as the sociocultural context of occupation so that occupational therapy can be nurtured. It should be made clear that any research that elucidates basic knowledge about occupation has the potential of falling within the conceptual boundaries of this new academic discipline.

Occupational science's legacy of return to occupational therapy: therapeutic application

We have stressed that the academic discipline of occupational science grew out of the foundations, ethics, and assumptions of occupational therapy. Its legacy of return to occupational therapy will consist of knowledge that will become available for therapists to draw on to enhance the potency of their treatment approaches. It is expected that occupational science will generate a shift in the emphasis of practice, not a reconstruction. Techniques currently used will continue to be used, but may be reframed in a context that unmistakably gives occupation the central position.

Some applications of concepts emanating from occupational science have already been published, but these must be regarded as tentative. Yerxa et al. (1990) propose that knowledge about the flow experience will enable therapists to assist patients in creating a satisfying round of daily activity. Increased understanding of the developmental progression of time use will foster therapists' ability to help their patients become competent in directing and organizing their activity spectra. Additionally, they claim therapists will be in a better position to recommend particular occupations for children for the purpose of building adult competence. Finally, they believe, occupational science findings will enable therapists to have a clearer sense of when patient activities do not constitute a balance of work, rest, and play and to know of multiple ways through which patient self-esteem can be fostered, identity constructed, and a sense of satisfaction attained through choice of occupation. For Yerxa et al. (1990), the availability of this knowledge will, in short, enable therapists to take better advantage of the full therapeutic valence of occupation in practice.

Jackson (1990) more concretely delineates how specific concepts from occupational science, based largely on the work of Reilly (1958, 1962, 1966a 1966b, 1969) and also Csikszentmihalyi and Larson (1984), were used in the development of a curriculum designed to foster the transition of adolescents with disabilities from school to independent living. Originally implemented at Savanna High School in Anaheim, California, through OSERS Grant #600840076, the program focused on occupations and occupational roles, the environment, the concept of independence, and the degree of harmony between activity demands and the perceived abilities of the students. Instead of focusing on dysfunction, the program encouraged the students to develop knowledge about themselves, their abilities, and their options and the skill and problem-solving and decision-making abilities to attain their goals.

Occupational science constructs have also been applied to program development for people with AIDS (Clark & Jackson, 1990). Once again, instead of focusing on the disease process or pathology, the program described by Clark and Jackson (1990) emphasizes the therapist's role in helping patients achieve a sense of life finish, of accomplishing their life goals within a truncated expected lifespan. The meaning which patients impart to occupation, their sense of what their life is about, and where they are in its narrative are given the central position in the therapeutic plan. Temporal rhythms, the health-promoting effects of occupation on the immune system, occupational role, and the building of a sense of community in the therapeutic milieu are also included in the treatment program.

Finally, in an article on conflict between the mothering and student roles of teenage mothers, Hermann (1990) illustrates how data gathered through occupational science can provoke thoughts on therapeutic approaches. She found that high-conflict mothers articulated plans for college, felt uncomfortable depending on others for child care, and filled out time logs documenting their daily activities accurately and completely. Low-conflict mothers, on the other hand, were unable to articulate educational or vocational goals, depended on others for the bulk of child care, and failed to complete the time log. Based on these findings, Hermann (1990) suggests that programs for teenage mothers should include,

(a) building self-esteem and confidence to facilitate emancipation from family . . . ; (b) offering . . . training to facilitate the occupational choice process; (c) stressing efficient use of time . . . to achieve role balance; and, (d) utilizing meaningful activity to teach problem solving and future planning skills. (p. 65)

Concrete methods for achieving these goals are also specified, including (a) having the mothers keep diaries on their time use; (b) exploring career interests; (c) outlining realistic plans for the future; (d) and assisting the students in achieving a sense of success in both their caretaking and student roles.

Although only a limited number of therapists to date have published papers on the therapeutic application of occupational science, we can speculate on the form that therapy would take if it were molded further using occupational science concepts. Clearly, of utmost concern to therapists would be evoking personal narratives from their patients that reveal the meaning the patients derive from particular occupations, how they chunk or enfold their occupations, and how their occupational patterns flowing through the stream of time fit into a framework of how they understand their lives. To elicit the narratives that would give these insights, therapists might begin to be trained in hermeneutic interviewing methods (Packer, 1985). Therapists would therefore need to understand the moral, emotional, spiritual, ethnic, and cultural dimensions of their patients.

Therapists may also begin to reframe their understanding of illness and catastrophic injury, by seeing them not as isolated circumstances but as a discontinuity within the framework of a total life. Such an approach is consistent with Bateson's idea of life as a compositional art form or symphony. The time spent in occupational therapy might be viewed as a transitional movement, with a distinct form and tempo, but containing many of the themes that had always characterized the patient's life. These themes might be recycled in the new situation so that the patient is inspired to reconstruct a sense of self that preserves elements of what he or she had always been with what he or she will become in the next phase of life.

Bateson (in press) believes that occupation is a "central element of human completeness and health" (p. 15). She has written that "If someone gains the capacity to do something useful for themselves or others, that is the key to personhood, whether it involves the ability to earn a living or cook a meal or to put on shoes in the morning. . . . Whatever skill needs to be mastered at this moment" (p. 14). Papers such as this produced by scholars from other disciplines who are contributing to occupational science encourage therapists to more fully value their impact on patients' lives.

Goldstein (in press), a renowned scholar in international relations, has written about the correspondence between the rules of childhood games and those that govern global international relations; Dear (in press), whose discipline is geography, has analyzed the power of place on occupation. An elaborated interdisciplinary understanding of occupation is bound to equip therapists to better use it therapeutically.

The knowledge produced by occupational scientists may generate frustration in therapists who may feel increasingly constrained by fiscal and other concerns of practice. Appreciating the complexity of occupation and the central place it has in people's lives, occupational therapists may insist that their roles be expanded and redefined. They may want to do in-depth hermeneutic interviews, to co-develop daily itineraries of occupation with their patients, to analyze the diaries of patients on their occupational patterns and their emotional reactions to them, and to go with their patients to their homes and places of work and leisure.

Occupational science may also assist therapists in understanding the complexity of occupation. Pierce (in press), in her study of the occupations of scholars, found that to be productive, scholars needed to be sensitive to daily and annual temporal rhythms, to be fueled by emotional excitement, to have established routines for apportioning their reserves of energy, and to have a support system. It is interesting that the scholars felt that they could not do their work at just any time, that they needed to be in the mood. They described themselves as submerging and surfacing from tasks. These notions may be true not only of the occupations of scholars, but of any productive activity requiring energy and concentration. They may imply guidelines for the use of occupation in the occupational therapy context. Do therapists need to be more sensitive to patient temporality, affective states, project orchestration, and the agency role of patients in directing the therapeutic plan?

Summary

This chapter has traced the links of occupational science to occupational therapy. Occupational science is a new social science that is expected to nurture occupational therapy, while resting on its ethical and philosophical foundations. Its focus is on the study of the human being as an occupational being. The Model of the Human as an Occupational Being was presented as an heuristic for organizing the interdisciplinary knowledge that contributes to an understanding of occupation. Research approaches to be taken in occupational science were discussed in relation to the ethics and values of occupational therapy. Some preliminary reflections were made on the ways in which occupational science may contribute to a shifting emphasis in occupational therapy.

The preparation of this manuscript was partially supported by the U.S. Department of Health and Human Services, Maternal and Child Health Bureau, Grant #MCJ009048.

The authors wish to acknowledge the following USC Occupational Science doctoral students: Erna Blanche, Linda Florey, Bonnie Kennedy, Valerie O'Brien, Ruth Segal, Betty Snow, John White, and Wendy Wood for contributing their ideas to the treatment application section.

References

Ayres, A. J. (1972). *Sensory integration and learning disorders.* Los Angeles: Western Psychological Services.

Bach-y-Rita, P. (1990). Thoughts on the role of the mind in recovery from brain damage. In E. Roy, et al. (Eds.), *Machinery of the mind: Data, theory and speculation about higher brain function.* Boston: Birkhauser.

Bateson, M. C. (1989). *Composing a life.* New York: Penguin Books.

Bateson, M. C. (in press). Occupation in the service of composing a life. *Proceedings of selected papers of occupation science symposia I–IV.* Philadelphia: F. A. Davis.

Beer, S. (1975). *Platform for change.* New York: John Wiley & Sons.

Belenky, M. F., Clinchy, B. M., Goldberg, N. R., & Tarule, J. M. (1986). *Women's ways of knowing: The development of self, voice and mind.* New York: Basic Books.

Ben-Ze'ev, A. (in press). What is an occupational activity? *Proceedings of selected papers of occupation science symposia I–IV.* Philadelphia: F. A. Davis.

Bockoven, J. S. (1963). *Moral treatment in American psychiatry.* New York: Springer.

Boulding, K. E. (1956). General systems theory—the skeleton of science. *Management Science, 2,* 197–208.

Bruner, J. (1990). *Acts of meaning.* Cambridge, MA: Harvard University Press.

Carlson, M., & Clark, F. (1991). The search for useful methodologies in occupational science. *American Journal of Occupational Therapy, 45,* 235–241.

Chandler, M., Fritz, A. S., & Hala, S. (1989). Small scale deceit: Deception as a marker of two-, three-, and four-year-olds' theories of mind. *Child Development, 60,* 1263.

Christiansen, C. (1981). Toward resolution of crisis: Research requisites in occupational therapy. *Occupational Therapy Journal of Research, 1,* 115–124.

Clark, F. A., & Jackson, J. (1990). The application of occupational science negative heuristic in the treatment of persons with human immunodeficiency virus infection. *Occupational Therapy in Health Care, 6,* 69–91.

Clark, F., Parham, D., Carlson, M., Frank, G., et al. (1991). Occupational science: Academic innovation in the service of occupational therapy's future. *American Journal of Occupational Therapy, 45,* 300–310.

Clark, P. N. (1979). Human development through occupation: Theoretical frameworks in contemporary occupational therapy practice, part 1. *American Journal of Occupational Therapy, 33,* 505–514.

Clark, P. N. (1979). Human development through occupation: Theoretical frameworks in contemporary occupational therapy practice, part 2. *American Journal of Occupational Therapy, 33,* 577–585.

Csikszentmihalyi, M. (1975). *Beyond boredom and anxiety: The experience of play in work and games.* San Francisco: Jossey-Bass.

Csikszentmihalyi, M., & Larson, R. (1984). *Being adolescent: Conflict and growth in the teenage years.* New York: Basic Books.

Csikszentmihalyi, M. (1991). Foreword. *Occupational Therapy in Health Care, 6,* xv–xvii.

Csikszentmihalyi, M., Larson, R., & Prescott, S. (1977). The ecology of adolescent activity. *Journal of Youth and Adolescence, 6,* 281–294.

Dear, M. (in press). Space, time and the geography of everyday life. *Proceedings of selected papers of occupation science symposia I–IV.*

Dunton, W. R. (1919). *Reconstruction therapy.* Philadelphia: W. B. Saunders.

Edelman, G. M. (1987). *Neural Darwinism: The theory of neuronal group selection.* Basic Books.

Edelman, G. M. (1989). *The remembered present: A biological theory of consciousness.* New York: Basic Books.

Geertz, C. (1973). *The interpretation of cultures.* New York: Basic Books.

Gergen, K. (1982). *Toward transformation in social knowledge.* New York: Springer-Verlag.

Goldstein, J. (in press). International relations and everyday life. *Proceedings of selected papers of occupation science symposia I–IV.*

Goodall, J. (1986). *The chimpanzees of Gombe: Patterns of behavior.* Cambridge, MA: Belknap Press of Harvard University.

Gritzer, G., & Arluke, A. (1985). *The making of rehabilitation.* Berkeley: University of California Press.

Harms, E. (1964). Beginning of psychotherapy in America. *American Journal of Psychotherapy, 18,* 287.

Harré, R., Clark, D., & De Carlo, N. (1985). *Motives and mechanisms: An introduction to the psychology of action.* New York: Methuen.

Heard, C. (1977). Occupational role acquisition. *American Journal of Occupational Therapy, 31,* 243–247.

Herrmann, C. (1990). A descriptive study of daily activities and role conflict in single adolescent mothers. *Occupational Therapy in Health Care, 6,* 53–68.

Holland, D., & Eisenhart, M. (1990). *Educated in romance: Women, achievement and college culture.* Chicago: University of Chicago Press.

Homans, G. (1967). *The nature of science.* New York: Harbinger.

Hopkins, H. (1988). An historical perspective on occupational therapy. In H. Hopkins & H. Smith (Eds.), *Willard and Spackman's occupational therapy* (7th ed., pp. 16–37). Philadelphia: J. B. Lippincott.

Jackson, J. (in press). Meaning in the occupations of the well elderly. *Proceedings of selected papers of occupation science symposia I–IV*. Philadelphia: F. A. Davis.

Kielhofner, G. (1980). A model of human occupation. Part 2. Ontogenesis from the perspective of temporal adaptation. *American Journal of Occupational Therapy, 34,* 657–663

Kielhofner, G., & Barris, R. (1986a). Organization of knowledge in occupational therapy: A proposal and a survey of the literature. *Occupational Therapy Journal of Research, 6,* 67–83.

Kielhofner, G., & Barris, R. (1986b). A response to commentary: Organization of knowledge in occupational therapy: A proposal and a survey of the literature. *Occupational Therapy Journal of Research, 6,* 67–83.

Kielhofner, G., & Burke, J. (1977). Occupational therapy after 60 years: An account of changing identity and knowledge. *American Journal of Occupational Therapy, 31,* 675–689.

Kielhofner, G., & Burke, J. (1980). A model of human occupation, part 1. Conceptual framework and content. *American Journal of Occupational Therapy, 34,* 572–581.

King, L. J. (1978). Toward a science of adaptive responses. *American Journal of Occupational Therapy, 32,* 429–437.

Krishnagiri, S. (in press). Mate selection as an occupation. *Proceedings of selected papers of occupation science symposia I–IV*. Philadelphia: F. A. Davis.

Kuhn, T. S. (1970). *The structure of scientific revolutions* (2nd. ed.). Chicago: University of Chicago Press.

Labovitz, D., & Miller, R. (1986). Commentary: Organization of knowledge in occupational therapy: A proposal and a survey of the literature. *Occupational Therapy Journal of Research, 6,* 85–92.

Langness, L. L., & Frank, G. (1981). *Lives: An anthropological approach to biography*. Novato, CA: Chandler & Sharp.

Lincoln, Y. S., & Guba, E. A. (1985). *Naturalistic inquiry*. Beverly Hills, CA: Sage Publications.

Llorens, L. (1970). Facilitating growth and development: The promise of occupational therapy. *American Journal of Occupational Therapy, 24,* 93–101.

Llorens, L. (1984). Theoretical conceptualizations of occupational therapy: 1960–82. *Occupational Therapy in Mental Health, 4,* 1–14.

Matsutsuyu, J. (1969). The interest checklist. *American Journal of Occupational Therapy, 31,* 243–247.

Matsutsuyu, J. (1971). Occupational behavior—a perspective on work and play. *American Journal of Occupational Therapy, 25,* 291–293.

Meyer, A. (1922). Philosophy of occupational therapy. *Archives of Occupational Therapy, 1,* 1–10. (Reprinted in *American Journal of Occupational Therapy, 31,* 639–642, 1977.)

Moore, A. (1991). *Reflexivity, an imperative in productive systems*. Unpublished manuscript.

Mosey, A. (1985). Eleanor Clarke Slagle lecture, 1985: A monistic or a pluralistic approach to professional identity. *American Journal of Occupational Therapy, 39,* 504–509.

Neisser, U. (1976). *Cognition and reality, principles and implications of cognitive psychology*. New York: Freeman & Co.

Occupational therapy and its relationship to physiotherapy. (1932). *Physiotherapy Review, 12,* 146.

Ornstein, R., & Sobel, D. (1989). *Healthy pleasures*. New York: Addison-Wesley.

Packer, M. J. (1985). Hermeneutic inquiry in the study of human conduct. *American Psychologist, 40*(10), 1081–1093.

Pierce, D. (in press). The occupation of scholars. *Proceedings of selected papers of occupation science symposia I–IV*. Philadelphia: F. A. Davis.

Polkinghorne, D. (1988). *Narrative knowing and the human sciences*. Albany: SUNY Press.

Reilly, M. (1958). An occupational therapy curriculum. *American Journal of Occupational Therapy, 12,* 293–299.

Reilly, M. (1962). Occupational therapy can be one of the great ideas of the 20th century medicine. *American Journal of Occupational Therapy, 16,* 1–9.

Reilly, M. (1966a). A psychiatric occupational therapy program as a teaching model. *American Journal of Occupational Therapy, 20,* 61–66.

Reilly, M. (1966b). The challenge of the future to an occupational therapist. *American Journal of Occupational Therapy, 20,* 221–225.

Reilly, M. (1969). The education process. *American Journal of Occupational Therapy, 23,* 299–307.

Reilly M. (1971). The modernization of occupational therapy. *American Journal of Occupational Therapy, 25,* 243–246.

Reilly, M. (1974). *Play as exploratory learning*. Beverly Hills: Sage Publications.

Report of the Baruch Committee on Physical Medicine, April 1944 (pp. 53, 77).

Robinson, A. (1977). Play: The arena for acquisition of rules for competent behavior. *American Journal of Occupational Therapy, 31,* 248–253.

Sameroff, A. J. (1982). Development and the dialectic: The need for a systems approach. In A. W. Collins (Ed.), *The Minnesota symposium on child psychology* (Vol. 15, pp. 83–103). Hillsdale, NJ: Erlbaum.

Schutz, A. (1976). Making music together: A study in social relationship. In A. Brodersen (Ed.), *Collected papers II—study in social theory* (pp. 159–178). The Hague, Netherlands: Martinus Nijhoff.

Serret, K. (1985). Another look at occupational therapy's history: Paradigm or pair-of-hands. *Occupational Therapy in Health Care, 5,* 1–31.

Stone, L. (1979). The revival of the narrative: Reflections on a new old history. *Past and Present, 85,* 3–23.

University of Southern California, Department of Occupational Therapy. (1982). *Self-study of an educational program for the occupational therapist*. Unpublished manuscript.

University of Southern California, Department of Occupational Therapy. (1989). Proposal for a doctoral dissertation in occupational science. Unpublished manuscript.

von Bertalanffy, L. (1968). *General systems theory*. New York: Braziller.

Wertsch, J. V. (1979). From social interaction to higher psychological process: A clarification and application of Vygotsky's theory. *Human Development, 22,* 1–22.

Wertsch, J. V. (1985). *Vygotsky and the social formation of mind*. Cambridge, MA: Harvard University Press.

White, D. (1991). Human activity systems and the theory of cultural evolution. Presented at the annual meeting of the Society for Applied Anthropology, Charleston, SC, March 1991.

Wood, W. (in press). Gender and the work of non-human primates: Implications for occupational science. *Proceedings of selected papers of occupation science symposia I–IV*. Philadelphia: F. A. Davis.

Wright, H. B. (1915). In W. R. Dunton (Ed.), *Occupational therapy: A manual for nurses*. Philadelphia: W. B. Saunders.

Yerxa, E. (1966). Authentic occupational therapy. *American Journal of Occupational Therapy, 21,* 1–9.

Yerxa, E. (1980). Occupational therapy's role in creating a future climate of caring. *American Journal of Occupational Therapy, 34,* 529–534.

Yerxa, E. (1981). A "developmental assessment" of occupational therapy research in 1981. *American Journal of Occupational Therapy, 35,* 820–821.

Yerxa, E. (1991b). Seeking a relevant, ethical, and realistic way of knowing for occupational therapy. *American Journal of Occupational Therapy, 45,* 199–204.

Yerxa, E. (1991c). *Searching for an ethical, realistic and relevant foundation for new models of occupational therapy practice*. Presentation November 15, 1991, VA Hospital, Los Angeles, CA.

Yerxa, E., Clark, F., Frank, G., Jackson, J., et al. (1990). An introduction to occupational science, A foundation for occupational therapy in the 21st century. *Occupational Therapy in Health Care, 6,* 1–17.

Zajonc, R. B. (1980). Feeling and thinking: Preferences need no inferences. *American Psychologist, 35,* 151–175.

Zemke, R. (in press). The relevance of Edelman's neurobiological theories for the study of occupation. *Proceedings of selected papers of occupation science symposia I–IV*. Philadelphia: F. A. Davis.

CHAPTER 4

Current basis for theory and philosophy of occupational therapy

SECTION 1

Philosophical base of occupational therapy

HELEN L. HOPKINS

LEARNING OBJECTIVES

Upon completion of this section the reader will be able to:

1. *Describe philosophy and its relationship to occupational therapy practice.*
2. *Describe the philosophical base of occupational therapy.*
3. *Identify the major knowledge bases needed for occupational therapy practice.*
4. *Identify the relationships between philosophical base, theory base, and knowledge bases as related to occupational therapy practice.*

Philosophy is concerned "with the meaning of life and the significance of the world in which man finds himself" (Randall & Buchler, 1960, p. 5). The **philosophy** of occupational therapy represents the profession's view of the nature of existence and gives meaning to and guides the actions of the profession. It also provides the fundamental set of values, beliefs, truths, and principles that guide the action of the profession's practitioners (Shannon, 1986).

The "Philosophical Base of Occupational Therapy," adopted in April 1979 by the Representative Assembly in Detroit, provides a foundation for the theory and practice of occupational therapy,

> Man is an active being whose development is influenced by the use of purposeful activity. Using their capacity for intrinsic motivation, human beings are able to influence their physical and mental health and their social and physical environment through purposeful activity. Human life includes a process of continuous adaptation. Adaptation is a change in function that promotes survival and self-actualization. Biological, psychological, and environmental factors may interrupt the adaptation process at any time throughout the life cycle. Dysfunction may occur when adaptation is impaired. Purposeful activity facilitates the adaptive process.
>
> Occupational therapy is based on the belief that purposeful activity (occupation), including its interpersonal and environmental components, may be used to prevent and mediate dysfunction, and to elicit maximum adaptation. Activity as used by the occupational therapist includes both an intrinsic and a therapeutic purpose. (Resolution 532–79, 1979, p. 785)

As an additional guide to education and practice, in April 1979 the Representative Assembly affirmed,

> . . . that there be a universal acceptance and implementation of the common core of occupational therapy as active participation of the patient/client in occupation for purposes of improving performance. The use of facilitating procedures is only acceptable as occupational therapy when used to prepare the patient/client for better performance and prevention of disability, through self-participation in occupation. . . . Increased emphasis should be placed "on more creative involvement of the patient/client in purposeful, motivating and constructive occupation based on individual behavioral evaluations and treatment." (Resolution 532–79, 1979, p. 785)

The definition of occupational therapy, the philosophical base statement, and the affirmation of occupation as the common core of occupational therapy place parameters on the scope of occupational therapy. They provide guidance for education and practice and for the development and validation of theoretical propositions through research.

Theory base

Throughout its history, the focus of the occupational therapy profession has been on the nature of the total person in relation to society and the world in which the person lives. The body of knowledge in occupational therapy and its theoretical base are derived from several broad scientific areas, including biologic and behavioral sciences, sociology, anthropology, and medicine. Knowledge in these areas is continually expanding and being modified, making it mandatory for occupational therapy to change. Occupational therapy uses the broad **knowledge areas** as its theoretical underpinnings and can be effective only in proportion to the accuracy of these knowledge bases. Theoretical propositions are being built on these broad knowledge areas to form the beginning of occupational therapy's unique body of knowledge.

At the University of Southern California, a doctoral program has been established in "Occupational Science" and another doctoral program has begun at Texas Woman's University in "Occupational Adaptation" (see Chapter 3 and Chapter 4, Section 3). The research being conducted through these doctoral programs now provides a potential for the development of an **academic discipline** that will provide occupational therapy with its own **theory base** from which to operate (Clark et al., 1991; Yerxa, 1991, pp. 680–681). See Chapter 4, Section 2 for a further discussion of the theory base of occupational therapy

Occupational therapy knowledge base

The occupational therapy process requires that students have in-depth knowledge from the biologic, behavioral, and medical sciences in order to identify theoretical formulations that will serve them in the development of frames of reference for practice. The nature of the individual and the function–dysfunction continuum, along with pathologic processes that impinge on function, must be understood so that appropriate occupational therapy intervention procedures may be determined. Thus, one of the knowledge bases for occupational therapy must be identified as the *neurosciences*. Moreover, because occupational therapy is concerned both with human function throughout the lifespan and with the uniqueness of the individual, it is essential that practice be based on the normal development process. The impact of occupation or purposeful activity on the human organism also must be understood so that age-appropriate activities may be used. These knowledge bases are discussed in Chapter 5.

References

Clark, F. A., Parham, D., Carlson, M. E., et al. (1991). Occupational science: Academic innovation in the service of o occupational therapy's future. *American Journal of Occupational Therapy*, 45:300–310.

Mosey, A. C. (1981). *Occupational therapy—configuration of a profession*. New York: Raven Press.

Randall, T. H., & Buchler, J. (1960). *Philosophy: An introduction* (p. 5). New York: Barnes & Noble.

Resolution 532–79. (1979). Occupation as the common core of occupational therapy. Representative Assembly minutes. April 1979, Detroit, Michigan. *American Journal of Occupational Therapy*, *33*, 785.

Shannon, P. D. (1986). Philosophical considerations for the practice of occupational therapy. In Ryan, S. E. (Ed.), *The occupational therapy assistant: Roles and responsibilities* (p. 37). Thorofare, NJ: Slack.

Yerxa, E. J. (1991). Occupational therapy: An endangered species or an academic discipline. *American Journal of Occupational Therapy*, *45*, 680–685.

SECTION 2

Theory base

LINDA L. LEVY

Behaviors Indicative of Function or Dysfunction	*Philosophical Base*
Case Method	*Postulates Regarding Change and Intervention*
Frame of Reference	*Practice Model*
Frame of Reference: Structural Hierarchical Components	*Practice Theory*
Function–dysfunction Continua	*Profession's Model*
	Theoretical Approaches for Practice
Levels of Knowledge	*Theoretical Base*
Paradigm	*Theory*

LEARNING OBJECTIVES

Upon completion of this section the reader will be able to:

1. *Identify the essential function of a theory.*
2. *Identify the essential function of a frame of reference.*
3. *Recall different methods that have been used to conceptualize the relation between theory and practice.*
4. *Recall the differences between a profession's model and a frame of reference.*
5. *Recall the structural components of a frame of reference.*
6. *Outline the relation of theory and practice.*

It has now become axiomatic to the profession for clinical practice to be grounded in a sound theoretical base. There is no longer a place for doing "whatever might work," or doing things "on faith." Whatever we do must have a basis in reason and the probability of success. To this end, therapists use theoretical principles and apply them to conditions for which they are appropriate. This is one of the distinguishing features of a professional.

Transition of theory to treatment

The transition from theory to viable treatment strategies is not direct. An intermediary mechanism is required. Theories form the scientific bases for occupational therapy practice and are derived from a number of disciplines, including the biologic sciences, psychology, sociology, medicine, and occupational sciences. The essential function of a **theory**, however, is to explain, describe, and predict behaviors. Ours is a practice profession, and explanations and predictions are not enough. We need to understand how best to *change* behavior. For this purpose, theories must be transformed. Theoretical knowledge must be systematically *re*organized to provide guidance on how to produce desired changes in behavior and to contribute to our understanding of function, dysfunction, evaluation, and treatment. In this way, theories become linked to practice.

A number of different methods have been proposed for conceptualizing this intervening mechanism between theory and practice. Examples are *frame of reference* (Ford & Urban, 1963; Mosey, 1970; Mosey 1981), *case method* (Line, 1969), *practice theory* (Argyris & Schon, 1984; Williamson, 1982) *practice model* (Reed, 1984a, 1984b), *paradigm* (Christiansen, 1981; Kielhofner & Burke, 1983 Kuhn, 1970), and *levels of knowledge* (Kielhofner & Barris, 1986).

Basically all agree that **theoretical approaches for practice** refer to sets of concepts, assumptions or postulates, evaluation instruments for assessing a function–dysfunction, and intervention strategies with well-defined outcomes that should enable research to demonstrate the effectiveness of intervention.

The intent of this section is not to argue the relative merits of various conceptual schemes but rather, by selecting one approach, to provide a consistent structure for comparing multiple content areas.

The frame of reference is the tool that will be used here because of its clear structure, its longevity within the profession, and its familiarity to most practitioners. Conceptually, however, it is similar to the methods just mentioned.

Another important issue needs to be addressed here. Although debate continues about the specific structure and *content* of the model for occupational therapy, it is nonetheless important to underscore the relation of a theoretical base of a frame of reference to the *concept* of the **profession's model**. According to Mosey (1981), a model of a profession is inherently broad in focus. It serves to provide unity and identity within a profession and defines the relation of the profession to the society to which it is responsible. A model might be conceptualized as the reservoir of all the profession's beliefs, philosophical assumptions, knowledge, and skills.

Frames of reference are derived from a profession's model, but they are much narrower in focus and different in intent. Frames of reference make use of only those theoretical principles relevant to a specific area of human functioning that, at the same time, are consistent with the philosophical assumptions of the model of the profession. The intent is to formulate treatment strategies directed to specific areas of practice.

Thus, a model defines the profession generically. Frames of reference describe varying treatment techniques used within a profession and specific to health problems encountered in practice. All treatment techniques are derived from frames of reference; they must be consistent with the profession's definition of itself—that is, with its model.

Frame of reference

A *frame of reference consists of four hierarchical components* (Mosey, 1970):

I.   Theoretical base (propositions)
II. Function–dysfunction continuum
III. Behaviors indicative of function–dysfunction
IV. Postulates regarding change and intervention

These components generate evaluation, activity analysis, and treatment principles, and they define expected outcomes of treatment.

The theoretical base of a frame of reference serves as the basis from which all of the components are derived. It is founded on concepts, definitions, and postulates from one or more theories that have been reformulated to provide guidelines for evaluation and intervention.

The theories selected are relevant to a specific area of human functioning addressed by the frame of reference and they relate to the potential effect of the human and nonhuman environment on that area of human functioning. It is important to recognize the sources of these theories because the resulting frame of reference is only as strong as the theories that make up its theoretical base.

To adequately account for the relatively complicated issue of change, components from a number of different theories are usually synthesized. White's concept of competence (1971), for example, is often integrated with less dynamic theories such as neuroanatomy or Piagetian cognition to account for change from dysfunction to function in a given area of human performance. Theoretical components that are selected, however, must be explicitly combined and related to each other to construct a logical and internally consistent framework. These components must also be congruent with the **philosophical base** of the profession (defined at the AOTA Delegate Assembly, 1979) and, once accepted, its model.

Function–dysfunction continua use the concepts from the theoretical base to identify the nature of the dysfunctional behaviors that are targeted for change by the frame of reference.

A gradation is implied from total inability to engage in a particular function to complete mastery of that function.

The term *continuum* emphasizes that function can be understood only in relation to a patient's age, cultural background, physiologic status, and environmental circumstances. Function–dysfunction continua specify what the therapist will assess during evaluation and the goals or expected outcomes of treatment. A frame of reference may have one or several function–dysfunction continua, depending on the scope of the area addressed by the frame of reference.

Behaviors indicative of function or dysfunction operationally define the behaviors that demonstrate function or dysfunction within each continuum. They serve as the basis for evaluation tools and activity analysis related to evaluation. Evaluative activities are selected in relation to their potential to elicit the behaviors to be observed that differentiate between function and dysfunction. When these definitions are specific and objective, evaluation procedures and expected outcome measures can be standardized more easily.

Postulates regarding change and intervention state the nature, quality, quantity, and sequence of interaction with the human and nonhuman environment that can potentially effect change in the dysfunctional behaviors previously defined. These postulates guide the therapist in selecting short- and long-term goals and in sequencing the treatment process. They also form the conceptual framework for analyzing the activities prescribed for treatment. For example, activities in frames of reference that use developmental postulates are selected based on their potential for being graded in accordance with the maturational levels of dysfunction defined by the function–dysfunction continua. Postulates regarding change guide the therapist in the design of appropriate activities and environments to promote change, and serve as the conceptual basis for therapeutic modalities and techniques.

Final comments

Some final points should be remembered. Practice based in a solid theoretical foundation provides orientation and direction to the treatment process, defines an individual's professional identity, and is one of the distinguishing marks of a professional.

A well-understood frame of reference guides the action of occupational therapists and helps to ensure that their activities are consistent and efficient. Each frame of reference has advantages and disadvantages, contributions and limitations, however. The question in selecting a frame of reference is not which one is right or wrong, but which one is most useful in which settings with which patients in helping to effect change in the dysfunctional behaviors encountered in practice. Ultimately, frames of reference can be evaluated only in terms of their usefulness, that is, how efficiently they can generate predictions about behaviors that later turn out to be true. Frames of reference for occupational therapy, however, all suffer from relative newness; they are only beginning to generate the refined instruments and empirical research that are necessary to demonstrate their validity for specific populations and environments.

Notwithstanding, the foundations for molding the profession into a theory-based discipline have been laid. Research to build a body of knowledge for the profession and to validate occupational therapy frames of reference is already serving to further the development of frames of reference in contemporary practice.

The generation of frames of reference and the hierarchical components are depicted in Figure 4-1.

Summary

It is important for occupational therapy practice to be based on theory, to be rooted in the philosophical base of the profession, and to be organized using a specific frame of reference to guide the choice of appropriate evaluation and treatment procedures so that our practice can be explained and refined. Frames of reference currently being used in practice are described in Chapter 4, Section 3.

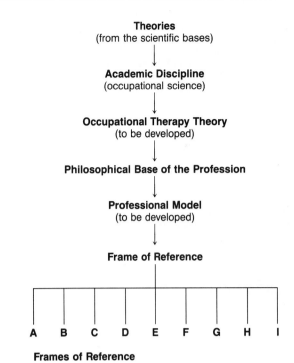

Theories
(from the scientific bases)

Academic Discipline
(occupational science)

Occupational Therapy Theory
(to be developed)

Philosophical Base of the Profession

Professional Model
(to be developed)

Frame of Reference

A   B   C   D   E   F   G   H   I

Frames of Reference

I. Theoretical base (propositions)
Conceptualization of man's purpose for interacting with the environment
Areas addressed within occupation therapist's domain of concern
Target populations

II. Function–dysfunction continuum
Definition of function
Definition of dysfunction
Treatment expectations/outcomes
Evaluation content/treatment focus

III. Behaviors indicative of function–dysfunction
Behaviors to be elicited in evaluation
Representative evaluation methods
Behaviors to be changed in treatment
Outcome measures
Guidelines for analysis of evaluative activities

IV. Postulates regarding change and intervention
Rationale for conceptualizing process of change
Sequencing of treatment strategies
Representative change techniques
Guidelines for activity analysis
Short-term and long-term treatment goals

FIGURE 4-1. *Relationship of theory, philosophy, and practice.*

The content of this section was adapted from Linda L. Levy. (1986). Frames of reference in mental health. In S. C. Robertson (Ed.), Strategies, concepts and opportunities for program development and evaluation (SCOPE). Rockville, MD: American Occupational Therapy Association.

References

Argyris, C., & Schon, D. (1984). *Theory in practice: Increasing professional effectiveness.* San Francisco: Jossey-Bass.

Christiansen, C. J. (1981). Editorial: Toward resolution of crisis-research requisites in occupational therapy. *Occupational Therapy Journal of Research, 1,* 115–124.

Ford, D., & Urban, H. (1963). *Systems of psychotherapy.* New York: John Wiley & Sons.

Kielhofner, G., & Barris, R. (1986). Organization of knowledge in occupational therapy: A proposal and a survey of the literature. *Occupational Therapy Journal of Research, 6*(2), 67–84.

Kielhofner, G., & Burke, J. P. (1983). The evolution of knowledge and practice in occupational therapy: Past, present and future. In G. Kielhofner (Ed.), *Health through occupation: Theory and practice in occupational therapy* (pp. 3–54). Philadelphia: F. A. Davis.

Kuhn, T. S. (1970). *Structure of scientific revolutions* (2nd ed.). Chicago: University of Chicago.

Line, J. (1969). Case method as a scientific form of clinical thinking. *American Journal of Occupational Therapy, 23,* 308–313.

Mosey, A. (1970). *Three frames of reference for mental health.* Thorofare, NJ: Slack.

Mosey, A. (1981). *Occupational therapy—configuration of a profession.* New York: Raven Press.

Reed, K. L. (1984a). Understanding theory: The first step in learning about research. *American Journal of Occupational Therapy, 38,* 677–682.

Reed, K. L. (1984b). *Models of practice in occupational therapy.* Baltimore: Williams & Wilkins.

White, R. (1971). The urge toward competence. *American Journal of Occupational Therapy, 25,* 271–272.

Williamson, G. (1982). A heritage of activity: Development of theory. *American Journal of Occupational Therapy, 36,* 716–722.

SECTION 3

Frames of reference in occupational therapy: introduction

REBECCA DUTTON, LINDA L. LEVY, and CAROLE J. SIMON

LEARNING OBJECTIVES

Upon completion of the following sections the reader will be able to:

1. *Identify the general principles of each of the frames of reference.*
2. *Identify various clinical applications of the basic principles in each frame of reference.*

Eleven frames of reference currently used in occupational therapy practice are described in the parts of this section that follow. Mosey's structural components for a frame of reference are used as an organizational scheme for all frames of reference. They are theoretical base: function–dysfunction continua (domains of concern or problems being addressed); behaviors indicative of function–dysfunction (targets of evaluation used to assess prob-

lems); postulates regarding change (links between presenting problem and goals), and postulates regarding intervention (links between goals and treatment–therapeutic activities).

The frames of reference that are described are behavioral, biomechanical, cognitive disability, developmental, neurodevelopmental, sensory integration, model of human occupation, rehabilitation, psychodynamic, spatiotemporal adaptation, and occupational adaptation. Table 4-1 summarizes the components of these frames of reference.

References

Mosey, A. (1970). *Three frames of reference for mental health.* Thorofare, NJ: Slack.

Mosey, A. (1981). *Configuration of a profession.* New York: Raven Press.

Mosey, A. (1986). *Psychosocial components of occupational therapy.* New York: Raven Press.

SECTION 3A
Behavioral frame of reference

LINDA L. LEVY

KEY TERMS

Adaptive Behaviors	*Modeling*
Backward Chaining	*Parsimony*
Biofeedback	*Operant Conditioning*
Classical Conditioning	*Rewarding Consequence*
Environmental Event	*Shaping*
Environmental Reinforcers	*Situational Specificity*
Learning Theories	*Token Economy Systems*
Maladaptive Behaviors	

Theoretical base

The behavioral frame of reference in occupational therapy is based on theories from the work of experimental psychologists such as Thorndike (1898), Pavlov (1927), and Skinner (1938, 1953). These theories have already been reformulated to develop intervention strategies to bring about behavioral change. As a result, they have undergone little transformation in their incorporation into the theoretical base of the behavioral frame of reference in occupational therapy; they are, however, applied in accordance with the philosophical base of the profession.

The central assumption of behavioral theories is that learning is the basis of all behavior. In addition, learning is always inferred from behavior and it leads either to more effective behavior, known as *adaptive behavior*, or to maladaptive behavior. When learning is applied to occupational therapy, the patient is seen as having developed a repertoire of behaviors, both adaptive and maladaptive, which determines his or her

TABLE 4-1. *Frames of Reference in Occupational Therapy Practice*

Frame of Reference	Theoretical Base	Function–Dysfunction Continua	Behaviors Indicative of Function–Dysfunction (Evaluations)	Postulates Regarding Change and Intervention (Treatment)	Proponents
Behavioral	Psychology: learning occurs through interaction with a reinforcing environment	Lack of skills	Skills checklist Observation	Instruct in skills needed to promote learning; provided through reinforcement: shaping, chaining, task analysis, feedback	Watson, Skinner, Sullivan, Thorndike, Pavlov
Biomechanical	Physical sciences: kinetics, kinematics, medicine	Deficits in structural stability, range of motion, strength and endurance	Assessment of range of motion, manual muscle testing, endurance testing	Reduce deficits through direct cause and effect treatment process—exercise and activity	Trombly, Pedretti
Cognitive disability	Biologic psychiatry, neurosciences, cognition underlies all behavior. A cognitive disability reflects impairments in the cognitive functions that guide motor action.	Cognitive levels describe difference in information processing capacities of individuals affected by brain pathology in terms of sensory cues, sensimotor associations and motor actions	Task analysis: selection and modification in range of patient's ability (ACL, RTI)	Provide tasks to match level of cognitive abilities—environmental compensations	Allen
Developmental	Psychology: human growth and maturation occur sequentially in a supporting environment.	Developmental lag, stress-induced regression	Assessment of developmental levels, adaptive behaviors, and range of functions	Alter activity components of environment to achieve appropriate behavior; create environment to promote development	Liorens, Ayres, Moser, Piaget. Erickson, Havinghurst, Gessell
Neurodevelopmental	Neurosciences: normalization and integration of biologic processes	Deficits in axial control, automatic reactions, limb control	Assessment of muscle tone, limb synergies, automatic reactions, gross and fine motor movement strategies	Inhibit or excite neural mechanisms; use special techniques and equipment to normalize biologic processes	Bobath
Sensory integration	Development, neurosciences: relation between sensory input and neural integration	Perceptual motor deficits, inability to integrate sensory stimuli and produce motor response, abnormal motor and learning problems	Perceptual testing, observation	Use body movement, gross motor and sensory integrative activities	Ayres, Wilbarger. Rood, King, Huss, Farber, Knickerbocker, Fiorentino, Brunnstrom
Model of human occupation	General systems theory, sociology Occupational behavior	Difficulties with roles, habits, and skills needed to function in society—viewed in terms of volitional, habituation, and performance subsystems	Interviews, time and activity inventory, observation in tasks, case analysis	Establish environment that allows exploration and development of competence and mastery; provide counseling and problem solving to identify and alter maladaptive occupational lifestyle	Boulding, Bruner. VonBertalanffy. Reilly, Kielhofner, Burke
Rehabilitation	Medicine, physical sciences: total capabilities of each individual based on examination of the parts	Dysfunction in basic and instrumental ADL, work and leisure	Assessment of deficits and capabilities in basic and instrumental ADL, work and leisure, and access to the environment	Compensate for disability by learning to live with one's capabilities in all aspects of life; adapt environment to obtain independence	Spackman, Trombly. Pedretti
Psychodynamic	Psychiatry, psychology: striving for need fulfillment	Symptom-producing unconscious content	Identification of symptom-producing unconscious content	Bring symptom-producing unconscious content to consciousness and intergrate with conscious content	Freud, Jung, Sullivan
Spatiotemporal adaptation	Neurosciences: biologic processes	Maladaptation to environmental demands	Movement skills available from a stable base and past experience	Engage in purposeful, developmental activities to stimulate maturation	Gilfoyle, Grady. Moore
Occupational adaptation	General systems theory: occupation and adaptation	Inability to adapt to changing expectations occurring from internal and external influences: occupational dysfunction	Identification of occupational and environmental influences and evaluation of adaptive responses	Focus on occupational activity of persons within environmental contexts: person and occupational environment interact through occupation. Relative mastery over environmental challenges	Schkade, Schultz. Spencer, Davidson

ACL, Allen Cognition Level Test; ADL, activities of daily living; ROM, range of motion; RTI, routine task inventory.

ability to function in activities of daily living, work, and leisure. In therapy, the patient is actively engaged in a learning process to develop the specific behaviors necessary for functioning in his or her environment.

The learning theory approach is differentiated from other approaches by its adherence to the principle of **parsimony**, its emphasis on the external environment, and its focus on the situational specificity of human behavior. **Learning theory** is parsimonious in that a single set of assumptions is used to explain a large variety of different behaviors. From a learning theory perspective, dysfunctional behavior can be understood in terms of only a few basic assumptions. In addition, learning theory looks to the environment, rather than within the individual, for the determinants of behavior. The learning theorist believes that behavior can best be predicted and controlled by attending to environmental influences. Learning theory adheres to the **situational specificity** of behavior. The learning theorist believes that people behave the way they do in response to the characteristics of the particular situation that they are in at the moment; as a result, a person's behavior is usually not consistent across situations. From this perspective, a person would not be perceived as aggressive dispositionally; rather, aggressive responses would be understood in relation to the specific situation.

Learning theorists differ with respect to the form of learning that they emphasize. There are two main approaches in behaviorism: classical conditioning and operant conditioning. The **classical conditioning** (or respondent) approach (Pavlov, 1927; Thorndike, 1898) focuses on how people learn new responses by coming to associate a set of circumstances that previously did not elicit a particular reaction with another set of circumstances that already led to that reaction.

For example, a student who did so poorly in an examination given in a specific room that he or she was fearful of failing the course, may experience fear when walking into that same room again. Or, with antabuse, an alcoholic patient is conditioned to associate alcohol ingestion with nausea rather than with the psychological high. The basic principles of classical conditioning have been demonstrated to hold from the smallest one-cell organisms to man, although they are generally limited to reflexive or involuntary behaviors.

Classical conditioning, however, has become increasingly important in understanding the relationship between stress and the functioning of the autonomic nervous system (Miller, 1969). It is also thought to be the basic process by which certain early fears are learned. Some specialists in psychosomatic medicine believe that the groundwork for psychosomatic diseases is laid in the very young infant by this process.

Operant conditioning applies to the more general situations of learning and is the most common theory of learning incorporated into the theoretical base of the behavioral frame of reference in occupational therapy. Operant conditioning affects all voluntary behavior, as well as that of the autonomic nervous system. According to the operant (or instrumental) learning approach (Skinner, 1938, 1953), behavior is learned as a result of the environmental consequences a person receives when performing the behavior. If positive consequences follow a behavior, the probability that the behavior will be repeated is increased. The *operant* is a behavior resulting in a reinforcement. The person emits a response that results in an **environmental event**, which is a **rewarding consequence**. Hence, the environment is seen to cause and to control behavior by teaching the person to behave as he or she does.

For example, when an autistic child imitates a sound from a therapist, the therapist reinforces the desired response by giving the child some candy. In operant conditioning, therapists are concerned with what in the environment serves to reinforce, and thereby maintain, both adaptive and maladaptive behaviors. **Maladaptive behaviors** are seen to have been learned through selective reinforcement from the environment in the same way that adaptive behaviors have been learned.

In treatment, therapists most often seek to change maladaptive behaviors by presenting desired environmental reinforcers to elicit more adaptive behavioral responses. **Environmental reinforcers** are usually one of three types: consumable (eg, candy, cigarettes, coffee), social (eg, attention, hugs, smiles, verbal praise), or participatory (the opportunity to participate in a favored activity). Initially, an immediate reward schedule of reinforcement is necessary to elicit the desired behavioral response. After a response is established, however, intermittent reinforcement (reinforcing every nth response) serves to effectively stabilize the response. Responses can also be **shaped** by reinforcing successively closer approximations of the desired response. A variation of this is **backward chaining**, wherein components of the task are learned by starting with the final step and working backward to the first step. The therapist may also model the behavior and receive reinforcement in the presence of the client. The client may then be reinforced for successful imitation of the behavior.

Operant conditioning principles are applied in **token economy systems** (Ayllon & Azrin, 1965). Patients in institutional environments receive tokens that can be traded for something they desire (eg, candy, television time, opportunities for privacy) if they produce certain types of behavioral responses (eg, grooming, laundering, food preparation). At first, any behavior is reinforced by a token, but later the behavior must be more adaptive (shaped) to be rewarded. Another application of operant principles is **biofeedback**, wherein the person is given reinforcement for emitting some type of physiologic response such as lowered heart rate, blood pressure. In biofeedback, reinforcement can often be as simple as a smile, a frown, keeping a light on, or success in creating change in the desired direction.

Prominent leaders in the development of the behavioral frame of reference (Diasio, 1968; Smith & Tempone, 1968; Seig, 1974; Jodrell & Sanson-Fisher, 1975; Trombly & Scott, 1977; Stein, 1982) have made convincing arguments that operant learning principles are especially applicable to occupational therapy because learning theorists and occupational therapists share the same philosophical assumption, that is, that the primary referent for the study of humans is behavior—what they *do*. Furthermore, they point out that the primary concerns of learning theorists are behavior and the environment in which it is maintained; these concerns are at the same time primary considerations in the occupational therapy treatment process.

Function–dysfunction continua

Function–dysfunction continua in behavioral frames of reference are vaguely defined. Some continua identify a wide spectrum of observable behaviors necessary for satisfactory functioning in activities of daily living, work, and leisure. The most comprehensive of these have been delineated by Mosey (1986) in her recently articulated role acquisition frame of reference. Here, seven major categories of function–dysfunction continua are identified, including task skills, interpersonal skills, family interaction skills, activities of daily living skills, work skills, play/leisure/recreation skills, and temporal adaptation skills. In a previous work entitled *Activities therapy* (Mosey, 1973), she presented a less global list of observable behaviors to be targeted for change. These include basic skills (task skills, group interaction skills), the "public self" (activities of daily living, work, recreation, and intimacy), and the "private self" (cognitive system, needs, emotions, and values). Function–dysfunction can also be conceptualized in terms of the specific skills that a physically disabled client must develop to maximize functional independence within the environment (Trombly & Scott, 1977). In these instances, the client is engaged in opportunities to learn the requisite adaptive techniques or modifications in the procedures for carrying out previous activities to enable him or her to compensate for specific physical limitations that compromise functional abilities.

In general, however, a state of function exists when the person has the requisite kinds and amounts of functional skills to attain maximal independence within his or her environment. Hence, function is conceptualized as a high incidence of adaptive behaviors required within the person's environment and a low incidence of maladaptive behaviors. Conversely, dysfunction is conceptualized as a low incidence of adaptive behaviors required within the person's environment and a high incidence of maladaptive behaviors. Both functional and dysfunctional behaviors are highly individualized and specific in this frame of reference, and are relative to the demands of the person's environment.

Behaviors indicative of function–dysfunction

Specific, definable, and observable behaviors that compromise functional abilities are targeted for change in the behavioral frame of reference. The frequency with which these behaviors occur within the environment is indicative of the degree of function and dysfunction. Task situations are used as naturalistic settings to observe typical behaviors and the environmental reinforcers that serve to maintain those behaviors. Hence, evaluative activities are conceptualized in terms of their potential for providing opportunities to elicit and observe specific behaviors targeted for change.

Postulates regarding change and intervention

After functional and dysfunctional behaviors are identified, the client is provided with opportunities to learn the specific behaviors necessary to maximize functional independence within the environment. Dysfunctional behaviors can be changed by manipulating environmental variables so that adaptive behaviors are reinforced and maladaptive behaviors are not reinforced.

Reinforcement methods include shaping, backward chaining, and ***modeling*** of desired behaviors. Activities are analyzed in terms of their potential for eliciting and providing reinforcement for behaviors targeted for change.

The following sequential steps that are considered in conceptualizing therapeutic activity programs have been delineated by Seig (1976).

1. Identify the terminal behavior, or the operationally defined treatment goal. Note that in order for the behavior to be assessed, it must be observable and quantified.
2. Determine the baseline performance, that is, the frequency of occurrence of the behavior before the onset of the occupational therapy program. The baseline performance is used to measure changes in behavior.
3. Design a data collection format. The occupational therapist selects an objective procedure for counting and recording the behavior such as the use of a counter, or charting behavior on a graph.
4. Select a reinforcer. The therapist identifies the principal reinforcers that are supporting the behavior. Positive reinforcers to be presented are most often consumable items, social reinforcement, or activity opportunities.
5. Determine the reinforcement schedule. The therapist determines when the patient should be reinforced, that is, immediately, intermittently, or after each activity session.
6. Chart the data. This provides clear information about the rate over a period of time.

References

Ayllon, T., & Azrin, N. H. (1968). *The token economy: A motivational system for therapy and rehabilitation*. New York: Appleton-Century-Crofts.

Diasio, K. (1968). Psychiatric occupational therapy: Search for a conceptual framework in light of psychoanalytic ego psychology and learning theory. *American Journal of Occupational Therapy, 22,* 400–414.

Jodrell, R. & Sanson-Fisher R. (1975). Basic concepts of behavior therapy: An experiment involving disturbed adolescent girls. *American Journal of Occupational Therapy, 29,* 620–624.

Miller, N. (1969). Learning of visceral and glandular responses. *Science, 163,* 434–445.

Mosey, A. (1986). Role acquisition. In *Psychosocial components of occupational therapy*. New York: Raven Press.

Mosey, A. (1973). *Activities therapy*. New York: Raven Press.

Pavlov, I. P. (1927). *Conditioned reflexes*. New York: Dover.

Seig, K. W. (1974). Applying the behavioral model to the occupational therapy model. *American Journal of Occupational Therapy, 28,* 421–428.

Skinner, B. (1938). *The behavior of organisms*. New York: Appleton-Century-Crofts.

Skinner, B. (1953). *Science and human behavior*. New York: Macmillan.

Smith, N., & Tempone, B. (1968). Psychiatric occupational therapy within a learning theory context. *American Journal of Occupational Therapy, 22,* 415–420.

Stein, F. (1982). A current review of the behavioral frame of reference and its application to occupational therapy. *Occupational Therapy in Mental Health, 2,* 35–62.

Thorndike, E. L. (1898). Animal intelligence: An experimental study of the association processes in animals. *Psychological Monographs, 2,* 1–5.

Trombly, C., & Scott, A. (1977). *Occupational therapy for physical dysfunction*. Baltimore: Williams & Wilkins.

SECTION 3B
Biomechanical frame of reference

REBECCA DUTTON

KEY TERMS	
Endurance	*Strength*
Range of Motion	*Structural Stability*

Theoretical base

Before World War I, purposeful activities were used strictly for diversional purposes (Reed, 1984). Baldwin was the first health care professional to analyze the use of joints and muscles during purposeful activity. He also developed methods for evaluating activities to see whether they were achieving their goal of increasing range and strength. Dr. Licht added the concern of work tolerance, which is referred to as endurance training.

The biomechanical frame of reference has four assumptions (Dutton, in press). The first assumption is the belief that purposeful activities can be used to treat loss of **range of motion** (ROM), **strength**, and **endurance**. The second assumption is the belief that after ROM, strength, and endurance are regained, the patient automatically regains function. The third assumption is the principle of rest and stress. First, the body must rest to heal itself. Then, peripheral structures must be stressed to regain range, strength, and endurance. The fourth assumption is the belief that the biomechanical frame of reference is best suited for patients with an intact central nervous system (Pedretti, 1990). Patients may have limited range, strength, and endurance but have the ability to perform smooth, isolated movements.

Function–dysfunction continua

The six function–dysfunction continua that are domains of concern for the biomechanical frame of reference are (1) structural stability, (2) low-level endurance, (3) edema control, (4) passive ROM, (5) strength, and (6) high level endurance (Dutton, in press).

Therapists used to be able to assume that **structural stability** was present before stressing peripheral structures. Changes in the length of hospital stay require therapists to treat patients very early while they still have partially healed bones and soft tissue. It is dangerous to separate structural stability from biomechanical issues. Endurance has traditionally been placed at the end of the biomechanical treatment sequence because therapists used to get well-rested patients with the ability to tolerate sedentary activity. Today, treatment can begin immediately at bedside so that even the ability to tolerate sitting up with support may not be present. Early use of resistance and repetition can be dangerous if low-level endurance is not addressed first.

Edema control has been separated from passive ROM because so many techniques have been developed specifically for this problem and because the long-term effects of uncontrolled edema can be devastating. Therapists are aggressive about treating edema even before they can range a swollen limb. The last three concerns—increasing passive ROM, strength, and high-level endurance—have been associated with the biomechanical frame of reference since Baldwin and Licht.

Behaviors indicative of function–dysfunction

A patient's behavior can be placed on the six continua (mentioned in the preceding text) by behaviors indicative of change found by using evaluation tools. Only the physician is allowed to evaluate the status of structural stability (Dutton, in press). Therapists have formal evaluation tools such as volumetry for edema, goniometry for ROM, and manual muscle testing for strength. These formal tests are supplemented by clinical observation such as the skin's appearance, end feels during range of motion (Clarkson & Gilewich 1989), and grip strength. Evaluation tools for endurance include cardiac step charts and metabolic equivalents (MET) charts, which sequence activities according to their endurance requirements. Informal assessment of endurance can also be done by timing the duration of an activity or counting the number of repetitions the patient can perform.

Postulates regarding change and intervention

Postulates regarding change identify links among the presenting problem, biomechanical goal, and functional outcome in a specific format (Dutton, in press). For example, the patient, a gardener, has burned her left hand.

General deficit is loss of ROM of the burned left hand.
Stage-specific cause is hypertrophic scarring.
Measurable biomechanical goal is metacarpal phalangeal (MP) flexion to 70 degrees, proximal interphalangeal (PIP) flexion to 50 degrees, and distal interphalangeal (DIP) flexion to 15 degrees.
Functional outcome is the ability to close her hand on gardening tools.

It is vital to link the biomechanical goal of increased finger flexion to gardening. Third-party payors require it to justify the need for therapy (Allen & Foto, 1991; Dahl, 1990; Pinson, 1991). The patient also needs to know why he or she is participating in stressful and sometimes painful treatment. In the above example, increasing finger flexion by 10 degrees is not what the patient cares about. She wants to know whether she can take care of her garden again.

The link between biomechanical goals and functional outcome must be established before the patient goes home. The ability to generalize biomechanical gains cannot be assumed even in cognitively intact and well-educated patients. Patients may believe that doing exercises twice a day at home will maintain gains achieved in the hospital despite constant disuse (Dutton, 1989). A patient may not even be aware of having developed the habit of using lateral trunk flexion to reach for clothes in the closet after having regained full shoulder motion. A brief rehearsal of a few functional activities may be needed to detect and change these compensatory strategies.

Three biomechanical goals are grouped together in the postulate just mentioned. Making each finger joint a separate goal produces an overwhelming list of biomechanical goals. A common way to chunk these goals is by shared method (Dutton, in press). Since all three joints will receive heat, stretch, and splinting to increase range of motion, why not group them together?

Postulates regarding intervention create links between biomechanical goals and therapeutic activities in a specific format (Dutton, in press). For example:

Measurable biomechanical goal of MP flexion to 70 degrees, PIP flexion to 50 degrees, and DIP flexion to 15 degrees will be achieved by a general method.

General method consists in heat, manual stretch, and splinting, which (*rationale*) increases elasticity of the skin, elongates collagen fibers, and positions the joints and soft tissue in one functional position.

Specific activity includes wearing a pressure garment to build up body heat, distracting the patient while stretching by closing her hand around a 1-inch dowel rod, and wearing a splint.

It is helpful to name the general method before selecting a specific treatment modality (Dutton, in press). This step allows you to argue for and against several methods, such as whether to use isometric or isotonic contractions to strengthen. It also narrows the choices you have to make about specific modalities. For example, if you use active stretch to increase range of motion, you should avoid activities that require maximal resistance. Resistance does not relax tight tissues and can confuse the patient by asking for maximal muscle contraction and maximal joint excursion at the same time.

It is easy to develop measurable biomechanical goals because this frame of reference uses quantitative evaluation data such as degrees of range of motion. Nevertheless, biomechanical goals are often confused with service goals. Biomechanical goals describe what deficits will be remediated. Service goals describe what the therapist will do (Denton, 1987). Today service goals are called treatment methods. As the above postulate regarding intervention shows, heat, manual stretch and splinting are not treatment goals, but methods for increasing range of motion.

References

Allen, K. A., & Foto, M. (1991). Reporting occupational therapy outcomes with the ICIDH codes. *Physical Disabilities Special Interest Section Newsletter, 14*(2), 2–3.

Clarkson, H. M., & Gilewich, G. B. (1989). *Musculoskeletal assessment.* Baltimore: Williams & Wilkins.

Dahl, M. (1990). *Money and reimbursement versus OT practice.* Pennsylvania manual muscle testing. Occupational Therapy Association Workshop, Philadelphia.

Denton, P. L. (1987). *Psychiatric occupational therapy: A workbook of practical skills.* Boston: Little, Brown & Co.

Dutton, R. (in press). *Clinical reasoning in physical disabilities.* Philadelphia: F. A. Davis.

Dutton, R. (1989). Guidelines for using both activity and exercise. *American Journal of Occupational Therapy, 43*(9), 573–580.

Pedretti, L. W., & Pasquinelli, S. (1990). A frame of reference for occupational therapy in physical dysfunction. In L. W. Pedretti & B. Zoltan (Eds.), *Occupational therapy practice skills for physical dysfunction* (3rd ed.). Philadelphia: C. V. Mosby.

Pinson, C. C. (1991). Work programs reimbursement: What is happening across the nation? *Physical Disabilities Special Interest Section Newsletter, 14*(2), 4–5.

Reed, K. L. (1984). *Models of practice in occupational therapy.* Baltimore: Williams & Wilkins.

SECTION 3C
Cognitive disability frame of reference

LINDA L. LEVY

KEY TERMS	
Allen Cognitive Level Test	*Information Processing*
Change in Capacity	*Motor Actions*
Changing the Environment	*Routine Tasks*
Cognitive Disability	*Routine Task Inventory*
Cognitive Levels	*Sensorimotor Associations*
Environmental Compensations	*Sensory Cues*

Theoretical base

The cognitive disability frame of reference in occupational therapy was developed by Claudia K. Allen (1982, 1985, 1987, 1988, 1992; Allen et al., 1989) throughout two decades of intensive observation and empirical research in the field of psychiatry. It has undergone continuous development and modification since its inception. As defined by Allen (1985, 1992), a **cognitive disability** represents a physiologic or biochemical restriction in the information processing capacities of the brain, which produces observable, measurable limitations in routine task behavior. Diagnostic categories that can produce a cognitive disability are cerebrovascular accidents, traumatic brain injury, dementia, cerebral palsy, developmental disabilities, drug/alcohol abuse, schizophrenic disorders, primary affective disorders, and AIDS. The cognitive disability frame of reference was developed to conceptualize intervention strategies for persons who, as a result of brain pathology, are not able to carry out their normal life activities. It was designed to provide a sound theoretical basis to enable occupational therapists to further "informal" understandings of the relationships between brain pathology and functional abilities by means of rigorous, empirical research.

Although founded on empiricism in the field of occupational therapy, the cognitive disability frame of reference derives its theoretical underpinnings from research in the fields of neurosciences, information processing, cognitive psychology, and biologic psychiatry, and from concepts of activity in the Soviet psychology literature. Its theoretical base is grounded in the following assumptions:

1. Cognition underlies all behavior.
2. Brain pathology compromises cognitive processes in a manner that can be observed in normal life activities. Just as a physical disability restricts the physical ability to perform a motor action, a cognitive disability restricts the person's cognitive ability to perform a motor action. Hence, a cognitive disability reflects impairments in the cognitive functions that guide motor actions; these impairments are manifested in difficulties in performing normal life activities.
3. Primary data for the assessment of the cognitive disability can be obtained by observing the performance of **routine (everyday) tasks** that the person wants to do. As he or she performs routine tasks, data emerge regarding the quality of performance. From this data inferences can be made about the cognitive (**information processing**) capacities and limitations of the individual.
4. The qualitative differences in routine task behaviors that a therapist observes are clarified by hierarchy of cognitive levels. The six **cognitive levels** operationally define the observable restrictions in the information processing capacities of persons affected by brain pathology. These levels provide the conceptual basis for assessing the impacts of brain pathology on those information processing capacities of the brain that are required for normal life activities. They also identify the varying qualities of environmental stimuli that serve to elicit motor responses (routine task behaviors) at different cognitive levels of functioning.
5. In medically unstable conditions (as in diseases of the brain in which recovery can be expected), the reorganization of cognitive capacities follows a predictable and hierarchical sequence. The reacquisition and stabilization of ontogenetically earlier processes are necessary for the emergence and stabilization of more complex information processes. In diseases marked by deterioration in which recovery cannot be expected (most notably in dementia), the disorganization and loss of cognitive capacities generally follow a predictable, reversed sequence.
6. With stable medical conditions, or with long-term disabilities that produce residual cognitive limitations (as in cerebral vascular accidents, traumatic brain injuries, developmental disabilities, schizophrenias, and dementias), the most viable intervention strategies are environmental compensations. **Environmental compensations** seek to offset the impairments produced by brain pathology by modifying the task environment to compensate for deficient information processing capacities.
7. Occupational therapists approach normal life activities for disabled persons from a unique perspective: the activities that patients choose to include in their daily lives are modified through application of activity analysis to allow them to succeed despite their disabilities. This frame of reference proposes a rigorous method of cognitive activity analysis to enable therapists to match activities more accurately and precisely to the capacities and preferences of the cognitively disabled. Desired activities are analyzed by the therapist to determine specific components in the typical procedure that the patient can and cannot do. Then activities are modified to maximize use of intact cognitive capacities and

to compensate for the cognitive processes that are deficient. The activity analysis suggested by this approach is intentionally designed to be applicable to *any* activity content that the person chooses (crafts, play, work, or self-care; Levy, 1987).

Information processing dimensions

The cognitive disability frame of reference seeks to identify the information processing capacities that need to be assessed to determine whether a person can perform a desired activity successfully, and that need to be compensated for in the event of cognitive limitations. To this end, Allen has proposed a hierarchy of six cognitive levels that define the information processing demands of normal life activities, as well as qualitative differences in functional capacities and limitations. Allen views three dimensions of thought as stages of an information processing model, which need to be assessed at each of the following six hierarchical cognitive levels:

1. **Sensory cues**. All information processing begins with sensory input from the environment. Allen identifies two sources of sensory cues that capture and sustain attention: those that arise from the person's inner world, including subliminal and proprioceptive cues; and those that arise from the environment, including tactile, visual, auditory, and finally, complex symbolic cues. At primitive cognitive levels, persons can attend only to internal cues, such as musculoskeletal sensations. At more advanced cognitive levels, persons can respond to progressively wider ranges of cues, including internal cues as well as those from the environment.
2. **Sensorimotor associations**. Sensorimotor associations are the interpretive processes that follow from sensory cues. This term refers to the goals implicit in performing an action. Allen's cognitive disability frame of reference demonstrates that the implicit goal of the person performing an action may not be consistent with the explicit goals of a given activity. Persons pursue activities with varying goals in mind, ranging from the simple pleasure of moving, to an interest in the effects of actions, to an investment in producing a high-quality end product. The problem is that at more primitive cognitive levels, a person may be able to comprehend only the motions involved in a desired activity, such as the motion of pushing a vacuum cleaner back and forth, and would not be able to comprehend the goal—or the result—that would be expected from someone with higher cognitive capacities, that is, the goal of a clean rug. Consequently, at more primitive cognitive levels, unintentional results become commonplace. Hence, it is important to recognize that the inability to comprehend traditional goals and expectations reflects a cognitive limitation that must be compensated for within the structure of an activity.
3. **Motor actions**. Motor actions are the final stage of Allen's information processing model. Actions are elicited by sensory cues, guided by sensorimotor associations, and can be observed in activity performance. There are two types of motor actions: spontaneous (self-initiated) and imitated (copied from another person). At more primitive cognitive levels, persons are able only to initiate and imitate motor

actions that are already very familiar behavioral actions. At more advanced cognitive levels, self-initiated motor actions are more diverse and persons are able to participate freely in desired activities.

A critical contribution of the cognitive disability frame of reference is that it provides a means for analyzing the relative difficulty of any desired activity in terms of requisite information processing demands. From this analysis, environmental factors can be identified that facilitate or constrain the production of each dimension of thought. Intervention strategies are derived from understanding how the environmental cognitive elements might best be modified within the structure of a desired activity to reinforce and capitalize on cognitive capacities and to compensate for cognitive limitations. As a result, desired activities are placed within a patient's range of comprehension and control. Specifically, therapists modify the structure of a desired activity in relationship to (1) the sensory cues that the patient is able to attend to while doing an activity at any given cognitive level; (2) the quality of sensorimotor association that the patient is able to comprehend, or the goal that motivates him or her to engage in activity at any given level; and (3) the degree of assistance required to enable the patient to most effectively complete a desired motor action at any given level (ie, whether the desired motor action is best imitated from the therapist or caregiver or can be successfully self-initiated; Levy, 1989).

Cognitive levels

To conceptualize a basis for intervention, the therapist must identify the patient's cognitive capacities and limitations, and the environmental factors that can be modified to enable successful participation in activities that support desired social roles. The discussion that follows provides a brief overview of the three dimensions of information processing that reveal cognitive capacities, limitations, and associated environmental factors. It provides guidelines for the design of environmental modification strategies required to capitalize on cognitive capacities and compensate for limitations at each of the cognitive levels (Levy, 1989). This discussion is summarized in Table 4-2, which delineates the sensory cues, sensorimotor associations, and motor actions and their functional implications at each of the cognitive levels. Therapists will find it useful to note that cognitive levels 1 and 2 are most often associated with conditions such as severe hemiplegia, severe dementia, and acute head injuries. Levels 3, 4, and 5 are associated with moderate hemiplegia, moderate and mild dementia, and major mental disorders.

Cognitive level 1: reflexive

At the first cognitive level, attention is directed to subliminal internal cues, such as hunger, taste, and smell, and persons are largely unresponsive to external stimuli. There is no goal, or reason, for performing motor actions; hence, few motor actions are being performed. Motor actions are limited to the potential to follow near-reflexive one-word directives such as "sip" or "turn." With little (if any) purpose and few (if any) motor actions available, the person has few cognitive capabilities to capitalize on. It is unrealistic to attempt to modify activities.

Cognitive level 2: movement

At the second level, attention is directed to proprioceptive cues from muscles and joints that are elicited by the person's own highly familiar body movements. The goal in performing a motor action is to repeat the one-step motor action component of the

TABLE 4-2. *Allen's Cognitive Levels*

	Level 1: Reflexive	Level 2: Movement	Level 3: Repetitive Actions	Level 4: End Product	Level 5: Variations	Level 6: Tangible Thought
Sensory Cues	**Subliminal**	**Proprioceptive**	**Tactile**	**Visible**	**Concrete Relationships**	**Symbolic**
Attention	Internal	Position and movement sense	To objects that can be manipulated	What is not clearly visible is ignored	Between two or more objects	Abstract, intangible
Example	Hunger, thirst, taste, smell	Movements of muscles and joints	Surfaces of objects	Concrete samples of end products	Space, depth, blending	Visual images, words
Sensorimotor Associations	**Arousal**	**Comfort**	**Interest**	**Compliance**	**Self-control**	**Reflection**
Goals/purposes	To alerting stimuli	Moves for pleasure or to reduce distress	Relationship between movement and effect on environment	In following procedure to reach goal	Initiates actions to produce desired effects	Imagines new possibilities and alternatives prior to action
Motor Actions						
Spontaneous	Automatic actions	Postural actions	Manual actions	Goal-directed actions	Exploratory actions	Preplanned actions
Imitated	None	Approximates gross body movement	Single, familiar, manual actions	2- to 3-step familiar directions	Several steps at a time	Not necessary
Example	Eating, drinking, standing, walking	Pacing, bending, stretching	Single repetitive actions	Familiar goal-related actions: simplified crafts	Alternative actions for producing different effects	Autonomous actions preceded by reasoning

activity for the pleasure of its effect on the body alone (ie, on the person's sense of position and balance or on sensory input to muscles and joints). Motor actions are limited to the ability to imitate, albeit inexactly, a one-step direction only if it involves the use of a highly familiar near-reflexive gross motor pattern. New learning is not possible.

Activities that can be successfully accomplished at this level are those that are adapted to capitalize on the capacity to imitate one-step familiar repetitive gross motor actions and that compensate for the inability to comprehend a purpose beyond the sensation of movement. Therapists and caregivers will find that providing opportunities to imitate simple movement, calisthenics, and modified sports activities are most often useful, but one-step activities (such as folding laundry, chopping vegetables, and polishing furniture) can be imitated if these activities were near habitual prior to the disability. Similarly, most instrumental activities of daily living (IADL) can be accomplished provided that the person has a model to follow.

Cognitive level 3: repetitive actions

At the third cognitive level, attention is directed to tactile cues and to familiar objects that can be manipulated. The goal in performing a motor action is limited to the process of discovering the kinds of effects a person's actions have on the environment. These actions are typically repeated to verify that similar results occur. Motor actions are limited to the ability to follow a one-step, highly familiar, action-oriented direction that has been demonstrated for the patient to follow. It is unrealistic to expect the patient to learn new behavior.

Activities that can be successfully accomplished at this level are those that are adapted to capitalize on the person's capacity to imitate one-step familiar, repetitive actions that provide predictable tactile effects and that compensate for the inability to follow multistep directions or conceptualize a predictable result. The patient should be provided with opportunities to participate in adapted activities that reinforce the relationship between actions and predictable tactile effects on the environment. Some possibilities are sports activities (such as swimming, biking, and playing catch); household maintenance activities (such as washing the car, mowing lawns, cultivating gardens, hand-washing laundry); and kitchen activities (such as washing and drying the dishes, peeling and chopping vegetables, and cleaning countertops); and IADL activities that are demonstrated one step at a time. As in level 3, functional performance can be maximized by teaching the caregivers how to present activities to the patient in a manner that will best promote productive motor actions.

Cognitive level 4: end product

Attention at the fourth cognitive level is directed to tactile as well as visible cues and is sustained throughout short-term activities to their completion. The goal in performing a motor action is to perceive cause-and-effect relationships between a tangible cue and a desired outcome. Motor actions are limited to the ability to follow a two- to three-step highly familiar motor process that leads to the accomplishment of familiar goals. At this level, patients can learn two- to three-step procedures that have visible and predictable results.

Activities that can be accomplished successfully at this level are those that are adapted to capitalize on the capacity to use two-to three-step familiar motor actions that have predictable visible results and those that compensate for the patient's inability to comprehend unpredictable results or notice mistakes when they occur. At this level, patients should be provided with opportunities to engage in simple, relatively error-proof, concrete activities that support desired social roles. This goal is best accomplished by incorporating into the person's daily routine yardwork, household chores (laundry, simple meal preparation, shopping for a few familiar purchases), familiar sports and dance activities, simple board games and puzzles, letter writing or typing, and walks to familiar destinations.

Despite significant cognitive impairment, the patient appears to be less confused at this level because activities are pursued with specific outcomes in mind. Caregivers and therapists should encourage these patients to engage in comprehensible concrete activities that will protect personal dignity and enable social role retention. Therapists should not expect the patient to notice mistakes or solve problems when they occur, to retain directions out of context, to plan beyond the immediate situation, to generalize learning to new situations, or to anticipate safety hazards, however. Patients at this level are more easily engaged in activities and therapeutic regimens than those at earlier levels because the goal is to achieve a desired outcome (eg, "to get the job done"). Desired outcomes, however, are restricted to those that are concrete and predictable and that entail no more than a three-step process.

Cognitive level 5: variations

At cognitive level 5, attention is captured and sustained by the interesting properties of concrete objects. The goal of action is to explore the effects of self-initiated motor actions on physical objects and to investigate these effects through the use of overt trial-and-error problem solving. Motor actions are exploratory to produce interesting effects on material objects, and they extend to the ability to follow through on a four- or five-step concrete process. The patient is now able to learn through doing.

Many activities can be accomplished successfully at the fifth level because in concrete activities (those involving familiar four- to five-step motor actions with visibly perceivable results), persons function relatively independently. The cognitive limitations experienced by persons at this level become apparent when they attempt activities that require attention to abstract and symbolic cues (such as those that involve spoken and written instructions, diagrams, or drawings). Activities requiring attention to these cues will accentuate the disability and should be avoided. (Allen, 1985, 1988; Levy, 1986; 1987, 1989).

Cognitive level 6: tangible thought

Attention at the sixth cognitive level is captured by abstract and symbolic cues. The goal is to use abstract reasoning to reflect about the range of possible actions, including reconsidering old plans and creating new ones. Spontaneous motor actions are those that have been planned in advance and on which there are no restrictions on performance. Learning uses symbolic thought and deductive reasoning, and can be generalized to new situations. Theoretically, this level represents the absence of cognitive disability. Activity adaptations to compensate for cognitive limitations are not required (Allen, 1985).

Function–dysfunction continua

A state of function exists when a person's information processing capacities match the routine task demands of the environment. A state of dysfunction exists when a person's information processing capacities are restricted such that he or she is unable to perform routine tasks. The six cognitive levels describe the severity of the disability from profound disability at level 1 to normal acquisition and adjustment at level 6. The levels are hierarchically organized within a continuum that differentiates dysfunction in terms of the characteristics of the information processed while the person is doing a desired activity: sensory cues, sensorimotor associations, and motor actions.

Behaviors indicative of function–dysfunction

Behaviors indicative of function–dysfunction are defined in terms of information processing capacities at each of the cognitive levels. Each level has assets that can be capitalized on and limitations that must be compensated for. These assets and limitations reflect behaviors indicative of function and dysfunction related to each of the cognitive levels.

Therapists use a number of tools to assess behaviors indicative of function and dysfunction in this frame of reference. One tool, the **Allen Cognitive Level Test** (ACL; Allen, 1985) is a standardized leather-lacing task that can be used to screen and assess cognitive levels 3, 4, 5, and 6. Another tool is the **Routine Task Inventory** (RTI; Allen, 1985), which was designed as a practical observational measure to describe and assess qualitative differences in the performance of a variety of routine tasks, such as bathing, grooming, and managing money. It also provides a comprehensive list of behaviors indicative of function and dysfunction to be observed in the performance of physical and instrumental daily living tasks that are specific to each of the cognitive levels.

Postulates regarding change and intervention

The cognitive disability frame of reference identifies two primary sources of change in cognitive level and functional performance. Change can occur in the capacity of the patient and within the patient's environment (Allen, 1987). **Change in capacity** can be influenced by a variety of external factors, such as medical intervention, psychotropic medications, and the natural healing process. Change can also occur when occupational therapy intervention aims to teach the patient to perform routine tasks; however, since brain pathology can impede the ability to learn and remember, this goal is restricted to those who are capable of functioning at cognitive levels 4 and 5.

Change in environment is accomplished primarily through occupational therapy intervention such as modifying task procedures, directions, and settings, and offering assistance to the patient. Although the patient's capacity may remain unchanged, the ability to experience success in performing routine tasks can increase. To this end, the therapist (1) evaluates the disability, (2) identifies how the procedures of the activity can best be adapted to reinforce the patient's cognitive capacities and to compensate for limitations, and (3) teaches caregivers to make the necessary environmental modifications indicated by the disability. Hence, the treatment focus in the cognitive disability frame of reference is to enable the disabled to make maximum use of residual functional assets while preventing or minimizing the interference of residual functional limitations. The primary intent is to facilitate the patient's best performance by changing the *activity* rather than attempting to change the person. This represents a major conceptual shift from other frames of reference in occupational therapy.

References

Allen, C. A. (1982). Independence through activity: The practice of occupational therapy. *American Journal of Occupational Therapy, 36,* 731–739.

Allen, C. A. (1985). *Occupational therapy for psychiatric diseases: Measurement and management of cognitive disabilities.* Boston: Little, Brown.

Allen, C. A. (1987). Activity: Occupational therapy's treatment method. *American Journal of Occupational Therapy, 41,* 563–575.

Allen, C. A. (1988). Cognitive disabilities. In S. Robertson (Ed.), *Focus: Skills for assessment and treatment.* Rockville, MD: American Occupational Therapy Association.

Allen, C. A. (1992). Cognitive disabilities. In N. Katz (Ed.). *Cognitive rehabilitation: Models for intervention in occupational therapy.* Boston: Andover Medical Publishers.

Allen, C. A., Foto, M., Moon-Sperling, T., & Wilson, D. (1989). A medical review approach to Medicare outpatient documentation. *American Journal of Occupational Therapy, 43,* 793–800.

Levy, L. L. (1986). A practical guide to the care of the Alzheimer's disease victim. *Topics in Geriatric Rehabilitation, 1,* 16–26.

Levy, L. L. (1987). Psychosocial intervention and dementia. Part 2. *Occupational Therapy in Mental Health, 7,* 13–36.

Levy, L. L. (1989). Activity adaptation in rehabilitation of the physically and cognitively disabled aged. *Topics in Geriatric Rehabilitation, 4* (4), 53–66.

SECTION 3D
Developmental frame of reference

CAROLE J. SIMON

KEY TERMS	
Facilitate	*Horizontal (Simultaneous)*
Growth Interruption	*Longitudinal (Chronologic)*

Theoretical base

After many years of clinical practice, research, and education, Lela Llorens framed a common sense vision of growth and development, which she presented to the occupational therapy profession in her 1969 Eleanor Clarke Slagle lecture (Llorens, 1970). Her views carefully encompassed all the parameters considered by occupational therapists, including the domains of physical, social, and psychological health. She acknowledged cultural context, mastery, competence, and coping skills to be important components of these considerations. Simply stated, her thesis is that occupational therapy is a facilitation process that assists the individual in achieving mastery of life tasks and the ability to cope as efficiently as possible with the life expectations made of him or her through the mechanisms of selected input stimuli and availability of practice in a suitable environment (Llorens, 1970). In the clinical setting this theory is applied when the occupational therapist *facilitates*, or assists, the adaptation process of the client within his or her environment.

Function–dysfunction continua

Llorens constructed 10 premises that fit together in a sequential and fundamental statement to support her vision of growth and development:

1. That the human organism develops horizontally in the areas of neurophysiological, physical, psychosocial, and psychodynamic growth and in the development of social language, daily living and sociocultural skills at specific periods of time;
2. That the human organism develops longitudinally in each of these areas in a continuous process as he ages;
3. That mastery of particular skills, abilities and relationships in each of the areas of neurophysiological, physical, psychosocial and psychodynamic development, social language, daily living and sociocultural skills, both horizontally and longitudinally is necessary to the successful achievement of satisfactory coping behavior and adaptive relationships;
4. That such mastery is usually achieved naturally in the course of development;
5. That the fundamental endowment of the individual and the stimulation of experiences received within the environment of the family come together to interact in such a way as to promote positive early growth and development in both the horizontal and longitudinal planes;
6. That later the influences of extended family, community, social and civic groups assist in the growth process;
7. That physical or psychological trauma related to disease, injury, environmental insufficiencies or intrapersonal vulnerability can interrupt the growth and development process;
8. That such **growth interruption** will cause a gap in the developmental cycle resulting in disparity between expected coping behavior and adaptive facility and the necessary skills and abilities to achieve same;
9. That occupational therapy through the skilled application of activities and relationships can provide growth and development links to assist in closing the gap between expectation and ability by increasing skills, abilities and relationships in the neurophysiological, physical, psychosocial, psychodynamic, social language, daily living, and sociocultural spheres of development as indicated both horizontally and longitudinally.
10. That occupational therapy through the skilled application of activities and relationships can provide growth experiences to prevent the development of potential maladaptation related to insufficient nurturance in neurophysiological, physical, psychosocial, psychodynamic, social language, daily living and sociocultural spheres of development both horizontally and longitudinally. (Llorens, 1970, p. 93)

Behaviors indicative of function–dysfunction

A key feature of this view is the suggestion of "snapshot" moments in time to examine the mastery of skills available to the growing child at stage-specific developmental periods across all domains. Growth occurs simultaneously in many areas. At critical times one growth experience may be emphasized at the expense of refinement in another area. For example, as the child is achieving a more upright position, he or she may need to forego fine motor hand development while using the upper extremities for needed stabilization. Llorens' framework allows appreciation for specific maturational and developmental growth each step of the way (horizontal) while the gains made over time (longitudinal) for attainment of the highest potential level of skill are recognized. This holistic approach found support in the literature of other developmentalists (Piaget, Erickson, Ayres, Havinghurst, Gessel) from whom Llorens drew and led her to construct a schematic representation of facilitating growth and development (Llorens, 1976). The interweaving of each important area of development supports future growth of the child.

In her book published subsequent to the initial presentation of this theory, Llorens (1976) clarified the terms **horizontal** and **longitudinal** as related to the concepts of **simultaneous** and **chronologic**. Both sets of terms give credence to the breadth and length of development and give rise to more specific considerations required in a function–dysfunction continuum. **Horizontal** growth specifically refers to gains made in all the developmental domains that appear **simultaneously** at a given age. For example, what are the skills demonstrated by a 5-year-old? **Longitudinal** growth is related to growth over time, observing the **chronological** age increments of the child, for example, observing growth over the span of zero to 21 years.

Postulates regarding change and intervention

After disruption to the normal progression of growth and development—either through physical or psychological trauma related to disease, injury, environmental insufficiencies, or intrapersonal vulnerability—gaps may occur in the developmental cycle with demonstrable disparities between the expected coping behavior and adaptive skills and the necessary prerequisite skills and abilities to support desired growth (Llorens, 1970). This **growth interruption** may cause a wide variety of problems for the child and his or her ability to interact with the environment. The identification and understanding of the importance of these deficiencies have implications for practice. The therapist may recognize that the client is functioning at an earlier level of skill than that required for successful task accomplishment. This indicates the need to gain or regain the deficient skills through the client's participation in tasks or purposeful activities that are appropriate yet challenging to the level of attainment to **facilitate** growth and development. This approach includes an element of prevention when problem areas can be addressed before they present major obstacles and maladaptive behavior in growth and development.

The role of the occupational therapist, who has a strong knowledge base regarding normal growth and development, is to identify the gaps in development and to provide selected tasks and relationships to promote the continuance of progression both simultaneously and chronologically. This frame of reference is particularly applicable to the child but has inherent usefulness for treating adults when regression or chronic conditions exists. Attention is specifically directed toward achievement of developmental tasks and ego-adaptive skills guided within the person's limitations and geared to a realistically attainable level (Llorens, 1970).

References

Llorens, L. A. (1970). Facilitating growth and development: The promise of occupational therapy. *American Journal of Occupational Therapy, 24*, 93–101.

Llorens, L. A. (1976). *Application of a developmental theory for health and rehabilitation.* Rockville, MD: American Occupational Therapy Association.

SECTION 3E
Neurodevelopmental frame of reference

REBECCA DUTTON

KEY TERMS

Axial Control   *Limb Control*
Automatic Reactions

Theoretical base

Berta and Karel Bobath created the neurodevelopmental (NDT) frame of reference as part of their work in the 1940s and 1950s with patients with cerebral palsy and cerebrovascular accidents. These were exciting decades when several sensorimotor theories were emerging. As the title implies, the theoretical base for NDT frame of reference comes from normal development and neurophysiology. It is not a pure developmental frame of reference, however, which the assumptions make clear.

There are five assumptions of the NDT frame of reference. The first assumption states that teaching normal motor milestones is NOT the proper focus for treatment (Adams, 1982). Normal development is important because it identifies the un-

derlying foundation skills that make motor milestones possible. For example, if midline symmetry is achieved, a minimum of practice is needed to achieve independent sitting. The second assumption is the belief that you cannot impose normal movement on abnormal muscle tone (Bobath, 1978). Spasticity and hypotonia both produce abnormal movements that become more pronounced with practice. The third assumption states that damage to higher centers in the brain produces a release phenomenon (Adams, 1982). Lower centers generate mass, obligatory, stereotyped movements in the form of hyperactive phasic and tonic reflexes and pathologic limb synergies. The fourth assumption is the belief that normal movement is learned by experiencing how normal movement feels (Adams, 1982). The Bobaths refer particularly to proprioceptive and tactile sensation. The final assumption states that the brain is very plastic and capable of remarkable recovery. Research has substantiated and explained central nervous system recovery (Moore, 1986).

Function–dysfunction continua

The three function–dysfunction continua that are the domains of concern for the NDT frame of reference are **axial control**, automatic reactions, and **limb control** (Dutton, in press). Axial control of the neck and trunk was ignored by other frames of reference until the Bobaths pointed out the importance of postural adjustment that accompanies all limb movement (Bobath, 1978). **Automatic reactions**, which include righting and equilibrium reactions, were part of evaluations before the NDT frame of reference, but it took the Bobaths to explain their importance in treatment. These reactions enable us to risk movement without the fear of falling (Adams, 1982). Without them, safety exists only in rigidly holding a posture. Finally, the Bobaths made us understand the importance of proximal limb structures, like the shoulder and pelvic girdles, to distal limb function (Adams, 1982). These proximal limb structures provide essential proximal stability during the early part of limb motion and contribute a significant number of degrees of range of motion when distal segments are moving in midranges (Norkin & Levangie, 1989).

Behaviors indicative of function–dysfunction

A patient's behavior is placed on these three continua by behaviors indicative of change found by using evaluation tools. Formal evaluation exists for reflex development and automatic reactions (Fiorentino, 1973), pathologic limb synergy (Sawner & LaVigne, 1992), and muscle tone (Dutton, in press). Clinical observation is needed to assess deficits that are ignored by formal tests, such as placing and eccentric control (Bobath, 1978). Clinical observation is also needed to evaluate deficits that are tested with poor sensitivity by formal tests, such as automatic reactions (Dutton, in press). These reactions are traditionally scored as present or absent.

Normal gross and fine motor trends are a valuable source of information about the primitive, transitional, and mature stages that identify underlying motor skills. For example, a gross motor trend entitled "flexor to extensor tone" tells us that mature extension is preceded by a transition behavior called extension with retraction (Dutton, in press). Extension with retraction is characterized by limb extension combined with neck and trunk hyperextension, scapular and pelvic retraction, and shoulder and hip abduction. This transition behavior is safe for normal infants but very dangerous for brain-damaged infants and adults.

Finally, the NDT neck, shoulder, and pelvic blocks are the hidden agenda in NDT evaluation and a good way to double check evaluation results. These blocks are stereotyped movements that produce deformities if treatment is omitted or delayed (Bly, 1983).

Postulates regarding change and intervention

Postulates regarding change identify links between presenting problems, NDT goals, and functional outcomes in a specific format (Dutton, in press). For example, the patient has suffered a cerebrovascular accident resulting in partial hemiplegia.

General deficit is poor axial weight shift.
Stage-specific cause is spastic lateral trunk flexors.
Measurable NDT goal is active weight shift onto the hemiplegic leg with elongation of the trunk on the weight-bearing side.
Functional outcome is the ability to hike up the hemiplegic hip for bathing with minimal assistance while sitting on a tub-seat.

It is vital to link the NDT goal of axial weight shifts with a functional outcome like bathing. Third-party payors require it (Allen & Foto, 1991; Dahl, 1990), and the patient needs to know why shifting from side to side is important. It is difficult for brain-damaged patients to understand the value of mat activities, especially if cognitive deficits are present.

You can see from the previous example that NDT goals are often made measurable with a qualitative rather than a quantitative approach. It is important to include these qualitative descriptions because these are often what we are trying to change with treatment. We do not necessarily want the patient to sit for longer periods of time. We want the patient to sit symmetrically with both shoulders level, equal weight on both hips, hips symmetrically abducted, and feet flat.

Postulates regarding intervention create links between NDT goals and therapeutic activities in a specific format (Dutton, in press). For example:

Measurable NDT goal of active weight shift onto the hemiplegic leg with elongation of the trunk on the weight-bearing side will be achieved by the general method.
General method consists of passive trunk elongation and proximal key points of control during active weight shift sideways, which (*rationale*) gives the sensation of how normal tone feels and inhibits spasticity while the patient initiates weight shift.
Specific activity is reaching across the midline with the sound hand to turn a newspaper page.

The neurodevelopmental frame of reference has eight *general methods* that inhibit spasticity: passive elongation, limb dissociation, normal weight shifts, normal limb movements free in space, positioning, orthotics, and reflex-inhibiting patterns (RIPs) (Dutton, in press). These methods are administered in three stages. The first stage is to use handling techniques to give the sensation of what normal tone and movement feel like. The second stage is to let the patient initiate movement during a purposeful activity while the occupational therapist (OT) maintains inhibition or facilitation. The third stage is for the OT to fade control from proximal key points of control, like the scapula or pelvis, to distal key points of control, like the hand or foot.

Every neurodevelopmental method must be applied in all three stages. It is especially important to achieve stages 1 and 2 within a single treatment session. The sensation of what normal feels like is very fleeting in the beginning. If you do not ask the patient to use the normal feeling right away by initiating his or her movement, you will not see any carryover.

References

Adams, M. (1982). *Eight week Bobath certification course*. Memphis, TN.

Allen, K. A., & Foto, M. (1991). Reporting occupational therapy outcomes with the ICIDH codes. *Physical Disabilities Special Interest Section Newsletter, 14*(2), 2–3.

Bly, L. (1983). *The components of normal movement during the first year of life and abnormal motor development*. Monograph of the NDT Association.

Bobath, B. (1978). *Adult hemiplegia: Evaluation and treatment* (2nd ed.). London: William Heinemann Medical Books Limited.

Dahl, M. (1990). *Money and reimbursement versus OT practice*. Pennsylvania Occupational Therapy Association Workshop. Philadelphia.

Dutton, R. (in press). *Clinical reasoning in physical disabilities*. Philadelphia: F. A. Davis.

Fiorentino, M. R. (1973). *Reflex testing methods for evaluating CNS development* (2nd ed.). Springfield, Il: Charles C Thomas.

Moore, J. C. (1986). Recovery potentials following CNS lesions: A brief historical perspective in relation to modern research data on neuroplasticity. *American Journal of Occupational Therapy, 40*(7), 459–463.

Norkin, C. C., & Levangie, P. K. (1989). *Joint structure and function*. Philadelphia: F.A. Davis.

Sawner, K. A., & Lavigne, J. M. (1992). *Brunnstrom's movement therapy in hemiplegia* (2nd ed.). Philadelphia: J. B. Lippincott.

SECTION 3F
Sensory integration frame of reference

CAROLE J. SIMON

KEY TERMS

Convergence	*Sensory Integration*
Elicit	*Syndromes of Sensory*
Sensory Dysfunction	*Dysfunction*

Theoretical base

Grounding her theoretical constructs in neurobiology, A. Jean Ayres relied on information known in neuroscience, neuropsychology, and neurophysiology to develop an approach to treatment that has had a major impact on the profession of occupational therapy. Her initial investigations with learning-disabled children yielded postulates about brain function that enabled further elaboration of her theory. Subsequently, Ayres and other therapists expanded the use of the frame of reference to other patient populations, including adults.

Ayres' conviction that the brain worked as a whole was based on phylogenetic and ontogenetic developmental principles. Older anatomic portions of the brain developed and functioned earlier than the more recently evolved components. Newer evolutionary brain segments relied on information from lower structures to function, and in addition, modulated the activity of those lower structures. Thus, a great interdependence existed in the hierarchy of the central nervous system. Tactile, proprioceptive, and vestibular systems mature early *in utero*, being older phylogenetically. Dysfunction in these systems may then have a deleterious effect on the function of higher cortical structures.

Some major neural structures, such as the brain stem and the thalamus, process sensory input from many sources. Acknowledging the interdependence of brain function, it is then presumed that these structures have a major impact on the functioning of the child. **Convergence** (coming together) of sensory information that comes from many sources to the brain stem and thalamus, suggests integration of input at that level. The brain's ability to filter, organize, and integrate masses of sensory information is critical to learning (Ayres, 1968). Thus, in the late 1960s Ayres began to use the term **sensory integration** and continued to apply her theory to the clinical problems she encountered (Ayres, 1968).

Function–dysfunction continua

Ayres proposed a model of child development that cited the senses, the integration of their inputs, and their end products (see Figure 13-33). It denotes the importance of vestibular, tactile, and proprioceptive input in the development of postural control, body schema, bonding, nourishment, coordination, emotional stability, language, and perception. It adds the visual and auditory senses as supplementary for later development. The end products are those that support academic learning, such as concentration, organization, self-control, self-esteem, self-confidence, abstract thinking, and specialization of each side of the brain and body. In addition, Ayres identified syndromes of dysfunction, which she postulated could be treated using selected sensory input with emphasis on the identified dysfunctional system. The reader is referred to Chapter 13, Section 4 for further information.

Behaviors indicative of function–dysfunction

To evaluate **sensory dysfunction**, Ayres devised the Southern California Sensory Integration Test in 1972, which was revised in 1980. In 1975, she introduced the Southern California Postrotary Nystagmus Test to assess vestibulo-occular function. The Sensory Integration and Praxis Tests became available in 1985 to offer a psychometrically sound and expanded evaluation tool.

Postulates regarding change and intervention

Treatment parameters for this frame of reference include control of sensory input through selected activities that emphasize subcortical intersensory integration. The therapist is seeking an adaptive response evoking motor behavior that supports effective interaction with the environment, especially in response to gravity and tactile input. Movement is an implicit component of therapy. A variety of equipment (such as scooter boards and bolster swings) that provides movement experiences is used. The child's response is carefully monitored to determine whether a maturing adaptive response appears, to assess whether signs of overstimulation or understimulation are present, and to determine the level of nervous system interpretation of the stimuli.

Each child has an innate drive to mature. Children usually self-select activities to support that maturation and express pleasure in experiencing that activity. Ayres (1979) described the "art" of therapy as using an approach that was pleasurable and that invited the child to initiate engagement with selected equipment or activities geared to improve dysfunctional systems and promote desired adaptive behaviors. Eliciting responses rather than imposing activities or tasks is considered to be more integrating.

This neurobiologically based frame of reference recognizes the hierarchical and interdependent qualities of the function of the brain, and focuses on convergence and integration of sensory stimulation. Evaluation tools identify areas or syndromes of sensory dysfunction and treatment relies on movement and tactilely based activities that promote successful adaptive responses to the demands of the environment.

References

Ayres, A. J. (1968). Sensory integrative processes and neurological learning disability. *Learning Disorders, III*, 41–58

Ayres, A. J. (1968). Reading—a product of sensory integrative process. In H. K. Smith (Ed.), *Perception and reading. Proceedings of the Twelth Annual Convention International Reading Association*. Part 4. (p. 12). Newark, DE.

Ayres, A. J. (1979). *Sensory integration and the child.* Los Angeles: Western Psychological Services.

SECTION 3G
Model of human occupation frame of reference

LINDA L. LEVY

KEY TERMS

Achievement

Adaptive Cycle

Competency

Exploration

General Systems Theory

Habituation Subsystem

Maladaptive Cycle

OCAIRS

Occupational Behavior Model

Occupational Behaviors

Occupational Role Dysfunction

Open System

Performance Subsystem

Volition Subsystem

Theoretical base

The model of the human occupation frame of reference in occupational therapy is based on theories that had their beginnings in the philosophical assumptions articulated by the founders of the profession in the early 20th century. It was immeasurably influenced by the works of Mary Reilly (1962, 1974), who developed the *occupational behavior model* in the late 1960s and 1970s. It was introduced to the profession in 1980, when Gary Kielhofner and Janice P. Burke proposed a comprehensive occupational therapy theory to reorganize the profession's body of knowledge and reaffirm its traditional principles, entitled the model of human occupation. This model, or paradigm as it was originally termed, has undergone continuous development and refinement since its inception. The focus of this discussion is the components of the model that have evolved into a frame of reference.

The model of the human occupation frame of reference draws heavily on the tenets of the occupational behavior model developed by Reilly and her students at the University of Southern California. In the late 1960s, Reilly called for a recommitment to the original philosophical premises of the profession that had been developed by Adolph Meyer (1922) and Eleanor Clark Slagle (1922). Reilly's model reinforced principles of moral treatment that espoused *habit training* (Slagle, 1922) and a balance of work, play, and rest (Meyer, 1922). She refocused the emphasis on habit training and the *work–play–rest continuum* to *occupational roles* (such as worker, student, housewife, retiree, or preschooler) because she believed that roles provide the context for organizing one's time for work, play, and rest. Occupational roles became conceptualized as *occupational behaviors*. A central premise of Reilly's model was that the primary purpose of occupational therapy was the remediation of *occupational role dysfunction* (Reilly, 1958). As such, Reilly sought to encourage occupational therapists to transcend what was considered to be the limited concerns of the biomedi-

cal approach of the time (a focus on disease and disability) and to address the larger biopsychosocial concern of promoting life satisfaction through occupational roles. Occupational therapy was seen to restore, increase, or maintain health by engaging the person in activities (occupations) that promoted desired social roles. Roles, therefore, were considered to be fundamental to the restoration and maintenance of health.

A number of central themes were inherent in the occupational behavior model. One was the concept of competency. *Competency*, as defined by White, is the capacity both to interact effectively with the environment and to be sufficient or adequate to meet the demands of the situation or task (White, 1959, 1971). To perform occupational roles effectively, a person must experience a sense of competency. The model also placed emphasis on the utility of play in developing the skills necessary for competent participation in occupational roles. Play was viewed as a subsystem of the learning system that itself comprised a hierarchy of three subsystems: *exploration*, competency, and *achievement* (Reilly, 1974). Play was used to remediate dysfunction because it provided a safe arena to experience competency and to acquire the necessary skills to support occupational roles. The model also emphasized the need for an appropriate balance of work, play, and rest to support competent functioning in occupational roles. This balance was viewed in a quantitative sense (time for work, play, rest, and sleep) as well as in a qualitative sense (opportunities to pursue interests and goals) (Shannon, 1970).

Reilly's oft-quoted hypothesis, that "man, through the use of his hands as they are energized by mind and will, can influence the state of his own health" (Reilly, 1962, p. 2) underscored two major premises of the occupational behavior model. The first premise is that engaging in activities (occupations) is essential to the maintenance and restoration of health; the second is that the person has an inherent need to explore and master the environment and to be competent.

The occupational behavior model served as the foundation for the model of human occupation that emerged in the 80s. The model of human occupation sought to more closely link Reilly's occupational behavior model with the demands of clinical practice. The intent was to provide means to conceptualize the occupational nature of the individual, to identify concepts critical to the understanding of occupational dysfunction, and to articulate the value of activities (occupations) as therapy.

The central premise of the model of human occupation is,

> All human occupation arises out of an innate, spontaneous tendency of the human system—the urge to explore and master the environment. The model is based on the assumption that occupation is a central aspect of the human experience. It is man's innate urge toward exploration and his consequent ability to symbolize that makes him unique among animals. (Kielhofner & Burke, 1980, p. 573)

Here, human occupation is defined as the innate, spontaneous tendency of the human system to explore and master the environment. In a later work, occupational behavior is defined as

> . . . behavior which is motivated by an intrinsic conscious urge to be effective in the environment in order to enact a variety of individually interpreted roles that are shaped by cultural tradition and learned through the process of socialization. (Burke & Kielhofner in Kielhofner, 1983, p. 136)

Inherent to these definitions is the concept of *intrinsic motivation*, both in terms of understanding human development and conceptualizing the process of change. That is, the person grows and changes because of a need to explore and be active. (In contrast, extrinsic motivation, ie, the demand for growth and change by external forces or for external rewards, is inconsistent with the tenets of this frame of reference.) These definitions also emphasize that the human occupation frame of reference is primarily concerned with action that is consciously motivated rather than action that might be conceived as unconsciously motivated.

General systems theory provides the structural framework for the model of human occupation (Kielhofner & Burke, 1980; Kielhofner, 1983, 1985). The model conceptualizes the individual as an *open system* that evolves and undergoes different forms of growth, development, and change through an ongoing interaction with the external environment. The human system simultaneously functions as a whole, with its own internal subsystems, and as a part of the larger social system. The cycle of interaction with the environment includes four phases: input, throughput, output, and feedback. *Input* refers to the importation of energy or information into the system. *Throughput* refers both to the transformation of the energy or information for assimilation by the system and to the transformation of the system to accommodate the incoming energy or information. *Output* refers to the external action or the behavior of the system and results in feedback to the system about the process and the consequences of the action. This ongoing cycle is responsible for the process of self-maintenance and self-change.

When applied to treatment, this model conceptualizes occupational therapy as an organizing process involving the input of information necessary for activity performance, the translation and use of that energy for performance (throughput), and the actual act of performance (output), which results in positive feedback to the system. Both input and feedback bring new information into the system, which results in changes in the system. Stated another way, information (input) enters the system and is processed by the throughput process to produce output, or the person's occupational behavior. Output (the person's occupational behavior) gives feedback in the form of information or experience to the person and the cycle is reinitiated. Hence, the system maintains itself through its own action, and successful participation in activities (occupations) produces behavioral change (Kaplan & Kielhofner, 1989). Learning in this frame of reference is viewed as a continuous process that occurs through experience (feedback), given the system's ability to organize and process new information.

As an open system, the human is further conceptualized as consisting of three subsystems: volition, habituation, and performance subsystems, which are hierarchically ordered from the highest to the lowest (Figure 4-2). Each subsystem has its own structure and function, and the interaction of the three subsystems constitutes the throughput of the system. The highest subsystem is referred to as *volition*; this subsystem is responsible for freely and consciously choosing participation in occupations. Its function is to enact behavior. The middle subsystem is *habituation*; it is responsible for organizing behavior into routines or patterns. Its function is to maintain behavior. The lowest subsystem is *performance*, which consists of the basic capacities for action (skills). Its function is to produce the action of the system.

Volition

The volition subsystem is composed of both an underlying energy source and a set of internal images that determine the motivation to enact occupational behavior. The energy source is believed to be the human's innate urge to explore and master the environment. The motivation to act is determined by internal images that a person holds about himself or herself as a participant in the external world. These images have been identified as personal causation, valued goals, and interests.

Personal causation refers to the person's belief that he or she has skills that can be used effectively, and that he or she is in

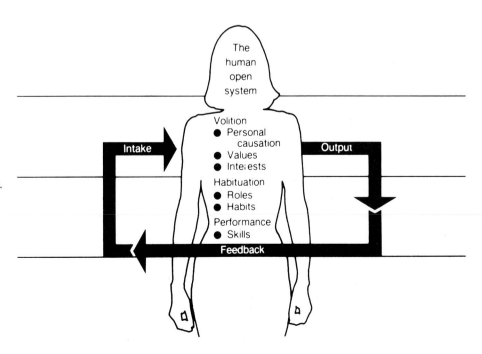

FIGURE 4-2. *The open system representing human occupation. (From* Kielhofner, A Model of Human Occupation, Williams and Wilkins, 1985)

control and is capable of achieving success, or expects failure, in the future. *Valued goals* are a person's internal images concerning what is good, right, and valuable. They provide a sense of obligation to participate in certain occupations that are culturally sanctioned, and help the person experience a sense of connection to the social group. *Interests* are the person's preferences for occupations based on prior experiences of pleasure and satisfaction while participating in those activities. From a person's value system, interests emerge that are transformed into goals. The authors of this model believe that clarifying values and interests is a necessary first step when a person has difficulty establishing goals.

Habituation

The habituation subsystem is made up of two sets of images that serve to maintain occupational behavior: roles and habits. Roles and habits organize, regulate, and maintain behavior to help the person meet socially approved standards and allow him or her to adapt to the environment (Kielhofner, 1983). Roles are images that persons hold about the positions they occupy in various social groups and of the obligations that go along with these positions. As such, they have an internal and external component. The *internal component* refers to the way in which a person perceives and acts on his or her roles. The *external component* refers to expectations that society identifies with the role. Role balance is the degree to which the person is able to integrate life roles into a satisfying and meaningful pattern of living. Habits are images that trigger automatic routines that organize behaviors according to social norms. The habituation subsystem organizes patterns of behavior that build on and make use of the underlying skills of the performance subsystem.

Performance

The performance subsystem is composed of skills and the constituents of skills that produce occupational behaviors. There are three types of skills: perceptual motor skills, process skills (behaviors such as planning and problem solving), and communication/interaction skills. *Constituents of skills* are the underlying structures used for skilled performance. Again, there are three types: symbolic, neurologic, and musculoskeletal. *Symbolic constituents* are the person's internalized rules for performance. The *neurologic* and *musculoskeletal constituents* refer to the nervous system and the musculoskeletal system, which take in sensory information and effect motor action.

Environment

The interaction of the individual with the environment is influenced by the status of the three subsystems, which in turn influences the subsystems. Barris (in Kielhofner, 1985) has conceptualized the human as a system performing in an environment composed of four concentric layers: culture, social groups, tasks, and objects. Each layer influences occupational performance. *Culture* determines the groups that are available to and valued by the individual. *Social groups* select and organize the tasks that individuals perform when they become members. *Tasks* define what objects will be used and how they will be used.

Finally, *objects* refer to the materials and artifacts that individuals use to perform tasks.

According to the model of human occupation, occupational behavior can be understood by examining the variables of the model and the way in which they contribute to an ongoing process of change. In an **adaptive cycle**, positive experiences support the person's desire to explore, master, and fulfill environmental demands. The person's choices, routines, and skills promote behaviors that lead to increased organization of the system. In a **maladaptive cycle**, the person repeatedly experiences disorganization, poor performance, and anticipation of future failure: his or her poor choices, poorly organized routines, and deficient skills lead to increased disorganization in the system and a state of occupational dysfunction. The primary goal of occupational therapy is to enable individuals to organize their occupational behavior so that adaptive cycles are learned or restored (Kielhofner, 1985; Kaplan & Kielhofner, 1989).

Function–dysfunction continua

Adaptive cycles result in a state of occupational function. Maladaptive cycles result in a state of occupational dysfunction. Individuals are occupationally functional when they meet both society's expectations for productive and playful participation and their own need for exploration and mastery. Conversely, individuals are occupationally dysfunctional when societal demands for productive and playful participation are not met or the individual's behavior does not fulfill the urge to explore and master (Kielhofner, 1985).

Recognizing that everyone exhibits degrees of adaptive or maladaptive occupational functioning, Kielhofner proposed an occupational function–dysfunction continuum made up of six levels of adaptation and maladaptation in occupational behavior. The three levels of occupational function—exploration, competence, and achievement—are derived from Reilly's theory and represent states of optimal arousal and involvement with the environment. The three states of occupational dysfunction—inefficacy, incompetence, and helplessness—represent stress and lack of involvement with the environment.

Inefficacy is conceptualized as the initial level of occupational dysfunction. Inefficacy results when there is an interference with performing meaningful activity accompanied by a dissatisfaction with performance. It is also often accompanied by a reduction in a sense of personal causation, and a negative impact on the person's interests, values, roles, and habits. **Incompetence** is conceptualized as the second state of occupational dysfunction. Incompetence is characterized by a major loss or limitation of skills, a failure or disruption of self-confidence and satisfaction, and an inability to routinely and adequately perform tasks of everyday living. It is often accompanied by a major reduction in personal causation and impairment in interests, values, roles, and skills. **Helplessness** is the third stage of occupational dysfunction and is characterized by a total or near-total disruption of occupational performance together with extreme feelings of ineffectiveness, anxiety, depression, or all three. It is accompanied by loss of personal causation, interests, and values; absent habits and roles; and highly deficient skills (Kielhofner, 1985).

Behaviors indicative of function–dysfunction

Occupational functioning is assessed by the Occupational Case Analysis Interview and Rating Scale (OCAIRS; Kaplan & Kielhofner, 1989). The **OCAIRS** identifies a series of 10 conceptual questions that enable the therapist to formulate an assessment of function and dysfunction. The primary questions provide focus for a semistructured interview designed to elicit information about the influence of each variable in the model on the person's adaptive functioning. The 10 questions are:

1. Does the person anticipate successful outcomes of action?
2. Does the person have valued goals?
3. Does the person have interests?
4. Does the person have primary occupational roles?
5. Does the person have organized habit patterns?
6. Does the person have the performance skills to carry out valued activities?
7. Does the person use performance skills competently and consistently?
8. Does the physical environment support competent and consistent use of skills?
9. Does the social environment require occupational roles that the person enjoys and performs well?
10. Does the social environment support successful occupational behavior?

In general, a negative answer to any of the 10 primary questions is indicative of dysfunction; however, descriptors are provided for each question to enable therapists to assess degrees of dysfunction by a five-point ordinal rating scale. Answers to these conceptual questions are also derived by interpreting and synthesizing data from a variety of assessment tools, including the Occupational Performance History Interview, play assessment, interest checklist, Role Change Assessment, Occupational Role History, adolescent role assessment, inventory of occupational choice skills, time and activities inventory, Comprehensive Evaluation of Basic Living Skills, activities of daily living checklists, decision-making inventory, environmental questionnaire, role checklist, sensory integration assessment, Bay Area Functional Performance Evaluation, and so on.

Postulates regarding change and intervention

Change is brought about by organizing occupational behavior so that adaptive cycles are learned or restored. Change is facilitated when the environment allows for the expression of the individual's innate urge for exploration, competency, and achievement. Through enactment of this innate urge in a facilitating environment, the individual can acquire the skills, habits, and roles required for occupational function.

After a source of occupational dysfunction has been identified, change in the system must be initiated within the volitional subsystem. The lowest level of motivation in the volitional system—exploration—is aimed at generating skills. The next level—competency—presents greater demands for performance and develops habits. The highest level—achievement—

prepares the person for occupational roles. Occupational therapists remediate occupational dysfunction by directly providing an occupation in which the person engages as therapy, counseling and problem solving with the person to identify and alter a maladaptive occupational lifestyle, and facilitating engagement in occupation by improving the fit between the person and his or her environment.

References

Kaplan, K., & Kielhofner, G. (1989). *Occupational case analysis interview and rating scale.* Thorofare, NJ: Slack.

Kielhofner, G. (1983). *Health through occupation: Theory and practice in occupational therapy.* Philadelphia: F. A. Davis.

Kielhofner, G. (1985). *A model of human occupation: Theory and application.* Baltimore: Williams & Wilkins.

Kielhofner, G., & Burke, J. P. (1980). A model of human occupation. Part I: Conceptual framework and content. *American Journal of Occupation Therapy, 34,* 572–581.

Meyer, A. (1922). The philosophy of occupational therapy. *Archives of Occupational Therapy, 1,* 1–10.

Reilly, M. (1958). An occupational therapy curriculum for 1965. *American Journal of Occupation Therapy, 12,* 293–299.

Reilly, M. (1962). Occupational therapy can be one of the greatest ideas of 20th century medicine. *American Journal of Occupation Therapy, 16,* 1–9.

Reilly, M. (1974). *Play as exploratory learning.* Los Angeles: Sage Publications.

Shannon, P. D. (1970). The work-play model: A basis for occupational therapy programming in psychiatry. *American Journal of Occupation Therapy, 24,* 215–220.

Slagle, E. C. (1922). Training aides for mental patients. *Archives of Occupational Therapy, 1,* 11–20.

White, R. W. (1959). Motivation reconsidered: The concept of competence. *Psychological Review, 66,* 297–328.

White, R. W. (1971). The urge toward competence. *American Journal of Occupation Therapy, 25,* 271–274.

SECTION 3H
Rehabilitation frame of reference

REBECCA DUTTON

KEY TERMS

Activities of Daily Living   Work
Leisure

Theoretical base

The rehabilitation frame of reference teaches patients to compensate for underlying deficits that cannot be remediated (Pedretti & Pasquinelli, 1990). This frame of reference became a national reality when the philosophy of rehabilitation was included in legislation (Dutton, in press). The Vocational Rehabilitation Amendment Act of 1954, the Social Rehabilitation Act of 1963, and the Architectural Barriers Act of 1968 are examples.

The rehabilitation frame of reference has five assumptions (Dutton, in press). The first assumption states that a person can regain independence through compensation. The second assumption states that motivation for independence cannot be separated from the volitional and habituation subsystems. Motivation for independence is influenced by lifelong values, future roles, and a renewed sense of purpose. The third assumption states that motivation for independence cannot be separated from environmental context. The demands of the discharge setting, the patient's financial status, and the family's emotional resources are examples of environmental influences on motivation for independence. The fourth assumption is that a minimum of emotional and cognitive prerequisite skills are needed to make independence possible. The fifth assumption is the belief that clinical reasoning should take a top-down approach. The five steps in this top-down hierarchy are identifying (1) environmental demands of the discharge setting such as a second floor bathroom, (2) current functional capability such as dependence in toileting, (3) task demands the patient cannot perform such as standing balance, (4) type of rehabilitation method such as adaptive devices, and (5) specific modalities such as long-handled reachers and one-handed techniques.

Function–dysfunction continua

The three function–dysfunction continua that are the domains of concern for the rehabilitation frame of reference are **activities of daily living** (ADL), **work**, and **leisure** tasks. ADL are further divided into self-care and homecare activities (Pedretti, 1990b). Self-care encompasses a wide range of skills including eating, dressing, bathing, and toileting. Homecare includes homemaking, childcare, and home maintenance tasks such as simple home repair. Leisure and work tasks are highly varied and constantly changing.

Behaviors indicative of function–dysfunction

A patient's behavior can be placed on these three continua (mentioned above) by behaviors indicative of change found by using evaluation tools. Test scores indicate the levels of assistance needed. Assistance formerly referred to the levels of physical assistance such as minimum, moderate, and maximal assistance. Today, Medicare guidelines for levels of assistance have added levels of supervision needed (Health Care Financing Administration, 1989). This documents the needs of cognitively impaired patients who can place a significant burden on caretakers.

Momentum has been growing for all hospitals to adopt one standardized self-care evaluation to provide uniform classification. Several standardized tests have been developed, but they exhibit little consensus (Dutton, in press). The skills they test vary considerably, with bed mobility, bowel and bladder control, skin care, communication, and environmental hardware such as doorknobs, most frequently omitted. Their scoring system also varies from a 2-point scale to a 7-point scale.

Tests that evaluate leisure skills are limited to interest checklists for adults and play evaluations for children. Work evaluations are available to assess work behaviors like punctuality, general work traits like grip strength, work tolerance, that is, the ability to sustain effort, and specific work skills like welding (Dutton, in press). Specific work skills can be evaluated using actual job samples or simulated work samples (Jacobs, 1985).

Postulates regarding change identify links between presenting problems and functional outcomes in a specific format (Dutton, in press). For example, the patient has suffered a cerebrovascular accident resulting in a flaccid left hemiplegia.

General deficit is dependence in toileting.
Stage-specific cause is flaccid left hemiplegia, hemianopsia, hemianesthesia, and shoulder pain.
Functional outcome is toileting with minimum physical assistance and intermittent verbal cuing by the patient's wife at home.

It is essential to identify the stage-specific cause of the dysfunction. If you omit this link in your thought process, you don't know whether you should use positioning devices that inhibit spasticity or compensate for lack of structural stability during the flaccid stage of recovery. The cause also identifies deficits such as pain, hemianesthesia, and hemianopsia, which will not respond to compensatory one-handed techniques.

Postulates regarding change and intervention

Postulates regarding intervention create links between functional outcomes and specific adaptive devices, modifications, and procedures in a specific format (Dutton, in press). For an example, see Table 4-3.

There are seven general rehabilitation methods: adaptive devices, upper extremity (UE) orthotics, environmental modification, wheelchair modification, ambulatory devices, adapted procedures, and safety education (Dutton, in press). The rationales for these methods identify the task demands that each method compensates for. Some method rationales are well established, such as the rationale for using a long-handled reacher, which is lack of sufficient reach. Some rationales need to be updated. For example, environmental modifications to improve safety have gone beyond grab bars and other strategies for the physically impaired. They now address safety issues on the job like low back and repetitive motion injuries. Some method rationales need to be identified. For example, wheelchair modifications are usually discussed by grouping wheelchair parts into categories such as armrests. Wheelchair equipment should be ordered because it facilitates transfers and proper positioning, overcomes architectural barriers, and permits self-propulsion and transportation of needed objects (Dutton, in press).

After you have used rationales to select the rehabilitation method that meets your patient's needs, you still need to critique the advantages and disadvantages of each method (Dutton, in press). For example, adapted procedures like one-handed techniques have the advantage of relatively low cost. The therapist's

TABLE 4-3. *Functional Outcome*

General Method	Rationale	Specific Activity
Adaptive devices	Compensate for lack of a stabilizing hand	Zipper pull
Adapted procedure	Substitute for loss of lower extremity ROM	Propel W/C using sound arm and leg
W/C modification	Facilitates W/C transfers	Detachable legrests
	Facilitates W/C proper positioning	Arm trough for left upper extremity
Environmental modification	Facilitates safety	Grab bars in private bathroom
Safety education	Compensates for hemianopsia	Use verbal cues to attend to left side
	Compensates for sensory loss of limbs	Turn on cold water before hot

time to teach adaptive procedures costs less than some wheelchairs and environmental modifications. Adapted procedures also have the advantage of low visibility. These procedures are not highly noticeable unless someone is really scrutinizing how a task is performed. People are likely to stare at a person who is using a rocker knife in a restaurant. Adapted procedures have the disadvantage of not providing external prompts to remind the cognitively impaired patient to perform activities a new way, however. Adapted procedures can also elicit strong negative emotions. Many feel resentment when their personal habits are scrutinized. Instead of the halo effect associated with technologic solutions like electric wheelchairs, adapted procedures often elicit comments like "I've done it my way for 40 years." Postulates regarding intervention in the rehabilitation frame of reference are the culmination of a complex interaction of therapist, patient, and current knowledge.

References

Dutton, R. (in press). *Clinical reasoning in physical disabilities*. Philadelphia: F. A. Davis.

Health Care Financing Administration. Outclient Occupational Therapy Medicare Part B Guidelines (DHHS Transmittal No. 55). In *Health insurance manual*, Baltimore, 1989.

Jacobs, K. (1985). *Occupational therapy: Work-related programs and assessments*. Boston: Little, Brown, & Co.

Pedretti, L. W., & Pasquinelli, S. (1990a). A frame of reference for occupational therapy in physical dysfunction. In L. W. Pedretti & B. Zoltan (Eds.), *Occupational therapy* practice skills for physical dysfunction (3rd ed.). Philadelphia: Mosby-YearBook.

Pedretti, L. W. (1990b). Activities of daily living. In L. W. Pedretti & B. Zoltan (Eds.), *Occupational therapy practice skills for physical dysfunction* (3rd ed.). Philadelphia: Mosby-YearBook.

SECTION 3I
Psychodynamic frame of reference

LINDA L. LEVY

KEY TERMS

Defense Mechanisms

Drive Control

Economic Theory

Ego

Id

Instinctual Drives

Interpersonal Relationships

Psychic Conflict

Object Relations

Pleasure Principle

Reality Principle

Reality Testing

Structural Theory

Superego

Symbolization

Transference

Unconscious Forces

Theoretical base

The psychodynamic frame of reference in occupational therapy is based on theories that had their modern beginnings with the work of Freud (1900, 1942, 1949) in the late 19th and early 20th centuries. It has undergone continuous development and modification since its inception, most notably by interpersonal psychiatric theorists such as Sullivan and, more recently, by the ego and object relations theorists (Hartmann, 1964; Fairbairn, 1952; Winnicott, 1958; Klein, 1959; Mahler, 1968; Kernberg, 1976). These theories, as reformulated to develop therapeutic intervention strategies, have undergone little change in their transformation into the theoretical base of the psychodynamic frame of reference in occupational therapy. When they are applied in occupational therapy, they are in accordance with the philosophical assumptions of the profession.

Psychodynamic theory is designed to help us understand ***interpersonal relationships***. It conceives of the mind as a system of forces in motion. These forces may be biologic, social, or most frequently, a combination of the two. The cornerstone of psychodynamic theory is the proposition that **unconscious forces** determine our behavior as much as, or even more than, conscious ones. The theory is primarily concerned with the person's attempts to establish some sort of equilibrium between its internal forces and those of the environment. Its concern, therefore, is with adaptation.

Two main aspects of psychodynamic theory are incorporated into the theoretical base of this frame of reference. The first considers **instinctual drives** (forces); the second considers concepts of the developing self as a mental apparatus to deal with those drives (psychic conflict).

Freud's theory of instinctual drives

Freud's theory of instinctual drives assumes two primary instinctual impulses that demand gratification. He identified these two primary drives as sexual and aggressive. To understand best what he meant by these drives, the broadest definitions of the terms sexual and aggressive are necessary. **Sexual drives** reflect those needs for gratification that exist in all positive aspects of human and nonhuman relationships and that result in pleasurable sensations to the individual. These drives are considered to be the constructive element in motivation for most human activities. **Aggressive drives** reflect the needs to relate with, adapt to, and master the external environment. They can take on destructive qualities in response to frustration and conflict. Both sexual and aggressive drives are used for the satisfaction of man's basic needs—affectional and material. They also serve as the wellsprings of all human behavior. Freud developed a number of theories to explain the functioning of the mental apparatus in dealing with the expression and gratification of instinctual drives. The first is the economic theory.

The **economic theory** states that the drives, and the wishes, fantasies, and needs of a person that are derived from these drives (**drive derivatives**), are associated with increments in psychic tension that disturb that state of minimal tension or emotional equilibrium that the person seeks to maintain. Because this psychic tension is unpleasurable and because the person strives to minimize such sensations, he or she responds with behaviors aimed at reducing the tension or, from a different perspective, satisfying the need or requirement. The problem is that, although drives require satisfaction or gratification, the demands of the external world often prohibit their direct expression, and to return to a state of emotional equilibrium, the person must develop a set of mechanisms by which the drives can be neutralized. To explain how this occurs, Freud developed the structural theory. Freud's **structural theory** defined the mind as consisting of three structures, referred to as the id, the ego, and the superego.

Id

The **id** is that portion of mind, unconscious by definition, that represents the source of the instinctual drives that continually strive for expression; it also serves as the locus of powerful unconscious, affect-laden wishes and fantasies that are derived from those needs. The id was seen to handle the individual's drives and wishes in accordance with what Freud referred to as the **pleasure principle**. The human organism strives to maximize pleasurable sensations and to minimize unpleasurable or painful ones. Internal drives and needs are associated with an increase in psychic tension. This is unpleasurable, and the mind seeks to reduce the tension by gratifying the need. At the level of the id, however, there is no concern for external reality constraints.

The id was also seen to proceed in accordance with primary process. Primary process is a mode of thinking dominated by affect-laden, wish-fulfilling fantasies derived from the drives. At this level, these fantasies are expressed in images, the earliest form of cognition. It is only when these fantasies, or their derivatives, reach the level of the ego that they are translated into words. The concept of symbolization is intimately related to this form of cognition. **Symbolization** is the uniquely human process in which one mental representation stands for another. The symbol is seen to have a conscious manifest form, but it also is derived from, and latently represents, unconscious mental content. Freud also understood symbols to result from unconscious, primary process mental activity, which served to displace wishes from forbidden objects onto substitute objects, thereby permitting some form of gratification. Although he believed that a symbol was best understood within a person's past and present context, he also acknowledged that knowledge of the common unconscious meanings of symbols, cautiously applied, can be useful in understanding the patient's conflicts.

Ego

The second structure of the mind is referred to as the **ego**. The ego develops out of the need to discriminate between the internal (id) drives and the constraints of external reality. Freud saw the ego as functioning as a mediator between external reality and the needs and demands of the id. The ego was seen to operate on the **reality principle**. That is, this aspect of mental functioning concerns itself primarily with the nature and constraints of the external environment rather than the id-based needs for pleasurable immediate gratification. The ego is realistic; it is tuned toward the outer world as well as toward the inner drives. It controls the drives by delaying, inhibiting, and restraining them in the interests of achieving their aims realistically. The ego aims to secure the maximum amount of gratification of affect-laden fantasies, compatible with internal morality and the environment. Its functioning, if effective, results in attainment of the aims of the drives. It is also the ego's role to mediate between the needs of the third mental structure in this theory, the superego.

Superego

The **superego** is that portion of the mental apparatus that represents the prescriptions and proscriptions of the outside world: the "thou shalts" and "thou shalt nots." It develops in response to interactions between the infant and the caretakers in his or her environment as they are intended to guide and modify the infant's behavior through the use of reward and punishment. The superego is that aspect of mental functioning that corresponds in a general way to what we ordinarily call conscience. It contains the internalized parental attitudes and moral values that serve to control the sexual and aggressive drives. Contrary to the ordinary meaning of conscience, however, the functions of the superego are largely unconscious.

The ego, in addition to the regulation and control of instinctual drives and needs and the role of mediating the demands of the superego, is said to serve several other functions (Kaplan & Sadock, 1988). These include the following.

Object relations

The capacity for developing mutually satisfying relationships (object relationships) is one of the fundamental functions of the ego. Object relations theorists considered this capacity as the primary function of the ego. The evolution of the child's capacity for relationships with others, which progresses from total involvement with self in early infancy to social relationships within the family and then the peer group, depends on the establishment of trust in the constancy of need fulfillment by the primary caretakers in the early stage of infantile development. Freud emphasized that the choice of a loved individual (object relationship), the love relationship itself, and all interpersonal and nonpersonal relationships (human and nonhuman object relationships) in all other spheres of activity would depend largely on the nature and quality of the child's object relationships during the earliest years of life.

Transference is an important type of object relationship; it is the displacement of patterns of feelings, thoughts, and behavior, originally experienced in relation to significant "objects" during childhood, onto a person involved in a current interpersonal relationship. Insofar as every object relationship is a reenactment of the first childhood attachments, transference is universal. It is also inherent in all therapeutic relationships.

The object concept was derived from Freud's instinctual drive theory. In his conception, the goal or intent of the instinctual drive was the relief of tension or the attainment of pleasure via the object. Object relations theorists, however, conceive of the primary goal of the drive as the establishment of satisfying interpersonal (object) relationships, in lieu of tension relief or pleasure seeking. Regardless of theoretical orientation, it is essential to recognize that objects are a critical part of the satisfaction of the instinctual drive, and that all drives exist within the context of interpersonal (ie, object) relationships. The development of object relationships is often used to distinguish between healthy and pathologic behaviors.

Regulation and control of instinctual drives

The development of the capacity to delay immediate discharge of wishes and impulses is essential if the ego is to fulfill its role as mediator between the id and the outside world. **Drive control** implies the ability to wait, to delay satisfaction, and to withstand anxiety and frustration. The development of the capacity to delay or postpone instinctual discharge is closely related to the progression from the pleasure principle to the reality principle, and parallels the development of logical thinking (secondary process) that aids in the control of drive discharge.

Synthesis and coordination

The ego's task is to promote mastery of experience and to guide action in such as way that a certain wholeness, or synthesis, is created between the diverse and conflicting aspects of life: between impelling wishes and compelling demands, between the most private and the most public aspects of existence. To do this job, the ego develops modes of synthesis as well as screening mechanisms of defense to enable the person to feel, think, and act in an organized and direct manner. This function is apparent

when the person experiences activities that satisfy drives, ego interests, and social demands in a harmonious manner.

Defensive functions

Critical elements of ego function, defense functions prevent the individual from being overwhelmed by anxiety emanating from conflicting instinctual drives and superego demands. **Defense mechanisms** are used by the ego to force out an awareness of sexual and aggressive impulses that would arouse anxiety. The ego, perceiving an impulse being aroused, experiences anticipatory anxiety (signal anxiety) and attempts to protect itself by instituting defenses. Among the more important defense mechanisms are intellectualization, rationalization, identification, introjection, projection, denial, repression, reaction formation, isolation, undoing, displacement, and regression.

The operation of the defense mechanisms is unconscious. Their effect, however, is observable in behavior and is open to direct investigation. Characteristic modes of coping behavior and adaptation, therefore, reflect the activity of the defense mechanisms.

Reality testing

The ego's capacity for objective evaluation and judgment of the external world and its generally accepted meanings is reality testing. Adaptation to reality means adjusting to the changing external world, whether it involves things, objects, or situations. The development of the capacity to test reality and to distinguish fantasy from actuality occurs gradually and is subject to regression and temporary deterioration in children in the face of anxiety. In general, the preservation of reality testing distinguishes relatively normal and neurotic individuals from psychotic ones.

Autonomous functions

Although most ego functions are easily disturbed by instinctual impulses and drives, autonomous functions have been conceptualized as relatively resistant to such forces (Hartmann, 1964). These ego functions develop outside of conflict with the id or superego, unlike such functions as object relations, synthetic functions, drive control, defenses, and reality testing. Autonomous functions are perception, intuition, thinking, language, certain phases of motor development, comprehension, learning, and intelligence.

Psychic conflict

The concept of *psychic conflict* is most simply defined as an internal struggle between the wish to express sexual or aggressive impulses (or both) on the one hand and the internal prohibition against expressing them on the other. In this sense, the clash is an internal struggle between id impulses and superego demands, a struggle that is regulated by the ego as an unconscious mental process. In this dynamic clashing of impulses, the individual is in conflict between drives and wishes, loves and hostilities, fears and longings, urges and resistances. It becomes the task of the organism, specifically the function of the ego, to establish a compromise that will allow for some expression of wishes and drives, but not so much as to engender intense guilt, anxiety, or social disapproval. As will be seen, pathology (dysfunction) in this frame of reference is an attempt to come to terms with unconscious intrapsychic conflict and its attendant anxiety.

In conflict, an unconscious affect-laden impulse or fantasy, disagreeable to the demands of the superego or society, threatens to rise into consciousness, raising the possibility that it might be translated into action. The unconscious ego experiences this as an imminent danger situation. To prevent the feared response from superego or society, anxiety is generated, which may not be perceived by the conscious ego. This anxiety is called **signal anxiety** and is unpleasurable. Since the psyche moves toward pleasure and away from pain, it works as a defense mechanism and is unconsciously set in motion to ward out awareness of the offending impulse and to remove the need for anxiety.

If the defensive maneuver is successful, a certain equilibrium is established and it is said that the ego defenses are intact—not overwhelmed—and effective. In most cases, the principle defense mechanism used is repression, which prevents the emergence of the drive into consciousness. Thus, the most favorable outcome of intrapsychic conflict occurs when a stable relationship exists between drive and defense, and the conflict has little or no intrusive impact on conscious life. When the defense mechanism fails, however, and the strength of the instinctual drive threatens to overcome the capability of the ego to provide an adequate defense, symptoms are likely to emerge. It is thought that symptoms can be explained as the unfavorable outcome of an intrapsychic conflict that has resulted in an ineffective compromise between expression of the drive impulse, disguise of the final expression of the drive, and the imposition of psychic punishment for the expression of that drive. When the defense or the symptom is unsuccessful, however, the signal anxiety (which is unconscious) becomes experienced as the well-known effect "anxiety." (In this sense, anxiety is related to a danger that is unconscious; it should be distinguished from fear, which is a response to a realistic danger.) Hence, psychodynamic theory sees the formation of intrapsychic conflict in terms of a sequence: Instinctual wishes come into conflict with internal or external prohibitions; the ego is threatened and produces signal anxiety; defenses are mobilized; and the conflict is resolved by compromise formations, which result in pathologic symptoms or adaptation.

Intrapsychic conflict is inevitable and universal. It is considered to be the most important dynamic factor underlying human behavior. Most conflicts are shared by virtually all of us. Significant differences exist in our ways of coping with these conflicts, however. That is, *individuals differ with regard to their abilities to handle conflict*. Ultimately, the outcome of conflict determines the basis of pathologic symptoms as well as wide variations in normal and abnormal behaviors. For example, persons who display psychotic symptoms are either those who apparently have no defense mechanisms to deal with those conflicts or those whose defense mechanisms are not adequate to cope with the conflicts. Those who develop neurotic symptoms are handling conflicts by using defense mechanisms at an unconscious level that are ineffective in mediating the conflict. It is generally agreed that a mentally healthy person is relatively reasonable and balanced in his or her attitudes and behavior, and adaptive ego functioning predominates over the drives of the id. Brenner (1982) presents clinical evidence that successful, adaptive compromise formations, even those containing some degree of conflict, are the hallmark of mental health.

The cornerstone of the psychodynamic treatment is insight into the unconscious. Essentially, treatment aims to provide for a safe interpersonal situation in which the patient's unconscious solutions to conflict can be explored, based on the assumption that since early childhood he or she has perceived certain impulses, wishes, fantasies, and emotions too dangerous to manage at a conscious level. The goal of such exploration is intended to lead to the inclusion of previously warded-off components of the personality and to help the patient achieve increasingly mature conscious solutions to his conflicts. This occurs within the context of a secure relationship between therapist and patient, known as the **therapeutic alliance**.

Function–dysfunction continua

Criteria for the definition of function and dysfunction within the psychodynamic frame of reference are only vaguely described and are relative to the subjective affective state of a person. Areas reflecting dysfunction frequently overlap even though they all are derived from conflicts related to the expression of instinctual drives. The continuum concept is not useful to determine relative states of health within this frame of reference because no logic or order can be superimposed on the mechanisms of the unconscious. Ultimately, a state of dysfunction is seen as a manifestation of an unfavorable outcome of intrapsychic conflict; that is, the person is not able to find means to express and gratify instinctual drives in a manner that is both satisfying to the self and acceptable to the demands of the social environment. Stated another way, dysfunction is defined as the presence of anxiety, the signal of unresolved unconscious conflicts. Conversely, a state of function exists when the person has learned to balance the expression of drives in ways that are self-gratifying and acceptable within his or her social environment.

Conflict areas that are assessed and most often serve as the focus of treatment represent what Mosey (1986) has described as the eight universal difficulties related to the expression of instinctual drives that are an intrinsic part of life. She provides a comprehensive description of these areas of potential conflict and dysfunction in her recently articulated "Reconciliation of Universal Issues" frame of reference (Mosey, 1986). They include issues related to intimacy, trust, dependence/independence, reality, aggression, sexuality, feelings of adequacy, and loss.

Behaviors indicative of function–dysfunction

The psychodynamic frame of reference looks *beneath* behavior and recognizes that the same observable unit of behavior may be determined from different directions, may serve different purposes, may be present for different reasons, and may have different meanings, depending on the individual. Behaviors indicative of function–dysfunction cannot be specifically defined because any given unconscious conflict can generate countless variations in behaviors. The nature of the conflicts that produce the dysfunction (anxiety or symptoms) are identified through the exploration and interpretation of nonverbal symbols elicited by unstructured, projective activities. The reader is referred to Mosey (1986) for a broad-based list of behaviors that tend to be associated with each of eight conflict areas. Behavior indicative of function is not identified because in most cases it is simply the absence of behavior indicative of dysfunction.

Postulates regarding change and intervention

Change takes place by bringing symptom-producing unconscious content to consciousness. The goal is to resolve the conflict, to allow for the satisfaction of needs in a manner acceptable to the social environment, and to help the person to learn new, more satisfying behavior with conscious insight. This process occurs primarily through the exploration and interpretation of symbols in projective media, through interaction in a safe, supportive, empathic relationship, and through examination of transference (object relationships) within the therapeutic relationship. The occupational therapist uses activities primarily as tools for nonverbal communication. The individual is encouraged to use such unstructured media as paints, clay, and collage to facilitate the expression of internal feelings, experiences, fantasies, and personal unconscious symbols. Activities are also selected to help determine the ability of the ego to integrate new information, to organize, and to problem solve.

Task groups (Fidler, 1969) are frequently used to help the person learn more self-satisfying and acceptable behaviors and communication skills in a supportive social setting. In addition, the **therapeutic use of self** (Frank, 1958) is of major importance. The information gathered by the therapist is shared with the individual and the treatment team. In this frame of reference, the psychiatrist or psychologist works closely with the therapist in directing the client to new behaviors through experiences in selected activities. Fidler and Fidler (1963) and Mosey (1970, 1986) are prominent leaders in the articulation of the psychodynamic frame of reference for occupational therapy.

References

Brenner, C. (1982). *The mind in conflict.* New York: International University Press.

Fairbairn, W. R. D. (1952). *Psychoanalytic studies of the personality.* London: Routledge & Kegan Paul.

Fidler, G. S. (1969). The task oriented group as a context for treatment. *American Journal of Occupational Therapy, 23,* 43–48.

Fidler, G. S., & Fidler, J. W. (1963). *Occupational therapy: A communication process in psychiatry.* New York: Macmillan.

Frank, J. (1958). The therapeutic use of self. *American Journal of Occupational Therapy, 12,* 215–225.

Freud, S. (1900). *The interpretation of dreams.* New York: W. W. Norton & Co.

Freud, S. (1942). *Beyond the pleasure principle.* New York: W. W. Norton & Co.

Freud, S. (1949). *An outline of psychoanalysis.* New York: W. W. Norton & Co.

Hartmann, H. (1964). *Essays on ego psychology.* New York: International Universities Press.

Kaplan, H., & Sadock, B. (1988). Sigmund Freud: Founder of classical psychoanalysis. In *Synopsis of psychiatry* (5th ed.) Baltimore: Williams & Wilkins.

Kernberg, D. (1976). *Object relations theory and clinical psychoanalysis.* New York: Aronson.

Klein, M. (1959). On the development of mental functioning. In M. Klein (Ed.), *Envy and gratitude.* London: Delacorte Press

Mahler, M. S. (1968). *On human symbiosis and the vicissitudes of individuation.* New York: International University Press.

Mosey, A. (1970). Object relation analysis. In A. Mosey (Ed.), *Three frames of reference for mental health.* Thorofare, NJ: Slack.

Mosey, A. (1986). Reconciliation of universal issues: An analytical frame of reference. In A. Mosey (Ed.), *Psychosocial components of occupational therapy.* New York: Raven Press.

Sullivan, H. (1953). *The interpersonal theory of psychiatry.* New York: W. W. Norton & Co.

Winnicott, D. W. (1958). *Collected papers.* New York: Basic Books.

SECTION 3J
Spatiotemporal adaptation frame of reference

CAROLE J. SIMON

KEY TERMS

Accomodation	*Assimilation*
Association	*Differentiation*
Adaptation	*Spiraling Continuum*

Theoretical base

The essence of the theory of spatiotemporal adaptation can be identified as a strong focus on the development of motor behaviors with an implicit understanding that competence in motor skills subserves development of other facets of the child. Gilfoyle et al. (1981) advanced the concept that **adaptation**, the continuous adjustment of bodily processes to the demands of the environment, occurred as an interaction between an individual and an environment of time and space. This is accomplished through an effective sensorimotor system (SMS) that uses all craniospinal sensory receptors, effectors to muscles and glands, and sensory re-afferents or circuits for feedback. The feedback loop allows the body processes to readjust in an ongoing way to each new piece of sensory information, much of which is a result of some motor behavior. In addition to the **sensorimotor–sensory process**, two other properties of adaptation included are its developmental nature and its purposeful nature. The *developmental nature* refers to the hierarchical properties of the central nervous system, the concept of neuroplasticity, and the growth, maturation, and integration of neuromuscular properties of movement. The *purposeful nature* of adaptation is reflected in strategies of posture and movement that allow activation or mobility (movement) to emanate from a base of control or posture (stability) for performance of desired actions. Postural strategies control movement, and movement strategies give rise to purposeful action (Holt, 1975).

In addition to movement, environment, and adaptation, a fourth category called **spiraling continuum** is a major construct inherent in the theory of spatiotemporal adaptation (Gilfoyle et al., 1990). The concept of spiraling continuum encompasses the sensorimotor–sensory feedback process, the maturation and modification of the maturing nervous system, and the integration of old with new development.

Like Llorens, Gilfoyle et al. blended their concepts with Piaget, Gesell, Erikson, and others. One example of this is a variation of the use of terminology from Piaget of assimilation, accommodation, association, and differentiation. **Assimilation** refers to the "taking in" of stimulus information, and **accommodation** denotes adjustment of the body to react to incoming stimuli. **Association** relates sensory information with the motor act being experienced as well as relating knowledge of past experience to the current experience. **Differentiation** is the process of discriminating the qualities of the specific behavior pertinent to the given situation that requires modification or alteration (Gilfoyle et al., 1990). Imagine a large beach ball being tossed to a child. The child sees the ball approaching (assimilation), adjusts his or her arms to capture the large ball (accommodation), remembers playing catch in the past (association), and recognizes the timing and the size of the ball require modified body responses (differentiation). Use of this concept assists in adapting lower level primitive patterns of posture and movement to higher level complex skills.

Function–dysfunction continua

Four important principles support the spiraling continuum of spatiotemporal adaptation:

1. A child's adaptation process with new experiences is dependent upon past acquired behaviors.
2. With integration of past experiences with new experiences, the past behaviors are modified in some manner and result in a higher level behavior.
3. Integration of higher level behaviors influences and increases the maturity of lower level behaviors.
4. Lower level functions or performance patterns may emerge during adaptation whenever the environmental demands exceed the functional capabilities of the child, resulting in a spatiotemporal stress reaction. (Gilfoyle et al., 1990. p. 23)

Stress to the system is created when the environment makes new demands that must be responded to effectively. This can be a positive growth experience challenging the child to use old knowledge and skills to support new attempts to interact with more complex situations. The child reverts to old strategies when the situation calls for more skill than is available or when the child is summoning learned skills to cope with the new demands. If a child has atypical development, challenges from the environment may have a negative impact, resulting in spatiotemporal distress. Higher levels of functioning may be blocked while the child repeats lower levels of adaptation. Repetition of purposeless lower level behaviors may lead to maladaptation in other developmental domains and has important implications for treatment.

Behaviors indicative of function–dysfunction

Gilfoyle et al. articulate a sequence for development of purposeful activity by describing a primitive phase, a transitional phase, and a mature phase. The primitive phase may have its base in reflex responses, the transitional phase incorporates voluntary components of movement, and the mature phase demonstrates skill. Thus, the key behaviors of walking, for example, would include primitive phase (primary standing, primary walking); transitional phase (pull to stand, supported standing, supported walking); and mature phase (squatting, standing, walking) (Gil-

foyle et al., 1990). It is evident that the new behaviors are based on previously acquired behaviors and that complex adaptation processes are required for this high-level, upright, skilled behavior.

Premises of the spatiotemporal adaptation theory have been expanded to include the following:

1. Development is a function of nervous system maturation, which occurs through a process of person–environment adaptation.
2. Adaptation is dependent upon attention to and active participation with purposeful events within the spatiotemporal dimensions of the environment. Without active participation the self-system is deprived of certain forms of sensation (sensory feedback) about self and the environment which, in turn, affects maturation.
3. Purposeful events (occupations) provide meaningful experiences for enhancement of maturation by directing a higher level adaptive response on the part of the "doer."
4. Higher level responses result from integration with and modification of acquired lower level functions; thus, adaptation of higher level functions and purposes is dependent upon a certain degree of association/differentiation of specific components of acquired lower level actions.
5. Adaptation spirals through primitive, transitional, and mature phases of development occurring at the same time within different body segments. The concurrent development of phases considers the adaptation of posture and movement strategies to developmental and purposeful sequences and of linking strategies and sequences for adaptation to skilled performance.
6. Environmental experiences may present situations of spatiotemporal stress. With stress, the system calls forth past acquired strategies and sequences to act upon the demands of the environment and maintain the system's homeostasis. Thus, acquired strategies and sequences are adapted with the present situation to direct higher level adaptive responses.
7. Spatiotemporal distress provokes dysfunctioning behaviors, resulting in maladaptation. With distress a child repeats purposeless lower level strategies and sequences and these actions are not linked to higher level behaviors. Repetition of purposeless strategies and sequences results in regression.
8. The developing nervous system has capacity to compensate for impairments by forming new connections during the early periods of maturation. Plasticity or flexibility of the formative nervous system enhances its capacity for sensorimotor-sensory adaptation processes to facilitate nervous system modification, e.g., changes in degree of myelination, dendritic growth, formation of new synapses.
9. An intervention program based on a spatiotemporal adaptation process of active participation with purposeful events provides appropriate sensory stimuli necessary to help mature synaptic connections.
10. An intervention program providing appropriate sensory input, motor output, and sensory feedback, and employing the spiraling process of linking strategies and sequences, enhances previously unresponsive brain cells, influences neural organization, establishes new engrams, and thus facilitates maturation. (Gilfoyle et al., 1990, p. 275)

Postulates regarding change and intervention

Spatiotemporal adaptation concepts provide a background for intervention practices that can incorporate all the media, modalities, and methods used in occupational therapy practice. The therapist uses positioning, selected tasks and relationships, active participation, technology, and equipment to promote developmentally appropriate adaptive responses within the framework of building blocks of neuromuscular maturation plus the intermingling of sequential levels of development. The sensorimotor–sensory feedback circuit, posture and movement stategies, adaptation within a spiraling continuum, primitive, transitional and mature phases, neural organization, and stress–distress function can be used effectively to enhance function and interaction of the child. These concepts can also be extrapolated to be useful with the adult client.

References

Gilfoyle, E. M., Grady, A. P., & Moore, J. C. (1981). *Children adapt.* Thorofare, NJ: Slack.

Gilfoyle, E. M., Grady, A. P., & Moore, J. C. (1990). *Children adapt* (2nd ed.). Thorofare, NJ: Slack.

Holt, K. (1975). Movement and child development. *Clinics in Developmental Medicine, 55*, 2–5.

SECTION 3K
Occupational adaptation: an integrative frame of reference

JANETTE K. SCHKADE and SALLY SCHULTZ

KEY TERMS

Adaptation Gestalt   Occupational Functioning

Occupational Adaptation   Occupational Response

Occupational Challenge   Relative Mastery

Occupational Environment

Theoretical base

Occupation and adaptation have been accepted concepts of occupational therapy since its origin (American Occupational Therapy Association, 1979; Kielhofner & Burke, 1977; Meyer, 1922). Numerous occupational therapy publications give credence to the significance and lasting importance of these two concepts (Bing, 1981; Fidler & Fidler, 1978; Fine, 1990; Gilfoyle et al., 1990; Johnson, 1973; King, 1978; Kleinman & Bulkley, 1982; Llorens, 1970, 1984, 1990; Nelson, 1988; Reed, 1984; Reilly, 1962).

The occupational adaptation frame of reference (OA) provides an additional dimension to the understanding of occupation and adaptation and their relationship to health. In this frame of reference, occupation and adaptation are treated as a single integrated phenomenon that describes an innate human process, and the patient's occupational adaptation process becomes the focus of therapy. Given this focus, the OA framework hypothesizes that it is the idiosyncratic process of occupational adaptation which is the essential vehicle through which occupational

therapy affects occupational functioning (Schkade & Schultz, 1992; Schultz & Schkade, 1992).

Occupational adaptation concept

Occupation is one of the most critical features of human growth and development throughout the lifespan. The activities associated with occupation enable persons to adapt to changing expectations that occur naturally from both internal and external influences. **Occupational adaptation** characterizes the interactive nature of occupation and adaptation that is present in the internal process by which persons respond to the demand for change.

A brief discussion of the basic conceptual framework follows. A more complete explanation is presented in Schkade and Schultz (1992) and Schkade (1991). Figure 4-3 shows the relationships among the constructs. The OA frame of reference focuses on the occupational activity of persons within environmental contexts. Individuals are viewed as person systems (sensorimotor, cognitive, psychosocial), uniquely configured for each person as a result of genetic, environmental, and experiential/phenomenologic subsystems. The environmental context is viewed as **occupational environment** (work, play/leisure, self-maintenance). Each occupational environment is uniquely configured by the physical, social, and cultural subsystems present in that environment (Spencer, 1987). These subsystems represent the complex of stimuli that impinge on an individual and set the stage for the **occupational response**. Thus, the person and the occupational environment interact through occupation.

Function–dysfunction continua

Relative mastery

An important aspect of the OA framework is that individual development proceeds through attempts at relative mastery over occupational challenges. **Occupational challenges** are situations that are new to the person and may require patterns of action not yet experienced by that person; therefore, these challenges present the need for some change in the person (adaptation) if **relative mastery** is to be experienced. A fundamental assumption is that the individual is endowed with a *desire for mastery*, the occupational environment has a *demand for mastery* and together these internal and external motivational forces provide an interactive *press for mastery*. When an occupational challenge occurs, both person and occupational environment contribute to the occupational role expectations consistent with an expected outcome of relative mastery.

Adaptive response generation subprocess

The individual, operating with a perception of the occupational role expectations, engages an internal feed forward process (adaptive response generation subprocess), which functions to produce the occupational response. One feature of this subprocess is the *adaptive response mechanism*, which selects components for the occupational response. This mechanism consists of the energy (adaptation energy) necessary to fuel the occupational response (Selye, 1956); the patterns of responses in the person's repertoire as a result of experience and maturation (adaptive response modes); and specific classes of behaviors that can be used (adaptive response behavior). The adaptation en-

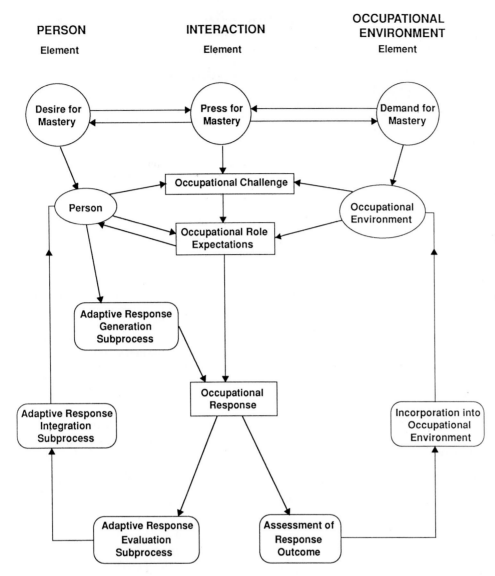

FIGURE 4-3. *Schematic representation of the relationships among constructs. From Schkade, J., & Schultz, S. (1992). Occupational adaptation: toward a holistic approach to contemporary practice. Part I.* American Journal of Occupational Therapy, 46(9). *Copyright 1992 by the American Occupational Therapy Association, Inc. Reprinted with permission.*

ergy has two levels: primary (active attention with relatively high energy expenditure) and secondary (sophisticated, creative with relatively low energy expenditure). Adaptive response modes may be existing, modified, or new. Adaptive response behaviors may be hyperstabilized (primitive), hypermobile (transitional), or modulated with a blend of mobility and stability (mature). After the adaptive response mechanism selects these components, they are configured into a plan called the **adaptation gestalt**, which will guide the occupational response. The adaptation gestalt represents the formatting of the sensorimotor, cognitive, and psychosocial systems perceived by the person to be appropriate to the occupational challenge.

Behaviors indicative of function–dysfunction

Adaptive response evaluation subprocess

After expression of the occupational response, the individual engages another internal process (adaptive response evaluation subprocess) to assess whether relative mastery was experienced.

As a result of answers to questions regarding whether the occupational response was efficient, effective, and satisfying to self and society (the components of relative mastery), the outcome of the occupational response is placed on a continuum ranging from occupational dysadaptation to occupational adaptation.

Adaptive response integration subprocess

Engagement of the third internal subprocess, adaptive response integration subprocess, follows. In this subprocess, the person integrates into the person systems the learning that has occurred and modifies the response repertoire for use with subsequent challenges. As a result of this learning, one of three states of **occupational functioning** is reinforced: occupational adaptation, homeostasis, occupational dysadaptation.

The occupational environment also assesses the outcome of the occupational event, and the external occupational role expectations are subject to potential modification or intensification as a result of that assessment. Thus, for both the person and the occupational environment, feedback functions provide the possibility of modification.

Summary

The occupational adaptation process just described reflects certain critical assumptions:

1. Every occupational response involves all person systems—sensorimotor, cognitive, psychosocial. The adaptation gestalt is a representation of the relative extent to which each system is involved. When a discrepancy exists between perceived and actual demands of a particular occupational challenge, the programming of the gestalt becomes imbalanced and the systems inadequately programmed for relative mastery.
2. For occupational functioning to be enhanced, all three OA subprocesses of the person systems must be operational.
3. Disruption at any point in the OA process results in occupational dysfunction.

Postulates regarding change and implementation

Therapeutic climate

The occupational adaptation frame of reference was developed with the practicing therapist in mind. (See Figure 4-4 for a model of the therapeutic process.) It is intended to be readily applicable to everyday treatment situations. Therapy based on the OA framework results in a distinct therapeutic climate. The therapist assumes the role of the primary facilitator of the therapeutic climate and functions as the agent of the patient's occupational environment(s). The patient functions as the agent of his or her unique person systems. This unique interdependency produces the therapeutic climate. The climate defines the role of each party, the goal of therapy, and the expected outcome. The therapeutic climate inherent in the OA frame of reference empowers both parties to make their optimal contribution to the outcome.

There are four generic steps in practicing from the occupational adaptation frame of reference. The first step is the *initial data gathering and evaluation*. In this phase of therapy, the occupational therapist's task is to collaborate with the patient and others who are significant in the patient's daily life. Through both formal and informal methods of data gathering, the patient's occupational environment(s) and related occupational challenges are identified. The initial data, along with the reason for referral, indicate the type of patient assessment and specific evaluation instruments to be used. The results of the assessment and the initial data gathering serve as the framework for introducing occupational therapy.

In *treatment planning and implementation*, the goal of the therapist throughout each stage of the therapeutic relationship is to positively influence the patient's internal occupational adaptation process. This is an overriding premise that guides therapy with even the most acute patients. The goal of therapy is improvement in the patient's internal occupational adaptation process, rather than functional independence. It is believed that such therapy will result in greater relative mastery as the patient experiences each successive occupational challenge after discharge.

The treatment plan consists of a program of relevant occupational readiness and occupational activity. The treatment program should specifically address both the patient's presenting problems and the patient's occupational environment(s)/role expectations. The more profound the presenting problems, the greater the need for occupational readiness (eg, strengthening exercises, passive range of motion, social skills training). The use of a certified occupational therapy assistant (COTA) to provide occupational readiness services allows the occupational therapist to concentrate on developing and monitoring the overall occupational adaptation program. As is tolerated by the patient, the therapist introduces occupational activities. Such activities have three properties: action, meaning, and process with a product that may be tangible or intangible (Schkade & Schultz, 1992). Although occupational readiness may improve functional independence, occupational activity has greater potential to influence the patient's occupational adaptation process.

The patient's occupational adaptation process cannot be objectively measured. It is possible to *measure outcome effect,* however. This is accomplished by quantifying the patient's experience of relative mastery. As the patient makes gains in his or her occupational adaptation process, relative mastery increases as a byproduct. There are three key points to remember in measurement of outcome effect (Schultz & Schkade, 1992): (1) the effect of therapy is measured by the patient's change in relative mastery of a critical task over time; (2) the critical task must have been identified by the occupational therapist and the patient and must be relevant to his or her idiosyncratic occupational environment; and (3) the patient must not be trained to do the critical task. This would defeat the goal of measurement; however, similar activities may be part of the treatment plan.

Throughout treatment planning and implementation the therapist assumes a questioning posture. The therapist periodically *evaluates the occupational adaptation program.* Programming must be continually questioned as to whether it is providing the patient with the optimal opportunity to improve his or her internal occupational adaptation process. The therapist must continually work to engage the patient in therapy that meets this goal. The therapist frequently assesses not only the patient's response to therapy but the quality of the therapeutic climate. Though the patient–therapist relationship is collaborative, the therapist assumes primary responsibility for creating and modifying the therapeutic climate to promote positive outcomes.

Implications for treatment: an example

The occupational adaptation frame of reference requires the therapist to be flexible, to be highly creative, and to approach the therapy relationship from a nontraditional perspective. As with all frames of reference, occupational adaptation has greater applicability in some situations than in others. The applicability of this frame of reference is not defined by type of practice domain, that is, physical dysfunction or psychosocial dysfunction, however. The following case illustrates application:

CASE STUDY

Jane is a 45-year-old woman who received a closed head injury in a motor vehicle accident. Before the accident, she had been employed for 15 years as an elementary school teacher. Her teaching area is writing and spelling. She is a single

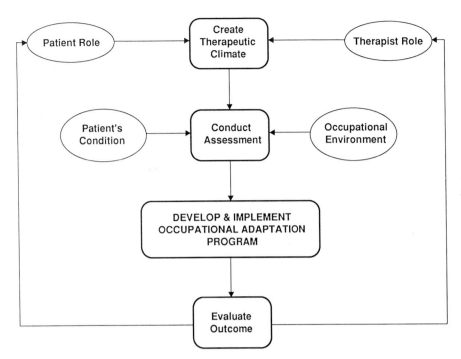

FIGURE 4-4. *Model of therapeutic process.*

mother of two teenagers. Jane has been in the rehabilitation unit for 2 weeks. She presented with classic symptoms of memory loss, word-finding difficulty, impaired speech, and right-sided weakness. She is right-handed.

The therapist might report on the patient's progress in a treatment team meeting in the following manner.

In our initial interview, Jane stated that her greatest concern was being able to get back to work. Not only did she need the income, she enjoyed her work. Occupational therapy has focused on enhancing her potential to again experience relative mastery in her work environment. I assessed her occupational environment and identified several significant occupational challenges to guide treatment. I initially started her with a basic upper extremity movement and exercise program. She progressed rapidly but questioned her ability to carry out tasks associated with her work. The patient and I discussed her concerns. Based on this, her treatment program was changed to include occupational activities that she thought were more relevant to her work. This change really excited her. Although her progress has been slow by her standards, I am very encouraged. I have noted that she is beginning to make her own modifications and generate new ways of doing tasks associated with teaching. She is becoming increasingly independent in this process. I plan to progressively upgrade the challenges presented by her occupational activities. The occupational readiness training program will be discontinued, providing more opportunity for occupational activity. Based on her present status and continued therapy, Jane has a good prognosis for successful and satisfying performance within her occupational environment.

Summary

Guidelines for use of occupational adaptation frame of reference in treatment applications reflects its unique perspective. First, it is a treatment approach designed to make an impact on the client's internal process of occupational adaptation. Second, the treatment focus is the idiosyncratic occupational adaptation necessary for the patient to experience relative mastery over occupational challenges. Third, the therapeutic roles assumed by both patient and therapist empower them to maximally affect the patient's occupational functioning. The patient serves as his or her own agent, whereas the therapist functions as an agent of the occupational environment. Finally, the goal of treatment is to improve occupational functioning as a result of occupational adaptation. Research is underway to continue to develop and refine this frame of reference (Spencer & Davidson, 1989).

References

American Occupational Therapy Association (1979): The philosophical base of occupational therapy. *American Journal of Occupational Therapy, 33,* 785.

Bing, R. (1981). The 1981 Eleanor Clarke Slagle Lecture. Occupational therapy revisited: A paraphrastic journey. *American Journal of Occupational Therapy, 35*(8), 499–518.

Fidler, G., & Fidler, J. (1978). Doing and becoming: Purposeful action and self-actualization. *American Journal of Occupational Therapy, 32,* 305–310.

Fine, S. (1990). Resilience and human adaptability: Who rises above adversity? 1990 Eleanor Clarke Slagle Lecture. *American Journal of Occupational Therapy, 45,* 493–504.

Gilfoyle, E., Grady, A., & Moore, J. (1990). *Children adapt* (2nd ed.), Thorofare NJ: Slack.

Johnson, J. (1973). The 1972 Eleanor Clarke Slagle Lecture. Occupational therapy: A model for the future. *American Journal of Occupational Therapy, 27,* 1–7.

Kielhofner, G., & Burke J. (1977). Occupational therapy after 60 years: Changing identity and knowledge. *American Journal of Occupational Therapy, 31*(10), 675–689.

King, L. (1978). Towards a science of adaptive responses. *American Journal of Occupational Therapy, 32,* 429–437.

Kleinman, B., & Bulkley, B. (1982). Some implications of a science of adaptive responses. *American Journal of Occupational Therapy, 36,* 15–19.

Llorens, L. (1970). Facilitating growth and development: The promise of occupational therapy. *American Journal of Occupational Therapy, 24,* 93–101.

Llorens, L. (1984). Theoretical conceptualizations of occupational therapy: 1960–1982. *Occupational Therapy in Mental Health, 4*(2), 1–14.

Llorens, L. (1990). Forward. In E. Gilfoyle, A. Grady, & J. Moore, *Children adapt* (2nd ed.), pp. xi–xii. Thorofare, NJ: Slack.

Meyer, A. (1922). The philosophy of occupational therapy. *Archives of Occupational Therapy, 1,* 1.

Nelson, D. (1988). Occupation: Form and performance. *American Journal of Occupational Therapy, 42*(10), 633–641.

Reed, K. (1984). *Models of practice in occupational therapy*. Baltimore: Williams & Wilkins.

Reilly, M. (1962). Occupational therapy can be one of the great ideas of 20th century medicine. *American Journal of Occupational Therapy, 16,* 1–9.

Schkade, J. K. (1991). Occupational adaptation as a model of professional development: Transition from student to clinician. Unpublished manuscript.

Schkade, J. K., & Schultz, S. (1992). Occupational adaptation: toward a holistic approach to contemporary practice. Part I. *American Journal of Occupational Therapy, 49*(9).

Schultz, S., & Schkade, J. K. (1992). Occupational adaptation: toward a holistic approach to contemporary practice. Part II. *American Journal of Occupational Therapy, 49*(10).

Selye, H. (1956). *The stress of life*. New York: McGraw-Hill.

Spencer, J. (1987). Environmental assessment strategies. *Topics in Geriatric Rehabilitation, 3,* 35–41.

Spencer, J., & Davidson, H. (1989). *Community adaptive patterns assessment*. Houston, TX: Texas Woman's University.

CHAPTER 5

Knowledge bases of occupational therapy

SECTION 1

Neurosciences

SHEREEN D. FARBER

KEY TERMS

Functional Neuroanatomy	Neurochemistry
Heterarchy	Neuropathology
Hierarchy	Neurophysiology
Homeostasis	Neurosciences
Neuroanatomy	Plasticity
Neurobiology	Therapeutic Intention

LEARNING OBJECTIVES

Upon completion of this section the reader will be able to:

1. *Comprehend the relevance of neuroscience as a knowledge base necessary to interpret human behavior in its cultural and environmental context.*

2. *Survey a selection of current neuroscientific assumptions and apply these assumptions to occupational therapy practice.*

3. *Stimulate neuroscientific and occupational therapy critical thinking by facilitating conceptual transfers from the context of pure neuroscience to occupational therapy.*

Purpose

What motivates an occupational therapist to learn about the nervous system in its extraordinary complexity? For many students, their initiation to the neurosciences consists of memorizing alien vocabulary, mastering neural tracts that connect multiple unfamiliar structures, and studying details that seem insignificant to human behavior. Inadequate numbers of students and clinicians uncloak "the secret" that by exploring nervous system functions, they can acquire a common denominator essential to interpretation and comprehension of typical and pathologic human behavior (Farber, 1989). Ideally, those who instruct occupational therapy students in neuroscientific and related areas should require conceptual understanding of the relationships between optimal nervous system function and quality occupational performance. The primary objective of this section is to provide information that will initiate meaningful dialogue among therapists, basic scientists, physicians, and other members of the treatment team. It is hoped that resourceful action plans will be designed not only to assist those afflicted with neurologic diseases but all clients who need occupational therapy services.

Basic definitions

When students are exposed to structures and locations within the central, peripheral, or autonomic nervous systems, they are learning **neuroanatomy**. **Neurophysiology** emphasizes the basic functions of neural structures, ranging from individual cell membranes to the cerebral cortex. Neuroanatomy unaccompanied by and not integrated with neurophysiology provides an incomplete neuroscientific foundation for therapists; many instructors compromise by teaching courses entitled **functional neuroanatomy**. Such courses often include the development of the nervous system; a superficial unit on **neurochemistry**, the actual communication systems of the brain; regional and systemic overviews of the nervous system; and a cursory exposure to **neuropathology**, the diseases of the brain. Relatively few occupational therapy students, however, are introduced to the comprehensive subject of **neurobiology** or the **neurosciences**, a discipline that includes all the terms defined above and is constantly evolving to incorporate other pertinent scientific areas.

Current status of neurobiology in the United States

The 1990s have been declared "the decade of the brain" by the United States Congress, which supplied the neuroscientific research community with a $1.2 billion annual budget intended to expand the neuroscientific knowledge base. This decade has the potential to help us understand, prevent, and treat the more than 1000 conditions related to nervous system dysfunction (Carey, 1990). Ninety percent of what we currently accept as valid information regarding nervous system function has been learned in the last decade. With this minuscule neuroscientific knowledge lifespan, it is necessary to be flexible to "new wisdom" and to be ready to integrate it with older but still valid concepts. In keeping with this perspective, the American Occupational Therapy Association initiated a self-study series, entitled *Neuroscience Foundations of Human Performance*, comprising 12 lessons, ranging from an interdisciplinary perspective of the brain and human performance to assessment of human performance related to brain function. Its editor, C. B. Royeen, invited as contributors occupational therapists with advanced degrees in neuroscience, master occupational therapy clinicians in neurorehabilitation, and scientists knowledgeable in our profession (Royeen, 1990). By studying this series at their individual learning rates, therapists can update neuroscientific assumptions, learn to formulate new applications to practice areas and, most importantly, ask knowledgeable questions regarding the proficiency of occupational therapy treatment in goal attainment. The American Occupational Therapy Association has also been involved with and continues to plan a series of continuing education programs to parallel the decade of the brain.

Neuroscience and occupational therapy are relatively young fields of study, both of which are aimed at comprehending the single organ that orchestrates all aspects of our lives. Each discipline operates with unique styles reflective of diverse philosophical bases. Leaders in the field of neuroscience have targeted a number of major areas to investigate during the decade of the brain, including homeostatic mechanisms of the brain; information storage and usage; expression of drives, rhythms, and emotions; and alterations that occur during neurologic and mental disorders (Carey, 1990). Occupational therapists who are prepared to collaborate in research related to these priorities, or to suggest additional questions reflective of crucial functional problems, will likely establish vital connections with neuroscientists that will persist long beyond this decade.

Current assumptions regarding the nervous system and its application to occupational therapy

The purpose of examining neuroscientific assumptions is to challenge the learner to investigate the relationships between contemporary findings in neuroscience and occupational therapy practice. Think of this as a reality test in which, if we accept a given assumption, we must examine the way in which we are using or not using it in occupational therapy. It is impossible to select all the current assumptions being investigated in neuroscientific research projects; however, each assumption that has been chosen will serve as a model for critical thinking and as a potential research proposal in the occupational therapy field.

Assumption 1

Although every brain has similar structures, the way in which each brain functions is totally unique (Maguire, 1990). Many hospitals use protocols to treat patients with given diagnoses. Unquestionably, patients with certain diagnoses or lesions demonstrate at least a few common behaviors and problems, but each patient has lived a unique life resulting in diversity of responses to identical stimuli. The way a person perceives a situation, solves a problem, or plans an action reflects that person's genetics and life experiences. Treatment protocols must be constantly modified as mandated by the individual responses of the patient. This is the only way to achieve optimal occupational performance or adaptive responses.

Assumption 2

There is a reciprocal connection between the mind and the body (Kandel et al., 1991; Farber, 1989; Ornstein & Sobel, 1987; Kielhofner & Fisher, 1991). Transdisciplinary acceptance has been expressed that for every mind state, there is a body reaction. The reciprocal condition is also accepted and expected. If this assumption is valid, why do we divide occupational therapy practice by diagnostic categories such as physical disabilities or psychosocial dysfunction? Should we be testing our practice premises and beliefs across all practice areas because it is impossible to categorize one human being into a physical or mental condition? One core belief of occupational therapy is that the therapist must address occupational performance problems across the continuum of mind, body, and environment. How many facilities are available that we can send students to that routinely practice mind–body–environment integration? Perhaps it is time to examine and adjust our educational and clinical philosophies?

Assumption 3

The human nervous system has the capacity to reorganize itself after injury, and that capacity persists for long periods. This reorganization is referred to as ***plasticity***. Plasticity is more potent during the early years of life, but does exist throughout the lifespan (Kandel et al., 1991; Cowan et al., 1991, Bach-y-Rita et al., 1988; Cotman & Nieto-Sampedro, 1984; Boyeson & Bach-y-Rita, 1989). An exhaustive literature review of plasticity will yield countless resources that demonstrate that the nervous system can and does reorder itself after injury.

Many factors may influence this reorganization, including the age of the patient; the degree of injury; the rate of injury; the skill of the therapeutic staff; the environment; the hopes and belief systems of patients, families, and health care professionals; and other ill-defined phenomena. In fact, Wolpaw et al. (1991) refer to a concept called activity-driven plasticity wherein learning (or relearning) results from experientially produced changes in synaptic connections. Many of the changes produced are short term, but it is surprising that some modifications are of long duration. Discovering the most efficacious agents to expedite plasticity should be a high priority of those who work with the brain-injured population.

Assumption 4

The manner in which we use and understand a therapeutic approach may ultimately be as important as the actual therapeutic technology (Farber, 1989). The biology of hope includes therapeutic intention, therapeutic and patient beliefs, and rapport between patients and therapists. Benson and Proctor (1987) believe that self-healing is often possible. If this is true, therapists should probe their own beliefs and purposes to maximize their positive therapeutic intention. If therapists do not realize that their personal, unresolved wounds may disrupt the therapeutic process, their ability to problem solve with their patients will be impaired. In addition, therapists must internalize and customize the therapeutic system they embrace, so that they can make automatic adaptations in the methodology to enhance patient performance. Failure to understand the underlying assumptions of a frame of reference for treatment or inability to modify that treatment system to flow with the therapists' beliefs and abilities may further hamper critical problem solving and positive patient outcomes.

Assumption 5

The brain is the major organ of adaptation. The nervous system requires internal stability and works hard to preserve that stability while maintaining flexible responses. **Homeostasis** (a state of equilibrium) and adaptation are not contradictory terms. Subtle changes in behavior or in the environment may be the best method of producing positive occupational performance and preventing rebound from large changes in homeostasis (Farber, 1989; Ornstein & Sobel, 1987). During evolution, some animals moved from water environments to land. These terrestrial creatures had to adapt over long periods of time. The lessons of evolution should guide and direct those who use sensory stimulation for the purpose of eliciting adaptive responses. The larger and more rapid the change from baseline, the greater the likelihood of rebound; the smaller and less rapid the change from baseline, the greater the opportunity to build adaptation. Testing and validating this assumption within an occupational therapy context would add immeasurably to the scientific foundation on which we operate.

Assumption 6

The development and activation of the sensory systems may produce behavioral consequences when developmental progression is abnormal (Ayres, 1972; Farber, 1982; Dunn, 1991). Numerous studies demonstrate formation, myelination, and interaction among the various sensory systems. The touch/tactile and vestibular systems develop early, whereas functional development of the visual system takes much longer. In one scenario, a type of vestibular dysfunction may impair ocular motility if the connections from the vestibular nuclei to those of the cranial nerve nuclei responsible for eye motility are lesioned. Therapists should examine patients' responses to all sensory input to determine whether the early evolving sensory systems show signifi-cant pathology. Occupational performance may be enhanced when sensory integration of the early developing systems is promoted, thus forming a meaningful context for sensations of the systems that develop later. This hypothesis was introduced to occupational therapists by Dr. A. Jean Ayres and remains to be further validated.

Assumption 7

Early postnatal movements are based on reflex hierarchies, whereas skilled movement requires a distributed heterarchy (Brooks, 1986; Carr & Shepherd, 1988, Carr et al., 1987; Turvey, 1977; Farber, 1991; Poole, 1991). Our knowledge about the motor system is changing rapidly with new technology. During the last two decades, intense modification of motor learning concepts has occurred. Those of us schooled in the 1960s were taught about the reflex hierarchy and several other obscure neural structures that contributed to our ability to move. Now we are learning that countless variables influence motor control and learning, that multiple theories exist regarding how normal persons learn activity, and that there is a lack of agreement regarding rehabilitation using motor learning theories.

The term **heterarchy** is commonly associated with new motor information because it refers to multiple centers, with distinct tasks, which are called on under certain circumstances. Assumptions made in each motor learning theory should be questioned, and any new theories must be comprehensive enough to integrate old but valid concepts with new findings. Invalid notions must be purged. It is beyond the scope of this treatment to review all the motor learning theories. See the bibiography for additional sources. Many of the motor learning theories were formulated based on data gathered on normal subjects; therefore, knowledge is inadequate regarding how the brain-damaged person relearns movement (although progress is being made).

Conclusions

Neuroscience is a valuable foundation for understanding human behavior. Knowledge of neuroscience is already necessary for the competent practice of occupational therapy. Both students and neuroscience instructors must work together to make neuroscience come alive for the occupational therapist.

You are challenged to review your neuroscience texts and look for further assumptions that should be presented to your peers, be integrated with occupational therapy core values, serve as a basis for development of new theories and intervention strategies, and inspire you to embrace this material as an integral part of your body of knowledge. It is often helpful to seek mentors who have successfully navigated the neural pathways and incorporated this knowledge into occupational science.

References

Ayres, A. J. (1972). *Sensory integration and learning disorders*. Los Angeles: Western Psychological Services.

Bach-y-Rita, P., Lazarus, J-A. C., Boyeson, M. G., Balliet, R., & Mayers, T. A. (1988). Neural aspects of motor function as a basis of early and post-acute rehabilitation. In J. DeLisa (Ed.), *Rehabilitation medicine* (pp. 175–195). Philadelphia: J. B. Lippincott.

Benson, H., & Proctor, W. (1987). *Your maximum mind*. New York: Avon Books.

Boyeson, M. G., & Bach-y-Rita, P. (1989). Determinants of brain plasticity. *Journal of Neurological Rehabilitation, 3*, 35–37.

Brooks, V. B. (1986). *The neural basis of motor control*. New York: Oxford University Press.

Carey, J. (Ed.). (1990). *Brain facts: A primer on the brain and nervous system*. Washington, DC: Society for Neuroscience.

Carr, J. H., & Shepherd, R. B. (1988). *A motor relearning programme for stroke*. Rockville, MD: Aspen Publications.

Carr, J. H., Shepherd, R. B., Gordon, J., Gentile, A. M., & Held, J. M. (1987). *Movement science: Foundations for physical therapy rehabilitation*. Rockville, MD: Aspen Publications.

Cotman, C. W., & Nieto-Sampedro, M. (1984). Cell biology of synaptic plasticity. *Science, 225*, 1287–1294.

Cowan, W. M., Shooter, E. M., Stevens, C. F., & Thompson, R. F. (Eds.). (1991). *Annual Review of Neuroscience* (Vol. 14). Palo Alto, CA: Annual Reviews.

Dunn, W. (1991). Sensory dimensions of performance. In C. Christiansen & C. Baum (Eds.), *Occupational therapy overcoming human performance deficits* (pp. 230–257). Thorofare, NJ: Slack.

Farber, S. D. (1982). *Neurorehabilitation: A multisensory approach*. Philadelphia: W. B. Saunders.

Farber, S. D. (1989). Neuroscience and occupational therapy: Vital connections—Eleanor Clarke Slagle Lectureship. *American Journal of Occupational Therapy, 43*, 637–646.

Farber. S. D. (1991). Neuromotor dimensions of performance. In C. Christiansen & C. Baum (Eds.), *Occupational therapy overcoming human performance deficits* (pp. 258–282). Thorofare, NJ: Slack.

Fisher, A. G., Murray E., & Bundy, A. C. (Eds.). (1991). *Sensory integration theory and practice*. Philadelphia: F. A. Davis.

Kandel, E. R., Schwartz, J. H., & Jessel, T. M. (Eds.). (1991). *Principles of neural science* (3rd ed.). New York: Elsevier.

Kielhofner, G., Fisher, A. G. (1991). Mind-brain-body relationships. In A. G. Fisher, E. Murray, & Bundy, A. C. (Eds.), *Sensory integration theory and practice* (pp. 30–44). Philadelphia: F. A. Davis.

Maguire, J. (1990). *Care and feeding of the brain: A guide to your gray matter*. New York: Doubleday.

Ornstein, R., & Sobel, D. (1987). *The healing brain*. New York: Simon & Schuster.

Poole, J. (1991). Motor control—Lesson 11. In C. B. Royeen (Ed.), *Neuroscience foundations of human performance*. Rockville, MD: American Occupational Therapy Association.

Royeen, C. B. (Ed.). (1990). *Neuroscience foundations of human performance*. Rockville, MD: American Occupational Therapy Association.

Turvey, M. T. (1977). Preliminaries to a theory of action with reference to vision. In R. Shaw & J. Bransford (Eds.), *Perceiving, acting, and knowing*. Hillsdale, NJ: J. Erlbaum.

Wolpaw, J. R., Schmidt, J. T., & Vaughan, T. M. (Eds.). (1991). Activity driven CNS changes in learning and development. *Annals of the New York Academy of Science, 627*, 115.

Bibliography

Barr, M. L., & Kiernan, J. A. (1988). *The human nervous system: An anatomical viewpoint* (5th ed.). Philadelphia: J. B. Lippincott.

Curtis, B. A. (1990). *Neurosciences: The basics*. Philadelphia: Lea & Febiger.

Gazzaniga, M. S. (1989). Organization of the human brain. *Science, 245*, 947–950.

Hutchinson, M. (1986). *Mega brain: New tools and techniques for brain growth and mind expansion*. New York: Ballantine Books.

Jackson, C. (Ed.). (1990). *How things work the brain*. Morristown, NJ: Time-Life Books.

Klivington, K. (1989). *The science of the mind*. Cambridge MA: MIT Press.

Littell, E. H. (1990). *Basic neuroscience for the health professions*. Thorofare, NJ: Slack.

Noback, C. R., Strominger, N. L., & Demarest, R. J. (1991). *The human nervous system introduction and review* (4th ed.). Philadelphia: Lea & Febiger.

Romero-Sierra, C. (1986). *Neuroanatomy: A conceptual approach*. New York: Churchill Livingstone.

SECTION 2A
Human development across the life span

CAROLE J. SIMON and MARY MARGARET DAUB

KEY TERMS

Adolescent	*Infant*
Adulthood	*Maturation*
Childhood	*Operant Conditioning*
Classical Conditioning	*Prenatal*
Cognitive Development	*Reflexes*
Human Development	

LEARNING OBJECTIVES

Upon completion of this section the reader will be able to:

1. *Understand the value of a knowledge base of human development to the therapeutic process.*

2. *Recognize influential factors that either support or interrupt human growth and development.*

3. *Understand theoretical foundations of growth and development as a base for occupational therapy practice.*

4. *Develop an awareness of the interplay of various developmental spheres in both the child and adult.*

5. *Recognize stage-specific issues and tasks to be accomplished throughout the lifespan.*

Importance of knowledge base

A broad view of human growth and development suggests that the ability to learn, adapt, and cope with the world has its ultimate genesis in movement and emotions. These two entities are linked because movement must come from an organism that feels secure enough to risk attempts to move and interact with the environment. The motor and socioemotional status of humans carries paramount importance to their well-being. Movement represents one of the first ways that humans learn about their world. If that learning channel is interrupted through dysfunction or trauma, a trickle-down effect will have an impact on many other developmental areas of function. Concomitantly, the sense of self that can come from a secure emotional base allows exploration of the world because one feels comfortable venturing forth. Thus, the availability and nurturance of these areas are critical to subsequent development of skill in the child, since development progressed sequentially from such building blocks.

Human development can be defined as changes in the structure, thought, or behavior of a person that occur as a function of both biologic and environmental influences (Craig, 1976). These changes may be quantitative or qualitative. Quantitative changes, such as height, physical skills, and vocabulary, are easily understood and measured. Qualitative changes are not so easily measured because they include a subjective element: there is no scale on which to weigh the influence of social interactions, the significance of dreams, or the level of a child's self-awareness. These quantitative and qualitative changes are part of developmental continuum, an ongoing, orderly process that lasts from conception to death.

During this process certain tasks are expected to be accomplished along the way. Mastery of specific skills or interactions at certain stages of development lays the groundwork for more mature behaviors to unfold. A developmental task arises at an approximate period in a person's life. Successful achievement of these tasks leads to happiness and success with later tasks, whereas failure leads to personal unhappiness, societal disapproval, and difficulty with later tasks (Havighurst, 1972). Three sources guide developmental tasks: (1) physical maturation, such as myelination of the neural mechanism for walking or toilet training; (2) cultural or societal pressures, such as schooling or responsible citizenship; and (3) personal values and aspirations derived from personality, temperament, and self-concept, such as honesty, intimacy, and occupation.

There are certain critical or sensitive periods when a person is able to learn best (Havighurst, 1972; Short-DeGraff, 1988). Critical periods are of limited duration and represent a period during which certain experiences must occur if they are to become an integral part of the person's repertoire. The concept of readiness emerges within this framework. Havighurst (1972) discusses "the teachable moment" when some developmental tasks may occur at ages of special sensitivity for learning them. For example, when the body is ripe (physical), society requires (culture), and the self is ready (aspirations, values), the child will learn to read. These concepts are important to occupational therapists, who must recognize and act on the readiness exhibited by their patients. Children have an innate drive to progress to the next level of skill. If this drive has been diminished or complicated by pathology, the occupational therapist can supplement and enhance function by recognizing what should occur next developmentally. Efforts will be wasted if emphasis is placed on tasks that are beyond reach due to immature physical, societal, or personal status.

This chapter is devoted to the developmental aspects that contribute to creating that miraculous and complex entity known as a human being: physical, sensory, perceptual, cognitive, emotional, social, and cultural. Figure 5-1 depicts the holistic view of each of these aspects as inherent in child development. As the person grows, these aspects mature and expand along a developmental continuum. Although they differ in content, their emphasis and focus are dynamically interrelated and interdependent. One aspect can strengthen another; a secure self can promote motor exploration. At certain critical periods one aspect may gain importance over another. If the occupational therapist fails to pay attention to all aspects of the develop-

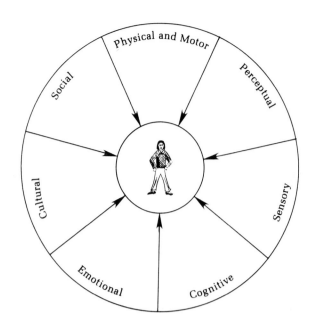

FIGURE 5-1. *The developmental aspects.*

mental wheel at all times, however, the best potential of the child may be circumvented.

There are several important reasons for occupational therapists to acquire a sound knowledge base about human growth and development. First, the primary focus of occupational therapy is on those who have had an interruption in one or more of the developmental aspects somewhere in the life continuum. These may require *habilitation* for aspects that have never or minimally been acquired, or *rehabilitation* for aspects lost through disease or trauma. The therapist may be able to capitalize on recognized strengths of the child who developed normally until meningitis at 3 years of age left him or her with poor stability and choreiform movements. Another 3-year-old born with athetosis may look somewhat similar, but need more attention to basic skills never experienced in his or her short lifetime. To provide meaningful service to these children, the occupational therapist must understand the underlying principles of growth, function, and the sequences of growth and behavior that are somewhat predictable for normal human development.

A second justification for the use of a solid knowledge base occurs when working with adult patients. Often the sequence of return of function takes place in a similar manner to the initial acquisition of the skill in infancy and early childhood. Thus, the astute therapist has a map to follow for rehabilitation of the stroke patient. The motor development may return through stages that replicate primitive, transitional, and mature stages of development.

As an agent of change, the occupational therapist can influence the changes a client must make to adapt to his or her life situation. To accomplish this change effectively, the therapist must know the range, potential, and readiness for change evident in the patient. Therefore, the therapist must have a working knowledge of the concepts of change, adaptation, and maturation inherent in the study of human development. By knowing normal developmental sequences and aspects, the therapist can recognize abnormal function and implement procedures to "normalize" the pathologic and dysfunctional interruptions.

Factors that influence growth and development

At birth children are biologic beings with inherited genes and characteristics. They then enter a world full of experiences that act on their biologic heritage. Scientists have long debated the relative importance of biologic versus environmental influences on the ultimate developmental make-up of each person. Biologic components include stages of growth, maturation, and aging. Growth refers to increase in size, function, or complexity up to some point of optimal maturity. Maturation reflects the emergence of an organism's genetic potential and consists of a series of preprogrammed changes that comprise alterations not only in the organism's structure and form but also in its complexity, integration, organization, and function. Aging is biologic evolution beyond the point of optimal maturity (Craig, 1976). Environmental factors include all human and nonhuman experiences that the developing child encounters, or the lack of such experiences, and the learning that results from such encounters.

The traditional debate regarding the relative effects of inheritance or learning on development is referred to as the *nature–nurture controversy* (Short-DeGraff, 1988). The contention is that behavior is primarily inherited (nature) or acquired (nurture). Many names have been applied to this concept including *maturation versus learning, nativism versus empiricism, innate versus acquired, preformed versus epigenetic, heredity versus environment,* or *biology versus experience* (Kagan, 1984; Lerner, 1976). Occupational therapists can reflect on the contribution of biology, environment, or both on the function of their clients. The innate endowments of the child or adult can be coupled with the therapeutic milieu to maximize performance. The important view for clinicians involves understanding that in every organism, internal and external forces interact in unique and often unpredictable combinations to produce behavior (Short-DeGraff, 1988). The goal of therapy is not to identify limiting factors, but to implement special interactions between the therapist, the environment, and the patient to enhance his or her unique potential for change.

The biologic make-up of the child is also the result of the chromosomal attributes of the sperm and the ovum. Genetic defects can occur that affect the viability of the embryo and the outcome of the fetus. Most severe chromosomal abnormalities are spontaneously aborted (Milansky, 1979). There are, however, those infants who survive and are born with defects that will need therapy. A widespread variety of birth defects may have a genetic origin including mental retardation, limb deficiency, sensory impairments, metabolic disorders, malformation of organs, structural abnormalities, and others. Mutations may also occur as a result of environmental factors. Drugs, tobacco, alcohol, irradiation, pollution, poor prenatal care, infection, and faulty nutrition may contribute to the appearance of developmental disorders or birth defects.

General principles of human development

There are some general principles and issues of human growth and development that must be understood before looking closer at specific areas of normal human growth.

1. *Development is orderly, predictable, sequential, and cumulative.*

2. *Each child develops at a different pace.* There is a wide range of individual differences along the normal continuum.
3. *The expectations of others affect a child's behavior.*
4. *At any one stage of development, a child might be placing particular emphasis on one aspect at the expense of another.*
5. *The behavior of a child does not consistently "improve"; it seems to alternate between periods of equilibrium (a good balance) and disequilibrium (less balance).*

Principles of maturation

In addition to these general principles of development, there are certain principles of maturation that tend to be relatively independent of environmental influences. These can be considered as anatomic directions of growth.

1. *Cephalocaudal pattern of development.* Muscular development, control, and coordination progress from the head to the feet. That is, head control precedes that of the trunk and lower extremities.
2. *Proximal-distal and medial (rostral)-lateral patterns of development.* Parts of the body closest (proximal), to the spine tend to be controlled in a coordinated manner before the parts farther away (distal) from it. Thus, the shoulder and elbow gain some control before the hand. Additionally, the hand held in anatomic position develops from the ulnar border (medial) to the radial border (lateral).
3. *Mass to specific pattern of development.* Initially, much of the motor activity of the infant consists of whole-body movement. With maturity, these undifferentiated and generalized mass responses become more specific.
4. *Gross-motor to fine-motor pattern of development.* Since control of proximal musculature precedes that of distal musculature, it follows that mastery of the larger muscles precedes mastery of the smaller muscles. This mastery must then become even more refined and definitive to permit acquisition of skills.

These four principles governing growth are not static but are continuously influencing motor development. All of the principles of growth and maturation can be applied to the habilitation and rehabilitation of clients.

Llorens (1970) refers to horizontal and longitudinal growth of the developing child. With this approach one considers development in all the aspects of the developmental wheel as it occurs simultaneously at stage-specific sensitive periods across all domains. This is horizontal growth and may represent refinement of one area at the expense of another for the moment. Over time the skills that have been mastered are built on to promote even higher levels of competence and skill. This is called longitudinal or chronologic growth. Such a view of the developing child allows the holistic approach to be supported over time. For further information, see Chapter 4, Section 3.

The concept of readiness is an important factor influencing growth and development. The maturational level of the child, cultural expectations, and personal aspirations and motivations contribute to possible progress. School readiness is responsible for success in that realm. Other readiness levels support motor and social skills.

Theoretical foundations

Theories are connected ideas or concepts that serve to explain a phenomenon. They are a way to think about the justification for an approach to treatment. That approach to treatment, known as a frame of reference, is the bridge between theory and clinical practice. Theories of human development are important to the occupational therapy process because

1. Theories serve as an organizing mechanism: they attempt to sort out some of the complex factors in development.
2. Theories provide a basis for frames or reference from which one can develop therapeutic program objectives and treatment.
3. Theories are a basis for research that is needed in the field of occupational therapy.
4. Knowledge of different theories extends insight into human behavior, presenting alternative explanations of behavior on which to base treatment goals.
5. Theories provide the bases for justification and accountability. In essence, a theory becomes the rationale for the treatment process.

In adhering to a single theory to the exclusion of others, the therapist must keep the following in mind.

1. No one theory accounts for every aspect of the developmental process; therefore, the therapist must fully understand the parameters of any chosen theory.
2. The therapist must be able to translate the theory effectively into occupational therapy application.
3. Strict adherence to just one theory does not always allow for individual differences and may indeed limit the repertoire and potential for therapy.
4. A single-theory approach may narrow a therapist's perspective and limit professional growth potential.

Conversely, when a therapist chooses an eclectic approach, that is, bases a rationale on varied sources of theories, caution is advised because to be truly eclectic, the therapist must be thoroughly versed in each theory. The therapist must know the advantages and limitations of the theories to present a clearly defined rationale for client treatment.

No matter which approach is chosen, it is imperative that everyone involved in the treatment process (1) know what rationale is being used, (2) understand how the rationale can be translated into occupational therapy practice, (3) be clear about how this treatment can be adapted to the individual client's needs, and (4) concur with the adoption of this rationale as a basis for treatment. Consistency in treatment approach from all personnel and disciplines allows for stability and consistency in patient response, thus avoiding confusion.

Learning theory

Learning is the basic developmental process by which an individual's behavior is changed by the environment. Learning is defined as a relatively permanent change in behavior or in having the capacity for behavior resulting from either experience or practice (Craig, 1976). There may be temporary changes in behavior as a result of behavioral states, fatigue, or drugs that do not fulfill the definition of relatively permanent change and are not therefore representative of learning. Since therapists have goals to change ineffective behavioral strategies, either motor or social, to aid acquisition of new skills, to promote developmental task execution, and to adapt to environmental demands, it is important to understand how learning takes place.

Behavioral theory

Behaviorists view learning as a function of stimuli and responses. These learning theorists are oriented toward the experimental investigation of observable, measurable behaviors. They see the person as a purely responsive being, a mechanistic result of present and past environments. There is little attention to interpreting underlying reasons for responses to stimuli; behavior is seen as a function of immediate stimuli. They suggest that learning takes place by means of respondent (classical) or operant conditioning.

In *classical conditioning*, two stimuli are presented at the same time. One is reinforcing (eg, food); the other is irrelevant (eg, sound of refrigerator door). This leads to the expectation of reinforcement and a concomitant automatic response (eg, salivation) associated with the irrelevant stimulus (ie, learning has taken place). Thus, even when the irrelevant stimulus is presented without the reinforcing stimulus, there is a response.

In *operant conditioning*, reinforcement (eg, praise or candy) is presented after behavior. Therefore, reinforcement is associated with the behavior (ie, learning has taken place). Thus, behavior is repeated. This is the basis of the technique of behavior modification, in which either positive or negative reinforcement is provided immediately after the behavior that is desired or that is to be extinguished.

Conditioning is one explanation of how learning occurs and may be useful to the therapist. Behaviorists believe learning is a direct result of the processes of classical or operant conditioning. In reality, even within the limitations of this theory, most learning would probably combine the two processes.

Ayres (1980) suggests that learning is a change in neural organization brought about through use and practice. In her theory of sensory integration, she states that some developmentally immature clients who exhibit learning disorders may benefit from meaningful sensorimotor experiences that gradually mature the neurologic connections between nerve cells known as synapses (Ayres, 1973). Thus, the connections between nerve cells are strengthened with use, and learning occurs.

Social learning theory

Social learning theorists expand learning theory to include the concept that learning takes place through observing behavior and the effects of behavior. This explains the use of models to learn social traits and a socially acceptable repertoire of behaviors.

Bandura (1977a) formulated social learning observations that extend the behavioristic theoretical base. This dimension has important implications for use in occupational therapy. He maintains that

1. Learning is acquired through observation and modeling.
2. There is a continuous reciprocal interaction between environmental, behavioral, and personal determinants of behavior.

3. The environment is not an autonomous force. It is regulated by its own contingencies, of which human behavior is only one.
4. Learning occurs by means of vicarious reinforcement (learning from observed positive and negative consequences of a model's behavior) and self-reinforcement.
5. Self-reinforcement yields self-efficacy or the ability of a person to cope with stress (Bandura, 1977b).
6. One's ability to judge how to deal with stress comes from
   a. The performance mode, that is, how similar situations were handled in the past.
   b. Vicarious information gained from observing the success or failure of others.
   c. Social persuasion, that is, the undermining of reinforcement of one's sense of efficacy by others.
   d. The person's perception of his or her physiology and its vulnerability in stressful situations (Bandura, 1977a; Davis, 1985).

The occupational therapist must develop sensitivity to the learner's needs. The learner may demonstrate a preferred sensory channel or mode of learning. Often optimum learning occurs when there is reinforcement through multiple sensory channels, for example, providing a visual, auditory, and movement component to the learning process.

Cognitive theory

Whereas learning theories focus on stimulus–response associations, cognitive theory includes intelligence, reasoning, learning, problem solving, memory, information processing, and thinking. These are the mediators that are used for interpretation of stimuli from the environment.

Jean Piaget

Jean Piaget has made a significant contribution to the development of cognitive theory. As a biologist and epistemologist, he investigated the origin, nature, methods, and limits of human knowledge. He synthesized nativism (innate) and empiricism (acquired) to suggest that each child develops his or her own way of thinking by using innate abilities in interaction with the world. In contrast to the learning theorists, Piaget saw the human as active, alert, and capable. That is, he believed that a person processes information rather than merely receiving it, and does more than respond to stimuli; he gives structure and meaning to stimuli. Piaget postulated that until a certain age, children form judgments through their perceptual world rather than by principles of logic. If the child's perceptions and experiences fit a structure within his or her mind, they are assimilated or understood, whereas if the information received does not fit an existing structure, the mind must change to accommodate the new experience. The schemata of a child—his or her methods of processing information—expand as the child grows. A person continuously adjusts his or her schemata to assimilate and accommodate new information. The human mind seeks equilibrium between assimilation and accommodation just as the human body seeks biologic homeostasis. The display on page 100 shows the major tenets of Piaget's continuum of cognitive development.

As the child grows, his or her structural abilities to accommodate new information grow also. Piaget saw this as occurring in four major steps with different modes of learning: the sensorimotor period—body and movement; the preoperational period—imagery; the concrete operational period—concrete human/nonhuman environment; and the formal operational period—abstraction.

Some researchers criticize Piaget for not giving enough credence to the preexisting presence of a fundamental, innate, perception-based orientation to the world. Piaget proposes that infants must act on the world to gradually come to understand the nature of objects through sensorimotor actions. Others argue that the existence of depth perception or perceptual constancies early in life allows understanding of the nature of objects to occur. Piaget's primary contribution to cognitive theory is his depiction of the child's ability to build on each stage and to progress through the cumulative sequence of cognitive development irrespective of specific chronologic ages associated with it.

Jerome Bruner

Jerome Bruner is another cognitive theorist who investigates the human as an artist (aesthetic being) and as a scientist (problem solver). Like Piaget, he sees the qualitative changes in the cognitive structures corresponding to biologic growth. Both scientists also see the mind as developing in stages, but they differ on the role of language in development. Piaget sees thought as preceding language skill, whereas Bruner sees language as a causative factor in acquiring problem-solving ability. Language acquisition may facilitate the use of effective thinking strategies and therefore clearly interacts with the development of cognition (Short-DeGraff, 1988). Additionally, cognitive and social development have a strong relationship. Language strengthens that bond as the means for people to communicate their needs and interact with others.

Ethologic theory

Ethologists emphasize innate, instinctual qualities of behavior as distinct from the stimulus–response approach of learning theorists. They focus on stereotyped, innate, unlearned behavior and consider predispositions to behaving a certain way. Their methodology for investigating behavior includes studying humans and animals in their naturalistic settings. They view species as having similar behavior traits and think that humans, like other animals, have inherited behavior patterns. According to ethologists, releasers and fixed action patterns are found in all animal species, including humans (Short-DeGraff, 1988). Actions such as smiling, laughing, and reflexes are included as human fixed action patterns or instincts.

Ethologists do not ignore the history and situation of behavior patterns, but essentially they look at behavior in terms of preserving the person or the species within the evolution of civilization. It is an interesting and relatively new way of studying human behavior and presupposes that animal behavior is a valid indicator of human behavior. Growing interest in its methods and principles indicates that ethology will play an increasing role in the study of human development. Because the areas of study undertaken by ethologists include physiology, development, ecology, function, adaptation, and purposefulness, their findings may have some real significance to occupational therapists.

SUMMARY OF PIAGET'S STAGES OF COGNITIVE DEVELOPMENT

The Sensorimotor Stage (Birth to 2 Years)

The infant operates almost exclusively with overt schemes and actions. Learning occurs in six substages, as the child learns about the world in terms of what he or she can do with objects and with abundant new sensory information.

Substage 1—Practice with reflexes. Reflex accommodation is a result of experience.

Substage 2—Primary circular reactions. Chance movements lead to interesting results, which the child reproduces by trial and error. The infant does not distinguish between body and outside events.

Substage 3—Secondary circular reactions. The child makes interesting things happen. He or she begins to coordinate two types of sensory information. The connections between actions and results are perceived and the actions are repeated.

Substage 4—Coordination of secondary schemes. The infant combines actions to attain a goal. Familiar strategies are used in combination and in new situations.

Substage 5—Experimentation. The infant tries new ways of playing, moving, and manipulating objects and begins to understand the concept of cause and effect.

Substage 6—Beginning of thought. Objects now have permanence. The child uses images, words, or actions to represent objects.

The Preoperational Stage (2 to 6 Years)

The child uses symbols and internalized actions in everyday activity and thinks in images. The content of the thought is magical. In the beginning of the stage, the child is "centered": he or she can focus on only one aspect of a thought or situation at a time. Ginsburg and Opper (1969) summarized the preoperational child accurately:

> The [preoperational] child decenters his thought just as in the sensorimotor period the infant decentered his behavior. The newborn acts as if the world is centered about himself; and must learn to behave in more adaptive ways. Similarly, the young child thinks from a limited perspective and must widen it. (p. 111)

Concrete Operational Stage (6 to 12 Years)

The child's logic is basic and inductive. He or she is still tied to specific experience but can do mental manipulations as well as physical ones (Bee, 1985).

Formal Operations (12 Years)

Abstract and hypothetical deductive reasoning emerges. The child can manipulate images and objects in the mind and can think about things that have not been experienced or have not yet happened. The child can organize and systematize thought deductively.

Psychoanalytic theory

Sigmund Freud

Sigmund Freud is considered the father of psychoanalysis. His contribution derives from a specific technique of psychotherapy, a method for gathering data and studying behavior, and a theoretical system for understanding human personality development. Some later theorists endorsed his work, some opposed it, and some have modified it to blend with more contemporary thinking. The theories of Freud, Erikson, and other neo-Freudians deal primarily with emotional and personality development.

Freud's theory sets forth basic assumptions about personality and psychosexual development.

1. All behavior is energized by fundamental instinctual drives: sexual drives or libido, life-preserving forces, and aggressive drives.
2. Throughout the lifespan, gratification and strategies to obtain gratification are the focal points of psychosexual development.
3. The type of gratification and the method of attaining it change with age, but the instinctual drive to obtain it remains constant.
4. Three basic structures of personality (id, ego, and super-ego) develop in childhood and function to assist in gratification of instincts.
5. If conflict arises between the different structures of personality, anxiety results. Defense mechanisms are automatic and unconscious strategies for dealing with anxiety.
6. A series of distinct psychosexual stages of personality development evolve during childhood. The first three, the oral, anal, and phallic stages, center on areas of the body that at each stage become a center for pleasure. These stages are followed by the latency and genital stages, during which the personality is influenced by degrees of sexual interest, socialization, and an evolving focus on life goals. Freud sets the stage for the explanation of development of the unconscious mind and its relationship to the ability to function.

Freud's beliefs were based on instincts but in a different context than those studied by ethologists. Freud viewed basic human instincts as primarily sexual and aggressive unconscious forces that shape human personality.

Erik Erikson

Other psychoanalytic theorists include Erik Erikson, a neo-Freudian who expanded Freud's work to include the societal environment. His approach focuses on human psychosocial de-

TABLE 5-1. *Comparison of Erikson's and Freud's Stages of Psychosocial Development*

Erikson		Freud	
Stage	*Age (years)*	*Stage*	*Age (years)*
Trust–mistrust	0–1	Oral	0–1
Autonomy–shame	1–3	Anal	2–3
Initiative–guilt	4–5	Phallic	4–5
Industry–inferiority	6–11	Latency	6–12
Identity–role diffusion	12–18	Genital	13–18 and adulthood
Intimacy–isolation	Young adult		
Generativity–stagnation	Middle adult		
Ego integrity–despair	Later adult		

velopment. Erikson sees personality development as unfolding progressively throughout the life cycle. This is in contrast to Freud, who placed paramount importance on childhood experiences. Erikson's eight stages of development are delineated by eight emotional crises or issues that must be resolved. Table 5-1 aligns Erikson's and Freud's stages of psychosocial development. The resolution of these issues is the balance between the negative and positive poles of each stage. This resolution and its importance at any one point in life is a function of the person's relationship to his or her place in the social and cultural environment. How a person resolves a crisis directly affects the quality of his or her ability to deal with a subsequent developmental issue. Furthermore, Erikson believes that these crises may emerge throughout life.

The basic strength of theorists such as Freud and Erikson is their willingness to look at the whole person and at the conscious and unconscious factors of emotional development. They deal with interpersonal relationships, particularly as they relate to childhood experiences. Erikson's theory recognized the significance of developmental tasks at stages throughout life. Freud, like Piaget, proposed theories that pertained through adolescence.

Other psychoanalytic theorists

Other theorists include Anna Freud, daughter of Freud, who extended the tenets of psychoanalysis to the study of children and education. She was concerned primarily with psychopathology rather than the normal sequences of personality development and focused much needed attention on the adolescent years. Harry Stack Sullivan expanded the original psychoanalytic orientation to include an interpersonal theory of psychiatry. He proposed that the "self system" matures through six stages of development through social interactions (Table 5-2). Peter Bios expanded psychoanalytic concepts, particularly in relation to adolescence. His theory centers on the process of individuation from parents and the development of significant relationships with others, tasks also emphasized by Havighurst.

The weakness of psychoanalytic theory lies in the difficulty of defining parameters of development and of validating research. Most data are gleaned from adults, whose subjective reconstruction of their childhood experiences may lead to invalid or vague conclusions.

Social–emotional theory

Social–emotional growth begins in infancy as the newborn expresses his or her reactions to the environment and receives a response that is either nurturing and growth producing or negative and restrictive. The social self develops through processes described by Freud and Erikson that aid in creating a secure self-identity. The trust in the world that occurs when early needs are recognized and met by the caregiver allows the infant to grow with a base of feelings of safety.

The social system of mother, or caregiver, and child begins an attachment process that is made up of each participant's responses to stimuli from the other. The pattern of social interaction here is a result of several forces that include the child's temperment; the effectiveness and strength of the baby's signals to the mother; the caregiver's own style, behavior, and temperment; and possibly some hormonal or physiologic triggering system in the mother, which may be stronger for some mother–infant pairs than for others (Connor, Williamson, & Siepp, 1978).

Emotions are feelings expressed using terms such as sadness, joy, anger, and jealousy. They differ from personality, which is represented by a more stable and enduring pattern of traits. Emotions are more fleeting, but may be part of the overall type of personality that develops. Greenspan and Greenspan (1985) describe the origins of emotional growth and highlight six emotional milestones.

TABLE 5-2. *Sullivan's Stages of Personality Development*

Approximate Age	Stage	Child's Social Needs
Birth–2 years	Infancy	Security
2–6	Childhood	Adult attention and validation of experiences
6–10	Juvenile	Peer relationships
10–12	Preadolescent	Interpersonal intimacy in an isophilic relationship
12–16	Early adolescent	Intimacy; sexual gratification; personal security in heterophilic relationship
16–20	Late adolescent	"Special" heterophilic relationship and place in society

1. *Organizing sensations.* The infant should feel tranquil and calm, and at the same time reach out toward the new world of sights, sounds, movement, touch, tastes, and smells. Another term for this is self-quieting behavior; it begins at birth.
2. *Taking a highly specialized interest in the human world.* Now the world beyond the stimuli appears most enticing to the infant. The 3- to 4-month-old will become enraptured with exploring faces.
3. *Entering into "dialogue" by responsive smiling.* Gutteral voice sounds in response to reactions by others will occur. The 3- to 10-month-old will express pleasure, anger, and protest.
4. *Learning to connect small units of feeling and social behavior into large, complicated, orchestrated patterns.* The 10- to 15-month-old will talk on a toy telephone, use gestures to communicate, and demonstrate understanding of the meanings of things.
5. *Being able to create objects in his or her mind's eye.* The 2-year-old is able to construct ideas and communicate an internal life, dream, and create his or her own experiences.
6. *Expanding his or her world of ideas into the emotional realms of pleasure and dependency, curiosity, assertiveness, anger, self-discipline, empathy, and love.*

The domains overlap as strong positive attachments in the social aspect and provide advantages in cognitive growth and learning capabilities. Social–emotional growth occurs within a rich blend of innate and environmental influences and is enhanced by concepts from the learning and social learning theorists.

Motivational theory

Motivation is described as arousal to action, initiating, molding, and sustaining specific action patterns (Cratty, 1973). The importance of the experience of success to promote feelings of efficacy and motivate further performance has been given power by terms such as *competence motivation* (White & Held, 1963) and *pleasure in mastery* (Hendrick, 1943). Motivating factors arise from an innate drive, curiosity, novelty, complexity, competition, need to interact with the environment, cooperation, survival, pleasure principle, issues of dependence–independence, social pressures, control, anxiety, and fear. Reinforcement principles can enhance or diminish motivation. Intrinsic satisfaction is often a more effective motivator than external rewards. Gerson (1978) found that too plentiful external rewards were likely to blunt the pleasures derived from sports participation and engaging in vigorous recreational activities.

Humanistic theory

Theorists such as Abraham Maslow and Carol Rogers set forth *humanistic approaches* for human interaction in an effort to separate from the strict biologic and mechanistic approaches of Freudian and behavioral models. Their focus is on human values in relationships and on the person, rather than on the person–environment interaction. The shift of terminology from "patient" to "client" occurred within the context of the humanistic movement to denote a human encounter with a collaborative relationship (Mosey, 1981).

Maslow stresses that each person has an innate need for self-actualization. It is possible to attain this goal only when a well-integrated person has satisfied "lower needs" such as safety, love, food, and shelter. Rogers is concerned with helping each person realize his or her potential by creating an interpersonal climate for growth with characteristics such as empathy, unconditional willingness to accept a person as he or she is, and a genuine involvement in the person's growth.

Humanistic psychologists focus on the person's concept of self, with humans viewed as self-determining and creative. Their aim is to maximize human potential, viewing each act optimistically as a function of the person's self. The strength of this approach is its concern with real-life situations and the value of the self.

Maturational theory

Maturation is related to behavioral and physiologic descriptions of development. Evolutionary principles have been applied in this theory, including the concept of recapitulation. This asserts that each person's development (ontogeny) proceeds through the same stages as the species did during evolution (phylogeny), hence, the phrase "ontogeny recapitulates phylogeny" (Gould, 1977). The maturational aspects of this concept are applied to treatment that guides patients through sequences to repeat normal development.

Hierarchical development is also based on maturation. Phylogenetically older, lower levels of the brain are organized for regulating early behavior in the neonate. After neuromuscular maturation, higher level behaviors appear. Fiorentino (1973) used this concept to test **reflexes**, recognizing that specific levels of the central nervous system regulate motor behaviors in a hierarchical manner (Table 5-3).

Arnold Gesell emphasized maturation as the primary influence of growth and development due to innate and endogenous factors. He did acknowledge that environmental and external factors contributed to development, which addresses a caution

TABLE 5-3.   *Hierarchical View of Normal Sequential Development*

Level of CNS Maturation	Corresponding Level of Reflex Development	Resulting Level of Motor Development
Spinal and/or brainstem	Apedal Primitive reflexes	Lying prone Lying supine
Midbrain	Quadrupedal Righting reactions	Crawling Sitting
Cortical	Bipdeal Equilibrium reactions	Standing Walking

From Fiorentino, M.R. (1973). Reflex testing methods for evaluating CNS development (2nd ed.) (p. 5). Springfield, IL: Charles C. Thomas.

that must be applied to dogged allegiance to this theoretical model. If sequence and hierarchy are so rigidly viewed, the significant factors of the unique self, human individuality, and the importance of the whole person may be overlooked (Bing, 1968). Nevertheless, Gesell produced age-related standards for motor, language, and social skills that are the basis of many developmental assessments. These parameters can help detect developmental delay and provide a baseline for treatment. Normative data such as this must be updated continually and used cautiously. It is important to know the type of population on which the scale was standardized and when it was developed. Many scales are not cross-cultural and may be invalid for certain groups of children. Additionally, "ages and stages" may not be the most appropriate view to take with children in our care because therapists are more interested in developmental levels than chronologic expectations.

Ecologic theory

Bronfenbrenner is credited with insisting that developmental psychology look beyond the dyad of mother and child into the cultural and personal relationships that form the ecologic niche in which the child grows. He explored the ecology of development.

The totality of child development includes parental behaviors such as emotional tone, methods of discipline, patterns of communication, and type and extent of cognitive enrichment. Other major influences include the impact of other institutions on the child; the support systems available to the family; and the types of play activities, social interactions, and other forms of cognitive stimulation to which the child is exposed (Bronfenbrenner, 1977a, 1977b). The value of the ecologic perspective is found in its realistic inclusion of all the variables in a person's life, including multiple, interacting, individual, social, and cultural factors.

Specific developmental areas

All of the developing systems of the infant and child are interrelated. Some take precedence over others at varying stages of development. Nevertheless, it is important to continue to view development as a whole to maintain a holistic approach to the child and family (see Figure 5-1). The following sections will highlight the developmental systems and the expectations of developmental sequences.

Physical/motor development

Physical development

In the first year of life, babies rapidly gain weight and length. Generally, the infant will triple his or her weight and add 10 to 12 inches in length within the first year. By age 2, most toddlers are already half as tall as they will be as adults. After 2, growth slows to a steady rate of 2 to 3 inches and 6 pounds a year until adolescence.

Body shape and body parts do not grow at equal rates. Hands and feet mature earliest, followed by arms, legs, and trunk. Bone growth follows a similar pattern, with the most rapid development and ossification occurring within the first 2 years.

The development of the brain and central nervous system is incomplete at birth. The cortex is the least developed area; cortical development is about half complete at 6 months and 75% complete by age 2 (Bee, 1985). The process of hemispheric specialization continues at least until adolescence. Likewise, although myelinization of the brain is thought to be almost complete by age 2, the process probably continues into adolescence.

The endocrine system is functional from about the fourth month of gestation. Thyroxine and the pituitary growth hormone are most active in the early years, then level off until pubescence (Tanner, 1978).

Respiration and breathing follow a predictable and orderly progression. Breathing patterns affect not only the child's ability to survive outside the uterus but also his or her feeding and speech patterns.

Other physical attributes—facial features, teeth, hair, skin—develop and change at a slower and more steady pace. Changes are usually complete by the end of adolescence. It is important to note that some of these changes may affect sensory ability. For example, as the face broadens, auditory localization becomes more accurate.

Gross and fine motor development

At birth, the child demonstrates orderly and predictable movement patterns. The development of muscle tone, posture, and motor responses allows the child to survive and adapt within his or her environment. The child first gains control of the head, neck, and trunk. Gradually, he or she is able to roll, sit, crawl, creep, kneel, stand, and free him- or herself from the forces of gravity in locomotion. The continuing effort of the growing infant is to get the body upright against gravity, maintain the head and eyes parallel to the horizon, and maintain balance when the center of gravity is changed.

The wonder of the developing child is that none of these developing patterns occurs in isolation; rather, they are interactive and interdependent on all senses and developmental systems. The child learns and develops more motor patterns in the first year than will be developed over the rest of his or her lifetime.

The beginning of motor development is found in reflexive movement. The neural network begins functioning prenatally and primitive movement occurs as a result of sensory input such as tactile, vestibular, and proprioceptive stimulation. The fact that these sensory modalities are functioning prenatally lends strength to the concept of their importance as a foundation for skill development.

A reflex is an automatic movement performed without conscious volition, usually initiated by sensory stimulation. It is an immediate, stereotyped, obligatory response, but its strength may vary depending on the state of arousal or previous learning of the infant. As a building block of movement, it provides the first change in distribution of muscle tone. The full-term newborn is dominated by physiologic flexion; reflexes offer the opportunity for extensor tone to come into play. As higher centers of the central nervous system mature, reflex activity evolves to volitional movement. The reflexes become integrated at anticipated times during the first year of growth. They never totally disappear, however, and may emerge in times of stress to the system. By 4 to 6 months most primitive reflexes have been modified (integrated) and no longer bring about a stereotypic response. Reflexes are clinically significant to the occupational therapist, who can assess the maturation of the central nervous system through observation of these primitive movement patterns.

In addition to primitive reflexes, other automatic movements include righting reactions, equilibrium reactions, and protective arm extension. Whereas reflexes are responses to specific stimuli and are integrated within the first months of life, reactions respond to more global stimuli and last a lifetime to support movement and balance. Righting reactions support positioning the head vertically in space, alignment of the head and trunk, and alignment of the trunk and limbs. Both head righting, which aligns the eyes with the horizon and aligns the head with the trunk, and body righting, which contributes to movement around the body axis, are used to assume antigravity positions.

Equilibrium reactions provide balance when the center of gravity is disturbed. They are more mature responses to regain balance than righting reactions, and include counterrotation of the head and trunk away from the direction of the displacement and the use of the extremities as they abduct and extend automatically. Maturation of higher centers of the central nervous system is essential before equilibrium reactions become available to the child, beginning at approximately 6 months and maturing at about 4 years.

Protective arm extension is used to prevent injury if the equilibrium reactions are unable to restore balance. Thus, slipping on the ice evokes extension of the upper extremities to prevent crashing to the ground. Protective extension emerges first to the front, then the side, then backwards. It also may be used to assess the maturation of the central nervous system and begins to be displayed at about 6 months in conjunction with attempts at sitting. Table 5-4 provides an overview of some important reflexes and reactions.

Gross motor control refers to the coordination of the large muscles of the body and may include the following:

Head and trunk control: muscle tone, segmental rolling versus log rolling, voluntary control of movement versus reflexive motor response.
Coordination of large body parts: crawling, creeping, jumping, kicking, skipping, galloping, hopping.
Balance/equilibrium: response to balance challenges in sitting, creeping, kneeling, standing.
Body awareness: awareness of position in space and movement.
Motor planning: sequencing of movement, movement problem solving.
Response to gross motor activities: enjoyment, experimentation, anxiety, cooperation.

Fine motor control begins with visual fixation, reaching, ulnar palmar, palmar, radial palmar, raking, radial grasp, release of objects, and pincer grasp, followed by refinement of each skill (Table 5-5). Components of fine motor control may include:

Eye movement: smooth, coordinated in horizontal, vertical, diagonal, and rotary planes.
Hand and finger movement: reach, grasp, dexterity, coordination, and control (based on the gross motor control and stability of trunk, shoulder, and elbow).
Eye/hand coordination: bilateral use of upper extremities, dominance, implement control of pencil, crayon, scissors.
Sensory awareness: temperature, touch, proprioception, stereognosis.

Motor planning: sequencing of fine movements, movement problem solving.

Children treated by occupational therapists should not be expected to perform fine motor tasks if they do not have the gross motor base of control and stability necessary as a foundation for the skill development. Judicious positioning of the infant or child can supplement gross motor stability. For example, a child who is positioned in a corner seat gains trunk support and shoulder protraction to aid in bilateral hand use.

Sensory development

Sensory modalities include systems for tactile, vestibular, proprioceptive, visual, auditory, gustatory, and olfactory awareness. Sensory stimuli must be received or registered by the brain for a response to be evoked. When any of the sensory systems are dysfunctional, responses to the stimulation may be diminished, aberrant, or absent. Interruption of sensory reception may occur peripherally, such as poor visual or auditory acuity, or may take place once the information gets to the brain, causing a central processing problem.

Tactile information is both protective and discriminative. Initially the infant reacts in a gross, protective manner to touch stimuli, then becomes more discriminative in relating to these experiences. The baby learns about his or her external world through touch, from the hands that nurture and cuddle to exploration of his or her body to acquaint him- or herself with body parts and their potential for movement. The baby "mouthes" items in the environment to learn sizes and shapes through his or her lips and mouth as well as hands and fingers. The tactile system is functioning in utero and is fundamental for learning about self and the environment. Montagu (1978) suggests that the deep touch pressure of vaginal birth is instrumental in promoting the functioning of the touch system. Sensitivity to light touch is dramatically demonstrated by an infant's reflexive response. With maturation and experience, this sense of touch becomes more refined.

The vestibular system is also functioning in utero and matures early, indicating its primacy as a sensory modality. Its function is to modulate movement. It accomplishes this through its close connections to oculomotor control; muscle tone; reflexes; righting and equilibrium reactions; protective extension; and movement awareness of acceleration, deceleration, up, down, gravity, and spatial orientation. The sensory receptors for vestibular information are located in the inner ear and consist of the semicircular canals, which process information about gravity, motion, and rotation of the head, and the utricle and saccule, which process motion with respect to the position of the head.

The system for proprioception receives information from special receptors in the joints, muscles, and tendons to provide knowledge about the body's position in space. This is usually at an unconscious level. Kinesthesia is a more conscious awareness of the body's movement and position in space. The vestibular and proprioceptor systems function jointly to supply and react to information about gravity, movement, and position in space.

Contrary to past beliefs, vision is functioning at birth. The neonate is able to visually follow stimuli from the periphery to the midline. Infants have early preference for sharp contrast, ie, black and white stimuli, as well as for faces. When searching for

(*Text continues on page 112*)

TABLE 5-4. *Neurophysiologic Reflex Processes and the Influence on Movement and Adaptation*

Reflex (See references below)	Position	Stimulus	Location	Responses	Adaptation	Origin	Reflex Age Range Initiation	Reflex Age Range Inhibition
Primitive Reflexes								
1. Rooting (15, 33)	Supine	Light tactile	Mouth	Opens mouth; rotation extension, and flexion of head follow	Search for breast or bottle in the direction of the stimulus	Pons	28 weeks' gestation	3 months
2. Sucking (12, 33, 37, 39)	Supine	Light tactile	Oral cavity	Close mouth, suck, and swallow	Obtain nourishment, develop tongue movement, and, later, produce sound	Trigeminal nerve	28 weeks' gestation	2–5 months
3. Traction (46)	Supine	Proprioception	Forearms	Total flexion of upper extremities	Momentary grasp with total flexion of UE leading to voluntary reach and grasp	Pons	28 weeks' gestation	2–5 months
4. Moro (1, 2, 5, 9, 19, 20, 34, 35, 36, 37, 39, 41, 46)	Supine	Sudden change of head position >30° extension (proprioception)	Head and trunk	1st: UEs extend and abduct; hands open and LEs may extend. 2nd: Flexion and adduction of UEs; hands close; may cry	If persists, will interfere with head control, sitting equilibrium, and protective reactions affecting adaptability of child for movement in space	Brainstem; medulla 1	28 weeks' gestation	5–6 months
5. Crossed extension (1, 4, 11, 24, 28)	Supine	Noxious tactile	Ball of foot	1st flexion, then extension and adduction of opposite LE	Preparation for reciprocal LE use; persistence indicates pathology and interference in reciprocation and in walking	Spinal	28 weeks' gestation	1–2 months
6. Flexor withdrawal (1, 2, 4, 16, 27, 34, 37, 39, 45)	Supine	Noxious tactile	Sole of foot	Withdrawal with flexion of hip and knee; dorsiflexion of foot with toe extension	Protection or defense. If persists, will interfere with weight bearing in standing	Spinal	28 weeks' gestation	1–2 months
7. Plantar grasp (31, 47)	Supine	Firm pressure	Ball of foot	Grasps with toes (flexion)	If persists, interferes with standing and walking; may evoke toe walking	Spinal	28 weeks' gestation	4–9 months
8. Galant (8, 38)	Prone	Noxious tactile	Along paravertebral column from 12th rib to iliac crest	Incurvature of spine to same side	Organizes for trunk adaptation. If persists, interferes with symmetric stability of the trunk, independent sitting, standing. May lead to scoliosis	Spinal	32 weeks' gestation	2 months
9. Neonatal neck righting (6, 27, 30, 31, 33, 37, 38, 41)	Supine	Proprioception to neck rotators	Neck rotators	Log rolling—supine to side	Rolling on body axis from back to right and left sides. Persistence delays segmented rolling and other developmental milestones, especially bilateral integration	Medulla	34 weeks' gestation	4–5 months
10. Plantar placing of legs (21)	Vertical	Proprioceptive	LEs; dorsum of feet (stretch)	Placing of feet; flexion of hips/knees; dorsiflexion at ankle followed by LE extension & support on surface	Correlates to spontaneous stepping—primitive form of ambulation and stepping over objects	Spinal	35 weeks' gestation	2 months
11. Neonatal positive support (1)	Vertical	Proprioceptive	LEs; soles of feet	Partial weight bearing with hips & knees flexed & ankle plantar flexion in contact with floor surface	Prerequisite for stepping. Preparation for motion; not static. Weight bearing	Spinal	35 weeks' gestation	1–2 months
12. Spontaneous stepping (1, 40)	Vertical	Proprioceptive and tactile	LEs with body inclined forward	Positive support then walking (coordinated & rhythmic with heel touching first)	Prerequisite for walking	Spinal and brainstem	37 weeks' gestation	2 months
13. Tonic labyrinthine (3, 17)	Prone	Head/face down in relation to gravity	Prone; head midline	Increases flexor tone of neck, UEs, & LEs	Contributes, when integrated, into a supportive framework of nonstressful movement	Inner ear—otototic utricle maculae	Birth	6 months

(continued)

105

TABLE 5-4. *Neurophysiologic Reflex Processes and the Influence on Movement and Adaptation (continued)*

Reflex (See references below)	Position	Stimulus	Location	Responses	Adaptation	Origin	Reflex Age Range	
							Initiation	Inhibition
Primitive Reflexes								
14.	Supine	Head/face up in relation to gravity	Supine; head midline	Increases extensor tone of neck, UEs, & LEs	If persistent, interferes with head control, coming to sit, rolling, creeping, and standing	Intermedulla		
15. Plantar arms placing (21, 34, 43)	Vertical	Proprioceptive (stretch)	UEs; dorsum of hands	Placing of hands: Flexion of shoulder and elbow, then fingers and wrist abduct and extend. Followed by extension of elbows & shoulders for UE support (infants may remain fisted)	Requisite for supporting body weight on forearms and extended arms	Spinal or brainstem	Birth	2 months
16. Asymmetrical tonic neck (3, 6, 8, 17, 22, 23, 25, 28, 42, 44–49)	Supine	Proprioceptive (stretch) visual for infants	a) Neck muscles (rotation) b) Gaze to induce neck rotation	a) Extension of UEs and LEs on face side; flexion on skull side b) As above, but not obligatory	Contributes to the supportive framework of nonstressful movement. Persistent obligatory presence indicates pathologic state, inducing lack of symmetrical posture, reach and grasp, normal rolling, unsupported sitting, and a deficiency in walking. Globally, a lack of ability to develop motorically. Structural deformity (ie, scoliosis); hip subluxation (skull side). Nonobligatory presence interferes in motor planning, bilateral integration, and reading comprehension.	Atlanto-occipital and axial joints to upper cervical roots, integrating at medulla	Birth	4-6 months
17. Symmetrical tonic neck (10, 28, 30, 31, 41)	Prone	Proprioceptive	Neck muscles, flexion and extension of neck	With neck flexion, UEs flex and LEs extend; with neck extension, UEs extend and LEs flex	Works strongly with asymmetrical tonic and tonic labyrinthine reflexes to influence tonic postural stability. Prolonged influence interferes with reciprocal creeping, sitting, standing, and walking	Same as for asymmetrical tonic neck reflex	4-6 months	8-12 months
Prehension Reactions								
18. Palmar grasp (42, 47)	Supine	Proprioception (palmar pressure)	Pressure on ulnar surface of palm	*"Catching phase,"* quick flexion and adduction of fingers. *"Holding phase,"* sustained finger flexion	Primitive precursor to coordinated voluntary grasp. If persists, will interfere with releasing and the development of prehension and hand skills	Subcortical	Birth	4-6 months
19. Avoidance (43)	Supine, sitting or standing	Light tactile stroke	Dorsum or ulnar surface of hands	Fingers open; move away from stimulus	May cause overpronation of forearms, flexion of wrist, abduction extension of fingers. If persists, will strongly reduce tactile exploration and hand usage	Subcortical	Birth	6-7 years
20. Instinctive grasp (19, 28, 30, 31, 41)	Supine, sitting or standing	Light tactile proprioception	Ulnar or radial border of hands	Orientation of hand and fractionation of total grasping reflex for voluntary grasping patterns	Facilitates radial palmar grasp, thumb-2-3 finger grasp, and voluntary pincer grasp	Subcortical	4-11 months	Persists

Righting Reactions

	Position	Stimulus	Response	Description/Function	Neural level	Onset	Persistence
21. Labyrinthine head righting *prone* (8, 28, 29, 37, 41)	Prone	Otoliths of the labyrinthine	Neck, without vision	Orients head (in space and to ground) in an upward position by neck extension	In general, automatic reactions that allow for normal standing position and preserve balance in the process of changing from prone or supine to fully upright position. Prerequisite for head control in the normal upright position. Initially, infant uses this reaction to clear the head in the prone position. In general, suppresses primitive abnormal reflexes and facilitates normal movement for sitting, creeping, standing, and walking	Red nucleus midbrain	Birth–2 months	Persists
22. Labyrinthine head righting *supine* (8, 28, 29, 37, 41)	Supine	Otoliths of the labyrinthine	Neck, without vision	Orients head (in space and to ground) in an upward position by neck flexion				
23. Labyrinthine head righting *tilting* (8, 28, 29, 37, 41)	Vertical	Otiliths of the labyrinthine	Neck, without vision	Orients head (in space and to ground) in an upward position by tilting of head				
24. Optical righting *prone* (8, 26, 37, 39, 43)	Prone	Vision versus labyrinthine	Neck, with visual receptors	Orient head in space in an upright position in extension	As in labyrinthine head righting, need the subsequent motor development requiring head control in the normal upright position	Cerebral cortex, especially occipital	2 months	Persists
25. Optical righting *supine* (8, 26, 37, 39, 43)	Supine	Vision	Neck, with visual receptors	Orients head in space in an upright position in flexion				
26. Optical righting *tilting* (8, 26, 37, 39, 43)	Vertical	Vision	Neck, with visual receptors	Orients head in space in an upright position in lateral tilting				
27. Neck righting (11, 30, 31, 34, 41)	Supine	Proprioceptive (stretch)	Neck–lumbar rotation	Body alignment in rotation on axis with segmentation. Shoulder–thorax rotation followed by trunk–pelvic rolling	Facilitates rolling for pursuits and for proceeding with head control to sitting, creeping, standing, and walking. Deficiency may indicate poor bilateral integration	Midbrain	4–6 months	5 years
28. Body righting (11, 30, 31, 37, 40)	Supine	Proprioceptive (stretch) and tactile	Pelvis rotation with hip flexion	Trunk (thoracic rotation) on body axis with segmentation; pelvic–trunk rotation followed by shoulder–thoracic rotation on body axis	Facilitates rolling for pursuits and for proceeding to sitting, creeping, standing and walking. Deficiency indicates diminished bilateral integration	Red nucleus of the midbrain	4–6 months	5 years
29. Landau (3, 8, 13, 18, 30, 31, 34, 37)	Prone	Proprioceptive (stretch)	Neck extensors	Increases prone extension tone	Dissociates flexor posture and assists neck extension in prone (especially pivot prone) coming to sit, and standing. Absence is associated with motor weakness and mental retardation. Early or exaggerated Landau is associated with spasticity or increased muscle tone. Delay in Landau will retard the development of prone extension, sitting and standing, and related developmental adaptations	Diffuse	3–4 months	12–24 months

(continued)

TABLE 5-4. *Neurophysiologic Reflex Processes and the Influence on Movement and Adaptation (continued)*

Reflex (See references below)	Position	Stimulus	Location	Responses	Adaptation	Origin	Reflex Age Range	
							Initiation	Inhibition
Equilibrium Reactions								
30. Visual placing arms (34, 43)	Vertical	Visual (advance UEs/hands toward supporting surface)	Hands	Flexion of shoulder/elbow followed by extension of elbow/wrist/fingers for support	Needed for weight bearing on forearms and extended arms; also for accurate placing of hands, creeping, and visual reaching and grasping	Cortical	3–4 months	Persists
31. Visual placing legs (8, 34, 43)	Vertical	Visual (advance LEs/feet toward supporting surface)	Feet	Hip and knee flexion followed by dorsiflexion of the ankle and LE extension for support on surface	Needed for LE weight bearing on knees and feet and for accurate placing of LEs in creeping, knee activity, and standing/walking	Cortical	3–5 months	Persists
32. Protective extension *forward*	Sitting	Vestibular and proprioceptive	Displace body forward	Flexion of shoulder with elbow, wrist, and finger extension	In general, protects body from harm when center of gravity of the body is displaced. Facilitates support with extended arms in sitting and is used to attain weight-bearing activities with UEs	Midbrain, basal ganglia, brainstem with cortical input	6–9 months	Persists
33. Protective extension *sideways* (1, 8, 14, 29, 30, 31, 34)	Sitting	Vestibular and proprioceptive	Displace body sideways	Abduction of shoulder with elbow extension and extension and abduction of the fingers	Sitting with arm support and protection against falling sideways. Needed for rotation in sitting		7 months	Persists
34. Protective extension UEs *backward* (34)	Sitting	Vestibular, proprioceptive, and visual	Displace body backward	Total extension of shoulder, elbow, wrist, and fingers with finger abduction	Sitting with arm support, rotating body on its axis, and protection from falling backward. Prolonged Moro may interfere with this development		9–10 months	Persists
35. Positive support (6, 7, 28, 34, 43)	Vertical	Proprioceptive, vestibular	Ball of feet	Hip abduction with external rotation, knee extension with dorsiflexion of ankles (cocontraction)	Facilitates weight bearing/standing and provides generalized support (not rigid) for activity and movement. Increased obligatory extensor tone with hip abduction and plantar flexion of ankle indicates pathologic influence and prevents normal gait, sitting, and stair walking. Structured deformity may occur secondarily to increased extensor tone	Midbrain or thalamus	6–9 months	Persists
36. Equilibrium *prone* (6, 29, 30, 31, 32)	Prone	Vestibular, proprioceptive, and visual	Displace the body, in prone laterally	Curvature of the spine, concave to the side being stressed or upward side, with abduction & extension of the extremities. Head turns toward upward side	In general, equilibrium reactions are automatic reactions which preserve body's center of balance when the supporting base is unstable. Also, equilibrium facilitates movement and postural adaptation to different gravitational changes	Cortical	5 months	Persists

Reaction	Position	Sensory Systems	Stimulus	Response	CNS Level	Age of Onset	Integration
37. Equilibrium *supine* (31)	Supine	Vestibular, proprioceptive, and visual	Displace the body, laterally in supine			7–8 months	Persists
38. Equilibrium *sitting* (31)	Sitting	Vestibular, proprioceptive, and visual	Displace the body, to the right and left, forward and backward	Curvature of the spine, concave to the side being stressed or upward side, with abduction and extension of the UEs. Stable, prone, and supine with beginning sitting equilibrium are necessary for sitting without support		7–8 months	Persists
39. Equilibrium *quadruped* (31)	Quadruped	Vestibular, proprioceptive, and visual	Displace the body on all fours	Curvature of the spine, concave to the side being stressed with increased UE and LE extension on stressed side. Stable prone, supine, and sitting equilibrium with beginning equilibrium in quadruped are needed for creeping	Cortical	9–12 months	Persists
40. Equilibrium *standing* (31)	Biped	Vestibular, proprioceptive, and visual	Displace the body in standing	Curvature of the spine, concave to side being stressed with abduction and extension of UEs and LEs. Stable equilibrium in quadruped and beginning biped standing reactions are needed for standing and walking. Delayed or deficient equilibrium reactions will interfere with all forms of volitional movement and restrict mobility and adaptability.	Cortical	12–21 months	Persists
41. Staggering reaction (protective) (14, 16, 29, 42)	Biped	Vestibular, proprioceptive, and visual	Displace the body in biped position forward, backward, and sideways	One or more steps in direction of displacement to maintain balance. Perfected staggering ensures safe independent walking and recovery from loss of balance in concert with protective reactions of UEs.	Brainstem, midbrain, basal ganglia with cortical input	15–18 months	Persists

Development of Prehension

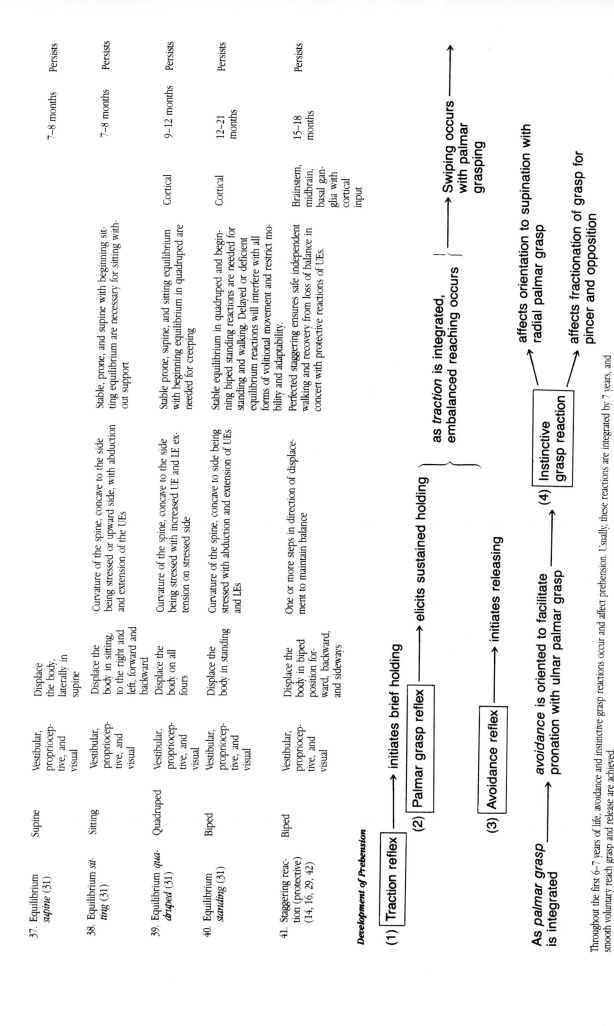

(1) Traction reflex → initiates brief holding

(2) Palmar grasp reflex → elicits sustained holding

(3) Avoidance reflex → initiates releasing

As *palmar grasp* is integrated *avoidance* is oriented to facilitate pronation with ulnar palmar grasp → (4) Instinctive grasp reaction

as *traction* is integrated, embalanced reaching occurs → Swiping occurs with palmar grasping

affects orientation to supination with radial palmar grasp

affects fractionation of grasp for pincer and opposition

Throughout the first 6–7 years of life, avoidance and instinctive grasp reactions occur and affect prehension. Usually, these reactions are integrated by 7 years, and smooth voluntary reach grasp and release are achieved.

(continued)

TABLE 5-4. *Neurophysiologic Reflex Processes and the Influence on Movement and Adaptation (continued)*

Reflex (See references below)	Position	Stimulus	Location	Responses	Adaptation	Origin	Reflex Age Range	
							Initiation	Inhibition

Reflex References

1. Andre-Thomas, Chesni Y, Saint-Anne Dargassies S: *The Neurological Examination of the Infant. Clin Dev Med, No. 1, 1960*
2. Andre-Thomas, Autgaerden S: *Locomotion from Pre to Post Natal Life. Clin Dev Med, No. 24, 1963*
3. Ayres AJ: *Sensory Integration and Learning Disorders. California, Western Psychological Services, 1972*
4. Beintema DJ: *A Neurological study of Newborn Infants. Clin Dev Med, No. 28, 1968*
5. Bench J, Collyer Y, Langford C, et al: A comparison between the neonatal sound-evoked startle response and the head-drop (Moro) reflex. *Dev. Med Child Neurol 14:308, 1972*
6. Bobath B: A study of abnormal postural reflex activities in patients with lesions of the central nervous system. *Physiotherapy 40:259, 1954*
7. Bobath B: *Abnormal Postural Reflex Activity Caused by Brain Lesions. London, William Heinemann Medical Books, 1971*
8. Bobath B: The very early treatment of cerebral palsy. *Dev Med Child Neurol 9:373, 1967*
9. Bobath B: Motor development, its effect on general development, and application to the treatment of cerebral palsy. *Physiotherapy 57:526, 1971*
10. Bobath K: The Motor Deficit in Patients with Cerebral Palsy. *Clin Dev Med, No. 23, 1969*
11. Bobath K, Bobath B: Cerebral Palsy. In Pearson P, Williams C (eds): *Physical Therapy Services in the Developmental Disabilities, pp 31–185. Springfield, IL, Charles C Thomas 1972*
12. Connor FP, Williams GG, Siepp J: *A Program Guide for Infants and Toddlers with Neuromotor and Other Developmental Disabilities, Experimental Edition. New York, United Cerebral Palsy Association, 1976.*
13. Capps C, Plescia MG, Houser C: The Landau reaction: A clinical and electromyographic analysis. *Dev Med Child Neurol 18:41, 1976*
14. Easton TA: On the normal use of reflexes. *Am Sci 60:591, 1972*
15. Farber S: *Sensorimotor Evaluation and Treatment Procedures for Allied Health Personnel. Indianapolis, Occupational Therapy Curriculum, Indiana University Medical Center, 1974*
16. Fiorentino MR: *Reflex Testing Methods for Evaluating CNS Development. Springfield, IL, Charles C Thomas, 1963*
17. Fukuda T: Studies on human dynamic postures from the viewpoint of postural reflexes. *Acta Otolaryngol (Suppl 161) 1960*
18. Gilfoyle E, Grady A: A developmental theory of somatosensory perception. In Henderson A, Coryell J (eds): *The Body Senses and Perceptual Deficit. Boston, Boston University, 1973*
19. Goldstein K, Landis C, Hunt W, et al: Moro reflex and startle pattern. *Arch Neurol Psychiatr 40:322, 1938*
20. Gordon MG: The Moro embrace reflex in infancy: Its incidence and significance. *Am J Dis Child 38:26, 1929*
21. Halsay HJ, Allen N, Chamberlin HR: Chronic decerebrate state in infancy. *Arch Neurol 19:339, 1968*
22. Hellebrandt FA, Waterland JC: Expansion of motor patterning under exercise stress. *Am J Phys Med 4:56, 1962*
23. Hirt S: The tonic neck reflex mechanism in the normal human adult. *Am J Phys Med 46:362, 1967*
24. Humphrey T: Some correlations between the appearance of human fetal reflexes and the development of the nervous system. *Prog Brain Res 4:93, 1964*
25. Ikai M: Tonic neck reflex in normal persons. *Jpn J Physiol 1:118, 1950*
26. Illingworth RS: *The Development of the Infant and Young Child: Normal and Abnormal, 6th ed. Edinburg, E & S Livingstone, 1975*
27. McGraw MB: *The Neuromuscular Maturation of the Human Infant. New York, Hafner Publishing, 1974*
28. Magnus R: Physiology of posture. *Lancet 2:531; 585, 1926*
29. Martin JP: *The Basal Ganglia and Posture. Philadelphia, JB Lippincott, 1967*
30. Milani-Comparetti A, Gidoni EA: Pattern analysis of motor development and its disorders. *Dev Med Chil Neurol 9:625, 1967*
31. Milani-Comparetti A, Gidoni EA: Routine developmental examination in normal and retarded children. *Dev Med Child Neurol 9:631, 1967*
32. Mohrar G: Motor deficit of retarded infants and young children. *Arch Phys Med Rehab 55:393, 1974*
33. Mueller HA: Facilitating Feeding and Prespeech. In Pearson P, Williams C (eds): *Physical Therapy Services in the Developmental Disabilities, pp 283-310. Springfield, IL, Charles C Thomas, 1972*
34. Paine RS: Evolution of postural reflexes in normal infants and in the presence of chronic brain syndromes. *Neurology 14:1036, 1964*
35. Paine RS: Neurological examination of infants and children. *Pediatr Clin North Am 7:471, 1960*
36. Parmelee AH: A critical evaluation of the Moro reflex. *Pediatrics 33:773, 1964*

37. Peiper A: Cerebral Function in Infancy and Childhood. New York, Consultants Bureau, 1963

38. Robinson RJ: Assessment of gestational age by neurological examination. Arch Dis Child 41:437, 1966

39. Saint-Anne Dargassies S: Neurological maturation of the premature infant of 28–41 weeks' gestational age. In Falkner F (ed): Human Development, pp 306–325. Philadelphia, WB Saunders, 1966

40. Saint-Anne Dargassies S: Neurological symptoms during the first year of life. Dev Med Child Neurol 14:235, 1972

41. Schaltenbrand G: The development of human motility and motor disturbances. Arch Neurol Psychiatr 20:720, 1972

42. Tokizane T, et al: Electromyographic studies on tonic neck, lumbar and labyrinthine reflexes in normal persons. Jpn J Physiol 2:130, 1954

43. Twitchell TE: Attitudinal reflexes. Phys Ther 45:411, 1965

44. Twitchell TE: Minimal cerebral dysfunction in children and motor deficits. Trans Am Neurol Assoc 91:353, 1966

45. Twitchell TE: Normal motor development. Phys Ther 45:419, 1965

46. Twitchell TE: Reflexes and normal development. Presented at the Pediatric Symposium, University of North Carolina at Chapel Hill, Chapel Hill, 1970

47. Twitchell TE: The automatic grasping responses of infants. Neuropsychologia 3:247, 1965

48. Twitchell TE: Variations and abnormalities of motor development. Phys Ther 45:424, 1965

49. Waterland JC, Hellebrandt FA: Involuntary patterning associated with willed movement performed against progressively increasing resistance. Am J Phys Med 43:13, 1967

LE, lower extremity; UE, upper extremity.

111

TABLE 5-5. *Fine Motor Development in the First Year*

Approximate Age (months)	Vision	Hand Position	Grasp
1	Follows object to midline; regards object when brought to or just past midline when object is only 8–9 inches from face	Hands fisted; forearm pronated; occasionally brings hand to mouth (primary circular reaction)	Grasp reflex; no release; object placed in hand drops immediately
2	Prolonged visual regard of objects; follows past midline; regards out-stretched arm (ATNR influence); follows object 180° in supine position	Brings hands to midline; hands may open at sight of object	Grasp reflex; no voluntary release
3	Glances at object in hand; shifts glance between two objects; regards object at midline	Holds hands loosely opened or closed; symmetrical arm/hand movement in supine position	Grasp reflex decreasing or absent; holds object briefly; attempts at swiping at object
4	Occular convergence; regards object held in hand; regards hand	Bilateral arm movement; waves arms and moves body at sight of object	Attempts to play with own fingers; palmar grasp emerges; temporary active grasp; attempts to reach object but misses target; object-to-mouth in supine position; lightly scratches or clutches at clothes
5	Looks momentarily after object dropped	Reaches for and grasps object with both hands; thumb to mouth	Holds block with one hand and regards second block; ulnar palmar grasp when given object
6	Eye–hand coordination emerges (arms used asymmetrically); prolonged regard of objects	Visually directed reaching; reaches for dropped object; supination of forearm in supine position	Radial palmar grasp with flexed wrist; rakes at pellet with fingers (no thumb); holds object in each hand; reaches for block beyond reach
7	Looks after object	Thumb opposition	Grasp in supine position with thumb adducted; poor active release; bangs, shakes, and pats objects; transfers one object hand to hand; retains one object when given another and regards both; radial palmar grasp with extended wrist; inferior scissors grasp with metacarpophalangeal joints flexed
8		Still rakes with entire arm	Inferior pincer (thumb, second, and third fingers); continues to drop objects; scissor grasp with thumb (metacarpophalangeal joint joint extended)
9		Extended reach and grasp; forearm use between midposition and pronation	Pokes with extended index finger; neat pincer grasp between thumb and index finger emerging; voluntary release emerging
10			Spontaneously notices pellet and pokes at it; voluntary release; good superior pincer; holds crayon with crude palmar grasp
12			Smooth grasp; precise release of object into cup of 2-inch diameter (concept of container and contained); pulls ¼-inch pegs from pegboard; removes and replaces pellet in bottle on command

Adapted from Gilfoyle, E.M., & Grady, A.P. (1982). Children adapt. *Thorofare, NJ: Slack*; Clark, P.N., & Allen, A.S. (1985). Occupational therapy for children. *St. Louis: CV Mosby*; The Mecklenburg Center of Human Motor Development Evaluation, Mecklenburg, NY, unpublished, 1970; Gesell, A. (1940). The first five years of life. *New York: Harper & Row.*

objects, babies generally demonstrate visual preference for their edges (sharp contrasts) rather than their features. The infant can and does attend to the features of a face, however. It also appears that the child can differentiate a photograph of a human face from the face itself (Goren, Sart, and Wu, 1975). Skills that develop to enhance vision include stabilization of the head and neck for fine motor use of the eyes; dissociation of the eyes from the head for independent use of oculomotor muscles; visual following, fixation, and attending; localization; convergence and divergence; and smooth, coordinated use of the eyes together. By 6 months of age these basic skills are present and ready for refinement.

Auditory acuity develops and improves until adolescence. At first the baby responds to hearing with a total body reaction of movement or quieting. Subsequently the infant orients to the sound and seeks its source. Current research suggests that within the general range of pitch and loudness of the human voice, infants hear as well as adults, although adults are more sensitive to quiet sounds (Sinnott, Pisoni, & Aslin, 1983).

Gustatory and olfactory senses have not been studied as

extensively as the others. These senses are interrelated and interdependent. Study of the development of the sensed of taste (sweet, sour, bitter, and salt) indicates that infants react differently to at least three basic flavors and prefer sweet tastes to others. When given a variety of pleasant and noxious olfactory stimuli, the infant consistently responds more definitively to noxious smells.

Interaction of many of the sensory modalities enhances their function. The sense of taste diminishes when the sense of smell is limited. The vestibular and tactile systems can be strong organizers for other functions of the body.

Perceptual development

Once a sensation has been registered in the brain, the infant or child must derive meaning from it. This is accomplished by relating the current experience to learning that has already occurred. Thus, the child can perceive the ball as part of a game because he or she has already had experience with round objects that are thrown. Over time the infant builds a repertoire of knowledge about the world that is based on visual, auditory, motor, and cognitive perceptions. The child explores new things, relates them to an earlier experience, and modifies his or her existing concepts while integrating the new experience into an old schema.

Emotional development and theories of personality

The emotional responses of children are related to the development of personality; that is, the person's unique, individual, relatively enduring pattern of relating to others and responding to the world (Bee, 1985). Several theories have been used to describe the development of personality.

Temperament theory

Temperament theory is predominantly, but not exclusively, a biologic theory of personality development. Some basic concepts of this theory are:

1. Each person is born with characteristic patterns of responding to the environment.
2. These temperamental characteristics affect the way the child responds to people and things around him or her.
3. The child's temperament also affects the way others respond to him or her.

Social learning theory

This theory states that patterns of social behavior (what we normally call personality) are learned through modeling and can be specific to particular situations. If these patterns of personality are situation specific, then personality patterns may not be consistent across situations or over time. The child's cognitive capacity may affect his or her ability to understand or attend to a model's behavior.

Psychoanalytic theory

Psychoanalytic theory considers both inborn qualities and particular environmental needs. The most well known of the psychoanalytic theorists, Freud and Erikson, dealt with the developmental aspects of the origins of personality in childhood.

As was discussed earlier in this chapter, Freud identified three basic structures of personality in childhood: the id, ego, and superego. The *id* is the storehouse of basic energy, continually pushing for immediate gratification. The *ego* organizes, plans, and reality-tests the personality. Thought and language are ego functions. The *superego* is the conscious portion of personality; it contains parental and societal values and is developed by means of the identification process. When conflict arises between the id, ego, and superego, anxiety results. The child develops defense mechanisms (normal automatic and unconscious strategies) for reducing stress when faced with intense anxiety. He or she also goes through distinct psychosexual stages, each of which focuses on sexual gratification in a specific erogenous zone.

Erikson concentrated on ego development throughout the lifespan. He was concerned with societal and social demands on the child and referred to "psychosocial" stages of development. The four stages in childhood are summarized below.

Basic trust versus mistrust

The first ego challenge occurs during the first year of life within the context of the relationship with the primary caregiver (usually the mother). The challenge is to establish a sense of *basic trust* in the world and in oneself. This sense develops when the caregiver accommodates him- or herself to the needs of the infant. The infant then learns that the caregiver is separate from the self but can be counted on to reappear even if he or she leaves temporarily. To the extent that the caregiver is unreliable and mutual regulation does not occur, a sense of *basic mistrust* may develop. In the adult, residues of basic mistrust may show up as extreme denial of needing anyone else or an inability to tolerate separation from those one depends on. The favorable outcome of this challenge to trust is the development of drive and hope. (Huyok & Hoyer, 1982).

Autonomy versus doubt and shame

The second challenge emerges from the increasing capacities for cognitive discrimination and self-control and is confronted during the second and third years of life. The young child relates importantly with both parents and can differentiate them from each other and from himself. The ego challenge is to establish a firm sense of *autonomy*, and of self as a distinct person capable of internal self-regulation and not ruled only by external forces. The risk at this stage is that the child will be incapable of self-regulation or will be given too little opportunity for self-regulation; in this case, a sense of *doubt* about the self and *shame* in one's impulses may overwhelm one's sense of autonomy. Adult manifestations of the sense of doubt and shame include an excessive preoccupation with issues of control—either keeping too much control over oneself or yielding too much control and direction to others. Establishing the right balance between autonomy and doubt results in the development of self-control and willpower (Havighurst, 1972).

Initiative versus guilt

The third challenge is to establish a sense of *initiative* and overcome excessive *guilt*. These issues are most crucial between the ages of 3 and 6 years, and they link the child in mutual regulation to the wider family unit. A special challenge involves the competition between the child and the same-sex parent for the attention and affection of the opposite-sex parent; this is traditionally referred to as the *Oedipal situation*, or the *family romance*. The favorable outcome of this period is to become capable of direction and purpose.

Industry versus inferiority

The fourth ego challenge links the child to the wider world of peers and adults outside the family. This phase usually begins with entrance into formal education at the age of 6 or 7 years and ends with puberty. The challenge is to establish a sense of *industry*—the sense that one is a worker who can develop whatever skills and competencies are needed to be productive and admired in that particular culture. The risk is that the child will not acquire the necessary skills to relate effectively outside the family and will develop a sense of *inferiority*. Some adults have a lingering sense of incompetence; they fear they cannot achieve anything well enough to be evaluated by an impartial judge. They may have great difficulties in work settings that are not "familial."

The emotional world of the child is a complex interaction of personality development, self-concept, bonding, attachment, family interactions, and personal relationships. Childhood is the testing ground for emotions and behaviors that will be the cornerstones of adaptive behaviors.

Social development

The concept of self

Any discussion of children's social relationships must proceed from an understanding of the concept of self and how it develops. The emerging concept of self has several elements, including:

1. *The I or existential self:* awareness of self as separate. This sense of self occurs with self-recognition at approximately 15 to 18 months of age.
2. *The me or categorical self*, arrived at by comparing the self to others in one or more categories.
3. *Self-esteem:* the dimension of self-concept that includes a negative or positive sense of self. Studies have demonstrated that the child with high self-esteem does somewhat better on school achievement tests; sees him- or herself as responsible for success or failure; has more friends; and has a positive view of parental relationships. (Damon & Hart, 1982).

Sex-role development

By the age of 2 or 3 years, the child generally identifies him- or herself as a boy or girl (gender identity). By age 4, he or she understands that gender is stable throughout life; and by age 5 or 6, the child has the concept of gender constancy (gender does not change by appearance change). Sex-role concepts and stereotyping appear to be strongest at 6 to 7 years of age.

There are many theories of sex-role development. Mischel, a social learning theorist, emphasizes the role of reinforcement and modeling as the basis of sex-role acquisition. Freud's explanation rests on the concept of identification, by which the child imitates the same-sex parent. Kohlberg proposed a cognitive-developmental model: the child imitates the same-sex model only after gender constancy is confirmed. Current research proposes that the child begins to develop rules about what a boy or girl does after he or she understands gender differences (Bee, 1985).

Social relationships

As the child develops a sense of self, he or she interacts with others to form social relationships. Bowlby and Ainsworth describe the basic sense of attachment in infancy. They see attachment as an invisible, internal affectional bond demonstrated by attachment behaviors that allow the child to retain closeness to a significant person. Attachment begins with initial bonding and continues with mutual attachment behaviors. Although research by Klaus and Kennel suggested that initial bonding (12 to 24 hours after birth) and early contact were vital for the development of parent–child relationships, more current research indicates that early contact may be only partially potent or critical for long-term parent–child relationships (Lamb, 1982).

The meshing of attachment behaviors is much more critical for parent attachment. The child develops attachment to both the mother and father. The child sends out signals and the parent responds. By 4 to 5 months of age, most infants have formed strong attachment to a primary caretaker (usually the mother). A father who was present at the birth of his baby bonds more strongly to the child than a father who was not present.

The attachment process occurs in several phases, according to Ainsworth:

Phase 1—initial attachment. During the first 4 months, the infant displays proximity-promoting behaviors (behaviors that bring people closer). There is no consistent attachment to one parent or the other.

Phase 2—attachment-in-the-making. At about 3 months of age, the infant can distinguish between familiar and unfamiliar faces and dispenses attachment behaviors more discriminatingly. There is no complete attachment to a single person.

Phase 3—clear-cut attachment. By about 6 to 7 months, attachment is directed toward one person. The mode of attachment changes—it becomes proximity-seeking. The child literally moves toward the caregiver.

Phase 4—multiple attachments. Single attachment occurs between 6 and 12 months. After that time, attachments spread to others (Ainsworth, 1982).

Patterns of attachment

In general from 7 to 8 months of age, the child shows strong attachment to either the father or the mother in preference to a stranger. He or she typically turns to the mother rather than the father when under stress. The older child seems to form a stronger attachment and identification with the same-sex parent. The securely attached child uses the adult as a safe base for exploration. Secure attachment is fostered by attentive and loving interaction between child and parent.

Relationships with other children

Relationships with other children become more central from the age of 1 to 2 years. By 4 to 5 years, children have formed individual relationships. Friendships become stable in elementary school. Peer interaction becomes increasingly important, reaching a climax during adolescence.

Development of social cognition

The child's thinking has an impact on his or her relationships with people and objects. In particular, the child's perspective-taking ability is central to his or her emerging understanding of other people and relationships. Selman's theory of social understanding indicates the relation of social perspective thinking to the development of social relationships. The level of social understanding can be seen in the child's understanding of friendships, groups, and parent–child relationships. The two key levels in early childhood are the reciprocal level (7 to 12 years) and the mutual level (10 to 15 years). In the reciprocal level, the child understands that others either feel and see things differently than he or she does or that others feel and see things in the same way. Relationships are seen as two-way interactions. In the mutual level, the youngster understands that relationships require constant mutual adjustment (Bee, 1985).

Moral development

Social understanding also requires the child to think about and explain other people's actions. The child must develop a sense of morality. Kohlberg has delineated six stages of moral reasoning (see display).

The development of the social world of the child is a complex process. Self-concept, bonding, attachment, social relationships with others, the understanding of social interactions—as well as the broader world of judgment and morality—all interact for the child to become socially competent.

Cognitive development

Major views

There are three major views of cognitive development.

Intellectual power approach

The intellectual power approach measures individual differences in intelligence by various tests. The intellectual quotient, originally a comparison of the child's chronologic age with his or her mental age, is no longer used. Now the child's performance is compared with the performance of a large group of children of the same age. The most commonly used tests are the Bayley Scales of Infants, the Stanford–Binet, and the Wechsler Intelligence Scales for Children. Both IQ tests and school achievement tests measure *performance*, not underlying intellectual ability or competence.

Cognitive developmental approach

The focus of the cognitive development approach is on the development of cognitive structures rather than of intellectual power. Patterns of development that are common to all children rather than to individuals are studied.

Jean Piaget described four major stages of **cognitive development** (see the display on p. 100 and Table 5-6).

Current research concerning Piaget's stages indicates that imitation of behaviors may occur in substage I rather than substage II (Meltzoff & Moore, 1983), that deferred imitation may occur 1 year earlier than Piaget predicted (Kastenbaum, 1972), and that infants remember what they see and organize their memory as early as age 8 to 10 months (Caron & Caron, 1982).

Research on the preoperational period indicates that children from the age of 2 to 6 years are more skillful than Piaget originally thought. For example, a child as young as 2 or 3 years has at least some ability to understand that other people see or experience things differently (Flavell, 1982). The preoperational child may understand identities and do simple classification as

---

SUMMARY OF KOHLBERG'S SIX STAGES OF MORAL REASONING

Level I

Pre-Moral (4 to 10 years). Primary emphasis is on external control and ideas of others. These standards are followed either to avoid punishment or to gain reward.

Type I—Punishment and obedience. The child obeys to avoid punishment.

Type II—Naive instrumental hedonism. Conformity to rules is out of self-interest.

Level II

Morality of Conventional Role Conformity (10 to 13 years). The child wishes to please others and internalizes some of the standards of those persons deemed important to him or her. The child now decides if some action is good by his or her standards.

Type III—Maintaining approval of others. The child judges the intentions of others and yields an opinion.

Type IV—Authority maintaining morality. The child shows respect for authority and maintenance of social order.

Level III

Morality of Self-Accepted Moral Principles (13 years to adulthood). True morality: the person recognizes the possible conflict between standards and realizes that conduct and reasoning about right and wrong are a result of internal control.

Type V—Morality of contract, of individual rights, and of accepted democratic law. People think in logical terms, valuing the will of society as a whole. These values are for the most part substantiated by obeying the law.

Type VI—Morality of individual principles of conscience. The individual does what he or she thinks is right as a result of his or her internalized values.

Adapted from Kohlberg, L. (1968). The child as a moral philosopher. Psychology Today, 2, 25.

---

early as 3 years (Bee, 1985; Marlcham, Cox, & Machida, 1981).

The latest research on Piaget's concrete operational stage focuses on the sequence of the development of concrete operations and on whether the child's skills are consistent across tasks. Carol Tomlinson-Keasey and others found that there are definitive sequences in operational thought and that a child in the concrete operational stage performs at or about the same level consistently on a wide series of tasks (Tomlinson-Keasey et al., 1978).

Information processing approach

A third approach, known as information processing, has emerged (Sternberg, 1981; Sternberg, 1982). This approach searches for the fundamental processes or strategies that constitute cognition. Once these processes are known, one can investi-

TABLE 5-6.   *Continuum of Cognitive Development*

Modality of Intelligence	Phase	Stage	Approximate Chronologic Age
Sensorimotor	Sensorimotor	1. Use of reflexes	0–1 month
		2. First habits and primary circular reactions	1–4.5 months
		3. Coordination of vision and prehension, secondary circular reactions	4.5–9 months
		4. Coordination of secondary schemata and their application to new situations	9–12 months
		5. Differentiation of action schemata through tertiary circular reactions, discovery of new means	12–18 months
		6. First internalization of schemata and solution of some problems by deduction	18–24 months
Represenative by means of concrete operations	Preconceptual	1. Appearance of symbolic function and the beginning of internalized actions accompanied by representation	2–4 years
	Intuitive thought	2. Representational organizations based on either static configurations or on assimilation to one's own action	4–5.5 years
		3. Articulated representational regulations	5.5–7 years
	Concrete operational	1. Simple operations (classifications, seriations, term-by-term correspondences, etc.)	7–9 years
		2. Whole systems (Euclidian coordinates, projective concepts, simultaneity)	9–11 years
Representative by means of formal operations	Formal operational	1. Hypothetico-deductive logic and combinatorial operations	11–14 years
		2. Structure of "lattice" and the group of 4 transformations	14 years +

From Maier HW (Ed.) (1969). Three theories of child development: The Contributions of Erik H. Erikson, Jean Piaget and Robert R. Sears, rev ed. (p. 15). New York: Harper & Row. Reprinted with permission. The source was Piaget's paper: Les Stades du developpement intellectuel de l'enfa et de l'adolescent (1956). Adapted from Table 1, Intelligence is an ultimate goal, in Décarié TG: Intelligence and Affectivity in Early Childhood, p 1 New York, International Universities Press, 1965. Reprinted with permission.

gate whether they change with age and whether children differ in their speed of acquiring cognitive skills. This approach seems to skillfully combine concepts of cognitive power with structural approaches to cognitive development.

Language development

An overview of cognition would be incomplete without a discussion of the acquisition of language skills. Language is the expression of the child's thoughts and the understanding of the world. Children's language is complex, productive, creative, and governed by rules. It is an arbitrary system of symbols that allows one to understand myriad messages. During the first year of the child's life, he or she goes through several prelinguistic phases: crying, cooing, babbling (see the display).

At approximately 1 year of age the first words emerge. After the first word is spoken, it takes 3 to 4 months to add the next ten words (Nelson, 1973). Vocabulary increases rapidly thereafter, and by 2 years of age, the child typically has a 300-word vocabulary. Language becomes more complex with the addition of plurals, past tense, auxiliary verbs, and prepositions. There appears to be a language sequencing in a predictable order, as the child progressively adds questions, negatives, superlatives, and so forth. Semantic development follows a predictable course. A child seems to have concepts or categories before he or she has words for them. By the time a child is 5 or 6 years old, his or her language is much like an adult's, but the child does not develop language skillfully until 8 or 9 years of age. The meaning of words for children seems to center on the function and the perceptual properties of objects and people.

There are individual differences in rate of language and grammar development, as well as in language style, that are influenced by both heredity and environment. Current theory focuses on the child's general cognitive development and the impact of the language heard by the child (Bee, 1985).

Cultural development

It is impossible to include all aspects and nuances of cultural influences in this overview of development. Instead, we will look beyond the primary attachments of mother and child to the family and the intricate network of relationships that form the child's ecological system or niche.

1. The family, with parental behavior, control, and emotional tone, has a most significant effect on the child's adaptive response. It appears that parents who are warm and affectionate foster in the child more secure attachments and peer relationships (Bee, 1985).
2. Parents who are autocratic instead of authoritarian or permissive in expressing parental control tend to influence positive self-esteem and competence. This positive sense of self extends to school and to a variety of social situations (Baumrind, 1973; Patterson, 1975).
3. Parents who provide a rich nonhuman environment, enriched language, and developmentally appropriate play activities seem to have a closer relationship with their child. The child also tends to show more rapid growth in cognitive ability (Wachs & Gruen, 1982).

There are many institutional and societal influences on a child's development. For example, the socioeconomic level influences family interaction, degree of stress tolerance, health, and availability of support systems to the family. Parents living in poverty tend to talk less frequently to children; they provide a less

SEQUENCES OF LANGUAGE DEVELOPMENT

Prelinguistic Speech

Before a child says his or her first real word, he or she goes through the following six, and perhaps seven, stages of speech:

1. *Undifferentiated crying*. With "no language but a cry," babies come into this world. Early crying is a reflexive reaction to the environment produced by the expiration of breath.
2. *Differentiated crying*. After the first month of life (and of crying), the close listener can often discriminate differences in a baby's cries and can identify their causes.
3. *Cooing*. At about 6 weeks, chance movements of the child's mechanisms produce a variety of simple sounds called cooing. These squeals, gurgles, and bleats are usually emitted when he or she is happy and contented. The first sounds are vowels, and the first consonant is "h".
4. *Babbling*. These vocal gymnastics begin at about 3 or 4 months, as a child playfully repeats a variety of sounds. Again, the child is most likely to babble when he or she is contented and when he or she is alone. As he or she lies in the crib or sits in the infant seat, he or she loquaciously, and often loudly, spouts forth a variety of simple consonant and vowel sounds: "ma-ma-ma-ma-ma," "da-da-da-da-da," "bi-bi-bi-bi-bi-bi," and so forth. While most children babble, a few seem to skip this stage. Deaf children babble normally for the first few months of life, but then appear to lose interest when they cannot hear themselves.
5. *Lallation or imperfect imitation*. Some time during the second half of the first year, a child seems to become more aware of the sounds around him. He or she will become quiet while listening to some sound. When it stops, he or she babbles in excitement, accidentally repeating the sounds and syllables heard. Then the child imitates his or her own sounds.
6. *Echolalia or imitation of the sounds of others*. At about the age of 9 or 10 months, a child seems to consciously imitate the sounds made by others, even though he or she still does not understand them.

7. *Expressive jargon*. During the second year, many children use *expressive jargon*. This term, coined by Gesell, refers to a string of utterances that *sound* like sentences, with pauses, inflections, and rhythms. However, speech is not yet communicated verbally on a consistent basis.

Linguistic Speech

1. *One-word sentence (holophrase)*. At about a year, a child points to a cracker, a toy, a pacifier, and says "da." Parents correctly interpret the command as "Give me that" or "I want that." He or she points to the door and says, "out." His or her single word thus expresses a complete thought, even though listeners may not always be able to divine what that complete thought may be.
2. *Multiword sentence*. Some time about the age of 2, a child strings together two or more words to make a sentence. When he or she wants to feed him- or herself with no interference, he or she says imperiously, "Mommy 'way."

   The child may develop a combination of sounds that mean something to him or her but may not necessarily be understood by the listener. Usually this communication style occurs at the time the child is learning nouns. The sounds or syllables are attached to the newly learned nouns.

   The earliest multiword sentences are combinations of nouns and verbs. Other parts of speech, such as articles, prepositions, and adjectives, are lacking. Although these sentences are far from grammatical, they do communicate. This is *telegraphic speech;* it contains only words that carry meaning.
3. *Grammatically correct verbal utterances*. At about the age of 3, the child has an impressive command of the language. He or she now has a vocabulary of some 900 words, speaks in longer sentences that include all the parts of speech, and has a good grasp of grammatical principles. His or her grammar is not the same one used by adults because the child makes little allowance for exceptions to the linguistic rules assimilated. Thus he or she says, "We goed to the store."

Adapted from Eisenson, J., et al. (1963). The psychology of communication. *New York: Appleton-Century-Crofts; Leneberg, E.H. (1967). Biological function of language. New York: John Wiley & Sons; Clifton, C. (1970). Language acquisition. In T.D. Spencer, N. Kass (Eds.),* Perspectives in child psychology: Research and review. *New York: McGraw-Hill.*

stimulating or age-appropriate learning environment. Poverty often causes the parent to be less available to the child. The parenting style appears to be more authoritarian and more physical in the approach to discipline (Baumrind, 1973). A child from this lower economic situation also tends to not do as well in school and to have lower IQ scores. Fewer students from poor families participate in higher education.

Research also points to the importance of a secure support system for parents. For example, Hetherington found that children of divorced parents tend to have closer and more secure

relationships with the parent who had continued support from friends and family (Hetherington, 1979). A social network takes time to cultivate, but the outcome for both child and parents seems positive.

Beyond family and social networks, the type and method of education have a major impact on the developing child. Attending school fosters information processing, but it is the qualities of the school and the teacher that affect the child's attitude toward school, academic achievement, and future educational pursuits. Effective schools and teachers are authoritative and they demonstrate excellent communication skills, shared goals, and high levels of control without strong punitive responses. They also emphasize academic importance and achievement (Rutter, 1983).

The play environment, television, and the types of aggressive activities engaged in also influence the effectiveness of the child's adaptation.

Throughout all the transitions of childhood, the child who experiences excitement, joy, pleasure, and mastery of developmental tasks shows positive adaptive behaviors. Parents also experience a feeling of self-satisfaction and delight in watching their children's development. The result can only be positive personal growth for child and parent.

Play in child development

As a child progresses from infant to adult, his or her major focus of activity evolves along a play–work continuum. At each developmental period, the balance between play and work shifts. For the preschool child, play is the central activity. The structure of the early school years teaches the child to balance work and play activities. As a child approaches adolescence, he or she becomes increasingly involved in structured and work-oriented activity. This work focus increases through the teen years. For adults, work and career development are balanced with either active or passive leisure time activities.

Over the years, educators and developmentalists have developed many definitions for the word *play*, but inherent in all of these definitions is the concept that play is an activity voluntarily engaged in for pleasure. This activity is significant because it helps the child adapt within his or her environment or culture. A child's play develops through several stages from passive observation to cooperative, purposeful activity (see display).

Functions of play

Through play, the child learns to explore, develop, and master physical and social skills.

Social

During play, the young child tests family, adult, and gender roles at his or her own pace, free from the limits of the adult world. Play teaches a child to relate to others, first as an observer and later as a participant in cooperative or competitive and group endeavors. Play provides a means by which the child gains an insight in the mores of his or her culture. As the child comes to an understanding of what is acceptable and not acceptable, he or she begins to develop a sense of social morality.

Physical/sensory/perceptual

Children love to repeat activity. They will engage in seemingly endless repetition of both gross and fine motor skills for the pure joy of mastery. As his or her skills proliferate, a child can integrate more complex and coordinated activities. Sensory and motor activity teach the child the physical realities of the world as well as the capabilities and limitations of his or her own body. Play also provides a release for excess energy, which restores body equilibrium, freeing the child for new endeavors. It heightens a child's perceptual ability: events or objects in the play environment allow the child to perceive forms and spatial and temporal relationships. He or she begins to classify objects and relate them to other objects, forming the basis for logical thought.

PLAY BEHAVIOR

Unoccupied Play Behavior. The child seems not to be playing but momentarily watches activity in the environment. When not attending, the child plays with his or her body, engages in gross motor behavior (eg, climbing up or down from chairs, following people around), or just sits looking around the room.

Onlooker Play. The child watches others play and engages in conversation with those playing. He or she definitely is observing the children rather than events, although he or she does not engage in actual play.

Solitary Independent Play. The child pursues play activities alone and independently from the other children playing. Although the child often positions him- or herself close to others, he or she makes no reference to what they are doing.

Parallel Play. The child plays with toys similar to those used by other children near him or her but plays beside rather than with the children.

Associative Play. The child plays with others. There is no organization of play activities in his or her peer group, no division of labor, and no product. Each child acts individually; his or her interest focusing on the association rather than the play activity.

Cooperative or Organized Supplementary Play. The child plays with other children in an organized manner for a purpose (eg, making something, formal games). There is a marked sense of belonging to the group, which is now directed by one or two leaders. Each child finds some role in the new organization, his or her efforts augmented by the other members of the group.

Adapted from Parten, M.B. (1932). Social play among preschool children. Journal of Abnormal Social Psychology, 27, 243.

Emotional

Play allows the child to discover a sense of self, an internal stability. The child begins to trust the constancy and consistency of the environment. This trust forms the basis for ego identity. Play lets a child test the reality of inner and outer worlds. It enables him or her to express feelings without fear of punishment and, conversely, helps him or her learn to control frustrations and impulses. This control provides the basis for ego strength, self-confidence, and potential adaptation to future needs. Play is fun—it opens a world of joy, humor, and creativity.

Cognitive

Play activities are closely related to the child's level of cognitive development. Through play, the child learns to manipulate events and objects in the internal and external environment. This manipulation and combination of novel events lay the foundation for problem solving. Representational thought emerges as the child engages in symbolic and dramatic play; abstract thought has its basis in activities that allow for classification and problem-solving ability. The concrete experiences of play allow the child to make a more accurate assessment of the environment and his or her role in it.

Content and structure of play

To gain a real insight into a child's world, we must look intently at his or her play. The classifications that follow are descriptive rather than theoretical.

Elizabeth Hurlock delineates four general stages of play:

1. *The exploratory stage (infant).* Once control of the upper extremities is attained, the infant can more determinedly explore his or her body and the objects within the environment.
2. *The toy stage (1 to 7 to 8 years).* Constructive play begins at 3 years and culminates in the development of hobbies. During the school years, hobbies and collections serve as social and status agents.
3. *The play stage (school years).* In this period, which overlaps with Stages 2 and 4, the development of productive construction, games, and sports occurs.
4. *Adolescent play/work stage.* Preadolescent play and work activities become more complex. The young person begins to project future goals and activity plans into his or her creative endeavors. The elements of introspection and daydreaming reach a peak (Schuster & Ashburn, 1992).

Sara Smilansky (1968) focuses only on dramatic play, defining four specific types:

1. *Functional play.* This includes all simple verbal and behavioral play and allows the child to explore the immediate environment.
2. *Constructive play.* At about 2 years of age, a child begins to demonstrate dramatic skill. "Making believe" in reality-oriented play helps the child make the link between his or her world and the adult world.
3. *Dramatic play.* The two main elements of dramatic play are imitation of an adult (the real world) and a "pretend" situation (the unreal world). The highest level of dramatic play is sociodramatic play, in which at least two children engage in play-acting activity, imitating the real speech and gestures of others in an imaginary situation.
4. *Games with rules.* This stage begins during the school years and culminates in adulthood.

Piaget (1953) identified the structure of play according to the cognitive complexity of activities. (See the display on p. 100 for a listing of sensorimotor substages.)

Practice games

Practice games include any activity that the child repeats for pure pleasure, such as pure sensorimotor practice and mental exercise.

These practice games appear in Piaget's Substage 2 of the sensorimotor period.

Symbolic games

Symbolic games appear in Substage 6 of the sensorimotor period. Symbolic games are difficult to differentiate from practice games; the main difference is the introduction of make-believe.

Games with rules

As the child grows and interacts with peers, sensorimotor and symbolic games become "games with rules." These games require mental organization and operations.

Constructional games

This fourth category is identified by Piaget (1953) although he specifies that it does not occupy its own space. Constructional games are found in all three structural types, but they occupy space "half-way between play and intelligent work, or between play and imitation" (p. 68).

Theories of play

Erikson

Erikson discusses play as a sequential unfolding of psychosocial relationships (Schuster & Ashburn, 1992).

Stage 1—the Auto-Cosmic Stage. From birth to 15 months, the child focuses on his or her own body. During the first phase of this stage, the self is the center of exploration. Kinesthetic sensations and sensual perceptions are repeated. In the second phase, the child starts to explore other people or objects. Although the focus of his or her actions is still sensual pleasure, the actions may now be directed to cause and effect (for example, crying for attention).

Stage 2—the Microcosmic Stage. From 15 months to 3 years, the child uses small toys and objects to play out themes, and he or she begins to master the environment.

Stage 3—the Macrosphere Stage. From nursery school to 7 years, the child's play revolves around other children. This interaction begins with minimal communication. Initially, a child may view other children as objects, but as his or her experiences increase, the child learns to participate in cooperative role taking.

Stage 4—Industry versus Inferiority. From 7 years to preadolescence, the school-age child learns the skills and tools of his or her culture. Mastery of tasks and the development of competency are intrinsic rewards.

Stage 5—Identity versus Role Confusion. During the adolescent years, the focus of play and activities is role identification. Work-oriented tasks play a major role in the child's life situation.

Anna Freud

To Anna Freud (1965), the ability to work is related to the pleasure of achievement, which has a basis in early play activity. A person's ability to work is related to his or her ego development and ability to (1) control and modify impulses, (2) delay gratification, (3) carry out preconceived plans even when frustration intervenes, (4) neutralize energies of instinctual drives through sublimated pleasures, and (5) be governed by a reality principle rather than a pleasure principle.

Jean Piaget

Piaget believed that activity or play may be an end product for a child. What is play at one stage may be work at another. Once the child learns an activity, it is repeated for the sheer joy of mastery. Piaget (1965) defined play as pure assimilation—the repetition of a behavior or a scheme solely for the pleasure of conquering a skill. He believed that the types and evolution of play activities a child chooses reflect the child's level of cognitive development. To Piaget, play and cognitive development are parallel and interdependent. Play fosters the child's ability to master and to become competent within his or her world.

Reilly

Reilly (1974) believes that in play, children require rules that give meaning to the environment (Clark & Allen, 1985). The three phases of play behavior that follow facilitate imagination, curiosity, and need fulfillment.

1. *Exploratory behavior:* the child's attempt to test reality; satisfy his or her basic needs; and search for the meaning of movements, objects, and people within his or her environment.
2. *Competency behavior:* environmental feedback and developmental sequences that facilitate acquisition of competence. The child learns to adapt behavior to develop a sense of mastery and self-confidence.
3. *Achievement behavior:* guided by societal standards, this behavior facilitates risk-taking ability and the development of a sense of competition.

Reilly believes that through play, the child acquires a variety of role behaviors and masters many skills. The play behavior of the child is an antecedent of adult competence.

Role of play in the occupational therapy process

Play is the "occupational" performance of childhood and thus is the medium of intervention in the pediatric occupational therapy process. The occupational therapist must understand the developmental sequences of play to facilitate appropriate play behavior. Observational skills, a play history, knowledge of developmental sequences, and activity analysis provide a baseline for pediatric assessment. Play serves as the main modality to facilitate change in the developmental level(s) of children. Roles and adaptive behaviors can be learned through the play process. The total life experiences of self-care, family, school performance, and social interaction can be enhanced by use of play in the treatment process. The occupational therapist adapts play activities to facilitate appropriate developmental sequences.

Takata (1980) and Florey (1971) provided a taxonomy and classification of play that forms a basis for establishing play history and developmental sequences of play behaviors. These schema provide a basis for organizing and assessing play behavior.

Stage-specific issues

Prenatal development

Periods of prenatal development

After fertilization of the ovum, there is a gestation period of 266 days (with a grace period of 11 days). The first phase (2 weeks) of **prenatal** growth is the *germinal period*. This is primarily a time of cell division and differentiation. Once the growing cell mass is fully implanted in the wall of the uterus, the *embryonic period* begins. During this period (8 weeks), structures and organs are formed and differentiated. Approximately 12 weeks after conception the *fetal period* begins: the first bone cells are developed, and growth continues until birth.

These first several weeks of development are marked by the emergence of physical characteristics. Approximately 26 days after conception, a body form is evolving, and there is the beginning of arm and leg buds. Two days later, the arms are developing

at a greater rate than the legs. By the end of the first month, the details of the head—rudimentary eyes, ears, mouth, and brain—are seen faintly. The brain already shows primitive specialization. There is also a primitive heart and an umbilical cord as well as organs such as the liver, kidney, and stomach. The primitive embryo is now 0.25 to 0.5 inches long, the size of half a pea. In 1 month's time the embryo is 10,000 times larger than the fertilized egg.

By the end of the second month, the embryo has familiar features: face, eyes, ears, nose, lips, tongue, muscles, and skin covering. The arms have discernible fingers and thumbs, and the legs have knees, ankles, and toes. All organs in the body are formed. The brain sends out impulses, the muscles and nerves are working together, and the heart is beating regularly and steadily. The endocrine system is functioning and so are the stomach, liver, and kidneys. Isolated reflexes can be elicited. In several months, these primitive systems will be truly functional.

The third month after conception traditionally marks the beginning of the fetal period. By the end of this month, the fetus has become active. It can kick, turn, close fingers, move its thumb into opposition, and open its mouth, although its eyelids are still closed. This period is marked by refinements of facial and extremity features. The palate and lips are formed and fused. Sexual differentiation is beginning.

The fourth month is a period in which the lower body parts develop more rapidly. The fetus weighs approximately 4 ounces and is 6 inches long. Its muscles and reflexive capabilities are maturing. The mother can now feel a "quickening" movement.

The fifth month is a stage of continued refinement. There is an increase in spontaneous activity. Fetal movements are markedly perceived by the mother. The fetus sleeps and wakes. However, its respiratory system is still too immature for life outside the uterus.

In the sixth month the eyelids of the fetus open. Its eyes are formed and capable of movements (lateral and vertical). Taste buds have developed, as have eyelashes and brows. The fetus has a marked grasp reflex. It now weighs approximately 1.5 pounds and is 12 to 14 inches long. But its breathing patterns are irregular; it can usually survive for only 24 hours outside the womb.

During the seventh month, the cerebral hemispheres cover almost all the brain, and the organism can make specialized responses. If born now, the child can survive in a sheltered environment.

The eighth and ninth months are periods of refinement of function. The immune system of the fetus begins to mature, enabling it to sustain independent life more safely when it is born.

Reflex development begins in the intrauterine environment. Reflexive behaviors are the building blocks of sensorimotor behaviors and the foundation of future sensorimotor patterns. As the central nervous system develops, reflexes/reflexive reactions are integrated and adapted for appropriate sensorimotor behaviors and skills to emerge. The absence or delay of reflex integration behaviors may indicate developmental delay or dysfunction.

Inherited and environmental influences

Genetic make-up delineates the parameters for development. Environmental factors influence the quality and extent to which heredity affects the potential for growth.

Although the uterus is a relatively safe and stable environment, it is not immune to environmental factors. The seriousness of the effect of these factors depends on the type of influence, the intensity of the influence, and the time the influence is introduced.

Since the germinal and embryonic stages are formation and differentiation periods, the first trimester of pregnancy (first 12 weeks) is critical in development. If normal growth is interrupted during this time, defects can arise.

Hereditary factors also contribute to the integrity of the growing organism. Therefore, it is imperative that the therapist understand the basis of genetic functioning, the implications of genetic malfunctioning for the developing organism, and those dysfunctions that are a direct result of genetic inheritance. Increased understanding of deoxyribonucleic acid (DNA) has shed light on those developmental traits that have specific hereditary components.

Early childhood

Accomplishments occur quickly for the **infant** and young child. The first year of life is full of developmental tasks that transform a relatively helpless infant into a baby with abilities in independent locomotion through sequential events of rolling, crawling, creeping, and perhaps even walking. Communication skills are present through meaningful sounds and gestures. Self-feeding is beginning, initiated first by holding the bottle and progressing to simple finger foods. A definite personality and temperament emerge.

Postural stability is a prerequisite to locomotion as well as fine motor skills. Early movement begins on a reflexive basis, ie, when the infant turns his or her head, neck righting aligns the trunk and limbs with the head and neck, which initiates a spontaneous roll. Thus, the skill of rolling begins. The infant manages crawling, which is forward progression with the abdomen touching the supporting surface, by pushing forward with leg extension, possibly facilitated by a positive support reaction as tactile stimulation to the sole of the foot occurs. Creeping, or four-point mobility with the abdomen above the supporting surface and only the hands and knees on the floor, requires dynamic stability at the shoulders and hips to allow movement that is controlled. Soon the infant has matured enough to be able to pull him- or herself up to stand. This progresses to lateral cruising as the child moves sideways, supporting him- or herself on a couch, coffee table, or toy box. By practicing using flexors and extensors to "bounce," experimenting with upright positions, and carefully letting go of the supporting surfaces, enough postural stability emerges to stand independently and then walk. The first tentative steps are taken with a wide-based gait and the arms held in "high guard," or abducted enough to provide additional balance. Learning to walk can occur sometime between the ages of 9 to 15 months. Biologic readiness must be present; the bones, muscles, and neural structures must be mature enough to support the activity.

The concept of "readiness" is applied to each developmental task. It is clear that the 1-week-old would not be ready to walk. There is a critical period within which environmental factors and bodily maturity create an optimum moment for learning. If occupational therapists recognize this moment, they can enhance the skills required.

The time period of 0 to 3 years represents the growth period from infancy to toddlerhood. The issues in this time period

include learning to walk, learning to take solid foods, learning to talk, and learning to control the elimination of body wastes (Havighurst, 1972).

The skills and issues of the toddler blend into those of the preschooler (ages 3 to 5 years). During this time the child is refining his or her motor skills, learning sex differences and sexual modesty, forming concepts and learning language to describe social and physical reality, getting ready to read, and learning to distinguish right and wrong and develop a conscience (Havighurst, 1972).

The period of birth to 5 years encompasses a strong sensorimotor period in which the child is learning through big activities how to handle his or her body. The child will learn more by participating in gross motor activities than he or she will through many fine motor, table-top activities. When the child is secure with his or her body and the spatial relations that gross motor activity have provided, skill in fine motor ventures will occur.

Middle childhood

Middle **childhood** is the period from about 6 to 12 years, or preadolescence. The child is becoming more independent, taking part in activities that take him or her out of the home and involve people other than family members. He or she makes friends with a peer group, becomes physical and athletic, sometimes taking part in organized sports. The child's maturing body has allowed refinement of motor skills; however, care must be taken not to overexert or damage the growing body.

School is important, as the child learns to follow rules, both implicit and explicit, while interacting in this new social setting. The child is also experiencing mental changes that allow him or her to make more complex connections with information at school as well as the outside world. It is an exciting time to grow, explore, make friends, nurture special skills and interests, and develop the self-awareness that will be available when entering the sometimes rocky teenage years.

Havighurst (1972) outlines the developmental issues and tasks of the middle years. They include learning physical skills necessary for ordinary games; building wholesome attitudes toward oneself as a growing organism; learning to get along with age-mates; learning an appropriate masculine or feminine social role; developing fundamental skills in reading, writing, and calculating; developing concepts for everyday living; developing conscience, morality, and a scale of values; achieving personal independence; and developing attitudes toward social groups and institutions. These prepare the child for the new issues of independence, social interaction, and productivity that will emerge in puberty and adolescence.

Adolescence

Adolescence is derived from a Latin word meaning *to come to maturity*. It begins at pubescence, a period of about 2 years before the onset of puberty. Pubescence is a time of physiologic changes: a growth spurt, a synchronous growth of body systems, and increased hormonal activity that triggers the emergence of primary and secondary sex characteristics. Pubescence culminates at puberty, when sexual maturity and reproductive capacity are complete.

It is not as easy to determine when adolescence ends and

TABLE 5-7.   *Theories of Adolescence*

Theorist	Theory and Hypothesis	Assumption(s)	View of Adolescence
C. Darwin	Evolutionary—laws of nature uniform throughout time	Natural selection, species variability adaptation	Maturation is result of adaptation; sexual behavior is influenced by learning
S. Hall	Evolutionary—theory of recapitulation of development	Simultaneous evolution of developmental aspects of adolescence with particular emphasis on biologic factor	Two distinct periods of adolescence (early, late) usually characterized by storm/stress. Adolescence is period of potential personal and societal changes
A. Gesell	Maturational—development is natural biologic unfolding	Predictable sequences and cycles of development (ages and stages)	Adolescence is transition toward maturity. There are specific descriptions of aspects of development during years 10–16
R. Havighurst	Normative—human behavior is learning	Each stage of development has specific learned tasks and there are teachable moments or sensitive periods for learning these tasks	The adolescent years (12–18) focus on eight developmental tasks: 1. Achieving new and mature relations with agemates of both sexes 2. Achieving appropriate sex-role development 3. Accepting one's physical development and using the body effectively 4. Emotional independence from primary caretakers 5. Preparing for marriage and family life 6. Career development 7. Value acquisition and development of personal ideology 8. Developing and achieving socially responsible behavior
S. Freud	Psychoanalytic—fundamental biological instincts; focus is on gratification of basic instincts in psychosexual stages of development	The unconscious; shifting sexual energy from the mouth to the anus to the genital area; id, ego, and superego as the three basic mental functions. Defense mechanisms, which protect ego from unacceptable wishes	Final stage of personality development in preadolescence; puberty results in re-emergence of infantile themes, especially Oedipal or Electra conflicts; patterns of impulse expression, defensive style, and sublimation crystallize into a life orientation; the genital stage
A. Freud	Same as S. Freud	Same as S. Freud	Time of increased libidinal energy associated with biological maturation; ego is in danger of being overwhelmed by instinct; emphasizes asceticism and intellectuality as two powerful adolescent defenses
P. Blos	Same as Freud	Adolescence is psychological adaptation to biologic maturation; the coping system	Three phases of adolescence: (1) early—the onset of puberty; (2) adolescence proper—autonomy from earlier objects of cathexis; (3) late—development of judgment, interests, and intellect; sexual identity established; consolidation of personal identity
E. Erikson	Neofreudian—focus on conscious self (ego development); psychosocial stages; social and cultural influences affect behavior	Eight stages of psychosocial development from infancy throughout adult life, with a psychosocial crisis or bipolar situation to be resolved during each stage. Developmental periods are defined partly by maturation	Identity versus role diffusion or confusion; adolescent reexamines identity and roles (sexual and occupational identities); resolution of crisis or task results ideally in reintegrated sense of self
H.S. Sullivan	Psychoanalytic/Social Psychology—all people exist in an interpersonal field with specific determinants of its own	Three kinds of experience: (1) sensations, perceptions, and emotions experienced before language; (2) private symbols, including fantasies and daydreams; (3) shared symbols. Dynamisms—patterns of interaction	Three phases of adolescence: (1) preadolescence—need for a close relationship with another person of the same sex; (2) early—interest in heterosexual relationships, conflict between needs for intimacy and needs for sexual gratification; (3) late—establishment of mature repertoire of interpersonal relationships, emergence of self-respect (see Table 5-2)

(continued)

TABLE 5-7.   *Theories of Adolescence (continued)*

Theorist	Theory and Hypothesis	Assumption(s)	View of Adolescence
J. Piaget	Cognitive/developmental—knowledge is based on action; structural properties of human brain, sense receptors, and nervous system provide universal bases for human cognition	Scheme: adaptation, which consists of assimilation and accommodation; stages of development: sensorimotor, preoperational, concrete operations, formal operations	Adult reasoning achieved during adolescence; thought governed by principles of logic; hypothesis raising and testing; simultaneous manipulation of more than two variables; consequences of actions anticipated; logical inconsistencies recognized; future computerized
L. Kohlberg	Cognitive/developmental—moral reasoning is reflection of level of cognitive development	Levels of moral reasoning: preconventional (ages 4–10); conventional (ages 10–16); postconventional (ages 16 on)	Period during which personal morality emerges; transition between conventional and postconventional levels may bring doubt, personal reflection, and confusion; period when new moral code or moral philosophy can emerge
K. Lewin	Social psychology—all behavior must be understood in context of field in which it occurs; every psychological concept can be expressed by a mathematical formula	Behavior is function of life space, which includes person and all facts or events in environment of which person is aware; person has a perceptual–motor region and an interpersonal region; environment is divided into regions that represent settings, relationships, and barriers to access	Adolescent as "marginal man" straddling of boundary between childhood and adulthood unstable; Greater uncertainty about regions of environment and about interpersonal and perceptual–motor regions
D. Ausubel	Integrated psychology of adolescent—adolescence is distinct developmental phase with changes that are biologic and social in origin	Adolescence is period of reorganization; biosocial changes are evident and discontinuous; changes are cross-cultural	Uniform elements of common psychological reactions, sexual maturation, sex roles combined with personality traits, changed states, and emerging adult roles
M. Mead and R. Benedict	Cultural anthropology	Degree of continuity between child and adult roles is central focus in cultural impact on personality development (Benedict). Relation between biologic and cultural determinants studied by Mead; was known as cultural determinants, which implied that culture was dominant factor in personality development	Gave cross-cultural perspective on adolescent behavior. Delineated operations of biology and culture in adolescent development and gave increased insight into our own and other cultures.
U. Brofenbrenner	Ecologic theory—child develops within context of ecologic systems	There is hierarchy of ecologic microsystems mesosystems, and exosystems overarched by macrosystem; these systems affect child's development and manner in which child perceives and deals with his or her environment; basis units of analysis are dyad, triad, etc.	Adolescent is seen individually in context of systems in which he or she is involved

Adapted from Bee, H. (1985). The developing child (pp. 330–339). New York: Harper & Row; Bronfenbrenner, U., & Crouter A.C. (1983). The evolution of environmental models in developmental research. In P. Mussen (Ed.), Handbook of child psychology, 4th ed., Vol. 1: History, theory and methods. *New York: John Wiley & Sons; Davis, I. (1985). Adolescence: Theoretical and helping perspectives (pp. 25–40). Boston: Kluwer & Nijhoff; Lloyd, M. (1985). Adolescence (pp. 9–26). New York: Harper & Row.*

adulthood begins. This depends on a combination of physical, emotional, social, legal, and cultural determinants.

Theories of adolescent behavior

At present, there is no single unified or comprehensive theory of adolescent behavior. Many theorists view adolescence from a specific aspect of the developmental continuum. Table 5-7 summarizes the theoretical orientations.

Developmental stages

Physical development

Bodily growth and sexual maturation are gradual processes brought about by androgens, estrogens, and other hormones. The first sign of puberty in girls is the appearance of "breast buds" (age 8 to 13 years). Puberty is completed within 3 years. Menarche (10 to 16.5 years) occurs at the end of this time after the peak of height spurt. Puberty in boys starts approximately 2 years later than girls. Pubic hair appears between 10 and 15 years; penis growth starts between 11 and 14.5 years, with ejaculation taking place a year after accelerated penis growth.

In addition to primary and secondary sex characteristics, other changes include:

1. Lungs and heart increase in size. The heart rate drops. This change is more pronounced in boys than in girls.
2. Boys experience greater growth in muscle and muscle mass in relation to body weight; girls have an increased ratio of fat tissue to body weight.
3. Facial structures begin to take on adult features.
4. Sex differences in the shape and proportions of the trunk become obvious.

5. Sex differences in strength (boy greater than girls) appear that seem to be related to the increase in muscle size, skeletal growth, body weight and neural organization (Lloyd, 1985; Tanner, 1970; Tanner, 1980).

6. Motor coordination shows little sex difference until approximately age 14. Boys continue to develop coordination after 14 years, whereas girls do not demonstrate marked changes after this age (Malina, 1975).

7. Some body organs and structures do not change appreciably during adolescence. For example, the brain reaches 95% of adult size and weight by age 10 (Tanner, 1970).

There is evidence that puberty is beginning earlier. This change is thought to be a result of better nutrition and a decrease in diseases. Another interesting hypothesis is the stimulation and stress factor theory, which states that such factors as stimulation, noise, crowding, and artificial light may effect these changes (Adams, 1981).

Sensory and perceptual development

The sensory and perceptual capabilities of the adolescent are negligible in contrast to his or her physical and cognitive changes. The perceptual world of the adolescent is enhanced by its interrelationship with expanding cognitive skill.

Cognitive development

Adolescence ushers in changes in cognitive processes. Piaget's period of formal operations emerges. Inhelder and Piaget characterize the adolescent's formal operational thought process as follows:

1. The capability of dealing logically with many factors at once.
2. The ability to use a secondary system, for example, trigonometry. This ability to manipulate symbols makes the adolescent's thought processes more flexible. He or she is now able to introspect and reflect on his or her own mental capacities.
3. The ability to construct ideal or contrary-to-fact situations.
4. The ability to deal with the possible as well as the real (Inhelder & Piaget, 1958).

One of the significant outcomes of formal operational thought is that the adolescent is freed from the cognitive limitations of the present. He or she now has a view of what is possible, of the future. This mode of thought is linked to the idealism of youth.

Social Cognition. Social cognition is the development of observations, information, and conceptualizations about our own and others' social roles and about relationships, thoughts, feelings, intentions, and moral or religious judgments. The adolescent's ability to make moral judgments seems to be related to his or her ability to see another's point of view and to relate it to him- or herself. Flavell and Ailman's view of social cognition parallels the adolescent's ability to reach formal operational thought (Flavell, 1977).

Adolescent Egocentricism. The concept of egocentricism is of special interest because it seems to be an important link between personality dynamics and cognitive processes. The freedom and flexibility of thought that come with formal operations can also cause the adolescent to be overly conscious of his or her thoughts, appearance, and feelings. He or she realizes that other people have their own thoughts and perceptions, but the adolescents' self-preoccupation persuades him or her that their thoughts are focused on him or her. Elkind (1967) describes manifestations of this egocentrism as follows:

1. *Imaginary audience.* The adolescent is constructing or reacting to an imagined audience. For example, when a student catches the eye of the teacher he or she wonders what the teacher is thinking about him or her at that moment.

2. *Personal fable.* The adolescent imagines that because so many people are interested in him or her, then he or she must be very special. For example, the adolescent knows that "no one ever has felt the way I do."

3. *Pseudostupidity.* The adolescent tends to interpret situations at a more complex level than is warranted. The obvious tends to elude him or her. For example, he may look for a lost sock, shoe, or book in the places he is least likely to find it.

Emotional development

Emotional responses are particularly significant in adolescence. Childhood feelings, coupled with new life experiences, affect personality and emotional development. Hormonal changes that accompany physical maturation cause frequent emotional lability. Cognitive changes allow for personal introspection and enable the young person to think about him- or herself in a more abstract manner. The focus of thought shifts inward. The adolescent is concerned with his or her own feelings as he or she responds to others and to his or her expanding world. This emotional awakening affects the evolving self-image and esteem of the adolescent. The teen must also adapt to new role behaviors and expectations within his or her environment. These changes often evoke strong emotional responses.

Concept of Self. Changes in self-concept are a reflection not only of physical and cognitive maturation but also of the search for a new understanding of self. Self-esteem (or how one perceives how others see him or her) is rooted in early family interactions. Self-esteem tends to increase from youth through late adolescence.

Sex Roles. Sex-role concepts are formed in early childhood. The adolescent's view of sexual identity depends a great deal on the kinds of models encountered. During adolescence, the young person's self-concept becomes more abstract and less dependent on external physical qualities. By late adolescence, the self-concept undergoes a kind of reorganization. The result is a new and future-oriented personal and ideological identity.

Social development

Peer relationships in adolescence are an essential part of the transition from dependent child to independent adult. Interaction with equals allows the teen to practice aspects of relationships that are critical to later role development. The influence of the group seems to peak in the early adolescent years (12 to 14) and declines in later adolescence (Berndt, 1979).

The structure of groups changes in adolescence. Early cliques or small cohesive groups evolve into larger crowds made up of several cliques. At 13 to 15 years, the young person begins to try out new heterosexual skills in the protected environment of the crowd. Once feelings of self-confidence develop, heterosexual pair relationships begin. Individual friendships take on importance in the adolescent years. With his or her increased cognitive skill, the teen is able to understand more fully the viewpoints and feelings of others. This ability fosters more intimate sharing of feelings between friends. The development of close friendships evolves through adolescence, and, as Erikson suggests, peaks in the early adult years.

Family relationships in early adolescence are more complex than friendships. The teen now understands and desires the concept of a more intimate relationship based on mutual tolerance (Selman, 1980); however, he or she is also keenly aware of the fact that adults possess more power. Conflict is a natural consequence of these polarized concepts. This cycle of intimacy, interdependence, and autonomy causes fluctuations and continued struggle between the family and child throughout the life cycle (Selman, 1980).

Cultural development

Developmental psychologists have been struggling with the question, "Is adolescence a culture unto itself or just a subculture within society?" The evidence suggests that it is a subculture. There seems to be only a broad transmission of values and traditions from one generation of teens to another; for instance, dress customs, behaviors, and mutual leisure activities provide a superficial "shared culture." But the behavior of teens does not consistently influence their adult life. The peer subculture appears, instead, to be a vehicle for transition into the adult world.

Issues in adolescence

Need for and development of independence

The adolescent's need for and development of independence is often manifested in parent–child conflict. Elkind (1967) interprets this conflict as a function of the age of the adolescent and the maturity of the parent. He states that conflicts arise as a result of three kinds of arrangements: bargains, agreements, and contracts.

For Elkind, the parent–adolescent conflict is a stage in the process of self-differentiation. He hypothesizes that each arrangement has three complementary "invariant clauses" whose content varies with age level.

Responsibility–freedom. The parent demands that the adolescent fulfill certain social responsibilities in return for complementary freedoms. The content of this clause changes with age.
Achievement–support. This clause functions in the development of a sense of competence: in the adolescent's ability to meet social and academic standards and in the parent's ability to instruct, supervise, and reinforce his or her accomplishments.
Loyalty–commitment. This clause is closely related to the development of a value system. The parent expects the adolescent to give primary allegiance to the family, and the young person expects the parent to support him or her and make a commitment to his or her values and beliefs.

Group interactions and peer relationships provide the transient feedback necessary for the adolescent's development of social independence and self-worth. Peer interaction teaches the adolescent the norms of society, as well as how to contribute to and establish group goals. In peer relationships he or she tests and begins to understand various social roles while reinforcing his or her own identity.

Awakening of sexuality—need for and development of intimacy

Physical changes in the young adolescent force him or her to face or identify his or her concept of sexuality and body image. Sexuality is the totality of the person's attitudes, values, goals, and behaviors (both internal and external) based on, or determined by, his or her perception of his or her gender.

Sexual awareness begins in and develops from early childhood, but adolescence brings a heightened, often acute, awareness of gender difference, erotic sensations, sexual relationships, potential adult roles, and the need for intimacy.

Although there is no significant intellectual difference between a male and female adolescent, there are cultural and social pressures that may influence his or her self-concept (Schuster & Ashburn, 1992).

Emotionally, adolescents must attempt to come to terms with both their ideal and their real selves. They are forced to evaluate their masculine/feminine roles, reviewing their gender identity, orientation, and gender preference.

As the young person resolves the issues of the adolescent period, a feeling of well-being and self-identity emerges. This process of identity formation does not evolve smoothly for all adolescents. If the crisis is not resolved, role diffusion results. The young person is unable to respond to the demands of various role expectations. The youth beset by role diffusion wanders from one goal to another. Instead of constructive experimentation with options, this adolescent makes aimless and vague attempts at problem solving.

In a predominantly peer environment, charged with sexual curiosity, adolescents confront two major types of relationships: homosexual and heterosexual. Evidence suggests that a homosexual relationship is not uncommon in adolescence. Possibly this stems from the adolescent's sexual insecurity—the need to compare him- or herself with someone nonthreatening and sexually similar. The encounter, conducted in a "safe" and comfortable environment, may be his or her first extrafamilial attachment. The development of a meaningful heterosexual relationship is based on both physical and psychosocial intimacy. To develop true intimacy, the adolescent must be aware of his or her abilities and be able to share him- or herself with others. It is critical that his or her internal identity be secure to prevent identity diffusion and stress on his or her sexuality.

Development of a philosophy of life, a value system, and a humanistic attitude

According to Piaget (1948), the adolescent (12 + years) develops a "morality of reciprocity." When a child reaches formal operational thought, he or she is able to engage in the abstract thinking and introspection that help him or her to develop an internally monitored value system. The adolescent's ability to interpret and internalize rules enables him or her to "discover the boundaries that separate his self from the other person, but (he) will learn to understand the other person and be understood by him." Through this process the adolescent begins to develop an empathetic attitude toward others.

Many factors influence the development of an ideology—parents, peers, significant others, religious training, and cultural and social background. Some theorists speculate that from the time of adolescence the person is dealing with the "child of the past"; that each early experience in the child's social life and culture directly and indirectly affect his or her development of a philosophy of life. This philosophy comes about, finally, as a result of the interaction between the individual's society and culture and his or her internal learned responses.

Consistency of attitude is the most valuable commodity a parent can transmit to a child to help him or her form an intact value system. High self-esteem, internalization of expectations, and self-discipline are linked with parental style and are crucial for the formation of adult moral standards (Berkowitz, 1964; Coppersmith, 1967).

Peers and significant others (family members, teachers, friends) provide an avenue by which the adolescent can identify and test his or her capabilities and ideas. Through testing, he or she will eventually crystallize his or her self-image and value system. Religious training and experience add another dimension to the young person's ability to internalize and reinforce value systems. Religious exposure seems to be most effective when both parents follow similar standards and reinforce their value system.

Different cultures produce different value orientations. There are differences in values both within a culture and between cultures. The expectations of the individual are determined by the way people in a given culture view life roles. Some of the issues around which individual roles are determined include:

1. Responsibility versus nonresponsibility
2. Authority figures versus nonauthority figures
3. Dominance versus submission

Development of a career choice

From approximately 15 through 65 years of age, work occupies a large part of a person's life. The vocational decisions an adolescent makes affect his or her future social relationships, leisure activities, material gains, and marital and child-rearing attitudes.

Major influences on career choice include ability, gender, community (rural versus urban), parental occupation, expectations, and occupational attractiveness.

Planning for work is difficult for a young person, whose aspirations tend to be more idealistic than realistic. With increased maturity, the adolescent gains a more realistic view of career choice and his or her abilities and needs.

One might surmise that minority students, who sometimes encounter stiff barriers and resistance as they move toward status roles, would tend to lower their career expectations. Studies have proved that the opposite is true however (Cosby, 1974; Kuvleky et al., 1971). This increase in vocational aspiration may reflect three attitudes: (1) their efforts to conform to the American cultural emphasis on occupational success and status; (2) their substitution of future projections for their inability to move ahead in a success-oriented society; or (3) their exaggerated perception of the new horizons open to minority groups.

Gender also plays an important role in career decisions. The feminist movement has had a strong impact on society's view of women's career options. Introduced early in the socialization process, these attitudes toward female career possibilities extend a girl's job scope. Even a girl with traditional expectations should take the time to explore her real career potential.

Brief summaries of three theories concerning career choice and development are discussed below.

Self-Concept Theory (Super). Super states that as a person grows, he or she must integrate self-images into a self-concept that prevails in all daily activities, including his or her job. Occupational experiences culminate in work roles and career patterns that are consistent with the maturation of self-concept. Super identifies five vocational developmental tasks.

1. *Crystallization of vocational preference (14 to 18 years).* As their self-concept matures, adolescents develop ideas about work, and they begin to make educational decisions based on these ideas.
2. *Specification of vocational program (18 to 21 years).* Detailed vocational plans are set forth.
3. *Implementation of vocational preferences (21 to 24 years).* The young adult has completed his or her initial training phase and has secured a job.
4. *Stabilization of career (25 to 35 years).* The person enhances his or her talents, narrows his or her field of interest, and finds personal satisfaction in work.
5. *Consolidation of career role (35 up).* The person develops expertise, strengthens his or her skills, and acquires status (Super, 1963).

This developmental theory is valid only in that there is a progression of vocational tasks. The age range varies with socioeconomic conditions.

Cognitive Social Theory (Ginsberg). Ginsberg believes that vocational choice is related to a developmental process of decision making. A person makes continuous choices "between career preparation and goals and the reality of the world of work." (Ginsberg, 1972) This process is open-ended and is continuous throughout life; it is not confined to the adolescent and young adult.

Lifestyle Orientation (Holland). Holland focuses on the relationship between personality characteristics and vocational choice (a trait-factor theory). He believes that job choice is a reflection of personality—that a person chooses work environments that foster his or her personal orientation.

Adulthood

Developmental progression reaches its height in **adulthood**. As the person grows beyond childhood, he or she refines his or her self-image, develops sexual and psychosocial intimacy, becomes productive and effective in the world of work and family, and finally reaches an integrity and a sense of fulfillment that affirms life as a meaningful adventure.

The complexity of the modern world, society, and culture inhibit the smooth resolution of many issues of adulthood.

Issues in young adulthood

Psychological issues

Our society designates young adulthood (the ages between 20 and 40) as prime time—when life is most satisfying and rewarding. Those persons considered "happiest" by others are the middle aged. Cameron concludes that happiness is not determined by, or closely related to, age as such; it is relatively constant across the lifespan. In another study, Lowenthal also concludes that neither age nor life stage is relevant in measuring life satisfaction, although the sense of well-being is different for men than for women. Women tend to express more complex stages of feelings. The "happiest" women in the study are those who have both positive and negative experiences, especially in the recent past; the "happiest" men relate only positive experiences in the recent past (Lowenthal, 1975).

Erikson believed that young adults are involved in working toward the development of intimacy with others as opposed to isolation from them. This intimacy includes a sense of commitment to concrete affiliations and partnerships, the ability to abide by such commitments, and the experience of cooperating and sharing with others even when this necessitates sacrifice and compromise (Kastenbaum, 1972). A person who is unable to develop a sense of intimacy lives in a world apart, absorbed by him- or herself.

Stress is one factor that does seem relative to age and stage in adult life. Young newlyweds, for example, reported 2½ times the number of stressful situations than did middle-aged and older adults, although the type of stress encountered varies with sex. For men, stress is usually related to occupation; for women, it stems more often from health issues (their own and others) and interpersonal conflicts. Middle-aged and older adults seem to experience less stress than the young.

Physical issues

In early adulthood most of the growth processes have run their course. The body never remains static, however; the bright-eyed and sharp-eared young adult is already undergoing decremental changes in vision and hearing. The earliest change is in visual accommodation ability, which peaks in grade school and begins to decline even before a person's "prime." Other aspects of vision tend to remain unchanged.

The ability to hear high-frequency sounds begins to diminish in adolescence, whereas pitch discrimination (high tones) begins to decline in the mid 20s. These slight negative changes in early adulthood usually have little or no effect on the daily functioning of the young adult.

Cognitive issues

Intellectual development peaks in the early adult years. Two levels of mental ability are discussed: fluid and crystallized intelligence. *Fluid intelligence* refers to capabilities such as associative memory, inductive reasoning, and figural relationships. *Crystallized intelligence* refers to skills such as verbal comprehension and the handling of word relationships. The former skills are closely aligned to innate intellect; the latter are more dependent on learning and experience. Horn presented evidence that suggests that fluid intelligence may diminish slightly after adolescence, whereas crystallized intelligence increases with age (Horn, 1970).

Creativity seems to peak in the early 30s. In a historical study of thousands of creative men and women, Lehman found that the peak years of most people's creative ventures have been in their 30s. For example, the mean years for symphony writing were 30 to 34 years of age. Dennis found that creative persons usually continue to produce creative endeavors throughout their lives (Dennis, 1966).

In Piaget's description of cognitive development, formal operational thought is acquired unevenly during adolescence and early adulthood. The ability to use interpropositional thought, combinational analysis, and hypothetical deductive rea-

soning are a result of innate intelligence, education, and life experiences. Some adults never attain formal operational thought. When this level of cognitive development is reached in early adulthood, the young adult relies heavily on it in all areas of life (Piaget, 1953).

Vocational and life goal issues

Career choice remains a paramount issue in the 20s. A high school graduate usually experiments with several jobs before settling into stable employment. Those young people who choose careers that required further education tend to remain on the job longer and feel more secure in their commitment.

Most employment in our culture involves some level of on-the-job training. The process of establishing a career involves the development of job skills and interpersonal working relationships between employer and other employees. Job changes are most frequent during the early adult years, the average duration of employment for the young adult is 2 years.

Lifestyle issues

As the young person enters adulthood, he or she usually leaves his or her family of origin and establishes a new nuclear family.

Blood (1978) suggests five prerequisites for a successful marriage: compatibility, skill, effort, commitment, and support. Folkman and Clatworthy (1970) add two more characteristics: flexibility and love. Americans tend to choose mates with similar backgrounds. Studies indicate that race is the most critical factor in this choice, followed by social class, educational group, religious affiliation, and ethnic origin (Schuster & Ashburn, 1992).

Alternatives to marriage began to emerge in the 1960s and 1970s. More permissive sexual attitudes and greater social acceptance, together with the advent of the feminist movement, brought about an increase in the practice of cohabitation. In many ways, "live-in" relationships appear to be similar to marriage; however, the marriage license seems to have a subtle psychological effect on such a commitment.

Many are choosing single life as an alternative to marriage. A primary reason is career development. Single persons have the advantage of freedom in decision making, though they often spend a large amount of time seeking companions and nurturing relationships (Schuster & Ashburn, 1992).

Other types of relationships, including homosexual bonding, communal living, and being a "swinging single," exist as alternatives to traditional lifestyles. Choosing the direction of one's personal life pattern is a major decision of early adulthood.

Another major issue in the young adult's life is parenthood. Both cultural and personal influences affect this decision. The reasons for choosing parenthood are as varied as the couples involved in the choice. Children may be viewed as another outlet for one's creativity, as an opportunity to fulfill a life goal, or as another opportunity to share oneself with others. A growing number of young couples are opting not to become parents. Some reasons cited include complete fulfillment with a mate, career development, and socioeconomic factors. Maternal instinct is a myth: not all women experience loving and protective feelings toward children. Women who have good self-concepts and who enjoy their roles in life are more likely to be good mothers than are those who are dissatisfied with what they are doing (Freiberg, 1979). Children can be enriching and exciting additions to the young adult's life when he or she is ready for the responsibility of rearing them.

Social issues

During adolescence, a person uses the peer group as a sounding board for developing a self-concept. Once this concept becomes stable, the young adult usually develops a few meaningful relationships—friends who usually have parallel interests and who compliment his or her uniqueness and need system.

When the young adult leaves home, the relationship with his or her family of origin may either weaken or grow stronger. The direction this relationship takes strongly depends on his or her ability to understand and react to other value systems and lifestyles.

Many young adults today have a variety of options available that were not available to their parents and grandparents—more vocational opportunities, more leisure time, and many more life choice possibilities.

Today's young adults are conscious of the need for a balance in the work–play continuum, and they establish meaningful life goals that balance their physical and psychosocial needs.

Issues in midadulthood

Physical issues

There are vast differences among people in midadulthood (the ages between 40 and 60) in terms of physical changes. After a person is 40 years of age, physiologic changes occur in all body systems, but the extent of their manifestation depends a great deal on individual genetic and environmental influences.

Menopause refers to all the physiologic changes that occur when a woman's monthly menstrual function ceases. The female reproductive system changes with advancing age, and childbearing usually ceases during the late 30s or 40s. American women reach menopause at approximately 40 to 54 years of age (Freiberg, 1979). As the levels of estrogen decrease, some women experience vasomotor and other physical changes. The psychological changes associated with menopause are often exaggerated.

There is a great deal of debate about whether men undergo a parallel experience (the male climacteric). Most social scientists believe that men do experience a transition. The time of onset is variable, and the period may be accompanied by both physical and psychological changes.

Cognitive issues

As mentioned previously, fluid intelligence may diminish gradually from middle to later years, whereas crystallized intelligence may increase. Cross-sectional studies comparing people of different ages show generational differences in intelligence. Recent generations tend to be taller, heavier, stronger, and more intelligent (Schuster & Ashburn, 1992). This generational shift is known as the secular trend. Other studies indicate that intellectual ability peaks during the middle years and then remains stable throughout this period and into the beginning of old age (Schuster & Ashburn, 1992).

Psychological issues

Erikson sees midlife as a crisis of generativity versus stagnation. Unless a person continues to grow and change, he or she stagnates and regresses emotionally. This growth is evidenced in his or her creativity, interest in others, and concern with the next generation. Generativity is fostered through positive reciprocal contacts with the younger generation.

Social issues

Certain social issue are paramount during middle age. Havighurst identifies seven developmental tasks with this period:

1. Achieving adult civic and social responsibility
2. Establishing and maintaining an economic standard of living
3. Assisting young people to become responsible adults
4. Developing leisure activities
5. Relating to one's spouse as a person
6. Accepting the physiologic changes of middle age
7. Adjusting to aging parents (Havighurst, 1972).

Levinson and Gould find significant differences between the developmental adjustments of the 40s and the 50s; whereas the 40s are often years of unrest, toward 50, adults settle down again (Levinson, 1974).

During his or her 40s a person may experience many transitions. Parents who are undergoing physiologic and psychological changes themselves may be confronted by children in the throes of adolescent conflict. Reaching a psychological half-way point sets off reflection on past achievements and concern for future goals. The stress of this midlife transition can be an impetus for developmental growth and change, or it can cause a crisis of discontent.

Midlife is often a time when people redefine relationships with parents. Researchers indicate that the middle-aged adult seems to become more empathetic and sympathetic toward his or her aging parents. He or she begins to feel that he or she understands his or her parents' life situation. But when aging parents become physically or economically dependent on their children, problems may arise.

For women, midlife may be the beginning of a second career, an exciting renewal. For men, midlife is often the time of highest financial security. Their career power and prestige are usually at a peak. Men seldom make radical shifts or impulsive moves at this stage. Generally they remain in the same job until retirement. Usually the years between 50 and 65 are the most satisfying of a man's career.

Leisure activities expand during midlife. It is common for adults to pursue activities that they had established early in their adult lives. Neugarten notes an interesting change in the concept of leisure in America. A hundred years ago, the higher one's education and income, the more leisure one had. Now the best educated and most skilled professionals put in 60- to 80-hour work weeks, and it is the blue collar workers who have the most leisure time (Neugarten, 1974).

The postparental period for some couples is a time to enjoy the fruits of the hard work of earlier years. These couples find a new pleasure in marriage and a new intensity in their relationship (Isaacson, 1968). But while marital happiness increases for some, it evaporates for others. Some couples seek divorce soon after their children leave home, although they have long since lost contact with each other.

When children leave home, one or both parents may experience the empty-nest phenomenon—a feeling of loss. This syndrome usually coincides with the marriage (or a comparable declaration of independence) of the last child at home. The crisis is usually resolved through expanding nurturing experiences (parents, pets, etc.). But the "empty nest" can eventually lead to sexual problems or divorce.

As their children establish new nuclear families, parents

take on new roles as grandparents and in-laws. These new roles bring to midlife another potential for satisfaction and happiness or for frustration and despair.

The middle years do more than reflect the accomplishments of earlier years. They are characterized by development and change. The physical and psychological crises that occur hold out tremendous potential for growth. Middle age rings with productivity, generativity, and a high satisfaction with life.

References

Adams, J. F. (1981). Earlier menarche, greater height and weight: A stimulation stress factor hypothesis. *Genetic Psychological Monograph, 104,* 3.

Ainsworth, M. (1982). Attachment retrospect and prospect. In C. M. Parkes, and M. Stevenson-Hind (Eds.). *The place of attachment in human behavior.* New York: Basic Books.

Ayres, J. (1980). *Sensory integration and the child.* Los Angeles: Western Psychological Services.

Ayres, J. (1973). *Sensory integration and learning disorders.* Los Angeles: Western Psychological Services.

Bandura, A. (1977a). Self-efficacy: Toward a unifying theory of behavioral change. *Psychological Review, 84,* 191.

Bandura, A. (1977b). *A social learning theory.* Englewood Cliffs, NJ: Prentice Hall.

Baumrind, D. (1973). The development of instrumental competence through socialization. In A. D. Pick (Ed.), *Minnesota Symposium on Child Psychology* (Vol. 7). Minneapolis: University of Minnesota Press.

Bee, H. (1985). *The developing child* (4th ed.). New York: Harper & Row.

Berkowitz, L. (1964). *The development of motives and values in the child.* New York: Basic Books.

Berndt, T. (1979). Developmental changes in conformity to peers and family. *Developmental Psychology, 15,* 658.

Bing, R. K. (1968). Discussion of Mosey's recapitulation of Ontogenesis. *American Journal of Occupational Therapy, 22,* 433–435.

Blood, R. O. (1978). *Marriage* (3rd ed.). New York: Free Press.

Bronfenbrenner, U. (1977a). Toward an experimental ecology of human development. *American Psychology, 32,* 513.

Bronfenbrenner, U. (1977b). *The ecology of human development.* Cambridge, MA: Harvard University Press.

Caron, A. J., & Caron, R. F. (1982). Cognitive development in early infancy. In T. M. Field (Ed.), *Review of human development.* New York: John Wiley.

Clark, P., & Allen, A. (1985). *Occupational therapy for children* (p. 38). St. Louis: Mosby.

Connor, F. P., Williamson, G. G., & Siepp, J. M. (1978). *Program guide for infants and toddlers with neuromotor and other developmental disabilities.* New York: Teachers College Press.

Coppersmith, S. (1967). *The antecedents of self esteem.* San Francisco: Freeman.

Cosby, A. (1974). Occupational expectations and the hypothesis of increasing realism of choice. *Journal of Vocational Behavior, 5,* 53.

Craig, G. J. (1976). *Human development.* Englewood Cliffs, NJ: Prentice Hall.

Cratty, B. J. (1973). *Movement behavior and motor learning* (3rd ed.). Philadelphia: Lea & Febiger.

Damon, W., & Hart, D. (1982). The development of self-understanding from infancy through adolescence. *Child Development, 53,* 841.

Davis, I. (1985). *Adolescents: Theoretical and helping perspectives* (p. 36). Boston: Kluwer-Hifhuff.

Dennis, W. (1966). Creative productivity between the ages of twenty and eighty years. *Journal of Gerontology, 21,* 1.

Elkind, D. (1967). Egocentrism in adolescence. *Child Development, 38,* 1025.

Fiorentino, M. (1973). *Reflex testing methods for evaluating CNS development* (2nd ed.). Springfield, IL: Charles C. Thomas.

Flavell, J. H. (1977). *Cognitive development.* Englewood Cliffs, NJ: Prentice Hall.

Flavell, J. H. (1982). Structures, stages and sequences in cognitive development. In W. A. Collins (Ed.), *The concept of development: Minnesota Symposium in Child Psychology* (Vol. 15). Hillsdale, NJ: Erlbaum.

Florey, L. (1971). An approach to play and play development. *American Journal of Occupational Therapy, 25,* 275.

Folkman, J. D., & Clatworthy, N. M. (1970). *Marriage has many faces* (p. 80). Columbus: Merrill.

Freiberg, K. (1979). *Human development: A life span approach.* Belmont, CA: Wadsworth.

Freud, A. (1965). The concept of developmental lines. In *Normality and pathology in childhood: Assessment of development.* New York: International Universities Press.

Gerson, R. (1978). Intrinsic motivation: Implications for children's athletics. *Motor Skills: Theory into Practice, 2,* 111–119.

Ginsberg, E. (1972). Toward a theory of occupational choice as a restatement. *Vocational Guidance Quarterly, 20,* 169.

Ginsberg, H., & Opper, S. (1969). *Piaget's theory of intellectual development* (p. 111). Englewood Cliffs, NJ: Prentice Hall.

Goren, C. C., Sart, M., & Wu, P. K. (1975). Visual following and pattern discrimination of face-like stimuli by newborn infants. *Pediatrics, 56,* 544.

Gould, S. J. (1977). *Ontogeny and phylogheny.* Cambridge, MA: Harvard University Press.

Greenspan, S., & Greenspan, N. (1985). *First feelings: Milestones in the emotional development of your baby and child.* New York: Viking Press.

Havighurst, R. J. (1972). *Developmental tasks and education* (3rd ed.). New York: Longman.

Hendrick, I. (1943). The discussion of the instinct to master. *Psychoanalytic Quarterly, 12,* 561–565.

Hetherington, E. M. (1979). Divorce: A child's perspective. *American Psychologist, 34,* 851.

Horn, J. (1970). Organization of data on life span development of human abilities. In L. Goulet, P. Baltes (Eds.), *Life span developmental psychology.* New York: Academic Press.

Huyok, M. H., & Hoyer, W. J. (1982). *Adulthood and aging.* Belmont, CA: Wadsworth.

Inhelder, B., & Piaget, J. (1958). *The growth of logical thinking from childhood to adolescence.* New York: Basic Books.

Isaacson, L. (1968). *Career information in counseling and teaching.* Boston: Allyn & Bacon.

Kagan, J. (1984). *The nature of the child.* New York: Basic Books.

Kastenbaum, R. (1972). *Humans developing: A life span perspective.* Boston: Allyn & Bacon.

Kuvlesky, W., Wright, D., & Juarez, R. (1971). Status projections and ethnicity: A comparison of Mexican American, Negro, and Anglo youths. *Journal of Vocational Behavior, 1,* 137.

Lamb, M. E. (Ed.). (1982). *The development of attachment and affiliative systems.* New York: Plenum Press.

Lerner, R. M. (1976). *Concepts and theories of human development.* Reading, MA: Addison-Wesley.

Levinson, D. (1974). The psychological development of man in early adulthood and midlife transition. In D. Ricks, A. Thomas, & M. Roff (Eds.), *Life history research in psychopathology III.* Minneapolis: University of Minnesota Press.

Llorens, L. A. (1970). Facilitating growth and development: The promise of occupational therapy. *American Journal of Occupational Therapy, 24,* 93–101.

Lloyd, M. (1985). *Adolescence.* New York: Harper & Row.

Lowenthal, M. T. (1975). *Four stages of life.* San Francisco: Jassey and Bass.

Malina, R. M. (1975). Adolescent changes in size, build, composition and performance. In *Human Biology* (pp. 46, 117–131). Washington, DC: National Center for Health Statistics.

Markham, E. M., Cox, B., & Machida, S. (1981). The standard object sorting task as a measure of conceptual organization. *Developmental Psychology, 17*, 115.

Meltzoff, A. N., & Moore, M. H. (1983). Newborn infants imitate adult facial gestures. *Child Development, 54*, 702.

Milansky, A. (1979). Genetic counseling: Prelude to prenatal diagnosis. In A. Milansky (Ed.), *Genetic disorders and the fetus: Diagnosis, prevention, and treatment*. New York: Plenum.

Montagu, A. (1978). *Touching: The human significance of the skin.* (2nd ed.). New York: Harper & Row.

Mosey, A. C. (1981). *Occupational therapy configuration of a profession.* New York: Raven Press.

Nelson, J. (1973). Structure and strategy in learning to talk. *Monograph Social Research in Child Development, 38*, 149.

Neugarten, B. (1974). The roles we play. In *Quality of life: The middle years*. Acton, MA: Publishing Sciences Group.

Patterson, G. R. (1975). *Families: Applications of social learning to family life.* Champaign, IL: Research Press.

Piaget, J. (1948). *The moral judgement of the child.* (M. Gaban, Trans.). Glencoe, IL: Free Press.

Piaget, J. (1953). *The origins of intelligence.* (M. Cook, Trans.). New York: International Universities Press.

Piaget, J. (1965). *Play, dreams, and imitation in childhood.* (C. Gattegango, & F. M. Hudson, Trans.). New York: W. W. Norton Press.

Reilly, M. (1974). *Play as exploratory learning: Studies in curiosity behavior.* Beverly Hills, CA: Sage.

Rutter, M. (1983). School effects on pupil progress: Research findings and policy implications. *Child Development, 54*, 1.

Schuster, C., & Ashburn, S. (1992). *The process of human development: A holistic lifespan approach* (3rd ed.). Boston: Little, Brown.

Selman, R. L. (1980). *The growth of interpersonal understanding.* New York: Academic Press.

Short-DeGraff, M. A. (1988). *Human development for occupational and physical therapists.* Baltimore: Williams & Wilkins.

Sinnott, J. M., Pisoni, D. B., & Aslin, R. N. (1983). Comparison of pure auditory behavior in human infants and adults. *Infant Behavior Development, 6*, 3.

Smilansky, G. (1968). *The effect of sociodramatic play on disadvantaged youth.* New York: John Wiley.

Sternberg, R. J. (1981). The evolution of theories of intelligence. *Intelligence, 5*, 149.

Sternberg, R. J. (Ed.). (1982). *Handbook of human intelligence.* Cambridge: Cambridge University Press.

Super, D. (1963). Vocational development in adolescence and early childhood: Tasks and behaviors. In D. Super, R. Starishevsky, J. Matliln, (Eds.), *Career development: Self concept theory.* New York: College Examination Board.

Takata, N. (1980). Introduction to a series: Occupational behavior research for pediatric process. *American Journal of Occupational Therapy, 34*, 11.

Tanner, J. M. (1970). Physical growth. In P. H. Mussen (Ed.), *Carmichael's manual of child psychology*, Vol. 2 (3rd ed.), pp. 95–96. New York: John Wiley and Sons.

Tanner, J. M. (1978). *Fetus into man: Physical growth from conception to maturity.* Cambridge, MA.: Harvard University Press.

Tanner, J. M. (1980). Sequence, tempo and individual variation in growth and development of boys and girls aged 12–16. In S. J. Harrison, J. F. McDermott, Jr. (Eds.), *New directions in childhood psychopathology: Vol. 1. Development considerations* pp. 182–202. New York: International University Press.

Tomlinson-Keasey, C., Eisert, D. C., Kahle, L. R., Hardy-Brown, K., & Keasey, B. (1978). The structure of concrete operational thought. *Child Development, 50*, 1153.

Wachs, T. D., & Gruen, G. E. (1982). *Early experience and human development.* New York: Plenum Press.

White, B. L., & Held, R. (1963). *Plasticity of sensorimotor development in the human infant.* Paper presented at the American Association for Advancement of Science, Philadelphia, PA.

SECTION 2B
Late adulthood

LINDA L. LEVY

Ageism	*Gerontologic Tripartite*
Age-Grading Systems	*Integrity*
Age-Specific Roles	*Physical Maturity*
Biologic Aging	*Psychological Aging*
Epigenetic Principle	*Sociologic Aging*

LEARNING OBJECTIVES

Upon completion of this section the reader will be able to:

1. *Describe the gerontological tripartite.*
2. *Identify and define key concepts related to the biology of aging.*
3. *Identify major changes that occur in the sensory system with increasing chronologic age.*
4. *Identify major changes that occur in the organ systems with increasing chronologic age.*
5. *Identify and define key concepts related to psychological aging.*
6. *Identify age-related changes in cognitive function.*
7. *Explain Erikson's epigenetic principle and its relationship to personality development in later adulthood.*
8. *Identify and define key concepts related to sociologic aging.*
9. *Describe ageism.*
10. *Describe how role and status changes are conceptualized in aging.*
11. *Identify factors that contribute to life satisfaction in aging.*

Gerontologists define the ***aging process*** in terms of three distinct phenomena: the ***biologic capacity for survival***, the ***psychological capacity for adaptation***, and the ***sociologic capacity for the fulfillment of social roles*** (Birren & Renner, 1977). Collectively, these approaches to the study of aging are known as the ***Gerontological Tripartite***. Within these three spheres, developmental challenges are presented to older adults that occur at different times and different rates. For example, a 60-year-old who is unable to establish intimate relationships would be considered young psychologically, whereas a still-employed 70-year-old would be considered young and a 40-year-old grandmother would be considered old in terms of social age. As a result, vast variations in biologic, psychological, and social aging exist, which are only roughly related to chronologic age. Age, then, is best conceptualized in terms of the person's health and diverse psychological and sociologic challenges rather than by chronologic age. This perception is aptly expressed by the adage, "You are only as old as you feel."

At the same time, it cannot be overemphasized that any of the challenges of aging are approached by adults whose life experiences in confronting developmental crises have provided them with a rich and complex variety of **coping mechanisms**. Hence, it would be inaccurate to characterize any but a broad and heterogeneous view of "normal" aging. Older adults vary more in patterns of normal functioning than do persons at any other stage in the lifespan. One of the few generalizations that researchers are willing to make about older adults is that they tend to become less like each other and more like themselves; that is, they become increasingly individualistic as they age. With this appreciation of the tremendous variability that exists among older people, we can begin to explore the developmental challenges that are presented by the aging process.

Biologic aging

Biologic aging refers to the condition of the biologic organism with respect to the potential lifespan and is closely connected to physical health (Birren & Renner, 1977). The physical changes that occur with aging are a continuation of the decline that most researchers agree begins as soon as **physical maturity** is reached at about age 18 to 22 years. It is not yet possible to distinguish which changes are truly a result of aging (those that are determined by heredity) and which are a result of disease or a variety of environmental and physical factors. One of the most consistently documented changes, however, is a diminished capacity to maintain or regain homeostasis, an internal steady state that normally is maintained in the face of changing environmental circumstances. Although there is little change in homeostatic mechanisms under resting conditions, the rate of readjustment to normal equilibrium *after stress* is slower in older persons than in young persons.

For example, the capacity of the kidneys for removing waste, the ability to maintain body temperature during exposure to heat or cold, and the efficiency of blood sugar regulation decrease with age. Similarly, when an older person develops an infection, the body temperature does not rise as rapidly or as markedly as in a younger person and, once raised, it takes longer to return to normal. The stressors that disrupt these processes can be either physical (a virus or exercise) or psychosocial (loss of spouse or relocation). In either case, with advancing age, the **capacity for homeostasis** gradually declines, and the range of adjustment and adaptation becomes smaller and narrower. Accordingly, biologic aging results in increased vulnerability. For reasons that are not yet fully understood, it also results in decreases in the efficiency and function of a number of organs.

Before we address these diverse changes, there are a number of issues to be kept in mind. First, it should be emphasized that biologic changes occur at different times and rates in different organs, tissues, and cells; within different individuals, these changes occur at different times and rates. For example, visible signs of aging such as graying or baldness can occur at age 30 in one person and at age 70 in another. Second, although some biologic aging occurs naturally in body organs, biochemical pathways, musculoskeletal systems, and the central nervous system, it is largely unappreciated that the health and physical ability of most older persons do not decline precipitously, nor are the changes quickly disabling. Limitations in the activities of daily living are reported by only 13% of those aged 65 to 74, 25% of those between 75 and 84, and 46% of those 85 years and older (U.S. Senate, 1986). Hence, most who live into their 80s do not experience difficulties in carrying out major tasks or changes in their normal functioning due to biologic aging. Eighty-five percent of the population over 65 years of age experiences at least one chronic condition, however, with multiple chronic conditions such as arthritis, hypertension, and impaired hearing being commonplace (U.S. Senate, 1986).

A key implication here is that despite the prevalence of chronic impairments, most older persons have developed coping mechanisms and compensatory strategies that enable them to lead well-functioning lives (Lowenthal & Chiriboga, 1973). At the same time, it becomes apparent that criteria such as "absence of disease" are not useful when addressing the question of what it means for the aged to be healthy.

Finally, it should be acknowledged that there is not necessarily a direct cause-and-effect relationship between the degree of structural impairment within an organ and the presence of impaired function or disease. For example, it is not unusual to discover at autopsy extensive changes in the blood vessels in the brain even in elderly persons who had little clinical evidence of mental impairment (Tomlinson et al., 1970).

Having considered these issues, we can begin to summarize some of the major biologic changes associated with aging. Age-related changes in the *sensory systems* include the following:

Vision. Decreased pupil size and loss of transparency and increased thickness of the lens allow less light to reach the retina. Therefore, older persons need twice as much illumination as younger persons. Decreased elasticity of the lens results in presbyopia (farsightedness). Visual acuity and the ability to discriminate colors also decrease progressively with age.

Hearing. Decreased auditory acuity at high frequencies impairs the ability to discriminate words and to understand normal conversation.

Taste and smell. Decreased sensitivity in discriminating salty, sweet, and sour tastes as well as in the ability to discriminate food odors is typical.

Levy (1986) has provided a comprehensive discussion of these sensory changes and their implications for the practice of occupational therapy.

Age-related changes in the *organ systems* include the following:

Muscular structure. Muscle weight and strength decrease, the number and diameter of muscle fibers decrease, and hypertrophy occurs. The valves of the heart become thicker and less flexible. Atrophy increases.

Skeletal system. Skeletal mass decreases and bones become more porous and brittle as demineralization occurs, resulting in an increased vulnerability to fracture; the synovium in joints degenerates, resulting in decreased flexibility, joint stiffness, and pain.

Cardiovascular system. The heart and blood vessels become more rigid due to collagen changes, and blood vessels narrow due to arteriosclerotic changes. A decline is evident in the maximal heart rate, exercise stroke volume, cardiac output, maximal oxygen consumption, and capacity for responding to extra work. Peripheral vascular resistance increases. These changes result in a diminished supply of oxygenated blood, which becomes a major cause of decreased stamina and endurance.

Respiratory system. Expiration and inspiration decrease as a result of atrophy of the intercostal muscles and diaphragm and decreased expandability of intercostal bone, muscle, and pulmonary tissue. Thickening of pulmonary arterial walls and thinning of the alveolar walls occur. Consequently, a 10% to 15% decrease occurs in the oxygen content of the blood, and emphysema becomes common in very old age, which further contributes to limitations in stamina and endurance.

Excretory systems. In the urinary system, there is a decrease in kidney weight and ability to eliminate waste products. Urinary frequency increases. In the digestive system, ability to secrete adequate digestive juices is reduced and there is atrophy of gastrointestinal mucosa, decreased absorption from the gastrointestinal tract, and decreased muscle tone and peristalsis, resulting in indigestion and constipation.

Gallbladder/liver. An increased incidence of gallstones and decreased size and efficiency of the liver occur in older persons.

Psychological aging

Psychological aging refers to a person's ability to adapt to changing environments; it is primarily reflected in a person's intellectual skills and emotional well-being. As we have seen, some degree of biologic decline is virtually inevitable as we age. This is not the case with psychological aging, however; there is great potential for continuing growth and development, and most older people get better as they get older.

In regard to intellectual skills, the relationship between age and intelligence is insignificant. Any relationship that does occur involves memory, speed of response, and perceptual–integrative functions (possibly reflecting decreased efficiency of the central nervous system) rather than overall intelligence (Botwinick, 1977). In crystallized aspects of intellectual functioning, older persons continue to improve until at least age 55 or 60, with little apparent decline until their mid-70s or beyond (Schaie, 1982). On the Wechsler Adult Intelligence Scale (WAIS), this would be reflected on the information, vocabulary, and comprehension subtests—those that involve verbal abilities and are influenced by both experience and education.

Palmore (1947) provides data from seven long-term investigations that older persons with advanced education who are working without time pressure show little or no cognitive deterioration with age. Memory, particularly short-term and recent memory, shows some decline with age, but persons who exercise their memories are able to maintain both remote and recent memory well into old age (Atchley, 1977). Finally, although older persons often require a somewhat longer period of time to learn material, when given extra time, they learn as well as younger people (Botwinick & Thompson, 1966).

In addition, many older adults continue to be creative in later life (Butler, 1967). Dennis found that creativity remained high in many older persons who were creative in their earlier years; for example, literary scholars, historians, and philosophers were as productive in their 70s as they were in their 40s

(Dennis, 1966). The productivity of most scientists in their 70s declined from 25% to 50% from its peak, but inventors were most productive from ages 60 to 80. Numerous examples of creative contributions were made from persons in old age. For example, Tolstoy wrote *Resurrection* when he was in his 70s, Ben Franklin invented bifocals when he was 78 years old, and both Georgia O'Keefe and Pablo Picasso were creating important works of art at 90 years of age. Michelangelo completed the dome of St. Peter's Basilica in Rome when he was 70, Goethe was 82 when he finished *Faust*, and Verdi produced *Otello* at 74 and *Falstaff* at 80. A number of reviewers note that works of late life typically have a maturity, a complexity, and an insight into the interrelationships of things that the works of younger people lack (Schaie & Geiwitz, 1982).

At the same time, late adulthood provides a number of opportunities for psychological growth and expansion. Older people may come to accept and understand both themselves and others better as they age. This insight is key to the development of a number of the intervention strategies used with dysfunctional older persons.

A brief review of Erikson's **epigenetic principle** may begin to shed light on this issue (Erikson, 1959). This principle states that human growth and development progress through a number of stages that are invariant, each stage being a necessary precursor to its succeeding stage. Within any stage, age-specific psychological conflicts emerge and assume priority in accordance with normal physiologic maturity and psychological awareness. This is not to say that the conflict is ever fully resolved within the stage where it assumes priority; rather, resolution becomes a continuing process that proceeds at different paces within each person in response to changing environmental circumstances. Therefore, as a person's relation to his or her environment changes, so does his or her experience of each of the conflicts. Notwithstanding, conflicts within each stage of development must be dealt with to a certain degree for further psychological development to occur. Simply stated, the issue becomes one of the ratio between the favorable and unfavorable qualities of any given conflict that become integrated within the personality structure at any given stage.

If the preponderance of integration is directed toward the favorable components of the conflict, a firm basis is laid for the development of succeeding components of the personality. Conversely, if the preponderance of integration is directed toward the unfavorable components of the conflict, a weak and vulnerable base is laid for further psychological development. Again, these conflicts are never resolved once and for all. Remnants of both components of each conflict (trust and mistrust, for example) remain as important personality determinants within each of us.

The epigenetic principle is of particular importance for understanding psychological aging because it underscores the unceasing potential for personality growth and development throughout the lifespan. It proposes that the individual continues to work through each of these conflicts to a greater or lesser degree throughout the life cycle as his or her environmental context changes, and it conceptualizes the healthy personality as continually in the process of growth, expansion, and development even until death. This principle also maintains that a person's psychological resources are intimately connected to the levels of integration he or she has attained thus far within stage-specific conflicts. An important corollary here is that the chances of integrating the favorable qualities of a given conflict inadequately increases as time goes on, which inevitably impairs development in each succeeding stage. As a result, the pleasures inherent in the last phase of life (***integrity***) are necessarily the most difficult ones to attain. The displayed material on pages 134 and 135, an adaptation of Erikson's Analysis of Life Stages, presents the implications of his analysis for the older adult.

In summation, Erikson's developmental tasks, if successfully negotiated, result in emotional maturity, integrity, and profound life satisfaction. Mature psychological development is reflected in an autonomous person who is able to value himself or herself while achieving closeness and relatedness to others, who is able to look realistically at successes and failures and feel that life has been worthwhile, and who has come to a sense of peace with the prospect of death. This state is attained by a continuing process of progressive synthesis and integration of a number of personality components. Conflicts are never permanently resolved, however; they are continually in the *process* of resolution. The aging individual, then, is ever-learning, ever-adjusting, and ever-developing. Indeed, he or she can be working through conflicts derived from deficient learning early in life even up to death.

Sociologic aging

A dynamic interaction between individuals and society is also inherent in the aging process. ***Sociologic aging*** occurs as the roles and functions of a person change within society. It refers to the age-specific roles a person assumes within the context of the society in which he or she lives and is reflected largely in how the person behaves in light of the expectations of his or her social group. As will be seen, some of the most significant challenges of aging are presented by the social aging process.

First, an overview of some basic sociologic concepts is in order. *Roles* are the social structures through which persons are given opportunities to make contributions to society. Role opportunities are provided in the institutional spheres of the society: the economic, religious, educational, and family systems. Roles also prescribe specific ***norms and standards*** for appropriate and expected behaviors. In addition, all societies use ***age-grading systems*** to define and classify who is young, middle-aged, and old. ***Age-specific roles*** and expectations for behavior are ascribed in terms of these classifications (Cowgill & Holmes, 1972). Hence, "young," "middle-aged," and "old" people are expected to behave and to be treated differently from those not within their age classes in a society. This serves to create predictable age-related patterns of behavior and social interaction. The often-heard exhortation to "act one's age" means precisely to conform to these age-specific role expectations.

Age roles and the associated expectations for appropriate behavior differ from culture to culture and from era to era. All individuals are effectively socialized to the particular role prescribed for their age group in their society, however. Therefore, when they reach later adulthood, their attitudes and behavior reflect their earlier expectations regarding appropriate behavior for older people. A person who lives in a society that considers the elderly useless and expendable is likely to have a negative view of his or her own aging and would be given limited role opportunities to make meaningful contributions; conversely, a person who lives in a society that considers the elderly valuable

and useful citizens is likely to have positive feelings about his or her own aging and would be given ample role opportunities to make meaningful contributions. In similar fashion, a person may be made to feel old because society expects him or her to be or the person may act older than he or she feels to avoid violating social norms and expectation. Hence, the subjective experience of social aging is to a large extent determined by the expectations of society.

As indicated earlier, age-specific roles are largely determined by the age-grading system that all societies use to classify their members into various categories. The criteria that societies use for age grading vary widely and often relate to a specific organization or activity. For example, in some societies, a person becomes old when he or she becomes the oldest member of a family or when he or she is no longer able to hunt. In industrial societies, however, there appear to be no specific criteria such as social categories or ability to function (Atchley, 1978). Instead, people are arbitrarily assigned to an age category. In the United States, this is usually done by chronologic age, such as when an individual reaches 65 years of age—the age of retirement arbitrarily selected in 1935 under the ***Social Security Act***.

A significant problem with this arbitrary designation is that when most Americans think of old age, they think of stereotypical (and ageist) characteristics, such as declining health, energy, or mental capacities. They also are led to believe that older people are a homogeneous group. Yet, as discussed earlier, chronologic age is an especially poor indicator of the characteristics of aging for individuals because the older a group of individuals gets, the more *dissimilar* they become in terms of abilities. In recognition of this misperception, a number of sociologists maintain that many of the problems that older people experience in American society can be attributed to the injustices of an arbitrary system that implies that everyone over 65 is physically and mentally old (Atchley, 1978). Rosow states the problem another way: That older people have two kinds of problems—the kind they really have and the kind that other people think they have (Rosow, 1967).

Both of these perspectives underscore the unfortunate reality that societies ascribe to their aged those roles and privileges commensurate with its underlying philosophy, regardless of the facts. In particular, our society promotes significant stereotypes and negative attitudes that serve to age individuals prematurely and unfairly. This is tantamount to discrimination against older people on the basis of age, a phenomenon that Butler has aptly described as ***ageism*** (Butler, 1975).

Butler conceptualizes ageism as the protective mechanism that society uses to avoid confronting the difficult issues of aging, illness, and death. It is merely a poorly masked innate fear of our own aging and death. Although largely unconscious, ageism results in a perception of aging as a period of powerlessness, uselessness, disability, and disease (Butler, 1975). This problem is accentuated by the fact that older people have already been socialized into accepting these negative stereotypes at the same time that others are perceiving them negatively. As a result, these stereotypes and attitudes cannot help but undermine the self-concepts and sense of self-worth of older people.

A closely related effect of ageist attitudes is the role restrictions that our society imposes on older people. Our society devalues older people and assumes them to be nonproductive and noncontributing. Consequently, older people are provided with few role opportunities and are not given the prerogative of

ERIKSON'S ANALYSIS OF LIFE STAGES

1. In the first stage of development, the individual faces the conflict between **trust** and **mistrust**. The task is to learn that the world is a good place and that others are trustworthy and to acquire a sense of trustworthiness as far as the self is concerned. Out of trust develops *hope*, the ego strength of infancy. In the older adult, this is reflected as *faith* in personal religious beliefs or in ethical and moral systems. A successful resolution of this conflict becomes manifest as a sense of peace within the context of dying. A well-loved child retains that sense of infantile omnipotence which trusts that the world ultimately has satisfying things to offer, even those that are unknown.

   The impairment of basic trust is expressed in a basic mistrust: a tendency toward withdrawal, alienation, fear of strangers, and lack of affiliation, as well as a belief in being controlled by fate or chance. This is a conflict that is often revived in the face of chronic illness when the individual places his life in the care of others. The struggle of helpless dependency and allowing oneself to be cared for is recreated and must be worked through.

2. In the second stage, the individual first experiences the impact of socialization and begins to adapt his or her wishes and needs to those of society. The developmental crisis is the struggle of **autonomy** (or self-control) against **doubt** and **shame**, and the critical learning tasks become those of "holding on" *versus* "letting go." From a sense of self-control not associated with loss of self-esteem comes a lasting sense of dignity and pride. If autonomy predominates over shame, the basic strength of early childhood, a rudimentary *will* develops. Failure to reach such autonomy results in a sense of doubt and shame, a loss of face and dignity, and a tenuous capacity for self-control. The individual compensates by becoming "overcontrolled"; ie, compulsive, in matters of time, money, and affection.

   This struggle is highlighted by the process of leaving a legacy (letting go) when one's physical or mental capacities require it. Letting go without loss of dignity involves the critical element of *free will*—of *choosing* to let go—as well as **trust** that others will carry on with what one has created. Difficulties in letting go of money or possessions is especially reflective of difficulties derived from this stage.

3. In the third developmental stage, the individual builds on his or her sense of autonomy and is ready to develop **initiative**, a sense of direction or *purpose* derived from his experiences of venturing out, exploring, and discovering what potential the world has to offer. Feelings of **guilt** (versus shame) are now possible because of the maturation of the child's conscience. (Shame is externally induced, whereas guilt is internal.) Hence, failure in this developmental stage leads to an undue sense of doing wrong and guilt. The adult overburdened with guilt—essentially for "having dared to dream"—may become excessively inhibited, vindictive, or self-righteous. Rather than seeing possibilities in life, he or she becomes concerned with what cannot or should not be done.

   In the older adult, failure within this stage will undermine the individual's ability to conceptualize and create new alternatives. This skill is critical to successful adjustment to changing environmental circumstances or increasing disability.

4. In the fourth developmental stage, the individual learns to gain recognition by learning specific skills and acquiring knowledge and is ready to develop a sense of **industry**. If industry predominates, the individual will derive a basic sense that he or she can master the environment—*competence*. If the person feels that his or her skills are not up to the requirements of the physical and social world, a sense of **inferiority** develops.

   In the older adult, a sense of competence is likewise required in the face of disability. Healthy adjustment is derived from the ability to compensate for disabilities by creatively manipulating the environment to permit maximum levels of functioning.

5. Adolescence, the fifth stage, is particularly critical because it is during this period that a sense of **identity** develops. The task of this difficult period is to discover "who one is": what kind of man or woman to be, what career and roles to pursue, and what one's individual outlook on society and the world is. Once a basic sense of identity is established, *fidelity* can emerge. The individual is able to commit to some desired goal or cause. Failure in this stage leads to **identity diffusion**: the individual does not attain a feeling of security about who he or she is or would like to be, his or her gender identity, ability to master drives, attractiveness to others, and ability to make the right decisions.

   The search for identity continues throughout life. As Butler phrases it, "When identity is established or maintained, I find it an ominous sign rather than a favorable one. A continuing life-long identity crisis seems to be a sign of good health." (Aiken, 1976) An individual's new identity in old age comes from finding new uses for what has been learned during previous years and from developing new ways of coming to terms with reality. That reality consists of personal strengths and weaknesses as well as a changing world that is not always to one's liking.

6. In young adulthood, the task is to develop **intimacy**, a development that necessarily requires the prior establishment of some sense of identity or self. In intimacy, the individual is able to fuse his identity with another and commit himself to relationships that demand sacrifice and compromise. Successful resolution of this stage results in *love*, where the individual comes to see himself or herself as worthy of love as well as capable of loving. When the stage is not resolved successfully, a sense of **isolation** and self-absorption predominates. The individual's relationships lack warmth, spontaneity, and deep

   (continued)

ERIKSON'S ANALYSIS OF LIFE STAGES *(continued)*

emotional commitment. There may also be fear that fusion with another will weaken one's own sense of identity.

For the older adult, research has amply demonstrated that the maintenance of a stable intimate relationship serves a critical function in protecting the individual's morale and mental stability against the various social losses (eg, widowhood, retirement) that are associated with aging (Lowerthal G. Haven, 1968).

7. In middle adulthood, the struggle is between **generativity** and the forces of **self-absorption** and **stagnation**. Generativity relates primarily to establishing and guiding the next generation and can be expressed in the bearing and rearing of children, in contributing to the well-being of others, and in creating products and ideas of value to society. Giving must assume priority over getting. In addition, this stage requires a reappraisal of work and relationship goals in order to focus efforts in directions consistent with inner values. It also requires an elemental *faith* that the species should be preserved and that the individual's contributions are valuable and can ultimately make a difference. When generativity fails to predominate, a sense of stagnation pervades the individual's life: the individual has failed to come to terms with his or her values and priorities, and his or her efforts lose their meaning.

   Generative acts are characterized by *care*, and for care to develop, an individual must have attained strengths from all the previous stages: *hope, will, purpose, competence, fidelity,* and *love*. Erikson sees generativity as the driving power of human organization. (Perhaps if more individuals were able to attain it, world peace might become a political reality.)

8. The final stage of the life cycle is later adulthood, when the task is to develop **integrity**, a sense of the coherence and wholeness of one's life. A person accepts that life, sees meaning in it, believes that he or she did the best that could be done under the circumstances, and feels satisfied with the wisdom attained thus far. When integrity predominates, *wisdom*, the virtue of old age, can emerge. Again, this presupposes the more or less successful resolution of the previous stages and builds on all the previously developed strengths of *hope, will, purpose,*

competence, fidelity, love, and *care*. With wisdom comes a shift in identity: out of the sense of identity developed in adolescence emerges an existential identity, which comes from facing the border of one's life, realizing the relativity of one's own identity, and coming to terms with the world outside the self and with one's connection to the universe. It also enables a reconciliation with, and acceptance of, death. Stern offers the thesis that adaptation to death is necessary for full personality maturation, and deficiency in this adaptation is an integral factor in neurosis. (Stern, 1968). It is a key developmental task—to come to view one's own death as the appropriate outcome of one's life. At age 80, Bertrand Russell beautifully characterized the successful negotiation of this stage when he wrote:

> Psychologically, there are two dangers to be guarded against in old age. One of these is undue absorption with the past.... The other ... is clinging to youth in the hope of sucking vigor from vitality.... The best way to overcome it—so it seems to me—is to make your interests gradually wider and more impersonal, until bit by bit the walls of the ego recede and your life becomes increasingly merged with the universal life. An individual human existence should be like a river—small at first, narrowly contained within its banks, and rushing passionately.... Gradually, the river grows wider, the banks recede, the water flow more quietly, and in the end, without any visible break, they become merged in the sea. (Dangott & Kalish, 1979, pp. 167–168).

When integrity fails to predominate, a sense of **despair** pervades. A person fears death and wishes desperately for another chance, or may withdraw from all involvement with others in a gesture of defeat.

It should be emphasized that the development of integrity is very much undermined by stresses inherent in the aging process. The multiple physical and social losses that occur must be worked through in relation to their relevant developmental conflicts, so there is much psychologically to be learned. Otherwise, the losses of aging can indeed become overwhelming contributors to despair.

---

selecting new roles, even if they are physically and mentally able to fill them. In our society, the age role of older people has often been characterized as a **roleless role**, meaning that few if any roles are expected of or provided for older people that would enable them to make meaningful contributions. Instead, older people are expected to defer their acquired positions of power and leadership within the community to the young. Perhaps one of the most blatant examples of these restrictions is mandatory retirement. Conceptually, **mandatory retirement** is a form of age discrimination because it imposes retirement purely on the basis of age (Atchley, 1978). The law prohibits age discrimination

in employment for people between the ages of 40 and 64, but older people are denied such protection.

The problem of restrictions in role opportunities for older persons is compounded by the fact that it occurs at a time when they are already experiencing a diminished opportunity to engage in many of their most meaningful roles because of, for example, reduction in income from loss of job, the death of family and friends, and mobility of children. The grandparent role is one of the few new roles that becomes open to them, and it takes on special significance because so many other areas of role performance have become closed. It also is a role that has many positive connotations, in contrast to the few other new roles that are available, such as "widow," "new resident" (special living conditions often become necessary, requiring relocation to unfamiliar environments), "volunteer," and "retiree."

Most older adults are pleased to discover that, despite the social obstacles just discussed, the role of retiree can have pleasant connotations (Streib & Schneider, 1971). This outcome depends on factors such as the work *versus* leisure orientation of the individual, on whether the individual has health and money and is able to find meaningful ways to occupy his or her time in spite of the restrictions imposed by our social system.

The tragedy is that when such restricted role opportunities are provided to older people, both society and older people lose. Society loses the talents of older people, and older people are excluded from significant social participation and deprived of their social identity. The responses of older adults to these injustices range from complete resignation to militant resistance. To intervene effectively in the process by which older persons find themselves less useful to society requires a reorganization of the social system and its underlying values to provide older individuals with opportunities to make meaningful contributions.

It is apparent that the social aging process is fraught with undue hardships and significant challenges. This is not to say that older adults have not been able to find ways to cope with the difficulties. It is testimony to the adaptability of older people that so many of them continue to report high life satisfaction and high morale despite the despiriting social restrictions that they encounter in their day-to-day lives. In fact, successful adaptation in old age is the rule rather than the exception (Lieberman, 1978). Research in this area reveals that there are two key variables in retaining high morale and a feeling of life satisfaction: health and meaningful activity (Neugarten & Hagestad, 1976). It also suggests that successful adaptation to social aging is to a large extent determined by the ability to compensate; for example, by finding ways to increase activity in other areas, when roles are taken away as through retirement or loss of a spouse. Obviously, older persons can and do survive in our restricted social environment; the larger question to be addressed is whether they *must*.

Nonetheless, there is evidence that the age-grading system, which has led to the restrictions in the social role allocation experienced by older persons, may be breaking down. Neugarten proposes that the United States is becoming an **age-irrelevant society**, in which chronologic age is losing much of the meaning it once had (Neugarten, 1975). Middle-aged and older adults are returning to school; middle-aged adults may divorce, remarry, and start new families; and both men and women are starting new careers during middle and retirement age. It is unclear how the age-grading system will adjust to these changes, but it can be hoped that society will begin to recognize that there are many different but equally acceptable ways for people to behave at all ages.

Neugarten and Hagestad (1976) also caution, however, that our age-grading system appears to be going in contradictory directions. On the one hand, chronologic age is being used increasingly as an index for benefits such as medicare and social security. On the other hand, this trend is counterbalanced by efforts to do away with the notion that age itself should be the determining factor in how roles and privileges are allocated in adulthood.

Not incidentally, this rethinking of age roles is occurring at a time when American society is seriously questioning its ability to financially support a growing population of nonworking adults over the age of 65. The age at which individuals can be required to retire has already been raised to 70 years, and it is likely that further efforts will be made to maintain older people in the economic sector. This economic imperative may well be the impetus required to force society's recognition that older adults are able to make contributions that were previously thought inappropriate or even impossible. Now that their productivity is needed, older persons may finally be provided with role opportunities to make meaningful contributions that they were always entitled to by virtue of their capabilities. Consequently, the status, self-identity, and life satisfaction of all older people may be enhanced, and the stresses inherent in social aging might be significantly eased for future generations.

Conclusion

Aging is a dynamic process that cannot be understood without an appreciation of the ways in which biologic, psychological, and social aspects interact over the course of the life cycle. The changes that older persons experience are mediated by their health, their own psychology, and their interactions with society. Biologic decline is inevitable, but it may not affect the functioning of older people to a great extent until some threshold has passed, usually in late old age. By contrast, psychological growth is not restricted: there is no point where the psychological growth of older people ceases. Considerable social growth may also occur in old age. Despite stereotypical beliefs about older people that may restrict new learning opportunities and obstruct participation, a significant number of older people succeed in leading productive and worthwhile lives.

Aging, then, is not without its difficulties, but there are also redeeming features. This perspective has been validated by a number of researchers who, like Maas and Kuypers, find that:

> Old age merely continues what earlier years have launched. Finally, even when young adulthood is too narrowly lived or painfully overburdened, the later years may offer new opportunities. Different ways of living may be developed as our social environments change with time—and as we change them. In our study, we have found that *old age can provide a second and better chance at life* [author's italics]. (Maas & Kuypers, 1974, p. 215)

Regarding age, George Bernard Shaw reminds us, "There is only one alternative."

References

Aiken, L. (1976). *Later life*. Philadelphia: W. B. Saunders.

Atchley, R. (1977). *The social forces in later life* (2nd ed.). Belmont, CA: Wadsworth.

Atchley, R. (1978). Aging as a social problem: An overview. In M. Seltzer, S. Corbett, & R. Atchley (Eds.), *Social problems of the aging*. Belmont, CA: Wadsworth.

Birren, J., & Renner, V. (1977). Research on the psychology of aging: Principles and experimentation. In J. Birren & K. Schaie (Eds.), *Handbook of the psychology of aging*. New York: Von Nostrand Reinhold.

Botwinick, J. (1977). Intellectual abilities. In J. Birren & K. Schaie (Eds.), *Handbook of the psychology of aging*. New York: Von Nostrand Reinhold.

Botwinick, J., & Thompson, L. (1966). Components of reaction time in relation to age and sex. *Journal of Genetic Psychology, 108*, 175–184.

Butler R. (1967). The destiny of creativity in later life. In B. Levin & R. Kahana (Eds.), *Psychodynamic studies on aging*. New York: International Universities Press.

Butler R. (1975). *Why survive? Being old in America*. New York: Harper & Row.

Cowgill, D., & Holmes, L. (1972). *Aging and modernization*. New York: Appleton-Century-Crofts.

Dangott, L., & Kalish, R. (1979). *A time to enjoy: The pleasures of aging*. Englewood Cliffs, NJ: Prentice-Hall.

Dennis, W. (1966). Creative productivity between 20 and 80 years. *Journal of Gerontology, 21*, 1–16.

Erikson, E. (1959). Identity and the life cycle. In G. Klein (Ed.), *Psychological issues* (Vol. 1, No. 1.). New York: International Universities Press.

Levy, L. (1986). Sensory change and compensation. In L. Davis & M. Kirkland (Eds.), *Role of occupational therapy with the elderly*. Rockville, MD: American Occupational Therapy Association.

Lieberman, M. (1978). Social and psychological determinants of adaptation. *International Journal of Aging and Human Development, 9*(2), 115–126.

Lowenthal, M. F., & Chiriboga, D. (1973). Social stress and adaptation: Toward a life course perspective. In C. Eisdorfer & M. Lawton (Eds.), *The psychology of adult development* and aging. Washington, DC: American Psychological Association.

Lowenthal, M., & Haven, C. (1968). Interaction and adaptation: Intimacy as a critical variable. *American Sociological Review, 33*, 20–30.

Maas, H., & Kuypers, J. (1974). *From thirty to seventy*. San Francisco: Jossey-Bass.

Neugarten, B. (1975). The future and the young-old. *Gerontologist, 15*, 4–9.

Neugarten, B., & Hagestad, G. (1976). Age and the life course. In R. Binstock & E. Shanas (Eds.), *Handbook of aging and the social sciences*. New York: Von Nostrand Reinhold.

Palmore, E. (1974). *Normal aging II*. Durham, NC: Duke University Press.

Rosow, I. (1967). *Social integration of the aged*. New York: Free Press.

Schaie, K. (1982). The Seattle longitudinal study: A twenty-one year exploration of psychometric intelligence in adulthood. In K. Schaie (Ed.), *Longitudinal studies of adult psychological development*. New York: Guilford Press.

Schaie, K., & Geiwitz, J. (1982). Late life. In K. Schaie & J. Geiwitz (Eds.), *Adult development and aging*. Boston: Little, Brown & Co.

Stern, M. (1968). Fear of death and neuroses. *Journal of the American Psychoanalytic Association, 16*, 3–13.

Streib, G., & Schneider, C. (1971). *Retirement in American Society: Impact and process*. Ithaca, NY: Cornell University Press.

Tomlinson, B., Blessed, G., & Roth, M. (1970). Observations of the brain of demented old people. *Journal of Neurological Science, 11*, 205–243.

U.S. Senate, Special Committee on Aging. (1986). *Aging America: Trends and projections, 1985–1986*. Washington, DC: US Government Printing Office.

SECTION 3

Occupation as the major activity of humans

GARY KIELHOFNER

KEY TERMS

Daily Living Tasks	*Play*
Occupation	*Work*

LEARNING OBJECTIVES

Upon completion of this section the reader will be able to:

1. *Define occupation.*
2. *Identify activities that are primarily occupational in nature.*
3. *Describe the three areas of occupation generally recognized in occupational therapy.*
4. *Describe how occupation has been a central factor of human evolution.*
5. *Describe how a human's goal-directed use of time and energy affects basic biologic processes.*
6. *Describe the relationship between occupation and the psychological and social dimensions of living.*
7. *Discuss two implications of the characteristics of occupation for therapy.*

In 1910, occupational therapy was defined as the "science of healing by occupation" (US Government Printing Office, 1918). Although many other definitions have since been proposed to elaborate this simple theme and to reflect growing knowledge in occupational therapy, it still stands as the best reminder of what the occupational therapist is—an expert in the influence of occupation on health.

Although early occupational therapy leaders saw the necessity of understanding occupation (Johnson, 1981; Kielhofner & Burke, 1977), it is only more recently that occupational therapists have begun to recognize the necessity of having a clearer and deeper conceptualization of occupation and its influence on health (Finn, 1977; Reilly, 1971; Weimer, 1979). Reilly and many of her students began developing the thesis that successful application of occupation as a therapeutic medium required a thorough understanding of the nature of occupation (Florey, 1969; Kielhofner & Burke, 1980; Matsutsuyu, 1971; Reilly, 1962; Reilly, 1971; Watanabe, 1968; Woodside, 1976). Yerxa (1983) placed this relationship in perspective when she identified the study of occupation as the basic science of the field and the study of occupational therapy as the field's applied science.

Responding to the need for a science of occupation, this chapter draws together relevant information to conceptualize the nature of occupation in human life. An interdisciplinary view of occupation is presented; knowledge that has been accumulated in various fields to explain occupation is organized around the following proposed definition,

> Occupation is the dominant activity of humans that includes serious, productive pursuits and playful, creative, and festive behaviors. It is the result of evolutionary processes culminating in a biological, psychological, and social need for both playful and productive activity.

This definition points out some characteristics of occupation and opens possibilities for further elaboration. As knowledge accumulates, the definition should expand and become more comprehensive and integrated.

Occupation

Occupation refers to human activity; however, not all activity is occupation. Humans engage in survival, sexual, spiritual, and social activities in addition to those activities that are specifically occupational in nature. Survival and sexual activities are rooted in the biologic requirements of the individual and the species. Survival functions preserve the basic integrity of the organism; they include such activities as eating and avoiding pain and danger. Sexual activities bond relationships and serve the perpetuation of the species. Social activities refer to the forms of interaction and relations between individuals and their patterned order. The social characteristic of humans involves the affiliative or affective bond between members of the species, their ability to share meanings, and their capacity for integration of action. Social activities have their genesis in the requirement of a group for coordinated activities among members. Language is probably the most important dimension of social activity, since it is the medium for most human interaction. Spiritual activities are also a fundamental part of human existence. Every civilization has some expression of human belief in an incomprehensible and ultimate dimension and related ethical codes.

Placing certain activities into spheres of human activity is not meant to suggest that all human activities can be neatly categorized into one of these areas. Social relations and sexuality overlap, spiritual activities involve coordinated human interaction, and social processes are often deeply infused with the spirituality of the cultural group. Certain human activities fulfill particular needs, however, and it is possible to characterize activities as primarily or uniquely spiritual, social, or sexual.

In everyday life, occupation can be interrelated with sexual, survival, social, and spiritual activities; some activities (work, play, and self-care activities) are primarily occupational in nature. Similarly, we can identify occupational dimensions of activities and enumerate activities that are primarily occupational.

Occupational therapy is not concerned with all forms of activity; it focuses on that which is occupational in human life. Humans clearly work and play far beyond the immediate demands for survival. Such activities, done for their own sake, serve the basic urge for exploration and mastery.

To say that occupation is a major human activity does not mean it is more important than other areas of human behavior but rather denotes that occupation ordinarily entails most human time. Most waking hours are spent in play, self-care, and work. For all their other characteristics, humans are most definitely occupational creatures.

Forms of occupation

The study of occupation begins with identification and classification of different forms of occupation. Furthermore, to guide treatment, occupational therapy needs to develop its own system of classifying occupational dysfunctions (Rogers, 1982). Such a classification of dysfunction must be built on a previous taxonomy of healthy occupations. For example, the concept of a patient having a work or play dysfunction implies that work and play are defined behaviors for which there are criteria of adaptive and maladaptive functioning.

In occupational therapy, three areas of occupation are generally recognized: work, play, and daily living tasks (Meyer, 1977). These categories appear to have inherent validity and will serve as a starting place for defining different forms of occupational behavior. These occupational behaviors form an interrelated gestalt. For example, work and play exist in an important dynamic balance throughout life, the daily life tasks of self-care are a necessary part of having a work role, and adult leisure is earned through work. These examples demonstrate the interdependence of these activities, which supports the argument that they form a common domain of behavior.

Work

Work may be conceptualized to include all forms of productive activities, whether or not they are reimbursed. Productive activities are those that provide a service or commodity needed by another or that add new abilities, ideas, knowledge, objects, or performances to the cultural tradition. The productive activity of work thus maintains and advances society. An activity considered to be a person's work is generally organized into a *major life role*. Life roles are positions in life recognized by the social environment and by the role incumbent. Roles are not merely a means of organizing a person's activity into a position within society; they also are an important source of identity. Thus, activities engaged in to fulfill an individual's duties as a student, housewife, or volunteer are properly considered work. According to this definition, work is not limited to adults; it extends to school-aged children and the elderly. Such a broad definition of work is relevant to occupational therapy, since many of the field's clients and patients do not have access to marketplace labor.

Daily living tasks

Daily living tasks include self-care, chores, maintenance of living space and economic resources, and those behaviors required for access to resources (traveling, shopping, and so forth). Daily living tasks are expected of all capable members of the social group. Unlike work, daily living tasks do not contribute directly to the services or commodities of the social group. When a person cannot perform them, however, the productivity of another social member such as a family member or a caretaker is required. Thus, daily living tasks are indirectly productive for the social group.

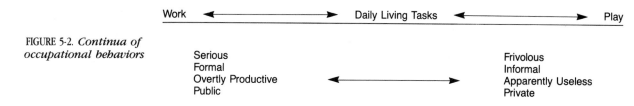

FIGURE 5-2. *Continua of occupational behaviors*

Play

A range of behaviors from childhood to old age constitutes play. In youth, play predominates in daily life and involves exploratory, creative, and game behaviors. In adolescence and adulthood, it decreases in amount and transforms into hobbies, social recreation, sports, cultural celebration, and ritual. In old age, play once again becomes a predominant occupational behavior; it is generally referred to as leisure—a way of life earned through the labor of adulthood.

Continuum of occupational behaviors

Occupational behaviors can be conceptualized as existing along a continuum. For instance, they range from serious to frivolous, from overtly productive to apparently useless, from private to public, and from formal to informal. On the one end of the continuum, we find playful behaviors that are typically perceived as frivolous, private, and apparently not productive, although it will be shown later that they have important use for individuals and social groups. On the other end of the continuum, we find the more serious, overtly useful, and public behaviors of work. Daily living tasks fall somewhere in between (Figure 5-2). Although this schema reveals something about the differences in these occupations, it also demonstrates that their characteristics may overlap. This points out the difficulty in establishing clear criteria to differentiate occupational behaviors. Additionally, some occupational behaviors such as hobbies or amateur pursuits appear to exist on the border between work and play. Thus, it is helpful not only to recognize the continuum of characteristics but also to note that the concepts of work, play, and daily living tasks are not always discrete and mutually exclusive.

The range of serious and frivolous activities and the formal and informal aspects of occupation can be a useful indication of someone's occupational adaptation. For instance, a person whose work is formal, serious, and highly productive may require play of the opposite character to counterbalance it.

Understanding more about the forms that occupations take enhances the ability of therapists to deal with the occupational problems of clients and patients as well as their ability to use occupation therapeutically. Further theory and research are needed to augment the field's understanding of occupation through the lifespan, its various forms in culture, and the overall dynamics of occupation in an individual's life.

Occupation as an evolutionary trait

Human behavior is a product of a long period of biologic and sociotechnical evolution. From the beginning of evolution, action was basic to survival; even the simplest organism is fundamentally spontaneous and active. The process of evolution, reflected in the phylogenetic scale, demonstrates a progressive increase in

organisms' requirements and capacities for more and more complex actions (von Bertalanffy, 1969). With advanced nervous systems came an increase in the amount and diversity of action needed and sought by the organism. This need first appears in the young, in whom spontaneous playful action is a means of learning basic skills that are biologically transmitted to members of lower, simpler species (Vandenburg & Kielhofner, 1982). As the nervous system of a species advances to a more complex and adaptable form, the rigidity of biologically encoded ability is progressively left behind. Thus, behavior that is innate in members of simpler species must be learned by the members of higher species. That is, animals that have very specialized behavior acquire much of it through genetic inheritances, whereas more complex animals that adapt through their behavioral variability are less endowed with inherent programming and have brains with a greater capacity to organize the information from experience.

Many theorists agree that play is the prerequisite for learning this flexible behavior. The play of young members of these more adaptable species is characterized by a greater urge to use capacity and by an exploratory urge that arises from the nervous system's requirement for experience as a learning process. Most mammals, in their immature period, romp, jump, run, engage in rough and tumble play, and explore objects and places, all with no apparent motive except the playing itself. Studies have supported the hypothesis that these animals learn to use their bodies and to deal with their environment through this early form of play, however (Cherfas & Lewin, 1980).

Primates

In primate species and in humans, play is more elaborate and includes social acts, fine motor manipulation, tool use, and imitation (Bruner, 1972). In these play forms, the individual learns complex behaviors that are part of the retinue of skills making up its species' typical approach to adaptation. Play enables this learning because it is a nonserious practice in which the organism can make mistakes, engage in trial and error, and try out new behaviors without serious consequences (Bruner, 1972).

Humans are at the apex of the evolutionary trend toward adaptation through flexible rather than specialized behaviors. The evolution of flexibility in human activity requires a highly plastic nervous system in the young, a behavioral mechanism to provide experience, a social system that supports and protects the young, and a process for storing the collective experience of members to provide a pool of information for the young to acquire.

The route to *generalization* (adaptation through flexibility rather than specialization) that humans followed in evolution is also reflected in the highly adaptive human hand and its intimate relationship to the brain. Together with the visual sense, they form a complex that greatly enhances the ability of the organism to explore and master its environment. The human hand is morphologically suited to extensive manipulation and exploration of objects in the environment. Consequently, there is a greatly enhanced capacity for gaining technologic control over the environment by using and elaborating this eye–hand–brain complex. This is first represented in the emergence of tool use and later in tool making.

Tools are primarily extensions of the hand (Washburn, 1960), and they represent elaboration of the urge to explore and to have effects on the world. Although many species exhibit some primitive kinds of tool use, only humans are spontaneous and extensive tool makers and inventors. The invention of tools, which is a central component of the tremendous growth of technology characterizing human work throughout history, is almost paradoxically an outgrowth or product of play (Bruner, 1973). Behavioral flexibility that is gained in play includes the production of extensions of biologic equipment, that is, tool production (Vandenburg & Kielhofner, 1982).

Observations of semidomesticated monkeys provide a model for how play was responsible for the evolution of tool making in human life (Kawai, 1956). In free-ranging monkey troupes who have a sufficient food supply provided by caretakers (hence, the term *semidomesticated*), play becomes more prevalent in the young. From this play emerges a plethora of new behavior forms. Most are idiosyncratic and eventually die out, but some of these behaviors, which include forms of tools use, prove adaptive. Older monkeys learn the new behavior by imitating it, and eventually the behavior is spread through the troupe and learned by successive generations in their play as they imitate older monkeys. This is a primitive version of the evolutionary complex of humans (including a plastic nervous system, a behavioral mechanism for learning, a pressure-free social group, and imitation as a means of spreading and preserving individual experience in the group). In addition to these primate studies, investigations of children have found evidence that play with objects is an important precursor to the inventive use of objects as tools (Dansky & Silverman, 1976; Sylva, Bruner, & Genova, 1976). Play is centrally important for the technologic abilities of both individual members and the entire social group.

Play, tool use, the human hand, and the brain all are important and interrelated factors in human evolution, wherein both behavior and physical morphology have been changed in concert. Each interrelates with and influences the selective advantage of the other. Bruner (1972) and Washburn (1960) propose the following explanation for how human evolution took place. As prehominids left the jungle for the savannas, they gained adaptive advantage by standing upright on the tall grassy plains. Eventually, they relinquished brachiation for ambulation as a mode of locomotion. Simultaneously, the pressures of hunting and of surviving predators on the savanna required coordinated group efforts. Individuals with more complex brains to initiate and interpret the communications had adaptive advantage.

This evolving animal with a larger brain had to be born through the smaller birth canal of the ambulator's stockier pelvis. Thus, the progeny of the changing prehominid were born more immature, with brains that would grow and mature substantially after birth. This more immature brain was more plastic and suited to learning. Concurrently, the growing complexity of the social group included a division of labor, with some individuals serving as caretakers of helpless (more immature) infants. This created an ideal environment for the emergence of more and more elaborate play forms. Young prehominids, protected by their mothers and whose survival needs were met by the work of the group, were freed to engage in whatever nonserious pursuits they wished. Unlike the young of other species, who had to locomote and perform many other adult skills soon after birth, these individuals remained immature for years, during which they played and acquired more and more behavioral flexibility. In time, this youthful play produced a more creative and inventive adult likely to contribute technical or social advancement to the group. Since group members could readily communicate, they could also acquire and impart these advances.

The end results of this evolutionary trend are the creative, aesthetic, and playful characteristics of the human and the flexible behavior that characterizes the species. It is no accident that humans play more than any other animal. In addition, humans have the unusual characteristic of elaborating their behavior far beyond what is required by survival. For instance, hunting and gathering societies that require only about 18 hours of weekly labor for food gathering and other survival needs manage a long week spent in ritual and festive behaviors that require substantial energy and investment. By evolving a more complex culture, and requiring new members to acquire it, human societies are constantly advancing the demands on individuals for adaptation. This is poignantly demonstrated in the situation in which persons who manage to fulfill their basic survival needs, but violate social norms of conduct, are judged to be maladaptive.

Not only has the human brain evolved to be able to learn these cultural behaviors, but its very structure and processes are intimately interrelated with these varied behavior forms. The human must acquire the complex behavior of culture to function at all (Kawai, 1956). In the course of evolution, the brain was programmed for exploration and mastery; consequently, individuals must engage in a wide range of occupational activities, especially early play, to use their biologic inheritance properly.

As human culture becomes more elaborate, its demands for all forms of occupation increase. Accumulated technology and knowledge make the requirement for learning to work ever more demanding. In human history, simple imitation was replaced by apprenticeship. More recently, the explosion of human knowledge and technique expanded apprenticeship to a long period of public tutelage, beginning with common knowledge and culminating (sometimes 20 or more years later) in specialized training. This process continues; just as mathematics and reading have become in a few generations almost essential for self-care and work, computer fluency will likely emerge as the new requirement for coming generations.

Thus, it can be seen that the process of human evolution has intimately involved occupation. Through evolution, the demands for both play and work have increased. Changes in the organism thrust the human species more and more toward both the capacity and the need for occupation. The human trait of occupation emerged in this evolutionary concatenation of a nervous system of growing complexity, increased playfulness, tool use, and increasing urge for action, and technical–social change and growth. The occupational nature of humans is reflected throughout the modern human situation. Humans begin life as players, go through a long period of preparations for productivity, enter worker roles, and eventually return to a play-dominated phase in retirement. This schema of daily human life has its origins in a complex interrelated set of factors that have unfolded over aeons. It is not by chance that humans work, play, and care for themselves; it is biologically and socially encoded in the species.

Because occupation has been a central feature of human evolution, it fills an important place in the adaptive capacity of the species and its individual members. Without occupational activities, individuals would regress and be disorganized, if they survived at all. Without the playful and productive contributions of members, social and cultural life would cease. Occupation is so central to adaptation that when it is absent or distorted in the individual or culture, there is great cause for alarm. The role of the occupational therapist centers on situations in which individuals' or groups' occupational capabilities are threatened or lost.

Biologic dimension of occupation

The complex nervous system of humans requires rich and varied stimuli achievable only through active engagement of the world (Reilly, 1962). Occupation is centrally important in the development of biologic features in childhood and their maintenance in adulthood. The nervous and musculoskeletal systems of the child receive constant use through the childhood occupation of play. Play is an important arena for the neurologic "programming" that the child's developing nervous system requires. Development is not just a predetermined change in the structures of the body; it includes the effects of experiences that become imprinted into the biologic structures (Bruner, 1973; von Bertalanffy, 1969). All those neurologic and musculoskeletal features that make possible functions such as coordinated movement and perception have much of their genesis in play.

In adulthood and in old age, occupation is important for maintaining biologic functions. For instance, a severe restriction of occupational activities is associated with the impairment of strength, endurance, mobility, cardiovascular function, metabolism, and nervous system function. Stress has long been recognized as a major etiologic factor in many biologic problems. It has also been recognized that boredom or a lack of satisfying and meaningful occupations produces stress and thus ranks as a physiologic threat. In addition, longevity and health in old age are related to maintaining meaningful work and leisure throughout adulthood and old age (Cousins, 1981).

The mechanism by which occupation maintains healthy biologic functioning is complex; only a little is understood about it. New relationships between occupation and biologic well-being are constantly being discovered. For example, it was noted a few years ago that running seemed to have a positive effect on depressed persons. Later, it was discovered that such physical exertion is a catalyst for the release of catecholamines in the brain, which are the organism's natural antidepressants (Leer, 1980).

It is theorized that the conscious functions of humans engaged in the purposeful activity of occupation have direct controlling effects on the brain's physiology (Furst, 1979; Sperry, 1970). Such proposals, which attempt to bridge the mind–body dichotomy, are paving the way to a deeper understanding of how a human's goal-directed use of time and energy reverberates throughout the organism, affecting basic biologic processes. In summation, it may be argued that when a human engages in meaningful occupation, mind and body function in an integrated and resonating manner. Thus, occupation plays a role in maintaining the biologic organization of the organism.

Psychological dimension of occupation

An intimate relationship exists between occupation and the psychological dimension of living; the latter is defined as the symbolic (temporal, meaningful, and purposive) and affective experience of the self and the world.

Experiences in childhood are an important determinant of children's growing sense of control over their world and their destiny; it is a source of their feeling of well-being. Children become aware of the effects they can have on the world, and they begin to develop a sense of personal causation—the belief that they have skills, can control events, and will succeed (Leer, 1980). Without positive play experiences, this image of personal competence does not develop.

Play is also central to children's symbolic development (Bruner, 1973). Their growing awareness of time and its role in structuring activities and their growing sense of meaning or purpose, which can define positive existence, all accrue from play experience (Robinson, 1977).

In play, children learn the basic symbolic skills that enable them to deal with motion, objects, people, and events. These have been referred to as the rules that children internalize about their actions and their environment (Robinson, 1977). These rules form an internal map of external reality and its potentials for action. Children deprived of play experiences are poorer practical problem solvers, are less creative, have less information about their environment, and exhibit less flexible and adaptive approaches to the environment (Dansky & Silverman, 1976; US Government Printing Office, 1918). In play, children learn a growing sense of time as they sequence events, take turns, and compartmentalize activities into meaningful episodes. Eventually, as the child's sense of time grows, there is an increasing future orientation. Children, in their fantasy, begin to bridge the transition to the future and, in so doing, create purposes and meanings for themselves about their own existence. The simple dramatic play of a child serves a deep purpose of allowing the child to experience some of the meaning of being a parent, firefighter, nurse, or other adult figure. Paradoxically, the fantasy of childhood is an important process for developing a healthy sense of reality and of how one can competently face and master the requirements of life.

As the child develops, the growing necessity of being productive slowly emerges. The child first learns tasks of self-care, advances to chores, and, by adolescence, begins entry into work situations. The less serious productive roles that children and adolescents perform in the home are important precursors of competence in adult life (Kielhofner, 1980). In the transition from childhood to adulthood, the individual also undergoes the important process of occupational choice (Webster, 1980). The combined experiences of dramatic play, childhood activities yielding interests and a growing sense of meaning and value, and realistic experiences of older childhood and adolescence culminate in the consequential choice to enter or begin preparation for a kind of work. As might be expected, children with poor play experiences and little opportunity for chores and recognition by adults may fail in this occupational choice process, and they may enter into a vicious cycle of dissatisfaction and failure in their adult work careers (de Renne-Stephen, 1980).

Daily living tasks and work are critical adult activities. For most adults, they are a means of earning a living and contributing to the maintenance of a household. The work role is valued by society, so that working is often the primary source of self-esteem and feelings of control and competence. Work is a means of pursuing personal interests and of developing personal abilities. Many persons who find they cannot meet these needs in work will seek to do so in their recreation or in more serious amateur pursuits. This reflects the fact that humans have a need for occupation far beyond that dictated by sheer survival.

Work is a major factor in the structuring of time throughout adult life. Daily and weekly routines are often dictated by the work schedule. The work career may imply a structured sequence of years of advancement through steps or positions in a given line of work. Individuals measure their own growth, and they progress by their advancement in time through a series of jobs, positions, or work titles. Failure to meet socially normative patterns of advancement can result in a loss of self-esteem and a sense of being out of control.

Satisfaction in work ordinarily requires that the person be able to exercise and develop skills he or she values, to find work interesting, and to see tangible results of his or her efforts. The satisfaction and sense of personal mastery that comes from work of whatever type is an important source of mental health in the adult. When people begin to fail in their work roles or when they cannot meet their needs for satisfaction in work, they may become candidates for mental illness (Shannon, 1970). The stress of not being able to find meaning in one's existence is being recognized increasingly as a significant etiologic factor in mental illness (Frankl, 1982). The growing trend in modern industrial societies toward impersonal, mechanized, and noncreative work has already initiated an epidemic of persons who exhibit maladaptive lifestyles.

As people become disengaged from the meaning of work and its potential for self-satisfaction, they become alienated from society, demonstrate deviant behaviors, and lead unhappy and often disorganized lives. As this trend continues, occupational therapy will have to address a whole new area of health problems that come directly from the disintegration of normal occupation. Such a demand will require occupational therapists to compel and encourage institutions and workplaces to make changes that would restore the health of individuals (Johnson & Kielhofner, 1983).

Although adult life is still largely dominated by work, a growing trend toward more leisure has occurred in modern society. Today, the leisure or recreational period of an adult's life is likely to be substantial and to have a large impact on life satisfaction. Vacations, weekends, and retirement are life spaces that the person literally earns through work. Adult life involves a dynamic balance of work, play, and sleep patterns. If balance is not preserved, the person may have a dysfunction of his or her occupational life with other consequences such as loss of life satisfaction and erosion of competence (Shannon, 1970).

Old age in modern society is marked by a major transition from working to enjoying leisure. This is often a period of adjustment; persons who have a well-developed leisure role before retirement (those who have hobbies or other avocational interests) generally have less difficulty adjusting to retirement. For many elderly persons, however, physical problems, lack of resources, and environmental constraints limit opportunities for engaging in sufficient occupational activities; when this is true, life satisfaction is less (Gregory, 1981).

Social dimension of occupation

The role of occupation in social life can be described in terms of the contributions of both work and play. As already noted, play was a central mechanism in the evolution of the human species, having been responsible for the elaboration and creation of new behaviors that eventually entered the cultural repertoire of the social group. It also serves to initiate the immature into the demands of the physical and social environment and to prepare the young for adult life in a particular social group. The special beliefs, values, ways of interacting, and technology of the social group are reflected in the play of the young who are thereby inducted into a way of living. For instance, social groups that stress competition in adult interaction have young who play competitive games, whereas social groups that stress cooperation in social interaction have a remarkable absence of competitive games in childhood (Gregory, 1981). Instead, children play to maximize everyone's status. In primitive tribes, children play with bows and arrows and the artifacts of that group; children in modern societies play with toy trucks, stoves, and other implements of modern culture. Play also keeps pace with the changes in the culture's technology. For instance, the appearance of electronic games in the play of today's young is an important precursor of a new generation for whom computer fluency will be highly desirable in adult adaptation. The games of each culture thus reflect its requirements so that the young learn how to participate in the culture through their play. The simple and seemingly unimportant play activities of children serve a vital function of maintaining the continuity of social knowledge and of bringing to the young the technology of the social system.

In human social life, play serves a vital role well beyond the childhood years. Adult play is important for reaffirming the culture's values, a way of stepping back and of affirming the fundamental tenets of a culture (Duthie, 1980). For instance, the football game has been analyzed as a metaphor for the competition, teamwork, and technical precision that characterize American work (Arens, 1980). Adult players and spectators become intensely involved in the emotion and meaning of the game at a symbolic level; this serves in subtle ways to cement their commitment to the way of life of their social group. The celebrative or festive and ritual forms of adult play are critical for the maintenance of social life. Graduation ceremonies, the 4th of July, religious rituals, Thanksgiving dinner, and other forms of celebration allow the individual to take account of accomplishments, worthwhile things in life, and central values. These forms of play are critical to the spirit of the culture.

When adult play forms begin to change, it may signal that cultural change is on the way (Lavenda, 1980). When such play becomes disrupted or when members of a group lose their affinity to such play forms, a culture may be in deep trouble. It is noteworthy that persons who find themselves alienated from social life (eg, the mentally ill) often find holidays intolerable and have difficulty celebrating. Despite its often frivolous and unproductive facade, the play of adult life is an important process in social life. It is a dynamic that maintains the morale, commitment, and value structure of the social group.

Work is a basic fact of all social groups. Human societies are characterized by a division in labor in which individuals take on specialized functions. Rarely do individual humans perform the whole range of labor necessary for self-preservation. Rather, tasks are traditionally divided according to age, sex, social position, and aptitude. Each worker depends in some important way on the contributions of others. In modern society, there is greater specialization of work than at any other time. The network of productive contributions in American society is almost unfathomable. From the perspective of social life, important contributions extend beyond paid labor. In fact, marketplace waged productivity is only a small portion of the actual work that keeps a society functioning. Everything from the household chores performed by the young through volunteer work, home-making, and mutual assistance in families and neighborhoods to the leadership jobs in government are necessary for the maintenance of social life. For this reason societies value the productive contributions of their members. The young are inducted into an ethic that defines social expectations for their work. In response, adults feel a sense of self-worth and affiliation with the social group by virtue of making productive contributions.

Some trends in modern life raise questions about the future of work in society. The substitution of mechanical and electronic process for human labor and thinking, as well as economic processes that do not demand everyone's contribution, may have ill effects for both the group and the individual. The social group not only needs the work of its members, but it owes them the opportunity to work. The reciprocity of the individual and the social group in productive exchange is a central feature of human life. Without work, neither the social group nor the individual can flourish.

One possibility for modern society is the emergence of new valued and valuable work forms. Volunteerism is an important factor in social life today, and it serves both individual and group needs. Hobbies have often been turned into productive pursuits that benefit others. In a society with increasing numbers of disabled, elderly, and unemployed persons, such emerging nontraditional work forms may well be a useful answer. To function, however, they must become part of the cultural fabric; thus, social change is required. For occupational therapists, the implication is involvement in social action as well as individual assistance. Functions such as organizing volunteer groups of disabled persons or running hobby shops for the elderly could be important types of socially based occupational therapy in the future.

Occupation and therapy

The previous sections examined several facets of the proposed definition of occupation. This final part discusses two implications of the characteristics of occupation for therapy: (1) since occupation is central to human adaptation, its absence or disruption (regardless of any other medical or social problem) is a threat to health; and (2) when illness, trauma, or social conditions have affected the biologic or psychological health of a person, occupation is an effective means of reorganizing behavior.

Although for conceptual clarity these two statements separate disruption of occupation from medical illness, it should be realized that many clients seen by occupational therapists show a complex of interrelated problems involving both a medical problem and a loss or disruption of occupation and the environmental conditions under which occupations are performed. Often the picture is complicated when the disorder is a developmental or longstanding one. For instance, children with neuromotor problems may be poor players because of their deficits. The paucity of play, in turn, slows the developmental process, exacerbating the original problem. Another example is the elderly person whose waning physical abilities force confinement to an institution where there are no opportunities to pursue some lifelong occupation; this deprivation may cause depression and lead to physical deterioration.

Sometimes a medical problem is not involved initially, as when a person loses an occupation by virtue of social circumstances; for instance, loss of a job or rearing in an environment that failed to nurture play. Such disruption of occupation can lead to psychological and biologic dysfunctions, however. Depression, physiologic correlates of the stress of boredom, and manifold other medical problems may have their etiology in the lack of normal occupation.

Occupational therapists intervene with carefully guided and organized activities. These occupational activities often influence both the occupational dysfunction and any extant medical problem. Since the two are likely to be intermingled to begin with, the use of occupation as therapy is often an especially efficacious approach. As in the previous examples, engagement of children in more rich and varied play not only allows them to acquire normal play behaviors but has an organizing and maturing effect on their nervous systems. Providing opportunities for elderly persons to pursue valued occupations not only restores morale but provides exercise of their physical capacities.

As the organizing influence of occupation is more fully understood, occupational therapists will become increasingly able to expand its therapeutic use. This will require careful study and the development of theories that explain the dynamics and characteristics of occupation.

A person must have a thorough understanding of any tool to use it effectively. Since an occupational therapists's unique and powerful tool is occupation, it behooves the field and the individual therapist to achieve a deep understanding of it.

References

Arens, W. (1980). Playing with aggression. In J. Cherfas & R. Lewin (Eds.), *Not work alone: A cross cultural view of activities superfluous to survival*. Beverly Hills, CA: Sage Publications.

Bruner, J. (1972). Nature and uses of immaturity. *American Psychology, 27*, 687.

Bruner, J. (1973). The organization of early skilled action. *Child Development, 44*, 1.

Cherfas, J., & Lewin R. (Eds.). (1980). *Not work alone: A cross cultural view of activities superfluous to survival*. Beverly Hills, CA: Sage Publications.

Cousins, N. (1981). *Anatomy of an illness*. New York: Bantam Books.

Dansky, J., & Silverman, I. (1976). Effects of play on associate fluency in preschool children. In J. Bruner, A. Jolly, & K. Sylva (Eds.). *Play—its role in development and evolution*. New York: Basic Books.

de Renne-Stephen, C. (1980). Imitation: A mechanism of play behavior. *American Journal of Occupational Therapy, 34*, 95.

Duthie, J. (1980). The ritual of a technological society? In H. B. Schwartzman (Ed.), *Play and culture*. West Point, NY: Leisure Press.

Finn, G. (1977). The occupational therapist in prevention programs. *American Journal of Occupational Therapy, 31*, 658.

Florey, L. (1969). Intrinsic motivation: The dynamics of occupational therapy theory. *American Journal of Occupational Therapy, 23*, 319.

Frankl, V. (1982). *Man's search for meaning: An introduction to logotherapy*. New York: Washington Square Press.

Furst, C. (1979). *Origins of the mind: Mind-brain connections*. Englewood Cliffs, NJ: Prentice-Hall.

Gregory, M. (1981). *Occupation behavior and life satisfaction among retirees*. Unpublished master's thesis, Virginia Commonwealth University.

Johnson, J. (1981). Old values—new directions: Competence, adaptation, integration. *American Journal of Occupational Therapy, 35*, 589.

Johnson, J., & Kielhofner, G. (1983). The role of occupational therapy in the health care system of the future. In G. Kielhofner (Ed.). *Health through occupation: Theory and practice in occupational therapy*. Philadelphia: F. A. Davis.

Kawai, M. (1956). Newly acquired pre-cultural behavior of the natural troop of Japanese monkeys of the Koshima Islet. *Primates 6*, 1.

Kielhofner, G. (1980). A model of human occupation 2: Ontogenesis from the perspective of temporal adaptation. *American Journal of Occupational Therapy, 34*, 657.

Kielhofner, G., & Burke J. (1977). Occupational therapy after 60 years: An account of changing identity and knowledge. *American Journal of Occupational Therapy, 31*, 675.

Kielhofner, G., & Burke J. (1980). A model of human occupation 1: Framework and content. *American Journal of Occupational Therapy, 34*, 572.

Lavenda, R. (1980). From festival of progress to masque of degradation: Carnival in Caracas as a changing metaphor for social reality. In H. B. Schwartzman (Ed.), *Play and culture*. West Point, NY: Leisure Press.

Leer, F. (1980). Running as an adjunct to psychotherapy. *Social Work,* January, pp. 20–25

Matsutsuyu, J. (1971). Occupational behavior—a perspective on work and play. *American Journal of Occupational Therapy, 25*, 291.

Meyer, A. (1977). The philosophy of occupational therapy. *American Journal of Occupational Therapy, 31*, 639,

Reilly, M. (1962). Occupational therapy can be one of the great ideas of 20th century medicine. *American Journal of Occupational Therapy, 16*, 1.

Reilly, M. (1971). Occupational therapy—a historical perspective: The modernization of occupational therapy. *American Journal of Occupational Therapy, 25*, 243.

Robinson, A. (1977). Play: The arena for the acquisition of rules of competent behavior. *American Journal of Occupational Therapy, 31*, 248.

Rogers, J. (1982). Order and disorder in occupational therapy and in medicine. *American Journal of Occupational Therapy, 36*, 29.

Shannon, P. (1970). The work-play model: A basis for occupational therapy programming. *American Journal of Occupational Therapy, 24*, 215.

Sperry, R. (1970). An objective approach to subjective experience: Further evaluation of a hypothesis. *Psychology Review, 77*, 585.

Sylva K., Bruner J., & Genova P. (1976). The role of play in the problem-solving of children 3–5 years old. In J. Bruner, A. Jolly, & K. Sylva (Eds.). *Play—its role in development and evolution*. New York: Basic Books.

Training teachers for occupational therapy for the rehabilitation of disabled soldiers and sailors. *Federal Board for Vocations Education Bulletin*, No. 6, (p. 13). Washington, DC: US Government Printing Office, 1918.

Vandenburg, B., & Kielhofner G. (1982). Play in evolution, culture, and individual adaptation: Implications for therapy. *American Journal of Occupational Therapy, 36*, 20.

von Bertalanffy, L. (1969). General systems theory and psychiatry. In S. Arieti (Ed.), *American handbook of psychiatry* (Vol. 3). New York: Basic Books.

Washburn, S. (1960). Tools and evolution. *Scientific American, 203*(2):63.

Watanabe, S. (1968). Four concepts basic to the occupational therapy process. *American Journal of Occupational Therapy, 22*, 339.

Webster, P. S. (1980). Occupational role development in the young adult with mild mental retardation. *The American Journal of Occupational Therapy, 34*:13.

Weimer, R. (1979). *Traditional and nontraditional practice arenas in occupational therapy: 2001 AD* (pp. 45–53). Rockville, MD: American Occupational Therapy Association.

Woodside, H. (1976). Dimensions of the occupational behavior model. *Canadian Journal of Occupational Therapy, 43*, 11.

Yerxa, E. (1983). *Oversimplification: The hobgoblin of occupational therapy*. Presented at the American Occupational Therapy Association Conference, Portland, OR.

CHAPTER 6

Specialized knowledge bases for occupational therapy practice

SECTION 1

The human and nonhuman environments

GLADYS MASAGATANI

LEARNING OBJECTIVES

Upon completion of this section the reader will be able to:

1. *Define environment.*
2. *Identify components of the human and nonhuman environments.*
3. *Understand the sciences of environmental psychology and occupational therapy as they relate to the concept of environment.*
4. *Understand the application of the concepts of human and nonhuman environments to the practice of occupational therapy.*

Consideration of the human and nonhuman environments is critical to the practice of occupational therapy. Although environment was not specifically identified as a concept by the founders of the profession, most current models of the domain of occupational therapy practice include the environment as an important component.

Environment and health

A fundamental belief held by occupational therapists is that humans can relate to human and nonhuman environments in a self-directed, purposeful, satisfying, and meaningful way and that by doing so, they achieve and maintain a state of health. *Health* typically is defined by occupational therapists as an adaptation process that demands day-to-day adaptive efforts directed at social situations or environments. This broad interpretation of health as adaptation suggests that the causes of health-related problems may be social, psychological, biophysical, or cultural. In addition, factors such as medical beliefs and practices, socioeconomic and legal status, political and religious ideology, racial and ethnic bias, and gender and age discrimination have a profound influence on the nature of a person's psychological state, physical condition, and perception of a social situation. These factors affect a person's ability to adapt and ultimately to achieve a state of health. These beliefs about and descriptions of health have resulted in the development of categories of environments for consideration and use by occupational therapists.

Environment and environmental psychology

Mosey (1986) defined **environment** as the aggregate of phenomena that surround a person and influence that person's development and existence. Environment includes nonhuman factors, such as physical conditions, things, and ideas, and human components, such as individuals and groups.

Consideration of the environment in occupational therapy practice paralleled the evolution of the science of environmental psychology. Environmental psychologists Proshansky, Ittelson, and Rivlin (1970) identified the following characteristics of *environmental science*: it deals with the human-ordered and human-defined environment; humans are identified as an integral part of every social problem; and, to a greater and lesser extent, all environmental science is concerned with the question of human behavior. These authors propose that living organisms engage in a complex interchange with their environment and, in the process, modify or are modified by that environment. The aim of environmental science is to study the interactional patterns between human behavior and the human-made modifications in the physical environment. Treshow (1976) suggests that the environment is a total of factors and forces, internal and external, biotic and abiotic, that influence an organism. Treshow also believes that people create the human environment and are themselves its most important element. Wagner (1972) believes that the features of environments are liable to stand for something and refer through time and distance to potential experiences. Wagner further suggests that physical activity within the environment must necessarily occur in humans as living organisms. Moreover, learning from such activity represents the articulation of behavior with circumstances. Leff (1978) suggests that the field of environmental psychology can be defined as the study of the interrelations between psychological and environmental variables. Psychological variables include characteristics of mental or behavioral events and can include interrelated activities, such as thinking, perceiving, feeling, imagining, manipulating, locomoting, and communicating. The environment encompasses the total physical surroundings, including everything that impinges on humans as physical, social, and psychological beings. Leff further suggests that the environment can be analyzed in terms of categories such as complexity, similarity to past surroundings of the organism, degree and type of human influence present, and number and type of other organisms present. The environment can be conceptualized in terms of physical and social content, structure, and dynamic properties. *Content* refers to all the actual things or ongoing events that are present, such as particular people, activities, buildings, vegetation, and weather conditions. *Structure* refers to the degree of diversity and complexity of these things, the ways in which they exist and are organized relative to each other, and other abstract dimensions of the total array of content. An example may be field workers (people) trying to save a field of crops (activity) from an unexpected hail storm (weather conditions). *Dynamic properties* refer to the process or cause-and-effect aspects of content and structure as exemplified by both natural phenomena and human-made laws. Interactions between humans and their environments produce some of the most important variables in environmental psychology because they contribute to the understanding of the meanings attached to environments, patterns of social behavior linked to special types of environments, and processes of modifying and designing environments. Such variables embody the interrelations of culturally and socially mediated patterns of thought, feeling, action, technology, and environment. It is in this context that processes of experience and meaning function. Proshansky, Ittelson, and Rivlin (1970) imply that environmental psychology is a multidisciplinary approach and that the potential for concept generation and theory building is far from complete. The contribution of occupational therapy to environmental science has been the development of a classification system and a unique method of applying the objects of the system to the practice of occupational therapy.

The human environment

Using the general systems approach and drawing from the science of environmental psychology, a system of occupational therapy classification would comprise the concepts of the human environment, including social and cultural environments, and the nonhuman environment, including the physical environment. These classifications are by no means mutually exclusive, nor is the total of the subcategories a final expression of the potential of the categories. This classification system is simply an attempt to capture a dynamic process for ease of identification and explanation.

Occupational therapy practitioners commonly define the ***human environment*** as individuals (the therapist and patient) and groups (the family, staff, and citizens of a community, state, or nation). The human environment also includes those variables that comprise the identity of a person: cognitive skills, biophysical status (age, sex, genetic and ethnic background), psychological make-up, religious and political ideations, economic status, and language. Human environments encompass human-made or human-ordered environments, such as social environments and cultural environments. Mosey (1986) defines a *social environment* as the matrix of people with whom a person presently relates and to whom a person will need to relate in the future. The *cultural environment* refers to the social structures, values, norms, and expectations that are known and shared by a group of people. These components of the human environment are significant to a person's level of awareness and self-definition, to the definition of a situation, and to the attainment of a state of health.

The nonhuman environment

Drawing from the early work of Searles (1960), occupational therapists looked at the interaction of the human environment with the nonhuman environment to identify how the nonhuman environment may foster or impede normal growth and development and how it may be a source of stress or anxiety. Searles explored, in depth, the kinds and qualities of meanings that people invest in their worlds of things, places, and spaces. Through this exploration process, the ***nonhuman environment*** was defined as the physical conditions, things, and ideas of a person's world. Mosey (1986) suggests that the nonhuman environment refers to all aspects of the environment that are not human. The nonhuman environment refers to those concrete and abstract components that surround a person and that may change a person or that a person may want or need to change.

Included in the nonhuman environment is the physical environment of objects and human-made or human-ordered ideas. The *physical environment* consists of things, (such as crafts, toys, furniture, equipment, food, housing or shelter, and clothing) and physical conditions (such a space, temperature, lighting, air, sound, and gravity). Human-made and human-ordered ideas include such variables as time, schedules, physical safety, architectural barriers, population pressures, resource scarcities, public hygiene, technology, temporal adaptation, and symbolism. The nonhuman environment contributes to the growth, development, and maintenance of humans by providing opportunities for object manipulation, the establishment of habitual patterns of behavior, and the organization of these patterns into lifestyles and expressions of emotions. For example, the infant may develop cognitive, psychosocial, motor, and sensorimotor skills by interacting with the nonhuman environment. Activities such as playing with toys, animals, or furniture provide the opportunity to touch, smell, and see objects and contribute to the development of a differentiation of self from nonself. The development and use of habit patterns in, around, and through the rhythms of the body and the physical environment help to establish a person's self-identity. The foods a person eats, the time and place a person eats and sleeps, the air a person breathes, and the time of day or year (the seasons) in which a person engages in these behaviors all help that person to become aware of purpose and pattern. The nonhuman environment also contributes to a person's sense of security and well-being and status within a group or community. Objects and ideas provide the sense of security, manifest a social role, and express emotions. A person may carry weapons or add locks to doors to feel safe in areas of overpopulation or high crime. Objects one carries (books or tools) or the way in which one dresses (in jeans or a uniform) help to affirm a social role (student or worker). Objects and style of dress are also used to express emotions and beliefs. A person may carry objects symbolic of love and safety (a quilt made by a family member, a stuffed animal) to make transitions from one environment to another (home to college or hospital). People also use objects to express emotions, such as by smashing things when angry or giving flowers when attracted to someone. Style of dress or the objects a person wears help to make a statement about a person's life or a condition in the environment. Hats, slogan T-shirts, or a pearl necklace provide the opportunity to express emotions, beliefs, and a particular lifestyle. The type or style of home or shelter may be the result of socioeconomic status, population pressures and density, resource scarcities (financial and structural), and architectural barriers. People may live in a box on the street, a log cabin in the woods, a publicly funded structure, or a house in suburbia because of preference or because of a lack of resources and community support to do otherwise. The nonhuman environment provides challenges for the development of skills and the experiences of competency and mastery. The nonhuman environment thus provides a practice ground for human interaction.

As noted previously, the categories of environment suggested above are not mutually exclusive. The occupational therapy practitioner must consider the interactive relations of the different parts of a person, including the environment, to understand behavior and assist the patient to adapt and live a full life.

The human and nonhuman environments and the occupational therapy process

The practice of occupational therapy may be characterized as a carefully orchestrated dance of the dynamic properties of the human and nonhuman environments to bring meaning and purpose to a person's life. Dunning (1972) has referred to occupational therapists as managers of space, people, and tasks. Perhaps even more than managers, occupational therapy practitioners are agents of environmental change. Within the limits of reality and probability, occupational therapists attempt to effect change by identifying, organizing, structuring, manipulating, and applying environmental components to achieve a state of health.

The view of the human and nonhuman environments dictates the nature of the service delivery model developed by the occupational therapy practitioner. The people to be served, how and where the services are to be delivered, who is to deliver the services, and what is the nature of the services to be provided may be conceptualized as the interrelation between the human and nonhuman environments. Because occupational therapy practice frames of reference typically include a "view" of the environment, the practitioner is always aware of the interface between the human and nonhuman environments. An understanding of this relationship is used to help determine the specific approaches, principles, and strategies to be used, the roles to assume, and the functions to perform to implement the therapy program.

The concepts of the human and nonhuman environments are used in all parts of the occupational therapy process: evaluation, treatment planning, implementation, and reevaluation. The occupational therapy practitioner routinely takes into consideration the content and structure of the person's human environment. The person's age, biopsychosocial status (diagnosis or condition), and sex are considered when selecting assessment methods or specific evaluation tools. The practitioner must decide what occupational performance areas or performance components are to be evaluated and what are the best methods to evaluate those components or areas. The practitioner must decide if using a specific activity (including objects and other people) or a particular instrument or process will evaluate the conditions and behaviors in question (validity of instrument or process) and where the evaluation can or should take place (in the clinic, classroom, patient's room or home). Answers to these questions give the practitioner a way to understand the dynamic properties of the social, cultural, and physical environments. Comparing the patient's scores against some norm or standard of performance often requires examining a matrix of environments, including social, cultural, and physical environments. Determining what the patient can achieve, how the patient did or did not achieve something, and what circumstances contributed to the success or failure on evaluation items is part of the process of analyzing the evaluation results. The interpretation of data should yield a list of patient strengths and weaknesses that is used as the foundation for the development of a treatment plan devised in conjunction with the patient.

The development of goal statements and the selection of methods to achieve those goals require integrating the dynamic properties of the content and structure of the human and nonhuman environments. The activity analysis process used by the occupational therapy practitioner involves identifying the content, structure, and dynamic properties of the social, cultural, and physical environments. The people, objects, conditions of the treatment area (temperature, space, lighting, air, and sounds), time of treatment, availability of the patient, and resources of the patient and department must be factored into the analysis process. The result of the goal-setting and methods-selection process is a clear statement of the correlation between all environmental components and a prediction of the outcomes of this correlation and how the entire process will be managed. The treatment plan represents a dynamic system of the total of factors and forces of the environment. The system also includes ideas and human-made and human-ordered components, such as safety, temporal adaptation, and symbolism. The practitioner is responsible for creating an environment that is conducive to learning and change and that is viewed by the patient to be safe, supportive, and facilitating. That which cannot be realistically created must be symbolically created as an *artificial environment*. The practitioner must then help the patient to make the transition from this artificial environment to an environment more consistent with reality. If the plan is correct and appropriate, the predicted results will occur. As the plan is implemented, the practitioner immediately starts the reevaluation process, and the cycle begins again.

The concepts of human and nonhuman environment can also be applied to the service management roles and functions of the occupational therapy practitioner. The depth and breadth of the occupational therapy program often depend on the political, economic, and legal resources of the institution, state, and health care system. Government or public policy and patient or guardian private resources are a part of the system of environments and must be considered when delivering occupational therapy services. The way in which services are defined may determine the amount or nature of the reimbursement for those services. The way in which the practitioner is credentialed or defined by law, assigned to practice arenas, and supervised are parts of the service management environment. The dynamic properties of the practitioner's administrative world have an impact on both what is done and how it is done.

Summary

The human and nonhuman environments are integral parts of the practice of occupational therapy. The social, cultural, and physical environments of the patient, the therapist, and the therapy process are uniquely choreographed into a complex and dynamic system. The occupational therapy practitioner is a manager and agent of change in the system. The practitioner identifies the components of the system, develops and changes its attributes when necessary, and clarifies the relations between its many parts.

References

Dunning, H. (1972). Environmental occupational therapy. *American Journal of Occupational Therapy, 26,* 292–298.
Leff, H. (1978). *Experience, environment, and human potentials.* New York: Oxford University Press.
Mosey, A. C. (1986). *Psychosocial components of occupational therapy.* New York: Raven Press.
Proshansky, H. M., Ittelson, W. H., & Rivlin, L. G. (1970). *Environmental psychology: Man and his physical setting.* New York: Holt, Rinehart and Winston.
Searles, H. E. (1960). *The nonhuman environment.* New York: International Universities Press.
Treshow, M. (1976). *The human environment.* New York: McGraw-Hill.
Wagner, P. L. (1972). *Environments and people.* Englewood Cliffs, NJ: Prentice-Hall.

Bibliography

Alonzo, A. A. (1968). Health as situational adaption: A social psychological perspective. *Social Science and Medicine, 21,* 1341–1344.
Bennett, R. J., & Chorley, R. J. (1978). *Environmental systems, philosophy, analysis and control.* Princeton, NJ: Princeton University Press.
Fidler, G. S., & Fidler, J. W. (1963). *Occupational therapy: A communication process in psychiatry.* New York: Macmillan.
Hopkins, H. L., & Smith, H. D. (1988). *Willard and Spackman's occupational therapy.* Philadelphia: J. B. Lippincott.
Levins, R. (1968). *Evolution in changing environments.* Princeton, NJ: Princeton University Press.
Stokols, D. (1977). *Perspectives on environment and behavior.* New York: Plenum Press.
Waitzkin, H. (1983). *The second sickness.* New York: The Free Press.

SECTION 2

Human sexuality and counseling

MAUREEN E. NEISTADT

KEY TERMS

Adaptations	*Sexual Response Cycle*
Awareness	*Sexuality*

LEARNING OBJECTIVES

Upon completion of this section the reader will be able to:
1. *Define sexuality.*
2. *List his or her sexuality developmental milestones.*
3. *Articulate his or her attitudes about sexuality and disability.*
4. *Describe the sexual response cycle.*
5. *Summarize the role of the nervous system in sexual functioning.*
6. *Explain how nervous, cardiac, and pulmonary system dysfunctions can affect sexual functioning.*
7. *Describe three levels of sexual counseling appropriate to occupational therapy.*
8. *List three different formats for providing patients with sexuality information.*

Adult *sexuality* is an important part of self-image and identity. It is more than genital sexual functioning. It is our sense of ourselves as men and as woman, as people capable of giving and worthy of receiving affection (Neistadt, 1986; Neistadt & Freda, 1987). This sense can be disrupted by physical or emotional illness or disability. As holistic caregivers dedicated to facilitating quality lives, occupational therapists should be prepared to address sexuality issues with their adolescent and adult patients.

This section provides guidelines and introductory information for sexuality counseling of adolescents and adults with disabilities. The information is designed to help occupational therapists counsel patients about their capacities for engaging in consensal and safe intimate relationships with peers. Issues of sexual abuse, family planning, and child-rearing are beyond the scope of this section; information on these issues may be found in the references and bibliography at the end of this section and in Chapter 15.

Sexuality counseling of adolescents and adults should include, at the least, acknowledgement of the patient's sexuality and provision of sexuality information at the level of the patients's understanding. For some patients, discussion of possible strategies for dealing with the functional sexuality problems associated with different disabilities may also be appropriate. Intensive sexuality therapy is not an appropriate level of counseling for occupational therapists (Annon, 1974).

As with all other areas of occupational therapy practice, therapists providing sexuality counseling need to have certain competencies. Sexuality counseling competencies fall into three categories: ***awareness***, *knowledge*, and *interpersonal skills*. Therapists need to be aware of their own and society's attitudes toward sexuality, sex roles, sexual preferences, and disability. In addition, therapists need to be aware of the emotional and physical needs of people with disabilities. Therapists must also have basic knowledge of the anatomy, physiology, and neurology of the human sexual system, of the ways different disabling conditions affect sexual functioning, and of ***adaptations*** that patients can make to overcome disability-related sexuality problems. In terms of interpersonal skills, therapists need to feel comfortable communicating with patients about sexuality issues and to have some specific counseling strategies (Neistadt, 1986; Neistadt & Freda, 1987).

Awareness competencies

Therapists who provide sexuality counseling are essentially bringing a personal topic into the realm of public discussion. This is true of other areas that occupational therapists address as well (eg, self-care and toileting), but sexuality is generally more emotionally charged than other issues for both therapists and patients. Therapists' personal attitudes about their own sexuality, sex roles, and sexual preferences influence their sexuality counseling. Therefore, it is important for therapists to be aware of these attitudes before they attempt to counsel patients about sexuality issues. One way therapists can become more aware of personal attitudes about sexuality is to think about their own development of sexuality.

The development of adult sexuality involves the interplay of genetics, hormones, intrauterine conditions, and social learning. This process can be divided into four phases: (1) chromosomal assignment at fertilization, (2) anatomic differentiation in utero, (3) development of sensuality and gender role behaviors from infancy through childhood, and (4) development of genital sexuality from adolescence through adulthood. Sex chromosome assignment at fertilization determines the ultimate sex of a child, with the XX combination resulting in females and the XY combination resulting in males. The sex chromosomes direct the manufacture of the sex-specific enzymes and hormones that cause gonadal differentiation in utero. During infancy and early childhood, children develop concepts of themselves as males or females by hearing themselves constantly referred to as "he" or "she." This process of gender identification is generally complete by the age of 2 or 3 years. Sexual preference is generally established by age 5 or 6 years, when children have had social experience with both same-sex and opposite-sex peers. During infancy and childhood, children also learn to appreciate the sensory experiences provided by their bodies. In adolescence, a surge of sex hormones causes the development of secondary sex characteristics and adult sexual drives. Through adolescence and adulthood, men and women strive to establish emotionally and physically intimate relationships with either same-sex or opposite-sex partners, if intimacy is important to them. The need for physical intimacy does not diminish with age or disability (Neistadt & Freda, 1987).

What sexuality-development milestones do you remember? What do you remember about childhood explorations of sensuality, your first experiences with masturbation, puberty, your first date, your first sexual experience? What feelings do you have about these memories? What were the reactions of peers, parents, and siblings to these events in your life? Making a list of positive and negative experiences and feelings in your development of sexuality might give you a sense of your comfort with your own sexuality. If you are uncomfortable with your own sexuality, then you will undoubtedly be uncomfortable discussing sexuality with your patients. If you blush at the mention of sexual concepts or terms, then you are not ready to discuss sexuality with your patients because your discomfort will make your patients uncomfortable as well (Neistadt & Freda, 1987).

Therapists also need to ask themselves about their attitudes toward sex roles and sexual preferences. How would you define male and female sex roles? How are your definitions and expectations different from or similar to those of friends, parents, or older relatives? Do you prefer same-sex or opposite-sex partners in intimate relationships? How do you feel about sexual preferences that are different from your own? Therapists who have strong prejudices against either heterosexual or homosexual preferences should not provide sexuality counseling. The therapist cannot predict the sexual preference of a patient and can do harm by reacting negatively to a patient's stated sexual preference.

Therapists need to be aware of their own attitudes toward disability and toward disability and sexuality. Do you see the establishment or reestablishment of intimate relations with significant others as a potential goal for your patients? Are you in touch with your patients' ongoing needs to be held and loved and to express affection?

Therapists need to be aware of all these attitudes so they can assess how comfortable they feel with their own senses of sexuality. Comfort with one's own sexuality is a prerequisite to developing comfort in discussing sexuality with patients.

Knowledge competencies
Anatomy

Therapists providing sexuality counseling need to know the location and function of the male and female sex organs. For the male, this includes the testicles, scrotum, efferent ducts, epididymis, vas deferens, seminal vesicles, ejaculatory duct, prostate gland, urethra, bulb, Cowper glands, penis, corpus spongiosum, corpus cavernosum, glans, and prepuce or foreskin. For the female, this includes the ovaries, uterine or fallopian tubes, uterus or womb, os, vagina, hymen, mons veneris, labia majora, labia minora, Bartholin glands, and clitoris. Therapists should also be familiar with the mechanisms of conception and contraception and with the process of adolescent development of secondary sex characteristics and reproductive capacity. Readers who are unfamiliar with any of these terms or processes should consult a biology or physiology text—some references are included at the end of this section.

The gonadal hormones of the endocrine system are important to normal development of adult sexual characteristics and to the maintenance of fertility and sexual desire, or libido. Readers are again referred to biology and physiology texts for details about the endocrine system.

Physiology

Masters and Johnson (1966) have described the physiologic changes of the body during the **sexual response cycle**. This cycle is divided into four progressive phases for both men and women: excitement, plateau, orgasm, and resolution. During the excitement phase, men and women experience initial swelling in breast and genital tissue—the latter results in erection in men and vaginal lubrication in women. These physical changes continue in the plateau phase. During orgasm, or climax, men ejaculate and women experience wavelike contractions down the length of their uterus and vagina. During resolution, all physiologic changes gradually return to their normal, preexcitement state. This cycle describes the body's response to sexual stimulation of any kind, that is, intercourse, masturbation, or oral sex.

The physiologic process underlying the first three phases is vasocongestion, caused by a combination of arterial dilation and venous constriction. Extra fluid in the congested blood vessels seeps into the surrounding soft tissue, causing the swelling of breast and genital tissues (Masters & Johnson, 1966).

Other physiologic changes also occur for both men and women during the sexual response cycle. Beginning in the excitement phase, blood pressure, pulse, breathing rate, and muscle tension rise, reaching a peak at orgasm and gradually returning to normal during resolution. Masters and Johnson (1966), working with subjects aged 21 to 40 years in a laboratory setting, found peak blood pressures of up to 220/130 for men and 200/120 for women, peak heart rates of 110 to 180 beats/min, and peak breathing rates of 30 to 60 breaths/min. These peak metabolic rates last for 10 to 20 seconds during orgasm and return to resting values within about 2 minutes after orgasm. Normal resting values for this age group would be 120/80, 60 to 80 beats/min, and 12 to 15 breaths/min for blood pressure, pulse, and breathing rate, respectively (Schottelius & Schottelius, 1973).

The peak orgasmic heart rates found by Masters and Johnson (1966) may have been unduly elevated secondary to the youth of their subjects and the environment of the laboratory setting (Neistadt & Freda, 1987). Other investigators, working with middle-aged men in their home settings, found peak heart rates of up to 117.4 beats/min (Hellerstein & Friedman, 1970). Masters and Johnson's peak blood pressure rates do not reflect the peak rates found in people with hypertension. Research has shown peak orgasmic blood pressure in people with hypertension to be as high as 237/138 for men and 216/127 for women (Staff, 1980 Science News).

Neurology

Control of sexual behavior involves the brain, spinal cord, and peripheral nerves (particularly the peripheral nerves for the genitalia and breasts). Both the somatic and autonomic divisions that use these anatomic pathways contribute to sexual functioning. The control of libido and sexual pleasure appear to be mediated by several areas throughout the cortex, midbrain, and brain stem. The initiation, self-monitoring, and performance of sexual behaviors requires the functioning of the motor strips (voluntary movement), sensory strips (somatic sensation), parietal lobes (perception), frontal and temporal lobes (cognition), limbic lobes (affect), and brain stem–midbrain reticular activating system (alertness and arousal).

The lumbosacral area of the spinal cord is involved in coordinating autonomic and somatic nerve impulses to and from the genitalia in women. In men, the sacral segments S2, S3, and S4 control erection and the wavelike, ejaculatory contractions along the length of the penis during orgasm by means of the parasympathetic and somatic nerves, respectively. The lumbar segments L1, L2, and L3 control the contractions of the seminal vesicles, prostate, and vas deferens that move the semen and sperm into the urethra just before ejaculation by means of the sympathetic nerves. The peripheral nerves, both somatic and autonomic, relay impulses between the spinal cord, the genital regions, and other body areas to effect the physical changes seen during the sexual response cycle. Sexual behavior can be initiated by either the brain, in response to stimuli or thoughts interpreted as sexual, or the peripheral nerves, as a reflex response to genital stimulation (Horn & Zasler, 1990; Neistadt & Freda, 1987; Noback, Strominger, & Demarest, 1991).

Disability effects and adaptations

Any change in physical appearance, roles, or cognitive or social skills can negatively influence self-esteem and sexuality. Adolescents and adults who have grown up with physical or mental disabilities may also have impaired senses of their sexuality because they are aware of looking different from able-bodied peers or of having relatively limited options in terms of life roles. In addition, the inaccessibility of many public places and private homes for people with physical disabilities can restrict their social contact. Occupational therapists can address these issues by promoting improved self-esteem and advocacy skills in their patients.

All disabilities, whether physical or psychological, can cause difficulties with sexuality, but some can cause problems with sexual functioning as well. Disorders of the nervous system can interfere with the control of sexual functioning. Disorders of the cardiovascular or pulmonary systems can affect the blood pressure, pulse, and breathing responses of the sexual response cycle. Any physical or medical problem that limits endurance or ease of movement can interfere with enjoyment of sexual activity.

Nervous system disorders

Brain

Diagnoses that affect brain functioning include cerebral palsy, epilepsy, head trauma, mental retardation, multiple sclerosis, Parkinson disease, stroke, and tumors. Generally speaking, brain lesions cause changes in libido and social behaviors but not in either fertility or the physical capacity to engage in sexual activity. There are, of course, exceptions to this rule. Some patients with traumatic head injury, for instance, may experience disturbances in gonadal hormone regulation as a result of injury to the hypothalamus, pituitary, or temporal lobes. This could result in impotence in men and infertility in women (Horn & Zasler, 1990). Lesions in the limbic system, brain stem, or cerebellum have also been associated with impotence in men (Schiavi, 1979). Some studies have found decreases in erectile and ejaculatory functioning in men and in vaginal lubrication and orgasm for women after stroke (Freda & Rubinsky, 1991).

Regarding libido, it is more common for men and women to experience decreased rather than increased libido secondary to brain injury (Berrol, 1981; Freda & Rubinsky, 1991). Some patients, however, may display sexual acting-out behaviors, such as public masturbation, during their recovery secondary to frontal lobe disinhibition. Patients in longer term settings who display publicly sexual behaviors may also be expressing frustration about having no social outlets for their normal sexual impulses.

Some of the medications prescribed for adults with brain lesions may interfere with sexual functioning. Some anticonvulsant medications, for instance, can cause decreased libido and can interfere with the gonadal reflexes involved in the sexual response cycle (Kolodny, Masters, & Johnson, 1979). It is important for patients to be aware of the sexual side effects of their medications so that they do not develop secondary, psychologically based sexual dysfunction in response to what they may perceive to be unexplainable failures in sexual performance. It is also important, however, that patients be advised to consult with their physicians if they suspect sexual side effects from their medications. Different medications have different effects on different people, so there is likely to be another medication without sexual side effects that can be substituted for one that is causing sexual problems. Patients who simply discontinue troublesome medications on their own run the risk of suffering further serious health problems.

Patients with brain lesions may also have to deal with other functional problems related to sexual functioning, including catheters, cognitive deficits, communication problems, contractures, incontinence, mobility loss, perceptual problems, sensation loss, tremor, and visual problems. Management of some of these functional sexual problems may simply mean applying general adaptive strategies to the specific situation of sexual activity. For instance, lessons patients have learned about bed positioning could be transferred to the concept of sex positions. Patients could be counseled to use positions that are physically comfortable and allow full use of unaffected extremities. A hemiplegic patient, for example, could lie on his or her affected side (provided that was comfortable), freeing up the unaffected side to caress a partner (Freda & Rubinsky, 1991; Neistadt & Freda, 1987). Other issues may require specific adaptations. Relative to indwelling catheters, for example, after erection, men can fold the catheter tube back over the shaft of the penis and secure it there with a lubricated latex condom. Women can keep the catheter tube out of the way during intercourse by bringing the tube back up over the stomach and securing it there with paper tape (Neistadt & Freda, 1987).

Spinal cord

Diagnoses that affect spinal cord functioning include amyotrophic lateral sclerosis, multiple sclerosis, spina bifida, trauma, and tumors. The degree of sexual dysfunction associated with spinal cord injury is dependent on the level and severity of the lesion. With incomplete lesions, voluntary control of sexual functioning by brain–spinal cord pathways might still be possible. With complete lesions, cortical input is eliminated. With cervical and thoracic lesions, reflex genital response is still possible through the lumbosacral reflex arcs that control erection and ejaculation in men and vaginal lubrication and orgasm in women. Reflex erection and vaginal lubrication are preserved more often with cervical than with thoracic lesions. The ability to ejaculate is more often preserved in men with lesions in the thoracic area. Lesions in the lumbosacral area can interfere with the genital reflex arcs, resulting in erectile and ejaculatory difficulties in men and lubrication and orgasmic difficulties in women.

Fertility is generally unaffected by spinal cord lesions. Those men who do not ejaculate normally frequently experience retrograde ejaculation, where the sperm and semen back up into the bladder instead of being emitted through the urethra. These sperm can be retrieved for artificial insemination, if the acidity of the bladder has been neutralized with either a medication course or an alkaline rinse before the retrograde ejaculation.

Patients with spinal cord lesions may also have to deal with other functional problems related to sexual functioning, including catheters, contractures, incontinence, mobility loss, and sensation loss. Again, management of some problems may simply mean applying general adaptive strategies to the specific situation of sexual activity, while other problems may require specific adaptations. Relative to mobility loss, for example, the patient might be counseled to use sex positions that do not require strong supporting movements by weakened muscles. Relative to sensation loss, emphasizing stimulation of body surfaces still sensitive to touch can be helpful since the last intact dermatome often becomes an erogenous zone. Even patients with complete loss of sensation below the cervical levels have reported a psychological sense of pleasure and release during sexual activity (Neistadt & Freda, 1987).

Peripheral nerves

Diagnoses that affect peripheral nerve functioning include alcoholism, diabetes, ileostomy, and prostatectomy. Any injury to the peripheral nerves innervating the genitals can interfere with sexual functioning by blocking the reflex arcs necessary for genital response to sexual stimulation. Men with damage to these nerves can experience difficulties with erection and ejaculation, while women may have difficulties with vaginal lubrication and orgasm. In cases of disruption of genital functioning, a person may have to use alternatives to coitus, such as manual manipulation, to gratify a partner. The importance of cuddling as an expression of affection may also need to be emphasized.

Cardiovascular disorders

Cardiovascular diagnoses include hypertension and myocardial infarction. Patients with these diagnoses often fear that the increases in blood pressure and heart rate that occur during sexual activity will trigger a stroke or heart attack. Research has shown that the risk of sustaining a myocardial infarction during sexual activity is relatively low (Ueno, 1969). Some investigators have suggested that the cardiac cost of sexual activity with a familiar partner is similar to the cardiac cost of activities such as driving a car or climbing one or two flights of stairs (Hellerstein & Friedman, 1970; Siewicki & Mansfield, 1977). Alternatives to coitus, such as masturbation, generally result in lesser peak heart rates and blood pressures during orgasm than does sex with a partner (Wagner & Sivarajan, 1979). Anal sex, however, may lead to irregular heart rhythms secondary to stimulation of the rectal muscle and mucus lining (Cambre, 1978).

Some medications prescribed for patients with hypertension or cardiac disease can interfere with sexual functioning. Some antihypertensives and antidepressants can cause impotence in some men and decreased vaginal lubrication in some women. Diuretics can cause erectile difficulties in some men. Some tranquilizers can interfere with ejaculation. Patients experiencing these difficulties should consult with their physicians about the possibility of trying alternative medications.

The main functional sexual problem experienced by people with cardiovascular problems is decreased endurance. Adaptations for this problem can include avoiding sexual activity when anxious or fatigued, waiting 3 hours after meals or ingestion of alcohol before engaging in sex, and avoiding sexual activity in extremely hot, cold, or humid settings. Anxiety, fatigue, digestion, and maintaining homeostasis all increase the cardiovascular costs of sexual activity. The vasodilation that accompanies alcohol ingestion can also trigger a reflex tachycardia in some people (Neistadt & Freda, 1987).

Pulmonary disorders

Pulmonary diagnoses include asthma, chronic obstructive pulmonary disease, and emphysema. The increase in breathing rate that accompanies the sexual response cycle may cause discomfort for some patients with pulmonary diseases. The suggestions for decreased endurance noted above would also apply for these patients. In addition, semireclined or seated sexual positions might make breathing easier during sexual activity (Neistadt & Freda, 1987).

Other diagnoses

A complete listing of all diagnoses commonly encountered in physical rehabilitation settings and their attendant functional sexual problems is beyond the scope of this section, as is a complete listing of specific suggestions for the major functional sexual problems. For further details, the reader is referred to the references and bibliography at the end of this section.

Sexually transmitted diseases

It is important for therapists providing sexuality counseling to understand that all people who engage in sexual behavior are at risk for contracting sexually transmitted diseases, including the human immunodeficiency virus (HIV) infection. Therefore, it is important for counseling to include cautions about high-risk behaviors, such as engaging in sexual activity without protective barriers. Protective barriers include latex condoms for coitus or anal sex and latex squares, such as dental dams, for oral sex. Vaginal spermicidal foams and gels add an extra measure of protection for women. These cautions are particularly important for people who do not expect to return to a long-standing monogamous relationship (AIDS Action Committee, 1989; American College Health Association, 1990).

Interpersonal competencies

All occupational therapy interventions are grounded in a therapeutic relationship between the therapist and patient. Therapists need good interpersonal skills to establish and maintain that relationship. Sexuality counseling poses some special challenges to those interpersonal skills. First, as mentioned previously, sexuality is a private topic for both therapists and patients. Therapists are not likely to have strong personal feelings about dressing techniques, but they will have strong feelings about sexuality. Therapists have to monitor those feelings during sexuality counseling sessions.

Second, sexuality counseling brings the therapist face to face with the patient's basic human losses. It is easier to deny the possibility of ever sustaining a spinal cord injury than it is to deny loneliness. Once the therapist acknowledges the patient's sexuality, the protective barrier of depersonalization, which all therapists use to some degree, is eliminated. Empathy about sexuality issues can bring therapists close to the emotional pain patients experience relative to their disabilities. Therefore, therapists providing sexuality counseling must be aware of their personal boundaries.

Third, sexuality counseling raises social issues for which there are no easy answers. Should adults with developmental disabilities be permitted to have conjugal relationships with other house residents? If not, why not? And if not, then what other social opportunities are available? Is there enough privacy for people to have intimate social relationships in rehabilitation hospitals, in long-term care facilities, in nursing homes, in group homes?

Finally, therapists providing sexuality counseling need to have some counseling strategies for dealing with this private and emotionally charged subject matter. Sexuality counseling can be viewed as having several levels: *acknowledgement* of a person's sexuality; provision of relevant *information* at the patient's level of understanding; and discussion of specific sexual *adaptations* patients can make relative to their disabilities. Intensive therapy for sexual dysfunction is not appropriate for occupational therapists; patients needing this level of counseling should be referred to sex therapists. Nor should occupational therapists attempt to provide counseling about long-standing relationship problems; patients needing this type of intervention should be referred to a psychologist or social worker.

Acknowledgement of sexuality

The therapist can acknowledge the patient's sexuality by providing positive feedback about the patient's physical appearance and by initiating discussion of sexuality issues. Complimenting a patient on a particular blouse or shirt, noting when a patient is well shaved, and noticing a new hair style, a new hat, or a new piece of jewelry are all ways of letting patients know that they are still attractive and appealing people.

Initiating discussions about sexuality issues is another way of letting patients know that they are still viewed as sexual beings. Research has shown that most rehabilitation patients have questions about sexuality but are too hesitant to ask those questions (Neistadt & Baker, 1978). Occupational therapists do not wait for their patients to initiate discussions about movement or activities of daily living problems, and they should not wait for patients to initiate discussions about sexuality concerns.

In general, occupational therapists feel most comfortable initiating discussions of sexuality with patients after they have worked with patients long enough to develop a therapeutic rapport and a picture of their patients' problems and strengths (Neistadt & Baker, 1978). It is also important to have a sense of how long the patient might remain in a rehabilitation or supervised living situation and whether the patient is involved in an intimate relationship. A married adult patient recovering from a stroke who is scheduled to return home within a few weeks will have different concerns than a single adult with a head injury who is likely to remain in a long-term facility for the foreseeable future. The latter patient's primary questions are likely to be about social opportunity, while the former patient may be more concerned with the physical logistics of having sex with a spouse.

One way for a therapist to initiate discussions of sexuality is to start with a general statement, such as, "People who have been in the hospital for a while or who are experiencing difficulties like yours often have questions about sexuality. I have some information about sexuality and disability, so I could try to answer your questions. If I do not have the answers to your questions, I will try to find the answers for you or refer you to someone on staff who knows more about this area than I do." (Neistadt & Freda, 1987). For patients with limited cognitive abilities, this introduction may have to be modified to, "Do you have any questions about sex?"

This general introduction raises the issue of sexuality and gives the patient permission to ask previously unspoken questions. The introduction also sets limits on the patient's expectations of the therapist's knowledge about sexuality issues. By saying that you have some information but may have to refer to others more expert than yourself, you are letting the patient know that your knowledge is limited. Patients usually respond to this matter-of-fact introduction with matter-of-fact responses. Some simply say they have no questions; others ask questions. There are several ways to provide sexuality information for those who want it.

Provision of information

It is important to be aware of the possible need for parental or guardian consent for sexuality counseling with patients who are under 18 or who are not their own legal guardians. Since sexuality is a highly charged, emotional issue, the provision of sexuality counseling may not be perceived by parents and guardians as a legitimate part of a general rehabilitation program. Parents and guardians can also limit the social opportunities of their charges if they choose to do so.

For patients who want sexuality information and have their guardians' permission to get it, information-sharing can be done in several formats: one-to-one counseling, group lectures and discussions, or formal sexuality programs. Information-sharing can also use several media: verbal, written information, or films and slide presentations. Given the emotionally charged nature of sexuality, it is wise to have administrative approval and backing for group and formal sexuality counseling formats.

One-to-one counseling is most appropriate for patients who are likely to have limited, focused questions about their own abilities to engage in sex or procreate. A combination of verbal and written information is most helpful for this type of counseling. Some patients may also want to include their significant others in these private counseling sessions.

Group lectures are most appropriate for sharing information common to particular disabilities with several patients. A lecture and discussion about the effects of cardiac disease on sexuality and sexual functioning is an example. This format offers the added advantage of peer support and sharing about sexuality difficulties. These lectures and discussions may include only patients with disabilities, patients and their significant others or families, or only significant others and family members, depending on staff time and the needs of patients and families. A combination of verbal presentation, written handouts, and film or slide presentations is helpful for group sexuality counseling sessions. The staff education departments or facilities are likely resources for up-to-date catalogs of audiovisual materials about sexuality. It is advisable for the group leaders to preview films and slide presentations to ensure that the media present relevant material in a tasteful manner.

Formal sexuality programs are most appropriate for patients who are likely to have both social and physical problems with sexuality as a result of their disabilities. Programs for patients with head injuries or developmental disabilities are examples. These programs usually involve a series of group meetings to cover the following: (1) development of sexuality, (2) sexual anatomy, (3) the human sexual response cycle, (4) the effects of specific disabilities on sexuality and sexual functioning, fertility, and child-rearing, and (5) contraception and safe-sex practices. In addition, these programs provide instruction about and practice in social behaviors and communication skills to address the social and communication skill deficits that might exist in these populations. Some combination of verbal presentation, written handouts, audiovisual presentations, and group activities is helpful for formal sexuality programs.

Sexuality adaptations

Information about sexual adaptations for different disabilities can be found in the references and bibliography listed at the end of this section. Patients and their partners are not the only people who can make sexuality adaptations—some thought also needs to be given to the adaptations that facilities can make to promote patient recovery or development of healthy sexuality. For example, all professionals should respect their patients' needs for privacy and modesty. This means never entering a patient's room without knocking and never leaving a patient in public view in an unclad or semiclad state. Some facilities also have privacy rooms where patients can share physical intimacies with significant others during lengthy hospital stays.

Summary

This section has provided an introduction to human sexuality and sexuality counseling for adolescents and adults with disabilities. Information about the physiology and neurology of sexual functioning and about the development of adult sexuality has been reviewed. The effects on sexuality of selected diagnoses have been discussed along with suggested adaptations. Levels of sexuality counseling have also been described.

Only therapists who are comfortable with their own sexuality and with discussing sexuality with patients should provide sexuality counseling. Those who are not comfortable with providing this counseling can develop comfort through further reading and by attending conferences about sexuality and disability. Becoming comfortable with sexuality counseling may take more time than becoming comfortable with other occupational therapy interventions, but the extra effort is well worth the quality therapists can add to their patients' lives by addressing sexuality issues.

References

Aids Action Committee of Massachusetts, Inc. (1989). *About aids*. South Deerfied, MA: Channing L. Bete.

American College Health Association (1990). *Safer sex*. Rockville, MD: American College Health Association.

Annon, J. S. (1974). *The behavioral treatment of sexual problems* (p. 1). Honolulu: Enabling Systems.

Berrol, S. (1981). Issues of sexuality in head injured adults. In Bullard, D., & Knight, S. (Eds.). *Sexuality and physical disability* (pp. 203–207). St. Louis: C. V. Mosby.

Cambre, S. (1978). *The sensuous heart*. Atlanta: Piedmont Hospital.

Freda, M., & Rubinsky, H. (1991). Sexual function in the stroke survivor. *Physical Medicine Clinics of North America, 2*, 643–658.

Hellerstein, H. K., & Friedman, E. H. (1970). Sexual activity and the post-coronary patient. *Archives of Internal Medicine, 125*, 987–999.

Horn, L. J., & Zasler, N. D. (1990). Neuroanatomy and neurophysiology of sexual function. *Journal of Head Trauma Rehabilitation, 5*, 1–13.

Kolodny, R. C., Masters, W. H., & Johnson, V. E. (1979). *Textbook of sexual medicine*. Boston: Little, Brown.

Masters, W. H., & Johnson, V. E. (1966). *Human sexual response*. Boston: Little, Brown.

Neistadt, M. E. (1986). Sexuality counseling for adults with disabilities: A module for an occupational therapy curriculum. *American Journal of Occupational Therapy, 40*, 542–545.

Neistadt, M. E., & Baker, M. (1978). A program for sex counseling the physically disabled. *American Journal of Occupational Therapy, 32*, 646–647.

Neistadt, M. E., & Freda, M. (1987). *Choices: A guide to sex counseling with physically disabled adults*. Malabar, FL: Robert E. Krieger.

Noback, C. R., Strominger, N. L., & Demarest, R. J. (1991). *The human nervous system*. Philadelphia: Lea & Febiger.

Schiavi, R. (1979). Sexuality and medical illness: Specific reference to diabetes mellitus. In Greene, R. (Ed.). *Human sexuality: A health practitioners text* (pp. 203–211). Baltimore: Williams & Wilkins.

Schottelius, B., & Schottelius, D. (1973). *Textbook of physiology*. St. Louis: C. V. Mosby.

Siewicki, B. J., & Mansfield, L. W. (1977). Determining readiness to resume sexual activity. *American Journal of Nursing, 77*, 604.

Staff. (1980, November 29). Love and hypertension. *Science News*, p. 344.

Ueno, M. (1969). The so-called coital death. *Japanese Journal of Legal Medicine, 17*, 333–340.

Wagner, N. N., & Sivarajan, E. S. (1979). Sexual activity and the cardiac patient. In Greene, R. (Ed.). *Human sexuality: A health practitioners text* (pp. 192–20l). Baltimore: Williams & Wilkins.

Bibliography and other sources

American Heart Association, 7320 Greenville Avenue, Dallas, TX 75231, (214) 373-6300, for information about sexuality and cardiac disease.

Arthritis Foundation, 1314 Spring Street NW, Atlanta, GA 30326, 1-800-283-7800, for information about sexuality and arthritis.

Berrol, S., Rosenthal, M., & Blackerby, W. F. (Eds.). (1990). Sexuality and head injuy (Special issue). *Journal of Head Trauma Rehabilitation, 5*, 92.

Conine, T. A., Carty, E. A., & Safarik, P. M. (1988). *Aids & adaptations for parents with physical or sensory disabilities*. Vancouver, British Columbia: School of Rehabilitation, University of British Columbia.

Hole, J. W. Jr. (1990). *Human anatomy and physiology*. Dubuque, IA: William C. Brown.

National Spinal Cord Injury Association, 600 West Cummings Park, Suite 2000, Woburn, MA 01801, 1-800-962-2722 or (617) 935-2722, for information about sexuality and spinal cord injury.

National Stroke Association, 300 East Hampden Avenue, Suite 240, Englewood, CO 80110-2654, 1-800-STROKES for information about sexuality and stroke.

Sex Information and Education Council of the United States, 130 West 42 Street, Suite 2500, New York, NY 10036, (212) 819-9770.

Schover, L. R. (1988). *Sexuality and cancer for the woman who has cancer and her partner*. Atlanta, GA: American Cancer Society.

Schover, L. R. (1988). *Sexuality and cancer for the man who has cancer and his partner*. Atlanta, GA: Anerican Cancer Society.

United Ostomy Association, Inc., 36 Executive Park, Suite 120, Irvine, CA 92714, (714) 660-8624, for information about sexuality and osteotomies.

SECTION 3

Interpreting culture in a therapeutic context

CHERYL MATTINGLY and DAVID W. BEER

KEY TERMS

Collaboration	*Individualization*
Communication	*Therapeutic Relationship*
Culture	*Values*

LEARNING OBJECTIVES

Upon completion of this section the reader will be able to:

1. *Recognize the importance of cultural sensitivity to the therapeutic process.*

2. *Perceive the subtleties of social communication, acknowledge the value of good communication with the patient to providing effective therapy, and convey the particular sensitivity required when the patient comes from an unfamiliar cultural background.*

3. *Reject a common-sense conception of culture as a static set of features or characteristics belonging equally to all members of a cultural group.*

4. *Recognize difficulties that arise when patients from different cultures are treated in ways that stereotype patients.*

5. *Recognize the need to check conceptions of the patient's concerns and values against cues given by the patient and become sensitive to mismatches between the therapist's expectations of the patient and the patient as he or she reveals him- or herself to be in the course of therapy.*

6. *Recognize the need to develop treatment goals and a process of treatment planning that takes the patient's values into consideration.*

7. *Recognize the complexities of negotiating with patients when values differ significantly between patient and therapist.*

The patient's world and its impact on therapy

Sometimes it is easier to consider a large abstract idea, such as culture, by beginning with a concrete example. This section opens with a story written by an experienced pediatric therapist about a difficult clinical experience.

CASE STUDY

The Case of Aaron

Elizabeth Creech

Aaron is a 10-year-old boy with sad blue eyes. Every morning when Aaron and I meet for our therapeutic occupational therapy session, he enters the room, slams the door shut, and grunts or mumbles something that sounds like "good morning." Rarely does he smile when he enters. Sometimes I get him to smile or laugh, and it is quite a beautiful smile. Even today, I do not know what causes the pain that I see in his face, or the sadness. Aaron has been labeled "learning disabled," and he has great difficulty with his handwriting. My evaluation showed that he has difficulty with head extension when prone on scooter-board, his upper-extremity strength is fair+, and his hand strength is fair+. He is unable to hold a pencil with a mature grasp. His handwriting is absolutely illegible.

Aaron is a very bright young man. He communicates well on the adult level. He enjoys discussing world events, such as the Berlin Wall coming down and war, and he enjoys warships. When slight pressure is placed on him ("Aaron, you can do five push ups"), he will state, "No, I can't," and become upset. He repeatedly informs me that he hates to be in the sessions.

For some time, I have changed my strategy with Aaron. Instead of giving him one activity, I set out three or four, and when he comes, he chooses whichever one he likes. He usually does all of them. This has decreased my telling him what to do, and he offers less opposition.

One particular morning, four stations were set up. Aaron did not say hello when he entered, and he avoided eye con-

tact, but there is nothing unusual about that. He began with the fine motor activity. As he quietly worked, I heard a noise, and the pennies he had placed in a wrapper had slipped out. I did not turn to look at him because I knew this was not pleasing Aaron.

Aaron: "I can't do this." (shouting, pause)

Elizabeth: "This is frustrating to you?"

Aaron: (bursting out, shouting) "Shut up! I hate my mother. I wish she were dead." (silence—a long silence, so it seemed)

Elizabeth: "Do you want to do some weightlifting?" (something Aaron enjoyed)

Aaron refused, just sat there, then he suddenly got up without a word and stormed out. I had given him a Valentine's Day card earlier.

Then, two sessions later, we had the following exchange:

Elizabeth: "Aaron, I would like to discuss something with you. If you had your choice to come to occupational therapy sessions or not, what would it be?"

Aaron: "I have no choice."

Elizabeth: "Why don't you have a choice?"

Aaron: "I don't."

Elizabeth: "Let's say you have a choice, you alone can make it, and you are the only one who can make that choice."

Aaron: "I don't have a choice. They won't let me."

Elizabeth: "Remember, Aaron, no one can make the choice for you but you."

Aaron: "What difference does it make? I have no choice."

Elizabeth: "Aaron, your dad told me you could choose."

No answer. We finished the session by talking about weightlifting.

Elizabeth: "Aaron, you can get instructions for weightlifting. I talked with the coach. You can practice with the football team or alone."

Aaron: "I don't have enough weight yet."

It seemed that Aaron sabotaged his own success at times.

This case reveals the puzzle of trying to understand one small boy. He has physical difficulties, but this is only part of a larger picture. This boy is terribly unhappy, terribly angry, and it is not clear why. He is not only extremely bright but also is willing to engage the therapist in discussions about a wide range of topics. The therapist has become attentive to some ways she needs to structure sessions to maximize his strengths and interests and to help him live with his limitations. She has learned to give him a range of activities so that he has a choice. His response is not only to choose one activity but, in the end, to do them all. In his own way, he is a cooperative patient, but enlisting his cooperation is a tricky affair.

The case study describes one particular session, when Aaron has difficulty with one of the activities. It is also a session when the therapist has given him a Valentine's Day card. When they boy gets angry at his failure and bursts out against his parents, the therapist responds by inviting him to choose, rather than be forced, to come to therapy. She also offers him the chance to do weightlifting with the school coach (which she mentioned had been an important wish he had confided in her about). She is trying to break a pattern of relationship to adults and the powerful sense this child has of living in a world where he cannot succeed and he cannot do what he most wants. The therapeutic problem, which might have begun with handwriting, has necessarily widened to larger issues that include not only the boy's internal psychology but also a puzzling and difficult family culture and set of family dynamics.

Even when therapists do not particularly want to enter into issues that relate to deeper social and psychological problems, often they are drawn in, as in the case above, because the success of the particular treatment activities depends on the patient's ability to use them to improve and grow. If the patient is too despairing or feels "chained" to therapy, it is unlikely that treatment will succeed. Even if Elizabeth can get the child to engage in a series of challenging motor coordination tasks in therapy, if he cannot endure failure, he is unlikely to seek out such tasks outside therapy. Yet, his ability to increase strength and coordination depends just as much on his tolerance for failure and his willingness to take risks as it does on his physical capacities. Because the therapist is well aware of this, she works to create an environment of trust in which the child can believe in himself and can take on the therapeutic challenges as his own rather than as something imposed on him from a hostile adult world.

The power of this case is that it ends in a puzzle, with the therapist finding herself blocked by the child's feelings and a family environment she cannot override. When we read this, we do not know whether she ever succeeds with Aaron, but we have the strong sense of how much clinical reasoning is involved in ferreting out the values, beliefs, and assumptions of patients—and their families—and how important this is to effective therapy. This boy's ethnic and socioeconomic background were not exceptionally different from the therapist's. Yet even with his cultural proximity, he remains a puzzle for her. If even culturally familiar patients are often mysterious, how much more is this true for culturally unfamiliar patients?

Culture and collaborative treatment

The case of Aaron illustrates a fundamental feature of good therapy: the need for the therapist to understand the patient well enough to create a treatment program that the patient values and trusts. This case also illustrates how difficult that process of understanding and collaborative treatment planning can be. Occupational therapists need to take the cultural backgrounds of their patients into consideration to provide good therapy, for two central reasons: (1) to develop a collaborative relationship with a patient, and (2) to individualize therapy. Each of these therapeutic goals depends on the other. Without **collaboration**, the therapist and patient cannot individualize goals. Conversely, without **individualization** of treatment goals, the therapist and patient are unlikely to develop a collaborative treatment process.

Culture matters for these two therapeutic goals because a person's character fundamentally is shaped by the cultural worlds the person inhabits. To belong to a **culture** is to have become socialized into a whole series of life worlds. What I care about, what I think my possibilities are, what I fear and love, and what I strive to become are deep **values** shaped by my life worlds. If I become disabled through injury or serious illness, a major impact of the disability is the need to rethink those deep

values, even my sense of identity, which I have cultivated as an inhabitant of a variety of life worlds. Sometimes, the worlds I once lived in can no longer be inhabited, or at least not in the same way. Disabled people may have to abandon professional cultures when they can no longer return to work. Entire family cultures may change when disabled members can no longer play the roles they once did and when the family must remake itself to accommodate. Basic values, often powerfully shaped by ethnic culture, often must be reconsidered in the face of serious disability. It is not merely a matter of readjusting roles or returning to previous roles with some adaptive equipment. When people become disabled, their whole life worlds often are turned upside down. Activities and values they took for granted, which were so obvious that they need not be mentioned or explicitly recognized, suddenly become a focus of attention.

Because occupational therapists often play pivotal roles in helping patients make the transition from clinic to home or to adapt to the "outside" worlds of home, school, or work, they often become engaged in helping patients think through what their new life will be like or what is worth valuing. This means that occupational therapy often demands that therapists try to understand the inner motivations, aspirations, and frustrations of their patients. Therapists must pay close attention to their patients because they must base treatment on more than their vision of how the patient should adapt to disability. Effective treatment is built on the dreams and fears of the patient. In addition, the therapist may see limitations the patient is not yet cognizant of or refuses to recognize. The therapist also may see possibilities that the patient is unprepared to realize, as Elizabeth did with Aaron. Therapy becomes a highly sensitive social interaction in which the wishes and frustrations of the patient, as well as the assessment of the therapist, are continuously negotiated.

Sensitivity to cultural background is required in this ongoing process of collaboration. In some professions, the client does not need to cooperate in a significant way to be provided service. For example, if I want to fly to New York, I must get myself on the plane. The success of the flight, however, does not depend on my capacities as an airline pilot or my vision of the destination. A good client, from the pilot's perspective, is a passive client, not someone who tries to fly the plane. Even in many health professions, patients do not need to participate in treatment in an ongoing, motivated way, as they must do in occupational therapy. When I go to the dentist to get a cavity filled, for instance, I must cooperate in the sense of actually getting myself into the dentist's chair. But once I climb into that chair, the primary cooperation required is to stay there and to move as little as possible. When I go to occupational therapy, on the other hand, I am asked to play an active role, to help create the treatment through my own efforts. I cannot lie back and simply endure therapy in the way I endure my visits to the dentist. Put another way, if my occupational therapist finds that I am only passively enduring therapy, it will soon become apparent that the treatment will not succeed. Occupational therapists need active, motivated patients who become committed to the therapeutic process.

This need for collaborative treatment, in which therapist, patient, and often the patient's family work together, makes it particularly important for the therapist to understand the meaning of the disability for the patient and what kind of life the patient values and expects to recommence. Creating a collaborative treatment relationship means building some level of trust and some shared sense that the patient and therapist confront this challenge together. This can be a difficult task that requires complex clinical reasoning, even when there is no significant cultural difference between the therapist and the patient, as in the case of Aaron.

One of the most subtle therapeutic tasks is creating a treatment approach tailored to the individual patient. Occupational therapists hold strongly that it is important to fit the treatment to the particular person. Pragmatically, a certain amount of tailoring is essential to the effectiveness of therapy because when goals and activities are too foreign or uninteresting to the patient, it is impossible to enlist the patient's active support in carrying out the treatment, even though the patient may passively comply. Taking the patient's cultural background into consideration can offer some information about what activities are more likely to be suitable in treatment. As an obvious example, it is less likely that a working-class Irish man will be interested in knitting as a treatment modality, although this might be just the thing for a 70-year-old Irish grandmother. These gender and age differences help create important cultural differences even within the same ethnic group.

Culture is not a thing

Therapists need to be attentive to the cultural backgrounds of their patients because this influences what form of social interaction therapy should take and what goals should be considered. Some of the most common ways to think about cultural differences, however, are more likely to exacerbate cultural misunderstandings than ameliorate them. The most common way of talking about culture turns it into a thing, an object that gets attached to a person. For instance, we often speak of culture as something we have, a kind of property, as we might talk about our old blue Ford or our black hair. We may speak of ourselves as being Mexican American or as having a mix of English and Italian blood. We also may speak of culture as though it were a kind of place we come from, such as being from Irish stock or, even more literally, as being a Brooklyn Jew. We may think in ethnic terms, such as thinking someone is Sicilian or African American, or in socioeconomic terms, such as thinking someone is a yuppie.

We speak and think in this way because it is handy, perhaps even necessary. To identify someone as a member of a culture gives us a quick first take on them. We seem to need a way to identify and understand one another not only as individuals but also as members of larger groups that have certain characteristics in common. Culture is one term we use to locate ourselves and others as belonging to recognizable groups. The word offers a shorthand that allows us to sum up a perfect stranger in a matter of seconds based on our past experience and stereotypes of that culture.

Reifying culture, that is, treating it as a thing that someone has, as one might have Alzheimer disease, is useful but problematic because it tends to promote typifying. Of course, in the real world, we operate with stereotypes all the time. The practical fact is that a therapist cannot spend a lot of time observing someone and asking endless questions before getting on with treatment. Even the initial assessment of a patient requires making a series of assumptions about the person that influence the phrasing of

questions and even the pitch of voice. The assessment stage involves more than gathering information; it is the beginning of a pattern of social interaction that will carry into the treatment phase. Getting off on the right foot is important to the success of any social encounter. Cultural and diagnostic stereotypes play a significant role in orienting a therapist to a new patient.

Viewing someone as just another member of a group—another preppie or another physical therapist or another Puerto Rican—has obvious disadvantages. In typing particular people with general class characteristics, it is easy to misread them or to presume to understand them better than is the actual case. At its worst, unreflective stereotyping, especially of negative characteristics, can lead to the worst form of prejudice. It often is extremely helpful to try to understand a person not only in psychological terms, as a singular unit, but in social and cultural terms, as someone who has attained a personal identity in part through growing up in a certain kind of family or in a certain kind of neighborhood or by joining a certain kind of profession. Put differently, seeing someone as an individual is helped by recognizing that person as having some beliefs, values, and assumptions derived from a cultural background.

This section discusses what comes after this initial stereotyping and how cultural sensitivity can help the therapist go beyond obvious stereotypes and generalizations to see the patient as a singular person with a unique life history. Recognizing someone as being from a particular culture can aid us in this process as we quickly note a situation that is foreign to us. For example, when we enter a new professional group, a new country, or even our spouse's family, we have an initial feeling of unfamiliarity that tells us we are on strange cultural ground. We begin watching for cues about how to act, how to speak, how to dress, how to sound intelligent, what, in other words, are the cultural "rules." We are aware of not knowing the rules, and if someone from a different culture says something that appears insulting or even unfriendly, we are more likely to hold the meaning of that action in question until we have a better grasp of the cultural rules, which will tell us what that behavior means.

The way cultural values influence a person's response to therapy is often much more subtle than the therapist might expect. Culture is a pervasive shaper of experience, but its influence often is hard to recognize. The following case study, written by a psychiatric occupational therapist, serves as a good illustration of the subtleties of cultural influence.

CASE STUDY

The Case of Levi

Thomas Swartwood

Levi is a patient in a long-term care psychiatric facility. He has a history of psychiatric admissions over the last 10 years. He is white, about 30 years of age, and a member of the Peachy Amish Order. His diagnosis is a schizoid-affective disorder, with depressed mood and right foot drop resulting from a gun shot wound to the head during a suicide attempt.

When I first met Levi, his presentation was guarded and withdrawn. He would not initiate conversation or participate in any therapy or groups. He became a special challenge for me as I got to know him and learned about his special cultural heritage. When approaching him, I found Levi to be pleasant and cooperative despite being very brief when responding.

Levi would not engage in any of the therapies or groups, either OT or others.

Levi had a sporadic work history, with long gaps surrounding his prior hospitalizations. His play history was limited, and his illness was evident in isolating behavior and apparent abnormal sensorimotor processing from childhood.

Levi was obsessed with a woman. He was certain they were meant for one another; he received that message in a vision from God. This woman totally rejected Levi and all his attempts at communication.

Levi's depression was a result of his inability to assume the roles and responsibilities that were well-defined by his Amish persuasion. Work and the family are the measure of a man in his society.

I spent time in the beginning with Levi establishing trust and rapport. We talked about Amish life in general and his life specifically. In an effort to engage him in some activity, we began playing basketball, and Levi became quite a foul-shooter. In time, he also agreed to participate in a vocational workshop three mornings a week. Since he expressed an interest in living independently, I arranged some other occupational therapy groups, including a transitional group that included cooking and house care. This was a radical departure from the role definitions in his culture. Levi was progressing apparently well when a family tragedy (my own) necessitated that I take a 2-week leave of absence. I explained to Levi what was happening and left.

After my return, I discovered that Levi was no longer attending occupational therapy groups and that no one had followed up, except to say that Levi was absent occasionally from the community dining group. This was a special dining group (family style). I tracked him to the vocational workshop, where he was spending all his time working. The workshop supervisors said he was doing very well. I was somewhat surprised when I saw him because he did not look well. He had lost weight, he was very thin, and he looked pale and agitated. I asked if I could speak with him and did. We talked about why he left all the other groups. He told me that the workshop people needed him because they had a contract deadline to meet and he wanted to help. I asked him if he wanted to return to the groups now or after helping with their deadline or at all. He agreed to return after the deadline was met and agreed not to miss any more meals.

Levi participated in a videotaping and in all his other groups for several weeks afterward. Then, he escaped one night and spent the night in a corn field. He returned the next day but would speak to no one except me. He explained to me that he needed time to think but would not share what he was thinking about.

Then came another change. One morning, Levi appeared dressed without his suspenders and in an AC/DC T-shirt. I asked him, "Why the change?" He responded, "It's O.K. if I dress this way, right?" I told him that he could dress any way he wanted, but it seemed out of character for him. Many of Levi's behaviors changed over several days, and then he fell into silence again and would speak to only me and only infrequently. He refused all group participation. One afternoon, he and I were engaged in a rare conversation, and I asked him if he missed any of the activities in which he had become involved. He said, "No. I did all that because you asked me. I did that for you."

Levi and I had some more conversations, and I tried to analyze the common ground between us and have him select activities that he wanted. He did reengage in a few groups—mostly male task-oriented. He eventually was transferred to a more chronic ward, where I kept in occasional contact with him until I left the hospital for another position. He is still there today. I believe Levi may have taught me more than I was able to teach him.

This case was an important one for Tom because it occurred early in his clinical practice and taught him how easy it is to misread a patient's motives and concerns, even when you try to be extremely attentive to them and to the cultural influences that helped shape them. Tom took Levi on as a special case, as a patient he felt he had some rapport with and might be able to help. He was immediately aware of Levi's particular cultural background and spent time talking about Amish life. Tom also became aware of the centrality of work to Amish life—that "work and the family are the measure of a man in his society."

Tom was also conscious of the limited nature of play in Levi's life and, thinking it would round out his life and give him new experiences, chose basketball as a treatment activity. He felt successful in his choice because Levi "became quite a foul-shooter." Tom had to leave the psychiatric facility for 2 weeks and discovered on his return that a thinner, paler Levi was spending all his time working in the vocational workshop. Levi had become withdrawn from Tom and all others in the facility. Tom was puzzled not only about his withdrawal but also about his lack of interest in going back to their basketball practice. He was finally able to ask Levi about it. Levi responded that he did not miss their activities, that he engaged in them only because Tom asked him. He said, "I did that for you."

Tom chose an activity that conformed to his own cultural view of the good life—one that balanced work and play. This choice of activity also conformed to his professional culture. Occupational therapy emphasizes the need for balance in the patient's occupational life, and occupational health tends to be equated with the ability to both work and play. When Levi participated with enough commitment to gain some skills at basketball, Tom presumed that he had also begun to value play. What was play from Tom's perspective was work from Levi's. Levi explained to Tom that he did it out of commitment and responsibility to Tom, out of a kind of obligation—a stance we associate more with work than with play, which should be fun, spontaneous, and definitely not a responsibility.

This case reveals something essential about the nature of culture. A person's culture does not simply define what that person chooses to do but also the meaning and interpretation of those actions and the actions of others. In a famous anthropologic essay, "The Interpretation of Culture," Clifford Geertz (1973) writes of the need to make "thick descriptions" of people's actions. What Geertz means by this is the need, particularly when trying to understand people from other cultures, to be able to interpret their outward actions in light of the cultural assumptions they themselves use to interpret their actions. Geertz cites a well-known philosophical example of the difference between twitches and winks. A twitch is not a cultural action, it is an animal behavior. A wink, on the other hand, while looking exactly like a twitch (from a behavioral point of view, if one just looks at the outward manifestation), is a cultural act, with particular cultural meanings. To determine whether a person has twitched or winked and, if it was a wink, what that wink means, requires knowledge of that person, the social context, and the cultural meanings that the action holds for the person.

To return to the case of Levi, playing basketball is like winking; it is a cultural action, and its meaning depends on how it is culturally interpreted. When Tom plays basketball with Levi, he believes that he is helping Levi to play. In Tom's culture, basketball is play, and a person plays out of desire, not obligation. Play is for fun. For Levi, interpreting basketball from his cultural perspective of the centrality of work and of family (and therefore, of social obligation), playing basketball is a kind of work. When Tom is on a leave of absence, Levi no longer plays basketball but returns to a more recognizable form of work in the vocational workshop, helping to meet a contract deadline.

The cases of Levi and Aaron show that a good therapist-patient relationship is not enough to ensure effective therapy. In both cases, it is clear that the therapists care a great deal about the patients. Yet each **therapeutic relationship** breaks down because at some basic level, **communication** breaks down. Therapists are not able to bridge the differences between their own worlds and those of their patients. In Aaron's world, the focus is on the family; it is a world defined by adults in which Aaron cannot succeed and cannot do what he wants most. Levi's world is defined by meaningful work and does not encompass the concept of play. Both therapists recognize these fundamental differences and make efforts to connect to their patients and discover what is blocking the channels of communication. They both are successful to the degree that they are able to understand their patients as members of powerful culture groups.

Seeing the individual through a cultural lens

One theme common to the cases of Aaron and Levi is the mysteriousness and singularity of the patient. In considering a patient's cultural background, it is wrong to presume that what is commonly true for a member of a certain cultural group holds true for a particular patient. Such culturally based assumptions must be held lightly as the therapist searches for clues to help modify those misreadings of a patient's interests and experiences that were based on stereotypes. Interest checklists and other assessment tools are imperfect in grasping a person's deepest life concerns, fears, loves, and commitments. Generally, it is during the course of treatment and the development of the therapist–patient relationship that what a person cares about becomes apparent. In subtle ways, expert therapists treat their assumptions about their patients' interests and concerns as hypotheses that are reevaluated during the course of treatment.

Rather paradoxically, the capacities to both collaborate with the patient and individualize the patient's therapy require the therapist to think beyond the patient's culture. Being culturally sensitive means being attentive to how the patient may respond differently than the therapist to a disability or a treatment activity because of differences in family, ethnic, professional, or social class. Knowing someone is different from oneself, however, is

only part of the task; the other piece is a concomitant reluctance to presume that there is some standardized response a person will have simply by virtue of belonging to a particular culture. Sensitivity to cultural differences alerts the therapist to pay more attention, to be wary of easy inferences, and to double check assumptions. It humbles the therapist into questioning actions that otherwise may appear obvious.

Sometimes this sensitivity can help the therapist to rethink cultural assumptions or to appreciate an unfamiliar way of life. The therapist who can become intrigued with unfamiliar cultural worlds is much more likely to be effective in treating a wide variety of patients. The following case describes one such experience for a home health therapist.

CASE STUDY

The Case of Elva

Sonja Sand

Each home health patient is always an anticipated challenge. The first contact provides me with an idea of who the patient really is and what my role will be in returning this patient to his or her original lifestyle. I enjoy entering the patient's world for a short amount of time. For me, visiting a patient at home is similar to traveling in a foreign country. I tune into a particular lifestyle, then adapt my approach according to the patient's daily routine. Often, the lifestyles of my ordinary patients contain something unique and valuable, even when they may be opposite to my own.

In the same way travel brochures capture only a few facets of a country, the cover sheet for a referral provides only a rough sketch of the patient. My last referral for an occupational therapy evaluation from the home health agency read: "A 70-year-old, white female with the primary diagnosis of osteoarthritis and left knee trouble. Need to assess for possible activities of daily living training." As I drove to her apartment, thoughts of effective pain management, range of motion, joint protection, and strengthening activities were on my mind.

Elva lived in a town-house apartment overlooking a busy street. As I entered her dark apartment, she sat poised in a wheelchair next to a Tiffany lamp. She waved her cigarette, which she held high in her right hand, in a cool gesture of greeting. I felt as if I had stepped into a 1940s bar room picture from *Vogue* magazine. An image of hard work and fast living surrounded this aging World War II model. Countless bottles of hard liquor clustered on the kitchen table and counters created a functional bar. A large wood and green velvet roulette table graced the entrance to her kitchen, where she sat. I introduced myself by name and purpose.

"Oh yes, I told my physical therapist that I needed to carry my drinks from the kitchen to the living room window, but I couldn't do it with my walker, wheelchair, or Canadian crutches," she said. Suspecting that she may need more occupational therapy than that, I answered, "Sure, there are ways to do that. Let me take a few minutes of your time to see if there are any other areas that I might be able to help you with. I would also like to look at your left shoulder since it has been fractured." She only seemed interested in the problem of transporting her drinks from the kitchen to the living room. "I'm a retired architect, and I did not even use my shoulder then. Why bother starting anything now?" She reluctantly let me proceed with the occupational therapy evaluation. I found a totally frozen shoulder with no scapular rotation. All planes of shoulder motion were severely limited. She had good strength within the limited range, which allowed her to use a walker and was sufficient enough for performing all grooming and hygiene activities. She was adamantly against increasing any range in her shoulder despite my suggestion that it could be improved.

Areas in which she did ask for further help included rearranging her kitchen so that she could prepare snacks independently; teaching her how to change the linens and make her bed independently; helping her to drive and get groceries independently. The logistics of adapting Elva's kitchen were made easy because of the adjustable cupboards. As I rearranged the overcrowded gallons and pints of wine, beer, vodka, and rum in her cupboard, I began to suspect that her primary diagnosis should have been alcoholism rather than the orthopedic injuries. Even the refrigerator served as a holding site for more liquids, mainly liquor. The contents of Elva's kitchen lacked even a semblance of the four main food groups. It appeared that her diet of alcohol was supplemented with crackers and peanuts.

Elva successfully learned how to make her bed in one session, despite the fact that she was chatty and woozy from a few strong drinks beforehand. "Onward," she cheered, "to the last goal in therapy. On Monday we will go shopping together." My level of concern for her drinking continued to rise. I vowed not to get in the car with her if I smelled alcohol on her breath but was undecided on approaching her on the subject. On the one hand, the evidence seemed overwhelming that alcohol was an important part of her life. A fall sustained on New Year's Day could easily be repeated. If she was an alcoholic, she appeared to be in denial.

During the grocery trip, my respect for Elva grew. Driving for the first time in 6 months, Elva was a changed woman. She proudly drove me by her community theater where she has worked part-time as a stage technician and actress for 40 years. She was now the treasurer and advisor. In the grocery store, other customers called her by name and stopped to ask how she was doing. Elva was obviously appreciated, and she was happy to have returned to the community from which she had been away for so long. She talked of cocktail parties, historic sites, and town politics. I chose not to intrude on her culture or lifestyle by voicing concern about her alcohol use.

Our last visit touched the subject of addictions, especially smoking. She started smoking and drinking during the war, when she worked in an ammunition factory. I am unsure that my lack of direct confrontation on the possibility of alcoholism was clinically sound. I suspect that Elva will continue to drink for the rest of her life. Should I have confronted the culture that she grew up in? In this case, I chose not to confront her.

Sonja is faced with a number of difficult decisions in treating Elva. Should she live with Elva's limited view of why she needed occupational therapy—to carry drinks from the kitchen to the living room? How far should she press Elva to work on her left shoulder despite Elva's apparent disinterest in increasing her range of motion? Of course, what should she do about Elva's drinking? The case reveals initial negotiations that lead to Elva's coming to identify a broader range of treatment goals than she began with and Sonja's abandonment of a treatment goal to improve her shoulder. Sonja ends her case story by asking herself—and the reader—whether she made the right decision.

There is nothing clearcut about Sonja's decision. Sonja insightfully recognized that drinking is not simply a disability or pathology for Elva but part of a way of life. To ask Elva to confront her drinking problem is also to ask Elva to rethink her own sense of self and her place in a particular cultural world. The beauty of this case is that Sonja reasons about what approach to take from a cultural perspective. She becomes a clinician-anthropologist, moving from her initial recognition that Elva is a woman who drinks (notice the description of Sonja's initial impressions on entering Elva's apartment) to a gradual awareness of the role of drinking in this woman's life. Although Sonja cannot approve of her probable alcoholism and is clear about the physical dangers it poses for a 70-year-old woman, she allows herself to become sufficiently acquainted with Elva's world to realize the cultural dimensions of her drinking. She learns something of Elva's history, including her strengths. In that trip to the grocery store in Elva's own community, she sees Elva's strength. Elva is much more than an old woman with physical difficulties and a drinking problem. She is a former architect and a current actress and stage technician, a woman of strength and strong social roots.

Sonja listens to her patient well enough to learn about her strengths as well as about the disabilities that initially brought Sonja to Elva's door. Sonja's capacity to see Elva as an individual is aided by her growing awareness of the social world Elva has inhabited for 40 years. She is able to place Elva within a life world that is unfamiliar and that probably carries different norms and values than Sonja's cultural world. What is so powerful about Sonja's cultural placement of Elva is that nowhere do we feel Sonja to be engaging in simple cultural stereotyping in this process. Rather, Sonja's ability to see Elva as belonging to a particular cultural world brings the patient into sharp relief, increasing Sonja's awareness of Elva's uniqueness and strength and helping her to sort out the extremely difficult problem of what therapeutic goals should be the focus of treatment.

Conclusion

It is essential that the therapist go beyond a view of culture as a collection of beliefs, values, and norms that the patient carries around like so much baggage. Because culture is not a thing or property that can be labeled or taken as given, the therapist must try to interpret the cultural world of the patient and decide how the patient's cultural background should influence treatment decisions.

Therapists do two things to learn about their patients' cultural backgrounds. First, they listen. Therapists are most likely to learn something valuable by listening to stories about a patient's past or present life, or about how a day was spent, than by directly questioning the patient about values. This is because most people cannot explicitly articulate their beliefs and values.

Part of the power of culture is its tacitness, the fact that it gives us a way to make sense of the world that seems natural. Anthropologists often say that one of the values of studying other cultures is that it gives us a chance to see ourselves differently. Our own culture becomes much more visible in the face of a different culture. Even short trips to other countries can provide a certain amount of culture shock—we are surprised at how differently people can act and feel. Culture shock also involves the recognition that how the people back home live is just one cultural variation. Therefore, when the therapist wants to understand what is valued and important to a patient, especially those values that are connected to deep cultural concerns, it is not easy to simply ask the patient to list them.

Anthropologists rely on participant observation to understand a particular culture. They not only talk to the people but also watch how people live and even live with them, cooking and dancing and going to religious ceremonies. This combination of participation and observation is the most effective way to reach this deep and tacit level of cultural knowledge.

Although therapists do not become immersed in the cultures of their patients, they tend to share experiences with patients during treatment as a way to understand what their patients value. Therapeutic activities can provide small experiences in which the therapist is able to both observe and participate with a patient in an activity. This clinical participant observation can provide an invaluable way to better understand the life world of the patient.

The second source of information therapists rely on, then, is observation, but observation alone can be deceptive. Cultural understanding is not easily gained by simply watching someone's behavior. Outward behavior must be understood by not only seeing someone do something but also by understanding the motives behind behavior. For this attribution of motive to be accurate, the therapist must have a reasonable grasp of the cultural background of the actor. Take, for example, the simple case of someone smiling. I find that when a good friend smiles, it is generally easy to interpret the meaning of the smile, that is, the motive behind the smile. It often is easy to distinguish a teasing smile or smirk from an encouraging smile from a smile that masks anger. The same outward behavior carries a completely different meaning. With a stranger, I am more likely to be mistaken in my interpretation of a smile, thinking that someone is encouraging me when they are actually bored and thinking about what they are going to have for dinner, for instance. With a stranger from a different culture, I can be more mistaken still. I see the behavior but, not knowing the culture, I cannot get a fix on what it means.

The culturally sensitive therapist moves between observation, often carried out by participation in an activity that holds special significance for the patient, and listening to what the patient says, which can help the therapist gain clues about why certain activities are significant.

Reference

Geertz, C. (1973). *The interpretation of cultures*. New York: Basic Books.

Bibliography

Anderson, P. P., & Fenichel, E. S. (1989). *Serving culturally diverse families of infants and toddlers with disabilities*. Washington, DC: National Center for Clinical Infant Programs.

Mattingly, C. (1991). What is clinical reasoning? *American Journal of Occupational Therapy, 45*(11), 979–986.

Mattingly, C. (1991). The narrative nature of clinical reasoning. *American Journal of Occupational Therapy, 45*(11), 998–1005.

Mattingly, C., & Gillete, N. (1991). Anthropology, occupational therapy, and action research. *American Journal of Occupational Therapy, 45*(11), 972–978.

Murphy, R. F. (1987). *The body silent*. New York: W. W. Norton.

Rosaldo, R. (1989). *Culture and truth*. Boston: Beacon Press.

SECTION 4

Family influences

HILDA P. VERSLUYS

KEY TERMS

Discharge

Family Adjustment

Family Dynamics

Family Roles

Family Stress

Family Support

Patient Motivation

LEARNING OBJECTIVES

Upon completion of this section the reader will be able to:

1. *Describe the importance of family support and involvement in the patient's motivation for recovery.*
2. *Understand the emotional reactions and stresses experienced by family members.*
3. *Explain functional and dysfunctional family behaviors and how these behaviors influence rehabilitation.*
4. *Describe the importance of family-centered evaluation and treatment.*

Importance of the family

The role of the family in the rehabilitation process is vital and enabling. The patient who receives ***family support*** and encouragement is more motivated to pursue difficult rehabilitation tasks, to tolerate painful procedures, to face unalterable losses, to adapt to lifestyle changes, and to pursue a productive daily life in the community. In fact, studies demonstrate that patients look first to their families for support and then to the professional staff (Power, 1985).

Family members, however, have their own emotional reactions and difficulties with acceptance and adaptation to the disability or illness of a family member. A family member's functional residual impairments may permanently alter the family structure and force change in individual *family roles*, use of time, personal interests, and goals (Power, 1985; Rohrer et al., 1980; Versluys, 1980a). Versluys (1985) and Zisserman (1981) state that therapists appear to understand patients' difficulties in accommodating to their disabilities but tend to expect the family to demonstrate instant ability in coping with the realities of having a disabled family member.

The contemporary family

During a period when hospital admissions are shorter, when modern technology saves more lives, and when there is less funding for community services, there is an increased expectation for family involvement in treatment and long-term caregiving after discharge (Zisserman, 1981). Availability of the American family as a support network for all its members has changed, however. The contemporary family model tends to have the following characteristics: the employment of both wife and husband; the socialization of women into serious career commitments; a reduction in the three-generation family network; and higher divorce rates with less long-term family stability (Versluys, 1985; Zisserman, 1981).

The contemporary family in the United States is represented by different ethnic heritages and religious beliefs. These beliefs may influence family understanding of the cause and meaning of patients' disabilities and the valuing of the rehabilitation process. Patients and families may believe that the illness was caused by supernatural forces and wish to rely on folk medicine and healing ceremonies as well as contemporary medicine. Patients may have difficulty with role change because of beliefs about appropriate gender roles. The therapist must understand the values and beliefs of the different ethnic populations they treat, communicate this understanding to the family, and use this information in the treatment planning process (Brantley, 1983; Queralt, 1984; Versluys, 1985).

Unfortunately, the typical medical system has not adapted to national, cultural, and social changes in the family but rather continues to practice in a traditional manner that tends to have unrealistic expectations for what the family can accomplish. The family routine is disrupted, and family members may face considerable sacrifice to attend hospital and educational meetings during the day and to manage the patient's long-term care. It is important for the occupational therapist to recognize that these conditions can exacerbate *family stress* (Versluys, 1980a; Versluys, 1985; Versluys, 1986; Zisserman, 1981).

How families differ

Families have different coping styles and strategies for managing family crises. It is important to identify a family's methods of coping with change and crises. A functional family tends to be more flexible, can prioritize family tasks, has effective communication patterns, values the rights and ideas of each family member, including the disabled member, has good time management skills, and can adapt to change over a period of time. With professional support, family members can see alternative solutions, solve problems, and make family lifestyle adaptations (Palmer, Canzona & Wai, 1982; Power, 1985; Versluys, 1980a). The

functional family can help the patient continue to carry out occupational and family roles, encourage the increase and maintenance of independent activities, and enable a child or adolescent to reach his or her developmental potential.

Some families, due to their own pathology or developmental problems, are more vulnerable to crisis and may experience continuous conflict and breakdown. A family that initially appears to be capable may be marginally functioning, and the occurrence of a medical crisis can exacerbate existing family anxiety and tensions. Some families have psychological problems, such as substance abuse or dependency problems, and some families lack organization as a family unit and thus are unable to work together to solve problems or to maintain consistent behaviors (Gans, 1983; Kaplan, Smith, Grobstein, & Fischman, 1977; Palmer et al., 1982; Versluys, 1980a).

A dysfunctional family reduces the patient's potential by overprotection and promotes regression by rejection, excessive control, and side-tracking the roles that the patient could carry out as part of an interactive family or as a community member (Dell Orto, 1984; Olsen & May, 1966; Power & Dell Orto, 1986; Versluys, 1980a; Versluys 1985; Zager & Marquette, 1981).

Family responses to crisis

The family and the patient experience similar emotional reactions to physical disability or illness. They may experience these reactions in a similar sequence, or their experience may differ in timing and in emotional intensity. Both the family and the patient may use adaptive mechanisms, such as denial, and experience emotional reactions, such as shock, disbelief, anger, anxiety, depression, mourning, and feelings of disassociation. These reactions can be temporary or continuous and can be re-experienced as an anniversary reaction (Versluys, 1985). Certain events in the rehabilitation process may herald an increase in the intensity of emotional reactions. For example, when the patient's progress stabilizes and functional improvement ceases or during the transitional period of *discharge*, both the family and the patient may show an increase in these emotional symptoms and behaviors (Cella, Perry, Kulchycky, & Goodwin, 1988; Versluys, 1985).

Emotional reactions to the medical incident and increased task demands may produce harmful stress experiences for family members. These stress reactions can be the root of maladaptive behaviors and influence the family's ability to provide emotional support and physical services to the patient. Families can feel powerless and insecure and have an unconscious need to have the rehabilitation staff share their pain and struggle. Emotional reactions to these feelings can be criticism, verbal attacks, and anger when fantasized needs are not met. This can occur even though the patient is making good progress in rehabilitation. Studies of stress syndromes in families of chronically ill patients show that family members can experience ongoing chronic stress with clinically significant symptoms of depression and anxiety (Cella et al., 1988; Gans, 1983; Moos & Schaefer, 1985). Spouses of chronically ill patients can develop symptoms such as fatigue, anxiety, role tension, and depression to a degree that equals that of the patient (Jaffe, 1978; Safilios-Rothschild, 1970).

It is important to recognize that the family members' emotional reactions are not necessarily synonymous with permanent dysfunctional behavior. Both the patient and the family need to express their grief and to mourn the physical or health-related changes and losses. This enables them to come to terms with altered future plans and lifestyles (Dell Orto, 1984; Versluys, 1985).

Threats to family adjustment

The following family problems complicate *family adjustment* and may compromise rehabilitation success: (1) denial that the changes are permanent; (2) feeling responsible for the injury or illness because of something they did or failed to do, such as getting into a fight or driving too fast (Gardner & Stewart, 1978); (3) fear that the patient will not be able to function adequately at home after discharge or plans for a separation or divorce may be interrupted (D'Afflitti & Weitz, 1977; Mastrangelo, 1990; Wepman, 1973); (4) tendency to be overprotective, to believe the patient is more disabled than is the actual case, and to encourage dependent behaviors so that the patient is unable to become independent, to engage in productive adult roles, or to maintain a positive self-identity (Frey, 1984; Versluys, 1980b; Versluys, 1985); (5) imposition of their own plans and beliefs without consideration of the patient's interests and goals (Versluys, 1985); (6) having opposing views concerning the patient's care, a different understanding of the long-term implications of the disability, and disagreement on the use of financial assets for the patient's welfare (Kaplan et al., 1977; Versluys, 1980a); (7) denial of the situation or rejection of the patient, leading to behaviors such as neglect to arrange home visits, to order equipment, or to keep appointments (Gans, 1983; Versluys, 1980a); and (8) engaging in denial, magical thinking, and believing that the patient is special and will recover—this may become an expectation of both the parent and the developing child that prevents good accommodation to the disability (Buchanan, LaBarbera, Roelofs, & Olson, 1985).

The family may feel anger and resentment toward the patient because the patient may have been noncompliant with health care rules, such as neglect of a diet, abuse of alcohol, or reckless driving. Examples of the outcomes of such an accident are spinal cord injury, burns, head injury, or exacerbation of medical problems, including myocardial infarction or diabetic crisis. This may mean that the family is faced with long-range caretaking commitments and depletion of personal time for things they enjoy. Because of the accident or the exacerbation of previous family problems, the patient may become a target for family hostility (D'Afflitti & Weitz, 1977; Gans, 1983; Power & Dell Orto, 1986; Versluys, 1985).

Treatment considerations

Hasselkus (1991) describes the importance of viewing the treatment process from the perspective of the patient and the family. This involves codevelopment of treatment goals and attention to those educational topics that have meaning for both patient and family.

A family-centered treatment approach begins with early identification of intrafamily difficulties so that intervention can reduce the incidence of family disorders and breakdown (Kaplan et al., 1977). The evaluation focus is on gathering information about family relationships, cultural background and values, the

psychological and physical home environment, and the family members' personal needs, including their own health care (Brady, 1978; Brantley, 1983; Mastrangelo, 1990; Power & Dell Orto, 1986; Power, 1985; Versluys, 1985). It is important to observe those situations in which family dysfunction tends to exacerbate or maintain an illness in the patient, the patient is at risk for abuse, or the family is noncompliant with health care rules related to the patient's well-being.

Family-centered treatment goals include (1) providing the family with knowledge about the physical dysfunction or illness and the effect on the patient's work, family, and social roles (Rohrer et al., 1980); (2) encouraging the family to value the patient's achievement of short-term goals (Versluys, 1980a); (3) assisting the family with understanding the purpose of the treatment procedures; (4) helping the family to increase positive communication with staff and the patient; (5) helping the family consider alternatives for family role taking and sharing of tasks; (6) encouraging the family to find interests, hobbies, or activities that they can do together and adapting hobby or recreational equipment; (7) encouraging the family to use appropriate community resources and support systems (Brady, 1978; Gallagher, Beckman, & Cross, 1983; Gardner & Stewart, 1978; Hasselkus, 1991; Wepman, 1973; Versluys, 1980a; Versluys, 1980b)

When the patient is a child or adolescent, family-centered treatment goals should involve helping the parents to: (1) facilitate social and cognitive development and independent behaviors (Rohrer et al., 1980); (2) use appropriate methods of discipline and set limits without feeling guilty (Buchanan et al., 1985; Gross, 1988; Mastrangelo, 1990; Murphy, 1982; Poznanski, 1984); (3) use intrafamily and community resources so that time will be available for other children and for personal needs; and (4) find enjoyment in the child's endearing and positive qualities (Kogan, Tyler, & Turner, 1974).

Discharge planning

Patients and family members are not usually psychologically or functionally prepared for discharge. During the transition from medical facility to home, families frequently have difficulty incorporating new information gleaned from the therapists into the home setting.

The delivery of quality rehabilitation must incorporate support and consultation for family members and provide educational and counseling programs to meet their needs. Family-focused hospital-based programs provide the family and the patient with education, counseling, and coaching and can reduce community emergencies and future admissions by increasing *patient motivation* and by involving family members in treatment decisions and discharge planning (Brady, 1978; Cella et al., 1988; Evenson, Evenson, & Fish, 1986; Power & Dell Orto, 1986).

The occupational therapist should evaluate and understand the family situation well in advance of discharge so that planning will be based on reality (Gans, 1983). The family needs information about the following topic areas: (1) the activities of daily living that the patient can carry out independently; (2) the activities of daily living that the patient needs to develop; (3) how to solve accessibility problems related to the home or business; (4) information on interior home design and how to purchase and care for adaptive equipment; (5) awareness of the availability of community resources, such as self-help groups, respite care, and independent living centers (Power & Dell Orto, 1986, Versluys, 1980a; Versluys, 1980b; Versluys, 1984; Versluys, 1985).

Group treatment has proved to be successful when used by occupational therapists for the treatment and education of physically disabled people and their families. A successful approach provides educational and experiential components, offers practical guidance and support in making changes, affords an opportunity to ask questions and to express feelings and concerns, and furnishes active assistance with the adaptation of household, hobby equipment, clothing, and toys and games for children (Democker & Aimpfer, 1981; Rohrer et al., 1980; Spitz, 1984; Versluys, 1980b; Versluys, 1984). Versluys (1980b) describes a series of task and experiential groups for hospitalized patients and their families, including a focus on maintenance of occupational and family roles, which fosters reintegration into the family and community. Group educational methods combine the use of readings and videotapes for problem solving and discussion, homework assignments at the hospital and in the community, and role playing about transitional experiences. These methods allow the patient and family to practice skills, solve problems, and experiment with role changes (Brady, 1978; Power, 1985; Versluys, 1980b; Versluys, 1984).

Summary

The family can be a major force in the adjustment and rehabilitation of a family member. Studies show, however, that family members often do not receive sufficient information about the physical, emotional, and social effects of the patient's functional impairments and do not understand the adaptive tasks facing the patient or how to provide meaningful support (Gardner & Stewart, 1978; Rohrer et al., 1980). Occupational therapists tend to be preoccupied with treatment of the patient. This may limit opportunities for communication, support, and teaching of family members. The family may not understand how the therapist can contribute to discharge planning or how they can use the therapist as a resource for improving the quality of patient and family life in the community. It is important that the occupational therapist understand *family dynamics* and system theory to develop a sensitivity for identifying and responding to each family's unique needs for services and thus to enhance the quality of family life.

References

Brady, G. P. (1978). Rehabilitation of spinal cord injured: A family approach. *Journal of Applied Rehabilitation Counseling, 9,* 70–76.

Brantley, T. (1983). Racism and its impact on psychotherapy. *American Journal of Psychiatry, 140,* 1605–1608.

Buchanan, D. C., LaBarbera, C. J., Roelofs, R., & Olson, W. (1985). In Moos, R. H. (Ed.). *Coping with physical illness: Vol. 2. New perspective* (pp. 145–158). New York: Plenum.

Cella, D. F., Perry, S. W., Kulchycky, S., & Goodwin, C. (1988). Stress and coping in relatives of burn patients: A longitudinal study. *Hospital and Community Psychiatry, 39,* 159–166.

D'Afflitti, J. R., & Weitz, G. W. (1977). Rehabilitating the stroke patient through patient-family groups. In R. H. Moos (Ed.). *Coping with physical illness* (pp. 323–332). New York: Plenum.

Dell Orto, A. E. (1984). Coping with the enormity of illness and disability. *Rehabilitation Literature, 45,* 22.

Democker, J. E., & Aimpfer, D. G. (1981). Group approaches to psychosocial intervention in medical care: A synthesis. *International Journal of Group Psychotherapy, 31,* 247–259.

Evenson, R. L., Evenson, M. L., & Fish, D. E. (1986). Family enrichment: A rehabilitation opportunity. *Rehabilitation Literature, 47,* 274–280.

Frey, J. (1984). A family systems approach to illness-maintaining behaviors in chronically ill adolescents. *The Family Process, 23,* 251–260.

Gallagher, J. H. J., Beckman, P., & Cross, A. H. (1983). Families of handicapped children: Sources of stress and its amelioration. *Exceptional Child, 50,* 10–19.

Gans, J. S. (1983). Hate in the rehabilitation setting. *Archives of Physical Medicine and Rehabilitation, 64,* 1775–1779.

Gardner, D., & Stewart, N. (1978). Staff involvement with families of patients in critical-care units. *Heart and Lung, 7,* 105–110.

Gross, A. L. (1988). The psychosocial impact of a handicapped child on the family. *Physical and Occupational Therapy, 8,* 97–110.

Hasselkus, B. R. (1991). Ethical dilemmas in family caregiving for the elderly: Implications for occupational therapy. *American Journal of Occupational Therapy, 45,* 206–212.

Jaffee, D. T. (1978). The role of family therapy in treating physical illness. *Hospital and Community Psychiatry, 29,* 169–174.

Kaplan, D. M., Smith, A., Grobstein, R., & Fischman, S. E. (1977). Family mediation of stress. In R. H. Moos (Ed.). *Coping with physical illness* (pp. 81–95). New York: Plenum.

Kogan, K. L., Tyler, N., & Turner P. (1974). The process of interpersonal adaptation between mothers and their cerebral palsied children. *Developmental Medical Child Neurology, 16,* 518–527.

Mastrangelo, R. (1990). It's all in the family. *Advance, 6,* 2-2, 15.

Moos, R. H., & Schaefer, J. A. (1985). The crisis of physical illness: An overview and conceptual approach. In R. H. Moos (Ed.). *Coping with physical illness: Vol. 2. New perspective* (pp. 3–25). New York: Plenum.

Murphy, M. A. (1982). The family with a handicapped child: A review of the literature. *Journal of Development and Behavior in Pediatrics, 3,* 73–82.

Olsen, J. Z., & May, B. J. (1966). Family education: Necessary adjunct to total stroke rehabilitation. *American Journal of Occupational Therapy, 20,* 88–90.

Palmer, S. E., Canzona, L., & Wai, L. (1982). Helping families respond effectively to chronic illness: Home dialysis as a case example. *Social Work in Health Care, 8,* 1–14.

Power, P.W. (1985). Family coping behaviors in chronic illness: A rehabilitation perspective. *Rehabilitation Literature, 46,* 78–83.

Power, P. W., & Dell Orto, A. E. (1986). Families, illness and disability: The roles of the rehabilitation counselor. *Journal of Applied Rehabilitation Counseling, 17,* 41–44.

Poznanski, E. O. (1984). Emotional issues in raising handicapped children. *Rehabilitation Literature, 45,* 214–218.

Queralt, M. (1984, March–April). Understanding Cuban immigrants: A cultural perspective. *Social Work,* 115–121.

Rohrer, K., Adelman, B., Puckett, J., Toomey, B., Talbert, D., & Johnson, E. W. (1980). Rehabilitation in spinal cord injury: Use of a patient-family group. *Archives of Physical Medicine and Rehabilitation, 61,* 225–229.

Safilios-Rothschild, C. (1970). *The sociology and social psychology of disability and rehabilitation.* New York: Random House.

Spitz, H. I. (1984). Contemporary trends in group psychotherapy: A literature survey. *Hospital and Community Psychiatry, 35,* 132–142.

Versluys, H. P. (1980a). Physical rehabilitation and family dynamics. *Rehabilitation Literature, 41,* 58–65.

Versluys, H. P. (1980b). The remediation of role disorders through focused group work. *American Journal of Occupational Therapy, 34,* 609–614.

Versluys, H. P. (1984). Community reintegration: The value of educational-action-training models. *Rehabilitation Literature, 45,* 138–145.

Versluys, H. P. (1985). Psychosocial accommodation to physical disability. In C. A. Trombly (Ed.). *Occupational therapy for physical dysfunction* (3rd ed., pp. 13–37). Baltimore, MD: Williams & Wilkins.

Versluys, H. P. (1986). Thuishulpcentrale: A dutch model for practical family assistance. *Rehabilitation Literature, 47*, 50–59.

Wepman, J. M. (1973). Rehabilitation and language disorders. In J. F. Garrett & E. S. Levine (Eds.). *Rehabilitation practices with the physically disabled* (pp. 329–362). New York: Columbia University Press.

Zager, R. P., & Marquette, C. H. (1981). Developmental considerations in children and early adolescents with spinal cord injury. *Archives of Physical Medicine and Rehabilitation, 62*, 427–431.

Zisserman, L. (1981). The modern family and rehabilitation of the handicapped: A macrosociological view. *American Journal of Occupational Therapy, 35*, 13–20.

Bibliography

Anderson, J., & Hinojosa, J. (1984). Parents and therapists in a professional partnership. *American Journal of Occupational Therapy, 38*, 452–461.

Bolodeau, C. B. (1971). Issues raised in a group setting by patients recovering from myocardial infarction. *American Journal of Psychiatry, 128*, 73–77.

Brown, H. N., & Kelly M. J. (1989). Stages of bone marrow transplantation: A psychiatric perspective. In R. H. Moos (Ed.). *Coping with physical illness: Vol. 2. New perspective* (pp. 241–252). New York: Plenum.

Callahan, D. (1988). Families as caregivers: The limits of morality. *Archives of Physical Medicine and Rehabilitation, 69*, 323–328.

DeLoach, C., & Greer, B. (1981). *Adjustment to severe physical disability: A metamorphosis.* New York: McGraw-Hill.

Dhooper, S. S. (1983). Family coping with the crisis of heart attack. *Social Work in Health Care, 9*, 15–31.

Doherty, W., & Baird, M. (1983). *Family therapy and family medicine.* New York: The Gilford Press.

Eisenberg, M. G., Sutkin, L. C., & Jansen, M. A. (1984). *Chronic illness and disability through the life span: Effects on self and family.* New York: Springer.

Hinojosa, J., Anderson, J., & Strauch, C. (1988). Pediatric occupational therapy in the home. *American Journal of Occupational Therapy, 42*, 17–22.

Krant, M. J., & Johnston, L. (1977). Family members' perceptions of communications in late stage cancer. *International Journal of Psychiatry in Medicine, 8*, 203–216.

Power, P. W. (1982, September). Family intervention in rehabilitation of patients with Huntington disease. *Archives of Physical Medicine and Rehabilitation, 63*, 441–442.

Power, P. W., & Sax, D. S. (1978). The communication of information to the neurological patient: Some implications for family coping. *Journal of Chronic Disability, 31*, 57–65.

Redman-Bentley, D. (1982). Parent expectations for professionals providing services to their handicapped children. *Physical and occupational therapy in pediatrics, 2*, 13–26.

Romano, M. D. (1974). Family response to traumatic head injury. *Scandinavian Journal of Rehabilitation Medicine, 6*, 1–4.

Rosin, A. J. (1977). Reactions of families of brain injured patients who remain in a vegetative state. *Scandinavian Journal of Rehabilitation Medicine, 9*, 1–5.

Singer, B. A. (1983). Psychosocial trauma, defense strategies and treatment considerations in cancer patients and their families. *American Journal of Family Therapy, 11*, 15–21.

Tyler, N. B., & Kogan, K. L. (1977). Reduction of stress between mothers and their handicapped children. *American Journal of Occupational Therapy, 31*, 151–159.

Zucman, E. (1982). *Childhood disability in the family.* The World Rehabilitation Fund, 400 East 34th Street, New York, NY 10016.

UNIT II

*Occupational therapy
assessment and treatment*

CHAPTER 7

Assessment and evaluation: an overview

HELEN D. SMITH

KEY TERMS

Assessment	Object History
Evaluation	Projective Tests
Nonstandardized Tests	Standardized Tests

LEARNING OBJECTIVES

Upon completion of this chapter the reader will be able to:

1. *Explain the difference between assessment and evaluation.*
2. *List and discuss four types of evaluations.*
3. *Describe the procedures for evaluating range of motion and muscle strength.*
4. *Discuss why it is important for the therapist to administer standardized tests according to the directions given in the test manual.*

The terms **evaluation** and **assessment** have been used with regard to procedures employed in fact-finding before and during treatment. In general, assessment refers to the sum of the results of the evaluation procedures used. Assessment yields a composite picture of the patient's functioning. Evaluation refers to the data gathered from specific procedures. Gillette (1971) referred to evaluation as a professional responsibility. She defined the functions of the evaluation process as (1) determining the baseline for objectives and providing the foundation for a treatment program, (2) identifying which problems can and cannot be remediated by occupational therapy, (3) giving some indication of the potential for change, (4) enlisting the cooperation of the patient in beginning to assess the patient's capabilities and dreams, and (5) helping the patient begin a course of action designed to master some of the difficulties the patient had previously tried to master alone.

> Evaluation also serves the purpose of keeping the therapist's work current, for it is a spiral, building process. Each treatment session should be assessed, and each target area should be reviewed in order to determine the effectiveness of the activity process and to revise the objectives as they are mastered or found to be unreachable. Treatment should not persist in a straight line. It is the system of evaluation that is built into the treatment process that ultimately determines the effectiveness of treatment. (Gillette, 1971, p. 79)

In occupational therapy, evaluation is a process of collecting and organizing the relevant information about a patient so that the therapist can plan and implement a meaningful, effective program of treatment. Several steps are involved:

Collection of data. This includes the selection and use of tools and methods by which information is obtained. The frame of reference for treatment determines the kinds of data sought. The participation of the patient in this process is critical to the success of the program.

Organization of data. Data are organized into a meaningful, dynamic description of the patient's strengths and limitations, with a focus on those areas in which occupational therapy can be of help. The patient, the therapist, and others should be able to understand this description readily.

Setting of treatment objectives. This involves the use of clinical judgment and predictive assumptions on the part of the therapist. Objectives must be based on the accumulated data, including the patient's goals, the therapist's knowledge about the clinical pathology, and the treatment frame of reference.

Commitment to continuing evaluation. As the occupational therapy plan is carried out, the original objectives and treatment plan need constant reassessment. Changes in the occupational therapy plan depend on the results of ongoing reevaluation.

The evaluation process thus represents an organized and systematic way of determining a patient's needs. It is essential for setting objectives, planning treatment, and assessing the effectiveness of the implementation of the treatment plan. Careful evaluation and reevaluation in occupational therapy also add significant information to the total treatment program of the team. This information then is used as an aid in setting overall goals and in monitoring the effectiveness of interventions such as medication or physical therapy.

Any fair and valid *assessment* of a patient must be based on several sources that yield a multidimensional picture of the patient's status. Assessment should focus on those data that are pertinent to the occupational therapy process. Any assessment procedure, moreover, should include a clear analysis of the context for treatment, the therapist's skills and resources, and the activities that can be used in treatment.

Types of evaluation

Evaluation procedures take many forms, ranging from tests for specific functions (eg, manual muscle testing) to more complex or comprehensive assessments that comprise data from several tests or procedures. Successful evaluation depends on the ability of the therapist to gain the trust of the patient so that a cooperative effort can be made. The therapist must observe and record data accurately and must make use of a wide range of appropriate information sources pertinent to the treatment process.

Medical records

The medical record provides valuable information about the patient and gives indications for precautions that must be considered when planning and carrying out treatment. Data gleaned from the medical record add to the baseline information necessary for effective treatment planning.

The past and present medical history, written by the physician, gives the therapist information on the patient's health status, former medical problems, present medical or physical findings, diagnoses, precautions, and prognosis. Daily notes by physicians and nurses list medications and treatments being given as well as the patient's responses. Reports and evaluations from other specialties (radiographic, dietary, social service, psychiatric, psychological, physical or speech therapy, vocational or rehabilitation counseling) are also included. With information from medical records as background, the therapist is ready to take the next step in the evaluation process.

Observation

A key to successful evaluation lies in the therapist's skills in observation. The abilities to see and to listen well must be accompanied by the abilities to sort through the mass of perceptual and conceptual data that may be presented and to focus on what is relevant to the process.

Humans communicate information about themselves in a great many ways. Verbal communication involves not only the choice of words and sentences but also their meanings and the quality of tone and inflection with which the words are said. Paralinguistic and nonverbal behaviors that accompany oral communication also reveal information through facial expressions, gestures, posture, and body movements. Attention to nonverbal communication is especially important for the occupational therapist because a large part of the occupational therapy process involves doing, not talking. Nonverbal expressions in humans are established earlier in life than verbal expressions and rely on older neurophysiologic structures (Freedman, Kaplan, & Saddock, 1976). A third mode of communication is the written form. It may be assumed that the written work has been more carefully considered and censored and thus is less spontaneous than verbal communication, although this is not necessarily true. What a patient writes may be useful as a representation of a desired or ideal self. The organization and form of the handwriting and its placement on the page have been considered to be clues to personality, feelings, and cognitive functioning at the time of the writing. Closely related to writing are other forms of psychomotor projection through which communication takes place, such as the behaviors connected with the use of media and the choice of clothing, colors, and objects. Over a longer period of time, a person communicates much information by the total effect of behaviors in a variety of circumstances, especially small, unconscious, and automatic behaviors.

The communication process that occurs between patient and therapist lays a foundation for rapport and trust. Patients need to believe that they have been heard and understood by someone who not only has some empathy but also has some knowledge and skill. Therapists' confidence in their abilities and in the profession may be crucial in setting the tone for all future transactions with their patients. Four filters affect interactions between people, and they are significant in their potential for distorting the observation process (Fidler 1976):

Perceptual—how sensory stimuli (color of clothing, perfume) affect the way the other person is perceived
Conceptual—the knowledge base brought to the interaction
Role—the way each person perceives the role he or she is to play in the interaction
Self-esteem—the way each person feels about himself or herself

It is useful for the therapist to consider these filters and the ways in which they might affect objectivity in observation.

The occupational therapist is in a position to observe the patient in a variety of structured and unstructured situations. The interview, formal testing procedures, and planned activities represent structured opportunities for observation. These usually involve some elements of prediction or expectation on the part of the therapist, and they are discussed in other chapters.

The therapist's opportunities to see and interact with patients in situations that are less planned vary with the setting. If it is possible for the therapist to interact informally and spontaneously with patients in situations in which role differentiation may be less clear, information may be available that otherwise might be difficult to obtain. For example, different perspectives on values, interests, and functional levels may be gained by seeing the patient in the snack shop, in the elevator, at recreational activities, or interacting with family or friends. It is desirable to build some opportunities for informal contact into the evaluation process whenever possible.

Interview

Occasionally, a health professional may wish to interview a patient formally or informally. Perhaps the most important occasion is the initial interview, undertaken as part of the process of evaluation. The initial interview serves several vital purposes. It provides for: (1) collection of information about the patient to help develop objectives and a plan for treatment, (2) establishment of understanding on the part of the patient about the role of the therapist and purposes of the occupational therapy process, and (3) an opportunity for the patient to discuss the particular situation and to think about plans for change.

Benjamin (1974) refers to important external and internal factors that require careful consideration when preparing for an interview. External factors include the room in which the interview is to take place and the extent to which the place is private and free of interruptions and other distractions. Internal factors are the attitudes, knowledge, and feelings that the therapist brings to the interview. It is important for the therapist to be clear about the purpose of the interview, to know the kinds of information specifically desired, to trust himself or herself, and to be honest.

Allen (1976) pointed out two requirements of the therapist for a successful patient interview: a solid knowledge base and skills in active listening. These requirements are not simple. They necessitate study, preparation, and practice. The solid knowledge base must underlie the therapist's selection of questions and areas to be covered in the interview. It is important that the interview reflect what the therapist knows as well as cover areas relevant to occupational therapy. Active listening means that the interviewer plays a deeply involved role that demonstrates genuine respect for the patient.

Benjamin (1974) delineated three parts to an interview: initiation, development, and closing. In the initiation phase, the therapist explains the purpose of the interview and the role of the therapist in relation to the patient. At this time, the therapist begins to establish mutual trust and understanding. During the initiation phase, the interviewer should define the parameters of the interview: the amount of time it should take, the kind of material to be discussed, and the uses to be made of the information.

During the development phase, the interviewer seeks information and explores issues with the person. If the initial interview is to encompass the evaluation procedure, the occupational therapist should bring an outline or list of planned questions to the interview to ensure that information vital to objective setting and treatment planning is covered. The kinds of questions the occupational therapist asks should allow the patient to respond with more than simply yes or no. The occupational therapist needs to be skilled in asking one question at a time, tolerating silence, listening carefully, observing both verbal and nonverbal responses, restating or clarifying questions when needed, and encouraging the patient to continue or to stay on track.

Clues marking the end of the interview are either the end of the time defined or the end of the list of questions or issues to be explored. It is important that both the therapist and the patient know that the interview is coming to a close. No new material should be brought up at this point. It is best to plan another time and place to discuss new material. Summarizing the material that has been discussed may be a useful way to terminate the interview as well as to double check the accuracy of the information gained.

The therapist should audiotape the initial interview or take notes during the interview so that it is unnecessary to relie on memory or on having time to record the interview later. The purpose of writing notes or using a tape recorder should be explained to the patient at the beginning of the interview. The patient should be allowed to read the notes or listen to the tape and should be informed that their sole purpose is to provide valid guidelines for the occupational therapy process.

Sometimes it is useful to have patients complete a simple questionnaire before coming to the interview. The use of a questionnaire has some advantages: it may save time in situations in which setting aside 30 to 45 minutes for an initial personal interview is not feasible; it can provide information about the patient's ability to read and to respond in an organized fashion in writing; and it may be used by the therapist as a discussion tool. The disadvantage is that some of the richness of detail and interaction may be lost. A written questionnaire can never completely replace a face-to-face interview.

The kinds of information that are best gained through an interview may vary somewhat according to the patient population and the general context for treatment. In general, the occupational therapist may learn about the patient's education; work experience; leisure interests and pursuits; the ways in which patients balance their work, sleep, and play and manage time; the quality and extent of their caring for their own personal needs (grooming, nutrition, laundry, housekeeping, hygiene); their families or significant people in households; friends or other family members who are supportive; the communities in which they live; their values and familiar objects; their own assessment of their current situations and problems; their personal goals; and their housing situations, including potential architectural barriers.

Knowledge about whether the patient's level of skill has been high enough to accomplish tasks and to fulfill expected social roles provides important clues to the kinds of experiences that should be provided in occupational therapy. The importance of collecting information about this history was outlined by Moorehead (1969):

> In gathering the occupational history, the investigator is concerned with discovering how and under what conditions the individual patient has learned to approach tasks and role expectations as he does; and whether he was ever more competent than he now appears. Can the therapist expect that the patient will be able to improve his role skills, and if so, how much? In other words, the investigator asks what a patient's particular life style is in terms of occupational function, so that therapy can be structured for him to build upon his experiences for improved function. (p. 331)

A terminal interview, undertaken just before the patient leaves treatment, serves other important functions. It gives the patient and therapist an opportunity to look together at what has taken place and to identify some of the things that have been learned in the process. Often the occupational therapy experience may be significant in helping the patient plan how to balance activities at home. A final interview helps to reinforce what the patient has learned—for example, which activities provide exercise or energy conservation and which are integrative and provide energy release.

Inventories and checklists

An adjunct to the interview is the checklist. The patient is asked to respond on paper to questions regarding interests, hobbies, and desires. Matsutsuyu (1969) developed the Interest Checklist, which has served as a prototype for many others. Another example is the Role Checklist developed by Oakley, Kielhofner, Barris, and Reichler (1986). Another useful inventory is the Activities Configuration developed by Watanabe (1968), which is used to identify the qualitative aspects of how a person uses time to meet particular needs.

Object history

One useful way to learn about a patient's values and cultural system is through the **object history**. The object history is a flexible evaluation tool that may be incorporated into the formal interview or used in informal conversation. Written object histories may also be solicited, either individually or in a group. The object history often helps to establish rapport among the people participating by permitting them to explore their respective backgrounds and experiences. It may also provide some important clues about the beginnings of the patient's pathology.

The object history simply asks the patient to try to remember something that was important or valued in an earlier period of life and to explain why it was important or valued. For example, a young man recalled a bush in front of his house where he went to hide as a child whenever he was scolded. From this statement, the therapist learned that the world of nature represented refuge to this person. Another person recalled an erector set with which he felt he could build anything mechanical. Thus, the therapist learned that mechanical things represented pleasure in accomplishment for this person. A young woman recalled a stereo set to which she used to dance. From this, the therapist learned that social dancing once was important to her. Through the exploration of important nonhuman objects, the therapist may learn about the kinds of things that may be integrative to the patient and about the patient's past ability to use the nonhuman world to meet emotional needs.

Over the years, occupational therapists have tended to develop tests, batteries of tests, checklists, and rating scales as the need arose. These tests helped to evaluate the requirements of their patients within their own contexts. In recent years, a need for reliable, standardized tools has become evident. Occupational therapists have found that they must identify and employ those tools that are in general use as part of the arduous process of establishing their legitimacy. At the same time, when occupational therapists use tools for which there are standard protocols and which require additional training or certification (eg, the Sensory Integration and Praxis Tests), it is essential that they be fully qualified to use them.

Evaluation of the patient's psychological or physical condition is indicated when a suspected or obvious problem exists. The therapeutic procedures chosen depend on the patient's diagnosis, medical reports, lifestyle, interests, and needs. Observations made by the therapist, checklists previously prepared by the patient, and information gained in interviews also suggest the best directions for treatment planning. Evaluation of special areas, such as cognition, perceptual motor function, activities of daily living (ADL), instrumental activities of daily living (IADL), and prevocational evaluation, may also be indicated. The remainder of this chapter deals with specific evaluation procedures used by occupational therapists in problem identification.

Psychological, psychiatric, and cognitive evaluations

Procedures have been developed in occupational therapy to assess psychological, psychiatric, and cognitive functioning. They supplement and specify, in occupational therapy terms, the data gathered by other members of the treatment team. The primary use of these procedures has been in the context of psychiatric treatment, but there are indications for their use in the wider range of primary disabilities because occupational therapy seeks to assess patients in terms of their total functioning. In choosing an assessment procedure, the occupational therapist must be clear about the nature of the data to be collected in terms of the frame of reference for treatment and the ways in which the specific data will relate to the subsequent therapeutic management of the patient.

Specific occupational therapy assessment procedures are listed in Table 7-1. General categories include **projective tests**, such as the Azima Battery (Azima, 1961 and 1982), the Comprehensive Assessment Process (Ehrenberg, 1982), the Goodman Battery (Evaskus, 1982), and the Shoemyen Battery (Shoemyen, 1970); *cognitive assessment*, such as the Allen Cognitive Level Test (Allen, 1985); and *batteries of tests*, which combine performance tasks, interviews, and checklists, such as the Bay Area Functional Performance Evaluation (1980), the Kohlman Evaluation of Living Skills (Ehrenberg, 1982), and the Comprehensive Occupational Therapy Evaluation (Brayman, 1982).

Projective tests used in occupational therapy exploit the rich potential of tapping into unconscious processes through the use of materials, supplies, and structures that permit free expression. These procedures have proved extremely useful in treatment settings that function on a psychoanalytic basis. Their use outside a psychoanalytically oriented treatment setting should be carefully and deliberately understood or avoided. The potential for free association and symbolic expression is high, but in short-term treatment contexts, the possibility of working productively with the material elicited is limited, and results may be counterproductive for the patient.

Tests geared to assessing specific functional areas may be valuable if the material elicited can be considered pivotal to the development of a treatment plan. This is the case in the Allen Cognitive Level Test (Allen, 1985), an assessment procedure developed to provide data to underlie the development of a therapeutic program based on clear knowledge of the patient's cognitive functioning.

Comprehensive batteries have been developed to assess a patient's total functional level. Because the data yielded in such batteries are extensive and frequently encompass a range of areas, their usefulness may be optimum in those situations in which the treatment program is extensive and in which occupational therapy is in a position to provide data that will support a number of different services. (See Chapters 14 and 17.)

(*Text continues on page 181*)

TABLE 7-1. *Sampling of Tests Used in Evaluation*

Name	Type	Description	Features	Source
Manual Dexterity and Motor Function Tests				
Jebsen–Taylor Hand Function Test	Individual test to evaluate functional capabilities	Seven subtests measure major aspects of hand function often used in ADL Equipment needed: stopwatch	Standardized tasks, objective measurements taken with stopwatch. Norms (360 normal subjects) included. Easy to administer. Test equipment and material are either made or easily available. Subtests are writing; card turning; picking up small objects; simulated feeding; stacking checkers; picking up large, light objects; picking up large, heavy objects Time: 12–15 min Age: child–adult	Jebsen et al., 1969 Sand P et al., 1974
Purdue Pegboard	Individual test to aid selection of employees for industrial jobs requiring manipulative dexterity	Measures gross movements of arms, hands, and fingers and fingertip dexterity Equipment: stopwatch	Two operations: rapid placing of pins in pegboard and assembly of pins, washers, and collars. Norms for male industrial applicants, veterans, college students, female college students, and industrial applicants Time: 12–15 min. Has face validity, low acceptable reliability	Science Research Associates, 259 East Erie St, Chicago, IL 60611
Minnesota Rate of Manipulation Test	Individual test of manual dexterity	Designed to measure dexterity	Five operations resulting in five scores: placing, turning, displacing, one-hand turning and placing, and two-hand turning and placing. Form board used—wells and round disks Time: 30–50 min Age: 7th grader–adult	American Guidance Service, Publishers Bldg, Circle Pines, MN 55014
The Lincoln–Oseretsky Motor Development Scale (Revised Oseretsky Tests of Motor Proficiency)	Scale of motor development. Individual test for hand and arm movements measuring speed, dexterity, coordination, and rhythm	First published in Russian, 1923; Portuguese adaptation, 1943; English translation, 1946; Sloan adaptation, 1948 Items sample variety of motor performances	Items arranged in order of difficulty. Instructions are concise, scoring is specific. Correlations of each item score with age and tentative percentile norms. Separate and combined scores given for sexes. Validated in relation to changes with age	CH Stoelting Co, 424 N Hohman Ave, Chicago, IL 60624
Pennsylvania Bi-Manual Work Sample	Individual test of bimanual dexterity: finger dexterity of both hands, gross movements of both arms, eye–hand coordination, and indication of use of both hands	Selection of a bolt with one hand and a nut with the other, assembling the two objects and placing in a receiving hole. Norms given for age, sex, blind, and partially blind	First part—assembly of 100 nuts and bolts. Second part—disassembly of nuts and bolts. Two scores, one for each operation Time: 10-min assembly and 5-min disassembly. Reliable. Validity not indicated	Educational Test Bureau, American Guidance Service, Publishers Bldg, Circle Pines, MN 55014
Crawford Small Parts Dexterity Test	Individual measure of fine eye–hand coordination and manipulation of small hand tools	10-inch-square board. Round wells for parts to be manipulated (ie, pins, collars, and screws); a metal plate containing 42 unthreaded and 42 threaded holes; two metal trays beneath the plate to receive the pins and screws	*Part I*—Examinee picks up pin with tweezers, inserts in small hole in metal plate, and places collar over it using preferred hand	Psychological Corporation, 304 East 45th St, New York, NY 10017

(continued)

TABLE 7-1. *Sampling of Tests Used in Evaluation (continued)*

Name	Type	Description	Features	Source
Manual Dexterity and Motor Function Tests				
		Tools: Tweezers and small screwdriver	*Part II*—Examinee picks up screw, starts it in threaded hole with fingers, then screws through metal plate with screwdriver, using both hands in operation. Six practice trials. Scored by time required	
			Time: *Part I*—5 min; *part II*—10 min	
			High reliability	
			Face validity	
Box and Block Test	Individual test of manual dexterity	Test has been used to measure gross manual dexterity and as a prevocational test for handicapped people. Test is timed. Subjects pick up one block at a time and place in second compartment	Normative data for adults, adults with neuromuscular involvement, and normal children 7–9 years old	Mathiowetz et al., 1985
		Equipment: Stopwatch; boxes; 150 colored 1-inch wooden cubes	Standardized instructions; reliability and validity data included	
Developmental Tests				
Bayley Scales of Infant Development	Individual scales of infant development	A three-part evaluation of a child's development in relation to other children of the same age. Scales include mental, motor, and behavior ratings	Well standardized. No data on validity of motor scale or predictive validity of mental scale. Reliability is satisfactory	Psychological Corporation, 304 East 45th St, New York, NY 10017
			Time: 45–90 min	
			Age: 2–30 months	
Brazelton Behavioral Assessment Scale	Individual score of infant interactive behavior	Evaluates the neonate's reaction to stimuli and responses to the environment	Best performance is scored. Photographs of testing procedures are included.	JB Lippincott, East Washington Square, Philadelphia, PA 19105
			Time: 20–30 min. Research in progress on test reliability and validity	Four training films available from Educational Development Corp, 8 Mifflin Place, Cambridge, MA 02138
Brigance Screen	Individual and group screening test for kindergarten and first grade	Adapted from and cross-referenced to readiness section of the Brigance Inventory of Basic Skills and Inventory of Early Development	Small group screening, individual screening added 2 or 3 min to the time	Curriculum Associates, 5 Esquire Rd, N, Billerica, MA 01862
			Cost for manual $19.95; pads of 30 forms, 25 cents per child	
		Identifies children needing referrals to special services and those needing further assessment; for program planning	Scoring—one scale, 100 points. Rank words to score	
			Time: 10–12 min	
Callier–Azusa Scale (1975)	Individual developmental scale for assessment of deaf, blind, and multihandicapped children	Designed to be used in a classroom, this scale is divided into five subscales: motor development, perceptual development, daily living skills, language development, and socialization. Subscales are made up of sequential steps describing developmental milestones	Examples of behavior are provided for many items (Behaviors were observed on deaf–blind children)	Robert Stillman, PhD, Callier Center for Communication Disorders, University of Texas/Dallas, 1966 Inwood Rd, Dallas, TX 75235
			Lists criteria	
			Observation to extend over a 2-week period	
			Reliability information available from author	

(continued)

TABLE 7-1.   *Sampling of Tests Used in Evaluation (continued)*

Name	Type	Description	Features	Source
Developmental Tests				
Denver Developmental Screening Test	Individual formalized observations of normal developmental behavior of infants and children	A screening tool for detecting infants and children with developmental delays. Areas evaluated: gross motor, fine motor, language, and personal–social development	Standardized on children aged 2 weeks–6.4 years in Denver. High percentage came from professional families. Inexpensive, quick, easy to use. Uses common items. Manual and scoring guide are clear Reliability and validity vary with age groups	Ladoca Project and Publishing Foundation, E 51st Av & Lincoln St, Denver, CO 80216
Developmental Screening 0–5 Years	Individual screening inventory of abnormal development	History and observation ratings in five areas: adaptive, gross motor, fine motor, language, and personal–social (selected items used from the Gesell Developmental Schedules)	Age: 1 year–18 months. No reliability data available Testing time: 5–30 min	Knobloch et al., 1966
The Gesell Developmental Tests	Individual scale of developmental levels	Scale of behavioral observations by age level (5–10 years) of the mental growth of the child to aid in determining school readiness	Qualitative measure of motor development, adaptive behavior, and personal–social behavior. Present functional level evaluated Time: 20–30 min	Programs for Education, Box 85, Lumberville, PA 18933
Sensory Integration Tests				
Developmental Test of Visual–Motor Integration (Berry K)	Used to detect problems in visual–motor integration in children	Subject is presented with 24 geometric forms arranged in order of increasing difficulty, which are copied into a test booklet	Standardized test that can be group administered. Emphasis is on preschool group. Directions are clear. Separate age norms for each sex. Two forms: ages 2–15 years (long form), ages 2–8 years (short form). Reliability and validity information appears to be incomplete Time: 10 min	Follett Educational Corporation, 1010 W Washington Blvd, Chicago, IL 60607
Marianne Frostig Developmental Test of Visual Perception	Individual and group test measuring visual perception	Five subtests of visual perception: eye-motor coordination, figure-ground, constancy of shape, position in space, and spatial relations	Five areas relate to preschool and early elementary academic performance. Group administration possible. Norms for ages 3–8 years. Reliability appears adequate. Validity information appears to be incomplete Time: Individual, 30–45 min; group, 40–60 min	Consulting Psychologists Press, 577 College Ave, Palo Alto, CA 94306
The Imitation of Gestures: A Technique for Studying the Body Schema and Praxis of Children 3 to 6 Years of Age	Individual test of perceptual–motor function			Berges & Lezine, 1965 Medical Market Research, 227 South 6th St, Philadelphia, PA 19105
Perceptual Forms Test	Individual and group testing for perceptual and readiness evaluation and training	Two parts: perceptual forms test and incomplete forms in which subject is required to complete partial drawings. Visual–motor coordination is required. Used to identify children who might have problems in school achievement	Geometric forms are copied. Templates are used. Formal scoring on the perceptual form test but not on the incomplete forms Age: 5–8 years. Reliability and validity information incomplete	Winter Haven Lions Research Foundation, PO Box 111, Winter Haven, FL 33880

(continued)

TABLE 7-1.   *Sampling of Tests Used in Evaluation (continued)*

Name	Type	Description	Features	Source
Sensory Integration Tests				
The Purdue Preceptual Motor Survey	Individual test of perceptual motor abilities	Identifies children with perceptual–motor problems that could interfere with learning of academic skills. Eleven subtests: rhythmic writing, walking board, jumping, identification of body parts, imitation of movements, obstacle course, chalkboard, Kraus–Weber, angels-in-the-snow, ocular pursuits, developmental drawing	Test based on theory. Easy to administer, and instructions and scoring keys adequate. Reliability and validity information are said to be good Time: 20 min Age: 6–10 years	Charles E Merrill Publishing, 1300 Alum Creek Dr, Columbus, OH 43216
Sensory Integration and Praxis Tests				
Tests for visualization; figure-ground perception; manual form perception; kinesthesia; finger identification; graphesthesia; localization of tactile stimuli; praxis on verbal command; design copy; constructional praxis; postural praxis; oral praxis; bilateral motor coordination; standing and walking balance; motor accuracy; and postrotary nystagmus	Battery of tests, given as a whole to identify sensory integrative dysfunction	Tests domains of sensory integration functioning: form and space perception, somatic and vestibular processing, praxis, and bilateral integration and sequencing	Administration requires training and certification through Sensory Integration International. Test results are computer scored by Western Psychological Services Time: 2.5 h Age: 4.6–10 years	Western Psychological Services, 12031 Wilshire Blvd, Los Angeles, CA 90025
Illinois Test of Psycholinguistic Abilities (ITPA)	Individual test of cognitive functioning	A test of language perception and short-term memory abilities to assist in diagnosing learning problems	Visual and auditory channels are used for input. Vocal and motor channels are used for output. Norms on children from slightly above average homes, aged 2–10 years. Reliability said to be moderate Time: 45–50 min	University of Illinois Press, Urbana, IL 61801
Intelligence Tests				
Goodenough–Harris Drawing Test	Individual or group test of conceptual and intellectual maturity	Tests accuracy of observation and development of conceptual thinking. The subject draws a man, a woman, and a self-portrait	A simple, nonverbal test. Norms were established on children aged 5–15 years from four major geographical areas and representative of various occupations. Reliability and validity information are said to be adequate Time: 10–15 min Age: 3–15 years	Harcourt Brace Jovanovich, 757 3rd Ave, New York, NY 10017
Peabody Picture Vocabulary	Individual test of verbal intelligence	Untimed test that estimates verbal intelligence by measuring hearing vocabulary. Subject chooses one of four pictures after hearing a word	No reading required. Standardized age range, 2.5–18 years. Content and item validity are good, and reliability is said to be adequate	American Guidance Service, Publishers Bldg, Circle Pines, MN 55014
Psychological Tests				
Adaptive Behavior Scales	Individual scale assessing adaptive behavior of the mentally retarded and emotionally maladjusted	Evaluation of subject's effectiveness to cope with environmental demands. Twenty-four areas of social and personal behavior are covered	Easy to administer, but hand scoring is complex. Norms based on institutionalized retardates beginning at age 3 years. Has face validity but no data on reliability Time: children, 20–25 min; adults, 25–30 min	American Association on Mental Deficiency, 5201 Connecticut Ave, NW, Washington, DC 20015

(continued)

TABLE 7-1.   *Sampling of Tests Used in Evaluation (continued)*

Name	Type	Description	Features	Source
Psychological Tests				
Vineland Social Maturity Scale	Individual performance scale of social maturity	Behavioral observations of self-help, self-direction, locomotion, occupation, communication, and social relations. Provides an evaluation of subject's social competency	Useful tool for evaluating mentally retarded individual. Includes 117 items Age: birth to maturity Time: 20–30 min	Educational Test Bureau, American Guidance Service, Publishers Bldg, Circle Pines, MN 55014
Bender–Gestalt Test	Individual or group projective evaluation of personality dynamics	Measures nonverbal gestalt functioning in perceptual–motor area. The subject copies designs	Evaluates perceptual–motor functioning, neurologic impairment, and maladjustment. Scoring system quantified and objective. Most validity research done on scoring system. No data on reliability Time: 10 min Age: 4 years and older	American Orthopsychiatric Association, 1790 Broadway, New York, NY 10019
Minnesota Multiphasic Personality Inventory (MMPI)	Individual and group nonprojective test measuring psychopathology	Assess the type and degree of emotional dysfunction in adults	Spanish edition is available. Normative and reliability data have not been changed since 1951 Time: Individual, 30–90 min; group, 40–90 min for complete form and 40–75 min for short version	The Psychological Corporation, 304 East 45th St, New York, NY 10017
Nurses' Observation Scale for Inpatient Evaluation (NOSIE)	Nonprojective individual rating scale measuring behavioral status and change	Highly sensitive ward behavior scale that assess subject's status and change over time	Seven scores: competence, social interest, personal neatness, irritability, manifest psychosis, and retardation. Easy to use. Norms based on adult male schizophrenics aged 55–69 years. Validity and reliability appear to be adequate Time: 3–5 min	Behavioral Arts Center, 90 Calla Ave, Floral Park, New York, NY 11001
Activity configuration	Pencil-and-paper schedule with clear legend	Client lists hourly activities for a typical week, with personal assessments of the nature of the activity (recreation, social, work, etc.), autonomy, pleasure, and adequacy Especially useful with clients who are depressed	Administration should be accompanied by discussion Promotes consideration of personal priorities, time management	Watanabe, 1968
Adolescent Role Assessment	Interview—individual or group administration	Semistructured dialogue with specific rating criteria to assess quality of childhood play, family interactions, chores, school skills, work attitudes, and fantasy	Specific questions to be explored with specific rating criteria so that role expectations may be consistent with values and skills	Black, 1976
Allen Cognitive Level (ACL)	Individual cognitive performance	Measures cognitive level through performance of prescribed tasks	Clearly delineated administration. Provides baseline for establishment of task expectations and ongoing monitoring of treatment effectiveness	Allen, C. (1985) *Occupational therapy for psychiatric diseases:* Measurement and management of cognitive disabilities. Boston: Little, Brown & Co.

(continued)

TABLE 7-1.   *Sampling of Tests Used in Evaluation* (*continued*)

Name	Type	Description	Features	Source
Psychological Tests				
Azima Battery	Projective battery	Assesses mood organization, organization of drives, ego organization, and object relations through client's performance in drawing, finger painting, use of clay and plastic media	Classic psychoanalytically based assessment, first presented in 1961 Valuable in treatment planning, detecting change, prognosis, effects of drug administration Heuristic considerations with regard to research, use in family therapy (comparative batteries)	Azima, 1982
Bay Area Functional Performance Evaluation (BAFPE)	Evaluation battery	Assesses functional performance in ADL with psychiatric clients Two subtests—Task Oriented Assessment (TOA) and Social Interaction Scale (SIS) Use of interview, structured and projective tasks, observation	Clear directions for assessment of ADL, motor skills, sensory motor function, sensation, endurance, cognition, appearance Rating scale and directions, research implications, and videotape available	Consulting Psychologists Press, 577 College Ave, Palo Alto, CA 94306
Comprehensive Assessment Process	Projective assessment process; includes structured interviews and group activities	Administration of initial interview and follow-up interviews, ADL questionnaire, and group activity sessions to yield observations of grooming, levels of awareness, orientation, affect, motor level, self-esteem, attendance, self-direction, task investment, independence, concentration, following instructions, problem solving, decision making, frustration tolerance, work tolerance, planning, workmanship, leadership, and more	Designed to evaluate overall client behaviors as basis for individualized plans in short-term, acute care psychiatric treatment facilities Indications for further research	Ehrenberg, 1982
Comprehensive Occupational Therapy Evaluation (COTE)	Evaluation scale	Assesses 25 identified behaviors in three areas: general, interpersonal, and task Provides guide to observation, interview, tasks, and recording methods	For use in adult acute care psychiatric setting to enhance observation, reduce subjectivity in reporting, and facilitate team communication; enables therapist to report a large volume of comprehensive and pertinent information quickly, in consistent format, and with defined terminology Grid with space for daily recording for 16 days	Brayman & Kirby, 1982
Goodman Battery	Projective battery	Evaluates cognitive and affective ego assets and deficits affecting function. Tasks presented represent decreasing structure—copying to freehand drawing to clay task	Very specific instructions retest environment, timing, and so forth Rating scales Further research implications	Evaskus, 1982
Interest Checklist	Interview with pencil and paper; checklist	Eighty activities listed with space for client to check interest level (casual, strong, no)	Administration should be accompanied by discussion Classic checklist, much adapted and widely used	Matsutsuyu, 1969

(continued)

TABLE 7-1.   *Sampling of Tests Used in Evaluation (continued)*

Name	Type	Description	Features	Source
Psychological Tests				
Kohlman Evaluation of Living Skills (KELS)	Structured interview with tasks	Gives indications of client's experience and interests Assesses psychiatric clients' skills in self-care, safety and health, money management, transportation and telephone, work, and leisure	Clear directions for observation, recording, and implications for community living or further treatment Protocol Videotape available	Health Sciences Learning Resources Center T 281 SB-56, Univ of Washington, Seattle, WA 98195
Lifestyle Performance Profile	Individual interview	Assesses performance skills and skill levels as determined by age, culture, and biology in the areas of self-care and maintenance; self-needs–extrinsic gratification; service to others	Data gathered yields information to aid description of skill deficits and strengths; sociocultural expectations for performance; lifestyle performance balance; nature of family; sociocultural, economic, and environmental resources or barriers; sensorimotor, cognitive, psychological and social skill deficits or strengths; individual characteristics; and interests that shape responses	Fidler, 1982
Schroeder Block S-I Evaluation	Comprehensive assessment tools	Assesses S-I in adult psychiatric clients using specific testing procedures and observation	Definite procedures, observations, scoring, work sheets, and summary sheets required Research implications	Schroeder et al., 1979
Shoemyen Battery	Projective battery (one to four clients)	Uses four activities: mosaic tile, clay figure, fingerpainting, sculpture media, and interview–discussion to gain information about attitudes, mood, cognitive and social skills, dexterity, attention, suggestibility, independence, and creativity	Information gained to aid in team treatment planning—to promote relatively natural therapist–patient relationship and collaborative planning and implementation of treatment	Shoemyen, 1982 Shands Teaching Hospital, U of Florida, Gainesville, FL
Stress Tools				
Holmes–Rahe Life Change Index	Individual evaluation of number of major life changes in past year	Self-assessment of stress level produced by major life changes	Age: adult	Holmes & Rahe, 1967
Type A Behavior Scale	Individual evaluation of number of Type A behavior traits in personality	Self-assessment of stress level produced by Type A behavior traits	Age: adult	AIM for Health, PO Box 182, Hanover St Sta, Boston, MA 02113, in study guide for slide–tape program, "Stress"
Stress Audit Questionnaire	Individual evaluation of patterns of stressors	Self-assessment of stress level produced by social and environmental stressors	Age: adult	Miller et al., 1982
Tests for Young Children and Their Families				
Miller Assessment for Preschoolers (MAP)	Level B developmental assessment for 3- to 6-year-olds, measuring cognitive, communication, motor, visual–perceptual, and social–emotional domains	35- to 40-min developmental assessment that is accurate in measuring ability in performance components of preschoolers. Includes numerous qualitative rating scales to enhance clinical observations. Can also be used as a comprehensive screening tool	Six scores: Total score and five index scores: foundations coordination, verbal, nonverbal, and complex tasks Based on neurodevelopmental and sensory integrative frame of reference but also includes cognitive items Standardized nationwide ($n = 1204$)	The Psychological Corporation, 555 Academic Court, San Antonio, TX 78204-2498

(continued)

TABLE 7-1. *Sampling of Tests Used in Evaluation* (*continued*)

Name	Type	Description	Features	Source
Tests for Young Children and Their Families				
Japanese MAP	Level B developmental assessment for 3- to 6-year-olds, measuring cognitive, communication, motor, visual–perceptual, and social–emotional domains	35- to 40-min developmental assessment that is accurate in measuring ability in performance components in preschoolers. Includes numerous qualitative rating scales to enhance clinical observations. Can also be used as a comprehensive screening tool	Excellent reliability, good construct, content, and predictive validity. Attractive materials, fun for children Translation, blind back–translation, and cultural review in Japan Numerous pilot studies completed including nationwide Try Out Edition Standardized nationwide in Japan with random, stratified sample All items are culturally and linguistically appropriate for Japanese-speaking children	Harcourt, Brace, Jovanovich, Ichibancho Central Bldg 22-1, Ichibancho, Chiyoda-ku, Tokyo 102 Japan
The First STEP (Screening Test for Evaluating Preschoolers)	Level A developmental screening for children ages 3 to 6 years, for five domains mandated by PL 99-457: cognition, communication, motor, social–emotional, and self-help	15-min screening tool that accurately identifies those children in need of follow-up diagnostic evaluations in five domains mandated by PL 99-457. Identifies children who are experiencing developmental delays or who are at risk for delay	Standardized nationwide ($n = 1433$) with extensive test–retest and interrater reliability studies. Concurred validity with five scales (WPPSI-R, TOLD-2, Bruininks, Walker, and Vineland) Short, fun for children, and inexpensive Easy to administer and score Designed for paraprofessionals as well as professionals	The Psychological Corporation, 555 Academic Court, San Antonio, TX 78204-2498
Primer Paso (translated version of The First STEP)	Spanish language Level A developmental screening test for children ages 3 to 6 years; for five domains mandated by PL 99-457: cognitive, communication, motor, social–emotional, and self-help	15-min screening tool that accurately identifies those children in need of follow-up diagnostic evaluations in five domains mandated by PL99-457. Identifies children who are experiencing developmental delays or who are at risk for delay	Intensive development of culturally and linguistically sensitive scale for Spanish–speaking preschoolers Translation and blind back–translation Review by experts in Cuban, Mexican-American, Puerto Rican, and Central and South American cultures Field tested on bilingual and monolingual Spanish children Funding pending for nationwide standardization	Research Edition available from The KID Foundation, 8101 E. Prentice Ave, Suite #518, Englewood, CO 80111
Miller Toddler and Infants Motor Evaluation (Miller TIME)	Comprehensive, diagnostic assessment of motor performance by children from birth to 42 months of age	Measures quality of movement in children demonstrating delays, or at risk of motoric dysfunction. Includes evaluation of variations within a position, transitions between positions, stability, motor organization, and dysfunctional positions	Extremely comprehensive, with small increments of change measureable Not based on motor milestones model Quantifiable scores in mobility, stability, organization, and dysfunctional positions Based on sensory integration and neurodevelopmental therapy constructs	Research Edition available from The KID Foundation, 8101 E. Prentice Ave, Suite #518, Englewood, CO 80111 Final Edition will be published in 1993 by Therapy Skill Builders, P.O. Box 42050, Tucson, AZ 85733

(*continued*)

TABLE 7-1. *Sampling of Tests Used in Evaluation (continued)*

Name	Type	Description	Features	Source
Tests for Young Children and Their Families				
Infant/Toddler Scale for Everybaby (ITSE, pronounced "itsy")	Developmental assessment (Level B) and screening (Level A) for children ages 3 months to 42 months. Evaluates five domains mandated by PL 99-457	This scale is administered by a partnership of parent and professional. Parent elicits play as examiner observes and scores child	Play-based, using naturalistic observations of children interacting with parents Parent-initiated play Based on mandate of PL 99-457 Play-based, using naturalistic observation Uses play house and other fun toys to elicit behaviors	Research Edition available from The KID Foundation, 8101 E. Prentice Ave, Suite #518, Englewood, CO 80111
The Family-Centered Interview	Individual family focused, open-ended narrative interview for gathering information about family resilience in families of children from birth to 42 months of age. Assesses both protective factors and risk factors in family	This nonintrusive methodology includes 40 questions plus a genogram and ecomap. It provides a linking process between the family and practitioner and is scored twice, once by the family to identify their resources, concerns, and priorities, and once by the examiner who uses the Family Assessment Interviewer's Rating (FAIR)	Focuses on families' resources, concerns, and priorities Oriented toward family resilience using a competency-based model Provides method for linking with family in a supportive manner Useful for developing Individualized Family Service Plan (IFSP)	Research Edition available from The KID Foundation, 8101 E. Prentice Ave, Suite #518, Englewood, CO 80111
Self-Help Assessment: Parent Evaluation (SHAPE)	Individual assessment of adaptive behavior for children from birth to 6 years of age	Uses a pictorial format to assess ADL, self-control, relationships and interactions, and functioning within the community	Oriented toward functional abilities Based on parents' perceptions of competencies Gathers information on parent satisfaction in each domain area Uses attractive illustrations of children accomplishing each task; parent indicates if child easily passes, is just learning, or is not yet able to complete each item	Research Edition available from The KID Foundation, 8101 E. Prentice Ave, Suite #518, Englewood, CO 80111
Test for Geriatric Patients				
Parachek Geriatric Rating Scale	Geriatric rating scale	Designed to help in planning treatment programs for the geriatric patient. Areas rated: physical capabilities, self-care skills, social interaction skills	Items arranged and rated in developmental sequence. Treatment manual attached Time: 3–5 min, once a month	Greenroom Publishing, 8512 East Virginia, Scottsdale, AZ 85257

From Buros, O.K. (Ed.). (1949–1978). The third-eighth mental measurement yearbooks. Highland Park, NJ: Gryphon Press.

Physical dysfunction evaluations

Numerous evaluation procedures are used to evaluate patients with physical dysfunction. These include but are not limited to evaluation of joint range of motion (ROM), muscle strength, muscle tone, reflexes, sensation, cognition, perception, coordination, and performance tasks such as ADL, IADL, play and leisure activities, and work (Trombly, 1989; Pedretti & Zoltan, 1990). These evaluations are performed to determine the patient's assets and limitations. The results are used to establish patient goals, to develop an effective treatment program, and to determine the functional capabilities of the patient in self-care,

leisure, and work skills. The initial test results become the baseline with which subsequent test results (during treatment and at discharge) will be compared to ascertain the patient's progress or lack of progress.

Therapists use both ***nonstandardized*** and ***standardized tests*** to evaluate patient performance. When using either type of test, the therapist should be competent in the test's administration. By developing a standard method for administering nonstandardized tests, reliability of the test results can be increased. It is important to follow the instructions in the test administration manual of standardized tests to ensure that the results are valid. Using these tests in a manner other than described in the test administration manual could result in an invalid assessment. (See Appendix I.) It is the responsibility of the therapist to develop skill in the administration of these tests. This takes time and practice. Some standardized tests require specialized training in their administration and interpretation (eg, the Sensory Integration and Praxis Tests).

Joint range of motion: goniometry

Joint ROM is measured in both upper and lower extremities to determine the existing freedom of motion at a joint. This is done either passively (part moved by an outside force, ie, the therapist) or actively (part moved by muscle contraction, ie, muscle power.) The causes of decreased ROM can be spasticity, joint disease, injury, muscle weakness, pain, edema, or bone block. A difference between active and passive ROM in the same joint usually indicates muscle weakness.

Measurement tools

The goniometer (Figure 7-1) is the tool most frequently used to measure joint ROM. Other tools used either alone or in conjunction with the goniometer include: a ruler to measure distance (used especially in hand evaluation); photographs of the patient performing the motion; outline drawings (eg, tracing the fingers while in abduction).

Procedure: 180-degree scale

1. Explain the procedure to the patient.
2. Check the noninvolved extremity for active and passive ROM. If no decreased motion is observed, it is permissible to record ROM as being within normal limits.
3. When measuring the involved extremity, use the anatomic position as the starting position when possible. The starting position is recorded as 0 degrees. Some exceptions to starting in the anatomic position are shoulder internal and external rotation and forearm supination and pronation.
4. Demonstrate the desired motion to the patient.
5. Prevent substitution by positioning and stabilizing the joint proximal to the joint being measured.

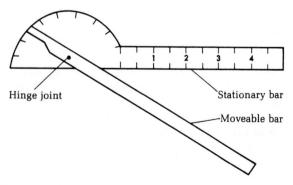

Hinge joint
Stationary bar
Moveable bar

FIGURE 7-1. *Goniometer.*

6. Apply the goniometer to the lateral side of the joint. Some exceptions are forearm supination and hip rotation.
7. Align the axis of the goniometer with the joint axis.
8. Align the stationary bar parallel to the long axis of the stationary bone.
9. Align the movable bar parallel to the long axis of the movable bone.
10. Have the patient perform the desired motion. Measure both the starting position and the maximal end range; this indicates the arc through which the part moves, thus measuring the freedom of motion at the joint. To determine passive ROM, carefully move the joint through its maximal passive range.
11. Record both the active and the passive degrees of motion on an ROM form (Figures 7-2 and 7-3). For example, 0 to 95 degrees indicates a limitation in flexion; 35 to 95 degrees indicates a limitation in both flexion and extension.
12. Indicate if any pain, swelling, or spasticity is present.
13. Sign and date ROM form.
14. To maintain reliability and accuracy, the same therapist should remeasure the patient at the same time of day, when possible.

Manual muscle testing

Manual muscle testing determines the strength of a muscle through manual evaluation. See the display for an example of a manual muscle evaluation form. Rating is done by having the patient move the involved part through its full ROM against gravity and then against gravity plus resistance. When the patient cannot perform the motion against gravity, the part is repositioned to eliminate gravity and the muscle power is reevaluated. Manual muscle testing should not be used when spasticity is present because the increased tone invalidates the results.

Grading Scale for MMT

0	0	*Zero:* No evidence of contractility
1	T	*Trace:* Evidence of contractility on palpation; no joint motion
	P−	*Poor minus:* Less than complete ROM with gravity eliminated
2	P	*Poor:* Complete ROM with gravity eliminated
	P+	*Poor plus:* Complete ROM with gravity eliminated, takes minimal resistance
	F−	*Fair minus:* Less than full ROM against gravity
3	F	*Fair:* Complete ROM against gravity
	F+	*Fair plus:* Complete ROM against gravity with minimal resistance
	G−	*Good minus:* Complete ROM against gravity with less than moderate resistance
4	G	*Good:* Complete ROM against gravity with moderate resistance
5	N	*Normal:* Complete ROM against gravity with full resistance

(*Text continues on page 189*)

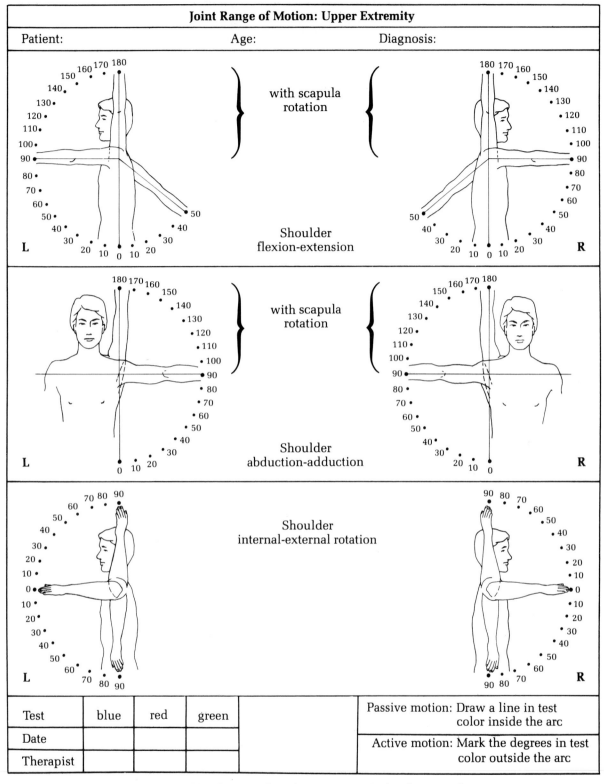

FIGURE 7-2. *Form for measurement of joint range of motion, upper extremity. Courtesy of Moss Rehabilitation Hospital, Department of Physical Therapy, Philadelphia, PA.*

(*Figure continues on next page*)

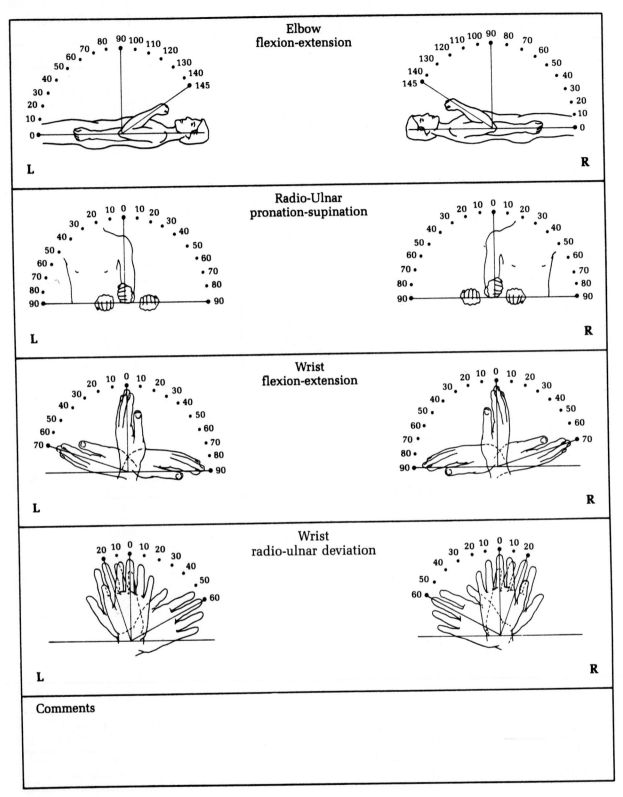

FIGURE 7-2. (*Continued*)

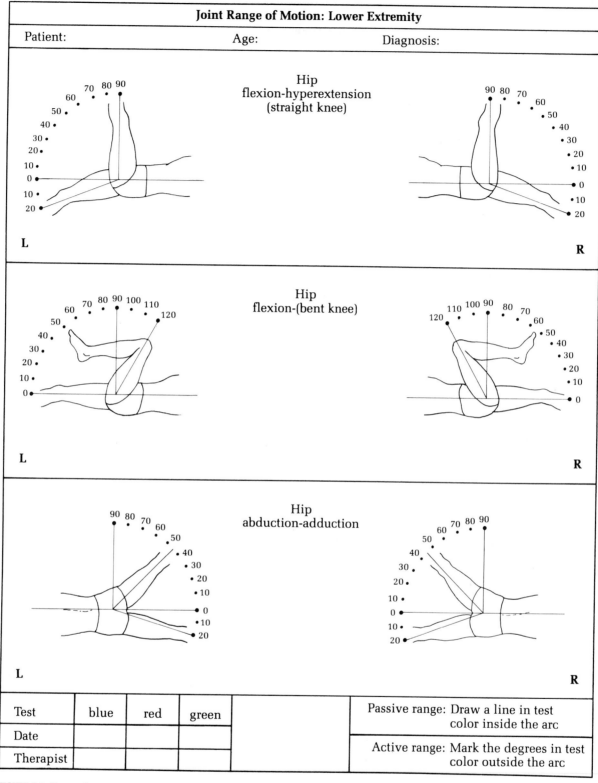

FIGURE 7-3. *Form for measurement of joint range of motion, lower extremity. Courtesy of Moss Rehabilitation Hospital, Department of Physical Therapy, Philadelphia, PA.*

(Figure continues on next page)

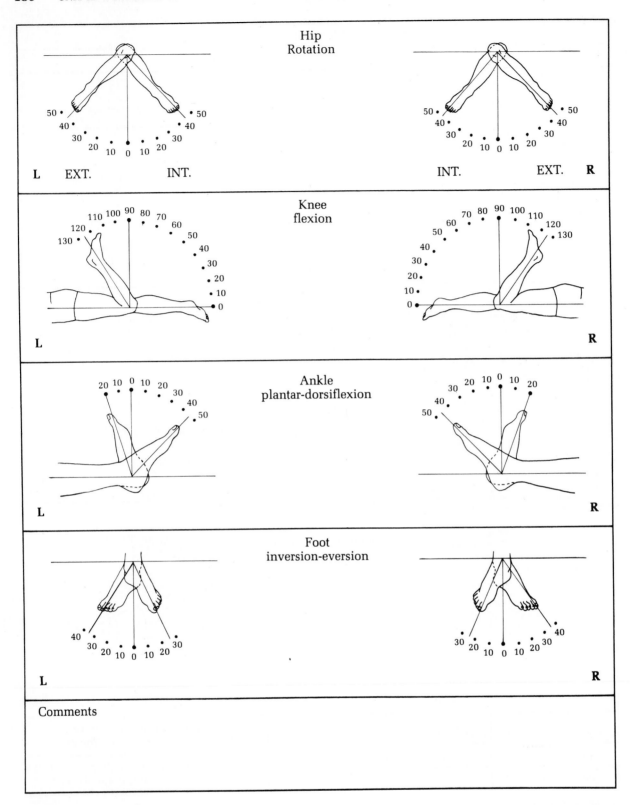

FIGURE 7-3. (*Continued*)

MANUAL MUSCLE EVALUATION FORM

CLINICAL RECORD—MANUAL MUSCLE EVALUATION

Name _____

Age _____

Diagnosis_____

LEFT   RIGHT

				ACTION	PRIME MOVERS	INNERVATION	SP. C. LEVEL				
					Examiner's Initials						
					Date						
		N E C K		Flexion	STERNOCLEIDOMASTOID	Spinal Accessory,	C 2-3	N E C K			
				Extension	EXTENSOR GROUP	Spinal Accessory,	C 1-8				
		T R U N K		Flexion	RECTUS ABDOMINUS		T 5-12	T R U N K			
				Rotation	EXTERNAL OBLIQUE		T 5-12				
					INTERNAL OBLIQUE		T 5-12				
				Extension	Thoracic	Post. Rami Spinal Nerves					
					Lumbar						
				Pelvic Elevation	QUADRATUS LUMBORUM		T 12 L 1-3				
		H I P		Flexion	ILIOPSOAS	Femoral	L 2-4	H I P			
					SARTORIUS	Femoral	L 2-4				
				Extension	GLUTEUS MAXIMUS	Inf. Gluteal	L 5 S 1-2				
				Abduction	GLUTEUS MEDIUS	Superior Gluteal	L 4-5 S 1				
					TENSOR FASCIA LATAE	Superior Gluteal	L 4-5 S 1				
				Adduction		Obturator	L 2-4				
				External Rotation			L 3 S 3				
				Internal Rotation			L 4 S 1				
		K N E E		Flexion	BICEPS FEMORIS	Sciatic	L 5 S 1-2	K N E E			
					SEMITENDINOSUS SEMIMEMBRANOSUS	Tibial	L 5 S 1-3				
				Extension	QUADRICEPS	Femoral	L 2-4				
		A N K L E		Inversion	ANTERIOR TIBIALIS	Deep Peroneal	L 5 S 1-2	A N K L E			
					POSTERIOR TIBIALIS	Tibial	L 4-5 S 1-2				
				Eversion	PERONEUS LONGUS	Sup. Peroneal	L 4-5 S 1				
					PERONEUS BREVIS	Sup. Peroneal	L 4-5 S 1				
				Plantar Flexion	GASTROCNEMIUS	Tibial	S 1-2				
					SOLEUS	Tibial	S 1-2				
		T O E S		Flexion	DIGITORUM LONGUS	Tibial	L 5 S 1-2	T O E S			
					DIGITORUM BREVIS	Tibial	L S 1-2				
				Extension	DIGITORUM LONGUS & BREVIS	Deep Peroneal	L 4-5 S 1				
		H A L L U X		Flexion	HALLUCIS LONGUS	Tibial	L 5 S 1-2	H A L L U X			
					HALLUCIS BREVIS	Tibial	L 5 S 1-2				
				Extension	HALLUCIS LONGUS	Deep Peroneal	L 4-5 S 1-2				

KEY: 5 N NORMAL   Complete range of motion against gravity with full resistance
         4 G GOOD   Complete range of motion against gravity with some resistance
         3 F FAIR   Complete range of motion against gravity
         2 P POOR   Complete range of motion with gravity eliminated
         1 T TRACE   Evidence of slight contractility. No joint motion
         0 0 ZERO   No evidence of contractility

(continued)

MANUAL MUSCLE EVALUATION FORM (continued)

Name _____ Age _____ Diagnosis _____

LEFT										RIGHT			
				Examiner's Initials									
				Date									
				ACTION	PRIME MOVERS	INNERVATION	SP. C. LEVEL						
			S C A P U L A	Elevation	UPPER TRAPEZIUS	Spinal Accessory	C 3-4	S C A P U L A					
				Adduction	MID TRAPEZIUS	Spinal Accessory	C 3-4						
					RHOMBOIDS	Dorsal Scapular	C 4-5						
				Abduction	SERRATUS ANTERIOR	Long Thoracic	C 5-7						
				Depression	LOWER TRAPEZIUS	Spinal Accessory	C 3-4						
			S H O U L D E R	Flexion	ANTERIOR DELTOID	Axillary	C 5-6	S H O U L D E R					
				Abduction	MIDDLE DELTOID	Axillary	C 5-6						
				Horizontal Adduction	PECTORALIS MAJOR Clavicular	Ant. Thoracic	C 5-8						
					Sternal		C 5 T 1						
				Extension	LATISSIMUS DORSI	Thoracodorsal	C 5-8						
				Horizontal Abduction	POST. DELTOID	Axillary	C 5-6						
				External Rotation			C 5-6						
				Internal Rotation			C 5-8						
			E L B O W	Flexion	BICEPS	Musculocutaneous	C 5-6	E L B O W					
					BRACHIALIS	Musculocutaneous	C 5-6						
					BRACHIORADIALIS	Radial	C 6						
				Extension	TRICEPS	Radial	C 5-8						
			FORE ARM	Supination	SUPINATOR	Radial	C 6	FORE ARM					
				Pronation	PRONATOR TERES	Median	C 6						
			W R I S T	Flexion	CARPI RADIALIS	Median	C 6	W R I S T					
					CARPI ULNARIS	Ulnar	C 8						
				Extension	CARPI RADIALIS L. & BREV.	Radial	C 6-7						
					CARPI ULNARIS	Radial	C 7						
			F I N G E R S	Flexion MP joint	LUMBRICALES 1,2	Median	C 7-8	F I N G E R S					
					3,4	Ulnar	C 8						
				Prox. IP joint	DIG. SUBLIMUS	Median	C 7 T 1						
				Dist. IP joint	DIG. PROFUNDUS 1,2	Median	C 8 T 1						
					3,4	Ulnar	C 8 T 1						
				Extension	DIG. EXT. COMMUNIS	Radial	C 6						
				Adduction	INTEROSSEI	Ulnar	C 8 T 1						
				Abduction	INTEROSSEI	Ulnar	C 8 T 1						
				Abduction, digit 4	DIGITI QUINTI	Ulnar	C 8						
				Opposition, digit 4	OPPONENS DIGITI QUINTI	Ulnar	C 8						
			T H U M B	Flexion MP joint	POLL. BREV.	Median	C 6-8	T H U M B					
				IP joint	POLL. L.	Median	C 8 T 1						
				Extension MP joint	POLL. BREV.	Radial	C 7						
				IP joint	POLL. L.	Radial	C 7						
				Adduction	ADDUCTOR POLLICIS	Ulnar	C 8						
				Abduction	POLL. L.	Radial	C 7						
					POLL. BREV.	Median	C 6-7						
				Opposition	OPPONENS POLLICIS	Median	C 6-8 T 1						

Courtesy of Moss Rehabilitation Hospital, Department of Physical Therapy, Philadelphia, PA.

Procedure

1. Explain the procedure to the patient.
2. Check the noninvolved extremity for muscle strength and use as a norm.
3. Check the patient's active and passive ROM before beginning manual muscle testing of the involved extremity.
4. Position patient so that the muscle will be tested against gravity (start in fair position).
5. Stabilize the joint above the one being tested to prevent substitution of incorrect muscles.
6. Have the patient perform the motion and observe the performance. If the patient cannot move the part against gravity, reposition to eliminate gravity.
7. Palpate the muscle performing the motion to be sure it is contracting.
8. Apply resistance into the opposite motion of the one being performed. (Resistance should be applied in the middle of the ROM.)
9. Grade the muscle strength.
10. Enter the results of each test, and sign and date the form.
11. To maintain reliability and accuracy, the same therapist should repeat this test on the patient at the same time of day, when possible.

Sensory testing

Sensory testing is frequently performed when evaluating patients with physical dysfunctions. Patients with burns, fractures, spinal cord injuries, or neurologic disease or damage often experience decreased ability to function in their environments due to impaired sensation. For example, decreased sensation in the hand impairs a patient's ability to manipulate objects successfully and is a safety factor. The hand could be injured while performing daily activities, for example, when cooking or using hot water.

Areas tested include but are not limited to light touch, pain, temperature, vibratory sense, moving touch, moving and stationary two-point discrimination, stereognosis, proprioception (position sense), and kinesthesia (movement sense).

General procedure

1. Sit opposite the patient.
2. Explain the procedure to the patient. Ask for feedback to be sure instructions are understood. Give instructions when the patient's eyes are not occluded and demonstrate on noninvolved extremity.
3. Occlude the patient's vision with a shield such as a file folder, screen, or cut-out box.
4. Test the nonaffected area first to be sure the patient understands your instructions.
5. Apply stimuli on both dorsal and ventral surfaces in an unpredictable pattern.
6. Ask if patient was touched. (If aphasic, the patient can nod head.)
7. Enter test results on specified form, date, and sign.

Sample rating scale

Intact—a quick, correct response
Impaired—an incorrect or delayed response
Absent—no response

Trombly (1989) suggests reporting the results by noting, for example, that "the patient was able to identify 9/10 common objects" during stereognosis testing; she believes this is a more useful method of communicating test results (p. 48). See Pedretti and Zoltan (1990) and Trombly (1989) for detailed information on sensory testing.

Coordination

Coordination is the working together of muscles or groups of muscles to perform a task. Both gross and fine coordination should be evaluated by the therapist. The tests listed in Table 7-1 under the heading Manual Dexterity and Motor Function Tests are recommended. All are standardized, and most have reliability and validity information. When these tests are not available, a task such as tossing and catching a bean bag or ball, playing a board game, or performing an ADL or IADL can assist the therapist in judging the patient's coordination.

Hand and pinch strength testing

Hand strength is measured with the patient gripping a dynamometer. The dial is calibrated in either pounds or kilograms, and the indicator stays at the highest reading until reset manually. An added feature in some dynamometers is an adjustable hand grip.

Pinch strength is measured on a pinch gauge. The dial is calibrated in pounds and measures finger prehension force. A quick reading of the dial must be made if the indicator does not stay at the highest reading point. Both the dynamometer and the pinch gauge can be purchased through suppliers of rehabilitation equipment.

Standardized positioning and instructions should be used for testing, as recommended by Mathiowetz, Weber, Volland, and Kashman (1984) in their study of grip and pinch strength reliability and validity. This study used a pinch gauge and a Jamar dynamometer and followed the American Society of Hand Therapists' recommendations for standardized positioning as well as established procedures and instructions for each test of strength (grip strength, palmar pinch, lateral pinch, and two-point and tip pinch). The authors found that higher interrater and test—retest reliability was achieved when standardized instructions and positioning were used. (See Appendix I.)

Endurance testing

Often, the patient is tested for the ability to reach or maintain the energy output necessary to perform an activity. This is especially important in ADL, homemaker retraining, and work-related activities. The amount of work and the time required to do the work are carefully noted, and work output and time are carefully increased according to the tolerance of the patient until either the desired or the maximal level is reached.

Functional assessment

Functional assessment is the evaluation of ordinary daily living demands and tasks. The patient's ability is observed during the performance of ADL and the more complicated IADL. ADL include bathing, toileting, dressing, eating, communication, transfers, and continence. IADL include taking medicine, shopping, preparing meals, doing housework, using the telephone, managing money, and traveling. Other performance areas that are assessed are play and leisure activities and work skills. (See Chapter 8.) These activities can be evaluated using standardized tests, such as the Katz Index of ADL and the Modified Barthel Index (Gallo, Reichel, & Anderson, 1988). Many nonstandardized tests for functional assessment are also available.

A computer-assisted functional assessment tool that integrates functional performance evaluations has been developed by the Trace Research and Development Center at the University of Wisconsin in Madison and is available from the American Occupational Therapy Association. This assessment tool, called the Occupational Therapy Functional Assessment Compilation Tool (OT FACT), takes evaluation data and creates an overall functional performance profile, which can be used to summarize patient performance, justify therapy plans, and document a patient's status over time (OT FACT workshop brochure, 1992).

Physical capacities evaluation

The physical capacities evaluation should summarize the patient's ability, endurance, speed, safety, and strength in all activities tested. The activities that the patient was unable to perform should be listed, along with why the patient was unable to perform each activity. The length of time the test took, the frequency of rest periods, the appliances used, the amount of pain or discomfort, and the patient's overall work endurance should also be included in the evaluation. The patient's emotional reactions, including emotional tolerance, ability to follow directions, appearance, and cooperativeness, are also important.

Standardized tests

Standardized tests of hand function, motor ability, intelligence, learning disability, development, sensorimotor ability, and personality have been incorporated into Table 7-1. Most of this information was obtained from Buros's *Mental Measurement Yearbooks* (Buros, 1978; 1972; 1965; 1959; 1953; 1949), with additional material from sources indicated in the table. The tests mentioned are referred to in various chapters of this book. This table is not intended to be a complete listing of all tests used by occupational therapists. See Appendix I for the Hierarchy of Competencies Relating to the Use of Standardized Instruments and Evaluation Techniques by Occupational Therapists.

The author thanks Elizabeth G. Tiffany for allowing use of portions of her material from the 7th edition of this book.

References

Allen, C. (1976, October). *The performance status examination*. Paper presented at the American Occupational Therapy Association Annual Conference, San Francisco.

Allen, C. (1985). *ACL*. In *Occupational therapy for psychiatric diseases: Measurement and management of cognitive disabilities*. Boston: Little, Brown.

Azima, F. J. (1961; 1982). Diseases of the nervous system (Monograph Suppl. 22) and in Hemphill, B. J. (Ed.). *The evaluative process in occupational therapy*. Thorofare, NJ: Slack.

Benjamin, A. (1974). *The helping interview*. Boston: Houghton Mifflin.

Berges, J., & Lezine, I. (1965). *Spastic Society medical education and information unit*. London: William Heinemann.

Black, M. (1976). Adolescent role assessment. *American Journal of Occupational Therapy, 30*, 73.

Bloomer, J., & Williams, S. (1982). *The Bay area functional performance evaluation*. In B. J. Hemphill (Ed.). *The evaluative process in occupational therapy*. Thorofare, NJ: Slack.

Brayman, S., & Kirby, T. (1982). The comprehensive occupational therapy evaluation. In B. J. Hemphill (Ed.). *The evaluative process in occupational therapy*. Thorofare, NJ: Slack.

Buros, O. K. (Ed.). (1978). *The eighth mental measurement yearbook*. Highland Park, NJ: Gryphon.

Buros, O. K. (Ed.). (1972). *The seventh mental measurement yearbook*. Highland Park, NJ: Gryphon.

Buros, O. K. (Ed.). (1965). *The sixth mental measurement yearbook*. Highland Park, NJ: Gryphon.

Buros, O. K. (Ed.). (1959). *The fifth mental measurement yearbook*. Highland Park, NJ: Gryphon.

Buros, O. K. (Ed.). (1953). *The fourth mental measurement yearbook*. Highland Park, NJ: Gryphon.

Buros, O. K. (Ed.). (1949). *The third mental measurement yearbook*. Highland Park, NJ: Gryphon.

Ehrenberg, F. (1982). Comprehensive assessment process. In B. J. Hemphill (Ed.). *The evaluative process in occupational therapy*. Thorofare, NJ: Slack.

Evaskus, M. G. (1982). Goodman battery. In B. J. Hemphill (Ed.). *The evaluative process in occupational therapy*. Thorofare, NJ: Slack.

Fidler, G. S. (1982). Lifestyle performance profile. In B. J. Hemphill (Ed.). *The evaluative process in occupational therapy*. Thorofare, NJ: Slack.

Fidler, G. S. (1976). Paper presented at Medical College of Georgia, Augusta.

Freedman, A., Kaplan, H., & Saddock, B. (1976). *Modern synopsis of comprehensive textbook of psychiatry* (2nd ed., p. 146). Baltimore: Williams & Wilkins.

Gallo, J. J., Reichel, W., & Anderson, L. (1988). *Handbook of geriatric assessment*. Gothersburg, MD: Aspen.

Gillette, N. (1971). *Occupational therapy and mental health*. In H. S. Willard, & C. S. Spackman (Eds.). *Occupational therapy* (4th ed., p. 79). Philadelphia: J. B. Lippincott.

Holmes, T. H., & Rahe, R. H. (1967). *Psychosomatic Research, 11*, 213.

Jebsen, R., Taylor, N., Trieschmann, R., Trotter, M., & Howard, L. (1969). An objective and standardized test of hand function. *Archives of Physical Medicine and Rehabilitation, 50*, 311.

Knobloch, H., et al. (1966). *Pediatrics, 38*, 1095.

Mathiowetz, V., Volland, G., Kashman, N., & Weber, K. (1985). Adult norms for the box and block test of manual dexterity. *American Journal of Occupational Therapy, 39*, 386.

Mathiowetz, V., Weber, K., Volland, G., & Kashman, N. (1984). Reliability and validity of grip and pinch strength evaluations. *Journal of Hand Surgery, 9A*, 222.

Matsutsuyu, J. (1969). The interest checklist. *American Journal of Occupational Therapy, 23*, 323.

Miller, L. H., Ross, R., & Cohen, S. I. (1982). *Bostonia Magazine, 56*(4), 5, 39–54.

Moorehead, L. (1969). The occupational history. *American Journal of Occupational Therapy, 23*, 331.

Oakley, F., Kielhofner, G. B., Barris, R., & Reichler, R. (1986). The role checklist: Development and empirical assessment of reliability. *Occupational Therapy Journal of Research, 6*(3), 157–170.

OT FACT workshop brochure. (1992). Madison: Trace Research and Development Center.

Pedretti, L. W., & Zoltan, B. (1990). *Occupational therapy practice skills for physical dysfunction*. Philadelphia: C. V. Mosby.

Schroeder, C. V., Block, M. P., Campbell, E. T., & Stowell, M. (1979). *Adult psychiatric S-I evaluation*. La Jolla, CA: San Diego VA SBC Research Association.

Shoemyen, C. (1982). The Shoemyen battery. In B. J. Hemphill (Ed.). *The evaluative process in occupational therapy*. Thorofare, NJ: Slack.

Shoemyen, C. (1970). Occupational therapy orientation and evaluation: A study of procedure and media. *American Journal of Occupational Therapy, 24*, 276.

Trombly, C. A. (Ed.). (1989). *Occupational therapy for physical dysfunction* (3rd ed.). Baltimore: Williams & Wilkins.

Watanabe, S. (1968). *Activities configuration* (1968 Regional Institute on the Evaluation Process, Final Report No. RSA-123-T-68). New York: American Occupational Therapy Association.

Bibliography

Christiansen, C., & Baum, C. (1991). *Occupational therapy: Overcoming human performance deficits*. Thorofare, NJ: Slack.

Hemphill, B. J. (Ed.). (1982). *The evaluative process in psychiatric occupational therapy*. Thorofare, NJ: Slack.

Hurff, J. (1974). A play skills inventory. In Reilly, M. (Ed.). *Play as exploratory learning*. Beverly Hills: Sage.

Knox, S. (1974). A play scale. In Reilly, M. (Ed.). *Play as exploratory learning*. Beverly Hills: Sage.

Llorens, L. (1967). Projective techniques in occupational therapy. *American Journal of Occupational Therapy, 21*, 266.

Oakley, F., Kielhofner, G. B., & Garris, R. (1988). The role checklist. In B. J. Hemphill (Ed.), (pp. 75–91, 250–253). *Mental health assessment in occupational therapy*. Thorofare, NJ: Slack.

Sand, P., Taylor, N., & Sakuma, K. (1973). Hand function measurement with educable mental retardates. *American Journal of Occupational Therapy, 27*, 138.

Sand, P., Taylor, N., Hill, M., Kosky, N., & Rawlings, M. (1974). Hand function in children with myelomeningocele. *American Journal of Occupational Therapy, 28*, 87.

Takata, N. (1969). The play history. *American Journal of occupational therapy, 23*, 314.

CHAPTER 8

Occupational therapy performance areas

SECTION 1

Activities of daily living

JUDY HILL

Role of the occupational therapist

The role of the occupational therapist in intervening in **activities of daily living** (ADL) is unique and specific (see the display). In different practice settings, including the patient's home, there may be many people who assist a patient with performing **self-care** tasks. These include nurses, nursing assistants, personal care attendants, home health aides, and family members. All these people have the potential to influence performance and to motivate or demotivate the patient. Among these interveners in self-care, however, only the occupational therapist is trained to assess and analyze the patient's performance to determine the degree and method of participation in self-care.

The occupational therapy assessment yields information about what factors are preventing performance, whether those impairments can be corrected, and whether the patient must learn to perform self-care tasks with adaptive equipment or techniques. The occupational therapist also identifies the importance to the patient of performing the activity independently, in light of the patient's home situation and occupational roles, and then bases intervention on this information. For example, a family member may be distraught to see the patient struggling with performing a self-care task and decide to assist more than is necessary. Or a family member may not understand why the patient is not performing a task and become frustrated and angry, blaming it on lack of motivation. Similar factors might influence how a home health aide assists, influenced by the aide's subjective judgment about the potential for independent performance.

The occupational therapist is trained to observe performance. In lower-extremity dressing, for example, the therapist may observe that the patient's hip range of motion is interfering with independent performance and plan a treatment program to improve hip range of motion. This treatment program would be based on knowledge about the patient's potential for improved range given the particular diagnosis. The occupational therapist also may observe that the patient is distressed by not being able to dress and would prefer to have no assistance in this task. The therapist then might determine that the patient is motivated to follow a treatment program to remediate the impairment in range. If, on the other hand, the condition was one in which

---

THE ROLE OF THE OCCUPATIONAL THERAPIST

- **Observe** performance
- **Situate** task performance within client's occupational roles and environment
- **Analyze** what is interfering with performance
- **Assess** level of impairment in component skills
- **Understand** medical and psychological conditions

---

improved range was possible but not ensured, and if the patient was motivated to return to the work role as quickly as possible, not wanting to concentrate on an exercise program for a number of weeks, the occupational therapist might determine that the treatment plan of choice would be to train the patient to use adaptive equipment.

Of those on the treatment team and in various practice settings, only the occupational therapist is trained to make these educated decisions and present them to the patient. The decisions are made based on assessment of psychosocial, sensorimotor, cognitive, perceptual, medical, environmental, and actual performance factors.

Relation between activities of daily living and role tasks

Activities of daily living include the self-care tasks of eating, grooming, dressing, bathing, and toileting. Mobility, communication, and home management frequently are included in this category (Hopkins & Smith, 1988; Pedretti, 1985; Trombly, 1987; Lawton & Brody, 1969; Chiou & Burnett, 1985; Halstead & Hartley, 1975). Chiou and Burnett (1985) extend the definition to include socializing, sexual activity, and exercise. There has been variation over the years in major occupational therapy texts, as well as articles referring to ADL, on exactly which tasks are to be included in the definition of ADL. New terms, such as *performance skills*, or tasks have been introduced to define the broad areas of function, self-maintenance, work, and play and leisure. In the context of performance tasks, the self-maintenance component plus mobility and communication are included in ADL (Trombly & Scott, 1987). Some centers have attempted to operationally define ADL as well. One such definition considers basic ADL as self-care and complex ADL or instrumental ADL (IADL) as homemaking, child or elder care, and community living skills (Rehabilitation Institute of Chicago, 1991). The most recent terminology situates ADL in the context of tasks that enable role performance (Christiansen, 1991). Role areas are defined along the lines of work, leisure, parenting, and volunteering.

Considering the relation of ADL to role tasks can be especially helpful in clarifying patient values (Chiou & Burnett, 1985). Once self-care competence is achieved, usually by 6 years of age, performance of these tasks is not a major motivating force in the day. The major rewards come more from role performance, that is, the challenges and successes of being a student, worker, partner, parent, sports participant, and so forth. When the ability

to perform basic self-care tasks is compromised by mental or physical illness, however, the resulting feelings of loss of competence can be devastating. A patient's display of a variety of reactions to loss of function in self-care indicates that the issues involved are complex and related to the value placed on their performance and their relation to other valued areas of performance, as the following case studies illustrate.

CASE STUDY

EV is a 36-year-old woman who sustained a spinal cord injury 1 year ago in a motor vehicle accident. She was not at fault in the accident and was wearing a seat belt and shoulder harness. At the time of her injury, EV was working full-time as a computer analyst, lived alone in an apartment, and enjoyed an active social life. Over the year since her accident, EV's incomplete injury has stabilized with C6 motor function on her dominant side and weak C8 function on her non-dominant side, including weak hand function. EV can feed herself, perform grooming and upper-body dressing, drain her leg bag, write, and use a phone and computer independently. She requires assistance with transferring to a bath bench for bathing and bowel and catheter management. EV can dress her lower body in 45 minutes but finds this tiring and impractical since it extends her total morning self-care time to 2.5 hours. EV has returned to her previous job, 6 hours a day, 3 days a week, and plans to gradually increase her work time. She tries to go out with friends at least once a week and would also like to increase gradually the amount of time she spends socializing. EV's occupational therapist feels that EV could achieve independence in dressing and bathing within 3 months if she would devote 2 to 3 hours per week to training and practice at these tasks. EV would like to be independent in these tasks but feels that her social and work roles are more important to her at this time. She has hired a trained personal care assistant to help her in the mornings and evenings and thinks she can afford to delay further self-care training for 6 months to a year, when she believes she will again be confident in her work and leisure roles.

CASE STUDY

LS is a 75-year-old woman who fell negotiating steep basement stairs while visiting her daughter 2 months ago and sustained a hip fracture. She has also suffered from chronic obstructive pulmonary disease for the past 10 years. She was living alone at the time, in an apartment in a senior living center. She enjoyed participating in some of the activities offered by the center, such as card games, community outings and crafts, 2 to 3 times per week. LS had been living in the center for 5 years and was feeling adjusted to the transition from her home of 30 years. After her injury, LS feared that she would not be able to care for herself well enough to stay in her current setting. She also was anxious about leaving her apartment because its closeness to her son's home allowed almost daily, brief visits from her grandchildren, which she enjoyed.

LS is able to feed herself, make a light meal, and perform grooming and upper-body dressing. She is independent in toileting but frequently needs to change clothes during the day because urinary urgency results in minor incontinence. She finds this, combined with her need for assistance in lower-body dressing, discouraging. LS requires only supervision to bathe, using a bath bench, hand-held shower, and long-handled sponge. Her occupational therapist feels that LS will be able to achieve independence in all self-care activities but that because of her weakness and chronic obstructive pulmonary disease, showering and dressing may take up to 1.5 hours and changing clothes 30 to 45 minutes if she is incontinent. Because LS has limited roles that require major time commitments, she feels she can spend a large part of her day in self-maintenance, especially if this will allow her to spend a small amount of time each day in her highly valued role of grandparent and some time each week in the card games and crafts that she enjoys. LS feels that she has lost some valued performance skills and roles already, and she has invested in maintaining those that remain as well as her ability to care for herself. The occupational therapist respects LS's values and establishes a treatment plan to achieve self-care independence. She is able to suggest the use of an incontinent pad during the day that easily can be changed to eliminate the need to change clothes.

These two examples illustrate the interaction between the performance of ADL and various roles and how individual patients may prioritize them differently. Similarly, a patient may prioritize tasks and roles differently at different times during the life cycle. Occupational therapists must be skilled in assisting patients to sort out these often emotionally difficult options, and therapists must remove their own values from this process. A discussion of values placed on roles and self-care tasks and assessment may be helpful.

This section addresses ADL treatments for the self-maintenance performance skills of eating, grooming, dressing, toileting, and bathing. When task accomplishment disability interferes with role performance, a handicap exists, and occupational therapy intervention can be used to remediate the impairment, enable task performance with adapted equipment and technology, or prevent handicap by delegation of the tasks to someone else. Christiansen (1991) refers to role performance taking place across the domains of self-maintenance, work, and leisure, with competent role performance often requiring accomplishment of tasks in all three domains. At times, for competent performance in the most highly valued domain, performance in other domains is delegated to others, such as paid assistants, family members, or friends. This does not occur only in cases of disability or handicap. For example, a patient may choose to have assistance with meal preparation to spend limited time and energy in the more valued leisure domain. Similarly, an able-bodied working parent may choose to have assistance with home maintenance to spend more time in the worker and parent roles. Thus, occupational therapy and the independent living movement intersect, with independence being equated with role performance, which can be accomplished by independent task performance or delegation. Role performance does not always require self-care independence.

Assessment of self-maintenance performance

Performance of self-care tasks can be evaluated through clinical observation of performance, patient interviews, and performance self-assessment by the patient. Clinical observation provides the most objective basis for assessing a patient's *ability* to perform tasks. Performance may be altered, however, as a result of having an observer present. For example, anxiety associated with modesty may result in less than optimal performance in bathing with a therapist observing. Conversely, an observing therapist may heighten patient motivation, resulting in improved performance. In the presence of an observer, patients often feel they should wait for instructions on how to do a task. In clinical observation, it is essential to make clear to the patient that the therapist wants the patient to do the task as well and as independently as possible without waiting for the therapist's instructions. Repeated observations to determine consistency of performance are also necessary. Patient interview and self-assessment can offer valuable information on the patient's *perception* of his or her ability to perform a task (Kielhofner & Henry, 1988). Some self-assessments also reveal patients' satisfaction with their performance of self-care tasks (Yerxa, Burnett-Bealieu, Stocking, & Azen, 1988).

Grading of self-care is done on a scale of dependent to independent function. The focus of grading scales is to reliably communicate the status of a patient to others involved in the care of that patient, including family members, other occupational therapists, other health care professionals, and reimbursers of health care services. Grading scales are used to justify further rehabilitation services by showing progress and estimated potential for further progress. They also are used to communicate to family members the amount of assistance the patient will need, to compare performance at different points in time and in different environments, and to estimate the amount of attendant care needed. Reliable, standardized self-care scales also are used for research. The grading must be *valid* for the performance skill it addresses and *sensitive* in detecting changes in performance.

The major, well-established scales of self-care performance include the Barthel Index (Mahoney & Barthel, 1965), the Klein-Bell ADL Scale (Klein & Bell, 1982), the Sister Kenny Self-Care Evaluation (Schoening et al., 1965; Iverson, 1983), and the Index of ADL, (Katz, Downs, Cash, & Grotz, 1970; Katz, Ford, Moskowitz, Jackson, & Jaffe, 1963) as well as others (Law & Letts, 1989). On these performance scales, the patient can be graded as dependent; independent; requiring the use of equipment, supervision, and various levels of assistance; or in the case of the Klein-Bell ADL Scale, able or unable. See Figure 8-1 for a sample self-care assessment form and grading scale (Rehabilitation Institute of Chicago, 1991).

During the past 10 years, an attempt has been made to establish universal scales to be used in all rehabilitation settings. These universal scales compile national data on performance outcomes in rehabilitation after disability and allow comparisons of outcomes across facilities. The Functional Independence Measure (FIM) is one such scale (Keith, Granger, Hamilton, & Sherwin, 1987; Guide to the Uniform Data Set, 1987; Granger, Hamilton, Keith, Zielezny, & Sherwin, 1986; Hamilton, Granger, Sherwin, Zielezny, & Tashman, 1987). Self-care is one of six areas addressed by the FIM.

Patient _____ RIC No. _____ Date _____

☐ Initial
☐ Re-eval
☐ Discharge

IV FUNCTIONAL SKILLS/ADL

KEY 7 = Independent
6 = Independent with equipment/modified environment
5 = Independent with set-up/distant supervision
4 = Minimal assistance/intermittent supervision (patient performs 75% or better)

3 = Moderate assistance/continuous supervision (patient performs 50 to 75%)
2 = Maximal assistance (includes dependent but can direct care) (patient performs 25 to 50%)
1 = Dependent (25% or less)
0 = Not applicable or patient not responsible for these tasks. Only selectable for certain items.

ALL CORE ITEMS NOTED WITH BOLD LETTERING MUST BE RATED. If skills vary within component groups, the more dependent rating is used for the core item functional level. If this is **NO goal**, or the patient is already at his/her expected level, rate the goal the same as the functional level. **Meal Preparation, Homemaking and Community Reintegration,** may be deferred until they may be appropriately addressed. On discharge, the date the goal was set shall be noted in the Date Column.

A = ADMISSION STATUS   G = DISCHARGE GOAL   CIRCLE = DISCHARGE STATUS

Feeding
Utensil Use
Finger Food
Drink/Straw
Cup Use
Cut Food

UE Dressing
UE On
UE Off
Fasteners On
Fasteners Off

LE Dressing
LE On
LE Off
Socks/Shoes On
Socks/Shoes Off
Fasteners On
Fasteners Off

Toileting
Manage Clothes
Empty Leg Bag
Change Leg Bag
Cathetorize/Irrigation
Digital Stim/Suppository
Hygiene

Grooming
Wash Face/Hands
Brush Teeth/Dentures
Comb/Brush Hair
Shave/Make-up
Apply Glasses/Contacts
Clean Glasses/Contacts
Dry/Set Hair
Floss Teeth
Apply Deodorant
Ear Care
Nail Care

Bathing
Bathe UES
Bathe Body
Bathe LES
Wash Hair

Communication
Writing
Telephone Use
Typing/Computer Use
Turning Page
Opening Mail

Date

Meal Preparation
Hot
Cold

Homemaking
Daily Clean-up
Vacuum/Mopping
Laundry
Ironing
Child Care

Community Integration
Planning
Resource Utilization
Money Management
Shopping
Safety Considerations
Home Access
Driving

Leisure Skills
Table Games
Crafts
T.V./Radio Use
Phonograph/Tape Recorder Use
Smoking

Equipment/Time Considerations

_____
_____
_____
_____
_____
_____
_____
_____

Distribution: White - Medical Records, Yellow - Physician
Pink - Department

FIGURE 8-1. *Self-care assessment form and grading scale. Courtesy of the Rehabilitation Institute of Chicago, Occupational Therapy Department.*

Factors to be taken into consideration in grading performance include consistency of performance under a variety of conditions, the time required for performance, and the type of assistance required, physical or verbal. These qualitative factors help to determine the amount and type of assistance necessary. Also important is determining the specific tasks for which assistance is required. A person requiring assistance in toileting may need help available 24 hours a day, whereas a person requiring assistance for bathing may require help only every other day. A person requiring bladder catheterization every 4 hours may require assistance at each catheterization time, whereas a person using an indwelling catheter might require assistance only once a month to change the catheter. Estimating the most logical balance of performance ability, care organization, care availability, and patient values is necessary in establishing treatment priorities and ultimate attendant care needs.

The treatment process

Once performance deficits in ADL that interfere with role competency are identified, treatment goals and plans can be established. Treatment goals should functionally describe patient performance, state expected performance in measurable terms, and be agreed on by both patient and therapist. A *functional* goal statement identifies the performance change that is expected. For a patient who is unable to perform lower-extremity dressing, a goal can be stated to reflect expected change in performance in terms of amount of assistance needed and task components. For example: Patient will be independent in pulling slacks from knees to waist and fastening them with minimal physical assistance. A *measurable* goal statement sets parameters for determining whether the goal has been met. The parameters must be measurable by patient report or by therapist observation using a defined scale. A measurable goal enables the therapist to state whether the goal has been met or not by comparing it to patient performance. In the example above, if the patient is unable to pull slacks from knees to waist with minimal physical assistance, the goal has not been met. Minimal physical assistance would need to be defined clearly using a reliable grading scale. An example of a goal statement that is measurable but not functional is: Patient will have 60 pounds grip strength in his left hand. Grip strength can be measured to identify whether the goal has been met, but the statement does not identify what functional performance is expected. Given 60 pounds of grasp, the patient still may not be able to accomplish lower-extremity dressing if other impairments interfere. An example of a goal that is functional but not measurable is: Patient will improve in ability to dress lower body. It may be difficult to say whether this goal has been met or not because this statement does not communicate expected performance. Improvement may range from being totally independent to being able to put on one shoe. Statements referring to what the therapist will do, such as evaluate upper-extremity strength, are plans, not goals.

Treatment plans are established to achieve goals. They include activities that remediate impairments underlying disability, adapt tasks to enable performance, and provide for task accomplishment with special equipment. Remediation components of the treatment plan address areas of impairment in sensorimotor, cognitive-perceptual, and psychosocial function that interfere with task accomplishment. This approach is used when it is reasonable to expect, based on medical information and the therapist's knowledge of the diagnosis and the patient, that sufficient improvement can be made in these areas to enhance goal achievement. Examples of remediation aspects of a treatment plan include:

- range-of-motion and reaching activities to enable reach to feet for lower-body dressing
- balance activities with hands-on guarding by therapist to reduce patient anxiety and fear of falling during dressing
- memory games and activities to improve patient's memory for precautions to take during dressing.

Specific remediation techniques are covered briefly later in this section and can be found in Units VI, VII, and VIII of this text.

Sometimes, remediation alone is not adequate to achieve the performance goal. In these cases, analysis of the task and knowledge of adaptive techniques enable the occupational therapist to establish treatment plans to teach the patient these adaptive techniques and have them practice. Examples of adaptive technique training treatment plan components include the following:

- Provide instruction and training in lower-body dressing in bed in long sitting using quadriplegic dressing techniques.
- Provide written instruction of lower-body dressing sequence to aid patient memory.
- Use reverse chaining to reduce frustration during lower-body dressing.
- Teach energy conservation techniques to be used in lower-body dressing.

Specific adaptive techniques are described later in this section.

When neither remediation nor adaptive techniques are likely to be sufficient to allow goal achievement, adaptive equipment provision and instruction in use is included in the treatment plan. Adaptive equipment usually is considered tertiary to remediation and adaptive techniques because of its cost, relative inconvenience, and acceptance factors. There are times when the occupational therapist's knowledge base indicates that treatment plans to provide adaptive equipment will result in the most efficient route to goal achievement. Examples of adaptive equipment plans include the following:

- Provide and instruct in use of dressing stick for independent trouser donning.
- Provide and instruct in use of long-handled shoehorn and sock donner to allow independent shoe and sock donning in 5 minutes.
- Provide and instruct in use of reacher to reinforce safe performance when retrieving objects from floor and closet.

Adaptive equipment used in overcoming performance deficits in ADL is discussed later in this section and in Chapter 9, Section 5.

Treatment interventions

The remainder of this section discusses occupational therapy treatment interventions used to reverse disabilities in ADL task performance. Disability is broken down into various task compo-

TABLE 8-1. *Diagnoses Associated with Impairments Causing ADL Disability*

Impairment	Common Diagnoses
Range of motion, strength and coordination of oral musculature impairment	Neurologic and neuromuscular conditions, including CVA, head injury, MS, ALS, CP
Upper-extremity passive and active range-of-motion impairment of UES (and LES)	Quadriplegia, burns, upper-extremity amputation, arthritis, MS, ALS, orthopedic and other traumatic injuries
Upper-extremity coordination impairment	Head injury, CP, CVA, MS, tumors, and other neurologic conditions
One upper-extremity or body side impairment	Hemiplegia (CVA or head injury) and unilateral trauma or amputation
Mobility impairment without upper-extremity impairment	Paraplegia, osteoarthritis, lower-extremity amputations, burns, hip and knee fractures and replacements
Cognitive, perceptual, or sensory impairment	Head injury, CVA, MS, Parkinson, and Alzheimer diseases, mental retardation, low vision, blindness, tactile sensory impairment with peripheral neuropathy or neurologic cause (MS, CVA, SCI, head injury)

CVA, cerebrovascular accident; ALS, amyotrophic lateral sclerosis; CP, cerebral palsy; LES, lower extremities; MS, multiple sclerosis; SCI, spinal cord injury; UES, upper extremities.

nents. Remediation, adaptive methods, and adaptive equipment techniques that may be used to enable task performance are suggested based on the impairment that limits function. Diagnoses associated with common impairments are listed in Table 8-1. Remediation techniques should be used only if the condition is likely to improve based on knowledge of the diagnosis and the patient's case history. Remediation techniques are based on impairment rather than being specific to a particular task. Table 8-2 lists general remediation techniques used for the types of impairment that cause ADL task disability. Remediation techniques also can be used during ADL adaptive technique training and should be incorporated in all aspects of treatment. For example, neurodevelopmental treatment principles and techniques can be incorporated in dressing training to maximize motor recovery and performance.

Interventions for performance deficits in feeding

Feeding disabilities can result from the inability to

- swallow food and drink safely
- reach the hand to the mouth
- pick up and hold utensils, finger foods, and beverage containers
- use both hands simultaneously to cut food
- attend to the activity, see the various items on the plate, locate them with the utensil, and then locate mouth with the utensil

These inabilities may result from impairments in

- passive range of motion in the upper extremities and oral area

TABLE 8-2. *General Remedial Techniques Associated with Impairments Causing ADL Disability*

Impairment	Remediation Techniques
Range-of-motion, strength, and coordination impairment of oral musculature	Oral motor stimulation, range-of-motion and strengthening exercises, and neurophysiologic treatment techniques (NDT, PNF, Rood)
Upper extremity passive and active range-of-motion impairment of UES (and LES)	PROM, static stretch, continuous passive motion, active assistive and resistive exercise, splinting and casting, and neurophysiologic treatment techniques
Coordination impairment	Neurophysiologic treatment techniques
One upper-extremity or body side impairment	PROM, static stretch, continuous passive motion, active assistive and resistive exercise, splinting and casting, and neurophysiologic treatment techniques for the affected upper extremity or body side
Mobility impairment without upper-extremity impairment	Balance, standing and ambulation activities, gross motor activities, and neurophysiologic treatment techniques
Cognitive, perceptual, or sensory impairment	Cognitive training or retraining, computer treatment for cognition and perception, perceptual retraining, sensory motor treatment techniques, and sensory reeducation

LES, lower extremities; NDT, neurodevelopmental treatment; PNF, proprioceptive neuromuscular facilitation; PROM, passive range of motion; UES, upper extremities.

- active range of motion (strength) in the upper extremities and oral musculature
- coordination in the upper extremities, neck, and oral musculature
- one upper extremity or body side
- cognitive, perceptual, and sensory abilities

Treatment interventions based on the area of impairment are listed below (Hopkins & Smith, 1988; Pedretti, 1985; Trombly, 1987; Ford & Duckworth 1987; Hill, 1986; Kovich & Bermann 1988).

Impairments in range, strength, and coordination of oral musculature

Adaptive techniques used with these impairments include

- head, neck, and body positioning to facilitate proper swallowing
- modification of food consistency

Adaptive equipment used with these impairments include

- positioning equipment to maintain the head slightly flexed and in midline, the trunk upright and in midline, the hips flexed at 90 degrees, and the feet supported (Kovich & Bermann, 1988)

Impairments in passive and active range of motion in the upper extremities

Adaptive techniques used with these impairments include

- using one upper extremity to assist the other in reaching to the mouth (lifting from the elbow)
- resting the elbow on a high surface to allow reaching to the mouth
- weaving utensil through weak fingers to hold it
- using both hands to hold a cup or glass
- using tenodesis (natural tightness of finger flexors when wrist is extended) to pick up glass, finger foods

Adaptive equipment used with these impairments include

- antigravity assistive arm placement devices (Swedish sling, deltoid aide, mobile arm support, over-head sling) for reach to mouth
- prostheses for reach to mouth and grasp
- mechanical grasp–release orthoses (wrist-driven flexor hinge, externally powered flexor hinge, cable-driven flexor hinge) when grasp is absent
- orthosis with utensil slot when wrist stability and grasp are absent
- utensil or universal cuff when grasp is absent or inadequate
- built-up handles on utensils when grasp is weak
- knife adapted to utensil cuff to secure to hand when grasp is weak or absent
- extended utensils (a right-angle pocket can be used to extend and alter the angle at which a utensil is held)
- swivel utensils if food slips off the utensil during reach to the mouth
- long straw and straw holder if cup cannot be lifted to the mouth
- drinking equipment set up on wheelchair (cup holder and extended long straw) or bedside to allow fluid consumption throughout the day and night
- nonskid place mat
- plate guard or scoop dish to prevent food from being pushed off the plate

Impairments of coordination in the upper extremities

Adaptive techniques used with these impairments include

- weighting the extremities
- use of one upper extremity to stabilize the other
- maintaining upper arms fixed against the trunk, or elbows or wrists stabilized on the table

Adaptive equipment used with these impairments include

- resistance-providing devices, such as the friction feeder for arm placement control
- weighted utensils (with severe incoordination a spoon is used rather than a fork for safety)
- nonskid place mat
- covered cup with straw or sipping spout for drinking or long straw and straw holder to enable drinking without picking up the cup
- drinking equipment set up on wheelchair or bedside
- rocker or regular knife to aid in cutting using a rocking motion, with both upper extremities used to stabilize if incoordination is not severe

Impairments in one upper extremity or body side

Adaptive techniques for this category are also called one-handed techniques and include

- using rocking motion with standard knife for cutting

Adaptive equipment used with these impairments include

- rocker knife
- plate guard or scoop dish if food is pushed off plate

Interventions for performance deficits in grooming

Grooming tasks include face and hand washing; hair combing, brushing, and styling; teeth brushing; glasses or contact lens care and donning; cosmetic application; shaving; deodorant application; and nail care.

Grooming disabilities can result from the inability to

- reach face, all areas of head, and faucets
- pick up, hold, and manipulate brushes, washcloth, razor, contact lenses, nail file, and other tools
- use both hands simultaneously to open containers or file nails
- attend to the activity, locate the items needed, and use them appropriately

These inabilities may result from impairments in

- passive range of motion in the upper extremities and neck
- active range of motion (strength) in the upper extremities and neck
- coordination in the upper extremities and neck musculature

- one upper extremity or body side
- cognitive and perceptual abilities

Treatment techniques are listed below (Hopkins & Smith, 1988; Pedretti, 1985; Trombly, 1987; Ford & Duckworth, 1987; Hill, 1986; Kovich & Bermann, 1988).

Impairments in active and passive range of motion in the upper extremities and neck

Adaptive techniques used with these impairments include

- assisting one extremity with the other to improve reach
- resting elbow on high surface to extend reach
- using mouth to open containers
- taping nail file down to hold it and moving nails across file if grasp is inadequate to hold file
- using both hands to hold glass, toothbrush, hairbrush, razor
- using liquid soap in push-button dispenser
- modifying hairstyle to eliminate need for setting
- setting dentures on wet face or hand towel in sink to prevent sliding when brushing
- using tenodesis to pick up glass and other items (tenodesis is usually not strong enough to hold toothbrush while brushing)

Adaptive equipment used with these impairments include

- antigravity assistive arm placement devices to reach face and head
- prostheses for reach to face and head and grasp
- mechanical grasp–release orthoses when grasp is absent
- orthosis with utensil slot when wrist stability and grasp are absent
- utensil or universal cuff when grasp is absent or inadequate
- built-up handles on hairbrush, toothbrush
- Velcro D-ring closure strap on hairbrush
- toothpaste dispenser
- deodorant spray adaptation
- deodorant holder to stabilize on hand
- make-up basket that secures cosmetics in place while opening
- razor holder
- shaving cream dispenser adaptation
- extended-handle toothbrush, hairbrush
- proximal interphalangeal (PIP) finger-joint stabilizer for holding finger stable to put in contact lens
- wash mit
- Octopus soap stabilizer
- extended faucet levers to allow reach and operation

Impairments of coordination in the upper extremities and neck

Adaptive techniques used with these impairments include

- choosing an easy-care hairstyle
- weighting the extremities
- using a towel in the sink when brushing dentures to prevent breaking
- using one upper extremity to stabilize the other or both upper extremities in task

- maintaining upper arms fixed against the trunk or elbows and wrists stabilized on sink or counter while washing face, combing hair, brushing teeth
- grasping hairbrush closer to bristles or on back where bristles are mounted
- using liquid soap in push-button dispenser

Adaptive equipment used with these impairments include

- resistance-providing device (friction feeder) for arm placement control
- mount toothbrush and razor on gooseneck or other stable mount and move head to accomplish task without upper extremities
- electric toothbrush, razor
- suction-cup, mounted brush for brushing dentures, cleaning nails
- make-up basket to hold cosmetics in place and prevent spillage

Impairments in one upper extremity or body side

Adaptive techniques used with these impairments include

- stabilizing containers between knees to hold them
- squeezing toothpaste onto brush that is sitting on counter
- changing hairstyle to one requiring no setting
- taping nail file down and moving nails of sound hand across file
- using a towel in the sink to hold dentures while brushing

Adaptive equipment used with these impairments include

- suction brush for nails, dentures
- make-up basket to stabilize cosmetics while opening and using

Interventions for performance deficits in upper-extremity dressing and undressing

Upper-extremity dressing disability can result from the inability to:

- reach to put arm in sleeve and lift garment over head or behind back
- grasp shirt to pull off and on, down in back
- manipulate buttons, zippers, snaps
- lift heavy clothing (eg, jackets)
- attend to tasks, perceive spatial relation between clothing and body parts, and understand and learn to use adaptive methods

These inabilities may result from impairments in

- passive range of motion in upper extremities and neck
- active range of motion (strength) in upper extremities and trunk
- coordination in upper extremities
- unilateral upper extremity use
- cognitive, perceptual, and sensory abilities

Treatment techniques are listed below (Hopkins & Smith, 1988; Pedretti, 1985; Trombly, 1987; Ford & Duckworth, 1987; Hill, 1986; Kovich & Bermann, 1988).

Impairments in passive and active range of motion in upper extremities and trunk

Adaptive methods used with these impairments include

- wearing loose, light clothing
- wearing front-opening as opposed to back-opening clothing
- leaving shirts partly buttoned (neck ties knotted) and putting them on and removing them over the head
- moving sleeve buttons to cuff edge to leave larger opening for donning and doffing without unbuttoning
- using support for weak trunk muscles or poor balance in sitting (sit in wheelchair, chair with arms, or hospital bed with back up for support)
- using an alternative method of putting on and taking off shirt (see the display)
- for bra donning, placing bra around waist with closure (Velcro or regular closure), closing, then turning bra to orient with closure in back, placing arms through straps and pushing straps onto shoulders, *or* leaving bra fastened and putting on and taking off as an over-head garment

Adaptive equipment used with these impairments include

- loop sewn in back of garment near collar to hook hand or short dressing stick and to lift garment over head for removal
- short dressing stick with rubber-coated hooks to push garment over shoulders or to hook sleeve near axilla to pull and allow arm to be pulled out
- Velcro closures (these can be difficult to manage because they stick when you don't want them to)
- zipper-pull loops or rings
- button-aide hook (can have large handle or handle with palmar strap for those with weak or absent grasp)
- prosthesis
- mechanical grasp–release orthosis
- front-closure bra with loops to pull closed if necessary

Impairments of coordination in the upper extremities and trunk

Adaptive techniques used with these impairments include

- wearing loose-fitting clothing
- avoiding small fasteners, opting for over-head clothing, or leaving clothing fastened and donning as over-head clothing
- ensuring that necessary fasteners are large
- keeping upper extremities close to body
- using alternative garment donning method 1 or 3 (see the previous display) and alternative bra donning methods under the section on impairments in passive and active range of motion

---

ALTERNATIVE METHODS OF PUTTING ON AND TAKING OFF SHIRTS FOR PATIENTS WITH IMPAIRMENTS IN PASSIVE AND ACTIVE RANGE OF MOTION IN UPPER EXTREMITIES

Method 1

1. Place shirt (over-head or cardigan) face down on lap, with sleeves and collar near knees.
2. Slide arms through shirt into sleeves, and push sleeves over elbows.
3. Gather shirt back and lift over head (may rest elbows on knees or table and bend head down to push through shirt collar).
4. Protract and retract and elevate and depress shoulders to get shirt over shoulders, or push shirt over one shoulder, then the other, with opposite upper extremity.
5. Retract shoulder while leaning forward slightly to get shirt down in back.
6. Pull shirt front panels near bottom to straighten and bring down fully (cardigans).
7. Place hands inside shirt front and pull slightly away from body, down, and toward sides, to bring shirt down fully (over-head clothing).
8. To remove garment over head, place hand inside shirt toward opposite sleeve, and pull sleeve opening over elbow. Repeat for other sleeve and remove over head.
9. To remove cardigan garment, push collar area back over shoulders, extend upper extremity, and retract shoulders to help sleeve drop below elbow arm from sleeve. *Or*, push one sleeve off shoulder, reach opposite upper extremity to sleeve hole, and hold while elevating shoulder, extending arm and

flexing elbow to remove arm from sleeve. Then pull shirt around back to other side with arm still in sleeve and slide arm out.

10. Unbutton using hand to stabilize shirt against body and thumb or knuckle to push button through hole while opposite thumb pushes fabric up over bottom.

Method 2

This method is available for patients with good trunk and lower extremity mobility but limited upper extremity strength and or range of motion (upper-extremity amputees, burn patients).

1. Place cardigan garment face up on bed.
2. Place one upper extremity in sleeve, and lie down using friction of shirt against bed to hold garment while sliding arm in.
3. Once one arm is all the way in and collar is up over shoulder, start other arm in sleeve and sit up to work arm into sleeve (garment must be loose for this method).

Method 3

This method is for use with over-head clothing.

1. Put head through neck hole first.
2. Place hand in sleeve, and push arm all the way into sleeve.

- weighting distal extremities
- ensuring postural stability by performing dressing in wheelchair, chair with arms, or bed with back support

Adaptive equipment used with these impairments include

- Velcro closures
- weighted button hook with large handle
- zipper-pull loops or rings

Impairments in one upper extremity or body side

Adaptive techniques used with these impairments include

- wearing loose, light clothing
- moving sleeve buttons to cuff edge to provide larger opening and to allow donning and doffing without unbuttoning
- using support in sitting if balance is poor
- using an alternative method of putting on and taking off clothing (see the display)

- putting on and taking off bra as an over-head garment, or fastening it in front at the waist, then moving it to proper position and pulling on the straps

Adaptive equipment used with these impairments include

- button hook to make buttoning faster
- Velcro and D-ring closure may make securely and tightly fastening a bra easier

Interventions for performance deficits in lower-extremity dressing and undressing

Lower-extremity dressing disability can result from the inability to:

- reach to feet
- stand to pull pants over hips
- grasp to pull clothing on and pull fabric together to fasten

---

ALTERNATIVE METHODS OF PUTTING ON AND TAKING OFF SHIRTS FOR PATIENTS WITH IMPAIRMENTS OF ONE UPPER EXTREMITY OR BODY SIDE

Method 1

1. Place cardigan garment on lap with front up, collar toward knees, and affected side sleeve opening exposed between legs.
2. Place affected upper extremity into sleeve, leaning forward to drop into sleeve as far as possible.
3. Pull sleeve up arm, at least above the elbow.
4. With unaffected hand, grasp collar and sleeve that are to be put on that side.
5. Lift unaffected arm over head, pulling shirt around back.
6. While pulling shirt around back, slip unaffected arm in sleeve, letting shirt fall onto arm, and pushing arm into sleeve as shirt is pulled around.

Method 2

1. Place cardigan garment on lap with front up, collar near thighs, and sleeve opening of affected side exposed between legs.
2. Place affected upper extremity in sleeve opening, leaning forward to drop it in as far as possible.
3. Pull sleeve up affected arm, at least above elbow, preferably up to axilla.
4. Place unaffected upper extremity in its sleeve.
5. Grasp collar, gather up back material, and lift over head.

Method 3

This method is used for over-head clothing.
1. Place shirt collar down on lap, and open bottom of shirt to expose sleeve openings.
2. Place affected upper extremity in its sleeve opening, and pull on to above elbow.
3. Place unaffected upper extremity in its sleeve opening.
4. Grasp back collar, gather back fabric with unaffected upper extremity, and lift over head.

Removing Cardigan Garment

1. Pull fabric toward unaffected side to make it as loose as possible.
2. Grasp unaffected side of unbuttoned cardigan garment, reach back and to the side to get it off shoulder, then pull it down and wriggle elbow out of shirt. Or, grasp sleeve of unaffected side with that hand, and gradually pull it down until elbow can be worked out of sleeve.
3. Pull fabric to affected side, and remove affected upper extremity.

Removing Over-head Garment

1. Pull fabric toward unaffected side to loosen.
2. Pull bottom of shirt on unaffected side down, squeeze elbow through sleeve hole, and remove unaffected upper extremity from sleeve.
3. Gather fabric, and grasp collar to lift garment over head. Or, grasp collar near nape of neck, gather back fabric with hand, and pull back over head.
4. Remove unaffected upper extremity from sleeve.
5. Remove sleeve from affected upper extremity.

- manipulate laces, zippers, snaps, and buttons
- attend to tasks, perceive spatial relation between garment and body parts, understand and learn adaptive methods

These inabilities may result from impairments in

- passive range of motion in upper extremities, lower extremities, and trunk.
- active range of motion (strength) in upper extremities, lower extremities, and trunk
- coordination in upper extremities, lower extremities, and trunk
- one upper extremity or body side
- mobility (without upper-extremity impairment)
- cognitive, perceptual, and sensory abilities

Treatment techniques are listed below (Hopkins & Smith, 1988; Pedretti, 1985; Trombly, 1987; Ford & Duckworth, 1987; Hill, 1986; Kovich & Bermann, 1988).

Impairments in passive and active range of motion in upper and lower extremities

Adaptive techniques are available for use with patients who have strength impairments. With passive range-of-motion impairments, equipment usually is needed to overcome lower-extremity dressing disability. Adaptive techniques used with these impairments include

- wearing loose, light clothing

- using an alternative method of putting on and taking off clothing (see the display)
- using thumbs to stretch a loose sock over the toes, and dampening the heel of the hand with saliva to provide friction to pull the sock onto the foot
- wearing loafers or shoes with Velcro closures that allow fastening without adaptive equipment
- avoiding wearing high tops and boots, which are difficult to put on
- putting on and taking off shoes and socks while in the wheelchair by lifting the foot over the opposite knee

Adaptive equipment used with these impairments include

- dressing loops attached to clothing, dressing stick hooks, and reachers (if adequate grasp is available) used to start pants over feet in bed or chair and pull up to within reach of hands and also to push off and pick up clothing, shoes, and socks
- suspenders substituted for loops, eliminating the step of removing or tucking away the loops
- long shoe horns and heel guards with extended handles or loops
- sock-donning aides
- button hooks—built-up handle or strap-on handle to secure to hand may be needed
- zipper-pull cuff or rings
- Velcro closures
- prosthesis
- mechanical grasp–release orthosis

ALTERNATIVE METHODS OF PUTTING ON AND TAKING OFF PANTS FOR PATIENTS WITH IMPAIRMENTS IN PASSIVE AND ACTIVE RANGE OF MOTION IN UPPER AND LOWER EXTREMITIES

Method 1

1. Sit with legs extended in bed, with or without back support, with clothing nearby on bed or chair.
2. Use weak grasp or drape garment over hand to hold it in preparation for putting it over foot.
3. Pull leg with forearm, lift under knee to bend leg, and bring foot up to opposite knee.
4. Drape garment over foot through leg opening, and pull it up to knee.
5. Lift leg and push on knee to extend.
6. Pull trousers over the foot and up to the knee during the same step as underwear, or use the same method for trousers as for underwear *after* underwear are pulled to the waist.
7. Once garment is pulled to the knees, pull it partly over the thighs by pulling on crotch of pants with forearm and pulling with hand in pocket of pants, or use both hands together to grasp and pull.
8. Lie down and roll side to side, pulling pants up over hip that is on top with each roll. Pull pants up using hand in pocket, thumb in belt loop, or hand inside pants under waistband.
9. Elastic waist bands can eliminate the need to use equipment to fasten the garment.
10. Reverse the process to remove the clothing.

Method 2

This method uses a different approach to get the clothing started over the feet and up to the knees but is otherwise the same as method 1.
1. Leave the legs extended in bed, separated slightly.
2. Reach forward to the feet, and place one wrist under the ipsilateral heel.
3. Drape the garment leg opening over the toes, and pull the garment over the heel while lifting the upper extremity under the heel slightly.

Method 3

This method offers another way to get the pants over the feet and up to the knees.
1. Place pants face up with the waist just above the knees and under the legs.
2. Lift legs up with the forearm one at a time, and place feet in leg openings.
3. Exert pressure on the knee to cause the leg to extend into the trouser.

Impairments in coordination of the upper and lower extremities and trunk

Adaptive techniques used with these impairments include

- wearing loose clothing
- performing dressing on stable surface with good support (bed, wheelchair, chair with arms)
- using one hand to stabilize while reaching to feet with the other
- stabilizing arms against legs when reaching to feet
- avoiding small fasteners, wearing elastic-waist clothing
- weighting on distal extremities

Adaptive equipment used with these impairments include

- Velcro closures
- zipper-pull loops or rings
- button hook
- elastic laces or Velcro closures on shoes

Impairments of one upper extremity or body side

Adaptive techniques used with these impairments include

- using an alternative method of putting and and taking off clothing (see the display)
- using a one-handed shoe-tying method (one method is illustrated by Trombly (1987); another is described in Figure 8-2)

ALTERNATIVE METHODS OF PUTTING ON AND TAKING OFF CLOTHING FOR PATIENTS WITH IMPAIRMENTS IN ONE UPPER EXTREMITY OR BODY SIDE

Putting on Clothing

1. Sit on bed at side or in chair or wheelchair that allows feet to be firmly positioned on the floor. Sitting on bed is preferable if unable to stand to pull up pants because patient can lie back down in bed to roll and pull pants over hips.
2. Cross affected leg over nonaffected leg.
3. Place garment over foot, and pull up to or over knee, making sure foot is through bottom of leg opening.
4. Replace foot on floor.
5. Hold garment near waist with unaffected upper extremity, and reach down to allow lifting of unaffected lower extremity into opening.
6. Pull garment up over thighs as far as possible while sitting.
7. Use affected upper extremity if possible to hold pants up while coming to stand, or hold pant waist with unaffected hand while using affected upper extremity as support while coming to stand.
8. Stand to pull pants over hips, leaning against wall, bed, or other stable object if necessary.
9. Attach fasteners while standing because clothing is looser if this can be done safely; if not, wear looser clothing and fasten while sitting.

Removing Clothing

1. Unfasten in seated position.
2. Allow garment to drop from hips while coming to stand.
3. Remove unaffected leg first, then affected leg by letting garment drop to floor and lifting affected leg out while holding garment on floor with unaffected leg, *or* by crossing affected leg over unaffected leg.

Putting on Socks and Shoes

1. Put on loose socks by putting unaffected hand in sock opening and spreading fingers to start sock over toes.
2. Place affected foot on a footstool or lift to the opposite knee to stabilize it during sock donning.
3. Once socks are over the toes, pull up using the unaffected upper extremity.
4. Put shoes on the unaffected side without adaptation.
5. Put shoes on the affected side by lifting the foot to the opposite knee or crossing the affected leg over the nonaffected leg, then using the nonaffected upper extremity to place the shoe on the foot. Some shoes may be able to be put on the affected lower extremity by placing the shoe on the floor and lifting the foot into the shoe, then pushing on the affected knee to push the heel into the shoe.

*Putting on and Taking off Ankle— Foot Orthoses**

1. Open the laces wide, and fold the tongue back over the laces.
2. Lay the brace on the floor between feet with shoe directly under knees.
3. Lift affected foot into shoe.
4. Pick up brace by calf band or metal upright, and slide shoe onto foot while moving it into position flat on the floor. Use the unaffected foot to prevent the heel of the affected foot from slipping backward out of the shoe.
5. Push on the knee of the affected leg to slide the heel into the shoe.

To remove orthosis:
1. Loosen straps and laces.
2. Hold heel of shoe down with unaffected foot while lifting affected heel out, then push on calf band to push shoe off. *Or*, cross affected leg over unaffected, and lever shoe off foot by pushing on calf band.

* *Other methods are suggested by Trombly (1987) and Malick & Almasy (1983, p. 261).*

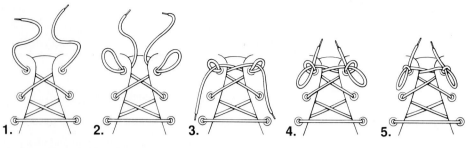

FIGURE 8-2. *One-handed shoe-tying method. From Jan Davis, OTR, NDT Certification Course 1977, Harmanville, PA.*

1. Lace laces in usual way.
2. Put both lace ends back through the holes they exited until the loops formed are small.
3. Put the lace ends through the opposite loops and pull to tighten loops, allowing just enough room to put the lace end back through the loop.
4. Put lace ends back through the loops, forming another loop.
5. Pull on these loops alternately to tighten.

Mobility impairments (without upper-extremity involvement)

Adaptive methods are used primarily with lower-extremity strength impairment; with passive range limitations, equipment must be used. Adaptive techniques used with these impairments include

- when lower extremities are very weak, using techniques listed under upper-extremity and lower-extremity passive and active range-of-motion limitations
- when a wheelchair is used for mobility, learning to dress from the wheelchair as well as from the bed (see the display)

Adaptive equipment used with these impairments include

- dressing stick or reacher to start garment
- long shoe horn
- sock donner
- slip-on shoes or elastic laces if unable to reach feet to tie

---

METHOD OF DRESSING FROM THE WHEELCHAIR FOR PATIENTS WITH MOBILITY IMPAIRMENTS

1. Sit on low bed, wheelchair, or standard chair with feet firmly planted on floor.
2. Cross one leg over the other to start garment and put on socks and shoes.
3. To pull garment over hips in wheelchair or bed (if unable to stand), lean far to one side to pull garment over opposite thigh and buttock; repeat for opposite side. *Or,* in wheelchair, support weight on elbows and lean on back of chair, bridging to lift buttocks from chair, and pull pants up.
4. To stand to pull up garment, stabilize with one upper extremity on ambulation aide or grab bar while pulling up garment with the other upper extremity, alternating sides. Or, stabilize against wall, bed, or grab bar while pulling garment up.

Interventions for performance deficits in bathing

Bathing disability can result from the inability to:

- get into tub or shower
- grasp and manipulate faucets, soap, sponge, washcloth, or towel
- reach all areas of body and faucets

These inabilities may result from impairments in

- passive and active range of motion in the upper extremities, lower extremities, and trunk
- coordination of the upper extremities, lower extremities, and trunk
- one upper extremity or body side
- lower extremity, passive and active range of motion (without upper-extremity impairment)
- cognitive, perceptual, and sensory abilities

Techniques and equipment used to enable bathing are similar regardless of type of impairment (Hopkins & Smith, 1988; Pedretti, 1985; Trombly, 1987; Ford & Duckworth, 1987; Hill, 1986; Kovich & Bermann, 1988). Adaptive techniques used with these impairments include

- for bed bathing, if access to bathroom is not possible, placing rubber sheet or flannel-backed tablecloth material on bed
- using mobility methods described under dressing to reach all areas of body to wash, rinse, and dry
- using separate cloths for washing and rinsing to keep rinse water cleaner
- using nonslip mat or strips in tub or shower bottom
- draping towel over back of shower chair to rub back against to cleanse; using dry towel in same manner to dry
- rubbing feet on soapy hand towel or washcloth in tub bottom to cleanse if feet can't be reached
- placing soapy washcloth over knee and bending forward to wash arms against it (for one upper-extremity impairment)
- using liquid soap dispenser

Adaptive equipment used with these impairments include

- roll-in shower and commode chair
- bath bench

- long-handled bath sponges
- wash mit or washcloth with loop if grasp is inadequate
- soap on a rope or soap bag on a rope
- loops on towels
- grab bars
- hand-held shower
- single-lever faucet

Many varieties of the bath bench are available, including models with back support and two legs inside and two outside the tub to allow sitting first outside the tub, then lifting the legs into the tub and sliding the rest of the body on the bench to a position over the tub (this type of bench offers the most support); stool models without backs that sit entirely inside the tub; short, footstool-height models that allow sitting down in the bath water or a step approach to the tub bottom; and hydraulic bath supports that allow lowering into the tub. Most commode shower chairs and bath benches can be modified with additional support straps for safety in cases of extreme incoordination or weakness.

Interventions for performance deficits in toileting

Toileting disability can result from the inability to

- access and get onto toilet
- move quickly enough to get to toilet
- reach perineum
- grasp and use toilet paper
- manage clothing
- manage urinal
- insert suppository
- empty colostomy, perform colostomy care

These inabilities may result from impairments in

- passive and active range of motion in upper extremities, lower extremities, and trunk
- coordination of upper extremities, lower extremities, and trunk
- one body side
- cognitive, perceptual, and sensory abilities

Techniques used to enable toileting are similar with the various types of impairment and vary depending on continence. Adaptive techniques used with these impairments include

- using adaptive lower-extremity dressing techniques for clothing management
- wrapping toilet paper around hand if grasp is weak

Adaptive equipment used with these impairments include

- extended-reach toilet paper holder or tongs (for limited reach)
- bidet for cleansing (for limited reach)
- grab bars for transfer to toilet and for stabilizing while reaching to cleanse (for weakness and incoordination)
- raised toilet seat
- bedside commode to eliminate need to navigate distance to bathroom during night
- incontinent pads for patients with occasional or minor incontinence
- bowel program and catheter for patients with loss of bowel and bladder continence, including: mechanical grasp–

release orthosis or other catheter insertion device; adapted urinary drainage bag valve; labia spreader; adapted urinal or other collection device; adapted Posey for male external catheter; leg abductor; suppository inserter; digital stimulator

Interventions used with impairments in cognitive, perceptual, and sensory abilities

These interventions are listed generally because they are similar for all tasks. Adaptive techniques used with these impairments include

- altering the environment to provide appropriate stimulation
- implementing chaining or reverse chaining to allow gradual assumption of task components
- ensuring consistency of environment, task structure, and sequence
- grading instructions into the number and complexity appropriate for the patient
- using written and pictorial lists to aid memory of task components
- choosing an adaptive technique that most closely approximates the way the patient used to perform the task to minimize need for new learning
- marking clothing to aid in proper orientation

For Patients with Visual Impairment

- providing proper lighting to maximize vision
- establishing predictable locations where necessary items will be located
- using braille or other labeling to identify different objects of same shape (clothing, various shades of lipstick)

For Patients with Tactile Impairment

- testing water temperature on sensate area before it contacts desensate area

Adaptive equipment usually is not indicated for enhancing self-care performance with cognitive and perceptual impairment. If adaptive equipment is needed because of impairment in other areas, it should be minimized because learning to use the equipment increases the complexity and decreases the familiarity of the task. Adaptive equipment used with tactile impairments include

- faucet temperature regulators or scald guards to prevent burns in patients with tactile sensory impairment

Ensuring maximal performance

Treatment to improve self-care performance inevitably begins with instruction and practice in performing individual tasks or even task components. It is important to keep in mind that these tasks are not performed in isolation in daily life. Various tasks are combined into routines that may be slightly different among patients. Bathing, grooming, dressing, toileting, and eating breakfast may all be combined in one patient's morning routine, while another may combine bathing with undressing and some grooming tasks in a prebedtime routine. It is important for occupational therapists to plan treatment with consideration for the routines into which tasks will eventually be combined. This allows the therapist to suggest equipment that can be used for more than one task in a routine, minimizing time taken for putting on and removing many different pieces of equipment. Evaluation of the patient's ability to perform entire routines can also indicate whether instruction in energy conservation is necessary to allow completion of the routine without causing fatigue. The occupational therapist can provide instruction in task organization, spacing, and allowing appropriate brief rest periods to prevent over-fatigue and frustration. Recommendations for the best way to combine tasks into routines to maximize efficiency and use of attendant care are also made.

Once a patient approaches the maximal level of independence in a routine, consideration is given to attendant care needs in terms of amount of time and type of assistance. If independent performance is expected, each task is scrutinized to ensure that the patient is consistently performing independently. This includes ensuring that the patient can manage all equipment independently and can access all necessary items for task performance in home, work, and community settings. Issues to be considered include retrieving clothing from the closet and setting it near the bed the night before if dressing is performed in bed, retrieving a backpack from the back of the chair to access feeding equipment at school, and carrying items while using a walker.

Summary

Activities of daily living include the self-maintenance tasks of feeding, grooming, dressing, bathing, and toileting, which support role performance. Assessment and treatment of disabilities in performance of these tasks is a component of occupational therapy in every setting. Adaptive remediation techniques and adaptive equipment interventions to enable task performance have been reviewed.

References

Chiou, I., & Burnett, C. (1985). Values of activities of daily living. *Physical Therapy, 65*(6), 901–906.

Christiansen, C., (1991). Occupational performance assessment. In C. Christianson, & C. Baum (Eds.). *Occupational therapy: Overcoming human performance deficits* (pp. 374–424). Thorofare, NJ: Slack.

Ford, J., & Duckworth, B. (1987). *Physical management of the quadriplegic patient.* Philadelphia: F. A. Davis.

Granger, C., Hamilton, B., Keith, R., Zielezny, M., & Sherwin, F. (1986). Advances in functional assessment for medical rehabilitation. *Topics in Geriatric Rehabilitation, 1*(3), 59–74.

Guide to the uniform data set (1987). Research Foundation, State University of New York.

Halstead, L., & Hartley, R. (1975). Time care profile: An evaluation of a new method of assessing ADL dependence. *Archives of Physical Medicine and Rehabilitation, 56,* 110–115.

Hamilton, B., Granger, C., Sherwin, F., Zielezny, M., & Tashman, J. (1987). A uniform national data system for medical rehabilitation. In M. Fuhrer (Ed.). *Rehabilitation outcomes: Analysis and measurement* (pp. 137–147). Baltimore: Paul H. Brooks.

Hill, J. (Ed.). (1986). *Spinal cord injury: A guide to functional outcomes in occupational therapy.* Rockville, MD: Aspen.

Hopkins, H., & Smith, H. (Eds.). (1988). *Willard and Spackman's occupational therapy* (7th ed.). Philadelphia: J. B. Lippincott.

Iverson, I. (1983). *The revised Sister Kenny self care evaluation.* Publication 722, Sister Kenny Institute. Minneapolis: Abbott-Northwestern Hospital.

Katz, S., Downs, T., Cash, H., & Grotz, R. (1970). Progress in development of the index of ADL. *Gerontologist, 10,* 20–30.

Katz, S., Ford, A., Moskowitz, R., Jackson, B., & Jaffe, M. (1963). Studies of illness in the aged. *Journal of the American Medical Association, 12,* 914–919.

Klein, R., & Bell, B. (1982). Self care skills: Behavioral measurement with Klein-Bell ADL scale. *Archives of Physical Medicine and Rehabilitation, 63,* 335–338.

Kielhofner, G., & Henry, A. (1988). Development and investigation of the occupational performance history interview. *American Journal of Occupational Therapy, 42*(8), 489–498.

Keith, R., Granger, C., Hamilton, B., & Sherwin, F. (1987). The functional independence measure: A new tool for rehabilitation. *Advances in Clinical Rehabilitation, 1,* 6–18.

Kovich, K., & Bermann, D. (Eds.). (1988). *Head injury: A guide to functional outcomes in occupational therapy.* Rockville, MD: Aspen.

Law, M., & Letts, L. (1989). A critical review of scales of activities of daily living. *American Journal of Occupational Therapy, 43*(3), 522–528.

Lawton, M., & Brody, E. (1969). Assessment of older people: Self maintaining and instrumental activities of daily living. *Gerontologist, 9,* 179–186.

Mahoney, F., & Barthel, D. (1965). Functional evaluation: The Barthel Index. *Maryland State Medical Journal, 14,* 61–65.

Malick, M., & Almasy, B. (1988). Activities of daily living. In H. Hopkins, & H. Smith, (Eds.). *Willard and Spackman's occupational therapy* (pp. 246–271). Philadelphia: J. B. Lippincott.

Pedretti, L. (1985). *Occupational therapy: Practice skills for physical dysfunction.* St. Louis: C. V. Mosby.

Rehabilitation Institute of Chicago Occupational Therapy Department basic self care and complex ADL assessment. (1991). Chicago: The Rehabilitation Institute of Chicago.

Schoening, H., Anderegg, L., Bergstrom, D., Fonda, M., Steinke, N., & Ulrich, P. (1965). Numerical scoring of self care status of patients. *Archives of Physical Medicine and Rehabilitation, 47,* 689–697.

Trombly, C. S. (1987). *Occupational therapy for physical dysfunction* (3rd ed.). Baltimore: Williams & Wilkins.

Yerxa, E., Burnett-Bealieu, S., Stocking, J., & Azen, S. (1988). Development of the satisfaction with performance scaled questionnaire. *American Journal of Occupational Therapy, 42*(4), 215–221.

Bibliography

Gresham, G., Phillips, T., & Labi, M. (1980). ADL status in stroke: Relative merits of three standard indexes. *Archives of Physical Medicine and Rehabilitation, 61*(8), 355–358.

Nixon, V. (1985). *Spinal cord injury: A guide to functional outcomes in physical therapy.* Rockville, MD: Aspen.

SECTION 2

Work

SECTION 2A
Home and family management

KATHLEEN HILKO CULLER

KEY TERMS

Caregiver

Complex Activities of Daily Living

Home Maintainer

Home and Family Management

Instrumental Activities of Daily Living

LEARNING OBJECTIVES

Upon completion of this section the reader will be able to:

1. *Identify tasks classified as complex ADL.*
2. *Describe the role of the occupational therapist in home and family management and in instrumental ADL.*
3. *Describe four areas in which the occupational therapist should obtain information to determine whether home and family management should be addressed in occupational therapy.*
4. *Describe four methods of assessing complex ADL.*
5. *Describe four instrumental ADL assessment tools (areas examined, population, distinguishing features).*
6. *Identify three criteria that should be present when setting complex ADL goals.*
7. *Identify and explain rationales for four strategies used in complex ADL treatment.*
8. *Given an impairment, describe one to two treatment interventions for each complex ADL.*
9. *Describe the purpose and procedure for conducting a home visit.*
10. *Describe the issues that need to be considered when assessing community integration skills.*

One of the major roles that a person may have during a lifetime is that of home maintainer. Oakley (1981) defines a ***home maintainer*** as a person who has responsibility, at least once a week, for the upkeep of the home such as housecleaning or yard work. ***Home management*** includes the tasks of clothing care, cleaning, meal preparation and cleanup, shopping, money management, household maintenance, and safety procedures (see

Appendix C). Lawton introduced the term ***instrumental ADL*** to recognize that a person needed to perform tasks beyond basic self-care skills to function independently at home and in the community. He noted that successful performance of ***complex ADL*** tasks (ie, cooking, cleaning, laundry, shopping, and housekeeping) requires higher-level neuropsychological organization than is required for performance of self-maintenance tasks (ie, bathing and dressing; Lawton & Brody, 1969). The role of caregiver often is closely related to that of home maintainer. Oakley (1981) defines a ***caregiver*** as a person who has responsibility, at least once a week, for the care of someone such as a child, spouse, relative or friend. A major focus of occupational therapy is to promote a patient's ability to return to these two roles.

Role of the occupational therapist in home and family management

The role of the occupational therapist in home and family management is similar to that with self-care ADL management (see Chapter 8, Section 1). As noted in the display below, however, the occupational therapist's role is further expanded to include complex ADL assessment and treatment. This is due in part to the inherent complexity of complex ADL performance, variable approaches of patients to task performance, and the degree of therapist knowledge and skill in patient assessment and treatment in these areas. (See the display on page 208.)

Task characteristics

Each complex ADL task contains numerous subtasks. *Subtasks* are the individual steps needed to perform the task. The display on page 208 lists the subtasks required to perform home management and caregiver tasks as outlined by the AOTA Uniform Terminology (1989). To be clinically useful, the therapist needs to perform a detailed activity analysis for each complex ADL task to identify the specific subtasks required for task performance. For example, the subtask of preparing food is listed in the meal

---

ROLE OF THE OCCUPATIONAL THERAPIST IN COMPLEX ADL ASSESSMENT AND TREATMENT

- Determine if the roles of **home maintainer** and **caregiver** are part of the patient's lifestyle.
- Determine which **tasks** and **subtasks** need to be performed by the patient in the roles of home maintainer and caregiver.
- Perform **activity analysis** of identified tasks to consider the degree of performance component skill and proficiency required for task performance.
- **Consider** whether the patient demonstrates adequate proficiency with component skills with basic ADL before assessing performance of complex ADL.
- **Observe** performance of relevant complex ADL.
- **Analyze** what is interfering with task performance.
- **Select** and **Implement** intervention strategies to improve patient task performance.

WHY ARE COMPLEX ADLS SO COMPLEX?

Task Characteristics

- They contain several subtasks.
- Varying levels of performance are possible within each complex ADL.
- They require higher level of proficiency in performance components compared with basic ADL performance.

Patient Characteristics

- Each patient has a unique approach to task performance.
- The patient's and therapist's perceptions of acceptable performance vary.

Therapist Background and Clinical Expertise

- Therapists' backgrounds and familiarity with home and family management tasks may vary.
- With lack of standardized complex ADL assessment, the therapist's ability to perform activity analysis, select level of task to assess, challenge patient during evaluation and treatment process, and identify interfering factors is more dependent on therapist judgment and expertise compared with basic ADL assessment and treatment.

HOME AND FAMILY MANAGEMENT TASKS AND SUBTASKS

Clothing Care: Obtain and use supplies, launder, iron, store, and mend.

Cleaning: Obtain and use supplies, pick up, vacuum, sweep, dust, scrub, mop, make bed, and remove trash.

Meal Preparation and Clean-up: Plan nutritious meals and prepare food; open and close containers, cabinets, and drawers; use kitchen utensils and appliances; and clean up and store food.

Shopping: Select and purchase items and perform money transactions.

Money Management: Budget, pay bills, and use bank systems.

Household Maintenance: Maintain home, yard, garden appliances, and household items, or obtain appropriate assistance.

Safety Procedures: Know and perform prevention and emergency procedures to maintain a safe environment and prevent injuries.

Caregiving: Provide for children, spouse, parents, or others, including the physical care, nurturance, communication, and use of age-appropriate activities.

Adapted from AOTA Uniform Terminology, 1989.

---

preparation and clean-up category. If a patient likes to bake, part of therapy may involve baking a cake. Specific subtasks of this task include stirring ingredients and pouring ingredients into a cake pan.

Since adults have varied lifestyles and responsibilities in the area of home and family management, varying levels of performance are possible for each complex ADL task. As an example, the Rehabilitation Institute of Chicago (RIC) protocol (1990) for meal preparation and clean-up recognizes five levels of performance (preparation of [1] self-serve; [2] cold meal; [3] hot beverage, soup, or prepared food; [4] hot one-dish meal; [5] hot multicourse meal). The five levels reflect increasingly complex tasks, ranging from preparing a self-serve meal, which requires the least amount of patient ability, to preparing a hot, multicourse meal, which requires the highest level of proficiency to perform. See the display for the RIC protocol for meal preparation and clean-up.

The therapist needs to obtain information about the patient's previous and anticipated levels of performance to aid in assessment, setting goals, and planning treatment. Figure 8-3 indicates the relation between the occupational roles of home maintainer and caregiver and the underlying skills or perfor-

---

REHABILITATION INSTITUTE OF CHICAGO FUNCTIONAL ASSESSMENT SCALE: SAMPLE PROTOCOL FOR MEAL PREPARATION AND CLEAN-UP

Levels

1. Self-serve. Access prepared meal (eg, Meals-on-Wheels, prepared lunch). Open thermos, unwrap food, pour liquid or use straw.
2. Cold meal. Plan, prepare, and serve cold meal.
3. Hot beverage, soup, or prepared food. Plan, prepare, and serve food, instant soup, drink, or packaged prepared food (eg, frozen pizza, packaged microwave dinner)
4. Hot one-dish meal. Plan, prepare, and serve one-dish convenience food (eg, casserole, cake mix).
5. Hot multidish meal. Plan, prepare, and serve multidish (specify number) meal.

Assessment Questions

- For hot food, indicate whether patient is using single or multiple sources for cooking (specify source: microwave, stove, range, toaster oven). Based on past lifestyle, patient may need varied experience with different cooking sources.
- In what environment is the food prepared (quiet and nondistracting versus multistimulatory)?
- Did the patient have to follow directions or recipes? How well does the patient perform this task?
- Is the meal preparation familiar or unfamiliar to the patient?
- How many appliances (specify: crock pot, blender, beaters) does the patient need to use, and how well does the patient manage these appliances?

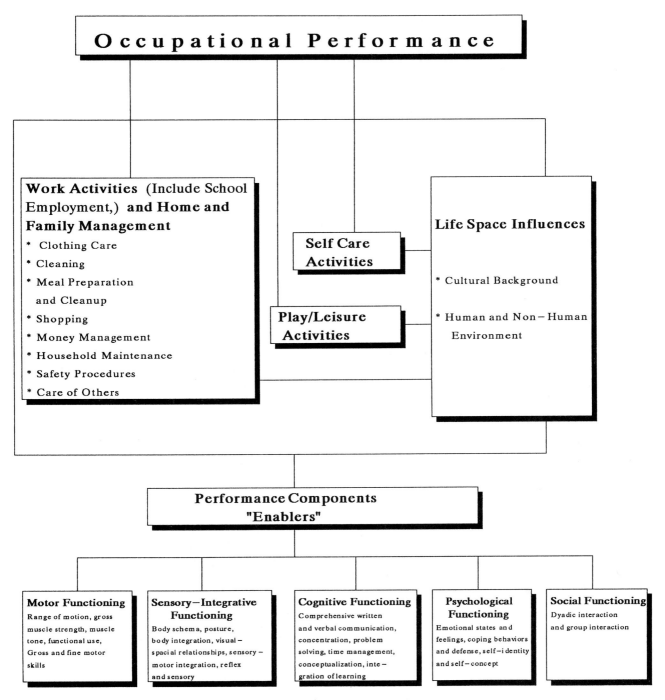

FIGURE 8-3. *Occupational performance frame of reference.* (*Adapted from AOTA,* [*1974*]. A curriculum guide for occupational therapy education. *Rockville: AOTA, p. 12.*)

mance components required for these roles. During the detailed activity analysis, the therapist must determine which performance components are required for task performance. For example, during the patient interview, the therapist may note that the patient often fixes a cup of coffee at home. The therapist could analyze this task to determine the performance components required. Examples of motor components involved in this task are standing balance and mobility to navigate in the kitchen, upper-extremity strength and range of motion to obtain a cup from an overhead cabinet, and fine motor coordination to open the coffee can and spoon coffee into the basket. Examples of cognitive components of this task are the ability to attend to the task while conversing with the therapist and remembering the procedure to fix coffee. Examples of sensory-integrative components are the figure–ground ability to distinguish a white cup in a white cabinet and motor planning to execute a familiar task. Examples of psychological components are positive self-esteem exhibited through task performance and adjustment to disability

TABLE 8-3.   *Occupational Therapy Approach to Home and Family Management*

Should the role of home maintainer or caregiver be a focus of occupational therapy?

Issues to Consider		Evaluation	Goal Setting	Intervention
		Pertinent Performance Areas		
Living circumstances	Cleaning	Which level of skill needs to be demonstrated?	A goal is set to reflect increased competency in performance of a subtask or performance area	Remediation
Are the roles valued by patient or family?	Meal preparation	Which subtasks are missing or deficient?		Compensation
Balance of activities and role responsibilities	Care of clothing			Techniques
	Shopping			Equipment
Available resources	Household maintenance			Modified environment
	Money management			Family and patient education
	Safety procedures		and/or	
	Care of others			
		Performance Components		
Areas of responsibility: past, present, and future	Motor	What are the major limiting factors to performing tasks listed above?	A goal is set to upgrade a performance component that is a major limiting factor to performance of complex ADL	
Prior, present, and anticipated patient status	Sensory-integrative			
	Cognitive			
	Psychological			
	Social			

by use of one-handed techniques to prepare coffee. An example of a social-functioning component of this task is interaction with the therapist while preparing and drinking coffee.

Patient characteristics

Unlike basic ADL, which have little variability in the steps required for task performance, patients may have their own method of performing complex ADL. As an example, in preparing vegetable soup, one patient may carefully peel and chop six or seven different vegetables before adding them to the soup stock. Another patient may use two to three vegetables and simply break them in half before adding them to the soup stock. It is useful to determine how the patient's present approach compares with previous task performance. If current task performance varies from the report of past performance, this may be an area of focus for occupational therapy. In addition, a patient's perception of successful or acceptable performance is colored by past experience and personal standards and will vary, ranging from the patient who needs only to fix a cup of coffee to the patient who is a gourmet cook.

Therapist background

Therapists' clinical experiences and personal backgrounds have greater impact on their roles with complex ADL than basic ADL assessment and treatment. As with any ADL, the therapist needs to be familiar with the task to accurately perform an activity analysis. For example, if the therapist is a mother, her depth of knowledge about child care responsibilities will be an asset in the comprehensive assessment of this role and in generating more effective intervention strategies. Since there are few standardized assessments of complex ADL, there is increased subjectivity. Therefore, increased therapist skills and judgment are required for performing a detailed activity analysis, for determining the appropriate level of task performance for the patient and structuring task performance accordingly, and for making com-

plete clinical observations of patient performance and using these to accurately identify performance components effecting task performance. In addition, the patient's background needs to be considered when a therapist is judging the quality of patient performance. As an example, the therapist would expect a gourmet cook's performance of meal preparation tasks to be much better than a patient's performance who did not have this experience. The final factor to consider is the therapist's standards for acceptable performance. One therapist may be more lenient and may judge patient performance to be adequate, whereas another therapist may consider it inadequate.

Table 8-3 lists the occupational therapy approach as it relates to home management and caregiver responsibilities. The remainder of this section further clarifies the role of the occupational therapist in determining whether the patient's roles of home maintainer or caregiver should be a focus of occupational therapy intervention. Also reviewed are methods of assessment and intervention for these areas.

Determining whether home and family management should be a focus of occupational therapy intervention

Because the diversity and range of home management and caregiver responsibilities vary greatly among adult patients, the therapist must determine whether evaluation and treatment will be done in these areas. To determine whether home or family management will be an appropriate focal area of treatment, the therapist interviews the patient or the patient's family to obtain information about the following areas:

Living circumstances: Where does the patient live? Is the home accessible? Are environmental adaptations required? Answers to these questions influence recommendations for home modification. For example, the patient who resides in a rental property is more likely to agree to bathroom modifications such as tub-mounted, removable grab bars than wall-mounted bars that require installation. The number of people in the household impacts the level of home management skills required by the patient. A patient living alone needs proficiency in many areas of household management to remain in an independent living situation as compared with the patient who resides with family or other people.

Patient and family background, goals, and values: What are the patient's previous and anticipated home management responsibilities? Did previous home management tasks require assistance? Does the patient have goals in the area of home or family management? The therapist must determine whether the patient's and family's culture and values are supportive of independence in home management because a person's value system can impact on motivation to maximize potential in this area. For example, a family member may be uncomfortable seeing a patient struggle to prepare a cup of coffee and therefore may do it for the patient.

Balance of activities in the patient's lifestyle: How did the patient previously value self-care, home management, work, and leisure activities? The therapist must determine how relevant to home and family management activities are to the patient to determine whether home management or caregiving responsibilities should be areas of focus. A patient who previously was a homemaker will most likely be motivated to learn adaptive methods to continue pursuing that role. A patient who is focused on returning to work, however, may opt to have a personal care attendant perform home management tasks so that time and energy can be used for the worker role.

Available resources: What resources (financial, emotional, social) are available to the patient? One patient may have the financial ability to make the home completely wheelchair-accessible, whereas another patient may need to consider less costly modifications to a portion of the living space. Obtaining information regarding the amount and type of available social support (from family members or from community services, such as Meals-on-Wheels) can affect the level of functional independence required to return to an independent living situation. Emotional support provided by family members and friends can also maximize patient potential in the role of home maintainer or caregiver.

Patient status: Is the patient's condition acute or chronic, temporary or permanent? This has implications for the types of treatment a therapist might plan for a patient. For a patient with newly diagnosed rheumatoid arthritis, a therapist may try to increase range of motion to perform ADL, whereas if the condition is chronic, the therapist may have the patient try an adaptive piece of equipment, such as a long-handled reacher to obtain objects from overhead cabinets and the floor. What strengths and performance component deficits are present? How do they impact the patient's ability to perform caregiver and home management tasks? Performance in home management and caregiver tasks requires greater physical and cognitive skills compared with routine self-care tasks. Therefore, the therapist must consider the patient's current and anticipated levels of functioning in the various performance components to determine whether the patient has adequate prerequisite skills for successful performance of home and family management. If the patient is dependent on others for routine self-care tasks, then it is not appropriate to address complex ADL with the patient unless the patient is interested in and capable of assuming a role that involved directing others to perform complex ADL tasks.

The following are descriptions of four tools that can be used to gather data related to the roles of home maintainer and caregiver:

The Role Checklist (Oakley, 1981) examines past, present, and future roles pertinent to the patient. It also evaluates the level of personal relevancy or value of home maintainer and caregiver roles to the patient. If the role of home maintainer or caregiver is identified as a present or future role and deemed to be of value by the patient, then it may warrant further consideration as a focus of occupational therapy intervention.

The Pie of Life Form (Simon, Howe, & Kirschenbaum, 1972) assists the therapist with obtaining information about the patient's lifestyle, including the amount of time spent in self-care, home management, work, and leisure activities. The patient completes one form each to signify past, present, and anticipated uses of time. The therapist then uses the three forms to discuss changes in the patient's use of time and whether further adjustments are required so that the patient is satisfied with the balance of activity.

The Activity Configuration Form (Mosey, 1973) assists the therapist in obtaining information about the patient's daily and weekly schedules. The patient's responses help the therapist to determine the types of activities performed (eg, heavy work versus light work; social versus solitary activities) as well as the frequency of performance of home management tasks. This information can assist both the patient and therapist to examine whether the current schedule maximizes patient ADL functioning.

The Occupational History Interview (Kielhofner, Henry, & Walens, 1989) includes questions about the patient's life roles, interests, values, and goals; acknowledgement of abilities and limitations; and effect of environment on ability to function (eg, funding, transportation, emotional climate of family and home).

Patients who communicate easily or who previously attempted home management tasks generally answer these questions easily. The patient who displays deficits that compromise communication (eg, aphasia, depression) or cognitive abilities (eg, traumatic brain injury or confusion) may be incapable of reliably responding to the interview questions. The medical chart, family members, or caregiver may be consulted to gain insight into the patient's past home management responsibilities, family goals, expectations, and the amount of support that can be provided to the patient at home. Obtaining information from other rehabilitation specialists working with the patient also may influence occupational therapy intervention. For example, in physical therapy, the patient's mobility status may be upgraded from using a wheelchair to a walker. The occupational therapist could then evaluate the patient's home management skills using the new mobility device to determine the patient's safety at home. Based on the results of interviews with the patient and caregiver, the therapist may initiate an assessment of home management and caregiver skills.

Assessment of home management and caregiver performance

Evaluation of different types of ADL is not done at one time. Initially, self-care, functional mobility, communication, and leisure skills may be assessed. As the patient gains skills in these areas, the therapist can evaluate ability to perform complex ADL (as they apply to the patient) and ability to access home and community. The therapist needs to consider whether the patient demonstrates adequate physical abilities, perceptual and cognitive skills, and the judgment to safely and effectively perform these tasks.

In comparison to the self-care area, the literature on home and family management assessments is sparse (Lawton & Brody, 1969; Intagliata & Sullivan, 1991). Because of the great variety of diagnostic categories of patients, the limiting factors affecting performance, and the range of home management activities that adults perform, home management assessments vary in content and focus.

There are four approaches to the assessment of home management and caregiver tasks. Formats for functional assessment include: (1) direct observation of specific patient performance, (2) self-administered questionnaire, (3) structured interview, or (4) evaluation of performance components. Advantages and disadvantages for each type of format are described in Table 8-4 (Law & Letts, 1989; Christiansen, 1991; Trombly, 1983; Yerxa, Burnett-Beaulieu, Stocking, & Azon, 1988). The first type of assessment is direct observation of patient performance areas critical to a patient's lifestyle (eg, meal preparation, laundry). The assessment can be either standardized (specific protocol has to be followed) or nonstandardized. It usually contains a listing of subtasks required to perform the task. For example, the meal preparation evaluation assesses whether the patient is able to perform tasks such as operating appliances and preparing and serving food. At the completion of the assessment, the therapist is aware of the subtasks that the patient is unable to perform, but the therapist may not know what performance components (eg, standing balance, memory, and problem solving) are major limiting factors to performance of home management and caregiver tasks. Through clinical observation of the quality of performance and approach to the task, the therapist needs to identify the performance component deficits interfering with task performance. Examples of assessments that evaluate performance areas are the Kohlman Evaluation of Living Skills (McCourtney, 1979) and the RIC Complex ADL Assessment Protocol (1990).

The second type of home management evaluation examines the performance components, such as standing balance and memory, required to perform complex ADL. With this type of evaluation tool, the therapist must clinically solve problems associated with the relation between the patient's apparent deficits and their impact on the performance of home management and caregiver tasks. An example of this second type of assessment is the Bay Area Functional Performance Evaluation (Bloomer & Williams, 1987). The Assessment of Motor and Process Skills (Fisher, 1991) is an example of an assessment tool that evaluates both the occupational therapy performance areas and the performance components.

The final types of assessment are the self-report questionnaire and structured interview. With both these assessments, the therapist relies on the patient to report ADL status. This may vary considerably from actual performance observed by the therapist.

TABLE 8-4.   *Complex ADL Evaluation Formats: Advantages and Disadvantages*

Format	Advantages	Disadvantages
Direct observation of specific behaviors (standardized or nonstandardized)	Most direct means of assessing functional performance	Costly due to professional time and judgment required to administer assessment
	Reliable and valid scores obtained when tests are standardized or protocol defined	Presence of examiner may impact results
	Can detect faulty or unsafe methods easily	Standardized tests are not designed for natural environments
	Can result in determining underlying components that affect task performance	Nonstandardized observation is a more subjective method of assessment; considered less reliable and valid as compared with criterion-referenced assessments
	With clinical or with nonstandardized observation, areas assessed can more accurately reflect patient lifestyle	With the nonstandardized observation, the therapist's experience/skill may affect interpretation of task performance
Self-report questionnaire	Can be used when observation is not allowed by patient or not needed because patient is reliable reporter	May not accurately reflect patient performance
	Least expensive means of gathering data	
	Patient satisfaction assessment recognizes that patient's perspective on quality of life is useful criterion for establishing treatment goals	
Structured interview	Can be used when observation is not allowed by patient or not needed because patient is reliable reporter	Interview/interviewer variation
	Increased reliability if training of interviewer done	Patient status (confused or communication difficulties) lowers reliability
	Less costly as compared with direct observation methods	
Performance component assessment	Means of obtaining more accurate information on status of performance component, which can effect functional performance	May not accurately reflect patient performance of complex ADL
		Costly due to professional time and judgment required to administer assessment

An example of a self-report questionnaire is the Satisfaction with Performance Scaled Questionnaire (Yerxa et al., 1988). The Functional Life Scale (Sarno, Sarno, & Levita, 1973) is an example of a structured interview.

Selected complex ADL assessments have been included in this section. Note that the focus, content, format, population, and amount of tool development (validity and reliability) vary with each instrument.

The Kohlman Evaluation of Living Skills (McCourtney, 1979) is designed to evaluate a psychiatric patient's ability to function safely and independently in the community. It examines six areas, including self-care, safety and health, money management, use of transportation and telephone, work, and leisure. The 18-item assessment is standardized and is a combination of interview and task performance. The ratings include whether the patient is independent or requires assistance in a selected area. The score obtained indicates whether the patient is capable of living in the community independently. This tool can be used with outpatient, long-term care, adolescent, and geriatric populations. Limited research data support the conclusion that the evaluation is reliable and valid.

The Bay Area Functional Performance Evaluation (Bloomer & Williams, 1987) is a standardized instrument designed to assess the performance components required for ADL. The evaluation consists of a preassessment interview and a task-oriented assessment, including sorting shells, money and marketing task, home drawing task, block design, kinetic person drawing, and a social interaction scale. Based on task performance, the therapist gains information about cognitive, affective, and performance functions. Each task is rated on a four-point rating scale, with specific qualitative criteria for each functional parameter of the task. The patient's social interaction is rated in five settings: one-to-one, mealtime, unstructured group, structured activity group, and structured verbal group. The areas rated include verbal communication, psychomotor behavior, socially appropriate behavior, response to authority figures, independence and dependence, ability to work with others, and participation in group or program activities. In addition, the evaluation includes an optional patient self-assessment of social behavior to assess patient insight into interactions with others. Substantial research suggests good reliability and consistent validity.

The Assessment of Motor and Process Skills (AMPS; Fisher, 1989; K. Bryze, personal communication, September 1991) is a criterion-referenced, objective, performance-based evaluation. AMPS allows for the simultaneous evaluation of complex ADL task performance in addition to the underlying motor and adaptive and organizational performance components necessary to those tasks. Motor skills include the performance components related to posture, mobility, coordination, and strength. Process skills include the attention, conceptual, organizational, and adaptive capacities required for task completion. The motor and process skills have been operationally defined and are scored on a four-point rating scale. Refer to Figure 8-4 for a sample of the rating and performance components assessed. A unique attribute of AMPS is that the patient chooses to perform 2 to 3 activities from a list of 31 complex ADL tasks. Examples of tasks include making a peanut butter and jelly sandwich; fixing eggs, toast, and coffee; and potting a plant. The task must be familiar to the patient and must require functional mobility. Fisher (1991) recognized that the complexity of instrumental ADL tasks varied, as did the raters' scoring of patient performance. Through the Rasch method of analysis, both these issues have been resolved.

Task selection and rater scoring have been calibrated in terms of task difficulty to allow the therapist to predict patient performance on complex ADL tasks in areas other than those assessed in addition to recalibrating scoring to account for therapist differences (leniency) in scoring. This instrument has been used with many populations, including adult psychiatric patients, adults with developmental disabilities, older adults (community living, frail, and well-elderly), and adults with orthopedic (arthritis and hip fracture) and neurologic deficits (cerebrovascular accident, CVA). Preliminary evidence of validity and reliability has been demonstrated with numerous populations (K. Bryze, personal communication, September 1991).

The Occupational Therapy Functional Assessment Compilation Tool (OTFACT; Smith, 1990) is designed to organize and document occupational therapy assessment results to generate a functional profile of the patient. OTFACT is designed to be hierarchic in nature and yields information about role balance, functional activities of performance, including personal care and occupational role–related activities (eg, home management), functional skills of performance (eg, motor integration skills, sensory integration skills), and the underlying components of performance (eg, neuromuscular components, cognitive components) in addition to the impact environment has on these components. Categories included in the area of home management are home acquisition, menu planning, care of clothing, cleaning, household repair and maintenance, household safety, and yard work. Other areas related to the role of home maintainer include consumer activities (purchasing and money management activities) and caregiving activities (physical and emotional nurturing activities). Each category is rated on a four-point scale defined in terms of no deficit, partial deficit, total deficit, and not examined. If a category receives a rating lower than no deficit, then subtasks required to perform the task are rated. As an example, under the category of cleaning are subtasks such as getting supplies, using supplies, and completing cleaning. If the rating for the category of cleaning is lower than a no deficit rating, then each subtask is rated. This built-in decision-tree structure is a key feature of this system and requires that the therapist report additional data only for areas in which deficiencies are noted. Once the subtasks receive a rating, the percentage of ability in that category is determined. The therapist continues in this manner, reporting status of the patient's integration skills and performance components. OTFACT integrates and reports the full range of functional performance, including both performance components and task performance. Thus, this approach aids the therapist in identifying the relation between occupational performance role deficits and performance components; it also aids in treatment planning. It can be applied to a wide range of patient groups, ranging from inpatient rehabilitation to mental health programs and home health care. Since OTFACT is a reporting mechanism, it offers no protocol for gathering information about patients. Although available in a paper-and-pencil version, the complexity of the system lends itself to the computerized version.

The RIC Functional Assessment Scale (RIC, 1991) is a seven-point rating scale that is used along with a protocol to assess physically disabled patients' proficiency in complex ADL tasks. It is recognized that normal adults have varied lifestyles and responsibilities in the area of home and family management. It is believed that an assessment and protocol are needed to capture the differences in a patient's lifestyle. The eight categories are

(Text continues on page 216)

AMPS SHORT SCORING FORM

DEMOGRAPHIC DATA

CLIENT:_____   EXAMINER:_____

TASK:_____   TASK#:_____

AGE:_____ DIAGNOSIS:_____

RACE: ___ WHITE ___ BLACK ___ HISPANIC ___ ASIAN ___ NATIVE AMERICAN

SEX: ___ MALE ___ FEMALE

AMPS MANUAL VERSION USED FOR SCORING: _____

OBSERVATION FORMAT: ___ DIRECT OBSERVATION   DATE:_____

                    ___ OBSERVATION OF VIDEOTAPE   DATE:_____

ADAPTIVE EQUIPMENT: ___ WHEELCHAIR ___ CANE ___ WALKER

___ OTHER (SPECIFY) _____

SETTING: ___ HOME/RESIDENCE ___ CLINIC

DEVIATIONS FROM SPECIFIED TASK: _____

OBSERVATION TASK NUMBER: ___ ONE ___ TWO ___ THREE ___ OTHER

CONSIDERING EVERYTHING YOU KNOW ABOUT THE CLIENT, HOW WOULD YOU JUDGE THE CLIENT'S OVERALL FUNCTIONAL ABILITY?

___ THE CLIENT CAN/COULD LIVE INDEPENDENTLY IN THE COMMUNITY

___ THE CLIENT NEEDS MINIMAL ASSISTANCE/SUPERVISION TO LIVE IN THE COMMUNITY

___ THE CLIENT NEEDS MODERATE TO MAXIMAL ASSISTANCE OR IS UNABLE TO LIVE IN THE COMMUNITY

AMPS SCORE SHEET

COMPETENT = 4   QUESTIONABLE = 3   INEFFECTIVE = 2   DEFICIT = 1

POSTURE

Stabilizes	4 3 2 1
Aligns	4 3 2 1
Positions	4 3 2 1

MOBILITY

Walks	4 3 2 1
Reaches	4 3 2 1
Bends	4 3 2 1

COORDINATION

Coordinates	4 3 2 1
Manipulates	4 3 2 1
Flows	4 3 2 1

STRENGTH AND EFFORT

Moves	4 3 2 1
Transports	4 3 2 1
Lifts	4 3 2 1
Calibrates	4 3 2 1
Grips	4 3 2 1

ENERGY

Endures	4 3 2 1
Paces	4 3 2 1
Attends	4 3 2 1

USING KNOWLEDGE

Chooses	4 3 2 1
Uses	4 3 2 1
Handles	4 3 2 1
Heeds	4 3 2 1
Inquires	4 3 2 1
Notices	4 3 2 1

TEMPORAL ORGANIZATION

Initiates	4 3 2 1
Continues	4 3 2 1
Sequences	4 3 2 1
Terminates	4 3 2 1

SPACE AND OBJECTS

Searches	4 3 2 1
Gathers	4 3 2 1
Organizes	4 3 2 1
Restores	4 3 2 1

ADAPTATION

Accommodates	4 3 2 1
Adjusts	4 3 2 1
Navigates	4 3 2 1
Benefits	4 3 2 1

FIGURE 8-4. *Rating and performance components of the Assessment of Motor and Process Skills (AMPS.) (From Fisher, A. G. [1991]. Assessment of motor and process skills [6th research ed.] Unpublished test manual. Chicago, IL: University of Illinois at Chicago, Department of Occupational Therapy.)*

AMPS SCORE SHEET

COMPETENT	QUESTIONABLE	INEFFECTIVE	DEFICIT
Competent performance that supports the action progression and yields good outcomes: Examiner observes no evidence of a deficit	Questionable performance that places the action progression at risk and yields uncertain outcomes: Examiner questions the presence of a deficit	Ineffective performance that interferes with the action progression and yields undesirable outcomes: Examiner observes a mild to moderate deficit	Deficit performance that impedes the action progression and yields unacceptable outcomes: Examiner observes a severe deficit (risk of damage, danger, or task breakdown)

POSTURE

Stabilizes   4 3 2 1

Aligns   4 3 2 1

Positions   4 3 2 1

MOBILITY

Walks   4 3 2 1

Reaches   4 3 2 1

Bends   4 3 2 1

COORDINATION

Coordinates   4 3 2 1

Manipulates   4 3 2 1

Flows   4 3 2 1

STRENGTH AND EFFORT

Moves   4 3 2 1

Transports   4 3 2 1

Lifts   4 3 2 1

Calibrates   4 3 2 1

Grips   4 3 2 1

FIGURE 8-4 (*Continued*)

meal preparation and clean-up, clothing care, cleaning, household maintenance, emergency procedures and household safety, money management, community skills, and care of others (child, older parent, or spouse). Each category is designed to be hierarchic in nature and reflects increasingly complex performance (ie, meal preparation contains levels ranging from self-serve meal preparation through multicourse, hot meal preparation). Since it is hierarchic in nature, it is assumed that the patient is capable of performing tasks within the lower levels. The protocol includes descriptions of subtasks to be assessed at each level, in addition to an activity analysis (see the display), which allows a therapist to examine the performance components that could be affecting patient performance. The instrument is considered to have face validity because there is evidence supporting occupational therapy concern with these tasks (Bloomer & Williams, 1987; Sarno et al., 1973). The advantages of the higher level ADL protocol is that it recognizes differences in a patient's lifestyle and allows a mechanism to incorporate these differences into a system for evaluation, goal setting, and treatment planning. Its reliability needs to be examined in terms of home maintainer and caregiver tasks.

The Comprehensive Evaluation of Basic Living Skills (Casanova & Ferber, 1976) evaluates three groups of basic living skills: (1) personal care and hygiene, (2) performance of high-level ADL tasks, such as meal planning, preparation, and clean-up, shopping, telephone and transportation use, and (3) reading, writing, understanding time, money management, and math ability. The evaluation contains direct observation of patient performance and nursing report of basic self-care status. Items are rated on a four-point scale. The evaluation is designed for

---

REHABILITATION INSTITUTE OF CHICAGO GENERAL ACTIVITY ANALYSIS FORM

For all ADL tasks the following should be considered as appropriate.

Task: _____

A. Planning (structuring the task before performance)

	Y	N	Comments
Sequences task correctly			
Displays adequate time management skills			
Anticipates possible problems			
Generates alternative solutions			
Shows good organization			
Interacts with other appropriately			

B. Task performance includes (1) task preparation (ie, gathering needed materials), (2) performance, and (3) cleaning up and putting away materials.

	Y	N	Comments
Sequences task correctly			
Manages time effectively for task performance			
Solves problems that occur			
Shows good organization			
Shows good safety awareness			
Interacts with others appropriately			
Demonstrates adequate physical abilities to perform task			
Is able to			
Bend			_____ height
Reach			_____ height
Lift			_____ weight
Carry			_____ weight
Uses good body mechanics			
Shows adequate coordination			
Shows adequate strength			
Shows adequate endurance			_____ time

From the Rehabilitation Institute of Chicago Occupational Therapy Department, 1990.

chronic psychiatric patients and can take up to 8 hours to administer. No reliability or validity data is provided by the authors.

The Functional Life Scale (Sarno et al., 1973) is intended to measure the effects of a patient's impairments on his or her ability to participate in day-to-day activities at home rather than in a rehabilitation setting. The instrument contains 44 items distributed among five categories: cognition, ADL, activities in the home, outside activities, and social interaction. Each item is rated on five-point rating scale (0—does not perform the activity at all, 1—very poor, 2—deficient, 3—approaches normal, 4—normal) for parameters of self-initiation, frequency, speed, and overall efficiency (as appropriate). An interview format is used to obtain information about patient status. A small sample demonstrated preliminary reliability, internal consistency, and validity.

The Assessment of Older People's Self Maintenance and Instrumental Activities of Daily Living (Lawton & Brody, 1969) contains a physical self-maintenance scale and an instrumental ADL (IADL) scale. The IADL section includes use of phone, shopping, food preparation, housekeeping, laundry, use of transportation, taking medications, and ability to handle finances. The instrument is intended for use with the elderly and uses interview to gather information from patient, family, friends, or institute personnel, as appropriate. A four-point rating scale is used. The IADL tool demonstrated 0.85 interrater reliability on a small sample group and adequate validity to warrant using this measure with other instruments to examine functioning in elderly patients. These assessments were later incorporated into the Multilevel Assessment Instrument (Lawton, Moss, Fulcomer, & Kleban, 1982), which assesses the overall well-being of older people.

The Satisfaction with Performance Scaled Questionnaire (Yerxa et al., 1988) was designed to measure a patient's satisfaction with performance of independent living skills. These skills include 24 home management tasks, such as washing pots and pans and using a vacuum cleaner, and 9 social and community problem-solving tasks, such as socializing with other people and going to an interview. The five-point rating scale asks patients to specify the percentage of time in the last 6 months that they felt satisfied with the way they performed the tasks. The authors believe that looking at patients' perspectives on the quality of their own performance is a useful criterion for establishing treatment goals. Although developed for use with disabled community college students, the authors believe this tool can be used with patients working on community living skills in settings such as outpatient hospital programs, independent living centers, schools, and home health care agencies. The authors also believe that the instrument has content validity and high reliability.

Goal setting for home management and caregiver tasks

After completing the assessment of complex ADL tasks pertinent to the patient's lifestyle and related performance components, the therapist can identify patient strengths and the factors that interfere with performance of home maintainer and caregiver tasks. Goals are then written to address factors that interfere with complex ADL performance. Goals are a prediction of the patient's functional status after therapeutic intervention. Goals can reflect either upgraded performance in complex ADL tasks or subtasks (eg, "the patient will perform three light homemaking tasks with minimal assistance") or upgraded performance in components required for complex ADL performance (eg, "the patient will demonstrate adequate cognitive ability to perform self-serve meal preparation independently," or "the patient will use the right upper extremity as a stabilizer consistently during meal preparation"). Goals should be functional, measurable, and objective. To be considered a functional goal, the outcome behavior needs to focus on occupational therapy–related areas—in this case, home maintainer or caregiver tasks.

To determine if the goal is observable, a pertinent question is whether another person could determine whether the goal was met. For example, "the patient will understand work simplification techniques for meal preparation" is not an observable behavior, but "the patient will incorporate three work simplification techniques during meal preparation" is an observable behavior. Objective or measurable criteria should be set for goal attainment. Examples of measurable criteria include

- the amount of physical assistance or supervision and cueing required for task performance (eg, minimal supervision implies that the patient performs three quarters of task safely and consistently and that the caregiver needs to provide physical or verbal assistance to complete one quarter of the task)
- the amount of time it takes the patient to perform the task (eg, patient completes three light housekeeping tasks within one half hour)
- the number of times a behavior is performed (eg, patient uses right upper extremity as a stabilizer three times during meal preparation)

The goal should include any conditions or modifications that must be present to obtain optimal performance. The following are some examples of conditions and modifications:

- The type of assistance (physical, cueing, written handout) required to perform the task reflects necessity of caregiver or therapist involvement in promoting patient function.
- The type of environment (nonstimulatory, multistimulatory, wheelchair-accessible) indicates whether environmental modifications are required to maximize patient functioning.
- Special techniques allow a patient to perform a task in a modified manner that maximizes function to perform complex ADL (one-handed strategies for CVA patients, memory compensation techniques for head-injury patients), improves quality of performance, or prevents disability (energy conservation, adherence to medical precautions such as hip precautions to prevent injury to the hip before healing).

Adaptive equipment compensates for impaired abilities and maximizes ADL independence. As an example, an adapted cutting board or rocker knife allows for performance of meal preparation by a stroke patient who has the use of only one hand to perform ADL tasks. Patient diagnosis and functional limitations relate to the selection of adaptive techniques and equipment.

The following are some examples of goals specifying conditions or modifications:

- The patient will prepare a two-course hot meal independently *using adaptive equipment*.

• The patient will incorporate *joint protection strategies consistently* during light homemaking tasks.

Using home and family management tasks as therapeutic treatment media

Home and family management tasks can be used as an occupational therapy tool in several different ways:

1. To upgrade performance component skills. A treatment medium identified as an interest area of the patient can be used to help the patient to improve performance component deficits. For example, if a patient needs or wants to cook or do laundry, then these tasks could be used to improve performance components, such as visual scanning, by finding objects in kitchen cabinets or at the grocery store, or standing tolerance, by cooking in the kitchen or doing laundry.
2. To determine if the patient can improve the quality of ADL performance by incorporating use of adaptive equipment or techniques; for example, using work simplification techniques during a cleaning task or using an adapted cutting board during a cooking task.
3. As a performance outcome measure. After using occupational therapy intervention strategies, the therapist reevaluates patient performance to determine whether patient performance has been upgraded. For example, if the patient previously required moderate assistance to perform two-course, hot meal preparation and now requires minimal assistance to perform the same task, then this indicates that occupational therapy intervention was successful.

Occupational therapy intervention strategies for home and family management

Treatment plans contain goals and activities or strategies that the therapist uses to achieve those goals. There are four types of intervention strategies that can be used with patients demonstrating deficits in the area of home management and caregiver responsibilities. The options for intervention include:

1. Remediation of deficits
2. Compensation for performance component deficits or task performance deficits
3. Environmental modifications
4. Education of patient or family to support the above approaches or as a means of preventing problems

Remediation

The focus of remediation is to improve or restore the patient's functional performance and performance components. (Refer to Table 8-2 in Chapter 8, Section 1, for suggested remediation strategies for performance component deficits.) This approach is used when a patient's condition or diagnosis (eg, generalized weakness, acute arthritis) or performance component deficits are likely to improve adequately to allow for task performance. As an example, a therapist may use a biomechanical approach to improve range of motion in the shoulder of an arthritic patient to allow the patient to perform meal preparation tasks, such as reaching into a cabinet for cooking supplies or dishes. Various parameters need to be considered when grading activities and measuring the effectiveness of treatment using a remediation approach. These parameters include the following:

Physical assistance. There should be an inverse correlation between the amount of ability demonstrated by the patient and the amount of assistance provided by the therapist or caregiver. Therefore, as a patient displays increased skill in completing a task, the therapist or caregiver should intervene less frequently.

Supervision and cueing can include the number of cues given in addition to the types (written materials, tactile and verbal cues) used. Written materials (booklets, handouts, written home programs with illustrations or pictures) can be used to reinforce teaching that has occurred during occupational therapy treatment. Tactile cues can be used effectively to modify or guide patient performance (eg, touch lower back of patient to obtain a more upright standing posture while vacuuming, or guide a stroke patient to use an involved arm to reach for a glass in a cabinet). Verbal cues include both direct and indirect cues. For example, while on a community outing to the grocery store, a direct cue provides the patient with a specific instruction, such as, "the spaghetti is here," as the therapist points to the aisle where spaghetti is located. An indirect cue provides assistance to the patient in a less directive manner, such as, "can you find the foods listed on you grocery list?"

Task demands (ie, the amount of cognitive and physical skill required to perform the task) affect quality of patient performance. In selecting the type of task, consider the complexity of performance skills demanded by the task. As a general rule, with neurologically involved patients, it is better to select a task with inverse cognitive and motor demands (Chapparo, 1979); that is, with low motor and high cognitive demands or with high motor and low cognitive demands, and then progress to increasing levels of both. As an example, for a stroke patient, participating in a community outing is an activity that requires high cognitive demand. In addition, the patient's mobility may become compromised. Thus, the patient may ambulate for a short amount of time, but as the quality of the patient's gait decreases, the patient may need to complete the community outing in a wheelchair. Increasing the number of steps or tasks that a patient needs to participate in can be indicative of increased proficiency. When using the RIC protocol, the task of meal preparation is graded from a self-serve meal to a multicourse hot meal. The protocol indicates the number of added skills required to safely and efficiently fix a multicourse hot meal. Cognitive tasks can be graded from routine familiar to unfamiliar or new. As an example, it is less demanding for a patient to cook a familiar recipe from memory than to follow a new recipe from a cookbook. A motor task performed from a seated position is less demanding than a task performed from a standing position or from a hands-and-knees position for an activity like scrubbing a floor. The amount of structure that needs to be provided for task performance can vary. The lowest level of patient performance is reflected in a situation in which all the organization and structuring of the environment for task performance is provided by the therapist; for example, for meal preparation, the therapist may obtain food for cooking and list step-by-step instructions for the patient to follow. The highest level of patient performance is in an unstructured situation in which the patient has total responsibility for organizing task performance and in which environmental conditions are not altered; for example, the patient has to deal with numerous interruptions and distractions while performing the task, such as conversing with the therapist, or with unanticipated occurrences, like burning food while cooking.

Environment plays a role in task performance. A familiar environment (eg, kitchen at home) is less demanding than a new environment (eg, clinic kitchen). In addition, the type of stimulation can vary from a quiet, nondistracting environment, such as a room with no noise or other people, to a distracting, busy environment, such as the community. For patients in wheelchairs, lack of wheelchair accessibility can prohibit the patient's ability to access services (banks, restaurants, stores) in the community.

By altering the various parameters, an activity can be upgraded or downgraded to provide a difficult but not overwhelming challenge that results in a failure experience for the patient.

Compensation

The compensation approach focuses on the use of remaining abilities to achieve the highest level of functioning possible in the areas of home and family management. If the patient cannot perform these tasks in the usual manner, then adapted techniques or equipment are used to maximize patient abilities. This strategy can be used when a patient's condition is temporary, such as for hip replacement, when precautions need to taken, when the condition is not amenable to remediation, or when task speed and proficiency are greatly improved by use of adaptive equipment or adaptive techniques. Use of adaptive techniques is preferable to use of equipment because techniques allow the patient more flexibility. Use of adaptive equipment is less preferable due to the cost incurred for purchase and maintenance and the inconvenience of having to transport the equipment for task performance. Table 8-5 outlines specific adaptive equipment and techniques that can be used for various impairments (Trombly, 1983; Hopkins & Smith, 1988; Pedretti, 1990; Klinger, 1978).

Energy conservation and work simplification techniques can be used with a number of physically disabled patients (Trombly, 1983; Hopkins & Smith, 1988; Pedretti, 1990; RIC, 1988; American Heart Association, date unknown). Because of a patient's disability, tasks may take much longer and require excessive amounts of energy. Therefore, these techniques are useful to incorporate into treatment. These techniques require that the therapist and patient address the following points:

1. Determine what tasks need to be improved, that is, according to the patient, what tasks take too long, cause fatigue, or take too much energy.
2. List all the steps of the task, including set-up, performance, and clean-up.
3. Analyze the task.
    a. Why is the task necessary?
    b. What is the purpose of the task?
    c. When and where should it be done?
    d. What is the best way for the patient to get it done?
4. Develop a new method of performing the task. Consider eliminating unnecessary steps, combining motions and activities, rearranging the sequence of the steps, and simplifying the details of the task by taking the following steps:
    a. Use correct work height to reduce fatigue and promote good posture. Correct work height in standing should be 2 inches below the bent elbow; in sitting, patient should avoid positions that require lifting the shoulders or "winging out" the elbows.
    b. Preposition supplies and equipment in work areas. Clear area of unnecessary items. As an example, to pay bills, obtain needed supplies, such as calculator, bills, and stamps, before beginning task.
    c. Organize work center. Having necessary supplies and equipment increases productivity with less effort. In kitchen, place the can opener near the canned goods. Place the most frequently used items within easy reach on counters or shelves immediately above or below counter height.
    d. Use labor-saving devices. This includes using wheels for transport; in the kitchen, using electric appliances, such as an electric mixer and food processor; for outdoors, using an electric garage door opener and self-propelled lawn mower. Transport heavy objects using wheels.
    e. Fatigue can result in poor body mechanics and reduced safety awareness. Regular rest breaks should be incorporated into the patient's schedule. The patient should alternate light and heavy tasks throughout the day and week. Heavy work tasks like cleaning the oven, stripping and waxing floors, or doing yard work should be delegated to another family member or done by a professional cleaning service.
    f. Use proper body mechanics. This includes use of a wide base of support, using both sides of the body and keeping objects close to the body, facing objects when reaching or lifting to avoid twisting, pushing rather than pulling objects, and alternating positions and motions to avoid fatigue.
5. Implement new methods.

Environmental modifications

Environmental modifications are considered a compensatory strategy. Compared with remediation and compensation, in which the therapist directly impacts patient functioning, the environment is seen as a means of indirectly maximizing patient function. This can range from extensive home modifications to make a home wheelchair-accessible, to low-cost strategies such as removing obstacles to make a household safer for an older person who has impaired vision and mobility. Additional information about this topic is included in Chapter 9, Section 6.

Education of patient and family members

The final type of occupational therapy intervention strategy is patient and family education. This is a key component to the occupational therapy treatment plan because the approaches of remediation, compensation, and prevention involve learning

(*Text continues on page 223*)

TABLE 8-5. *Adaptive Equipment and Techniques for Home and Family Management Activities*

ADL Area	Adaptive Equipment	Adaptive Techniques

Impairment

One upper-extremity or body side impairment

Common Diagnoses Resulting in This Impairment

Hemiplegia (cerebrovascular accident [CVA] or head injury), unilateral trauma or amputation, temporary conditions such as burns and peripheral neuropathy.

Rationale for Using Compensatory Strategies

To allow for safe, one-handed performance; to stabilize objects for task completion; with hemiplegia, to compensate for loss of balance and mobility

ADL Area	Adaptive Equipment	Adaptive Techniques
Meal preparation and clean-up	To stabilize objects, consider use of: • Adapted cutting board with stainless steel or aluminum nails for cutting or peeling food. Raised corners on the board can stabilize bread to spread ingredients or make a sandwich. • Sponge clothes, dycem or suction devices to stabilize bowls or dishes during food preparation • Pot stabilizer To allow for safe, one-handed performance, consider use of: • Adapted jar openers • Electric appliances such as food processor and hand mixer save time and energy. Note: patient safety and judgment need to be considered when electrical appliances are considered. • Rocker knife • Whisk to mix food To compensate for decreased standing tolerance and mobility, consider use of: • Utility cart to transport objects • If cooking is done at wheelchair level or seated, use angled mirror over the stove to watch food on the stove. For clean-up, consider use of: • Hand-held spray for rinsing dishes • Rubber mat at bottom of sink to reduce breakage • Suction-type brush to clean glassware	If balance is affected, it is recommended that the task be done in a seated position. • Objects can be stabilized by using the knees. • Pots and pans can be slid across counters rather than lifted. • To open a jar, place it in a drawer, then lean against it to stabilize it before opening. • Scissors can be used to open plastic bags. • Milk cartons can be opened by using the pronged portion of a fork. • An egg can be cracked by holding it in the palm of the hand, hitting the egg against the edge of the bowl, and separating the egg shell with the index and middle fingers. For clean-up: • Soak and air-dry dishes for easier clean-up.
Clothing management (hand laundry, machine laundry, ironing, and repair)	Laundry can be transported to and from the washer and dryer using a wheeled cart.	Incorporate energy conservation and work simplification into task. Can this be delegated to another member of the family or sent out to be done? Small loads are easier to handle.
Housecleaning	• A tank-type vacuum permits the client to sit and reach areas to be cleaned. • Long-reach duster • Long-handled dustpan and brush • Self-wringing mop	• Incorporate energy conservation by making bed up completely at each corner before progressing to the next corner. • No-wax floors are easier to care for. • If balance or ambulation problems are present, some floor care can be managed from a seated position.
Child care	For feeding use: • High chairs with one-handed tray release mechanism • Electric baby dish keeps food warm during the meal. • Tongs can be used to remove baby food from heated water. • Use screw top rather than plastic liner bottles. For bathing: • Strap the baby into a suction-based bath seat. For dressing: • Use a Velcro strap on dressing table to reduce squirming. • Use disposable diapers with tab closures. For transporting child: • Use a backpack child carrier (if balance is adequate).	For feeding, prop the infant on pillows, in an infant seat, or against arm of an upholstered chair. For bathing: • Turn on cold water before hot water. • Dry the baby off before lifting the baby onto another towel. For dressing: • Dressing can be done most safely on the floor. For transporting: • Carry the child on the hip on the side with the functional arm.

Impairment

Reduced upper-extremity range of motion and strength

(continued)

TABLE 8-5. *Adaptive Equipment and Techniques for Home and Family Management Activities (continued)*

ADL Area	Adaptive Equipment	Adaptive Techniques

Common Diagnoses Resulting in This Impairment

Quadriplegia, burns, arthritis, upper-extremity amputation, multiple sclerosis, amyotrophic lateral sclerosis, orthopedic and other traumatic injuries.

Rationale for Using Compensatory Strategies

To compensate for lack of reach or hand grip; to compensate for lack of strength or tolerance for prolonged activity; to allow gravity to assist; to compensate for decreased balance

ADL Area	Adaptive Equipment	Adaptive Techniques
Meal preparation and clean-up	Consider the use of: • Adapted jar opener • Foam or built-up handles on utensils • Universal cuff to hold utensils to compensate for reduced grip • Long-handled reacher to obtain lightweight objects from overhead or low places • Wheeled cart to transport objects • Adapted cutting board • Loop handles can be added to utensils to substitute for reduced grasp. • If using a walker, a walker basket can help to transport objects. For marketing: • Marketing by phone or mail is recommended since many objects may be out of reach.	• Joint protection measures for rheumatoid arthritis • Position electrical appliances within easy reach. This helps to conserve energy. • To conserve energy, work at a seated position. • Use teeth to open containers. • Purchase convenience foods to eliminate food preparation. • Tenodesis action (wrist extension and finger flexion; wrist flexion and finger extension) can be used to pick up lightweight objects. • Use a fork to open milk cartons. • Use lightweight pots, pans, and utensils.
Housecleaning	• Long-handled reacher allows for objects to be picked up from the floor. • Long-handled sponge to clean bath tub • Self-wringing mop • Use lightweight tools such as sponge mops and brooms for floor care.	• Use aerosol cleaners to dissolve dirt before cleaning surfaces. • When making the bed, do *not* tuck sheets in.
Laundry	• If patient is ambulatory, the preference is for a top-loading washer to avoid the need to bend. • Push-button controls on the washer and dryer are easier to use than knobs. If knobs are present, they may need to be adapted. • If patient chooses to iron, set iron at a low temperature setting. An asbestos pad can be placed at the end of the ironing board to eliminate the need to stand iron up after each ironing stroke.	• Use premeasured packages of soap or bleach to avoid handling large containers. It may be more economical to buy larger containers and have someone else measure soap or bleach into single packets. • Use energy conservation: Place hangers near dryer to hang permanent press items as they come out of the dryer. Remain seated to do ironing.
Child care	• If patient lacks mobility to get up and down from the floor, then a crib with a swing open side allows the mother in a wheelchair to wheel close to the baby. An ambulatory mother can sit on the crib mattress. • Feeding can be done with the child in an infant seat or propped up on pillows. • An electric baby dish can be placed in a convenient area and keep food warm throughout the meal. • Formula can be prepared by another family member and placed in bottles for use during the day. • Clothing should be large with closures that are easily handled. • Disposable diapers with tabs are easily manipulated.	Use energy conservation: • Have client do the more enjoyable tasks, delegate other tasks to a helper. • The safest place to handle an infant is on the floor, if the client can get up and down from the floor. All tasks, including sponge bathing, dressing, feeding and playing, can be done on the floor. • A method to obtain assistance in an emergency needs to be determined.

Impairment

Incoordination of upper extremities

Common Diagnoses Resulting in This Impairment

Head injury, cerebral palsy, CVA, multiple sclerosis, tumors, other neurologic conditions

Rationale for Using Compensatory Strategies

To stabilize proximal portion of limbs; to reduce movements distally by using weight; to stabilize objects for task completion; to provide a safe environment in which patient is safe and proficient; to avoid breakage or accidents with sharp utensils or hot food or equipment

(continued)

TABLE 8-5. *Adaptive Equipment and Techniques for Home and Family Management Activities (continued)*

ADL Area	Adaptive Equipment	Adaptive Techniques

Rationale for Using Compensatory Strategies

ADL Area	Adaptive Equipment	Adaptive Techniques
Meal preparation and clean-up	• Use heavy cookware, ironstone dishes to aid with distal stabilization. • Use pots and casserole dishes with double handles to provide greater stability. • Weighted wrist cuffs may reduce tremors. • Use nonslip materials such as dycem to provide stability. • Use adapted cutting board to stabilize food while cutting. • A serrated knife is less likely to slip than a straight-edged knife. • Using a frying basket to cook foods such as vegetable makes for safe removal and reduces chance of burns. • Free-standing appliances, electric skillet, and counter top mixer, are safer than transferring objects out of oven or using hand-held mixer. • Use a milk carton holder with handles to pour milk. • A stove with front controls is preferred so the patient does not need to reach over hot pots to the back of the stove. • A wheeled cart that is weighted is one alternative for transporting food. • Place a rubber mat or sponge cloth at the bottom of the sink to cushion fall of dishes.	• During food preparation, such as cutting and peeling, stabilize arms proximally to reduce tremors. • Start the stove after the food has been placed on the burner. • Sliding food and dishes over a counter is preferable to lifting to transport food item. • To avoid breakage, soak dishes, rinse with hand sprayer and drip dry—eliminate dish handling.
Housecleaning	• Heavier work tools are useful. A dust mitt is easier to handle than gripping a duster. • Fitted sheets on a bed are recommended.	• Eliminate excess household decorations or store to reduce dusting.
Laundry		• Premeasured soap and bleach eliminates spills that can occur during measuring. • Eliminate ironing through selection of no-iron clothing and materials.
Child care	• Use a wide safety strap on dressing table. • Use disposable, tape-tab diapers. • Use Velcro closures for infant clothing. • Feeding with a spoon is recommended only if incoordination is mild.	With mild incoordination: • Use stabilizing measures such as holding upper arms close to body and sitting while working. • It is safer to work on the floor while caring for the infant.

Impairment

Mobility impairment without upper-extremity involvement

Common Diagnoses Resulting in This Impairment

Paraplegia, osteoarthritis, lower-extremity amputation, burns, leg and knee fractures and replacement

Rationale for Using Compensatory Strategies

Mobility may be provided by a wheelchair. Wheelchair accessibility includes consideration of work heights, maneuverability, and access to storage, equipment, and supplies.

Other types of mobility devices (walker, crutches) may require increased endurance. Note that making an environment wheelchair-accessible is addressed in Chapter 9, Sections 5 and 6.

ADL Area	Adaptive Equipment	Adaptive Techniques
Meal preparation and clean-up	• Transport items using a wheelchair laptray. The laptray can be used as a work surface to protect lap from hot pans. • Stove controls should be in the front of the stove. • Use an angled mirror to see the contents of pots.	• Remove cabinet doors to eliminate need to maneuver around them. • Place frequently used items on easy-to-reach shelves, above and below countertop level. • Increase height of wheelchair to allow use of standard-height countertops.
Laundry	• Use front-loading washer and dryer.	
Housekeeping	• Use self-propelled, lightweight vacuums.	
Child care	For feeding: • Use plastic baby bottles with liners to eliminate the need to sterilize bottles.	

(continued)

TABLE 8-5. *Adaptive Equipment and Techniques for Home and Family Management Activities* (*continued*)

ADL Area	Adaptive Equipment	Adaptive Techniques

Rationale for Using Compensatory Strategies

Child care (continued)

- Position the baby in an infant seat. The seat can be held or placed on a table.
- For high chairs, select a chair with a safety belt and a swing-away tray with one-hand release.

For a playpen:

- Use an adjustable-height, portable crib with a hinged door for easy access.

For lifting, carrying, and transporting:

- A converted, lightweight car bed with straps sewn on the side of the bed can be secured to the wheelchair armrests.
- With an older child (4 to 5 months old), touch-fastener seat belt can be attached to the wheelchair.
- Select stroller with the following features: Single handle to allow for one-handed steering, brakes, and opening and closing of stroller should be managed easily.
- Attach a safety strap from handle of stroller to waist of parent to prevent stroller from pulling away on an incline.

---

new strategies and, more important, incorporating these strategies into patient and family habits and lifestyles. In some circumstances, the therapist may provide education to the family in addition to patient education or in place of patient education. The following issues are central to effective patient and family education (Bowling, 1981; Kautzman, 1991):

- *Have a clear plan about the purpose of the teaching session.* An observable goal for teaching can assist both the therapist and patient regarding expectations and anticipated outcome. Based on patient and family motivation, cognitive status and skill level that need to be achieved, and time availability for the teaching and learning process, the expected outcomes or goals may vary. The three levels of goals include knowledge, application, and problem solving. At the level of knowledge, a patient is asked to recall basic facts presented by the therapist. For example, the therapist may ask a patient to name the five techniques used for good body mechanics. At the application level, the patient and family are shown ways of incorporating this information into complex ADL. For example, the therapist may demonstrate how to use body mechanics when retrieving food from the oven during performance of meal preparation and then ask the patient to incorporate the same strategy while performing the task. At the level of problem solving, the patient is asked to use information in new situations that have *not* been demonstrated by the therapist. For example, the therapist may ask the patient to demonstrate how to use good body mechanics when shoveling snow.
- *The presentation of information needs to be appropriate to the patient's educational and emotional levels.* The choice of terminology used with a patient who has had a few years of formal education should vary from that used with a patient who has a college education. Patient readiness to receive information will vary. The patient may be overwhelmed with life changes caused by the disability and unable to concentrate on issues that the therapist feels

needs to be addressed. Therefore, for a task that a patient may not be concerned with but that will be needed at home, the inpatient therapist may try to increase patient awareness by introducing appropriate adaptive equipment. Once the patient has returned home, the motivation to perform in this area may increase. Then the outpatient therapist can promote patient application and problem solving in the occupational therapy treatment.

- *Instructions must be clear.* Clear instructions increase the possibility of patient compliance. For example, instead of telling a patient to use proper body mechanics for all activities, it is preferable and more realistic to begin with having the patient identify one to two activities that require these techniques. The patient may need assistance to do this. Another strategy to increase compliance is to explain the rationale for the therapy recommendations.
- *Ask open-ended questions to ensure patient understanding.* For example: Why is it important for you to incorporate proper body mechanics into your day-to-day activities?
- *Use patient response to determine the amount of information presented during a session.* If the patient's attention is waning or if the patient's learning ability is decreased, termination of the teaching session is recommended. If the amount of information is extensive, it may be preferable to present it in a number of sessions. Taking the added time to ensure patient competence in performance is time well spent.
- *Promote the highest level of learning possible, preferably the problem-solving level.* Get patients involved by asking questions about how information presented might impact their lifestyles. For example, a therapist may ask of an arthritic patient: Which joint protection techniques do you think you would use at home? How could you use these techniques while cooking? It is preferable to follow this up with patient performance of the complex ADL task to ensure that the patient has integrated the information into pertinent ADL tasks.

- *Illustrate or demonstrate the points being taught.* Using aids such as demonstration, pictures, videotapes, and handouts reinforces teaching and helps the patient and family to remember the information presented. A study of patient–doctor visits found that only half of the information covered was remembered by the patient (Ley, 1972). Therefore, some of the ways of reinforcing teaching include repeating information throughout the session and allowing adequate time for practice by the patient or family members to ensure that they are comfortable with and capable of using the information outside the therapy situation. If the patient or family member cannot gain adequate competency or perform the task in a safe manner, then other options such as paid caregiver or identifying community supports (eg, Meals-on-Wheels, home health aide) need to be considered.

Child care

For patients who have responsibility for infants, it may be useful to use a life-sized, weighted doll to simulate caregiver tasks. A parent whose ability to perform caregiver tasks safely is questioned should be advised to find help to care for the child.

Home visits

Often the question arises about whether the patient will be safe at home. The purposes of a home visit are to assess patient level of functional independence and safety at home and to provide the patient and family with recommendations concerning accessibility, safety, and home modification. A home visit is best done by an occupational and physical therapist.

It is important to explain the purpose of the home visit to family and patient. During the home visit, the patient should complete activities that typically are performed at home, such as making a bed, transferring in and out of the tub, getting on and off the toilet, and fixing something in the kitchen. The tasks should be relevant to anticipated home responsibilities as well as to patient and family expectations.

The results of the home visit should be discussed with the patient and family. Recommendations are then written up to reinforce the discussion. (Refer to the display for a checklist of home recommendations for use with patient or family members. For patients who use a wheelchair as a chief means of mobility, a more individualized list of recommendations probably is required.) Recommendations may vary based on patient circumstances (eg, preferences, financial support). When a home visit is not feasible, obtaining information from the patient or family member regarding the discharge environment is a useful option.

Training apartment

A training apartment, available in the health care setting, can be used to simulate the experience of returning home and confronting issues that may arise. The time spent in a training apartment may range from individual treatment sessions 1 hour long to 1- to 2-night stays. Based on the anticipated circumstances, the patient and family members (if appropriate) can attempt personal care and home management tasks required after discharge. This provides an opportunity to identify areas in which the patient and family members feel comfortable and to identify issues that

need further consideration. The occupational therapist then can intervene appropriately in preparation of discharge to home.

Regaining community skills

Frequently, patients need to access the community for home management tasks, such as grocery shopping and banking, and for returning to work and leisure pursuits. Areas that need to be assessed include planning, money management, path finding, community safety, use of transportation, mobility, time management, and psychosocial issues, such as exhibiting problem solving to overcome obstacles and interpersonal skills for social interaction. Although a therapist may pursue evaluation and training on an individual basis with a patient, community reentry groups are another mechanism that can allow patients to discuss and practice community skills required on discharge from a structured setting. It is helpful if the group is interdisciplinary, with the focus of occupational therapy generally being on tasks and performance components required for successful transition into the community. Activities may include setting goals to promote learning, problem solving, and adjustment through interaction with others with similar disabilities; practicing skills and using equipment introduced in individual treatment; developing behaviors appropriate and acceptable in social situations; developing psychomotor skills adequate for safe community mobility; and planning and organizing daily routines using sound judgment, problem-solving memory, and compensatory strategies. The focus will vary based on patient diagnosis. For example, for a stroke patient whose major limiting factors are in the perceptual and cognitive area, therapy may focus on safe ambulation (looking both ways before crossing the street), ability to attend to a task in a busy environment (finding items on a grocery list), and problem solving (what to do when unable to locate a food item). On the other hand, for a patient with a spinal cord injury whose major limitations are physical, the focus may be on dealing with accessibility and managing personal care tasks in the community (eg, changing a leg bag).

Summary

The occupational therapist plays a key role in facilitating a patient's return to the roles of homemaker and caregiver, and normal adults have varied lifestyles and responsibilities in these two areas. The therapist needs to consider the patient's previous involvement in these roles, patient and family goals, and knowledge of patient condition to determine whether this is a realistic area of focus for the patient. Assessments of complex ADL function vary based on patient population, complex ADL areas addressed, format, and level of development as an assessment tool (standardized, unstandardized protocol). Formats include direct observation, interview, and self-report questionnaires, and each has advantages and disadvantages. Most assessment tools used in occupational therapy involve observation of performance. A valuable skill the therapist brings to this type of assessment is clinical observation, which provides insight into both the ability and the process used to perform tasks. This information then forms the basis of the occupational therapy treatment plan. Treatment intervention strategies include remediation, compensation, environmental modification, and education. The therapist selects the treatment strategies based on factors such as patient

HOME RECOMMENDATIONS CHECKLIST

Entrances

Primary

_____ Handrails: _____ right _____ left _____ both sides

_____ Physical assistance will be required to negotiate stairs

_____ Ramp (general recommendations for construction)
- Ramp length: 1 foot of ramp for 1 inch of stair height (eg, 6-inch steps equals 6-foot ramp)
- 2- to 3-inch lip along sides of ramp
- Nonskid runner
- Construct with sturdy, weather-resistant material (eg, treated lumber or concrete)

Secondary

_____ Handrails: _____ right _____ left

_____ Ramp

Kitchen

_____ Place utensils within reach, reorganize cabinets

_____ Remove all throw rugs

_____ Appropriate chair available for safe transfer (ie, chair of correct height with armrests and back support)

Living Room and Dining Room

_____ Appropriate chair available (armrests, back support, correct height)

_____ Modification in furniture placement as specified in additional recommendations

_____ Remote-control television

_____ Programmable and portable telephones

Bathroom

_____ Chair at sink

_____ Grooming items within reach

_____ Over-toilet commode seat

_____ Toilet safety rails: _____ right _____ left _____ both sides

_____ Raised toilet seat

_____ Hand-held shower message

_____ Remove glass shower doors and replace with shower curtain

_____ Nonskid mat in/outside tub/shower

_____ Chair in shower stall (as specified in additional recommendations)

_____ Chair in tub

_____ Use tub-transfer bench

_____ Install grab bars as specified

_____ Remove bathroom door and molding

Bedroom

_____ Have light available at bedside

_____ Have phone available at bedside

_____ Bedside commode

_____ Dowel in closet to enable person to reach clothes from wheelchair

_____ Hospital bed

_____ Side rails on regular bed

Additional Recommendations

Form developed by Occupational Therapists at L.W. Blake Hospital (L. Hankinson, OTR/L).

---

and family goals, patient condition, anticipated length of treatment, interdisciplinary goals and treatment (eg, if the physical therapist upgraded mobility device to a cane, the occupational therapy would incorporate use into performance of complex ADL tasks), and the therapist's professional judgment about skills needed to perform pertinent complex ADL tasks.

References

American Heart Association. (Date unknown). *Five step plan for work simplification* (Handout).

American Occupational Therapy Association (1989). Uniform terminology for occupational therapy (2nd ed.). *American Journal of Occupational Therapy, 43,* 808–814

Bloomer, J. S., & Williams, S. K. (1987). *The Bay Area functional performance of evaluation* (research ed.). Palo Alto, CA: Consulting Psychologists Press.

Bowling, B. (1981). *Effective patient education techniques for use with aging patients.* Lexington, KY: University of Kentucky.

Casanova, J., & Ferber, J. (1976). Comprehensive evaluation of basic living skills. *American Journal of Occupational Therapy, 30,* 101–105.

Chapparo, C. (1979). Sensory integration for adults. Workshop sponsored by Illinois Occupational Therapy Association, Glen Ellyn, Illinois.

Christiansen, C. (1991). Occupational performance assessment. In C. Christiansen & C. Baum (Eds.). *Occupational therapy—Overcoming human performance deficits.* Thorofare, NJ: Slack.

Fisher, A. G. (1991). *Assessment of motor and process skills* (6th research ed.). Unpublished test manual. Chicago, IL: University of Illinois at Chicago, Department of Occupational Therapy.

Hopkins, H., & Smith, H. (Eds.). (1983). *Willard and Spackman's Occupational Therapy* (6th ed.). Philadelphia: J. B. Lippincott.

Intagliata, S., & Sullivan, B. (1991). Development and implementation of the Rehabilitation Institute of Chicago Functional Assessment Scale. *Occupational Therapy Practice, 2,* 26–37

Kautzman, L. (1991). Facilitating adult learning in occupational therapy patient education programs. *Occupational Therapy Practice, 2,* 1–11.

Kielhofner, G., Henry, A., & Walens, D. (1989). *A user's guide to the occupational performance history interview.* Rockville, MD: American Occupational Therapy Association.

Klinger, J. (1978). *Mealtime manual for people with disabilities and the aging* (2nd ed.). Camden, NJ: Campbell Soup Company.

Law, M., & Letts, L. (1989). A critical review of scales of activities of daily living. *American Journal of Occupational Therapy, 43,* 522–528

Lawton, M. P., & Brody, E. (1969). Assessment of older people: Self maintaining and instrumental activities of daily living. *Gerontologist, 9,* 179–186

Lawton, M. P., Moss, M., Fulcomer, M., & Kleban, M. H. (1982). A research and service oriented multilevel assessment instrument. *Journal of Gerontology, 37,* 91–99.

Ley, P. (1972). Comprehension, memory and the success of communications with the patient. *Journal of Instructional Health Education, 10,* 23–29.

McCourtney, L. K. (1979). *Kohlman evaluation of living skills.* Seattle, WA: KELS Research.

Mosey, A. (1973). *Activities therapy.* New York: Raven Press.

Oakley, F. (1981). *Role checklist.* Presented at Workshop on Enhancing Clinical Effectiveness: Practical Application of the Model of Human Occupation. University of Illinois at Chicago, July 24 and 25, 1989.

Pedretti, L. (1990). *OT practice skills for physical dysfunction.* St. Louis: C. V. Mosby.

Rehabilitation Institute of Chicago Occupational Therapy Department (1988). *Work simplification/energy conservation principles* (handout). Chicago: RIC.

Rehabilitation Institute of Chicago Occupational Therapy Department (1990). *Complex ADL assessment protocol.* Unpublished manuscript. Chicago: RIC.

Rehabilitation Institute of Chicago Occupational Therapy Department (1991). *RIC revised functional assessment scale.* Chicago: RIC.

Sarno, J., Sarno, M., & Levita, E. (1973). The functional life scale. *Archives of Physical Medicine and Rehabilitation. 54,* 214–220.

Simon, S., Howe, L., & Kirschenbaum, H. (1972), *Values clarification: A handbook of pictorial strategies for teachers and students.* New York: Hart.

Smith, R. O. (1990). *Administration and scoring manual: Occupational therapy functional assessment compilation tool (OTFACT).* Rockville, MD: American Occupational Therapy Association.

Trombly, C. (Ed.). (1983). *Occupational therapy for physical dysfunction.* Baltimore: Williams & Wilkins.

Yerxa, E., Burnett-Beaulieu, S., Stocking, S., & Azon, S. (1988). Development of the satisfaction with performance scaled questionnaire (SPSQ). *American Journal of Occupational Therapy, 42,* 215–221.

SECTION 2B1
Work assessments and programming

KAREN JACOBS

KEY TERMS

Americans With Disabilities Act

Career Theories

Commission on Accreditation of Rehabilitation Facilities

Essential Functions of a Job

Job Coach

Job Site Evaluation

Methods-Time Measurement

On-The-Job Evaluation

Physical Demands

Postoffer Screening

Psychometric Instruments

Reasonable Accommodations

Rehabilitation Workshop

Situational Assessment

Supported Employment

Work

Work Adjustment

Work Aptitudes

Work Behaviors

Work Hardening

Work Sample

Work Skills

LEARNING OBJECTIVES

Upon completion of this section the reader will be able to:

1. *Discuss the history of work practice.*

2. *Explain essential functions of a job and reasonable accommodations as defined in the Americans With Disabilities Act.*

3. *List the processes used by occupational therapists in work assessments.*

4. *List four types of work evaluations.*

5. *Define on-the-job, or job site, evaluation.*

6. *Name two commercially available work samples.*

7. *List four criteria used in selecting a work evaluation.*

8. *Define supported employment.*

9. *Discuss the role of the job coach.*

10. *List three theories of career development.*

11. *Define work adjustment.*

12. *Define Methods-Time Measurements.*

13. *Define work.*

Joshua attends second grade. Ariel is an occupational therapist. Matthew is a retiree who seriously collects coins. Laela is a homemaker who volunteers twice a week at a local hospital gift shop. What these four people have in common is that they are all workers. "***Work*** includes all forms of productive activity, regardless of whether they are reimbursed" (Jacobs, 1991, p. 17). These human occupations—student, homemaker, hobbyist, volunteer—constitute work regardless of whether they are reimbursed. Work is not limited to adults but is relevant throughout the lifespan and can be applied to a broad range of people, from school-aged children with emotional or physical disabilities, to adults in rehabilitation facilities, to people with industrial injuries in a work capacity evaluation center, to disenfranchised older adults.

Two important elements constitute the concept of work: work behaviors and work skills, aptitudes, and physical capacities. **Work behaviors**, also referred to as *prevocational readiness*, are those behaviors that are necessary for successful participation in a job or independent living. They include but are not limited to cooperative behavior, attention span, decision making, motivation, attendance, acceptance of supervision, appropriate appearance, punctuality, responsibility, organization, and productivity. Work behaviors are the antecedents to specific work skill development. Work skills, aptitudes, and physical demands, frequently referred to as *vocational skills*, are required to perform the tasks of an actual job. More specifically, **work skills** are capabilities that the worker has learned or has the potential to learn, such as typing, welding, drafting, soldering, and cooking. **Work aptitudes** are abilities that are, to one degree or another, possessed by nearly all workers. They include coordination, dexterity, and intelligence.

Physical demands are factors defined in the *Selected Characteristics of Occupations Defined in the Dictionary of Occupational Titles* (U.S. Department of Labor, 1981). Seven physical demands—standing, walking, sitting, lifting, carrying, pushing, and pulling—are expressed in terms of five levels of strength:

S—sedentary
L—light work
M—medium work
H—heavy work
V—very heavy work

Other physical demands include climbing, balancing, stooping, kneeling, crouching, crawling, reaching, handling, fingering, feeling, talking, hearing, acuity (far), acuity (near), depth perception, visual accommodation, color vision, and field of vision. (U.S. Department of Labor, 1979).

History

The 1980s heralded a renewed interest in work practice, and this trend is predicted to continue into the 21st century. In particular, the areas of **work hardening** and ergonomics have come to the forefront in practice.

Environmental trends have provided a conducive climate for occupational therapy practitioners to become more involved in work practice. The following are some of these trends:

- Increased number of industrial injury cases
- Lack of adequate comprehensive services
- Escalating prohibitive costs of supporting injured workers
- Regulatory agency guidelines
- Workers' Compensation and Public Laws (eg, PL 101–336 and PL 94–142; Jacobs, 1991)

For example, in 1989, the **Commission on Accreditation of Rehabilitation Facilities** (CARF) established "Work Hardening Guidelines" that are predicted to have a significant impact on work practice (CARF, 1989). Kentucky, Florida, and Ohio have incorporated these guidelines as mandatory for reimbursement in their workers' compensation systems (Toppel, 1990), and it is predicted that many states will follow suit. Since the release of the guidelines, 130 facilities have become accreditated by CARF, and about 200 should be accredited by the end of 1991 (CARF, 1991). A revision of the guidelines is forthcoming.

The **Americans With Disabilities Act** of 1990 (ADA; PL 101–336) will have a significant impact on work practice. Under this landmark legislation, people with disabilities receive comprehensive civil rights protection from discrimination in employment, transportation, public accommodations, telecommunications, and activities of state and local governments (Golden, 1991). This section focuses on the area of employment.

The ADA prohibits discrimination "against any qualified individual with a disability because of the disability of such individual in regard to job application procedures, the hiring, advancement, or discharge of employees, employee compensation, job training, and other terms, conditions, and privileges of employment" (ADA, 1990, pp. 13–14; Golden, 1991). According to the ADA, "the term 'qualified individual with a disability' means an individual with a disability who, with or without reasonable accommodation, can perform the essential functions" of the job that this individual holds or desires (ADA, 1990, p. 14; Golden, 1991). Two key terms within this definition are worthy of a more thorough explanation: **essential functions of a job** and **reasonable accommodations**. Essential functions of a job are job tasks that are fundamental, not marginal, to the job (ADA, 1990). For example, a job description for a secretarial pool of 20 workers lists a driver's license as a requirement, but the job entails no driving. Under the ADA, a driver's license would not be an essential function of the job and could no longer be included in the job description. "Reasonable Accommodation is any modification or adjustment to a job or work environment that will enable a qualified applicant or employee with a disability to perform essential job functions" (National Easter Seal Society, 1990, p. 15). For example, a reasonable accommodation might be restructuring a job, modifying work schedules, adapting equipment, or providing an interpreter. A reasonable accommodation could be as simple as allowing an employee to wear sneakers instead of shoes. According to Golden, "it is important to note that many individuals with disabilities do not require any reasonable accommodation whatsoever" (1991, p. 15).

Another provision of the employment section that is of particular importance to the occupational therapist is that no preoffer medical examinations or preemployment screening may be given (ADA, 1990).

The occupational therapist can play a key role in promoting compliance with the ADA and educating patients about their rights and responsibilities. As a professional interest, occupational therapists need to rally to this cause.

Occupational therapists have demonstrated renewed interest in and enthusiasm for the area of work practice. The following brief historical overview is presented so that the reader can appreciate more fully the scope and importance of this interest.

Precursors to current work practice

"Work is at the heart of the philosophy and practice of occupational therapy. In its broadest sense, work, as productive activity, is the concern in almost all therapy" (Jacobs, 1985, p. ix). Indeed, the area of work parallels the profession's development. (See Chapter 2 for a historical review.)

> [Occupational therapy] has been linked to vocational education and rehabilitation through legislation in response to war-generated needs and social change. The initial legislative thrust came in the World War I era. Soldiers were the first to receive vocational education and rehabilitation, then civilians. The second thrust came during World War II, when medical services became available.
>
> In the beginning, emphasis was placed on those people who could be returned to employment quickly. As the need for workers decreased, the social value of work was replaced by a social value of a humane response to disability itself: Everyone deserved a chance to work. Finally society decided that everyone also deserved to live as independently as possible. (Kirkland & Robertson, 1985b).

The accompanying display lists importance legislation that has affected work-related practice.

The American Occupational Therapy Association's (AOTA) members confirmed their commitment to work practice in 1986 through the establishment of the Work Programs Special Interest Section (WPSIS). In 1990, there were about 2900 members in the WPSIS (AOTA, 1990). During that same year, the 1987 to 1990 WPSIS Standing Committee completed the first demographic survey of work hardening programs in addition to an outcome study of over 40 programs. Results from both the survey and study have been disseminated through articles and lectures (Wyrick, Niemeyer, Ellexson, Jacobs, & Taylor, 1991).

The interest in work practice has been evidenced through an increase in the number of textbooks, professional articles, conferences, and workshops on this subject.

Current work practice

Many settings exist for employment in work practice. These include but are not limited to acute care and rehabilitation facilities, industrial and office environments, work evaluation and work hardening centers, sheltered workshops, transitional workshops, related transitional settings, psychiatric treatment centers, programs for the elderly, educational systems, and home environments.

Significant opportunities exist and others are being created in work practice. If occupational therapists are to play a key role, they must monitor environmental trends, keep their skills and knowledge current, develop marketing savvy, and be more visible as the primary advocates for their patients.

The work process

The following occupational therapy functions relate to work (AOTA, 1980; ADA, 1990; Hightower-Vandamm, 1981a, 1981b, 1982; CARF, 1989):

- Initial screening
- Support in exploration and identification of possible work interests, abilities, and needs
- Functional capacity evaluation (FCE), which may include baseline evaluation, job capacity evaluation, occupational capacity evaluation, and work capacity evaluation
- Evaluation of psychosocial, neurologic, cognitive, perceptual, and motor function
- Evaluation of work skills and tolerances
- Evaluation of work behaviors
- Evaluation of work-related capabilities, such as transportation, communication, and self-care
- Postoffer screening
- Work hardening
- Work adjustment and habit and behavior programs
- School programs
- Delineation of essential functions of a job and reasonable accommodations, such as task and environmental adaptations
- Job analysis and job site analysis
- Application of ergonomic principles
- Education and instruction in injury prevention, such as proper body mechanics, pain management, postural awareness, and safety
- Termination or follow-up care

From this list, it is possible to group the functions of occupational therapists related to work practice into four sequential categories that may be viewed as similar to the vocational rehabilitation process: *assessment, planning, treatment and programming,* and *termination and follow-up care* (Reynolds-Lynch, 1985a).

Within this process, the occupational therapist has the opportunity to work with a broad array of personnel. In the rehabilitation field, these may include rehabilitation engineers, ergonomists, rehabilitation counselors, work evaluators, work adjustment specialists, employment or vocational counselors, rehabilitation nurses, occupational health nurses, and risk managers. Other personnel that the occupational therapist may work with are teachers, administrators, employers, physicians, physical therapists, and social workers (Wright, 1980).

Assessment

Often, the term *assessment* is incorrectly thought to be synonymous with evaluation. Actually, assessment encompasses evaluation as one of its three phases, which are (1) intake interview, (2) general medical examination, and (3) evaluation. The following assessment processes are used by occupational therapists:

1. Review of medical, educational, and vocational records
2. Interviews with the patient, family, employer, teachers, and other personnel
3. Observation
4. Inventories and checklists
5. Standardized and nonstandardized evaluations (Reynolds-Lynch, 1985b)

Specifically, work assessment uses these processes in an attempt "to predict current and future employment potential by evaluating mental, emotional, and physical abilities along with limitations and tolerances. It focuses on the identification of a person's strengths and weaknesses in relation to general employability factors and specific vocational skills" (Reynolds-Lynch, 1985a, p. 176). Also important is the assessment of the patient's occupational interests and ancillary (indirect) job needs, that is, mobility skills.

The following discussion briefly reviews observation, inventories, and checklists and then focuses on standardized and nonstandardized evaluations.

SIGNIFICANT LEGISLATION RELATED TO WORK

1916—National Defense Act: Improved military efficiency and enabled soldiers to become more competitive in civilian life. The focus was educational, but no agency was established to carry out the directives.

1917—PL 64-347, Smith-Hughes Act (Vocational Education Act): Created the Federal Board for Vocational Education (FBVE)

1918—PL 65-178, Smith-Sears Act (Soldiers Rehabilitation Act): Enlarged the role of FBVE to provide programs for disabled veterans who were unable to succeed at gainful employment

1920—PL 66-236, Smith-Fess Act (Civilian Rehabilitation Act): Initiated rehabilitation for the general public. Provided funds for vocational guidance and training, occupational adjustment, prostheses, and placement services. Occupational therapy was reimbursed if it was part of medical treatment. No reimbursement for psychiatric or developmentally disabled people

1921—PL 67-47, Veterans Bureau Act: Established the Veterans Bureau as an independent agency with a director responsible to the President

1933—PL 73-2, Veterans Administration Act: Recognized the Veterans Bureau and designated this federal agency as the Veterans Administration

1935—PL 74-271, Social Security Act: Established unemployment compensation, old-age insurance, child health and welfare services, crippled children services, and public assistance for the aged, blind, and dependent children

1943—PL 78-16, Welsh-Clark Act (World War II Disabled Veterans Rehabilitation Act): Provided vocational rehabilitation for disabled veterans of World War II

1943—PL 78-113, Barden-LaFollette Act (Vocational Rehabilitation Act): Changed the original provisions of PL 66-236. Physically disabled, blind, developmentally delayed, and psychiatrically disabled were added to those served. Office of Vocational Rehabilitation (OVR) established. New emphasis on activities of daily living (ADL) and adaptation. Removed ceiling on appropriation

1944—PL 78-346, Servicemen's Readjustment Act (GI Bill): Provided for the education and training (tuition and subsistence) of individuals whose education or career had been interrupted by military service

1945—PL 79-176, Joint Congressional Resolution for a National Employ the Physically Handicapped (NEPH) Week: Established an annually observed NEPH week. In 1954, Truman changed it to President's Committee on Employment of the Physically Handicapped; in 1962, Kennedy changed it to President's Committee on Employment of the Handicapped

1954—PL 83-565, Hill-Burton Act (Vocational Rehabilitation Act Amendments): Greater financial support, research and demonstration grants, professional preparation grants, state agency expansion and improvement grants, and grants to expand rehabilitation facilities. Many occupational therapists received this money for training and education

1965—Vocational Rehabilitation Act Amendments of 1965: Increased services for several types of disabled and socially handicapped people. Construction money made available for rehabilitation centers and workshops

1968—PL 90-480, Architectural Barriers Act: Led the way to changes in access for disabled people

1970—PL 91-517, Developmental Disabilities Services and Facilities Construction Act: States were given broad responsibility for planning and implementing a comprehensive program of services to developmentally delayed, epileptic, cerebral palsied, and other neurologically impaired people

1973—PL 93-112, Rehabilitation Act: Expanded services to the more severely disabled. Also provided for affirmative action in employment (Section 503) and nondiscrimination in facilities (Section 504) by federal contractors and grantees

1975—PL 94-142, Education for All Handicapped Children Act: Provided educational assistance to all handicapped children in the "least restrictive environment." Occupational therapists included as "related personnel"

1978—PL 95-602, Amendments to the Rehabilitation Act of 1973: Expansion of rehabilitation to include independent living. Established the National Institute of Handicapped Research. Provided employer incentives for training and hiring disabled people

1983—PL 98-199, Education of the Handicapped Act Amendments of 1983: Established better transition from school to work

1984—PL 88-210, Carl D. Perkins Vocational Act: Authorized federal grants to states to assist them in (1) extending, improving, and maintaining existing programs of vocational education; (2) developing new programs; (3) providing part-time employment for youths who need earnings to continue their vocational training on a full-time basis; and (4) assisting people of all ages (secondary, postsecondary, and adult levels) to enter the labor market, upgrade their skills, or learn new ones. Provides funding for the following grant programs: Adult Training and Retraining, Career Guidance and Counseling, High Technology Training, Title II Basic Grants, Consumer and Homemaking Education, and Community-Based Organizations (CBO) programs

1986—PL 99-357, Carl D. Perkins Vocational Education Act Amendment: A technical amendment to rectify a problem with state allocation of funds, particularly for the Consumer and Homemaking Education program

1986—PL 99-457, Education of the Handicapped Act Amendments: Provides a significant increase in federal funds to encourage states to provide special education and related services to preschoolers aged 3 through 5 years. Federal funds for this age group will be terminated if this is not initiated by school year 1990–91. Also included is a mandate for a new comprehensive, interagency program to provide early intervention to infants and toddlers with handicaps, aged birth through 2 years

1990—PL 101-336, Americans With Disabilities Act: Provides comprehensive civil rights protection from discrimination in employment, transportation, public accommodations, telecommunications, and the activities of state and local government for people with disabilities.

Observation

Occupational therapists are trained to sharpen observation skills. Applying these observation skills in the assessment process represents the key to developing an accurate performance profile of the person (Kirland & Robertson, 1985). (See Chapter 7 for more information on observation.)

Inventories and checklists

Many inventories and checklists can be used to gain insight into the patient's interests, desires, and possible work objectives. These include the Activity Configuration (Watanabe, 1968), the Interest Check List (Matsutsuyu, 1969), the Vocational Behavior Checklist (Walls, Zane, & Werner, 1978), Reading-Free Vocational Interest Inventory (Becker, 1981), Assessing Your Work Values (Catalyst, 1980), Occupational Role History (Florey & Michelman, 1982), and the Occupational History (Moorehead, 1969).

The Reading-Free Vocational Interest Inventory provides a series of 55 rows of line drawings arranged in groups of three depicting various unskilled, semiskilled, and skilled tasks (Figure 8-5). The evaluee is instructed to selected one picture from each row of three. After all rows are completed, a profile is calculated based on percentiles of interest within the 11 interest areas (eg, automotive, animal care, laundry service) presented. Reading comprehension is not a variable of this inventory.

Assessing Your Work Values was developed as a checklist for women who want to plan, begin, change, or advance their careers and is used to help clarify motivations for working. Figure 8-6 provides examples of 3 of 13 work values that the patient may find important.

Additional inventories and checklists can be found later in this section in Figure 8-13, under the category of Volitional Subsystem, which is part of Kielhofner's model of the person as an open system (Kielhofner, 1983).

Evaluation

CARF (1987) composed the following list as a guideline for work evaluation:

Physical and psychomotor capacities
Intellectual capacities; emotional stability; interests, attitudes, and knowledge of occupational information; personal, social, and work histories; aptitudes

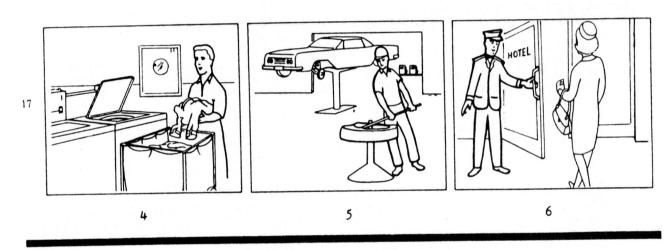

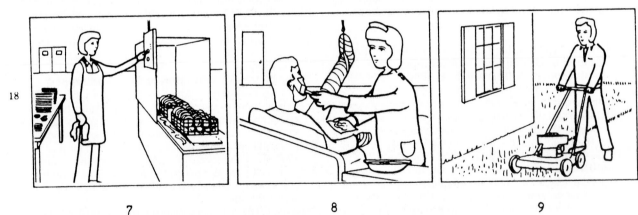

FIGURE 8-5. *An example of the Reading-Free Vocational Interest Inventory: M F devised by Ralph L. Becker. Evaluees are instructed to circle the picture in each row that they like best to ascertain work interests. The complete inventory contains 55 rows of pictures of people working at various jobs.* (Beckr R. L. [1981]. Reading-Free Vocational Interest Inventory: M F. *Columbus, OH: Elbern Publications.*)

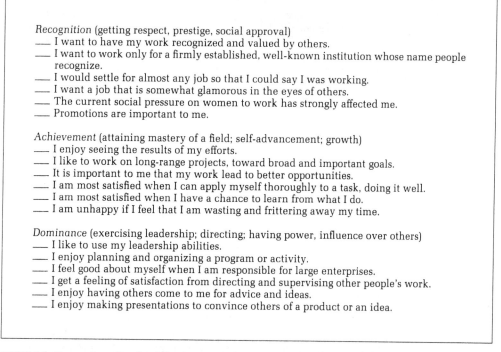

Recognition (getting respect, prestige, social approval)
___ I want to have my work recognized and valued by others.
___ I want to work only for a firmly established, well-known institution whose name people recognize.
___ I would settle for almost any job so that I could say I was working.
___ I want a job that is somewhat glamorous in the eyes of others.
___ The current social pressure on women to work has strongly affected me.
___ Promotions are important to me.

Achievement (attaining mastery of a field; self-advancement; growth)
___ I enjoy seeing the results of my efforts.
___ I like to work on long-range projects, toward broad and important goals.
___ It is important to me that my work lead to better opportunities.
___ I am most satisfied when I can apply myself thoroughly to a task, doing it well.
___ I am most satisfied when I have a chance to learn from what I do.
___ I am unhappy if I feel that I am wasting and frittering away my time.

Dominance (exercising leadership; directing; having power, influence over others)
___ I like to use my leadership abilities.
___ I enjoy planning and organizing a program or activity.
___ I feel good about myself when I am responsible for large enterprises.
___ I get a feeling of satisfaction from directing and supervising other people's work.
___ I enjoy having others come to me for advice and ideas.
___ I enjoy making presentations to convince others of a product or an idea.

FIGURE 8-6. *Examples of a checklist based on 13 work values, such as recognition, achievement, and money, which is used to clarify a person's motivation for working. The evaluee is instructed to check one statement within each value category that is important to him or her. (From* What to do with the rest of your life. *New York: Simon and Schuster, 1980.)*

Achievements (eg, vocational, educational)

Work skills and work tolerances

Work habits (punctuality, attendance, concentration, organization, and interpersonal skills)

Work-related capabilities (eg, mobility, communication, hygiene, homemaker, money management)

Job-seeking skills

Potential to benefit from further services specifically identified

Employment objectives that may involve either competitive or noncompetitive employment or programs in industry options

Ability to learn about oneself as a result of information obtained and furnished through the evaluation experience

Assessment of the most effective mode of understanding and responding to various types of instruction

Identification of the need for tool and job site modification or adaptive equipment that may enhance employability (CARF, 1987)

This list, although also composed of some secondary treatment goals, is consistent with occupational therapists' education, skills, and experience. Actually, many of the evaluations commonly used in occupational therapy practice to evaluate strength, endurance, coordination, dexterity, ADL, and interpersonal skills can be considered part of work evaluation (Thompson, 1987).

Botterbusch (1978, 1982) categorizes work evaluations within one of four techniques: (1) on-the-job evaluations, (2) situational assessment, (3) psychometric instruments, and (4) work samples. There is an inverse relation between the closeness of the technique to real work as viewed by the patient and the overall cost of the technique. Botterbusch notes that

tests . . . are the cheapest way of obtaining information about a patient. Job site evaluation requires a heavy staff investment in terms of the amount of time needed to develop the initial job site and to maintain a patient on the site. Situation assessment requires the existence of a workshop, production contracts, and staff for supervision. If "homemade" work sample techniques are used, they require staff time to develop as well as money and time to construct; commercial work sample systems can cost up to $20,000 for the initial purchase. All work samples eventually require replacement parts and many require expendable supplies. Tests have the advantages of:

1. being cheaper to buy,
2. usually being group administered, and
3. often having separate answer sheets which reduce the expense of expendable supplies. (1978, p. 1)

This can be visualized as in Figure 8-7.

Usually, combinations of these techniques are the most effective way to appraise a patient's work potential and future performance in job training and employment (Wright, 1980; Jacobs, 1991). Not all the evaluation techniques are used by occupational therapists, however, nor are they appropriate for every person. For example, a school-aged person with no work experience may be referred for an evaluation with the purpose of ascertaining occupational interests, whereas another person who has work experience but has been fired from a series of jobs may be referred for the purpose of evaluating work behaviors to find out what is causing job instability.

Technique:

On-the-job evaluation
Situational assessment
Work sample techniques
Psychological testing

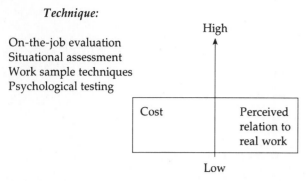

FIGURE 8-7. *A model that demonstrates the inverse relationship between the closeness to real work as viewed by the client of a work-evaluation technique and the overall cost of the technique.*

On-the-job evaluation

On-the-job, or **job site**, **evaluation** is used to assess the person's ability to perform successfully in a competitive employment situation. Under ideal conditions, before performing the job site evaluation, the occupational therapist has the opportunity to review the worker's job description and explore the *Dictionary of Occupational Titles* (DOT) and its companion publications for background information on the demands of the job. From this fact-finding, the occupational therapist may be better prepared for evaluating the actual job. On-the-job evaluations deal with the interaction of the worker to the environment. Most of the following information is assessed to some degree: physical demands, psychosocial factors, cognitive factors, analysis of the essential functions of the job, tools and machines used, description of the work environment, and hazards and stress factors.

Under the ADA, the occupational therapist can provide a **postoffer screening** only after the person has been offered employment. The evaluation should include assessing the person's ability to perform the essential functions of the job.

Situational assessment

Situational assessment involves placing the person into a realistic work situation. In contrast to on-the-job evaluation, variables such as production demands or stress factors can be systematically altered, and the person's performance under each circumstance can be observed (Marshall, 1983).

Psychometric instruments

Psychometric instruments include an almost endless variety of paper-and-pencil and apparatus techniques for measuring general intelligence, achievement, abilities, and related characteristics. These instruments typically are administered by psychologists (Botterbusch, 1978, 1982; Reynolds-Lynch, 1985b). Table 8-6 offers some of the most commonly used psychometric instruments.

Work samples

Work samples are the primary technique of work evaluation. They evolved "to meet the growing demand for vocational and special services to a variety of disability groups in traditional rehabilitation settings, clinics and public schools" (McCarron & Dial, 1986, p. 1). A work sample is a "well-defined work activity involving tasks, materials, and tools which are identical or similar to those in an actual job or cluster of jobs. It is used to access an individual's vocational aptitude, worker characteristics and vocational interests" (Rosenberg, 1973, p. 55). Work samples have the advantages of resembling actual work and providing an opportunity to observe work behaviors and physical functioning and a variety of work areas (Botterbusch, 1982). The four types of work sample correspond to actual jobs: actual job samples, simulated job samples, cluster trait samples, and single trait samples (Botterbusch, 1982).

The TOWER system and some of the work samples in the Valpar Component Work Sample Series (VCWS; eg, VCWS #15, drafting) are commercially available *actual job samples;* that is, they are samples of work that have been taken in their entirety from an employment setting and brought to a testing environment for the purpose of evaluating a patient's interest and aptitude. Some types of actual job samples include pipe-fitting, refrigeration, electronic assembly, baking and cooking, and cosmetology (Valpar, 1986).

A *simulated job sample* is a representation of the common critical factors of a job. It differs from an actual job sample in that all factors affecting the job are not replicated, for example, environmental stress (Wright, 1980). Figure 8-8 portrays a simulated job sample of grill work for a fast-food restaurant that has been constructed in a special-needs high school and used with learning disabled students. Another example of a simulated job sample is the Baltimore Therapeutic Equipment Work Simulator (Figure 8-9). This simulated job sample is composed of an adjustable shaft that accommodates a variety of tools that simulate jobs (eg, shoveling) and can be adjusted to different angles and heights with a computer console that displays the amount of

TABLE 8-6. *Psychological Tests Frequently Used in Work Assessment*

Category	Name
Achievement and reading	Adult Basic Learning Examination
	California Achievement Tests
	Gray Oral Reading Test
	Nelson-Denny Reading Test
	Peabody Individual Achievement Test
	Tests of Adult Basic Education
Personality	Minnesota Multiphasic Personality Inventory
	Draw-a-Person Test
	House–Tree–Person Test
Intelligence	Wechsler Adult Intelligence Scale
	Peabody Picture Vocabulary Test
Vocational aptitudes	General Aptitude Test Battery
	Non-Reading Aptitude Test Battery
	Purdue Pegboard
	Crawford Small Parts Dexterity Test
	Stromberg Dexterity Test
Vocational interests	Strong Vocational Interest Blank
	Geist Picture Interest Inventory
	Minnesota Importance Questionnaire
	Kuder Occupational Interest Survey
	Wide Range Interest–Opinion Test

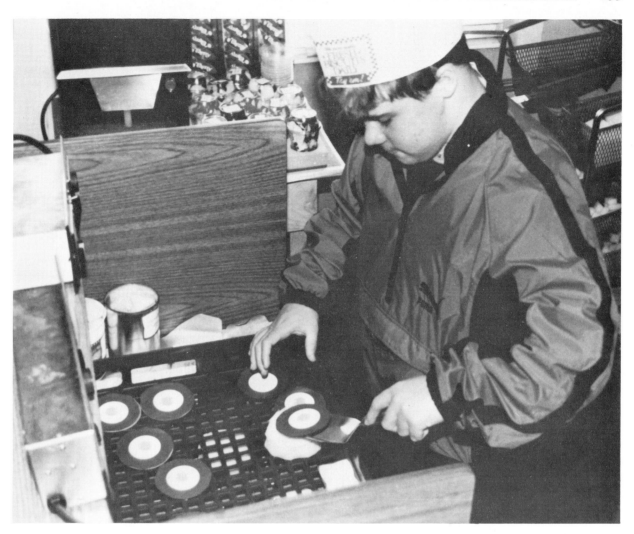

FIGURE 8-8. *Student working in a simulated job of a fast-food restaurant. Job simulation such as this can be used in both evaluation and treatment.*

resistance programmed by the therapist. After the completion of an activity, there can be a printout with data such as the amount of time spent on the activity and force exerted on the tool (Bettencourt, Carlstrom, Brown, Lindau, & Long, 1986).

The Work Evaluation Systems Technology (WEST; eg, WEST 7, Bus Bench; Figure 8-10) and some of the work samples composing the VCWS (eg, VCWS #4, upper extremity range of motion) are examples of a *cluster trait sample* because they assess a number of traits inherent in a job or various jobs, such as strength, endurance, range of motion, speed, and dexterity.

The Purdue Pegboard, Minnesota Rate of Manipulation, Crawford Small Parts Dexterity Test, O'Connor Dexterity Tests, Pennsylvania Bimanual Work Sample, Bennett Hand-Tool Dexterity Test, and Stromberg Dexterity Test are examples of *single trait samples*, which assess a single worker trait, in this case, dexterity (Wright, 1980; Thompson, 1987). These tests occasionally are included under psychological tests of vocational aptitudes.

Many standardized and standard work samples have been developed. Because of the high cost of many commercially available work samples, design of work samples by the therapist for a

particular population is often appropriate. An example of a therapist-designed work sample system is the Jacobs Prevocational Skills Assessment (JPSA) developed for a learning disabled adolescent population at the Learning Prep School in West Newton, Massachusetts. This 15-task battery relies heavily on observational skills to provide a profile of a patient's skills and behaviors. Table 8-7 provides the checklist for the JPSA, which actually is an activity analysis of each work sample. Examples of tasks include quality control, carpentry assembly, office work, and food preparation (Jacobs, 1985, 1991). Figure 8-11 is an example of Factory Work Task 7.

A number of additional work evaluation systems are commercially available (Botterbusch, 1982). Many of these are used completely or in part by occupational therapists as well as other professionals, such as work evaluators. The McCarron-Dial, Valpar, and TOWER systems are reviewed in more detail next.

McCarron-Dial System. The McCarron-Dial System (MDS) was developed in 1973 to determine the "prevocational, vocational and residential functioning levels of disabled individuals" (McCarron & Dial, 1986, p. 7), with the revision and expansion of

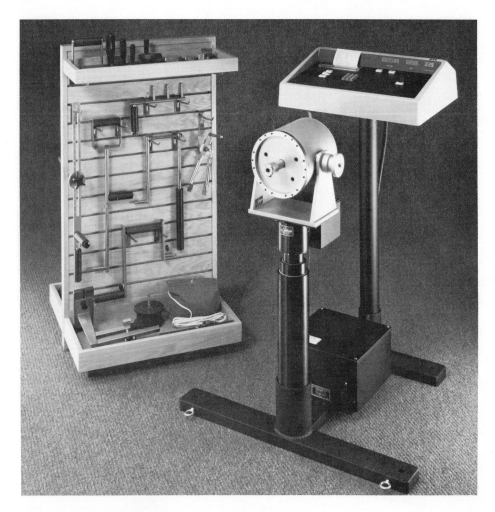

FIGURE 8-9. *Baltimore Therapeutic Equipment (BTE) Work Simulator, with attachments; the simulator is used in both evaluation and treatment. (Photography courtesy of Baltimore Therapeutic Equipment Co, Hanover, Maryland.)*

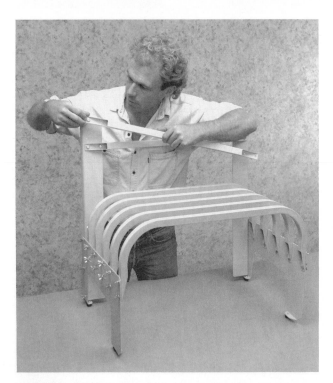

FIGURE 8-10. *Worker assembling the WEST-7 Bus Bench.*

the norm base to include the general population. The system is targeted for patients with learning disabilities, mental health problems, mental retardation, cerebral palsy, closed head injuries, social handicaps, or cultural disadvantages, with adaptations for use with the visually and hearing impaired. The MDS is based on a neuropsychological theoretic framework to assess five factors: (1) verbal, spatial, and cognitive abilities; (2) sensory ability; (3) motor ability; (4) emotion; and (5) integration, coping, and adaptive behaviors. The basic system consists of six widely accepted assessment instruments in combination with performance and behavioral observation. Table 8-8 contains a summary of MDS factors, definitions, and instruments. The system provides flexibility based on the needs of the patient or the setting, with the ability to add or substitute other instruments.

The MDS evaluation process begins with a preliminary screening through interview and referral information. The administration of assessment instruments (work samples) starts with factor 1 and proceeds through factor 5. Both a formal testing setting and a period of placement in a work or classroom setting are used. The formal testing can be completed in about 3 hours, and the systematic observation in a work or classroom setting can take up to 5 days.

The basic MDS is packed in three kits, each the size of a large briefcase, with the only expendable items being various answer sheets, behavioral observation forms, and report forms. Some tasks are timed, with the emphasis in scoring on the quality and

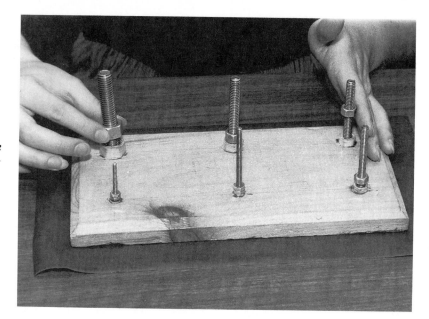

FIGURE 8-11. *Example of Factory Work Task 7 from the Jacobs Prevocational Skills Assessment (JPSA.)*

quantity of performance. The reporting format includes the various scores profiled for each of the five factors, strengths and weaknesses, programming priorities, and programming recommendations.

The producers of MDS require a commitment to pursue training as a prerequisite to purchasing the system. Each basic training workshop is 3 days long.

Valpar Component Work Samples. Valpar International Corporation has devised a diverse product line in vocational evaluation that includes self-reporting interviews; microcomputer evaluation and screening assessment; computer-based job-search program (which provides both a national job data base and training bank program and the capability to build your own local job data base and training bank); computerized self-reporting; the self-reporting Physical Functioning Questionnaire and work samples; and the Valpar National Training Institute. It is important to note that occupational therapists are among the target audiences for their products. Only the Valpar work samples are described in this section.

The various Valpar tools have been designed to meet the vocational evaluation needs of people ranging from nonhandicapped to profoundly handicapped or disabled (Rosenberg, 1973). VCWSs also have been used extensively with injured industrial workers.

The 18 VCWS involve a worker trait and work factor approach using task analysis:

1. Small tools (mechanical)
2. Size discrimination
3. Numeric sorting
4. Upper-extremity range of motion
5. Clerical comprehension and aptitude
6. Independent problem solving
7. Multilevel sorting
8. Simulated assembly
9. Whole-body range of motion
10. Trilevel measurement
11. Eye–hand–foot coordination
12. Soldering and inspection
14. Integrated peer performance
15. Electrical circuitry and print reading
16. Drafting
17. Prevocational readiness battery
18. Conceptual understanding through blind evaluation (CUBE)
19. Dynamic physical capacities (Valpar, 1986)

The work samples are intended for use as individual components, are packaged separately, and have minimal expendable materials. Although the company offers suggestions for use, the order and number of samples given to a person is left to the therapist's discretion.

The work samples most frequently used by occupational therapists are VCWS #1, small tools (mechanical); VCWS #8, simulated assembly; VCWS #9, whole body range of motion; and VCWS #19, dynamic physical capacities (Figure 8-12) (Mobray-Swallow, personal communication, 1987). VCWS #19 is used particularly in work evaluation and work hardening programs. It is composed of 28 individual tasks that are similar to those of a shipping and receiving clerk or parts-order clerk (eg, lifting, climbing and balancing, stooping). These tasks measure the physical demands factor of Worker Qualifications Profile of the DOT (Reynolds-Lynch, 1985a).

Scoring emphasizes quality and time. These scores can be converted to **Methods-Time Measurement** (MTM), an industrial standard, and to percentiles with one or more of the eight norm groups (Botterbusch, 1978; Kester, 1983). A five-point scale is used to rate patients on each of 17 worker behavior characteristics, such as ability to work alone, respond to change, communicate, and make decisions. Norms are available on various groups. Reliability coefficients are generally high, and descriptions of different types of validity are provided in each manual.

Training is not required as a condition of purchase, al-

(*Text continues on page 238*)

TABLE 8-7.   *The Jacobs Prevocational Skills Assessment (JPSA)*

Tasks	Fine Motor Coordination	Eye–Hand Coordination	Motor Planning	Figure–Ground	Sorting	Classification and Sequencing	Decision Making	Problem Solving	Organizational Skills
1. Quality control	✔			✔	✔		✔		✔
2. Filing A	✔				✔	✔	✔	✔	✔
B	✔			✔	✔	✔	✔	✔	✔
C	✔				✔	✔	✔	✔	✔
3. Carpentry assembly	✔	✔	✔	✔			✔	✔	
4. Classification	✔					✔	✔	✔	
5. Office work A	✔	✔	✔			✔	✔	✔	✔
B	✔	✔	✔			✔		✔	✔
C	✔	✔	✔			✔		✔	✔
6. Telephone directory A	✔	✔		✔		✔			✔
B	✔	✔							✔
7. Factory work	✔	✔	✔	✔			✔	✔	
8. Environmental mobility A	✔	✔	✔	✔				✔	✔
B								✔	✔
9. Money concept A									
B									
C	✔			✔			✔	✔	
D	✔			✔			✔	✔	✔
10. Functional banking A	✔	✔		✔			✔		
B	✔	✔		✔			✔		
11. Time concept A									
B				✔					
C									
12. Work attitudes A				✔		✔	✔		✔
B							✔	✔	
13. Body scheme	✔							✔	✔
14. Leather assembly	✔	✔	✔	✔		✔			✔
15. Food preparation	✔	✔	✔			✔	✔		

From Jacobs, K. (1985). Occupational therapy: Work-related programs and assessments. Boston: Little, Brown.

| Use of Tools | Ability to Follow Directions | | | | | Behavioral Observations |
	Visual	Written	Verbal	Conceptual Skills	Task Focus	
			✔		✔	
		✔		✔	✔	
		✔		✔	✔	
		✔		✔	✔	
✔					✔	
			✔		✔	
✔					✔	
	✔		✔		✔	
		✔		✔	✔	
			✔		✔	
			✔	✔	✔	
			✔		✔	
			✔		✔	
		✔			✔	
			✔	✔	✔	
			✔	✔	✔	
			✔	✔	✔	
		✔	✔	✔	✔	
✔			✔	✔	✔	
			✔	✔	✔	
			✔	✔	✔	
			✔		✔	
			✔		✔	
			✔		✔	
	✔		✔		✔	
✔	✔				✔	
✔	✔				✔	

TABLE 8-8. *McCarron-Dial System Factors, Definitions, Instruments, and Supplementary Measures*

Factor	Factor Definition	Instruments
Verbal, spatial, and cognitive	Language learning ability, achievement, memory	Wechsler Adult Intelligence Scale (WAIS or WAIS-R) or Wechsler Intelligence Scale for Children (WISC or WISC-R)*
		Peabody Picture Vocabulary Test (PPVT or PPVT-R)
		Perceptual Memory Test (PMT)†
		Wide Range Achievement Test (WRAT)†
		Peabody Individual Achievement Test (PIAT)
		Woodcock-Johnson Psychoeducational Battery†
		Booklet Category Test†
Sensory	Perceiving and experiencing the environment	Bender Visual Motor Gestalt Test (BVMGT)
		Haptic Visual Discrimination Test (HVDT)
		Haptic Memory Matching Test (HMMT)§
Motor	Muscle strength, speed and accuracy of movement, balance and coordination	McCarron Assessment of Neuromuscular Development (MAND)‡
Emotional	Response to interpersonal and environmental stress	Observational Emotional Inventory (OEI or OEI-R)
		Emotional Behavioral Checklist (EBC)†
Integration and coping	Adaptive behavior	Behavior Rating Scale (BRS)
		Street Survival Skills Questionnaire (SSSQ)
		Survey of Functional Adaptive Behaviors (SFAB)†

* Used in educational evaluation of patients under the age of 16 years

† Supplementary tests or procedures

‡ Used in clinical neuropsychological evaluation

§ Used instead of the HVDT for evaluating the blind

From the McCarron-Dial Systems Manual.

though it is available. Valpar International Corporation provides support to their customers, including a support line (800-528-7070), four regional training offices, newsletters called the *Valparspective*, and the Valpar National Training Institute, which offers yearly courses and workshops that supplement the use of their products.

In general, the work samples are appealing to the evaluee and are easy to administer and score.

TOWER. Work sampling began in 1936 with the development of the TOWER system by the New York Institute for Crippled and Disabled, now known as the International Center for the Disabled (ICD). TOWER is an acronym for testing, orientation, and work evaluation in rehabilitation. Originally developed for use with physical disability patients, TOWER is now used with all types of people, including those with emotional disabilities.

The system is composed of 110 work samples arranged into 14 occupational areas:

1. Clerical
2. Drafting
3. Drawing
4. Electronics assembly
5. Jewelry manufacturing
6. Leather goods
7. Machine shop
8. Lettering
9. Mail clerk
10. Optical mechanics
11. Pantograph engraving
12. Sewing machine operating
13. Welding
14. Workshop assembly

Each of the 14 areas is independent, with selection of areas at the therapist's discretion. Within each area, the work samples are arranged in order of complexity. For example, the work sample for jewelry manufacturing is composed of the following tasks, from simple to complex: use of saw; use of needle files; use electric drill press; piercing and filing metals; use of pliers; use of torch in soldering; and making an earring and broach pin (B. Rosenberg, Director of Vocational Rehabilitation Services, ICD, and one of the originators of TOWER, personal communication, 1987).

A list of hardware and equipment needs, purposes, and procedures is provided by the system manual and other accompanying literature. The use of a realistic work setting and atmosphere is recommended when administering the samples. Completion of the entire system by an average patient takes 3 weeks, but most samples usually are not administered to each patient.

Time and work quality are given equal weight in scoring, which is done on a five-point scale. Work factors and work behaviors are recognized by ICD as an essential part of the TOWER system. Although the evaluator rates these different factors and behaviors in the final report, they have not been described or incorporated formally into the TOWER manual (Botterbusch, 1982; Kester, 1983; Reynolds-Lynch, 1985a).

Selecting an evaluation

The state of the art in work evaluation is consistently refined and improved. External forces, such as reductions in funding, have forced decreases in the amount of time spent in evaluation and

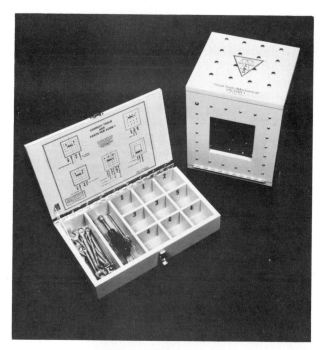

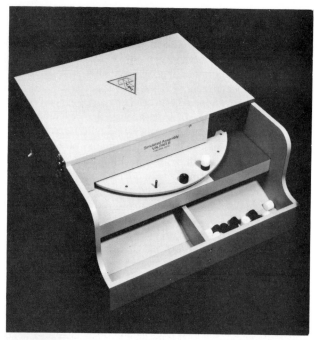

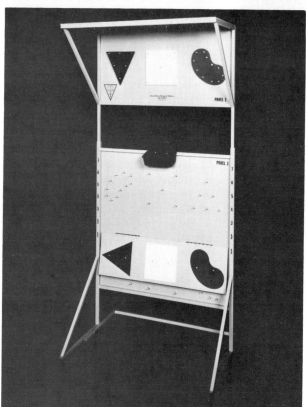

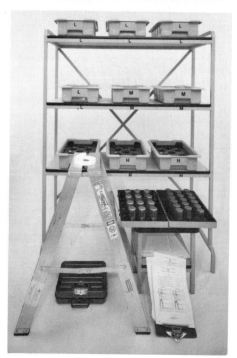

FIGURE 8-12. *Valpar Component Work Samples: A. No. 1, small tools (mechanical). B. No. 8, simulated assembly. C. No. 9, whole body range of motion. D. No. 19, dynamic physical capacities. (Photographs courtesy of Valpar International Corp, Tucson, Arizona.)*

the amount of money spent for tools. These same factors, however, have increased the need to obtain a large amount of data in a short time. Many of the well-known, commercially available work evaluation systems and work samples have been computerized to perform job-matching with the DOT in a matter of minutes (U.S. Department of Labor, 1977).

Of particular importance in selecting an evaluation is obtaining information regarding normative data, reliability, and validity. Ideally, the occupational therapist should look for evaluations that have MTMs. MTM is an example of a criterion-references procedure "which analyzes any manual operation or method into the basic motions required to perform it and assigns to each motion a predetermined time standard which is determined by the nature of the motion and the conditions under which it is made" (MTM, 1990). For example, an MTM rating of 100% is considered entry-level job readiness, and 150% represents a greater level of success. MTM is becoming more popular among developers of evaluations and can be found in VCWSs and in most WEST evaluations. Despite its popularity, there are some limitations. For example, MTMs do not take into account a worker performing in awkward or hazardous postures, such as overhead or with arms horizontally extended in front of the body, and analysis assumes the worker is not fatigued (Chaffin & Anderson, 1987). In addition, it is rare in industry to achieve 100% MTM consistently; most often, an overall production rate of 60% to 70% is considered acceptable if quality is maintained. MTM standards should be used only as a guide, never as an absolute, and they should be used in conjunction with behavioral observation (Jacobs, 1991; Niemeyer, 1991).

The following list is presented as a guide in the selection of appropriate evaluations:

- Investigate the range and type of jobs available in the local catchment area; determine the relevance of the evaluation to local jobs and training programs.
- Analyze the patient population, considering their assets and deficits.
- Review commercially available systems, either by visiting other facilities that have them or by borrowing them for a period of time. The Materials Development Center has many audiovisual materials that review vocational evaluation and may aid in the decision-making process (Botterbusch, 1978).
- Carefully review the evaluation manual, its answer sheet, and other parts to answer the following questions: What is its purpose? What is the reading level? How clear are the instructions and procedures? How much does it cost? How much time does it take to administer and score? Is training necessary? How much space is needed? For what population was the evaluation designed? Has the evaluation established reliability, validity, and norms or MTMs? (See Bolton, 1976, for an overview.)
- Investigate what resources already are available within your facility or a neighboring facility.
- Consider whether you need to purchase an evaluation. Can you borrow it or develop your own from existing subcontracted work, in-house jobs, or other sources?

A review of the literature indicates the need to base practice on a clear conceptual framework. Various frames of reference have been developed, including Clark's model of human development through occupation (1979), Mosey's three frames of reference (1970, 1981), and Kielhofner's paradigm of the future (1983), which is based on general systems theory. Creighton, however, believes that "no recent attempt has been made to identify the specific implications of various theoretical orientations for specialized areas of occupational therapy practice, such as vocational rehabilitation" (1985b, p. 331). Creighton selected Mosey's three frames of reference as one theoretic perspective on base planning, assessment, and treatment in the area of work practice.

Thompson has followed Kielhofner's model of the person as an open system to organize the classification of various work assessment tools (Kielhofner, 1980; Thompson, 1987). Figure 8-13 lists the different instruments within the three subsystems: volitional, habituation, and performance. Kielhofner describes the human being as a dynamic system composed of these three subsystems that interact and influence each other. The volitional subsystem, at the top, is composed of values, interests, motivation, and personal causation. The habituation subsystem, viewed as below the volitional subsystem, is composed of roles and habits. The performance subsystem (formerly called production), is at the base and is composed of aptitudes and skills (eg, sensory, motor, perceptual, cognitive, and social).

Planning

After the assessment process, the therapist and evaluee should plan programming priorities and establish short- and long-term goals. In this planning stage, many factors should be taken into account, particularly if the work program is new to the occupational therapy department. The following are some pertinent questions:

- What are the person's interests?
- What are the person's aspirations and interests regarding future employment?
- Are the person's job goals realistic?
- What is the extent of the person's job experience?
- What type of work is available to the person, particularly in the local community? Does the patient have the necessary skills to perform that kind of work?
- What resources are available in the therapist's facility and in the community for use as simulated job experiences?
- What kinds of budget limitations exist for developing and operating the program?
- Does the therapist have access to equipment and supplies that may relate to programming?
- How much physical space is available for the program?
- Does the therapist have the support of the administration and staff of the facility? (Jacobs, 1985, 1991)

Programming

Traditionally, the occupational therapist has been faced with people of varying ages who are either unsuccessful at work, are unable to work for a variety of reasons, or have never had the opportunity to acquire work behaviors and work skills. Such people may include a nurse with an acquired chronic back injury who now feels unable to ever return to work; an older adult who has been replaced by high technology, feels disenfranchised, and has become severely depressed; the institutionalized adolescent with developmental disabilities who has never been exposed to

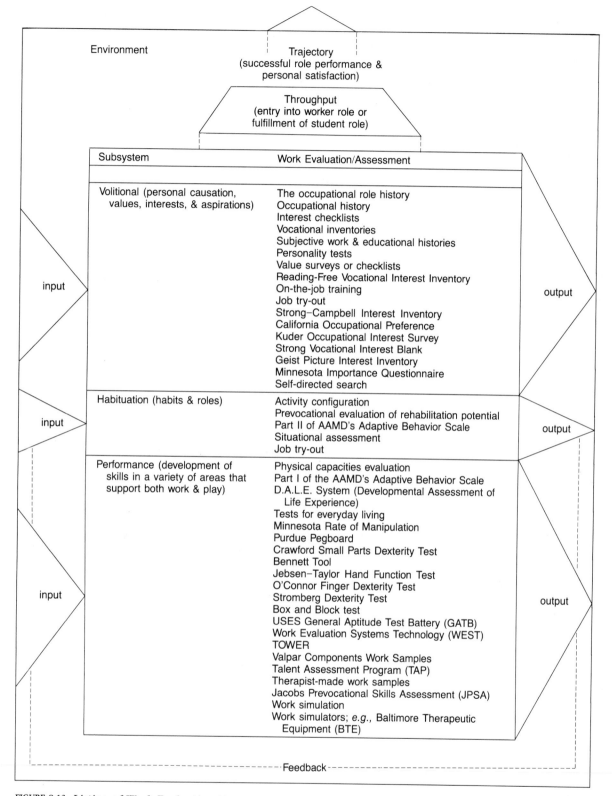

FIGURE 8-13. *Listing of Work Evaluations/Assessments categorized in Kielhofner's model of human occupation. (From Kielhofner G. [1980]. A model of human occupation, part 3. Benign and vicious cycles. American Journal of Occupational Therapy, 34, 731.)*

appropriate work behaviors; the homemaker who, after severe head trauma due to a car accident, has limited cognitive and physical functioning; and the upper-extremity amputee from a recent industrial accident.

From a functional standpoint, these people's dysfunctions can be viewed in two major categories: (1) lack of work behaviors and work skills, and (2) neurophysiologic impairments. The importance of work behaviors is emphasized by the fact that most unemployed workers are unable to obtain or keep jobs or have lost their jobs because of problems with interpersonal skills—that is, trouble getting along with coworkers and supervisors—rather than because of inadequate work skills, aptitudes, or physical demands (Distefano & Pryer, 1970; Jacobs, 1985, 1991; Kiernan & Petzy, 1982). In addition, "limited concentration, distractibility, or psychological pressures that limit tolerance for specific activities might preclude employment even though job skills are present" (Kiernan & Petzy, 1982, p. 251).

Assessment may point to one of the following types of programming:

- Direct competitive job placement
- Supported employment
- Educational training
- Remediation
- Rehabilitation workshop employment

As previously identified, the functions of occupational therapy related to work programming may include, but are not limited to, support in exploration or identifying possible work objectives; work hardening; work adjustment and habit and behavior programs; independent living skills programs; work placement; job site analysis; prevention and education; and task and environmental adaptation. Some of the functions provided by the occupational therapist within each type of programming are described next.

Direct competitive job placement

Although many consumers believe that occupational therapists get people jobs, the occupational therapist rarely does formal job placement. The therapist may, however, play an active role in the decision-making process by assisting in career exploration and identification of work objectives and by ascertaining when the person is ready for competitive employment, what type of job is feasible, and the extent, if any, of reasonable accommodations (eg, adaptations, work simplification, or modifications) that need to be made at the job site. Familiarity with references such as the DOT, the *Guide for Occupational Exploration*, and *Selected Characteristics of Occupations Defined in the Dictionary of Occupational Titles* can aid in the process (U.S. Department of Labor, 1977, 1979, 1981). Job site analysis also is a useful tool in assessing the person's work site needs.

Occupational therapists working in industry may play the additional role of researcher–practitioner, working to prevent initial work-related injury (Bear-Lehman & McCormick, 1985–1986). Many injuries that could be prevented "are caused by the use of poorly designed tools and work stations and improper work performance movements" (Bear-Lehman & McCormick, 1985–1986, p. 80). Bear-Lehman and McCormick, occupational therapists, remark that occupational therapists "can be influential in injury prevention by working with local safety and industrial groups to develop educational programs and to investigate

injuries" (1985–86, p. 81) The use of ergonomic principles by occupational therapists is important.

Another evolving population for the occupational therapist includes the disenfranchised workers or the "new poor." These are people who are unemployed due to modernization, lack of current skills, or sagging markets. The occupational therapist can be part of a consortium effort by providing retraining techniques, job site analysis, and occupational exploration (Small, 1986).

Supported employment

Supported employment is paid employment that is provided at integrated settings for people with severe disabilities for whom competitive employment has not occurred or for people whose competitive employment has been interrupted or intermittent as a result of a severe disability and who, because of this disability, need ongoing support services to perform job tasks. According to federal guidelines, for a program to be considered as supported employment, it must meet the following criteria:

Employment must average at least 20 hours per week over the course of the employee's normal pay period.

A competitive wage must be paid in accordance with fair labor standards.

The work site must provide an integrated work setting, where no more than eight persons who have disabilities work in the same area.

The employee who has a disability must be able to have frequent daily interactions with nondisabled employees.

Ongoing support—both on and off the job site—must be provided to the worker and the employer for an indefinite period of time through the use of a job coach. (Abberbock, 1991)

The ***job coach*** provides the on-the-job support and advocacy services to the worker and assists the worker to achieve independence in the employment setting. For example, a job coach may provide one-to-one assistance to the worker in the acquisition of the skills to perform the essential functions of the job. As the worker learns to perform these functions, the job coach spends less time on the job site. The role of a job coach is ideal for the certified occupational therapy assistant.

Four basic models of supported employment are available: (1) the Individual Placement Model, (2) the Enclave Model, (3) the Mobile Work Crew Model, and (4) the Small Business Model (Abberbock, 1991). The *Individual Placement Model* allows for diversity and works best with jobs that are available in service industries. This model uses a job coach to evaluate, place, train, and follow the worker at the job site. "The *Enclave Model* provides community employment in a small group setting of up to eight workers who receive permanent on-site supervision by one or two job coaches. This works best for individuals who require a high degree of job supervision and support" (Abberbock, 1991, p. 63). The *Mobile Work Crew Model* performs specialized services in the community on a contractual basis. Examples of some jobs are custodial work and grounds keeping for a local school. The ratio of job coach to worker is typically 1 : 3 or 1 : 4. In the *Small Business Model*, workers operate a small business to produce a product or provide a service. This model is most suitable for people who have problematic interpersonal skills or who require intensive job skill training.

Educational training

For some people, success on a job may be predicated on the need to receive vocational or academic training before job placement, for example, a work-study program in a secondary school or a vocational technical program. The implementation of Public Law 94–142, Education of the Handicapped Act, has made occupational therapy a well-recognized profession within the educational arena.

Career theories

Play is the work of children, but when they enter school, their work becomes studying. An understanding of **career theories** may be beneficial to the occupational therapist developing work programming for children and adolescents. There are five widely accepted theories of career development, which were originated by psychologists and sociologists and have been adopted by practitioners:

1. Trait-and-factor (Parsons, 1909)
2. Sociologic (Caplow, 1954; Miller & Form, 1951)
3. Psychodynamic (Roe, 1957)
4. Developmental (Ginzberg, Ginzberg, Axelrad et al., 1951; Super, 1957; Havighurst, 1964)
5. Systems (Kiernan & Petzy, 1982; Osipow, 1973)

Developmental theories are applied in occupational therapy educational programs as well as in schools for counseling and career education. Developmental theory views career development as a gradual process within human growth that takes place over the lifespan in predictable stages (Creighton, 1985a). Ginzberg and coworkers (1951), Super (1957), and Havighurst (1964), although developmental theorists, have different beliefs about how and why development occurs (Table 8-9).

Work is a dynamic process, and programming must begin at a young age with the introduction of career awareness and exploration of work capabilities and interests. Although this awareness and exploration must be reinforced with normal children, it is particularly critical for programming to be presented developmentally and initiated at an early age for children with special needs. The rationales supporting this are that these children have "fewer opportunities for free play experiences with other children" (Stephens & Clark, 1985, p. 281); they typically have a limited or lack of exposure to the world of work; and their parents and society have limited career expectations for them (Jacobs, 1985, 1991). In addition, too often people around these children tend to do things for them or assign others tasks that they could accomplish if expectations were not based on time, tolerance, or temperament (Stephens & Clark, 1985). It is important that "training materials and work performance requirements should increasingly approximate actual industrial demands and that training should move from the school to the actual work site as soon as possible" (Kiernan & Petzy, 1982, p. 4).

The creation of simulated business enterprises, such as a fast-food restaurant (see Figure 8-5), supermarket, cookie company, or library, can create a work environment within the confines of a classroom. Academic training and the reinforce-

TABLE 8-9.   *Three Theories of Career Development*

Ginzberg and Associates: Stage and Characteristics	Super: Stage and Characteristics	Havighurst: Stage and Characteristics
Fantasy Period Below age 11: Choices are governed by wish to engage in exciting adult activities	**Growth Stage** Ages 4–10—Fantasy: Needs are dominant; role-playing is important	**Stage I** Ages 5–10—Identification With a Worker: Identifies with significant people; concept of working is incorporated into egoideal
Tentative Period Ages 11–12—Interest: Choices are governed by likes and dislikes	Ages 11–12—Interests: Likes determine aspirations	**Stage II** Ages 10–15—Acquiring the Basic Habits of Industry: Learns to organize time and energy, put work ahead of play
Ages 13–14—Capacity: Begins to consider own abilities objectively	Ages 13–14—Capacity: Abilities are given more weight	**Stage III** Ages 15–25—Acquiring Identity as a Worker in the Occupational Structure: Chooses and prepares for occupation, gets work experience
Ages 15–16—Value: Attempts to clarify goals	**Exploration Stage** Ages 15–17—Tentative: Variety of factors are considered, choices tried out	
Age 17—Transition: Is suspenseful about future.	Ages 18–21—Transition: Gives reality more weight; attempts to implement self-concept	**Stage IV** Ages 25–40—Becoming a Productive Person: Masters skills and moves up ladder in occupation
Realistic Period Age 17—Young adulthood (stages not closely correlated with chronologic age)—	Ages 22–24—Trial: Beginning job is tried out as life work	**Stage V** Ages 40–70—Maintaining a Productive Society: Emphasizes societal aspects of worker's role
Exploration: Obtains information about various vocations	**Establishment Stage** Ages 25–30—Trial: Changes may be necessary before life work is found	**Stage VI** Age 70 on—Contemplating a Productive and Responsible Life: Withdraws from worker role and reviews and accepts productivity
Crystallization: Assesses all factors influencing choice and commits self	Ages 31–44—Stabilization: Career pattern becomes clear; attempts to make secure place in work	
Specification: Considers field of specialization, particular career objectives	**Maintenance Stage** Ages 45–64: Concern is to hold place in world of work	
	Decline Stage Ages 65–70—Deceleration: Pace or nature of work changes to fit declining capacities	
	Age 71 on—Retirement: Occupation ceases	

Adapted from Ginzberg et al., 1951; Super, 1957; Havighurst, 1964; and Creighton, 1985a.

ment of work behaviors and skills can be incorporated into this setting through the collaborative effort of the occupational therapist and teacher. For example, simple math problems can be designed around the purchase of a week's groceries or a hamburger and french fries while practicing appropriate interpersonal skills. The accompanying display, devised by Stephens and Clark (1985), is a composite list of play, leisure, and household activities promoting readiness for work that may be incorporated into classroom activities.

COMPOSITE LIST OF PLAY-LEISURE AND HOUSEHOLD ACTIVITIES THAT PROMOTE VOCATIONAL DEVELOPMENT

1. Construction sets: erector sets, Tinkertoys, Lego sets
2. Toy cars and trucks
3. Doll play
4. Household odds and ends
5. Toy tools
6. Handcrafts
7. Collections
8. Dress up
9. Cops and robbers
10. Doctor–nurse–patient
11. Space fantasy games
12. Other dramatic play
13. Races
14. Contests
15. Model building
16. Photography
17. Playing cards
18. Sketching
19. Drawing and coloring books
20. Painting
21. Scrabble
22. Dramatics
23. Musical instruments
24. Creative writing
25. Inventions
26. Experiments
27. Videogames and computer play
28. Soccer
29. Basketball
30. Baseball and softball
31. Aerobic exercises and dancing
32. Care for pets
33. Care for younger siblings
34. Help with housework
35. Clean own room
36. Make own bed
37. Wash and dry dishes; help load dishwasher
38. Remove trash
39. Help with yard work
40. Set dinner table
41. Prepare simple foods
42. Run errands for parents
43. Do chores for neighbors and teachers

Adapted from Goldstein & Oldham, 1979; Shannon, 1974; and Stephens & Clark, 1985.

Work programs particularly targeted toward students with special needs should include the following options, which can be visualized in a hierarchy: *regular vocational education; adapted vocational education; special vocational education; individual vocational training;* and *prevocational evaluation services* (Howard, 1979).

Regular vocational education

In regular vocational education, specific vocational and academic programming is provided. Training is dependent on the student's age, strengths and weaknesses, interests, motivation, and goals. The occupational therapist may work directly with the student in vocational classes, provide individual or group therapy, or act as a consultant to faculty.

Adapted vocational education

Regular vocational programs may be modified to meet the needs of the special students. The occupational therapist may act as a direct consultant to the vocational teacher by providing adaptive devices, work simplification techniques, or task analysis or by working directly with the student in class to implement these recommendations. In addition, individual or group treatment may be provided by the occupational therapist.

Special vocational education

For the student whose disability is so severe as to preclude success in a regular vocational program, a self-contained special education class or placement in a facility specializing in the student's needs may be a valuable option. Programming usually focuses on the development of work behaviors and skills that may be used in entry-level, semiskilled jobs or in vocational training programs. Rehabilitation workshops may be used for training. The occupational therapist may consult with the classroom teacher in developing appropriate tasks that facilitate work behavior and skill development or engage in direct programming with the student. Direct treatment is typically in the form of group activities related to work, for example, playing the role of a grocery bagger or babysitter.

Individual vocational training

Programming may also be tailored to meet the individual needs of each student because the level of functioning may vary greatly. Some students may be capable of performing rudimentary academic, work-related tasks and self-care activities; whereas others who are severely disabled may require constant supervision and intensive individual and group training. Programs may be offered in a variety of settings, such as school, community, work-study, and on-the-job training. The occupational therapist can assist in planning goals for the student, perform job site analysis, and provide direct and consultative care. Occupational therapy programming usually requires that the tasks be performed in highly structured environments under close supervision. Some commonly used work tasks may be categorized as independent ADL, for example, sweeping, mopping, dusting, folding clothes, washing dishes, setting tables, and handling and moving materials.

Prevocational evaluation services

Prevocational evaluation services are "designed to provide vocational assessment to students whose disability precludes the use of the regular education sequence" (Howard, 1979, p. 14) These services are usually provided by facilities under contract with the school, such as rehabilitation workshops and private vocational assessment centers. Subcontracted activities are often used in programming, for example, collating, packaging and labeling, envelope stuffing and stamping, and assembly.

Remedial services

When the person has been identified, through the assessment process, as having medical, psychological, social, or physical limitations, remediation is needed. Kester states that

> some conditions are temporary and do not prevent return to previous employment, even before remediation is completed. Other disabilities that are more permanent in nature might not preclude return to work if adaptive devices or environmental changes could compensate for the personal limitation. A third category involves the permanent . . . disability that is severe enough to prevent return to previous employment. . . . (1983, p. 251)

This third category may even include disability that is severe enough to prevent exposure to work in the first place. Direct treatment is typically used for the first two categories and work adjustment services for the third category.

Direct occupational therapy treatment and intervention

The occupational therapist has an almost limitless number of activities to use in treatment. Depending on the facility and its philosophy, treatment may involve support in exploring or identifying possible work objectives, independent ADL training, and preventive education training. Some modalities used are work simulations, work samples, and crafts, such as woodworking and leather crafts. Work hardening is a frequently used approach to intervention.

Often, success at intervention relies on the person's motivation to succeed at established goals and on addressing the psychosocial ramifications of the disability. Involving the person in planning intervention goals and using activities that are of interest to them (such as tasks from their work) may be the best course of action. For example, the occupational therapy department at the Liberty Mutual Medical Service Center in Boston uses various work samples, such as a multiwork station that resembles a two-story house under construction and a cross-section of truck cab, that are composed of job tasks common to their industrial-injury patients. In addition, they use the popular work simulator in treatment (Bettencourt et al., 1986; Jacobs, 1985, 1991).

For the person with psychosocial disabilities, the variety of treatment modalities also is almost limitless, although there may be specific safety precautions that eliminate some of the options. Some additional variables that may need to be considered in designing programming are that these people often have difficulty making transitions and tend to decompensate when adapting to change usually because of their fear of failure; and inconsistencies in behavior and work performance can be due to changes in medication or their inconsistent use or disuse (Jacobs, 1985, 1991). Activities that provide the opportunity for group interaction are highly recommended. The designing of a business enterprise, which allows for grading jobs in various

levels of difficulty, has been met with much success—for example, the establishment of a greeting card company whose jobs include stamping precut designs on paper, folding paper, wrapping and packaging, taking inventory, and bookkeeping.

Work adjustment

> ***Work Adjustment*** is an educational/training process utilizing individual and group work, and work-related activities, to assist individuals in understanding the meaning, value and demands of work; to modify or develop attitudes, personal characteristics, and work behaviors; and to attain a functional level of vocational development. (McCarron & Dial, 1986, p. 3).

Work adjustment services should focus on the following objectives:

- Development of work tolerance
- Motivation to do productive work
- Becoming self-reliant
- Accepting supervision
- Relating effectively to coworkers
- Developing safety habits
- Punctuality
- Developing concentration, accuracy, and speed on the job (McCarron & Dial, 1986)

Occupational therapists use some or a combination of the following techniques with these people: individual or group therapy, planned work experience, modeling and imitation learning, behavior modification, and individual and group instruction.

Rehabilitation workshop employment

Rehabilitation workshop employment offers assessment, training, employment, and other rehabilitative services in a controlled and protective setting that allows people to work at their own capacities and often to receive corresponding remuneration (Jacobs, Mazonson, Pepicelli, Clague, & Leekoff, 1985–1986). These facilities typically are privately operated and serve either the developmentally or emotionally disabled. Although generally called *sheltered workshops*, there are four categories under this model: transitional workshops, sheltered workshops, work activity centers, and avocational or day adult activity centers (Jacobs et al., 1985–86). Occupational therapists and certified occupational therapy assistants may be employed in rehabilitation workshops in full- and part-time capacities and as consultants. Typically, they work as consultants to rehabilitation staff and directly with patients to develop work behaviors and skills. Common activities used with patients include ADL, subcontracted piece work, and work simulations. In addition, the occupational therapist may use job analysis, work simplification, and adaptation techniques.

Termination and follow-up care

For some people, the vocational rehabilitation (work) process is finite and can be terminated after programming goals are attained. For others, this may be a lifelong process or one that is entered into periodically, with follow-up care provided.

Summary

The area of work practice provides many opportunities for the occupational therapist. This has been reflected through a review of its history and significant legislation related to work.

Work practice provides the occupational therapist with a variety of employment settings and contact with diverse professionals on an interdisciplinary team. The occupational therapist provides assessments, in particular work evaluations. There are a vast array of evaluations to choose from, and more are being developed and refined. Both the occupational therapist and the certified occupational therapy assistant provide work intervention and programming that is dependent on the individual patient's needs. This might include, for example, providing work hardening for a worker injured on the job, supported employment for a patient with a long history of mental health issues, or educational training to develop work behaviors for a student with developmental disabilities.

The area of work practice has greatly expanded in the 1980s, a trend that is predicted to continue into the 21st century. Prevention and the use of ergonomic principles will become key areas for practice. The occupational therapist who wants to keep a strong hold on this area of practice will need to anticipate change to be ready to meet the demands of the future (Jacobs, 1991).

CASE STUDY

J, age 59 years, was seen over a period of 4 months in occupational therapy at a local vocational rehabilitation center. J had been an assembly-line worker at a local factory for 40 years, since graduation from high school. When the factory was sold, the new owner modernized the factory, replacing J's job with high technology. Shortly thereafter, J was laid off and went on unemployment. For 3 months, he diligently looked for employment similar to his past job but found that all the jobs of a similar nature had been replaced by high technology. During this period of job searching, J became depressed and developed carpal tunnel syndrome in his left, nondominant hand. After seeing his family doctor for his physical complaints, he was referred to the local vocational rehabilitation center.

At the center, the vocational rehabilitation counselor coordinated J's assessment process. The occupational therapist was included in J's rehabilitation team. As part of the assessment process, the occupational therapist reviewed J's records and had the opportunity to interview his wife and son. An interest inventory was provided to explore and identify interests, desires, and possible work objectives. J was given the following three VCWSs: VCWS #1, small tools (mechanical), VCWS #8, simulated assembly, and VCWS #18, dynamic physical capacities, as well as a partial sensorimotor evaluation. J was cooperative and pleasant during the evaluation sessions. The interest inventory indicated that J enjoyed many activities that involved fine motor skills, use of tools, reading, and spectator sports.

J's confidence increased while his depression decreased as he was able to complete the work samples with an above-average speed, with no errors, and with average and above quality. He was able to lift the required weight and perform physical tasks required at each strength level. The only potentially limiting factor was revealed in the sensorimotor test-ing: paresthesia and some pain involving the first three fingers of his left, nondominant hand, the forearm, and wrist. Sensation was slightly diminished along the median nerve distribution. No edema was noted. J noted that his discomfort usually increased in the evening.

Evaluation results were shared with J's vocational rehabilitation team, who believed that J became aware of his capabilities through the evaluation process. With the support of the vocational rehabilitation team, J was able to make the transition from feeling disenfranchised to developing the confidence to make a commitment to learning a new job that required his previously developed work behaviors, physical capacities, and aptitudes. The team recommended that J try on-the-job training, which could be provided at a local air-conditioning repair company. The job placement specialist assisted J with the formal training period at this job. Follow-up care would be provided if needed. A prescription for a neutral position splint was obtained from J's physician, and the occupational therapist constructed a splint to be worn in the evenings.

References

Abberbock, E. (1991). Supported employment. *Independent Living, 6,* 63–64.

Americans With Disabilities Act of 1990. Public Law 101–336. (1990). Washington: Federal Register.

American Occupational Therapy Association. (1990). *Membership files.* Rockville, MD: AOTA.

American Occupational Therapy Association. (1986). *Work hardening guidelines.* Rockville, MD: AOTA.

American Occupation Therapy Association. (1980). *The role of occupational therapy in the vocational rehabilitation process.* Rockville, Md: AOTA.

Bear-Lehman, J., & McCormick, E. (1985–1986). The expanding role of occupational therapy in the treatment of industrial hand injuries. *Occupational Therapy in Health Care, 2,* 79–88.

Becker, R. L. (1981). *Reading-Free Vocational Interest Inventory.* Columbus: Elbern Publications.

Bettencourt, C. M., Carlstrom, P., Brown, S. H., Lindau, K., & Long, C.M. (1986). Using work simulation to treat adults with back injuries. *American Journal of Occupational Therapy, 40,* 12–18.

Bolton, B. (Ed.). (1976). *Handbook of measurement and evaluation in rehabilitation.* Baltimore: University Park Press.

Botterbusch, K. F. (1982). *A comparison of commercial vocational evaluation systems* (2nd ed.). Menomonie, WI: Materials Development Center, Stout Vocational Rehabilitation Institute, University of Wisconsin-Stout.

Botterbusch, K. F. (1978). *Psychological testing in vocational evaluation.* Menomonie, WI: Materials Development Center, Stout Vocational Rehabilitation Institute, University of Wisconsin-Stout.

Caplow, T. (1954). *The sociology of work.* Minneapolis: University of Minnesota Press.

Catalyst. (1980). *What to do with the rest of your life.* New York: Simon and Schuster.

Chaffin, D. & Anderson, P. (1987). *Occupational biomechanics.* New York: John Wiley & Sons.

Clark, P. N. (1979). Human development through occupation: Theoretical frameworks in contemporary occupational therapy practice, part 1. *American Journal of Occupational Therapy, 33,* 505–514.

Commission on Accreditation of Rehabilitation Facilities. (1989). Work hardening programs. In *Standards manual for organizations serving people with disabilities,* pp. 69–72. Tucson: CARF.

Commission on Accreditation of Rehabilitation Facilities. (1987). *Standards manual for organizations serving people with disabilities.* Tucson: CARF.

Creighton, C. C. (1985a). Career development theory. In M. Kirkland, & S. Robertson (Eds.). *Planning and implementing vocational readiness in occupational therapy.* Rockville, MD: AOTA.

Creighton, C. (1985b). Three frames of reference in work-related occupational therapy programs. *American Journal of Occupational Therapy, 39,* 331–334.

Distefano M. K. Jr., & Pryer, M. W. (1970). Vocational evaluation and successful placement of psychiatric clients in a vocational rehabilitation program. *American Journal of Occupational Therapy, 24,* 205–207.

Florey, L. L., & Michelman, S. M. (1982). Occupational role history: A screening tool for psychiatric patients. *American Journal of Occupational Therapy, 36,* 301–308.

Golden, M. (1991). The Americans With Disability Act of 1990. *Journal of Vocational Rehabilitation, 1,* 13–20.

Ginzberg, E., Ginzberg, S. W., Axelrad, S. et al. (1951). *Occupational choice: An approach to a general theory.* New York: Columbia University Press.

Goldstein, B., & Oldham, J. (1979). *Children and work: A study of socialization.* New Brunswick, NJ: Transaction Books.

Havighurst, R. J. (1964). Youth in exploration and man in emergence. In H. Borow (Ed.). *Man in a world of work.* Boston: Houghton Mifflin.

Hightower-Vandamm, M. (1981a). Nationally speaking: The role of occupational therapy in vocational evaluation, part 1. *American Journal of Occupational Therapy, 35,* 563–565.

Hightower-Vandamm, M. (1981b). Nationally speaking: The role of occupational therapy in vocational evaluation, part 2. *American Journal of Occupational Therapy, 35,* 631–633.

Hightower-Vandamm, M. (1982). Nationally speaking: To market, to market. *American Journal of Occupational Therapy, 36,* 293–299.

Howard, R. (1979). *Vocational education of handicapped youth: State of the art.* Washington, DC: National Association of State Board of Education.

Jacobs, K. (1991). *Occupational therapy: Work-related programs and assessments* (2nd ed.). Boston: Little, Brown.

Jacobs, K. (1985). *Occupational therapy: Work-related programs and assessments.* Boston: Little, Brown.

Jacobs, K., Mazonson, N., Pepicelli, K., Clague, I., & Leekoff, W. (1985–1986). Work center: A school-based program for vocational preparation of special needs children and adolescents. *Occupational Therapy in Health Care, 2,* 47–57.

Kester, D. (1983). Prevocational evaluation. In H. Hopkins, & H. Smith (Eds.). *Willard and Spackman's occupational therapy* (6th ed.). Philadelphia: J. B. Lippincott.

Kielhofner, G. (1980). A model of human occupation, part 3: Benign and vicious cycles. *American Journal of Occupational Therapy, 34,* 731–737.

Kielhofner, G. (1983). *Health through occupation: Theory and practice in occupational therapy.* Philadelphia, F. A. Davis.

Kiernan, W. E., & Petzy, V. (1982). A systems approach to career and vocational education programs for special needs students: Grades 7–12. In K. P. Lynch, W. E. Kiernan, & J. A. Stark (Eds.). *Prevocational and vocational education for special needs youth: A blueprint for the 1980s.* Baltimore: Paul H. Brookes.

Kirkland, M., & Robertson, S. (Eds.). (1985a). An overview of tests and measurements. In *Planning and implementing vocational readiness in occupational therapy.* Rockville, MD: AOTA.

Kirkland, M., & Robertson, S. (1985b). The evolution of work-related theory in occupational therapy. In *Planning and implementing vocational readiness in occupational therapy.* Rockville, MD: AOTA.

Marshall, E. (1983). [Notes on situational assessment.] Unpublished raw data. Loma Linda Department of Occupational Therapy, School of Allied Health Professions, Loma Linda University, Loma Linda, CA.

Matsutsuyu, J. (1969). The interest checklist. *American Journal of Occupational Therapy, 23,* 323–328.

McCarron, L., & Dial, J. G. (1986). *McCarron-Dial evaluation system: A systematic approach to vocational, educational and neuropsychological assessment.* Dallas: McCarron-Dial.

Miller, D. C., & Form, W. H. (1951). *Industrial sociology.* New York: Harper and Row.

Moorehead, L. (1969). The occupational history. *American Journal of Occupational Therapy, 23,* 329–334.

Mosey, A. C. (1981). *Occupational therapy: Configuration of a profession.* New York: Raven.

Mosey, A. C. (1970). *Three frames of reference for mental health.* Thorofare, NJ: Slack.

M.T.M. (1990). MTM (brochure).

National Easter Seal Society. (1990). *The Americans With Disabilities Act: An easy checklist.* Chicago: National Easter Seal Society.

Niemeyer, L. O. (1991). Procedural guidelines for the WEST standards evaluation, section 6: Methods-time measurements new normative data for use with the WEST 1, 1A, 2, 2A. Long Beach, CA: WEST.

Ogden-Neimeyer, L., & Jacobs, K. (1989). *Work hardening: State of the art.* Thorofare, NJ: Slack.

Osipow, S. H. (1973). *Theories of career development.* New York: Appleton-Century-Crofts.

Parsons, F. (1909). *Choosing a vocation.* Boston: Houghton Mifflin.

Reynolds-Lynch, K. (1985a). Prevocational and vocational assessment in occupational therapy. In M. Kirkland, & S. Robertson (Eds.). *Planning and implementing vocational readiness in occupational therapy.* Rockville, MD: AOTA.

Reynolds-Lynch, K. (1985b). Vocational assessment: The field in general. In M. Kirkland & S. Robertson (Eds.). *Planning and implementing vocational readiness in occupational therapy.* Rockville, MD: AOTA.

Roe, A. (1957). Early determinants of vocational choice. *Journal of Counseling Psychology, 4,* 216.

Rosenberg, B. (1973). The work sample approach to vocational evaluation. In R. E. Hardy, & J. G. Cull (Eds.). *Vocational evaluation for rehabilitation services.* Springfield, IL: Charles C. Thomas.

Shannon, P. (1974). Occupational choice: Decision-making play. In M. Reilly (Ed.). *Play as exploratory learning: Studies in curiosity behavior.* Beverly Hills: Sage.

Small, L. M. (1986, November). Disenfranchised worker strategies. *Occupational Therapy News,* 28.

Stephens, L. C., & Clark, P. N. (1985). Schoolwork tasks and prevocational development. In P. N. Clark, & A. S. Allen (Eds.). *Occupational therapy for children.* St. Louis: C. V. Mosby.

Super, D. E. (1957). *The psychology of careers.* New York: Harper and Row.

Thompson, G. (1987). Work-related assessment in occupational therapy: An overview. *Work Programs Special Interest Section Newsletter (AOTA), 1,* 1.

Toppel, A. (1990). *Work Programs Special Interest Section annual business meeting.* New Orleans: AOTA.

Uniform Terminology for Occupational Therapy. (1989). *American Journal of Occupational Therapy, 43,* 808–815.

U.S. Department of Labor. (1981). *Selected characteristics of occupations defined in the dictionary of occupational titles.* Washington, DC: Superintendent of Documents, U.S. Government Printing Office.

U.S. Department of Labor. (1979). *Guide for occupational exploration.* Washington, DC: Superintendent of Documents, U.S. Government Printing Office.

U.S. Department of Labor. (1977). *Dictionary of occupational titles* (4th ed.). Washington, DC: Superintendent of Documents, U.S. Government Printing Office.

Valpar International Corporation. (1986). *Valpar International Corporation brochure.* Tucson: Valpar International Corporation.

Walls, R. T., Zane, T., & Werner, T. J. (1978). *The vocational behavior checklist.* Dunbar, WV: West Virginia University Research and Training Center.

Watanabe, S. (1968). *Activities configuration.* 1968 Regional Institute on the Evaluation Process, Final Report RSA-123-T-68. New York: AOTA.

Wright, G. N. (1980). *Total rehabilitation.* Boston: Little, Brown.

Wyrick, J. M., Niemeyer, L. O., Ellexson, M., Jacobs, K., & Taylor, S. (1991). Occupational therapy work-hardening programs: A demographic study. *American Journal of Occupational Therapy, 45*, 109–112.

Bibliography and other sources

Ad Hoc Committee of the Commission on Practice (1980). The role of occupational therapy in the vocational rehabilitation process: Official position paper. *American Journal of Occupational Therapy, 34,* 881.

American Occupational Therapy Association. (1991). *Occupational therapy services in work practice.* Rockville, MD: AOTA.

Bailey, D. (1971). Vocational theories and work habits related to childhood development. *American Journal of Occupational Therapy, 25,* 298.

Brolin, D. E. (1976). *Vocational preparation of retarded citizens.* Columbus: Charles E. Merrill.

Cromwell, F. (Ed.). (1985/86). *Work-related programs in occupational therapy.* Occupational Therapy in Health Care. New York: Haworth.

Cromwell, F. S. (1976). *Occupational therapist's manual for basic assessment: Primary prevocational evaluation.* Altadena, CA: Fair Oakes Printing Co.

Cromwell, F. S. (1959). A procedure for prevocational evaluation. *American Journal of Occupational Therapy, 13,* 1.

Ethridge, D. A. (1968). Prevocational assessment of rehabilitation potential of psychiatric patients. *American Journal of Occupational Therapy, 22,* 161.

Fidler, G. S. (1966). A second look at work as a primary force in rehabilitation and treatment. *American Journal of Occupational Therapy, 20,* 72.

Granofsky, J. (1959). *A manual for occupational therapists on prevocational exploration.* Dubuque, IA: W. C. Brown Book Co.

Herbin, M. (1987). Work capacity evaluation for occupational hand injuries. *Journal of Hand Surgergy, 12A,* 5.

Hertfelder S., & Gwin, C. (1989). *Work in progress.* Rockville, MD: AOTA.

Jacobs, K. (Ed.). (1990a). Industrial rehabilitation. *Work: A Journal of Prevention, Assessment, and Rehabilitation, 1,* 5–77.

Jacobs, K. (Ed.). (1990b). Work: Occupational therapy interventions. *Occupational Therapy Practice, 1,* 1–87.

Materials Development Center. (1984). *Work adjustment program: An overview.* [Slide/tape]. Menomonie, WI: Materials Development Center, University of Wisconsin-Stout.

Materials Development Center. (1980). *Vocational evaluation: An overview.* [Slide/tape]. Menomonie, WI: Materials Development Center, University of Wisconsin-Stout.

Maurer, P. A. (1971). Antecedents of work behavior. *American Journal of Occupational Therapy, 25,* 295.

Occupational therapy benefits from CARF changes. (1987). *Occupational Therapy News, 41,* 1.

Reed, K., & Sanderson, S. R. (1980). *Concepts of occupational therapy.* Baltimore: Williams & Wilkins.

Wegg, L. S. (1960). Eleanor Clarke Slagle lecture: The essentials of work evaluation. *American Journal of Occupational Therapy, 14,* 65–69, 79.

Woodside, H. H. (1971). Occupational therapy. A historical perspective: The development of occupational therapy—1910–1929. *American Journal of Occupational Therapy, 25,* 226–230.

Recommended resources

Baltimore Therapeutic Equipment Co., 1201 Bernard Drive. Baltimore, Maryland 21223.

Journal of Rehabilitation, National Rehabilitation Association, 633 South Washington Street, Alexandria, VA. 223124.

Materials Development Center, Stout Vocational Rehabilitation Institute, School of Education and Human Services, The University of Wisconsin-Stout, Menomonie, Wisconsin 54751.

Methods-Time Measurement Association for Standards and Research, 1411 Peterson Ave., Park Ridge, IL 60068.

The National Center for Research in Vocational Education, Ohio State University, 1960 Kenny Road Columbus, Ohio 43210-1090.

Vocational Evaluation and Work Adjustment Bulletin, published by the Vocational Evaluation and Work Adjustment Association, a division of the National Rehabilitation Association.

SECTION 2B2
Industrial rehabilitation

SALLIE E. TAYLOR

KEY TERMS

Classification of Jobs According to Worker Traits

Cumulative Trauma Disorder

Dictionary of Occupational Titles

Dictionary of Occupational Titles Supplement

Ergonomics

Job Simulation

Physical Demands

Primary Limiting Factors

Product Line

Symptom Magnification

Work Station

Work Hardening

LEARNING OBJECTIVES

Upon completion of this section the reader will be able to:

1. *List seven potential sources of referral for an industrial rehabilitation program.*

2. *List the two product lines that have comprised the bulk of practice in industrial rehabilitation to date.*

3. *Name the two most promising growth areas in industrial rehabilitation for the 1990s.*

4. *Describe the components of a functional capacity evaluation.*

5. *List four types of functional capacity evaluations in a CARF-accredited work hardening program.*

6. *Compare the roles of the registered occupational therapist and the certified occupational therapy assistant in an industrial rehabilitation program.*

7. *List two changes that will contribute to the shaping of the practice of industrial rehabilitation during the 1990s in each of the following areas: the workplace, the economy, and the practice of industrial rehabilitation.*

The development of programs and services to facilitate the rehabilitation of the injured worker has enjoyed unprecedented growth during the past decade. Starting as an aggressive, multidisciplinary program called work hardening, industrial rehabilitation has rapidly grown into a cadre of services designed to meet the special needs of business and industry. Occupational and physical therapists have formed the cutting edge, establishing programs of injury prevention, safety education, worker selection, work station modification, and ergonomics consultation. By combining efforts, occupational and physical therapists have made industrial rehabilitation the fastest growing area of rehabilitation practice in the United States.

Historical overview

Occupational therapy's commitment to the rehabilitation and health concerns of the worker has roots that reach back to the 1920s. After World War I, restoration aides—some of whom were later to become occupational therapists—directed their skills toward helping wounded veterans achieve the functional level necessary to gain employment. With time, occupational therapists applied their skills in rehabilitation treatment and creative problem solving to a broader scope of functional tasks. Since the 1960s, most occupational therapists have practiced in hospital- or school-based rehabilitation programs. These programs have typically been directed toward independent function in the school, the home, and the community. The special needs of the injured worker in preparing for return to work after injury were de-emphasized and almost lost from occupational therapy practice. Even so, some occupational therapists always have directed their practice toward helping the injured worker regain independence on the job.

Conditions that created the opportunity for occupational therapy

When an employee is injured on the job, the cost of the injury can be astounding. Although state law guides the workers' compensation (insurance payment) system, injured workers are entitled to a percentage of their usual pay throughout the treatment and recovery periods. The employer must pay for all medical and physical rehabilitation expenses incurred in treating the injury. Sometimes, there are payments for psychological treatment as well as for transportation to and from medical and rehabilitation appointments. Finally, a settlement agreement is negotiated between the employer and the injured worker or an agent. The settlement usually includes compensation for the injury and for any residual disability, along with an additional amount for pain and suffering. There also are legal fees associated with reaching the settlement. All these out-of-pocket costs are born by the employer.

Until the early 1980s, payments connected with on-the-job injuries ran into millions of dollars annually. Costs of work injuries in the United States continued to escalate each year. Before the mid-1980s, these costs had always been considered an inevitable expense of doing business. The costs were simply added to the price of the industry's product. In the early 1980s, however, many companies found that they were in danger of pricing themselves out of business. As an alternative method of retaining profitability, management began a search for areas with potential for cost reduction. Costs incurred in connection with on-the-job injuries were a natural target for closer control.

Corporate interest in cost containment coincided with a major change in health care reimbursement practices. The medical community was adjusting to the economic impact of Medicare's 1983 shift away from fee-for-service payment to prospective payment for care provided to the nation's hospitalized elderly. The pressure on hospital-based occupational therapy departments caused by Medicare cutbacks provided the incentive for occupational therapy department directors and hospital administrators to examine the new, nontraditional practice of work hardening. At that time, specialized rehabilitation services for the injured worker were 100% reimbursable by workers' compensation insurance. Hospital and rehabilitation administrators quickly recognized that work hardening could provide a lucrative revenue base.

Dr. Leonard Matheson, a psychologist with training in vocational rehabilitation, provided significant impetus for occupational therapists to reclaim a major role in industrial rehabilitation. In 1983, Matheson initiated a series of workshops on work tolerance screening and work hardening. Assisted by Linda D. Neimeyer, OTR, Matheson described his highly successful program of assisting workers to reenter the work force. Matheson urged occupational therapists to apply their professional skills to the needs of modern industry. Meanwhile, Carolyn Baum, OTR, FAOTA, American Occupational Association President in 1982 and 1983, was simultaneously advocating the exploration of new opportunities for occupational therapy. Baum strongly supported occupational therapists' reentry into the workplace. Baum, Matheson, and Neimeyer provided the leadership that enabled occupational therapists to maximize their initial opportunity to build work-focused programs.

The transition

As occupational therapists began to envision application of their skills in the work environment, the transition from a hospital- or classroom-based model of practice to one of work-related service delivery occurred smoothly. Skills previously used to guide patients from dependence to independence in the school, hospital, home, or community were easily translated to guiding patients into functional independence in the job setting. Employers and their insurance carriers welcomed the new, aggressive work hardening therapy. Employers, insurance carriers, and physicians have continued to benefit from the variety of work-focused programs that industrial therapists (both occupational and physical therapists) have developed. Industrial therapists have rapidly expanded the scope of their services to meet the many specialized health care needs experienced in business and industry.

Interfacing with business: communication

The practitioner of industrial rehabilitation must communicate with employers and insurance carriers in terms that are familiar to them. The language of this market has been established by the United States Department of Labor and differs from the medical terminology in which occupational therapists have been schooled. The industrial rehabilitation therapist becomes bilingual in a very real sense. Information regarding a patient's performance during evaluation or treatment may be reported to the referring physician in one way and to insurance carriers, attorneys, Social Security administrators, judges, and employers in different nomenclature to provide the clearest meaning to the reader.

Reference materials

The United States Department of Labor has compiled several documents that provide excellent references for the therapist who wishes to develop a second language in work-related practice. The first of these is the **Dictionary of Occupational Titles** (DOT). The DOT, and its companion publications, the **Dictionary of Occupational Titles Supplement** and the **Classification of Jobs According to Worker Trait Factors** (COJ), provide generic information about the more than 20,000 jobs that exist in the United States economy. The DOT and its supplement contain the following useful information:

- An alphabetic listing of all occupational job titles
- A brief description and job title for most jobs encountered in the United States labor market
- An occupational listing of titles arranged by industry
- An analysis of requirements placed on a worker who performs the job

The COJ is used in tandem with the DOT and its Supplement. A full range of worker trait factors is cross-referenced in these documents for each job title listed in the DOT and its supplement. Worker trait factors include the following:

Environmental conditions surrounding the worker, such as extremes of heat or cold, noise, fumes, and hazards
General educational level or training required to perform the job proficiently
Aptitudes generally needed for successful job performance, such as intelligence, form perception, and manual dexterity
Interests and temperaments commonly found in workers who successfully perform the job, such as adaptability to accepting responsibility or to performing repetitive work
Physical demands of the job, such as seeing, hearing, feeling, handling, lifting, carrying, climbing, pushing, and pulling.

All jobs listed in the DOT fall into one of five work levels according to the United States Department of Labor's Work Level Classification System (see the display). This classification system is based on the amount of weight that must be lifted, moved, or handled on the job. Both the usual amount and the maximal amount of weight moved figure into the assignment of a work classification for a particular job. The COJ provides the work level at which a given job generally is performed. The usual and maximal amounts of weight moved in performing a given job is vital information for the industrial rehabilitation therapist, who is either evaluating a patient or guiding a patient's rehabilitation program toward specific job performance.

Referral sources

Referrals to the industrial rehabilitation program are generally made by someone who is seeking definitive information about a patient's capabilities and limitations. Often, a *physician* makes a referral to help determine a worker's readiness for return to employment after injury. Sometimes, an *employer* requests services that will help determine how effectively a worker may perform a new job. The employer may also seek services that will help prevent injury and promote safety and wellness in the workplace. The employer's *insurance carrier* or *administrator* may request rehabilitation services to return an injured worker to the job as rapidly as possible.

When an injury case is severe or when it takes undue time for a worker to recover from an injury, a *case manager* assumes direction of the case. The case manager often is a rehabilitation nurse employed by an insurance carrier. The case manager may refer a patient to the industrial rehabilitation program for evaluation or for therapy.

Attorneys make referrals to industrial evaluation and rehabilitation programs. Either the plaintiff's or the defendant's attorney may request a functional capacity evaluation (FCE) or treatment in personal injury or in workers' compensation cases. *Rehabilitation counselors* also may request an FCE. Data from the FCE may help establish a patient's potential to perform a certain job for which the patient was trained under the sponsorship of vocational rehabilitation services. Representatives of *educational institutions* may refer students to industrial rehabilitation programs for this same reason.

Industrial rehabilitation services

Whether the industrial rehabilitation program deals with patients with psychosocial or physical problems, many of the program services may be the same. Although industrial rehabilitation facilities typically include a variety of programs, the two **product lines** that have comprised the bulk of practice for most therapists to date have been *FCE* and *work hardening therapy*. *Work conditioning* is becoming increasingly popular and shows great promise as a program that facilitates an employee's early return to work. *Ergonomics consultation* is a product line with great appeal to many occupational and physical therapists. The demand for ergonomic services is expected to increase in the

---

CLASSIFICATION OF WORK LEVELS

Sedentary work requires a maximum lift of 10 lb, infrequently and occasional lifting or carrying of papers, small tools, or file folders. Sedentary work may require occasional walking or standing.

Light work requires a maximum lift of 20 lb, with frequent lifting or carrying of up to 10-lb objects. If a great deal of walking, standing, or pushing and pulling of arm or leg controls is required by the job, the job is classified at the light level even though the lifting requirements do not exceed 10 lb.

Medium work requires a maximum lift of up to 50 lb with frequent lifting and carrying of weights up to 25 lb.

Heavy work requires a maximum lift of 100 lb with frequent lifting or carrying of objects weighing up to 50 lb.

Very heavy work requires lifting objects greater than 100 lb with frequent lifting or carrying of objects weighing 50 lb or more.

decade of the 1990s. Before discussing these four areas in greater detail, let us briefly describe some of the other product lines commonly structured to form an industrial rehabilitation program.

Physical therapy

Injuries to the lower back, neck, shoulders, elbow, hand, hips, knees, and ankles are the most commonly seen in industrial rehabilitation programs. Strains, sprains, and fractures are the most frequently diagnosed problems. Early referral to treatment is an important factor in accomplishing rapid return to work. If a patient with a musculoskeletal injury can start physical therapy treatment within the first week after injury, the chances of fast recovery at a low cost are optimal. If the patient has not recovered sufficiently within a few weeks to return to work, the patient should be reevaluated medically. It may be appropriate at this point to transfer the patient into a more aggressive rehabilitation program, such as work conditioning or work hardening. Close communication with the physician helps the therapist know how hard to push the patient toward recovery.

Hand therapy

In most states, hand injuries constitute a large percentage of workers' compensation claims. Therapists with specialized training and certification in hand rehabilitation can effect an optimal return to work if they become involved in the management of the injury at an early stage. Specialized skills, good rapport with the patient, and close communication with the treating physician or surgeon, as well as with the employer and the insurance carrier, helps to ensure the best possible outcome for the patient and the employer. Types of injuries commonly treated by hand therapists vary from region to region depending on the risks of the industries located in the geographic area.

Postoffer job evaluation

Postoffer evaluation may be requested by an employer for a worker who has accepted a position with the company as a new employee or as a transfer to another job within the organization. The data collected in this evaluation help the employer to evaluate the match between the worker's demonstrated capabilities and the specific performance requirements of the new job. This service is usually purchased by a company in an effort to reduce risk of injury by ensuring that the worker is physically able to perform the most strenuous parts of the job.

Prevocational evaluation

Prevocational evaluation and treatment programs help patients achieve a level of mastery of self-care or general work skills before determining job placement. School-based occupational therapy programs, head trauma centers, pain management units, and rehabilitation centers provide a first step toward the long-term goal of entry or reentry into the work force.

Job modification

Company managers are increasingly cognizant of the importance of safe, efficient placement or location of job components in the design of a job to prevent occupational injuries. The occupational therapist may recommend job or equipment modifications to reduce the physical or psychological stress imposed on the worker. Sometimes, adjustment of the height of the work surface, the distance or angle of reach, or the seating arrangement can make a significant difference in the stress imposed on the worker by the task.

Physical injury prevention programs

Many companies have begun to recognize the value of offering injury prevention programs for their workers. The most common of these programs provided by industrial therapists are back schools and cumulative trauma prevention programs. Back schools demonstrate safe lifting techniques and methods of handling materials associated with a company's specific jobs. Back schools typically emphasize both the biomechanically and physiologically safest movements and lifts for the employee to use in a particular job.

Educational programs that inform the employee and supervisor about high-risk factors for **cumulative trauma disorders**, especially for carpal tunnel syndrome, are growing in popularity as an increasing number of jobs involve extensive use of computers and video display terminals. Cumulative trauma disorders (CTDs) are diseases that result from physical stress to the musculoskeletal or peripheral nervous system over a period of time. Repetition, force, vibrations, and cold temperatures are recognized as the primary factors in either work or leisure activities that most often result in CTDs. Industries that require fine hand and finger movements, such as the electronics industry, also expose workers to high risk for developing cumulative trauma disorder. Educational programs encourage the worker to identify and avoid positions and movements that are likely to result in physical injury. They also emphasize to the worker the importance of seeking medical treatment at the earliest signs of discomfort. This enables supervisory and medical personnel to begin to manage the problem before it develops into an injury of major proportions.

Expert witness testimony

Industrial therapists may be engaged to provide expert witness testimony in a court of law. The therapist may be hired by either the plaintiff's or the defendant's attorney to assess functional limitations and capabilities. In either case, the industrial therapist's testimony is usually based on an FCE administered to the plaintiff. The FCE must be conducted and documented in the same way for either situation, regardless of the focus the attorney gives the reported findings. The therapist must remain as objective and unbiased as possible, or the credibility of the testimony will be damaged.

Health promotion and wellness programs

Many companies offer their employees short training programs to assist them in taking responsibility for their own health behavior. The objective is to provide the worker with information and assistance in developing healthy lifestyles that minimize time lost from work due to physical or emotional stress. Among the most popular training programs offered by occupational therapists are stress management, development of leisure skills, relaxation, smoking cessation, energy-saving techniques for home or work management, and personalized exercise programs with emphasis on flexibility, muscle balance, and cardiovascular fitness.

Ergonomics consultation

Ergonomics consultation is rapidly becoming a popular specialty service for occupational and physical therapists in industrial rehabilitation. Smith (1989) defines *ergonomics* as "the study of the interaction or fit between workers and their total workplace environment" with the overall goal of improving worker safety and performances by maximizing this fit (p. 128). The ergonomist's role at the work site is to provide guidance in the physical arrangements of the various job components so that workers can perform all parts of their jobs with minimum physical stress. The ergonomics specialist may work with the company's industrial engineer, industrial hygienist, and perhaps representatives from management and labor in designing equipment layout, work flow, or work stations. The *work station*, or physical space and equipment required by a worker to perform the duties of the job, is of special interest to the ergonomics specialist. The ergonomics specialist may offer advice, such as appropriate height of work surface, so that a task may be done without the workers having to bend too far or reach too high. The ergonomist may suggest ways of adjusting the height of the work surface so that both short and tall people can perform the job without undue physical stress. Suggestions about modifying a work station may be offered so that the work is in good visual alignment. The ergonomist may recommend altering the positioning of a job task or changing the handle of a tool so that upper extremities may be well aligned while performing a task. The ergonomist may recommend chairs or stools that provide the worker with optimal back support.

The occupational therapist follows an injured or disabled worker into the workplace to recommend ways that the individual job, tools, or work station may be modified to enable the worker to attain or retain competitive employment. The ergonomist, in contrast, makes recommendations to companies on behalf of apparently healthy workers in the plant. These suggestions are focused on preventing injury and minimizing physical discomfort for all employees. Special training in ergonomics through university courses or continuing education is a prerequisite for the industrial therapist who offers consultation in ergonomics.

Work conditioning

Many industrial rehabilitation programs offer work conditioning as an alternative to work hardening. Work conditioning is a concentrated program of exercises and exercise activities individually prescribed to increase strength, flexibility, and aerobic capacity. The program is frequently set up on the basis of circuit training and aerobic conditioning activities.

Work conditioning is the program of choice if the patient needs more rigorous exercise than would be received in a typical physical therapy program and if the patient does not require job simulation activities before returning to work. Preceded by a brief course of physical therapy, this program is increasingly prescribed within the first few weeks of injury. Work conditioning may also be integrated into a program of work hardening if the patient has been off work for an extended period.

As companies try to keep pace with changing requirements of business, it may be necessary to transfer or reassign workers to different jobs. This could happen as a result of downsizing, retooling, or automating a job. Some companies have employees work in several different jobs during the course of a day or week. Many companies request that the industrial rehabilitation program provide work conditioning to help employees prepare for the physical demands of the new job.

Work conditioning is a natural extension of a physical or occupational therapy program. It forms a natural bridge between acute physical therapy and work hardening. Managed by a physical or occupational therapist or an exercise physiologist, work conditioning has become an important product line for industrial rehabilitation programs in the 1990s.

Functional capacity evaluation

The FCE stands alone as a one-time evaluation. It measures a patient's performance against given criteria to predict his or her potential to engage in work. The criteria against which measurements are made may be job-specific, as in the case of an injured worker who may eventually return to his or her job. Alternately, the test may be made using the general classification of work levels defined by the United States Department of Labor. In this case, the general work level in which the patient may successfully function is identified (see the display).

Reasons for referral

Functional capacity evaluations may be requested from a variety of sources. A physician may request an FCE to obtain data on which to base a patient's disability rating. The physician may also wish to receive objective performance data to help in prescribing appropriate treatment.

An insurance carrier may require data to assist in the settlement of a workers' compensation claim. An attorney in personal injury litigation may seek a clear definition of a patient's ability to function normally. A rehabilitation counselor may require physical performance parameters to develop an individualized employment plan with a patient.

The FCE findings are used to help the referring source make a decision that requires clear delineation of the worker's abilities and limitations.

Preparing for the evaluation

Preparation for evaluation begins several days in advance of the actual evaluation. The therapist must arrange for review of medical records, including the records of any therapy the patient has received relative to the reason for evaluation. Before the first measure is taken, the therapist should be acquainted with three factors from the patient's perspective:

1. What the patient perceives has happened
2. What the patient recognizes has been done about it
3. What the patient expects will happen in the future with regard to recovery and return to work

This information may be obtained by telephone contact with the patient. Use of a mailed questionnaire in advance of a work performance evaluation is highly desirable because it allows the patient to respond thoughtfully to queries. This permits the patient to consider the questions carefully, to refer to records, and to note names and dosages of present medications directly from the labeled containers. Generally, educational and work histories are more extensive if the patient prepares them in response to items on a questionnaire in advance of the appointment.

When the patient arrives for the initial visit, information may be obtained from the receptionist regarding the patient's manner and any physical limitations exhibited on entering the evaluation center. Any assistance required by the patient during the registration process is noted by the receptionist and related to the evaluating therapist.

The evaluation process

Interview

An interview, which can be accomplished in 15 to 30 minutes if the patient has brought a completed questionnaire to the appointment, allows the therapist and the patient to initiate their working relationship. In addition to obtaining subjective information from the patient, the therapist begins the objective evaluation by observing the patient's sitting tolerance for the duration of the interview.

Direct measures

With subjective reporting by the patient well covered, the evaluation moves into a second phase, a period of specific and direct measurement. The basic measures of muscle strength, joint range of motion, sensibility, coordination, balance, functional mobility, and endurance are performed and recorded.

Most industrial evaluation and treatment centers have computerized equipment for use in measuring lifting, pushing, and pulling strengths. Data from this equipment contributes to the overall objectivity of the FCE.

Standardized tests

A number of standardized tests may be employed in the data collection process at this point. Tests such as grip strength, the Minnesota Rate of Manipulation Tests, the Jebson-Taylor Test of Hand Coordination, and any combination of the many standardized instruments on the market provide useful information and normative data for comparison.

Standardized test results can add strength to the overall test findings if the patient is a member of the reference group on which the norms were based.

Job simulation

Finally, the FCE often has a work sample or simulated job task component (*job simulation*) that is individualized for each patient.

When the patient's job is specified, the therapist selects those factors that are essential to the job but that the therapist deems likely to challenge the patient's performance ability based on information concerning the nature and extent of injury in the medical record. These functions of the job are set up as nearly as the therapist can manage to require the same motion, pace, and resistance required on the job. Tests that give a good idea of the patient's cognitive as well as physical functioning are included in the various components of the total evaluation.

When there is no specific job targeted in testing the patient, a general FCE may be conducted. Testing follows the same pattern through the subjective, direct, and standardized measurements. For the job simulation component, however, the evaluation designates several tasks at the sedentary work level as defined by the U.S. Department of Labor in the COJ. After completion of sedentary work tasks, the patient is advanced through tasks at successive work levels (light, medium, heavy, and very heavy) until the patient's performance reaches a plateau. The level at which the patient can safely and comfortably perform both the frequent lifting and the maximal lifting requirements specified in the COJ is the work level classification at which the patient reasonably may seek gainful employment.

Evaluation findings

After the FCE is concluded, the therapist will have obtained considerable data regarding the limits of the patient's functional performance for the day of testing. Many tests will have been performed to the patient's point of maximal strength or endurance. Other tests will have provided data that allow the therapist to compare the patient's performance with that of a normative group.

After review of data collected in the work performance assessment, the therapist is able to identify the patient's strengths and weaknesses for job performance. The therapist can identify the factors that impede the patient's return to work at the time of testing, which are called *primary limiting factors* for the job. The therapist can also determine the extent to which the limitations prevent the patient from performing the job.

Calling on professional experience, the therapist is able to make a judgment regarding which of the limiting factors may yet be responsive to remediation, adapted devices, or adapted environments. The therapist also can identify the skills that the patient has to offer in the labor market and the skills on which alternative work may be based.

In discussion with the patient, and then in a written report to referral sources, it is appropriate for the evaluating therapist to recommend a course of action that may enable the patient to enter or reenter the work force. The recommendation may, for example, include a course of acute hand or physical therapy, a period of work conditioning, or entry into a work hardening program. In this case, the evaluation also specifies the estimated length of time that the recommended therapy program may be expected to last.

Work hardening program

Work hardening accounts for a large portion of the practice of occupational therapists engaged in industrial rehabilitation programs. The *CARF Standards Manual for Organizations Serving People With Disabilities* (1991) describes work hardening programs:

> *Work hardening* programs, which are interdisciplinary in nature, use conditioning tasks that are graded to progressively improve the biomechanical, neuromuscular, cardiovascular/metabolic and psychosocial functions of the person in conjunction with real or simulated work activities. Work hardening provides a transition between acute care and return to work while addressing the issues of productivity, safety, physical tolerances, and worker behavior. Work hardening is a highly structured, goal-oriented, individualized treatment program designed to maximize the person's ability to return to work. (p. 64)

Program accreditation

Industrial evaluation and rehabilitation services are provided most frequently through hospital-based, medically affiliated, or independent, free-standing facilities. Since 1989, CARF has provided guidelines for accreditation of work hardening programs that are applicable in any of these settings (CARF, 1991). Many consumers, especially the large workers' compensation insurance carriers and self-insured companies, have a policy of referring workers only to CARF-accredited work hardening programs. Accreditation by this national body provides the consumer with assurance of a high standard of rehabilitative care.

Program entry

Entry into work hardening occurs in one of two modes. The patient may enter a program immediately after an injury. Often, however, patients are referred to work-hardening programs some time after the injury has occurred. It is preferable for work hardening therapy to closely follow the completion of the acute phase of rehabilitation. Work hardening, then, becomes a progressive step in the total rehabilitation process. When little time is allowed to elapse between the injury and enrollment in an aggressive rehabilitation program focused on return to work, few changes in life roles for the patient or for family members are likely to occur.

Evaluation

The key to successful treatment in work hardening therapy, as in other occupational therapy treatments, is well-executed evaluation. A strong evaluation procedure provides the therapist with data on which to base treatment goals and to construct a strong treatment plan.

The evaluation should establish abilities and limitations within the framework of the demands of competitive work. Therefore, an FCE is the first step in the work hardening program. CARF guidelines establish the following specific types of FCE for work hardening programs:

Baseline evaluations: A baseline assessment of functional ability to perform work activities, which includes the U.S. Department of Labor's physical demand factors

Job capacity evaluations: An assessment of the match between the patient's capabilities and critical demands of a specific job

Occupational capacity evaluation: An assessment of the match between the patient's capabilities and the critical demands of an occupational group

Work capacity evaluation: An assessment of the match between the patient's capabilities and the demands of competitive employment (CARF, 1991)

As with the FCE, the testing time for each of these evaluations may vary from a half day to a week. The length of the assessment depends on the specific questions concerning the patient's rehabilitation that the test is designed to answer.

Preparation for treatment

Once the patient's abilities and limitations for work performance have been identified, the industrial rehabilitation treatment team formulates measurable, work-related rehabilitation goals. Goals are set for both long- and short-term treatment. Each of the rehabilitation goals must be realistic, attainable, and focused on the patient's reentry into the work force.

The work hardening program may be designed to challenge the patient to a higher level of physical or cognitive demand than demonstrated in the evaluation. A work hardening program of this type is appropriate for patients who have not yet selected or targeted a specific vocational or job goal.

Most often, however, work hardening is job-specific. In the case of a work injury, the patient usually attempts to return to the former job. The patient, of course, knows the requirements of that job well.

The employer usually is willing to provide the treating therapists with information about the job, including affording the therapists the opportunity to visit the workplace and see a worker actually performing the job. Job tasks that challenge the patient's physical or cognitive abilities are the focus of the job-specific work hardening program.

Treatment process

After acceptance into the work hardening program, treatment consists of graded activity to increase the patient's strength, aerobic capacity, and tolerance for tasks and postures required on the job. Exercise, activity, and simulated work tasks are fundamental to the treatment protocol. The therapy program is carefully designed to require the patient to move in the same planes across the same distances and to use the same muscle groups at the same pace and frequency required by the job. The therapist also designs simulated work tasks that require the patient to lift and carry materials of the same size and weight for the same distances as the job demands. Frequently, the employer lends significant items used in the patient's daily work to the therapists so that a job task can be closely simulated or practiced during work hardening.

The patient must be guided to progress to the next higher level of physical performance as soon as it is safe to do so. The goal of work hardening—returning the injured worker to work as quickly and safely as possible—must always serve as a guiding principle of the patient's rehabilitation.

Psychosocial considerations

Although the physical effects of the injury may be the primary focus of a work-hardening treatment program, the psychosocial needs of the patient should not be underestimated. Although these needs are not explored here, the following are some of the issues the injured worker faces during work-hardening therapy:

- Fear of reinjury on returning to the same job
- Concerns regarding supervisory response to returning to the job
- Concerns from peers regarding the patient's competence to perform job duties adequately, to carry a fair share of the work load, and, perhaps more important, to avoid injury to them
- Diminished financial settlement if the patient returns to work
- Concerns regarding the permanence of the job if the patient returns to work. In recent years, many companies unable to hold market position have simply gone out of business. As a result, some patients feel they must calculate whether they

will "come out better" with the maximal workers' compensation settlement they can obtain or whether they will be able to support their family better on unemployment benefits.

- Concerns regarding change in the role assignments within the family structure if the patient returns to a worker role

Although the patient may give fleeting thought to these issues on entry into a work hardening program, the initial focus of the program is primarily biomechanical. As the patient shows improvement in physical function and becomes aware of the possibility of returning to work, these psychosocial issues play a more dominant role in the total treatment process. The work hardening staff must provide the patient with sensitive assistance in working through these concerns.

Sometimes, psychosocial issues become a significant block to the rehabilitation process. In this event, the work hardening team typically refers the patient to a more specialized source of assistance for working through the problem. A referral to a psychotherapist, perhaps through the employer's Employee Assistance Program, often is appropriate.

Discharge

When the patient has demonstrated proficiency in accomplishing the job requirements over a 3- to 5-day period, the patient may be released to return to the physician for final disposition. At this point, it is appropriate for the therapist to recommend that the patient return to full duty without restrictions if the work hardening therapy performance has demonstrated the patient's ability to do so. Not all work hardening patients, however, are successful in meeting return-to-work requirements. When this is the case, the therapist may recommend a return to restricted work. The therapist specifies to the physician the demonstrated limitations or restrictions that will enable the patient to perform at maximal job capacity.

In preparation for a patient's return to restricted work duties, the industrial therapist may visit the worker's supervisor at the job site. Together, they may be able to design equipment or work station or task modifications that will enable the worker to do the job. There are many possibilities for work modifications. The most commonly practiced include instituting rest pauses and job rotation. The supervisor may even be able to relieve the worker of a task that the worker cannot yet perform and reassign it to another employee on a temporary basis. In this case, the supervisor usually appreciates receiving recommendations from the industrial therapist.

If return to former or modified work is deemed impractical, a referral to a vocational rehabilitation counselor is usually appropriate. The aim is to assist the patient in retaining gainful employment at maximal functional level.

Symptom magnification

One of the most difficult yet interesting challenges for the occupational therapist in industrial rehabilitation is the issue of symptom magnification. During the course of the evaluation and treatment processes, the therapist must be sensitive to *any* inconsistencies in the patient's performance. The patient who clings to the banister during direct testing of stair climbing but walks down stairs without holding hand rails at the end of the

evaluation or the simulated work day is demonstrating a performance inconsistency. The patient who cannot bend forward on direct testing but does so to obtain a soft drink from the soda machine is performing inconsistently. These inconsistencies often represent the patient's effort to impress staff with greater than actual impairment. This misrepresentation is commonly called *symptom magnification*.

This behavior is sometimes displayed by the worker to impress on the therapist the intensity of the injury. When this is the case, the patient is often able to set this behavior aside and get on with recovery when gently confronted. Occasionally, however, the magnified symptoms are an attempt on the part of the worker to prolong the time away from the job or to increase the amount of the workers' compensation case settlement. Although symptom magnification behavior may be observed and should be documented for referral and payment sources, the therapist must not make assumptions about motivations for the patient's behavior.

Impairment rating

After worker injury, rehabilitation, and recovery or stabilization, a physician performs an impairment rating examination of the patient. This examination results in the assignment of a percentage rating of the residual functional limitation sustained by the worker. Monetary settlements, sometimes of vast sums, are made on the basis of the assigned impairment rating. Typically, until the late 1980s, little or no consideration was given to the extent to which the patient's job performance was affected by the injury. Nor was it customary for the physician to determine whether or not job performance was affected at all by the injury. The advent of industrial rehabilitation programs in the early 1980s made new information available to the rating physician.

Many physicians now rely heavily on data obtained from an FCE or from a course of work hardening therapy in their final evaluation of the injured worker. This allows the physician to consider the patient's strengths and assets for job performance as well as limitations or disabilities when assigning an impairment rating.

Vocational rehabilitation and vocational evaluation

Sometimes a patient's job performance ability is permanently affected by accident or disease to the extent that the patient is unable to return to the previous work. Inability to meet job demands may be immediately obvious, as in the case of a barge deck hand whose leg is traumatically amputated in a motorcycle accident and who would be unsafe walking or hopping on a string of river barges in choppy water. The construction worker whose back is broken in a fall, resulting in partial paralysis of both lower extremities, provides another example. With other patients, limiting factors that prevent return to previous work may not show up until the FCE or even until a period of work hardening has been accomplished and the patient's functional limitation is consistently shown to interfere with the performance of simulated job tasks.

When the industrial therapist makes the judgment that the patient is unable to return to the original or modified work, a referral to a vocational rehabilitation counselor or to a vocational evaluator is appropriate. Members of these two professions, if at all possible, identify and match the patient's transferable skills with opportunities for employment in the local community.

Litigation

Because the question of financial settlement is often pending when patients enter an industrial rehabilitation program, many patients are not totally committed to attaining or to demonstrating complete recovery from their injuries. It is extremely important for the therapist to be sensitive to the implications of pending litigation, which include the following:

- The patient may put forth less than maximal effort in the FCE, work hardening, or work conditioning program. This is likely to reveal itself in inconsistencies in performance during the testing or treatment period.
- The patient's motivational level for return to work may be low.
- The patient may be sensitive to the fact that all documentation of performance in the industrial rehabilitation program will be reviewed by parties involved in the litigation.

The patient population treated by industrial therapists is likely to be more manipulative than many patients treated by occupational therapists in other areas of practice. It is not unusual for the patient to attempt to play one member of the rehabilitation team against another. For this reason, it is important for members of the industrial rehabilitation team to communicate frequently with each other and to present a coordinated approach to the patient's care.

It is not unusual for the industrial therapist to be called on to give legal testimony regarding a patient's performance in an evaluation or a patient's response to a rehabilitation treatment program. The close adherence to the evaluation or rehabilitation program's established protocols and accuracy in documentation will prove extremely helpful to occupational therapists who practice industrial rehabilitation in the event that they are called on to explain testing or treatment procedures in a court of law.

Role of the therapist

The practice of industrial therapy provides challenging opportunities for occupational therapists and for certified occupational therapy assistants. The occupational therapist conducts all job analyses, FCEs, work hardening evaluations, and testing in post-offer screenings. The occupational therapist considers the evaluation findings and formulates an assessment statement for all documentation. In addition, the occupational therapist establishes an appropriate treatment plan with specific short- and long-term goals.

Industrial rehabilitation provides many opportunities for the certified occupational therapy assistant. Early in the work hardening program, the assistant is encouraged to visit the work site to see the job to which the injured worker will return. This first-hand exposure allows the certified occupational therapy assistant to closely simulate job tasks in following through with the patient's treatment program. Under the supervision of the occupational therapist, the assistant implements the patient's

treatment plan and collects performance data by taking performance measures in the preparation of progress or discharge reports. If the patient returns to work with restrictions, the certified occupational therapy assistant may suggest and implement modifications at the work site. The assistant who knows the returning patient well and the progress made in the work conditioning or work hardening program can provide the company supervisor with information concerning the patient's capabilities. The supervisor will find this helpful as the recovered worker returns to the job.

Marketing and sales are an important part of the operation of an industrial rehabilitation program. Many occupational therapists and assistants enjoy the challenge of interacting with company representatives in a marketing or sales capacity. The positive experiences that patients have in the industrial rehabilitation program are extremely important in the continued viability and growth of the program. Cooperative, respectful relationships among staff, especially between occupational therapists and certified occupational therapy assistants, are important in creating an atmosphere in which positive rehabilitation can occur.

Future considerations

The phenomenal success of industrial rehabilitation therapists during the past decade in addressing the needs of business and industry has established this specialty area well into the 21st century. During the 1990s, industrial therapists may expect significant changes in the workplace, in the economy, and in the practice of industrial rehabilitation. Workplace changes are likely to include a moving away from jobs requiring heavy lifting and gross body movements to an increasing number of upper-extremity–intensive jobs. Many of these jobs are highly repetitive and frequently lead to the development of cumulative trauma disorders. Therefore, there may be an increased number of these cases. The number of jobs requiring heavy labor is decreasing due to increased automation in industry. Back injuries are becoming less prevalent.

As the American work force has grown older, interest in wellness and health promotion programs has increased and employers have become more willing to invest in education and injury prevention programs in an effort to keep workers' compensation costs from escalating beyond control. The economic environment of the 1990s shows that cost containment is key in conducting industrial rehabilitation practices; nevertheless, workers' compensation costs continue to climb. Escalating costs give insurance carriers greater power over companies to direct the spending of the insurance dollars. An effort may be made to establish a ceiling on workers' compensation payments. A number of health care providers may become members of preferred provider organizations and may discount fee-for-service payments to remain competitive in the delivery of occupational medicine services.

In the practice of industrial rehabilitation, occupational therapists will direct their energy in the 1990s toward refining their services to business and industry. Cost containment and quality service must be guiding principles for the most successful programs. Injury prevention and worker education will receive great emphasis. Accreditation for work hardening programs will become a significant factor in the selection of providers by consumers. Work conditioning may cut into the large work hardening referral base. Many occupational therapists will become ergonomics specialists. These many changes in the practice of industrial rehabilitation and the health care environment will be both challenging and rewarding to the occupational therapist and will result in improved service delivery to the worker.

Summary

Industrial therapy has captured both health care and corporate dollars. It continues as a growth industry as practitioners provide evaluation, rehabilitation, and training services to meet the specialized needs of business and industry. At this time, FCEs and work hardening programs comprise the major portion of industrial rehabilitation practice. Work conditioning and ergonomic consultation are increasingly in demand.

Worker education and injury prevention programs will become important product lines in the 1990s. Occupational therapists will be challenged to contain costs while improving health care services to the patient. As occupational therapists scrutinize and refine their programs on at least an annual basis, the practice of industrial rehabilitation will continue to evolve and to grow in step with changing business practices in a fluctuating economy.

References

Commission on Accreditation of Rehabilitation Facilities. (1991). Work hardening programs. In *Standards manual for organizations serving people with disabilities* (pp. 64–67). Tucson, AZ: CARF.

Field, J. E., & Field, T. F. (Eds.). *The classification of jobs according to worker trait factors.* Athens, GA: Elliot and Fitzpatrick.

Smith, E. R. (1989). Ergonomics and the occupational therapist. In S. Hertfelder & C. Gwin (Eds.). *Work in progress* (pp. 127–156). Rockville, MD: American Occupational Therapy Association.

U.S. Department of Labor. (1977). *Dictionary of occupational titles* (4th ed.). Washington, DC: U.S. Government Printing Office.

U.S. Department of Labor. (1986). *Dictionary of occupational titles* (4th ed.), supplement. Washington, DC: U.S. Government Printing Office.

SECTION 2C
Retirement planning

ELLEN DUNLEAVEY TAIRA

KEY TERMS

Arousal	*Naturally Occurring*
Cohort	*Retirement Communities*
Competence	*Role Continuity*
Environmental Press	*Role Discontinuity*
Instrumental ADL	*Life Expectancy*

LEARNING OBJECTIVES

Upon completion of this section the reader will be able to:

1. *Recognize elementary statistical concepts about life expectancy.*
2. *Recognize the role of environmental press in late life.*
3. *Incorporate preventive strategy into a treatment plan.*

I want to be thoroughly used up when I die.

GEORGE BERNARD SHAW

Shaw was 93 years old when he died. He lived a productive life and left us a rich legacy of his creative work, which continues to be presented on Broadway more than 100 years after his birth. Creative people usually have the good fortune to be able to do their work outside the constraints of the traditional schedule to which most of us are tied. They also have less job security, more freedom, and no need to heed mandatory retirement rules. Not surprisingly, then, people in the arts are often cited as examples of productive aging (Schechter, 1988). In fact, conductors like Toscanini and Fiedler have been studied to see if all their upper-extremity activity is a positive force in healthy aging!

Role continuity

What is most significant about the aging of people in the arts is that they are not required to stop abruptly and reverse their roles from active to passive. In other words, there is continuity from one stage of life to the next (Cox, 1988). Clark (1956) studied the leisure habits of retired men from different socioeconomic groups and found them to be consistent in their choice of leisure pursuits. Men from professional backgrounds with a high degree of education pursued more intellectual activities, such as reading, theater, and the arts, whereas men with occupations that taxed more physical than mental capacities chose fishing, hunting, and playing poker. According to Reitzes, Mutran, and Pope (1991) the more assets and education a retiree has, the more likely the retiree is to have an active social life. Marriage was also found to be a positive factor.

The theory of **role continuity** favored by sociologists is the process whereby people's activities and roles are adequate preparation for what will be expected at the next stage. Of greater concern is the strong tendency toward **role discontinuity** in American society, whereby passing from one stage of life to the next is not a smooth transition. The sudden offer of unlimited leisure to a person who had been engaged in daily work can have devastating physical and psychological effects. Most of us can reach into our family history and find a grandparent or great grandparent who died within a year of mandatory retirement.

Life expectancy

To plan for later years, a person must have a long-range view and a sense of confidence that the retirement years will offer pleasures that were unimaginable in youth. The idea of living to a ripe old age is relatively new. In 1900, the average **life expectancy**

TABLE 8-10. *Life Expectancy at Birth (in years)*

	1900		1990	
	Males	Females	Males	Females
Whites	48.2	51.1	73	78.9
Blacks	32.5	35	68.4	75.6

From U. S. Bureau of the Census, 1989; Hess, 1990.

was 50 years. In 1989, life expectancy was 79 years for women and 75 years for men (Table 8-10). The primary causes of death in the early part of the 20th century were infectious diseases that are now preventable because of advances in public health and the widespread availability of drugs, especially antibiotics.

Statisticians also consider a person's likelihood of living beyond age 65 because there is a presumption that if a person survives to that age, the chances of living to a very old age are good. A person who was 65 in 1987 can expect to live an additional 16.9 years, which is a 2-year increase from the 1979 to 1981 life expectancy tables. A great number of people will be over 85 years old in the next century since this is the fastest growing age group. This age group is also most vulnerable to functional disability (Kovar & Feinleb, 1991; Elston, Koch, & Weissert, 1991).

As life expectancy increases, planning for years without family or work responsibilities has become increasingly important. During the past century, most people were still working at the time of their death, except for the fortunate few who had good genes or perhaps good luck. Planning for old age meant helping with chores and assisting with the care of younger family members. Three generations under one roof was common. The idea of 25 years of leisure was novel.

Chronic diseases and the elderly

The most common causes of death among older people are heart disease, cancer, and stroke, which are responsive to preventive measures (U.S. Department of Health and Human Services, 1989). Public health professionals refer to a group of people of a certain age as a **cohort**. The cohort of older people now in their 60s and 70s did not grow up thinking about how to live a productive life when they were old since most did not expect to live this long. Yet these are the persons who will be coming to the attention of therapists for the next decade and into the next century.

CASE STUDY

A young therapist is working with an 80-year-old woman who has had degenerative arthritis since age 55. Gradual loss of function has brought her to the level of dependency that puts her at risk of nursing home placement. Reading her long history at the outpatient service, the therapist wonders why there was so little attention paid to her prognosis. The woman moved into a lovely house that had three stories and many steps when she was in her early 50s and has been struggling to stay ahead of the chores since her husband died 10 years ago.

Coming to terms in midlife with anticipated limitations is part of preretirement planning. People with mature coping skills are able to look honestly and objectively at their strengths and weaknesses in an effort to find the right amount of environmental press to support their later years.

Arousal and environmental press

As a person ages, the inevitable physical changes in sensory acuity, psychomotor speed, mobility, and social values require becoming more dependent on the physical environment. Urban or near urban seniors give up their cars and take buses or taxis. Women proud of their self-sufficiency agree to accept help with heavy housework. Younger home owners realize they need hand rails on their front steps as they watch their 75-year-old parents attempt to negotiate the steps.

Environmental psychologists discuss the delicate balance between arousal and environmental press. **Arousal** is the most primitive state of consciousness. **Environmental press** is defined by Lawton (1986) as expectations for certain behavior that stem from the setting. This environmental force can be physical, interpersonal, or social. A high level of personal **competence** increases an older person's ability to adapt to environments with varying degrees of press. Conversely, reduced competence leads to vulnerability to environmental influences and the potential for maladaptive behavioral outcomes (Lawton, 1986).

The physical limitations experienced with advanced age are the most devastating to an older person's independence but are also the most responsive to environmental interventions. Loss of strength and stamina makes stair climbing and carrying heavy bundles a primary consideration when planning for late life.

Barrier-free environments

The Rehabilitation Act of 1973 was landmark legislation that began the process of creating a barrier-free environment. Older buildings with small elevators and heavy entrance doors are reminders of how far we have come in our efforts to integrate people with physical and sensory limitations into our communities. This legislation, of course, included anyone who was handicapped without regard to age; older people as well as younger disabled people saw the Rehabilitation Act as a means of gaining access to buildings, services, and opportunities (Taira, 1984).

Although we have become accustomed to adapting the physical environment for disabled people, we will be required to do more because of the Americans with Disabilities Act (ADA). The improved accessibility of buildings, such as banks, theaters, and public transportation systems, mandated by the ADA will have a profound affect on accessibility issues confronted by our aging population.

A lifestyle change that late-middle-aged people may consider is a move to an apartment or retirement residence. This type of relocation can offer an environment that is sufficiently stimulating to provide activity but not so complex as to promote additional environmental press than can be supported by a person of gradually deteriorating competence.

CASE STUDY

A 68-year-old, recently widowed woman elected to sell her large, four-bedroom, colonial-style house in a residential neighborhood located in a medium-sized city not long after the death of her husband of nearly 50 years. This seemed unwise to her advisors, but she had experienced considerable environmental press in the brief time she was alone in the house. Although she could afford to pay for help, it was difficult to find people to do chores other than cleaning the house. In addition, she had been burglarized during her absence, and all her jewelry was stolen. A move to a condominium with other older people, good security, and the availability of assistance with repairs and household chores provided the supportive environment she needed in her advancing years.

Instrumental activities of daily living

When planning for the needs of the elderly, the principal means used to determine the functional level of an older person is assessment of ADL and instrumental ADL limitations. ADL tasks are customarily defined as eating, personal care, bathing, dressing, and mobility. **Instrumental ADL** tasks usually include shopping, meal preparation, laundry, light housekeeping, and money management.

Instrumental ADL tasks, especially shopping and laundry, are of particular concern to the occupational therapist when assisting an older person to plan for retirement years. Stone and Murtaugh (1990) found that 11% of their sample of community elderly needed assistance with shopping and that 8% percent had difficulty with mobility out of doors; this was considerably more assistance needed for these categories than for any other instrumental ADL category.

Need for activity

Since occupational therapy as a profession is solidly based in the need for purposeful activity throughout the lifespan, it follows that continued engagement in activity will contribute to life satisfaction (Barris, 1987 p. 43). Considerably more older people suffer from boredom and loneliness due to insufficient activity than from the excesses of a frantic social life.

Another important consideration when planning for retirement is the proximity of supportive friends and family. It is not surprising that older people contemplate moving closer to children and siblings when work or family obligations are reduced. Despite glamour stories of moves to sunbelt communities, less than 5% of older people live in retirement communities. Many move to condominiums and apartments that attract older residents known as **naturally occurring retirement communities** (Hunt & Ross, 1990).

Planning for a successful retirement is directly associated with functional independence. In a study of Canadians who were interviewed in 1973 and followed-up 12 years later, Roos and Havens (1991) found that remaining independent was the definition of successful aging and was associated with a higher level of life satisfaction and markedly less use of the health care system.

Summary

The burgeoning elderly population that is expected in the next century has implications for the practice of occupational therapy. Since the promotion of maximal functional independence is the primary goal of occupational therapy, assisting patients to plan for a purposeful, active, healthy retirement is an appropriate therapeutic intervention. Despite increases in life expectancy, there has not yet been a decrease in the prevalence of chronic disease. Planning for the consequences of physical aging and the inevitable wearing of the organism is an essential component of intervention. A retirement that includes sufficient stimulation and activity can be realized with skilled therapeutic intervention and attention to the strengths and limitations of mature years.

References

Barris, R. (1987). Activity: The interface between person and environment. *Physical and Occupational Therapy in Geriatrics, 5*(2), 39–49.

Clark, A. (1956). The use of leisure and its relation to levels of occupational prestige. *American Sociological Review, 21,* 301–7.

Cox, H. (1988). *Later life: The realities of aging.* Englewood Cliffs, NJ: Prentice Hall.

Elston, J., Koch, G., & Weissert, W. (1991). Regression adjusted small area estimates of functional dependency in the noninstitutionalized American population age 65 and over. *American Journal of Public Health, 81*(3), 335–343.

Hess, B. (1990). The demographic parameters. *Generations, 14*(3), 12–15.

Hunt, M., & Ross, L. (1990). Naturally occurring retirement communities: A multiattribute examination of desirability factors. *Gerontologist, 30*(5), 667–674.

Kovar, M., & Feinleb, M. (1991). Older Americans present a double challenge: Preventing disability and providing care. *American Journal of Public Health, 81*(3), 287–288.

Lawton, M. P. (1986.) *Environment and aging.* Albany: Center for the Study of Aging.

Reitzes, D., Mutran, E., & Pope, H. (1991). Location and well being among retired men. *Journal of Gerontology, Social Sciences, 46*(4), S195–S203.

Roos, N., & Havens, B. (1991). Predictors of successful aging: A twelve year study of Manitoba elderly. *American Journal of Public Health, 81*(1), 63–68.

Schechter, M. (1988). The music of productive aging, under the maestro's baton. In *Productive Aging News* (issue 25). New York: Mt Sinai Medical Center.

Stone, R., & Murtaugh, C. (1990). The elderly population with chronic functional disability: Implications for home care eligibility. *Gerontologist, 30*(4), 491–96.

Taira, E. (1984). An occupational therapist's perspective on environmental adaptations for the disabled elderly. *Occupational Therapy in Health Care, 1*(4), 25–33.

U.S. Bureau of the Census. (1989). *Projections of the population by age, sex and race: 1988–2080.* Current Population Reports, Series P-25, No. 1018. Washington DC: U.S. Government Printing Office.

U.S. Department of Health and Human Services. (1989). *Health United States and prevention profile.* DHHS Pub No(PHS) 90–1232. Washington DC:

Bibliography

Ager, C. (1986). Therapeutic aspects of volunteer and advocacy activities. *Physical and Occupational Therapy in Geriatrics, 5*(2), 3–11.

Dorfman, C., & Ager, C. (1989). Memory and memory training: Some implications for the well elderly. *Physical and Occupational Therapy in Geriatrics, 7*(1), 21–41.

Fazio, L. (1987). Sexuality and aging: A community wellness program. *Physical and Occupational Therapy in Geriatrics, 6*(1), 59–68.

Marino-Schorn, J. (1985). Morale, work and leisure in retirement. *Physical and Occupational Therapy in Geriatrics, 4*(2), 49–59.

SECTION 3

Play and leisure

SUSAN H. KNOX

KEY TERMS

Leisure	*Play*
Occupations	*Work*

LEARNING OBJECTIVES

Upon completion of this section the reader will be able to:

1. *Define the concepts of work, play, and leisure in terms of their form, function, meaning, and context.*
2. *Explain the stages of play and leisure throughout the life cycle.*
3. *Describe a variety of play assessments and determine their usefulness in evaluating children.*
4. *Differentiate play as a treatment method and play as treatment modalities and describe circumstances for the use of each.*
5. *Describe various leisure assessments.*
6. *Describe the importance of leisure theories in planning occupational therapy.*

Clark et al. (1991) define **occupations** as "the chunks of culturally and personally meaningful activity in which humans engage" (p. 310). People create or orchestrate their daily experiences by planning and participating in occupations (Yerxa et al., 1989). Occupational therapy generally considers work, self-care, leisure, play, and rest to be the major occupations of people. Since the inception of the profession, occupational therapy has always valued a balance of these occupations. It is not always clear, however, what is work or play or what constitutes a balance. This section addresses play and leisure but also clarifies work and its interrelation with play and leisure. The definitions of work, play, and leisure are explored; play and leisure throughout the life cycle is discussed; and play and leisure theories, assessment, and use in treatment are addressed.

Definitions

Occupations can be explained through the substrates of form, function, meaning, and context (Clark et al., 1991). Form includes products, activities, properties, and relations to time. Function includes process and experience. Meaning includes motivations and satisfaction. Context relates to changing definitions and views, historically and in different societies. These substrates form the basis from which work, play, and leisure can be defined.

Form

One of the foremost distinctions of activity is in relation to the availability of time within a day. Work time is often designated as paid employment and nonwork time as time spent outside work. Work is usually defined in terms of earning a living, either in paid employment or in productive activities (Parker, 1976, 1983). Work also includes nonsalaried activity that contributes to subsistence, such as homemaking, or reproduction, such as child care. Characteristics that distinguish work are: (1) extrinsic rewards, (2) formal duties and obligations, (3) performance within specified structure or time constraints, (4) task determined, and (5) predictability (Anderson, 1961; Neulinger, 1981; Parker, 1983; Brook & Brook, 1989).

Nonwork includes taking care of physiologic needs, nonwork obligations, and leisure. Often, nonwork time is equated with leisure. De Grazia (1962) counters this distinction:

> Work is the antonym of free time. But not of leisure. Leisure and free time live in two different worlds. Anybody can have free time. Not everybody can have leisure. . . . Free time refers to a special way of calculating a special kind of time. Leisure refers to a state of being, a condition of man, that few desire and fewer achieve. (p. 5)

Dumazedier (in Anderson, 1961) believes that leisure is time whose content is oriented toward self-fulfillment and is outside the needs and obligations of a person's occupation, family, and society. Kaplan (1975) notes seven characteristics of leisure: (1) leisure is self-determined, (2) it falls into free time, (3) it is viewed as leisure by the participants, (4) it is psychologically pleasant, (5) it has a range of commitment and intensity, (6) it contains norms and restraints, and (7) it provides opportunities for recreation, personal growth, and service to others.

Many play theorists (Caillois, 1958; Ellis, 1973; Cohen, 1987; Bergen, 1988) have categorized types of activities in which children engage. These include games, construction activities, social activities, imitation, practice play, and symbolic or dramatic play. There is no single characteristic common to all kinds of play, but among the qualities are the following: intrinsically motivated, spontaneous, fun, flexible, totally absorbing, vitalizing, an end in and of itself, nonliteral, and challenging (Huizinga, 1950; Ellis, 1973; Reilly, 1974; Cohen, 1987).

Function

Form and function are often combined when authors describe characteristics of work, leisure, and play, as can be seen in the aforementioned characteristics. Functions of work have been described as providing a livelihood, goal achievement, and production (Anderson, 1961; Neulinger, 1981; Parker, 1983; Brook & Brook, 1989). The functions of leisure can be described as personal development, enjoyment, entertainment, interaction with others, relaxation, free choice, challenge, and goal achievement (Dumazedier [in Anderson, 1961]; Kelly, 1983; Brook & Brook, 1989).

The values or benefits of play are many. Play contributes to development in giving children a sense of mastery over their own bodies and over the environment. It contributes to the development of sensory integration, physical abilities, cognitive skills, and interpersonal relationships. Play is one of the mediums through which children learn to express themselves and develop symbol formation. Through play, children practice adult and cultural roles and learn to become productive members of society (Reilly, 1974; Levy, 1978, Bergen, 1988). Takata (1971) cites the following principles of play: (1) play is a complex set of behaviors characterized by fun; (2) it is sensory, neuromuscular, mental, or a combination; (3) it involves repetition of experience, exploration, experimentation, and imitation; (4) it precedes within its own time and space boundaries; (5) it functions as an agent for integrating the internal and external worlds; and (6) it follows a sequential developmental progression.

A number of problems arise when one considers only form and function when attempting to differentiate work, play, and leisure. Often, activities that one person might consider work another might consider play. There often is an overlap of work and play or leisure, or a person may be involved in more than one activity at a time. Therefore, one must consider other factors when trying to determine the differences in the terms.

Meaning

Another way of classifying occupations is in terms of meaning of the experience. Parker, Brown, Child, & Smith (1977) cite three areas that affect the subjective experience of activities: attitude, motivation, and satisfaction. *Attitude* is the general approach that people have to activities as a result of their values and those of society. *Motivation* refers to the factors that pull people toward achieving certain goals, such as earning a living, fulfilling a duty, or self-esteem. *Satisfaction* is the relation between what one expects of a job or an activity and what is actually experienced. Brook and Brook (1989) state that satisfaction in work depends on the amount of recognition received for accomplishments and on the chance to use one's abilities and skills. They conclude that there are both intrinsic and extrinsic features present in work as well as factors related to stress, time constraints, and lack of free choice.

The reasons for satisfaction with leisure include the opportunity to recreate oneself; to gain new strength or to maintain good health, and to provide variety, self-actualization, self-reflection, and contemplation. Characteristics of the leisure experience are: (1) a sense of separation from the everyday world and a sense of timelessness, (2) freedom of choice in one's actions, (3) pleasurable involvement in the event, (4) spontaneity, (5) fantasy or creative imagination, (6) a sense of adventure and exploration, (7) self-realization, and (8) challenge (Anderson, 1961; Neulinger, 1981; Gunter, 1987).

Anderson (1961) states that different kinds of leisure have different values or meanings, and it is through this variety that people can derive satisfaction from their leisure activities. Neulinger (1981) states, "To one person it may mean something good, to another something bad, to one, something active, to another something passive, still to another something noble and

worthwhile, while to another something to be frowned upon, nay, immoral" (p. 1). However individual the leisure experience is, the most salient characteristics related to meaning appear to be the capacity for self-fulfillment, personal growth, creative expression, and personal autonomy.

Csikszentmihalyi (1975, 1990) has contributed a great deal to understanding the meaning and the motives for doing activities. He developed the concept of optimal experience and flow. Csikszentmihalyi describes optimal experience as happening when the challenge of an activity is congruent with a person's skills and abilities. He describes this state of psychic energy as flow. He states, "people become so involved in what they are doing that the activity becomes spontaneous, almost automatic; they stop being aware of themselves as separate from the actions they are performing" (1990, p. 53). Csikszentmihalyi believes that flow is a state of deep concentration in which consciousness is well ordered and that it leads to increased complexity of the self and increased integration of the self. Elements present during flow are a feeling of control, loss of self-consciousness, transformation of time, and concentration on the task at hand. Flow can occur in almost any type of activity, work or nonwork, and it provides motivation, satisfaction, and inner rewards. The flow experience contains many of the qualities described in play; however, Csikszentmihalyi makes a distinction in that play is often viewed as being removed from real life while flow has direct consequences to the person's everyday life.

Context

Work, play, and leisure obtain meaning through context. Iso-Ahola (1979, 1980) lists functions of leisure, related to context, that can also apply to work or play: (1) socialization of the young into society, (2) enhancement of one's performance by improving skills, (3) development and maintenance of interpersonal and social skills, (4) social entertainment, (5) enhancement of character and personality, (6) prevention of idleness and antisocial activity, and (7) development of a sense of community.

The value that the society places on activity influences individual interests. Historically, play and leisure were viewed as rare abnormal activities as opposed to the normal activities of work. And as the work ethic grew strong, play and leisure were regarded as undesirable. Play generally was viewed in terms of having to have a specific purpose to explain its existence, such as development of cognitive skills, and leisure was equated with recreation. It has only been in the postindustrial era that play and leisure have become more accepted (Cohen, 1987; Iso-Ahola, 1980; Kando, 1980; Neulinger, 1981; Mergen, 1977).

In primitive cultures and in some cultures today, there are not clear distinctions between work and nonwork or leisure. Anderson (1961) describes cultures in which all time is structured but not all time is work. In some farming or pastoral communities, work and leisure seem to be intertwined throughout the day depending on the rhythms and demands of the land or of the seasons.

Cultural perspectives also include the culture of the person's work place and how different work settings can influence one's work and leisure patterns (Epstein, 1990).

To summarize, **work** can be defined as activity done for production or reward as well as nonsalaried activity that contributes to subsistence or reproduction. It usually is constrained by time, space, or task, and it derives meaning through satisfaction, providing a livelihood and goal achievement. Work is usually driven by external motivation. *Leisure* usually occurs outside the obligations of one's work and provides opportunities for enjoyment, relaxation, recreation, personal growth, and goal achievement. Leisure is driven by internal motivation, implies freedom of choice, and is not usually constrained. *Play* is a developmental phenomenon, a type of activity and a way children interact with their environment. Play is the way children learn about the world through exploration, experimentation, and repetition. Play is spontaneous, intrinsically motivated, fun, totally absorbing, and performed for its own sake.

Play and leisure throughout the life cycle

The terms *play* and *leisure* are often used interchangeably and are usually differentiated by age, in that children play and adults engage in leisure activities. But play and leisure are not synonymous. Play has also been linked to work because the child learns skills and develops interests through play that later affect choices in work and leisure. Thus, play can be viewed as a continuum leading to both work and leisure. Children's play experiences lay the foundations for work and leisure through exploration; manipulation and investigation; learning; social interaction; competition, cooperation, and the learning of rules; and the development of competence, self-determination, and personality.

Throughout a person's life, the amount of time spent in activities defined as play, work, or leisure varies. In early childhood, most time is spent in play. As children mature, time is divided between school and free time, later work and nonwork. In older adults, leisure time predominates.

Stages of play and leisure have been summarized by Bergen (1988), Neulinger (1981), and others. In infancy, sensorimotor and exploratory play predominate. Infants develop mastery over their bodies and learn the effect of their actions on objects and people in the environment. The stages of this early sensorimotor play have been described by Piaget (1962), Rubin (1980), and others. By the end of the first year, infants are actively engaged in exploration, beginning to understand cause and effect, and interested in how things work. In the second year, play centers around combining objects and learning their social meaning. Children begin to classify objects and develop purpose in their actions. During the end of the first year and through the second, children begin to develop symbolic play and pretense. Social play begins very early with interaction between the infant and mother, and by age 3, children engage in complex social games.

Major changes in play occur from ages 3 to 5 years as children learn to adjust to the physical and social environment. Practice and exploratory play gradually shift into constructive play, and children become more interested in the outcome of the activity. Constructive play predominates in this period. Symbolic and pretense play are refined into dramatic and sociodramatic play. Children at this stage begin role play and thus learn about social systems. Garvey (1977b) describes four types of roles seen in group play: (1) functional roles (eg, doctor), (2) relational roles (eg, mother and baby), (3) character roles (eg, Superman), and (4) peripheral roles with no alternate identity. In addition to pretense play, social play continues to develop in two other forms: rough and tumble play and emergent games with rules (Bergen, 1988).

Play of the school-aged child has not been studied as extensively as that for other ages because school-aged children have more obligations on their time, namely school, and play is relegated to nonschool time. The major type of play seen at this stage is rule-governed games (Bergen, 1988), through which children learn reciprocity, or turn-taking. Social play and games with rules are particularly influenced by the culture. The physical environments available for play, peer groups, and the types of play encouraged by parents have changed as our society has become more urbanized (Neulinger, 1981). The current emphasis on organized sports (eg, Little League) and planned after-school activities illustrates some of these changes. In school-aged children, one can still observe practice and constructive play, but the difference lies in that the play appears to be ends-related rather than means-related. In other words, children practice to develop skills or construct to make a project. Symbolic play tends to be integrated into games with rules, such as Dungeons and Dragons, or transformed into mental games and language play, such as riddles or secret codes (Bergen, 1988). Fantasy play persists in secret clubs, daydreaming, or is substituted by television.

Adolescents are developing autonomy and becoming socialized into the adult role. This is a period of transition as obligations, time available for leisure, changes and refinements of interests, and family and peer pressures all affect teen activity (Neulinger, 1981). In a study by Csikszentmihalyi and Larson (1984), the largest single activity of adolescents was socializing; second was television and third was sports, games, hobbies, reading, and music.

The adult's predominant use of time is in work and raising a family. Multiple factors affect leisure patterns in adulthood, such as age, sex, marital status, work roles, and whether one has children and the children's ages. Time available for leisure and habits change as one goes through the stages of the adult. For example, single adults take part in a wider variety of activities outside the home than married people and, in particular, physical recreation or social activities vary between men and women of different ages. The impact of such innovations as television and computers has also changed leisure patterns through the years (Neulinger, 1981).

As people reach middle age and children leave home, time available for leisure increases. Neulinger (1981) states that the "general trend is for leisure interests and activities to become increasingly restricted with age, despite decreased responsibilities" (p. 580). A study by Nystrom (1974), however, showed that frequency of participation in activity and variety of activity chosen did not decrease with age, which reinforced the concept of maintenance of activity with aging.

Older adults are thought of as having a great deal of leisure. Broderick and Glazer (1983) found correlations between pre-retirement leisure participation and postretirement leisure, but age, health, mobility, and income played important roles in the amount of leisure and the quality of its enjoyment. Nystrom (1974) found that the most common activity for this age group was television; second was socializing, and then small handicrafts and reading. She found a slightly higher incidence of passive activities than active ones. Gregory (1983) found a relation between activity and meaning and life satisfaction.

Iso-Ahola (1980) cited research that shows that types of play in childhood affect adult leisure patterns but also that leisure patterns change continuously over the lifespan. He believed that this change is due to the person's need to seek novel and arousing leisure experiences. The acquisition of new leisure skills and replacement of old also shows the influence of socialization on leisure patterns. There tend to be changes in leisure activities rather than cessation as people age.

Play

Theories

Theories of play can be classified into four broad categories: evolutionary, physiologic, psychological, and sociocultural. They have been summarized by Reilly (1974), Ellis (1973), Parker (1976), and Neulinger (1981). Evolutionary explanations include such theories as Hall's recapitulation theory, Groos' view of play as preparation for life, and analogies between animal play and human play. Physiologic explanations include Schiller's and Spencer's idea of working off surplus energy, Patrick's view of recreation and relaxation, and Berlyne's theory of arousal. Psychological explanations include White's concept of intrinsic motivation and competence, Freud's unconscious processes, Erikson's development of ego function, cognitive development as described by Piaget and Bruner, and learning as summarized by Sutton-Smith. Sociocultural explanations include the development of social abilities as described by Parten, Huizinga's view of play and culture, symbolization and ritual, games as described by Caillois (1958), meaning and myth, and Reilly's rules and role development. Most of these explanations emphasize play's value in contributing to the child's development or to enculturation.

Assessment

Watching children play is like looking through a window into their lives since play is the way the child learns about the world. Analysis of children's play tells us much about their physical and cognitive abilities, social participation, imagination, independence, coping mechanisms, and environment (Brown & Gottfried, 1985; Bruner, Jolly, and Sylva, 1976; Ellis, 1973; Garvey, 1977a; Hartley & Goldenson, 1963; Bergen, 1988). Assessment of play and of the child's abilities as seen through play are necessary to provide the therapist with tools to analyze play and to plan treatment. Ellis (1973) believed that play could be defined in terms of motive or content. Motives are the reasons why or where play occurs. Content refers to the elements of play. Most of the play assessments examined developmental motives and looked at specific elements of play. This review of assessments includes those most often used in the occupational therapy literature. The reader is also referred to a comprehensive review of play and leisure assessments by Kielhofner and Barris (1984).

Kalverboer (1977) studied play as the relation of play organization to neurologic function. Descriptions were gathered on the child's behavior in relation to the physical and social environments. Levels of complexity of play were defined, and consistency and duration of play were designated. Kalverboer videotaped play observations with preselected play materials in a structured setting with a preset sequence.

Rosenblatt (1977) considered play to be a cognitive activity that contributes to children's knowledge of their relation to the world around them. Play and language are part of a continuum in the development of the meaning of symbols outside the child.

She observed children from 9 to 24 months of age in their homes with a standard set of toys using time sampling and classified the children's responses to toys in terms of types of play and quality of play.

Hulme and Lunzer (1966) were also interested in the relation of play, language, and reasoning. They observed the free play of children aged 2 to 6 years using an observation rating scale. The behavior was rated on each of two subscales: adaptiveness in the use of materials and integration of behavior. Adaptiveness in the use of materials considered the degree to which the child used the material appropriately and the extent to which the child adapted materials in other than obvious ways using constructive or imaginative purpose. Integration of behavior was a measure of complexity of behavior.

Smilanski (1968) elaborated on the stages of play development discussed by Piaget and others in her examination of sociodramatic play. She developed an assessment of six elements of sociodramatic play: (1) imitative role play, (2) make-believe in regard to objects, (3) make-believe in regard to actions and situations, (4) persistence, (5) interaction, and (6) verbal communication.

Rubin, Maioni, and Hornung (1976), Rubin, Watson, and Jambor (1978), and Sponseller (1974) developed similar observation models that feature the social play categories of Parten and the cognitive play categories described by Piaget and Smilanski. Behaviors were coded along the dimensions of social and cognitive play categories. These scales were used for observing toddlers and preschool-aged children.

Wolfgang and Phelps (1983) assessed children's preferences for play materials as reflecting development. They developed an inventory based on Piaget's categories of play. The inventory used pictures of play, and children were asked about play preferences.

Parten (1933) assessed social participation in play of preschool-aged children. She classified play into two dimensions: degree of participation and degree of leadership. Degree of participation included unoccupied, solitary, onlooker, parallel, associative, and organized supplementary play. Degree of leadership included independent pursuit, following some and directing others, sharing leadership with others, and directing alone.

Liebermann (1977) examined the relation of playfulness to divergent thinking. He observed kindergarten children on five playfulness traits: physical spontaneity, manifest joy, sense of humor, social spontaneity, and cognitive spontaneity. Each trait was measured for quantity and quality. Truhon (1983) examined playfulness in creative play by using Liebermann's categories along with tests of verbal and nonverbal creativity. Barnett (1990, 1991) and Barnett and Kluber (1982, 1984) further refined the concept of playfulness and developed a rating scale to assess the traits inherent in the definition of playfulness.

Although most of these assessments treat play as a developmental phenomenon, their focus has been on isolated aspects of play. Evaluation using one of them alone gives a biased view of the complexity of play. If one is only looking at cognitive or social context, the richness of the play experience is reduced. Linder (1990) developed a transdisciplinary play-based assessment that assesses the child in cognitive, social-emotional, language, and physical and motor development. The child is evaluated through observation of play in structured and unstructured settings, alone, with parents, and with peers.

In occupational therapy, the focus of therapy has been on

the whole child functioning within the environment. All aspects of development are considered important, and the developmental aspects of play have been the focus (Reilly, 1974; Takata, 1974; Florey, 1971, 1981). In the occupational therapy literature, two assessments explore play developmentally and consider the complexity of play: the Play History (Takata, 1969, 1971, 1974) and the Preschool Play Scale (Knox, 1968, 1974; Bledsoe & Shephard, 1982).

Takata (1969, 1971, 1974) looked at play as a developmental phenomenon, bounded by time and space, reflecting the interaction between the person and the external environment. She devised a semistructured interview and play observation to yield information about the child's daily activity schedule. She identified two elements of play: form and context. Form included the choice of play materials, amount and nature of playfulness, and organization in play and was thought to parallel changes in development. Context was the expression of the child's immediate needs, impulses, and physical and emotional states and reflected life's situations. Behnke and Fetokovich (1984) conducted reliability and validity studies on the Play History and found it to be a reliable and valid instrument for assessing children's play behavior.

Knox (1968, 1974) developed an observational assessment designed to give a developmental description of normal play behavior through the ages of 0 to 6 years. The assessment described play in terms of yearly increments and in terms of four dimensions: space management, material management, imitation, and participation. Space management was "the way in which the child learns to manage his body and the space around him; through the processes of experimentation and exploration" (p. 45). Material management was "the manner in that the child handles materials and the purposes for that he uses materials" (p. 46). Imitation was "the way in which the child gains an understanding of the social world around him and learns how to express and control his feelings through the processes of observation . . . imitation . . . and dramatization" (p. 46). Participation was "the amount and manner of interaction with persons in his environment, and the degree of independence and cooperation demonstrated in play activities" (p. 46). Children were observed indoors and outdoors and rated on all four dimensions.

Bledsoe and Shephard (1982) revised the scale and renamed it the Preschool Play Scale. They examined reliability and validity with normal children. Harrison and Kielhofner (1986) did the same with a disabled population. Both found the scale to be highly reliable and valid.

Two unpublished assessments have been designed to evaluate play in the middle childhood years. McDonald (1987) developed a self-report instrument designed to measure play activity and play style in 7- to 11-year-old children. Play activity was the chosen type and amount of time spent in specific play activities, and play style was the child's perceived style of play and frequency of participation in play behaviors. The instrument was tested on 77 children, and validity and reliability were established. Primeau (1989) developed an observation tool to assess game-playing behavior in preadolescent boys aged 9 to 11 years. The guide looked at violations of the social quality of game-playing behavior in the areas of obedience to rules, cooperation with other game players, and sense of fair play.

Recently, qualitative methods have been used to explore specific aspects of play. Pierce (1991) observed and analyzed the play of infants and toddlers to determine early object rule acqui-

sition. Three types of object rules were identified: rules of object properties, rules of object action, and rules of object affect. Knox (in press) observed the play of preschoolers to determine characteristics of playfulness and effects of caregivers and environments on playfulness. Qualitative methods offer much promise in examination of the complexity of play within natural environments.

Use of play in treatment

Play, especially in young children, is an automatic, integral part of existence. All children engage in some form of play, and it is through play that they develop an understanding of the world and competence in interacting with it. Play is an important treatment media in pediatric occupational therapy because of its importance to the child. Play activities are used in two ways: as a treatment method (play) and as treatment modalities (play activities).

The use of play as a treatment method has been described within the occupational behavior and sensory integration frames of reference. In occupational behavior, Reilly and her students (1974) first studied play systematically and studied the treatment effects of play on developing competent behavior. Reilly described play as the child's occupation and saw occupational behavior as the continuum of play and work. She defined play as a multidimensional system for adaptation to the environment and believed that the exploratory drive of curiosity underlies play behavior. This drive has three hierarchic stages: exploration, competency, and achievement. Exploratory behavior is seen most in early childhood and is fueled by intrinsic motivation. Competency behavior is fueled by effectance motivation and is characterized by experimentation and practice to achieve mastery. The third stage, achievement, is linked to goal expectancies and fueled by a desire to achieve excellence. Using an occupational behavior frame of reference, a goal of treatment would be the development of play behavior per se and the development of those elements of playfulness that would fuel competent interaction with the world through play.

Play is also valued as the arena through which sensory integration develops (Ayres, 1972, 1979). Successful play experiences depend on adequate adaptive responses to environmental demands that in turn are dependent on adequate sensory integration. In therapy, the therapist sets up and manipulates the environment (setting, objects, people) so that the child can choose among activities that potentially offer a challenge that is "just right" (Lindquist, Mack, & Parham, 1982). During treatment, the therapist constantly adjusts the environment, child, or activity to bring about successful adaptation. An excellent description of the role of play within a sensory integrative framework was provided by Bundy (1991):

> Play is a powerful tool for treatment. For many individuals, the most important byproduct of occupational therapy may be the improved ability to play. If it is carefully planned and conducted, therapy using the principles of sensory integration may be very helpful in facilitating the development of play. Likewise, play, as a part of a well orchestrated treatment plan, can result in improvements in sensory integration. (p. 67)

Mack, Lindquist, and Parham (1982) synthesized the communalities of play from the occupational behavior and sensory integrative viewpoints that relate to use of play in treatment and to the desired outcome:

In practice, both approaches deem the therapist responsible for structuring adaptive behavior from the child. Thus, the potency of the environment's influence on development is confirmed by both. But from neither perspective does therapy rely solely on environmental manipulation. The child's initiative and active involvement are critical to the therapeutic process. From both perspectives, the intrinsic motivation or self direction of the child is primary in guiding therapy, for importance is placed on the child's inner drive toward mastery. Play, then, is the process through that therapeutic goals are achieved. The ultimate goal of therapy—competence in daily life activities—is also shared by both perspectives. (p. 367)

What differentiates free play from therapeutic play? As described earlier, free play is intrinsically motivated, fun, and is performed for its own sake rather than having a purpose. In therapy, goals and objectives are established by the therapist. Rast (1986) described this apparent dichotomy and how play serves as the natural arena within which therapy goals can be achieved:

> Play offers a practical vehicle to enlist a child's attention, to practice specific motor and functional skills, and to promote sensory processing, perceptual abilities, and cognitive development. It also serves to support social, emotional, and language development. In the therapeutic setting, play often becomes a tool used to work towards a goal, despite the fact that the goal-oriented, externally controlled aspects of the therapy situation conflict with the essence of play itself. (p. 30)

For play to be used successfully in treatment, the child should feel responsible for choosing or directing the play episode. This is particularly important when the goal is to increase competence in play development. Research has shown that when external constraints are placed on play, it is perceived as work and no longer contains playful elements (Mogford, 1977, Wade, 1985, Rast, 1986).

There may be instances when the therapist needs to be more directive, such as with a child who has severe problems with self-initiation of activity, when a specific skill needs to be taught, or when a specific goal (such as increasing range of motion) needs to be met. Here, playful activities can be used in a more structured or defined sense. For example, a child's favorite toy might be positioned in such a way to improve the child's range of motion, or adapted to increase the child's strength. Conflict may arise when therapy goals or techniques require a more structured, hands-on approach, and it often requires skill and imagination on the part of the therapist to combine approaches successfully and creatively. Anderson, Hinojosa, and Strauch (1987) provide helpful suggestions for incorporating play into neurophysiologic treatment approaches.

Adapting toys and play equipment is also an important role of the occupational therapist, especially for the severely involved child. The therapist must know the properties of toys as well as how to adapt them appropriately. Switches, adaptive keyboards, or provisions for sensory impairment may be necessary for the child to benefit from and be more independent in play.

Working with parents in relation to play is vitally important. Parents of handicapped children often are so concerned with their child's disability that they view their roles as substitute therapists and try to structure therapy into every aspect of the child's day. Mogford (1977) presented a comprehensive review of the play characteristics of different handicapped groups. She particularly discussed studies dealing with parents' perceptions of and feelings toward play. Mogford cited a study by Shere and

Kastenbaum, who found that the parents had a preoccupation with their children's physical progress and speech development and failed to appreciate their need for play and exploration on their own or their own roles in encouraging play. Missiuna and Pollack (1991) discussed play deprivation in children with physical disabilities. They described four barriers to free play: limitations imposed by caregivers, physical and personal limitations of the child, environmental barriers, and social barriers. They proposed suggestions for intervention in providing support for free play, consultation with parents, consultation with teachers and caregivers, and recommendations about playthings.

In summary, assessment of play behavior in children and use of play in treatment is of great concern to occupational therapists. The challenge of successful accomplishment of therapeutic goals and using play can be rewarding to the therapist and the child.

Leisure

Theories

Leisure theories have not been as numerous or as well developed as those of play. Often, leisure is explained in relation to work behavior. Wilenski and Burch (in Neulinger, 1981) state that the qualities that one experiences in work are reflected in leisure in three ways: compensatory, familiarity, and personal community. Compensatory activities are those that are opposite to those experienced in work; familiarity refers to activities that are the same as in work; and personal community denotes the influence of the person's social circles on choice of activity. Amount of satisfaction with one's work influences those activities chosen outside of work.

Others attempted to classify activities according to characteristics that distinguish leisure from work. Neulinger (1981) identified factors that distinguished between leisure and nonleisure. He developed a paradigm describing leisure as a state of mind and identified two dimensions of leisure: (1) perceived freedom, a continuum between perceived degrees of freedom and constraint; and (2) motivation for the activity, a range from intrinsic to extrinsic. Intrinsic motivation occurs when the satisfaction stems from engaging in the activity itself, and extrinsic motivation occurs when there is some payoff from the activity.

Using these dimensions, activities could be described in terms of their likeness to leisure, work, and jobs. Pure leisure is an activity freely engaged in and done for its own sake. It requires freedom from both external and internal constraints and implies intrinsic rewards. Pure work is an activity engaged in under constraint while providing entirely intrinsic rewards; it provides perceived satisfaction but lacks perceived freedom. Pure job is an activity engaged in under constraint and with no reward in and of itself but through a payoff resulting from it. It is the opposite of pure leisure.

Gunter and Gunter (1980) developed a model of leisure that assumes that leisure is a combination of time free from work or other obligations, activity, and state of mind. Leisure is a continuous phenomenon, and there may be some leisure in virtually every activity. Their model is depicted along two dimensions: involvement and time/choice structure. The involvement dimension indicates the degree and type of the person's investment in a specific activity or situation, and it ranges from engagement to disengagement. The time/choice dimension ranges from structured and constrained time and obligation to relative freedom from such constraints.

Four styles of leisure can be determined with this model:

Pure leisure refers to activities that are high on both involvement and choice dimensions and represents an ideal. It includes "peak experiences," flow and, a "blending of the individual and the situation" (p. 368).

Anomic leisure refers to those conditions in which there is free time from social obligations but lack of adequate mechanisms for governing the time.

Institutional leisure occurs when involvement and enjoyment are maximal but involvement in institutions with structured constraints is present. An example of this type of leisure is epitomized by the "workaholic."

Alienated leisure occurs when there is little enjoyment or satisfaction plus maximal constraint. It is the closest to nonleisure but includes free time activity and the pursuit of activities out of duty or habit.

Assessment

Traditional approaches to the assessment of leisure have been in three areas, depending on the author's definition of leisure (Neulinger, 1981). There are measures of leisure activity in terms of time and money; interests; and the meaning of leisure. Most of the assessments reviewed measure a combination of these areas.

Matsutsuyu (1969) developed an interest checklist that examines the intensity of a person's interest in 80 different activities. Interests are classified in five categories: manual skills, physical, sports, social recreation, ADL, and cultural or educational.

Two assessments use history-taking. Potts (1969) developed a leisure history that contains questions on leisure and on use of leisure time. Activities are divided into five areas: manipulative-exploratory, practical-inventive, reflective-epistemonic, social, and communal. Florey and Michelman (1982) developed a screening device, the Occupational Role History, to explore the following areas: sequence and continuity of occupational roles and components; satisfaction with interests, people, tasks and environments; occupational roles; and expressed comfort, satisfaction, and competence in each; areas of skill and problem areas; and degree of balance between work, chores, and leisure.

Others evaluated activity patterns. Nystrom (1974) examined the activity patterns, leisure concepts, and meaning of leisure time activity among a group of elderly residents in a low-income, urban housing development. She developed a questionnaire that measures active participation and includes questions about the definition of leisure. Gregory (1983) examined the activities of a group of retirees in relation to life satisfaction. He adapted Nystrom's activity checklist to include questions related to the meaning of the activities and also asked questions related to life satisfaction. Medrich, Roizen, Rubin, and Buckley (1982) developed a questionnaire to describe children's activities when out of school. They examined opportunities and constraints on time use and explored attitudes, purposes, and meanings for nonschool time use.

Tickle and Yerxa (1981) developed a Need Satisfaction of Activity Interview to examine a person's two most important activities, the frequency of participation in them, and the type of

need (according to Maslow's hierarchy) each activity primarily satisfied.

Csikszentmihalyi and Larson (1984) used experience sampling methods to examine activities and their meanings in adolescents. The experience sampling method consists of using electronic pagers to send random signals to people. On receiving the signals, the person fills out a self-report related to current activities, companions, emotional feelings, and mood. This method enables in-depth examination of personal experiences (activities) and of thoughts and feelings about those experiences.

Neulinger (1981) developed a leisure attitude questionnaire that contains questions on leisure, work, sex, and background information. He identified five factors influencing leisure choices: (1) amount of work or vacation desired, (2) society's role in leisure planning, (3) self-definition through work or leisure, (4) amount of perceived leisure, (5) and affinity to leisure.

Qualitative methods have also been used to study leisure. Glancy (1986) used participant observation of sport-group membership to develop grounded theory associated with freedom, expressiveness, meaning, and motivation in leisure. Howe (1988) used structured interviews to explore the role of leisure with subjects in a senior adult fitness program and used case study design to describe emergent patterns. Krefting and Krefting (1991) described how ethnographic approaches may be applied to the understanding of leisure activity among disabled populations.

Use in treatment

People are usually referred to occupational therapy when their performance of daily occupations has been altered as a result of injury or illness. Therapists are also involved in prevention and wellness programs when there is the potential for disruption of occupation. A major goal of occupational therapy is to help the person achieve a balance of meaningful activities in daily life. As we have seen, the same activity may provide different meanings for different people, or different activities may provide the same meaning. To plan effective treatment, the therapist needs to examine leisure performance and its meanings. The therapist also needs to explore constraints to the successful performance of activities.

McGuire (1985) described constraints to leisure that occur across the lifespan, the effect of which limits the freedom of choice required for leisure. Constraints can result when there are too many choices and not enough time, thus causing a need to eliminate some choices. In this case, the person has some control over the extent of the limits. Second, attitudes held by the person result in self-imposed limits on leisure choice. In this case, the perception of options is reduced. Third, conditions beyond the person's control, such as health or economic factors, may limit options. The therapist's role is to explore all three of these types of constraints to assist the patient in making realistic leisure choices.

McDowell (1981), in discussing leisure counseling, described seven steps in the process by which one makes choices about his or her activities: (1) awareness, (2) knowledge, (3) skills, (4) resourcefulness, (5) strategies, (6) assertion (doing), and (7) reflection. These steps are all used by the occupational therapist in treatment. Therapists assist patients in their awareness of options and limits. They provide information regarding options, help develop skills, and provide resources, thus increasing and refining choices and building competencies. Therapists also help patients devise strategies for goal achievement and provide opportunities for assertion through performance of activities. Reflection involves evaluation of results by the patient and the therapist. Occupational therapy, with its emphasis on purposeful activity, is unique in its ability to provide all these steps within a treatment program.

Activities that are usually ascribed to leisure are also used by occupational therapists to achieve specific goals. Crafts and recreational activities provide opportunities for active involvement on the part of the patient and can be adapted to meet therapeutic goals. With adults, as with children, it is important to use activities that are meaningful to the person as well as therapeutic.

Summary

This section has reviewed definitions of work, play, and leisure. The relations among work, play, and leisure were viewed developmentally, with play leading to both work and leisure. Theories of play and leisure were also reviewed. The importance of assessment of play and leisure was stressed, and a review of various evaluation methods and tools was presented. Finally, the use of play and leisure in treatment was discussed.

References

Anderson, J., Hinojosa, J., & Strauch, C. (1987). Integrating play in neuro-developmental treatment. *American Journal of Occupational Therapy, 41*(7), 421–426.

Anderson, N. (1961). *Work and leisure*. New York: The Free Press of Glencoe.

Ayres, A. J. (1979). *Sensory integration and the child*. Los Angeles: Western Psychological Services.

Ayres, A. J. (1972). *Sensory integration and learning disorders*. Los Angeles: Western Psychological Services.

Barnett, L. (1991). The playful child: measurement of a disposition to play. *Play and Culture, 4*, 51–74.

Barnett, L. (1990). Playfulness: definition, design, and measurement. *Play and Culture, 3*, 319–336.

Barnett, L., & Kluber, D. (1984). Playfulness and the early play environment. *Journal of Genetic Psychology, 144*, 153–164.

Barnett, L., & Kluber, D. (1982). Concomitants of playfulness in early childhood: Cognitive abilities and gender. *Journal of Genetic Psychology, 141*, 115–127.

Behnke, C., & Fetokovich, M. (1984). Examining the reliability and validity of the play history. *American Journal of Occupational Therapy, 38*(2), 94–100.

Bergen, D. (1988). *Play as a medium for learning and development*. Portsmouth, NH: Heinemann Educational Books.

Bledsoe, N., & Shepherd, J. (1982). A study of reliability and validity of a preschool play scale. *American Journal of Occupational Therapy, 36*(12), 783–788.

Broderick, T., & Glazer, B. (1983). Leisure participation and the retirement process. *American Journal of Occupational Therapy, 37*, 15–22.

Brook, J., & Brook, R. (1989). Exploring the meaning of work and nonwork. *Journal of Organizational Behavior, 10*, 169–178.

Brown, C., & Gottfried, A. (Eds.). (1985). *Play interactions*. New Brunswick, NJ: Johnson and Johnson Baby Products Co.

Bruner, J. S., Jolly, A., & Sylva, K. (Eds.). (1976). *Play—Its role in development and evolution*. New York: Basic Books.

Bundy, A. (1991). Play theory and sensory integration. In A. G. Fisher, E. A. Murray, & A. C. Bundy (Eds.). *Sensory integration: Theory and practice* (pp. 46–68). Philadelphia: F. A. Davis.

Caillois, R. (1958). *Man, play, and games*. New York: The Free Press of Glencoe.

Clark, F., Parham, D., Carlson, M., Frank, G., Jackson, J., Pierce, D., Wolfe, R., & Zemke, R. (1991). Occupational science: Academic innovation in the service of occupational therapy's future. *American Journal of Occupational Therapy, 45*(4), 300–310.

Cohen, D. (1987). *The development of play*. New York: New York University Press.

Csikszentmihalyi, M. (1990). *Flow*. New York: Harper and Row.

Csikszentmihalyi, M. (1975). *Beyond boredom and anxiety*. San Francisco: Jossey-Bass.

Csikszentmihalyi, M., & Larson, R. (1984). *Being adolescent*. New York: Basic Books.

De Grazia, S. (1962). *Of time, work, and leisure*. New York: The Twentieth Century Fund.

Ellis, M. J. (1973). *Why people play*. Englewood Cliffs, NJ: Prentice-Hall.

Epstein, C. F. (1990). The cultural perspective and the study of work. In K. Erikson, & S. P. Vallas (Eds.). *The nature of work*. New Haven: Yale University Press.

Florey, L. (1981). Studies of play: Implications for growth, development and for clinical practice. *American Journal of Occupational Therapy, 35*(8), 519–524.

Florey, L. (1971). An approach to play and play development. *American Journal of Occupational Therapy, 25*, 275–280.

Florey, L., & Michelman, S. (1982). Occupational role history: A screening tool for psychiatric occupational therapy. *American Journal of Occupational Therapy, 36*, 301–308.

Garvey, C. (1977a). *Play*. London: Fontana/Open Books.

Garvey, C. (1977b). Play with language. In B. Tizard, & D. Harvey (Eds.). *Biology of play*. Philadelphia: J. B. Lippincott.

Glancy, M. (1986). Participant observation in the recreation setting. *Journal of Leisure Research, 18*, 59–80.

Gregory, M. D. (1983). Occupational behavior and life satisfaction among retirees. *American Journal of Occupational Therapy, 37*(8), 548–553.

Gunter, B. G. (1987). The leisure experience: Selected properties. *Journal of Leisure Research, 19*(2), 115–130.

Gunter, B. G., & Gunter, N. (1980). Leisure styles: A conceptual framework for modern leisure. *Sociological Quarterly, 21*, 361–374.

Harrison, H., & Kielhofner, G. (1986). Examining reliability and validity of the preschool play scale with handicapped children. *American Journal of Occupational Therapy, 40*(3), 167–173.

Hartley, R., & Goldenson, R. (1963). *The complete book of children's play*. New York: The Cornwall Press.

Howe, C. (1988). Using qualitative structured interviews in leisure research: Illustrations from one case study. *Journal of Leisure Research, 20*, 305–324.

Huizinga, J. (1950). *Homo ludens*. Boston: Beacon Press.

Hulme I., & Lunzer, E. A. (1966). Play, language and reasoning in subnormal children. *Journal of Child Psychology and Psychiatry, 7*, 107.

Iso-Ahola, S. E. (1979). Basic dimensions of definitions of leisure. *Journal of Leisure Research, 11*(1), 28–39.

Iso-Ahola, S. E. (1980). *The social psychology of leisure and recreation*. Dubuque, IA: William C. Brown.

Kalverboer, A. (1977). Measurement of play: Clinical applications. In B. Tizard, & D. Harvey (Eds.). *Biology of play* (pp. 100–122). Philadelphia: J. B. Lippincott.

Kando, T. (1980). *Leisure and popular culture in transition*. St. Louis: C. V. Mosby.

Kaplan, M. (1975). *Leisure: Theory and policy*. New York: John Wiley & Sons.

Kelly, J. R. (1983). *Leisure identities and interactions*. London: George Allen & Unwin.

Kielhofner, G., & Barris, R. (1984). Collecting data on play: A critique of available methods. *Occupational Therapy Journal of Research, 4*(3), 150–180.

Knox, S. (1968). *Observation and assessment of the everyday play behavior of the mentally retarded child.* Unpublished master's thesis, University of Southern California, Los Angeles.

Knox, S. (1974). A play scale. In M. Reilly (Ed.). *Play as exploratory learning.* Beverly Hills: Sage.

Knox, S. (in press). Playfulness in preschool children. *Proceedings of the Fourth Annual Symposium on Occupational Science.* Philadelphia: F. A. Davis.

Krefting, L., & Krefting, D. (1991). Leisure activities after a stroke: An ethnographic approach. *American Journal of Occupational Therapy, 45,* 429–436.

Levy, J. (1978). *Play behavior.* Malabar, FL: Robert E. Kruger.

Liebermann, J. (1977). *Playfulness: Its relationship to imagination and creativity.* New York: Academic Press.

Linder, T. (1990). *Transdisciplinary play-based assessment.* Baltimore: Paul H. Brooks.

Lindquist, J., Mack, W., & Parham, D. (1982). A synthesis of occupational behavior and sensory integrative concepts in theory and practice, part 2: Clinical applications. *American Journal of Occupational Therapy, 36*(7), 433–437.

Mack, W., Lindquist, J., & Parham, D. (1982). A synthesis of occupational behavior and sensory integrative concepts in theory and practice, part 1: Theoretical foundations. *American Journal of Occupational Therapy, 36*(6), 365–374.

Matsutsuyu, J. S. (1969). The interest check list. *American Journal of Occupational Therapy, 23,* 323–334.

McDonald, A. (1987). *The construction of a self-report instrument to measure play activities and play styles in 7–11 year old children.* Unpublished master's thesis, University of Southern California, Los Angeles.

McDowell, F. (1981). Leisure: Consciousness, well-being and counseling. *Counseling Psychologist, 9*(3), 3–31.

McGuire, F. (1985). Constraints in later life. In M. Wade (Ed.). *Constraints on leisure.* Springfield, IL: Charles C. Thomas.

Medrich, E. A., Roizen, J., Rubin, V., & Buckley, S. (1982). *The serious business of growing up: A study of children's lives outside school.* Berkeley: University of California Press.

Mergen, B. (1977). From play to recreation: The acceptance of leisure in the United States, 1890–1930. In P. Stevens (Ed.). *Studies in the anthropology of play.* West Point, NY: Leisure Press.

Missiuna, C., & Pollock, N. (1991). Play deprivation in children with physical disabilities: The role of the occupational therapist in preventing secondary disability. *American Journal of Occupational Therapy, 45,* 882–888.

Mogford, K. (1977). The play of handicapped children. In B. Tizard, & D. Harvey (Eds.). *Biology of play* (pp. 170–184). Philadelphia: J. B. Lippincott.

Neulinger, J. (1981). *The psychology of leisure* (2nd ed.). Springfield, IL: Charles C. Thomas.

Nystrom, E. P. (1974). Activity patterns and leisure concepts among the elderly. *American Journal of Occupational Therapy, 28*(6), 337–345.

Parker, S. (1983). *Leisure and work.* London: George Allen & Unwin.

Parker, S. (1976). *The sociology of leisure.* New York: International Publications Service.

Parker, S. R., Brown, R. K., Child, J., & Smith, M. A. (1977). *The sociology of industry.* London: George Allen & Unwin.

Parten, M. (1933). Social play among pre-school children. *Journal of Abnormal and Social Psychology, 28,* 136–147.

Piaget, J. (1962). *Play, dreams and imitation in childhood.* London: William Heinemann.

Pierce, D. (1991). Early object rule acquisition. *American Journal of Occupational Therapy, 45*(5) 438–449.

Potts, L. (1969). *Toward a developmental assessment of leisure patterns.* Unpublished master's thesis, University of Southern California, Los Angeles.

Primeau, L. (1989). *A description and comparison of game playing behavior of preadolescent boys 9–11 years of age with and without developmental dyspraxia.* Unpublished master's thesis, University of Southern California, Los Angeles.

Rast, M. (1986). Play and therapy, play or therapy. *Play: A skill for life.* Rockville, MD: American Occupational Therapy Association.

Reilly, M. (1974). *Play as exploratory learning.* Beverly Hills: Sage.

Rosenblatt, D. (1977). Developmental trends in infant play. In B. Tizard, & D. Harvey (Eds.). *Biology of play* (pp. 33–44). Philadelphia: J. B. Lippincott.

Rubin, K. H. (1980). *Children's play.* San Francisco: Jossey-Bass.

Rubin, K., Maioni, T. L., & Hornung, M. (1976). Free play behaviors in middle and lower-class preschoolers: Parten and Piaget revisited. *Child Development, 47,* 414–419.

Rubin, K., Watson, K., & Jambor, T. (1978). Free play behaviors in preschool and kindergarten children. *Child Development, 49,* 534–536.

Smilanski, S. (1968). *The effects of sociodramatic play on disadvantaged preschool children.* New York: John Wiley and Sons.

Sponseller, D. B. (1974). *Play as a learning medium.* Washington, DC: Association for the Education of Young Children.

Takata, N. (1974). Play as a prescription. In M. Reilly (Ed.). *Play as exploratory learning.* Beverly Hills: Sage.

Takata, N. (1971). The play milieu—A preliminary appraisal. *American Journal of Occupational Therapy, 25,* 281–284.

Takata, N. (1969). The play history. *American Journal of Occupational Therapy, 23*(4), 314–318.

Tickle, L., & Yerxa, E. (1981). Need satisfaction of older persons living in the community and in institutions, part 2: Role of activity. *American Journal of Occupational Therapy, 35,* 650–655.

Truhon, S. (1983). Playfulness, play and creativity: A path analytic model. *Journal of Genetic Psychology, 143,* 19–28.

Wade, M. (1985). *Constraints on leisure.* Springfield, IL: Charles C. Thomas.

Wolfgang, C., & Phelps, P. (1983). Preschool play materials preference inventory. *Early Child Development and Care, 12,* 127–141.

Yerxa, E., Clark, F., Frank, G., Jackson, J., Parham, D., Pierce, D., Stein, C., & Zemke, R. (1989). An introduction to occupational science, a foundation for occupational therapy in the 21st century. *Occupational Therapy in Health Care, 6,* 1–17.

CHAPTER 9

Tools of practice

SECTION 1

Therapeutic use of self

SHARAN L. SCHWARTZBERG

LEARNING OBJECTIVES

Upon completion of this section the reader will be able to:

1. *Explain the meaning and significance of therapeutic use of self in occupational therapy.*
2. *Describe the therapeutic relationship and use of self in occupational therapy.*
3. *Recognize and describe the ways occupational therapists employ themselves in a therapeutic or countertherapeutic way in individual and group treatment.*
4. *Explain the impasses to therapeutic use of self and how to modify these impasses in the therapeutic relationship through personal change and structural change in the relationship.*
5. *Specify some of the methods used to teach therapeutic use of self in occupational therapy curriculum.*
6. *Analyze current research on clinical reasoning of therapists regarding their use of self as occupational therapy practitioners.*

Occupational therapy consistently involves four tools: therapeutic use of self, purposeful activity, activity analysis, and activity adaptation. In this section, a profile of the therapeutic use of self is offered. It is presented as a generic component to all areas of practice. Detailed descriptions of restricted therapeutic use of self to achieve goals in specific occupational performance areas and component skills can be found in more specialized literature. The therapeutic use of group process incorporates principles from the four areas mentioned above. The use of group is described Chapter 9, Section 2.

Definition of therapeutic use of self

The therapist's use of self is critical to engaging the patient in occupational therapy. Three ingredients are essential to establishing a therapeutic relationship: understanding, neutrality, sometimes called empathy, and caring (Siegel, 1986). As Siegel explains these principles, the therapist accepts the patient as he or she is. In addition, the therapist is tolerant and interested in the patient's painful emotions. Finally, the therapist is able to communicate to the patient what the patient expects from the therapist. By remaining neutral but engaged, the therapist encourages the patient to interact (Siegel, 1986).

The therapeutic relationship in occupational therapy

Although the patient–therapist relationship is not ordinarily considered the central focus of occupational therapy, it is a primary and necessary ingredient in the therapeutic process. In occupational therapy the relationship with the patient is not the sole focus of treatment, but rather it is believed that the clinician's therapeutic use of self is a necessary requirement to the relationship. This is similar to the use of purposeful activity in occupational therapy. As single elements of a process, the activity and relationship are each insufficient when used alone. The unique emphasis in use of interpersonal process in occupational therapy is further explained when group treatment formats are compared in Chapter 9, Section 2.

Humanistic roots of the profession

The occupational therapist's role has always been that of a facilitator. In their description of the profession's founding identity, Kielhofner and Burke (1977) explain that "the theoretical base for treatment lay in the principles of moral treatment and the psychobiological theory of Adolph Meyer. Patients were viewed from the perspective of their productive roles in society and their rights to respectability" (p. 681).

To "adapt opportunities" and to "respect the native capacities and interests of the patient," two basic tenets of modern day occupational therapy were described by Meyer (1917/1922) over 70 years ago:

> Our role consists in giving *opportunities* rather than prescriptions. There must be opportunities to work, opportunities to do and to plan and create, and to learn to use material....
>
> It takes rare gifts and talents and rare personalities to be real pathfinders in this work. There are no royal roads; it is all a problem of being true to one's nature and opportunities and of teaching others to do the same with themselves.... It takes, above all, resourcefulness and ability to respect at the same time the native *capacities and interests* of the patient. Freedom from premature meddling, and tact in avoiding false comparisons or undue expectations fostering disappointment, orderliness without pedantry, cheer and praise without sloppiness and without surrender of standard—these may be the rewards of a good use of personal gifts and of good training. (pp. 641–642)

The same concepts are seen in approaches to conscious or therapeutic use of self in day-to-day communications with the patient, family members, and other people significant to the patient. Whether it be in the clinic, an office, on the telephone, or on a playground, the therapist remains a tool for helping. In all instances of interaction, there is an implicit or explicit therapeutic message, an implication for which the therapist bears responsibility.

Occupational therapy approaches

Yerxa (1967) identifies four key factors as features of the purpose of occupational therapy: "choice"; "self-initiated," "purposeful activity"; "reality orientation," and "perception." These are basic approaches to the therapeutic relationship. Yerxa explains that "this active role of the occupational therapist in helping the client delineate his choices takes more knowledge, skill and sensitivity plus more faith in the individual than an authoritarian role of 'you must do this because it is good for you' " (p. 4). Whether a patient is confronting the daily living effects of a head injury or major depressive disorder, for example, the therapist provides opportunities for the patient to adjust to the new self by restoring old capacities or substituting new capabilities to function.

> The authentic occupational therapist recognizes that although initial dependency might require a temporary suspension of the patient's right to choice, the therapeutic experience is primarily an opportunity for self-actualization. Therefore, the occupational ther-

apist does not force his value system upon the client. But rather, through using his skills and knowledge, exposes the client to a range of possibilities which constitute his external reality. The client is the one who makes the choice. (Yerxa, 1967, p. 8)

The occupational therapy environment

Conscious use of self

On the basis of the previous definition, one may wonder if a therapeutic relationship is like a paid friendship. For it to qualify as therapy, however, the therapist must do more than be tolerant and empathic. Therapists must also manage their own subjective responses or countertransference reactions.

Self-awareness

Both patients and therapists have personalities. It is the clinician's first job to understand his or her own vulnerabilities, biases, and wishes. This understanding is instrumental to therapist neutrality and objectivity.

Nonverbal and verbal communication

As therapists interact with patients, signals come from both verbal and nonverbal aspects of the communication. Paying attention to both areas provides clues to the patient's internal frame of reference as well as to the therapist's thoughts, feelings, and reactions. The therapist should look for mixed signals, a mismatch between verbal and nonverbal behaviors, and content emphasis of the verbal or nonverbal components.

Depending on the degree of trust and nature of the relationship, the therapist may choose to raise questions about observed discrepancies between verbal and nonverbal communication. A discussion may lead to a better understanding of areas of conflict or discomfort as well as to feelings of acceptance. This type of feedback, however, may be misinterpreted and met with resistance or confusion. Interpretation of nonverbal, as well as verbal, communication should be judicious and offered with great caution and sensitivity to the patient's need for privacy. Nonverbal communication may simply imply the request for physical assistance, for example, to relieve discomfort in a wheelchair due to an inability to shift position or to aid balance when it is difficult to walk down stairs without a railing. Patients may not ask for help verbally for a variety of reasons—they may be unaware of asking; they may feel embarrassed and think they should not need assistance; they may think they do not deserve the attention; or they may have physical difficulties with communicating. In these instances, it is best to simply be direct and offer assistance.

Empathy

When a person experiences **empathy**, he or she feels the other person's condition as if it were his or her own. Yerxa (1967) aptly describes this condition in her definition of therapeutic "**authenticity**:"

> Personal authenticity as an occupational therapist means that the therapist allows himself to feel real emotion as he enters into *mutual* relation with the client....
>
> "Being there" also means being able to separate his feelings for the client as a human being from projections of how *he* would

feel if he had experienced the client's disability. For the authentic occupational therapist knows that the client is the only one who can discover his own particular meaning. (p. 8)

Rapport

Empathy is commonly viewed as a necessary condition to therapeutic **rapport**, which occurs when the patient experiences the therapist's respect and regard as well as appreciation of the patient's uniqueness and capability. Participation in such a humanistic relationship in occupational therapy brings the patient hope in the potential for growth and change (Briggs, Duncombe, Howe, & Schwartzberg, 1979).

Monitoring objective observations and subjective responses

Objective observations are behavioral descriptions of perceived external characteristics. *Subjective observations* are descriptions of internal visions, feelings, and thoughts, which are based on a person's needs, past experiences, and assigned meanings. An example of an objective observation is: The patient was silent during the community outing to the Museum of Fine Arts. A subjective observation of the same incident might be: The patient's withdrawal from the group caused me to feel angry and confrontational.

Both objective and subjective observations are brought to the therapeutic relationship. Objective perceptions permit systematic analysis and reporting; subjective perceptions are useful for understanding reactions to a patient. Responses based on subjective perceptions, however, might not be in the best interest of the patient. For example, a therapist's unconscious anger may cause the therapist to be overly protective and to passively encourage the patient's nonparticipation in activities. To identify a subjective response, the therapist may ask questions such as: What nonverbal messages am I sending to the patient? Is my reaction to this situation or person exaggerated? Am I attempting to fulfill my own unmet needs? Clinical supervision, separate from the patient–therapist relationship, provides the therapist with an opportunity to discuss these reactions in a neutral and less emotionally charged environment.

Practice

The therapeutic relationship influences how and what one does in both individual and group therapy formats. The patient–therapist relationship in a group setting is discussed in more detail in Chapter 9, Section 2.

Individual treatment

Challenges to establishing and modulating a therapeutic relationship

A therapeutic relationship is a developmental process. The therapist constantly monitors and adjusts the amount and nature of support and gratification necessary to sustain the patient's health and well-being. These needs vary depending on the phase of the relationship. Establishing and maintaining trust is preliminary to any therapeutic relationship. Concerns related to termination of

therapy also vary. In more long-term and intense relationships, feelings of anger, sadness, and loss may be particularly acute during periods of separation, such as vacations or at termination of the relationship. Anxiety concerning the future is common in short-term therapeutic relationships. Each patient's unique history and set of problems require that the therapist respond on an individual basis.

Facilitating self-initiated communication and action

Patient involvement is key to occupational therapy. To encourage patient-initiated communication and action, the therapist establishes a physical and emotional environment that makes the patient feel cared for, understood, and masterful. The patient should be involved as much as possible in setting goals for therapy. A noncritical atmosphere with realistic expectations often inspires adaptive action. Pleasant physical surroundings and challenges within the patient's capabilities can foster feelings of self-respect and competence.

Benjamin's interview categories

Benjamin (1974) identified five types of communication in the therapeutic interview: "interviewee-centered responses and leads," "interviewer-centered leads and responses," "authority leads and responses," "open use of interviewer authority," and "humor." Each of these can be graded and structured to the nature of the therapeutic relationship.

Group treatment

Establishing and modulating a therapeutic relationship

The therapist is responsible for creating a helping atmosphere in group treatment as well as in individual treatment. In Howe and Schwartzberg's (1986) model of the "functional group" in occupational therapy, the leader acts to maintain a delicate balance between group maintenance or social-emotional roles and group task roles. Howe and Schwartzberg further identify leadership skills and responsibilities to include planning the group activity; conveying genuineness and empathy; modeling behavior; reality testing; and communicating (listening and responding, feedback, concreteness, confrontation, and self-disclosure).

Facilitating self-initiated communication and action

The group therapist also considers the developmental phase of the group and individual members' needs when planning and responding to the group. Activities are adjusted to encourage member participation and involvement. Establishing a caring climate and involving patients in setting group and individual goals are examples of strategies used to achieve this end. A variety of activities, both structured and unstructured, are adapted using a wide range of modalities, such as crafts, activities of daily living, and movement.

Toxic and benign environments

The interactive environment between the patient and therapist can be empathic, at best; benign, at the very least; or immobilizing or toxic, at worst.

Authoritative, punishing, and critical responses

Just as involvement of the patient in an active process increases self-initiated behavior, certain therapist behaviors are likely to create a negative response or environment. The following case study illustrates a therapist response that is authoritarian and nonencouraging of the patient's autonomy.

CASE STUDY

An Authoritarian Response

A social skills group is being formed for outpatients who recently survived traumatic head injury and are now receiving services in the community. The group leader is an occupational therapist, and the goal of the group is to decrease social isolation of the members. At the first meeting of the group, the therapist asks for a list of the names and phone numbers of the group members. A group member inquires if she might receive a copy of the list so she may call other members. The therapist responds quickly with: "No, this list is for the hospital records. I can't give you a copy."

In this example, the therapist cut off communication and established herself as the authority rather than supporting and positively reinforcing the patient's independent wish to initiate relationships and socialize. Due to her own anxiety about the successful functioning of the group, the therapist neglected the patient's healthy instincts and failed to show trust in the member's capabilities.

When therapists find that they are being critical, punitive, or dictatorial, they should ask themselves the following questions: What is creating this reaction? Does the interaction resemble a prior relationship? Is it time for a vacation? Should someone else be treating the patient? Is a consultation or discussion in clinical supervision indicated? All these questions should be answered with care, and the patient's needs should be given priority.

Creating dependency

For unconscious or conscious reasons, therapists may foster dependent relationships with their patients, creating a therapeutic environment that reinforces feelings of hopelessness and helplessness. Behaviors that signal this type of therapist behavior include making extra time for a patient at the expense of other patients, colleagues, or personal commitments; being argumentative or critical with other staff members when a patient's treatment is being discussed; avoiding usual channels of communication and bending institutional rules and requirements in the "best interests of the patient"; and "doing for" the patient. In the long run, the patient suffers a loss of trust with the therapist when the patient's unrealistic demands are not discussed in an open and caring manner. The following is a case example of a therapist acting on her own unconscious need to be needed and special.

CASE STUDY

A Therapist Acting on Her Own Needs

An experienced therapist who was recently separated from her husband finds she is taking on a much heavier case load than usual. She is repeatedly critical of other therapists in her department and has on occasion changed the department treatment schedule so that some of her favorite patients would be seen by her alone. The therapist felt these patients were being misunderstood.

In this situation, the therapist is unable to separate her feelings of loss in her personal life from her actions in the therapeutic relationship. The patients are held captive to the therapist's needs and are not receiving the most effective therapy.

Patient-centered involvement

Recent exploratory ethnographic research on clinical reasoning provides specific insights into the patient–therapist relationship in occupational therapy. These data lend support to the importance of orienting therapeutic interactions toward the patient's internal frame of reference.

In her study of the therapeutic relationship in occupational therapy, Langthaler (1990) found that "appropriate behavior is context-related, reasoned and person oriented. The therapist's and patient's behavior are matched according to each one's perception of a situation. Other influences on this matching are, the goal pursued, the requirements to increase or decrease stimuli, and the personality style of the therapist (p. v)." Langthaler further stressed "choice" and "future orientation" as components of participation in occupational therapy. "Being with a patient includes quality and responsibility in interaction. Whereas doing, with a patient relates to provoking the desire to engage, perform and evaluate activity. The content for doing with the patient should emerge from being with the patient" (Langthaler, 1990, p. vi).

Sperber (1989) examined active patient involvement in occupational therapy. Using an ethnographic design, she identified three theories to describe how in the therapeutic process therapists elicit active involvement: (1) "the therapeutic relationship is empowering," (2) "patients through partnership, storytelling, having choice, and humor become emotionally and intellectually involved," and (3) patients become active "through a process in which they distance from images of their pre-illness bodies and move in to their new bodies" (p. iii).

Siegler (1987) found four characteristic functions of humor in occupational therapy: (1) "maintaining the therapeutic alliance," (2) "distraction from pain and pain of understanding," (3) "clinical management" ("correcting performance," "reinforcing progress," and "pushing the patient harder"), and (4) "helping patient envision a life beyond the sick role" (p. iv).

Impasses to the therapeutic relationship

The reader is encouraged to examine occupational therapy frames of reference for background information on function and dysfunction continua related to the individual patient. This section examines only some of the impasses to the therapeutic relationship.

Noninvolvement of the patient

Patients may remain uninvolved in the therapeutic relationship for several reasons. To understand the absence of involvement, the therapist should look at both the patient and the therapeutic relationship. An understanding of the patient requires hypotheses or explanations from the biologic, psychological, social, and behavioral domains.

Overinvolvement of the therapist

The focus on *quality* of involvement is especially important in occupational therapy because of the profession's philosophical emphasis on patient involvement in choice-making, revision, and self-directed action. The therapist may become overinvolved, or as discussed next, noninvolved, by attempting to meet personal needs in the patient–therapist relationship. **Countertransference** occurs when the therapist's emotions are projected toward the patient. These emotions may be conscious or unconscious. Overinvolvement may be encouraged by the therapist who seeks love and attention because the patient makes the therapist feel needed. Patients may idealize the therapist because of a past history of deprivation or present pain and suffering. By overtaking the patient's autonomy, the alliance suffers. When the patient is slow to make progress, the therapist may take this as a personal attack. Typically, the patient experiences a sense of failure and becomes incapable of self-directed action.

Noninvolvement of the therapist

Fear of dependency, a difficulty with setting limits because of unresolved anger, or other personal anxieties may lead therapists to be overly concerned with their degree of involvement with the patient. Therapists may become overly attentive or may withdraw inappropriately from a patient. The therapist's continued lack of awareness may give rise to unexpressed anger in the relationship and may be expressed by forms of noninvolvement. Unconscious countertransference reactions may include boredom, missed or brief appointments, being critical of the patient, blaming the patient, or overinterpreting the patient's behavior. Typically, the patient experiences rejection, which often reinforces an already negative self-image common to those with illness or disability. The patient may also withdraw or direct actions at repeated failed attempts to please the therapist. Ultimately, by the patient's internalization of the therapist's projected emotions, the aims of self-directed and purposeful activity are thwarted. A case study follows.

CASE STUDY

Therapist Avoidance

An occupational therapist in his 40s finds himself forgetting to arrange transportation to the occupational therapy clinic for appointments with an elderly male patient who is severely depressed, extremely negative, critical, and demanding. The nurses have a difficult time finding the patient when it is time for the occupational therapy appointment. The patient feels that there is no hope and that no one cares for him.

In this situation, the therapist is withdrawing from the patient. By forgetting to arrange for the patient's transportation, the therapist avoids spending time with the patient. The therapist is having difficulty setting limits with the patient because he feels uncomfortable. His discomfort, when examined, reveals an unrealistic wish to please the patient as he never felt he had pleased his own father. The therapist's behavior reinforces the patient's self-fulfilling prophesy that no one cares for him.

Countertransference difficulties

Both the patient and therapist bring personal thoughts, feelings, and unconscious reactions to the therapeutic relationship. There are bound to be problems in the therapeutic process when therapists are unaware of their own perceptions and unconscious impulses or wishes. For example, Maltsberger (1985) explains that patients with borderline personality disorders make others hate them because they "need" to feel victimized and rejected. To acknowledge countertransference impulses, which are mostly unconscious, Maltsberger suggests that therapists be aware of their own feelings, such as nervousness or anxiety.

Countertransference responses occur in both individual and group therapy. A group leader perceives multiple combinations of personalities and forces acting on the therapeutic dynamics. It often is useful to work with another therapist to help sort out the many interactions and potential distortions.

Education of the therapist

The skilled clinician continually works to examine and perfect the therapeutic use of self. Supervision is an important tool in this educational process. Understanding the use of self as a therapeutic tool, however, begins in the classroom with the clinical education of the occupational therapy student.

Teaching therapeutic use of self

The selection and breadth of courses prepares an occupational therapist in particular ways to interact with a patient. Both classroom and clinic should be considered in planning a curriculum.

Classroom education and background liberal arts education

To engage the patient requires use of self and an understanding of others. In addition to studies in occupational therapy, courses in language, the arts, social sciences, and humanities are suggested. By understanding our patients as individuals and as members of diverse cultural groups, we become more aware and accepting of attitudes and expectations that may differ from our own.

Clinical education and supervision

Through supervision, it is possible to examine the structure and process underlying the care delivered through the therapeutic relationship. The opportunity to learn from a role model and to observe and discuss the actions and clinical reasoning of more experienced clinicians is particularly important in the clinical education of students. At its core, the therapeutic relationship always involves the patient and therapist as people. Therefore, supervision of the interactive facets of occupational therapy are important aspects of a therapist's basic and continuing education.

Improving therapeutic use of self

Individual, group, and peer supervision

Therapists should have the opportunity to discuss their feelings and countertransference reactions on a one-to-one basis with a supervisor as well as with colleagues in an institutional or peer group setting. This is essential since the occupational therapist's work is stressful and often entails intimate care (eg, teaching bathing, feeding, and grooming activities) of patients who are gravely ill or seriously disabled, some of whom may be dying. Forstein and Baer (1991), in their discussion of the suicidal patient with AIDS, observe how suicidal patients, especially those with advanced disease, challenge the purpose of the therapist's caregiving and sense of what is right and wrong. Forstein and Baer remark that, in these cases,

> many countertransferential issues emerge, including the difficulty watching young people lose function and experience increasing pain and/or realistic hopelessness about the future. Staff may have conscious or unconscious wishes that the patient die. Staff must feel free to discuss these matters with supervisors, in staff meetings, and as a part of the unit's didactic program. (p. 207)

Individual and group psychotherapy

Sometimes occupational therapists may benefit from involvement in group or individual psychotherapy. Personal psychotherapy allows clinicians to focus on themselves alone rather than on their patients' care and well-being. Psychotherapy may be indicated for the therapist when the therapist's personality prevents him or her from seeking or receiving peer support. Regular vacations, routine exercise, and a healthy diet are also important in minimizing stresses inherent in the work of the helping professions.

Research

Further studies in clinical reasoning are necessary to better understand how to facilitate a therapeutic relationship. Studies such as the one by Bradburn (1992) help to explain strategies used to engage patients in various specialty areas. Through qualitative and quantitative descriptions of the process of occupational therapy, patient outcomes can be better measured and procedures more carefully applied.

Summary

The therapeutic use of self in occupational therapy was described, and means of employing and blocking such a relationship were outlined. The historical significance of the therapeutic use of self to the profession and some preliminary recent findings of related studies in clinical reasoning were presented.

References

Benjamin, A. (1974). *The helping interview* (2nd ed.). Boston: Houghton Mifflin.

Bradburn, S. (1992). *Psychiatric occupational therapists' strategies for engaging patients in treatment during the initial interview*. Unpublished master's thesis, Tufts University, Medford, MA.

Briggs, A. K., Duncombe, L. W., Howe, M. C., & Schwartzberg, S. L. (1979). *Case simulations in psychosocial occupational therapy*. Philadelphia: F. A. Davis.

Forstein, M., & Baer, J. (1991). HIV Infection. In L. I. Sederer (Ed.), *Inpatient psychiatry diagnosis and treatment* (3rd ed.) (pp. 189–211). Baltimore: Williams & Wilkins.

Howe, M. C., & Schwartzberg, S. L. (1986). *A functional approach to groupwork in occupational therapy*. Philadelphia: J. B. Lippincott.

Kielhofner, G., & Burke, J. P. (1977). Occupational therapy after 60 years: An account of changing identity and knowledge. *American Journal of Occupational Therapy, 31*(10), 675–689.

Langthaler, M. M. (1990). The components of therapeutic relationship in occupational therapy. Unpublished master's thesis, Tufts University, Medford, MA.

Maltsberger, J. T. (1985, October). *Hospital treatment of borderline patients: Problems of suicide*. Paper presented at the 37th Institute on Hospital and Community Psychiatry, American Psychiatric Association, Montreal.

Meyer, A. (1977). The philosophy of occupational therapy. *American Journal of Occupational Therapy, 31*(10), 639–642. (Original work read in 1921 and published 1922.)

Siegel, A. (1986, April). *Prerequisites for engagement in psychotherapy: Implications for the therapist*. Paper presented at the Mount Auburn Hospital Department of Psychiatry Grand Rounds, Cambridge, MA.

Siegler, C. C. (1987). *Functions of humor in occupational therapy*. Unpublished master's thesis, Tufts University, Medford, MA.

Sperber, T. (1989). *An ethnographic study of active involvement in occupational therapy*. Unpublished master's thesis, Tufts University, Medford, MA.

Yerxa, E. J. (1967). 1966 Eleanor Clarke Slagle Lecture: Authentic occupational therapy. *American Journal of Occupational Therapy, 21*(1), 1–9.

Bibliography

Combs, A. W., Avila, D. L., & Purkey, W. W. (1971). *Helping relationships: Basic concepts for the helping professions*. Boston: Allyn and Bacon.

Egan, G. (1986). *The skilled helper: A systematic approach to effective helping* (3rd ed.). Monterey: Brooks/Cole.

Gazda, G. M., Walters, R. P., & Childers, W. C. (1975). *Human relations development: A manual for health sciences*. Boston: Allyn and Bacon.

Mosey, A. C. (1981). *Occupational therapy: Configuration of a profession*. New York: Raven Press.

Navarra, T., Lipkowitz, M. A., & Navarra, J. G. (1990). *Therapeutic communication: A guide to effective interpersonal skills for health care professionals*. Thorofare, NJ: Slack.

Purtilo, R. (1984). *Health professional/patient interaction* (3rd ed.). Philadelphia: W. B. Saunders.

SECTION 2

Group process

SHARAN L. SCHWARTZBERG

LEARNING OBJECTIVES

Upon completion of this section the reader will be able to:

1. *Describe the history and present role, types, purposes, and models of group work in occupational therapy.*

2. *Compare the use of group process in occupational therapy with the the use of group process in other formats of group therapy.*

3. *Explain the effects of basic group variables and dynamics on leadership and membership roles.*

4. *Relate the techniques and procedures for conducting a therapeutic group in occupational therapy.*

5. *Describe the value of group process in occupational therapy and specify selected problems requiring further investigation.*

Past and present trends in group therapy

Occupational therapy group treatment is the combination of structured, adapted group process and tasks or activities aimed at fostering change and adaptation in people with acute or chronic illness, impairments, or disability. The occupational therapist's use of group process requires knowledge of theories of group process and group dynamics, understanding of conceptual models that describe group principles and parallel therapeutic techniques, and knowledge of empiric research on variables related to the small, task-oriented group, both nonclinical and therapeutic. Group therapists must be able to use this information, along with their knowledge of pathology, wellness, and the use of purposeful activity, to reason about the individual patient in the group context. The group therapist incorporates principles of therapeutic use of self described in Chapter 9, Section 1 into procedures that are unique to a group interactive format.

Historical overview

A contemporary occupational therapy group consists of more than simply two or three people doing solitary activities in the same room. Nevertheless, it was not uncommon to find such parallel interaction constituting group treatment in the profession's early years (Howe & Schwartzberg, 1986). Today, it is incongruous to have occupational therapy conducted in groups without consideration of the unique properties of the group format. When occupational therapy groups are compared with verbal psychotherapy and peer support groups, the group properties receive different emphases (Table 9-1). Occupational therapy's unique perspective of the group as a format for service delivery is further understood with descriptions of past and current practices. Separate historical periods have been identified (Howe & Schwartzberg, 1986), and the focus of group involvement during these eras is outlined in Table 9-2.

Current status

The use of group treatment in occupational therapy is often mistaken as primarily restricted to practice in mental health or to the treatment of children or the elderly. Duncombe and Howe (1985), however, established that "60% of occupational therapists in all areas of practice lead groups in treatment" (p. 163). Undoubtedly this number is now much larger due to cost-containment measures in health care and growing occupational therapy services in schools and community-based settings.

Recent reports also specifically document the value of group occupational therapy for patients with physical problems such as Parkinson disease (Gauthier, Dalziel, & Gauthier, 1987), head injuries (Lundgren & Persechino, 1986), and rheumatoid

TABLE 9-1. *Comparison of Therapeutic Uses of Group Properties*

Group Properties	Occupational Therapy	Verbal Psychotherapy	Peer Support
Leader involvement	Very central	Not central	Not central
Purposeful activity	Very central	Not central	Not central
Structure and format	Very central	Not central	Somewhat central
Practice	Very central	Somewhat central	Not central
Teaching and learning	Very central	Somewhat central	Very central
Socialization and outside action	Somewhat central	Not central	Very central
There and then	Not central	Very central	Somewhat central
Here and now	Very central	Very central	Very central

TABLE 9-2.   *Eras of Group Work in Occupational Therapy*

Era	Focus of Group Involvement
Project Era, 1922–1936	Project completion
Socialization Era, 1937–1953	Social activity
Group Dynamics–Process Era, 1954–1961	Interpersonal dynamics
Ego Building–Psychodynamic Era, 1962–1969	Ego reconstitution
Adaptation Era, 1970–present	Social adaptation

Historical analysis is from Howe, M. G., & Schwartzberg, S. L. (1986). A functional approach to group work in occupational therapy. Philadelphia: J. B. Lippincott.

TABLE 9-3.   *Occupational Therapy Group Variables*

Setting
Therapeutic factors
Goals: short-term and long-term
Duration of group
Composition of group
Time frame and format
Population
Group size
Frame of reference
Open versus closed membership
Member selection and preparation
Contraindications

arthritis (Van Deusen & Harlowe, 1987). Projects like Trahey's (1991) study of services to patients with a total hip replacement demonstrate not only the therapeutic value but also the cost effectiveness of occupational therapy group treatment when compared with individual treatment as the primary format for care in physical disabilities practice.

Definitions and types of occupational therapy groups

In a survey of group practice, Howe and Schwartzberg (1986) identified 10 types of groups commonly used in occupational therapy: (1) exercise, (2) cooking, (3) tasks, (4) activities of daily living, (5) arts and crafts, (6) self-expression, (7) feelings-oriented discussion, (8) reality-oriented discussion, (9) sensorimotor or sensory integration, and (10) educational. In addition, they found a greater number of activity groups than verbal groups and more groups with 10 or less members.

At least 12 variables describe an occupational therapy group; these are listed in Table 9-3. Each needs to be considered in the formation and design of a therapeutic group. One of the most important of these variables, the group setting (inpatient or outpatient) has an impact on the group goals and techniques used. The relation between group orientation or format and therapeutic focus is given in Table 9-4.

Models in occupational therapy: roles of leader, group member, and activity

Several different group approaches are used in occupational therapy, and to varying degrees, each has its own articulated theoretical perspective. Selected occupational therapy group approaches are identified in Table 9-5. The roles of the leader, group member, and activity vary among the models. Each deserves attention when the models are applied to practice. The reader is referred to the original works for details about each approach.

The Functional Group Model (Howe & Schwartzberg, 1986, 1988; Kielhofner, 1992) is considered a generic group model in occupational therapy. It incorporates four key concepts: "purposeful activity," "self-initiated action," "spontaneous action," and "group-centered action." Howe and Schwartzberg (1988) explain how to enhance group process through group structure:

> To accomplish this result within the functional group model, the following factors should be considered in planning, running, and

reviewing the group: (1) maximum involvement through group-centered action, (2) a maximum sense of individual and group identity, (3) a "flow" experience, (4) spontaneous involvement of members, and (5) member support and feedback. These five major categories should be reviewed individually in terms of the parameters to be considered by the leader or co-leaders. It is suggested that the Group Session Plan Protocol be used to organize and formulate the clinical reasoning process for group interventions. (p. 3)

Leader techniques and procedures for conducting a group are described later in this section.

Comparison to group formats of other professions

As depicted in Table 9-1, the occupational therapy group format is significantly different from verbal psychotherapy groups conducted by other professionals, such as psychiatrists, psychologists, nurses, and social workers. In verbal group psychotherapy, for example, the emphasis is often on talking, insight, and understanding. In a psychodynamic or interpersonal model of group treatment, the ***there-and-then experience***, or past experience, which often is familial, is used as a means to understand present conflicts. The ***here-and-now experience***, or immediate experience, in the group is examined as a projection of the patient's past and provides members with an opportunity to test new and more adaptive interpersonal styles. These groups require members to have a fair degree of abstract capability and self-control over their behavior.

In contrast, as a general rule, occupational therapy groups focus as much as possible on shared "doing" and adjusted experience within the here-and-now experience. Groups are structured and graded so that members with modest to more advanced social and cognitive skills may participate. Mosey's (1973a) classification of group interaction skills is often used to designate the type and level of interaction required in an activity group. These levels are designated as (1) "parallel group," (2) "project group," (3) "egocentric–cooperative group," (4) "cooperative group," and (5) "mature group." They range from the parallel level, with maximal leader support and structure and with little expectation for interaction around a task, to the mature level, with minimal leader intervention and with a high degree of interaction required for task completion and social-emotional satisfaction.

A nonprogressing but multilevel scheme is the hierarchic task analysis developed by Allen (1985). This task analysis is used

TABLE 9-4. *Occupational Therapy Group Settings, Goals, and Techniques*

Group Orientation or Format*	Inpatient Goals and Techniques	Outpatient Goals and Techniques
Interpersonal and dynamically oriented	Support; containment	Social change; insight
Behaviorally and educationally oriented	New skills and attitudes; structure; here-and-now experiences	
Support groups	Acceptance	Legitimization; information; decreased isolation
Maintenance and rehabilitation groups	Safety; reevaluation; discharge planning	Adaptation; resources; minimization of stress

* These categories were adapted for this purpose from Vinogradov and Yalom's (1989) classification of outpatient groups.

to group patients according to their cognitive capabilities. Group tasks of varying complexity are chosen accordingly.

Theory and practice

The practice of group work in occupational therapy involves observation and interaction as well as the procedures of assessing, designing, planning and evaluating, analyzing and responding, and documenting.

Observation

The leader looks for information about the group's process in several areas. All aspects of the group are considered dynamic and therefore are constantly changing, which makes observation difficult and challenging.

Group as system: group process, phase, and dynamics

Groups progress through stages of development when therapeutic conditions have been achieved, such as clear, mutual goals and trust. **Group phases** indicating the phases of group development in terms of leader, group member, and activity roles are identified in Table 9-6. In observing the group's development, leaders look at the group's phase in relation to decision-making patterns, membership and leadership roles, and the level and type of participation patterns, such as who initiates communication, who talks to whom, and the tone of voice members and leaders use.

Individual member in system

In addition to the group as a whole, the leader observes the group member in relation to other members, the leader, and the group task. These observations of **group dynamics** may be informal or structured around a task designed to demonstrate certain skills and behaviors, such as cooperativeness, mobility, attention span, memory, concentration, and assertiveness. The observation task may also include functional activities, such as collaborative work, cooking, or other activities of daily living. Depending on the setting and length of treatment, when possible, the therapist may also conduct pregroup interviews as a means to observe, establish rapport, and gain information about a potential group member.

Leader and co-leader self-awareness

An equally important area of observation is the leader's own behavior and internal reactions. It is common practice for group leaders to write group process notes after each group meeting. In these notes, therapists describe their personal reactions, thoughts, and the critical events in the group. It is beneficial to share observations of the group and of each other with a co-leader. These observations are helpful in clinical supervision and in analysis of countertransference.

TABLE 9-5. *Selected Occupational Therapy Group Approaches and Theoretical Considerations*

Group Approaches
Task-Oriented Group (Fidler, 1969)
Functional Group Model (Howe & Schwartzberg, 1986)
Directive Group Therapy (Kaplan, 1988)
Activity Group (Borg & Bruce, 1991; Mosey, 1973a, 1973b)
Developmental Group (Mosey, 1970)
Psychoeducational Group (Lillie & Armstrong, 1982)
Integrative Group Therapy Structured Five-Stage Approach (Ross, 1991)
Peer Support Group (Schwartzberg, 1992)
Theoretical Considerations
Theoretical base
Function–dysfunction continuum
Behaviors indicative of function or dysfunction
Postulates of change

TABLE 9-6. *Sample Roles and Phases of Group Development*

Roles	Formation	Development	Termination
Leader	Set climate Provide structure Offer support	Grade actions Facilitate	Aid separation Reinforce gains
Member	Identify purpose	Collaborate Initiate	Evaluate Express reactions
Activity	Form goals Establish trust	Purposeful action	Review

Group, member, and leader observations

The observation of **group process** is conducted at the levels of (1) the group, (2) the individual members in relation to the group, (3) the individual members and the group in relation to the leader or co-leaders, and (4) all in relation to a task or activity. In addition, for purposes of feedback, the therapist may look for opportunities to observe the group member in functional contexts outside the group, such as in the community, school, work, or family environments.

Interaction

An important aspect of group therapy practice as well as individual therapy practice is the therapist's use of self in the group. Leaders serve particular roles and use techniques that they are continually attempting to perfect to achieve therapeutic goals.

Leader

The primary roles of the leader include observer, group designer, role model, and climate-setter (supporting and substituting actions as needed in the group). A skilled leader continually weighs individual and group needs and chooses techniques by considering past responses and immediate as well as long-term therapeutic goals. Techniques commonly used by the leader include therapeutic use of self, attending and listening, self-disclosure, empathy, feedback, confrontation, and activity analysis and adaptation (Howe & Schwartzberg, 1986). Particular use of these techniques is dependent on the group's goals and conceptual framework, the group's phase of development, and the therapist's relationship with the group members. The following case study is an example of the use of feedback and the group's response. This example illustrates the value of a clinical strategy such as encouraging feedback.

CASE EXAMPLE OF FEEDBACK

Elaine is 42 years old and has lived independently for 22 years after sustaining a head injury. She arrived at a group meeting with both eyes black and blue. Two weeks earlier the leader had expressed concern when she noticed a large bruise on Elaine's leg. This time the leader again asked Elaine what had happened. Elaine responded by telling the group her story. One evening the previous week she bumped her head on a table in her apartment. She woke up the next morning in bed with terribly bruised eyes and forehead. To encourage further exploration concerning Elaine's safety and judgment, the leader asked for more details about the incident and medical follow-up. Members followed by asking Elaine questions: "How and when did you learn of the bruises? What were you doing at the time of the fall? What resources are available to you in an emergency when you cannot reach the phone? Have you heard about Lifeline, an emergency call system?" Elaine's response was negative to the suggestion. It was too expensive. She wouldn't want to wear anything around her neck. She would forget it. The group would not accept her reply: "You can afford to buy the company (jokingly). You don't have to wear it in a visible place." This led to a group discussion about stigmatization and group conflict with another member concerning the

dangers of her wish to not reveal medical problems by wearing a medical alert bracelet. At the following group meeting, Elaine was the first to speak: "Can someone give me the phone number for that company, what do you call it?"

As Vinogradov and Yalom (1989) explain, "as with any affectively charged experience in the group, the therapist encourages reactions, active feedback, and consensual validation—a consensus of opinion on the true nature and meaning of the conflict—from all the group members" (p. 68).

Group members

The therapist and members of a group have work to accomplish in a group. Nevertheless, some problems commonly surface in group work, including difficulty establishing trust with the leader and other group members; dependency on the leader; difficulty setting goals; misdirected anger, competition among group members, subgrouping, and withdrawal from the group or task; lack of skill; absenteeism, members leaving the group meeting, and premature termination from the group; external conflicts and pressure (eg, from family); and interference from outside the group (eg, interruptions from other services, such as laboratory). When one of these problems arises, it must be examined separately and interpreted differently depending on the clinician's theoretical framework. A clinical example of a problem interaction in the development phase follows as an illustration of group work.

CASE STUDY

Interaction in the Development Phase

For 1½ years, the leader gave one of the group members a ride home from group meetings. They had a spoken agreement that unless notified otherwise, the leader would continue to drive the member home but could not drive her to the meetings. Nevertheless, the group member regularly called the leader to request a ride to the meeting, as she did on the day of the last meeting before a 2-month summer vacation.

    Leader: Hello.

    Member: Hello. (prolonged silence)

    Leader: I guess you're checking in to see about this afternoon.

    Member: Yes. By the way, can I have a ride?

    Leader: I can give you a ride home, as usual, but I can't take you there.

    Member: Okay (with despondency in voice).

    Leader: I'll see you this afternoon.

    Member: I suppose. As long as I haven't melted.

    Leader: Very funny (laughing). So I'll see you later and give you a ride home. Bye.

    Member: Byyyeh (jokingly with remorse).

In this group example, three themes appear: implied acceptance; testing the limits, with humor acting as an emotional cushion; and the need for reassurance in the face of absence or loss. Given the goals of the group, the therapist adopts a reality orientation to the here-and-now experience rather than an insight or interpretive approach. Although use of structure and direct support are primary considerations in the formative stage of a group, the often fragile self-esteem and cognitive impairments of patients seen in occupational therapy require that the leader pay particular attention to these elements throughout the group's existence.

Co-leaders

In working together, co-leaders assist in the physical and emotional management of the group. This is particularly important when the group is large or when members require considerable individual attention because of cognitive, physical, or social-emotional limitations. In addition, co-leaders are model participants in the group, demonstrating healthy interaction and ways of resolving conflict with others.

It is often useful to have supervision with both leaders present. These sessions help the leaders to work out differences of opinion, conflicts, and rivalry that inevitably exist when co-leading a group. When possible, a more experienced therapist co-leads with a beginning therapist. The experienced therapist serves as a model and can also provide peer supervision. Often, the co-leaders' relationship draws attention from the group. As model participants in the groups, the co-leaders provide members with an opportunity to observe a working, productive, teaching–learning relationship.

Procedures

Group leadership in occupational therapy requires time in designing the overall group plan and individual session plans. The leader also evaluates individual sessions and member progress and overall group progress.

Assessing individual members and the group

Assessment is an ongoing process that usually begins with meeting the patient before the first session. The therapist may have a formal referral or see a group member as part of a larger program. Groups may also be used for the sole purpose of evaluation. This is common in inpatient settings when patients are discharged rapidly and when the main goal of hospitalization is evaluation and discharge planning.

In some settings, the registered occupational therapist evaluates the patients and develops a plan and the certified occupational therapy assistant actually conducts the group. The registered therapist or experienced therapist may provide supervision as well. The arrangement of services varies from setting to setting.

Designing

The group's design has several components. The design is usually written in the form of a group protocol that includes: (1) group and, if possible, individual member short- and long-term goals; (2) selection criteria for membership; (3) group size and composition; (4) group methods, techniques, and activity modalities; (5) time and location of the group meeting and group leaders' names; and (6) referral procedures. Protocols aid therapists in communicating with other professionals and prospective group members.

Planning and evaluating

Evaluation is continuous throughout the group's existence. After evaluating each session, the leaders create detailed individual group session plans with categories similar to the overall, more generalized plan. When there is a major shift in patient population, the leader may also modify the general group plan.

Analyzing and responding

Each group situation is analyzed separately and continuously if the group is ongoing. To respond, the therapist uses the group's history as well as individual members' histories of strategies that were successful or unsuccessful. In an open group with a changing membership, the leader's experience with similar situations becomes particularly useful. In a closed group, the membership remains consistent from session to session. In these cases, the therapist can use prior experience for analyzing and responding, and the group can become its own control.

Documenting

Clinicians must consult their individual facilities, third-party payers, and state requirements for specific information concerning appropriate documentation of group evaluation and treatment. Therapists usually document each patient's progress separately after group sessions as well as keep records of the group's progress as a whole. As mentioned earlier, group protocols, session plans, and process notes are other forms of documentation commonly used in group practice.

Research and conclusions

Problems and strengths

Much remains to be understood about the use of group process in occupational therapy and about the best methods for teaching students and therapists how to use this important tool. A strength is the apparent value of the group to its members and to health care delivery as a cost-effective treatment.

Current research

Recent studies strongly suggest differences in outcomes when activity groups are compared with psychotherapy groups (DeCarlo & Mann, 1985; Klyczek & Mann, 1986; McDermott, 1988; Mumford, 1974; Schwartzberg, Howe, & McDermott; 1982). In contrast, although differences have been noted (Finn, 1989; Webster, 1988), similarities have also been found between members' perceptions of the therapeutic value of occupational therapy groups and the perspectives of members of psychotherapy groups (Falk-Kessler, Momich, & Perel, 1991; Webster & Schwartzberg, 1992). In addition, there appear to exist unique roles and helping factors when peer-led groups are compared with professional-led groups in occupational therapy (Sacenti, 1988; Schwartzberg, 1992).

Future research in all settings in which occupational therapists use group treatment should address both outcomes and patient perceptions of group treatment. Regardless of group format, it would be of interest to know, for example, if patient perceptions of therapeutic factors are related to functional outcomes, or vice versa. Further studies in activity group analysis and the meaning of restricted variables would also support the endeavor to explain the therapeutic use of group process in occupational therapy (Adelstein & Nelson, 1985; Henry, Nelson, & Duncombe, 1984; Kremer, Nelson, & Duncombe, 1984; Nelson, Peterson, Smith, Boughton, & Whalen, 1988; Steffan & Nelson, 1987; Steffan, 1990).

Summary

The past and present trends in group process as a tool of occupational therapy were introduced. Models of group treatment in occupational therapy were described and the procedural aspects of this practice highlighted. Some recent research on the use of group treatment was summarized, and as examples, a few principles in need of verification were identified.

References

Allen, C. K. (1985). *Occupational therapy for psychiatric diseases: Measurement and management of cognitive disabilities.* Boston: Little, Brown.

Adelstein, L. A., & Nelson, D. L. (1985). Effects of sharing versus non-sharing on affective meaning in collage activities. *Occupational Therapy in Mental Health: A Journal of Psychosocial Practice and Research, 5*(2), 29–45.

Borg, B., & Bruce, M. A. (1991). *The group system: The therapeutic activity group in occupational therapy.* Thorofare, NJ: Slack.

DeCarlo, J. J., & Mann, W. C. (1985). The effectiveness of verbal versus activity groups in improving self-perceptions of interpersonal communication skills. *American Journal of Occupational Therapy, 39*(1), 20–27.

Duncombe, L. W., & Howe, M. C. (1985). Group work in occupational therapy: A survey of practice. *American Journal of Occupational Therapy, 39*(3), 163–170.

Falk-Kessler, J., Momich, C., & Perel, S. (1991). Therapeutic factors in occupational therapy groups. *American Journal of Occupational Therapy, 45*(1), 59–66.

Fidler, G. S. (1969). The task-oriented group as a context for treatment. *American Journal of Occupational Therapy, 23*(1), 43–48.

Finn, M. (1989). Patients' perceptions of occupational therapy groups: Interview generated factors. Unpublished master's thesis, Tufts University—Boston School of Occupational Therapy, Medford, MA.

Gauthier, L., Dalziel, S., & Gauthier, S. (1987). The benefits of group occupational therapy for patients with Parkinson's disease. *American Journal of Occupational Therapy, 41*(6), 360–365.

Henry, A. D., Nelson, D. L., & Duncombe, L. W. (1984). Choice making in group and individual activity. *American Journal of Occupational Therapy, 38*(4), 245–251.

Howe, M. C., & Schwartzberg, S. L. (1986). *A functional approach to group work in occupational therapy.* Philadelphia: J. B. Lippincott.

Howe, M. C., & Schwartzberg, S. L. (1988). Structure and process in designing a functional group. *Occupational Therapy in Mental Health: A Journal of Psychosocial Practice and Research, 8*(3), 1–8.

Kaplan, K. L. (1988). *Directive group therapy: Innovative mental health treatment.* Thorofare, NJ: Slack.

Kielhofner, G. (1992). *Conceptual foundations of occupational therapy.* Philadelphia: F. A. Davis.

Klyczek, J. P., & Mann, W. C. (1986). Therapeutic modality comparisons in day treatment. *American Journal of Occupational Therapy, 40*(9), 606–611.

Kremer, E. R. H., Nelson, D. L., & Duncombe, L. W. (1984). Effects of selected activities on affective meaning in psychiatric patients. *American Journal of Occupational Therapy, 38*(8), 522–528.

Lillie, M., & Armstrong, H. (1982). Contributions to the development of psychoeducational approaches to mental health service. *American Journal of Occupational Therapy, 36*(7), 438–443.

Lundgren, C. C., & Persechino, E. L. (1986). Cognitive group: A treatment program for head injured adults. *American Journal of Occupational Therapy, 40*(6), 397–401.

McDermott, A. A. (1988). The effect of three group formats on group interaction patterns. *Occupational Therapy in Mental Health: A Journal of Psychosocial Practice and Research, 8*(3), 69–89.

Mosey, A. C. (1970). The concept and use of developmental groups. *American Journal of Occupational Therapy, 24*(4), 272–275.

Mosey, A. C. (1973a). *Activities therapy.* New York: Raven Press.

Mosey, A. C. (1973b). Meeting health needs. *American Journal of Occupational Therapy, 27*(1), 14–17.

Mumford, M. S. (1974). A comparison of interpersonal skills in verbal and activity groups. *American Journal of Occupational Therapy, 28*(5), 281–283.

Nelson, D. L., Peterson, C., Smith, D. A., Boughton, J. A., & Whalen, G. M. (1988). Effects of project versus parallel groups on social interaction and affective responses in senior citizens. *American Journal of Occupational Therapy, 42*(1), 23–29.

Ross, M. (1991). *Integrative group therapy: The structured five-stage approach* (2nd ed.). Thorofare, NJ: Slack.

Sacenti, L. (1988). Mastery and levels of participation in members of two groups for chronic pain: Self-help and professionally led. Unpublished master's thesis, Tufts University—Boston School of Occupational Therapy, Medford, MA.

Schwartzberg, S. L. (1992). *Helping factors in a peer developed support group for head injured individuals.* Manuscript submitted for publication.

Schwartzberg, S. L., Howe, M. C., & McDermott, A. (1982). A comparison of three treatment group formats for facilitating social interaction. *Occupational Therapy in Mental Health: A Journal of Psychosocial Practice and Research, 2*(4), 1–16.

Steffan, J. A. (1990). Productive occupation in small task groups of adults: Synthesis and annotations of the social psychology literature. In A. C. Bundy, N. D. Prendergast, J. A. Steffan, & D. Thorn (Eds.), *Review of selected literature on occupation and health* (pp. 175–281). Rockville, MD: American Occupational Therapy Association.

Steffan, J. A., & Nelson, D. L. (1987). The effects of tool scarcity on group climate and affective meaning within the context of a stenciling activity. *American Journal of Occupational Therapy, 41*(7), 449–453.

Trahey, P. J. (1991). A comparison of the cost-effectiveness of two types of occupational therapy services. *American Journal of Occupational Therapy, 45*(5), 397–400.

Van Deusen, J., & Harlowe, D. (1987). The efficacy of the ROM dance program for adults with rheumatoid arthritis. *American Journal of Occupational Therapy, 41*(2), 90–95.

Vinogradov, S., & Yalom, I. D. (1989). *A concise guide to group psychotherapy.* Washington, DC: American Psychiatric Press.

Webster, D. (1988). Patients' perceptions of therapeutic factors in occupational therapy groups. Unpublished master's thesis, Tufts University—Boston School of Occupational Therapy, Medford, MA.

Webster, D., & Schwartzberg, S. L. (1992). Patient's perception of curative factors in occupational therapy groups. *Occupational Therapy in Mental Health: A Journal of Psychosocial Practice and Research, 12*(1).

Bibliography

Benjamin, A. (1978). *Behavior in small groups.* Boston: Houghton Mifflin.

Bion, W. R. (1974). *Experiences in groups.* New York: Ballantine Books.

Bradford, L. P. (1978). *Group development.* San Diego: University Associates.

Bruce, M. A. (1988). Occupational therapy in group treatment. In

D. W. Scott, & N. Katz (Eds.), *Occupational therapy in mental health: Principles in practice*. Philadelphia: Taylor and Francis.

Bruce, M. A., & Borg, B. (1987). *Frames of reference in psychosocial occupational therapy*. Thorofare, NJ: Slack.

Cartwright, D., & Zander, A. (Eds.). (1968). *Group dynamics: Research and theory* (3rd ed.). New York: Harper and Row.

Cermak, S. A., Stein, F., & Abelson, C. (1973). Hyperactive children and activity group therapy model. *American Journal of Occupational Therapy, 26*(6), 311–315.

Corey, G., & Corey, M. S. (1982). *Groups: Process and practice* (2nd ed.). Monterey: Brooks/Cole.

Fidler, G. S. (1984). *Design of rehabilitation services in psychiatric hospital settings*. Laurel, MD: RAMSCO.

Hughes, P. L., & Mullins, L. (1981). *Acute psychiatric care: An occupational therapy guide to exercises in daily living skills*. Thorofare, NJ: Slack.

Kaplan, K. (1986). The directive group: Short-term treatment for psychiatric patients with a minimal level of functioning. *American Journal of Occupational Therapy, 40*(7), 474–481.

King, L. J. (1976). A sensory integrative approach to schizophrenia. *American Journal of Occupational Therapy, 28*, 529–536.

Knowles, M., & Knowles, H. (1972). *Introduction to group dynamics* (revised ed.). New York: Association Press.

Miles, M. B. (1981). *Learning to work in groups: A practical guide for members and trainers* (2nd ed.). New York: Teachers College Press.

Mosey, A. C. (1986). *Psychosocial components of occupational therapy*. New York: Raven Press.

Napier, R. W., & Gershenfeld, M. K. (1985). *Group theory and experience* (3rd ed.). Boston: Houghton Mifflin.

Posthuma, B. W. (1989). *Small groups in therapy settings: Process and leadership*. Boston: Little, Brown.

Ross, M. (1987). *Group process using therapeutic activities in chronic care*. Thorofare, NJ: Slack.

Ross, M., & Burdick, D. (1981). *Sensory integration: A training manual for therapists and teachers for regressed, psychiatric and geriatric patient groups*. Thorofare, NJ: Slack.

Sampson, E. E., & Marthas, M. (1981). *Group process for the health professions* (2nd ed.). New York: John Wiley & Sons.

Slavson, S. R., & Schiffer, M. (1975). *Group psychotherapies for children: A textbook*. New York: International Universities Press.

Yalom, I. D. (1983). *Inpatient group psychotherapy*. New York: Basic Books.

Yalom, I. D. (1985). *The theory and practice of group psychotherapy* (3rd ed.). New York: Basic Books.

SECTION 3

Use of activity and activity analysis

CAROLE J. SIMON

KEY TERMS

Activity	Occupational Performance
Activity Analysis	Performance Components
Activity Synthesis	Therapeutic Teaching and
Motivation	Learning Process

LEARNING OBJECTIVES

Upon completion of this section the reader will be able to:

1. *Explain the philosophical base for the use of activities.*
2. *Relate the historical foundation of manual skills and activities in occupational therapy.*
3. *Relate the significance of motivational factors.*
4. *Develop an awareness of cultural and lifestyle implications with regard to selection of activities.*
5. *Appreciate inherent characteristics of activities.*
6. *Describe the value of activities as a basis for occupational therapy.*
7. *Analyze and synthesize the component parts of an activity.*
8. *Recognize gradation capabilities of activities for adaptation to meet patient needs.*
9. *Understand how a client uses activities to move from dysfunction to function.*

Philosophical base

The affirmation of occupation, or ***activity***, as the common core of occupational therapy has been stated in the "Philosophical Base of Occupational Therapy" adopted in 1979 by the Representative Assembly,

> Man is an active being whose development is influenced by the use of purposeful activity. Using their capacity for intrinsic motivation, human beings are able to influence their physical and mental health and the social and physical environment through purposeful activity. Human life includes a process of continuous adaptation. Adaptation is a change in function that promotes survival and self-actualization. Biological, psychological, and environmental factors may interrupt the adaptation process at any time throughout the life cycle. Dysfunction may occur when adaptation is impaired. Purposeful activity facilitates the adaptive process.
>
> Occupational therapy is based on the belief that purposeful activity (occupation), including its interpersonal and environmen-

tal components, may be used to prevent and mediate dysfunction, and to elicit maximum adaptation. Activity as used by the occupational therapist includes both an intrinsic and therapeutic purpose. (Representative Assembly, 1979a, p. 785)

The Representative Assembly further advocated,

a universal acceptance and implementation of the common core of occupational therapy as active participation of the patient/client in occupation for purposes of improving performance. The use of facilitating procedures is only acceptable as occupational therapy when used to prepare the patient/client for better performance and prevention of disability, through self-participation in occupation . . . increased emphasis should be placed on more creative involvement of the patient/client in purposeful, motivating and constructive occupation based on individual behavioral evaluations and treatment. (Representative Assembly, 1979b, p. 785)

These statements acknowledge the existence of activity as a part of every person's life. Moreover, they emphasize the power that activities or occupation can have when used to help improve a person's functional capabilities. To be useful in aiding growth in skills and successful adaptation to the environment, an activity must be purposeful and provide meaning to the person engaging in the selected task.

Every person's life is filled with activities—some are boring, routine, and necessary, whereas others are playful, creative, and joyful. The main focus of an activity may be for survival, such as eating or finding shelter, or it may be expressive, offer comfort, or provide pleasure. Activities may be performed alone, or they may support social interaction. The scope and variety of activities in life allow for the idiosyncratic growth of a person and define who that person is by virtue of their choice of activities. Inherent in the pursuit of an activity is the concept of doing. Engaging in activity is not a passive act. One must make choices, use body parts, problem-solve, interact with others or the physical environment, and react to the outcome of success, failure, or perhaps frustration and anxiety.

Activity also has a temporal aspect. Within each 24-hour period, time is divided by participation in a variety of activities that support the function and competence of each person in the areas of self-care, work, and play and leisure. The extent of time needed and the skills available to accomplish the tasks and activities that occupy the hours in a day can provide insight into the occupational therapy needs of any adult or child. People experience themselves and come to know their strengths and weaknesses through the things they do (Hopkins & Tiffany, 1988). The occupational therapist can use activities to assess the skills and deficits of each client and to identify subsequent treatment planning rationales. Through collaboration of the patient and the occupational therapist, a plan can emerge that promotes the appropriate use of time and skill to successfully accomplish the highest potential in occupational performance for self-care, work, and play and leisure activities.

Environmental factors play a key role in determining engagement in selected activities. For example, the person whose wheelchair does not fit through the entrance door is unable to shop in a popular dress store. Cultural values suggest preeminence of some activities at the expense of others. For example, in some cultures, men are expected to do heavy labor but never cook or sew; in other settings, men are the premiere chefs and tailors. Human and nonhuman factors are also important. The human factors include men, women, and children and interactions at all levels among them. The nonhuman component of the environment refers to everything else. Space, sounds, tools, supplies, furniture, lighting, and smells are some of the elements of the nonhuman environment. The placement, availability, and amount of nonhuman elements can influence the therapeutic environment.

Cynkin (1979) suggests that activities in a field of action (or environment) can structure the therapeutic intervention so that experiences can simulate possible conditions the client may meet in the real world. Accordingly, if the interactive skills of a client are going to be tested in the real world, the client in therapy may need to learn to share a limited number of tools in an activity group. The life role that a person is expected to fulfill (eg, student, mother, father, breadwinner) also influences the activities required and the reasonable amount of time allotted to each activity.

In Figure 9-1, the backdrop of influences from life space, culture, and human and nonhuman environment colors the **occupational performance** of a person carrying out activities necessary for self-care, work, and play and leisure. Furthermore, the skills or levels of function and dysfunction of a person promote or diminish the quality of the **performance components** necessary to accomplish the total task. It is imperative, therefore, to learn about the needs of a client by examining the client's history, life roles, cultural values, activity configuration (amount of time spent daily on specific activities), and functional levels of neuromuscular, sensory integrative, cognitive, psychological, and social areas. A clear understanding of the interplay among these factors will aid in the appropriate collaborative selection of therapeutic activities to be used in the restoration or habilitation of the client.

Once an activity has been selected, the performance of it becomes paramount. At the outset, the *process* is more important than the ultimate *outcome*. The **motivation** of the client undergirds the client's engagement in the task; a client who is not motivated will not participate therapeutically in activities. Hence, the initial collaborative investigation of activities that are intrinsically meaningful to the client pays off. By observing the process of accomplishing the task, both the therapist and the client can gain insight into such areas as organizational skills, problem-solving abilities, work habits, muscle strength, fine motor skills, and coping behaviors. With enhancement of identified problem areas through experience in therapeutic activities, a satisfactory outcome or product can be anticipated. Emphasis on an artistic or perfect product is unrealistic since the journey to the end product carries the importance.

Defining crafts and activities

The reader should refer to Chapter 2 for an in-depth review of the history of occupational therapy. In this section, crafts are acknowledged to be one of the initial activities used to further patient performance.

When occupational therapy began in hospitals for the mentally ill, the women from the community worked on craft activities with the patients to ameliorate problems. Meyer (1922) stipulated that pleasure in achievement, a real pleasure in the use of one's hands and muscles in activities, and a happy appreciation of time began to be used as incentives in the management of

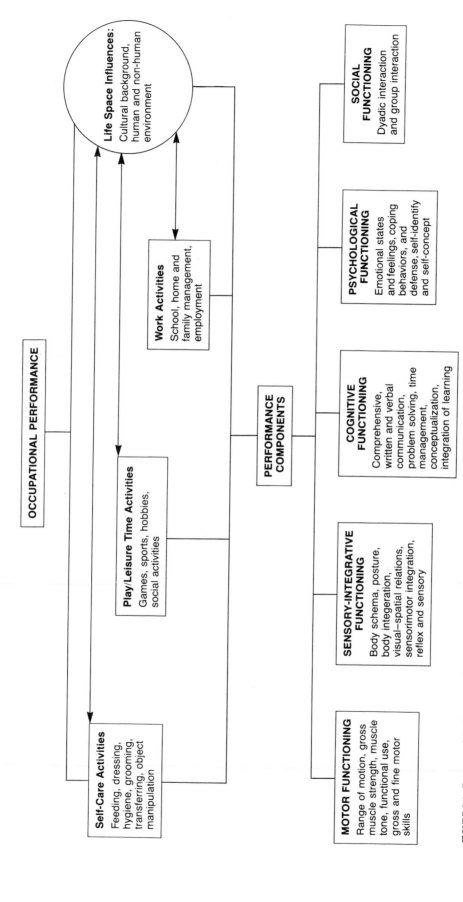

FIGURE 9.1. *Frame of Reference, Dimension Two, Content of Occupational Therapy Process (From Schnebly, M. E., Prendergast, N. D. [Ed.], Pasch, M. & Evans, K. A. [1974]. Rockville, MD: American Occupational Therapy Association.)* A Curriculum Guide for Occupational Therapy Educators.

patients. Occupational therapy health care during and after World War I followed this tradition. The occupational therapy profession has a rich heritage in the use of arts and crafts to foster patient progress.

Over time, occupational therapists have added to their repertoire as a result of burgeoning information in both the scientific and technologic arenas. As a result, occupational therapy practice has changed dramatically from the early days of arts and crafts. Nevertheless, our strong roots in the craft tradition need not be cast aside. In perspective, crafts can be a potent therapeutic tool. Remaining mindful that the client needs to value the activity to be pursued, the occupational therapist and client can select a meaningful craft or activity that can fulfill the required performance components. The creativity inherent in completing a craft may be the sole feature that engages the client's attention. Creativity is a basic urge within all of us, and stifling creativity leads to a decrease in problem-solving abilities and a decreased quality of life (Miller & Fox, 1988). Thus, through creativity, the client can practice skills and adapt as needed while achieving goals in a more holistic and satisfying manner than could be expected through exercise alone.

Swift (1981) noticed that many physical disability clinics have eliminated activities and concentrate only on exercise. He suggests that many occupational therapists have come to view humans in reductionist terms. In other words, they have become muscle- and joint-oriented in physical disabilities, group therapy–oriented in psychiatry, and biologically oriented in sensory integrative dysfunction. This not only does a disservice to the patient but also has allowed an erosion of basic occupational therapy tenets. At the same time, other professionals are recognizing the value of activities in therapy and are embracing these as "new" ideas.

By being fully cognizant of the relevance of activities, by articulating a clear rationale for their use, and by using the full range of preparatory activities and modalities available to the profession, occupational therapists can enhance their professional image. To justify the use of crafts and activities, the occupational therapist needs only to reflect on the ultimate purposeful activity the client must be able to accomplish and sustain to be functional in his or her life role. This can be coupled with the advanced technology that is available today in such a way that the unique vantage point that represents occupational therapy can benefit the client in a manner that no other discipline can offer. Emergence of exercise and other modalities has created a controversy regarding the legitimate tools of occupational therapy and the true role of the occupational therapist as part of the health care team (Bing, 1981; Reed, 1986; West, 1984). Dutton (1989, p. 574) states: "The controversy over the role of occupational therapists has persisted because activity and exercise have been seen as mutually exclusive, philosophically opposed treatment approaches. Activity and exercise are actually at complementary ends of the same continuum." Thus, the *application* of the increased strength or range of motion gained through exercise or other treatment techniques is the qualitative use of the effectiveness of occupational therapy treatment. For example, the client who has been actively playing a game with weighted pieces can then apply the increased upper-extremity strength to the activity of brushing teeth, and the client who has been the recipient of proprioneuromuscular facilitation techniques can proceed using those movement patterns for dressing to don a shirt.

Therapeutic implementation

In therapy, experiencing success is critical. The activity regimen must be styled to offer success, plus a challenge to spur the client on to the next level of competence. The observable actions of the client reflect his or her inner experience and can provide the alert therapist with information regarding the need to adapt the activity, increase or decrease the skill level required, or change to a more motivating format.

Csikszentmihalyi (1975) described the pleasurable sensation that an organism experiences when it is functioning according to its physical and sensory potential. A state of flow ensues that provides opportunities for action that can be undertaken without boredom or anxiety. Figure 9-2 provides a model to demonstrate the channel of flow that occurs when the skills of the client match the challenges or action opportunities offered in therapy. At any given point in the model, a person is aware of the challenge to act while at the same time being aware of his or her own skills and capacity to cope with demands imposed by the therapeutic environment. When skills are not compatible with demands, a state of anxiety ensues; when demands are fewer, but still more than the client feels capable of handling, the client expresses worry. Conversely, if the client's skills are greater than the opportunities available to use them, boredom quickly follows, and there may be little motivation to engage in the activity. A person with great skills and few opportunities to apply them will pass from a state of boredom to a state of anxiety. Whether the person is in a state of flow depends on the person's *perception* of the environmental challenges and available skills. This perception is more than the objective demands of the situation and may be positively influenced by the therapist's conscious use of self to motivate engagement by the client in the selected activity. Two factors can return those in a state of worry to a flow

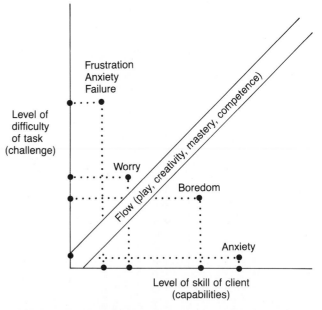

FIGURE 9-2. *Model of Balance Between Client Skill and Task Difficulty (Adapted from "Beyond boredom and anxiety: The experience of play in work and games" by M. Csikszentmihalyi [1975]. Cambridge, MA: Belknap Press of Harvard University Press.)*

status: decrease the challenge (downgrade the activity) or increase the skill (enhance performance components). Those who are bored can return to flow by increasing the environmental challenge or by decreasing the level of skill. Adaptation of an activity may be essential to promote success and challenge. This can be accomplished in many ways, from increasing the complexity of a leather tooling design to positioning the pottery to be glazed on a stand at a proper height. Adaptation of the tools to be used can also provide a more successful experience; for example, the handle of the fork can be enlarged to offer easier grasp.

Characteristics of occupational therapy activity

Occupational therapists become acquainted with many activities and crafts to use their inherent qualities to provide goal-directed "occupations" for clients. Activities are the core of occupational therapy and as such should fulfill at least the following characteristics:

1. *Be goal directed.* Activities should have some purpose or reason for their use to be considered occupational therapy activity. "Busy work," or just keeping the hands occupied, may be of some value to the client, but generally it is not chosen with a specific goal in mind.

2. *Have significance at some level to the client.* Activities should have value and usefulness to the client, even though the value may be realized only at some future date. That is, the activity may seem to have no immediate value in reaching a specified goal but will make it possible to reach that goal in a week, a month, or some time later. The activity should have some relationship to the roles the individual plays in society.

3. *Require client involvement at some level* (either mental or physical). Activities require "doing" or participation on the part of the client. The individual engaged in the activity should be involved in selecting the activity as well as in the performance of it and thus receives self-gratification from the results. He or she is not a recipient but rather a participant. Participation may be active or passive.

4. *Be geared to prevention of malfunction and/or maintenance or improvement of function and quality of life.* The choice and type of activity is dependent on the client's level of function and ability to participate; however, the goal is clear.

5. *Reflect client involvement in life task situations* (ADL, play, work). Activities are used to acquire or redevelop those skills essential for fulfillment of life roles. Activities develop competence in the performance of those tasks essential to the life roles of each individual.

6. *Relate to the interests of the client.* Involvement in the choice of activity is vital. Commitment to the tasks will be attained only if client goals and interests are considered and met.

7. *Be adaptable and gradable.* Activity must be age appropriate, be able to be increased or decreased in complexity, and be graded in time and strength required.

8. *Be determined through the occupational therapist's professional judgment based on knowledge.* Knowledge of human development, medical pathology, interpersonal relationships, and value of activity to the person are required to make the match between client problems and the activities that will be most meaningful and serviceable in reaching the therapeutic goals of occupational therapy. (Hopkins & Tiffany, 1988, pp. 93–94)

In addition to the overall characteristics to be considered for employing activities therapeutically, qualities specific to each activity must be analyzed. The materials used sometimes define the possibilities for treatment. For example, if a piece of lumber is cut to size, it will always be that size. On the other hand, clay is constantly remoldable until it is fired and hardened; fabric can be stretched or eased into a given space. Each of these qualities may lend itself to specific use in the treatment setting. The outcome for the patient who is quick and careless with measurements and work habits is clear when the wooden pieces prepared haphazardly do not assemble into the birdhouse the client had envisioned. The client can be encouraged to generalize this experience to gain insight into other areas of life that have been unsuccessful for similar reasons. The patient with weak hand muscles can model a piece of clay into an infinite number of shapes and enjoy the exercise available through this resistive material, thus responding to the inherent motivating quality of the medium. Another client can learn to adjust fabric to fit a specific area. Rather than viewing misjudgment as an outright failure, it becomes a problem-solving opportunity.

Activity analysis

Activity analysis consists of each activity being evaluated carefully to determine its therapeutic potential. With experience, the occupational therapist can quickly recognize the possibilities and pitfalls inherent in a given task. Also, the therapist can readily perceive ways to upgrade or downgrade the level of difficulty of the activity to individualize its characteristics for specific patient needs. The accompanying sample form on pages 268 and 287 depicts a general activity analysis based on explicit data that indicate the range of considerations possible for a given task (Hopkins & Tiffany, 1988).

After ascertaining precisely what movement, skill, or cognition the activity requires, the therapist must recognize what gain the activity can offer the client. Next, the therapist must decide what adaptations, either to the environment or the activity, will allow success or will challenge the client. Table 9-7 suggests ways to analyze components of leather and ceramic activities using the concept of gains the patient can achieve from the inherent requirements of the craft. The use of uniform terminology for occupational therapy will enhance clarity of thought in the process of activity analysis.

The dimensions of any activity include: the *analysis* of the adaptive skills required; the *skill level* needed to accomplish the activity at a minimal level; the *gradability* of the activity in terms of skill levels, time to accomplish, and repetition; its *flexibility* in terms of space, equipment, and supplies; its *cultural implications*; *age-appropriateness*; *safety considerations*; *and cost* (Hopkins & Tiffany, 1988).

Therapeutic application of activity

The application of an activity, or the making of the *match* between the activity and the client, is critical to the occupational therapy process. Mosey (1985) defines the process as **activity synthesis**, in which the therapist combines the component parts of the human and nonhuman environments to design an activity suitable for evaluation or intervention. It is at this point that the data collected regarding the activity and the client must be seen within the perspective of a *frame of reference* (Hopkins & Tiffany, 1988). The frame of reference defines the choice of activity and the aspects of that activity that will promote the goals

(*Text continues on page 289*)

ACTIVITY ANALYSIS FORM

Activity analyzed:
Average time required for completion:
Average number of sessions required to complete:
Brief description: (include criteria for determining success)

Activity Characteristics	Explanations		

A. MOTOR
    1. Position:
       a. activity
       b. patient/client
    2. Motion(s) components
       a. joints involved
       b. motion(s) involved
    3. Muscles utilized
    4. Direction of resistance

Activity Characteristics	Skill required ✓	Degree Low Medium High	Is activity gradable? How?
A. MOTOR (cont.)			
5. Action rather than position			
6. Repetition of motion(s)			
7. Rhythm developed			
8. Maintained contraction (static)			
9. Manual dexterity			
10. Gross motor			
11. Fine motor			
12. Bilateral			
13. Unilateral			
14. Endurance			
15. Rate of performance			
16. Grading adaptability			
a. R.O.M.			
b. resistance			
c. coordination			
d. substitution			
B. SENSORY			
1. Visual			
2. Auditory (impact on)			
3. Gustatory			
4. Olfactory			
5. Tactile			
a. temperature of material			
b. texture of material			
c. heavy to light touch			
C. COGNITIVE			
1. Organizational ability			
2. Problem solving ability			
a. planning			
b. trial and error			
3. Logical thinking			
4. Concentration			
5. Attention span			
6. Written/oral/demonstration directions			
a. complex			
b. simple			
7. Reading			
8. Seriation			
9. Interpret signs & symbols			
10. Multiple processing/steps involved			
11. Creativity			
12. Use of imagination			
13. Establish goal & carry out means to attain it			
14. Causal relationships involved (perceive cause & effect)			
15. Centering			

(continued)

Activity Characteristics	Skill required ✓	Degree Low Medium High	Is activity gradable? How?
16. Perceive viewpoint of others			
17. Test reality			
D. PERCEPTUAL			
1. Sensory integration required			
2. Differentiation			
a. Figure-ground			
b. Space relationships			
c. Object constancy			
d. Kinesthesia			
e. Proprioception			
f. Stereognosis			
g. Form constancy			
h. Color perception			
i. Auditory perception			
3. Tactile integration			
4. Motor planning			
5. Bilateral integration			
6. Body scheme			
7. Vestibular			
E. EMOTIONAL			
1. Passive or aggressive motion			
2. Destructive			
3. Gratification			
a. immediate			
b. delayed			
4. Structured			
5. Unstructured			
6. Allows control			
7. Success/failure possibility			
8. Independence			
9. Dependence			
10. Symbolism involved			
11. Reality testing			
12. Handle feelings			
13. Impulse control			
F. SOCIAL			
1. Interaction required			
2. Isolating activity			
3. Group activity			
4. Competition			
5. Responsibility involved			
6. Communication necessary			
7. Work in small groups			
8. Work in large groups			
9. Work with one other person			
10. Test reality			
11. Control—lead			
12. Follow—cooperate			
G. CULTURAL			
1. Relevancy to personal			
a. Value system			
b. Life situations			
H. COMMON TO ALL			
1. Age appropriateness			
2. Safety precautions & hazards			
3. Sexual identification			
4. Space required			
5. Equipment needed			
6. Vocational application			
7. Cost			
8. Adaptability			

TABLE 9-7.   *Analyzing an Activity*

Activity	Performance Components	Activity Requirements/Provisions	Patient Gains	Adaptations
Leatherwork	Motor	Cut leather with shears	Bilateral coordination Eye–hand coordination Manual dexterity	Many or few pieces for intricate or simple pattern
		Lace pieces together	Range of motion Fine grasp, dexterity	Short or long lengths of lacing Simple or complex stitch
		Use rotary hole punch	Strengthen hand Endurance	Thick or thin leather More or fewer holes
	Sensory–perceptual	3-D effect of design by tooling	Figure-ground perception	Simple or complex design
		Texture of various leathers, wet or dry	Increased tactile perception	Vary leathers
		Use of modeling tools	Proprioception Kinesthetic perception Motor planning	Vary complexity of design
	Cognitive	Directions	Oral, written, or diagram directions	Demonstrate or model task; one- or two-step directions; independent use of instructions
		Multiple steps: wet leather transfer-design, tool, finish	Organization Logical thinking	Structure for client
		Trial and error (*eg*, setting hardware)	Problem solving	Provide or withhold solutions
	Psychological	Success or failure probability when modeling design	Coping abilities	Provide more or less supervision and suggestions
		Hammer with mallet	Use of aggressive energy	Increase design or hardware
		Individual activity	Independence Control Pride	Vary amounts of intervention
	Social	Parallel activity	Ability to work in proximity to others	Arrange seating
		Share workspace, tools, supplies, or project	Responsibility Cooperation Group interaction	Limit number of available tools Assign clean-up tasks
Ceramic Tiles	Motor	Repetition of positioning tiles	Practice in grasp and release Endurance	Increase or decrease amount or size of tiles
		Application of glue	Bimanual hand use Coordination Practice with skilled hand	Use squeeze bottle of glue or stabilize surface for one-handed application
		Cut tiles to fit with tile cutter	Increased hand strength	Vary amount to be cut for design
	Sensory–perceptual	Design with colors and sizes	Color and size discrimination Visual–spatial relations Figure-ground discrimination	Single color Simple design Complex mosaic
		Tactile experience with tiles, glue, grout	Size, shape, and texture discrimination	Vary choice of tiles to select from one container Apply glue and grout with fingers
		Auditory input when searching in or emptying tile container	Auditory habituation	Use many or few tiles Situate near others making noise
	Cognitive	Learn to sequence task: glue, dry, grout, finish	Logical thinking Organization Judgment when to proceed to next step	Explain one step or several Assist or allow independence
		Concentration to make design	Attention span	Large or small project or units of project
		Problem solving to fill in spaces	Judgment about size to fit Conceptualize design	Simple or complex design or shapes

(continued)

TABLE 9-7.   *Analyzing an Activity (continued)*

Activity	Performance Components	Activity Requirements/Provisions	Patient Gains	Adaptations
	Psychological	Requires wait for glue and grout to dry	Delayed gratification	Explain and structure time
		"Destruction" of design with application of grout	Experience success following a "mess"	Use as an analog for life situations
			Coping skills	
		Structured or creative possibilities	Work independently	Vary supervision
			Trial and error	
	Social	Group project possible	Interaction with others to plan and execute design	Work in pairs or more
		Parallel project	Share and observe products of others	Ease and structure feedback
			Ability to receive compliments and criticism	

of the intervention. The frame of reference determines which dimensions of the activity are to be emphasized and the depth to which some of the dimensions are to be explored and exploited. For example, a biomechanical frame of reference will be most concerned with the motor aspects of the activity, whereas a psychoanalytic frame of reference will be concerned with its symbolic potential. Activity analysis based on a behavioral frame of reference is concerned especially with the specification and serialization of the component parts of the activity, their potential as, or the need for, reinforcement contingencies, and the measurability of the data. A sensory integrative frame of reference focuses on the sensory, perceptual, and physical aspects of the activity. A developmental perspective is concerned with the parallels between the levels of functioning required or expected and developmental levels. Within an occupational behavior perspective, the concern is for the potential of the activity to promote competence and balance within the client's life roles in society (Hopkins & Tiffany, 1988).

Given the emphasis provided by the frame of reference, additional considerations are necessary for physical and psychosocial dysfunction. Those activities selected for their physical restorative powers must never be separated from their psychological and psychosocial properties, which serve to enhance the physical treatment. The following criteria assist in meeting physical restoration requirements:

1. *Provide action rather than position.* Activity should provide for alternate contraction and relaxation of muscles. Activities should be analyzed from a kinesiologic point of view to determine their components, the motions required, the muscle power required, and the range of motion and strengthening the activity can provide.
2. *Require repetition of the motion.* Activity should permit repetition of the desired motion for an indefinite but controllable number of times.
3. *Permit gradation in the range of motion, resistance, and coordination.* Activity should allow a greater range of motion than is permitted by the limitation in the joint so the activity can allow for increase in *joint range. Resistance* is required in order to strengthen a muscle. Thus the activity should be gradable in the amount of resistance it provides so that resistance can be increased as power returns. When *coordination* is affected, the activity should be graded so that it provides exercise requiring gross coordination and working toward fine

coordination. The activity may also be varied or adapted through positioning or by changing the way the task is performed (Hopkins & Tiffany, 1988, p. 95). For example, the occupational therapist can change the size, shape, or texture of the materials, or add weights, springs, rubber bands or other apparatus to change the resistance encountered.

Keeping in mind that the psychosocial properties of activities are important in the treatment of all types of dysfunction, the following list illustrates psychodynamic properties that are primary in psychiatric occupational therapy (Norristown State Hospital, 1977).

- Property of materials (resistive, pliable, controlled, or messy) and sensory input provided (tactile, auditory, olfactory, visual, proprioceptive, vestibular, gustatory)
- Complexity of the activity—number of steps and repetition required
- Preparation—arrangement of supplies, adaptation of environment
- Amount and type of directions—oral or written, diagrams, demonstration
- Inherent structure and control (rules)
- Predictability of results—success experience
- Type of learning—old learning, adapted old learning, or new learning
- Decision making
- Attention span—minutes, hours, days
- Interaction—solitary; parallel; with peers, small group, large group; cooperation, sharing
- Communication—nonverbal, amount, oral directions, reading, writing
- Motivation—creative, gratifying, intellectually challenging, effect on others, relevance to life space and roles
- Time—completion of activity in one or many sessions, quick success, delayed gratification

Additional therapeutic considerations include special populations as delineated by Hopkins & Tiffany (1988). In working with children, a combination of psychosocial, psychodynamic, physical, and developmental factors must be considered. The activities may be required to provide specific aspects relating to normal growth and development and must be age-appropriate in complexity and dexterity required yet may need to provide some aspects that promote physical function and psychological well-being.

Prevocational activities are selected on the basis of their ability to contribute to work-related skills. They must be selected for their relation to the components of the actual work requirements, including physical performance, coordination, concentration, speed, accuracy, endurance, routinization and boredom factors, initiative, and decision making.

For people with sensory integrative problems (cognitive-perceptual-motor dysfunction), the sensory stimuli presented by the activity must be analyzed along with the "intersensory-integrative mechanisms involved and the motor response required" (Llorens, 1973, p. 453). Thus, tactile, kinesthetic, visual, auditory, and olfactory sensations must be analyzed for each activity along with the type of response required (motor, visual, and verbal). Activity analysis in this area requires analysis of the neurologic integration of the input from the senses and the muscular response to this stimulation and integration, and it is therefore called the *neurobehavioral approach* to activity analysis. Activities must be analyzed with all the components in mind to choose the one most appropriate to meet all therapeutic requirements (Llorens, 1973).

In selecting an activity to be used in the therapeutic process, the therapist must answer five basic questions (Hopkins & Tiffany, 1988):

1. *How* is the activity done? The therapist must know the components of the activity, the process involved, and the tools, equipment, and supplies needed. The therapist must know how to do the activity well enough to be able to teach it.
2. *What* activity is most appropriate for the requirements of the situation? The therapist must assess the problems involved—the needs, interests, preferences, and roles of the client—and, with the client, determine the activity that best meets the requirements for therapeutic intervention.
3. *Why* was a specific activity chosen? The therapist must be able to determine the reason for the choice of activity on the basis of a frame or reference that is consistent with the overall treatment rationale.
4. *Where* will the activity be performed? The therapist may be constrained in the choice of an activity by the location or situation within which the activity will be carried out. For example, if the activity is to be done by a person in bed, it cannot be too messy or require large tools or equipment.
5. *When* will the activity be carried out? The time of day or season of the year may influence the type of activity that is relevant. For example, self-care activities are most logically carried out at the time of day when they are usually done, such as bathing and dressing before breakfast. Relevance may be dictated by the time of year, for example, making decorations or presents for a birthday or holiday.

Tool use

Competence in handling tools is critical in accomplishing many activities. Human evolution has revealed anatomic perfection of the hand and enlargement of the brain, which allows refined manipulation and skilled tool use. Tools can be considered as extensions or aids to the hand that amplify human actions. Clients may find they are enabled to accomplish their required life tasks by using tools or adaptive equipment. For instance, a buttonhook can aid in dressing, and a reacher can provide independence in a variety of settings. In addition, tools can assist in restorative treatment: sawing with a cross-cut saw provides resistance and strengthens upper-extremity muscles; setting a screw with a screwdriver provides movement in supination and pronation. It is imperative that the occupational therapist become familiar and comfortable with tools and know the correct way to use each tool as well as how to select the right tool for the specific task. With this knowledge, the occupational therapist is equipped to teach the patient necessary skills. The therapist cannot serve the patient's needs if he or she cannot demonstrate proper use of tools when teaching skills.

The therapeutic teaching and learning process

The ***therapeutic teaching and learning process*** is a series of cues and responses. Both the therapist and the client learn from one another. The occupational therapist carefully determines the client's learning style. Can the client handle more than one or two simple directions at a time? Does the client respond better to verbal or visual cues? Is the client easily distracted by the surroundings? Does the client require many prompts and assistance? How much time does the client needed to accomplish the task or units of the task? Can the client learn in a group or does he or she need one-to-one instruction? What are the client's work habits? Creativity? Initiative? At the same time, the client may devise an innovative yet logical way to approach the task that the therapist can capitalize on for collaborative success.

The client can learn by hands-on demonstration, by observing and imitating, through pictures and diagrams, as well as from verbal instructions. The occupational therapist chooses the mode of transmitting information that allows the client to clearly understand the instructions, minimizes the amount of supervision and instruction, and optimizes opportunities for a successful outcome. The therapist determines the complexity of the activity to be certain it is within the ability of the client (see Figure 9-2). Special adaptations may be necessary for specific patient dysfunctions. Some patients, such as the visually impaired, learning disabled, or autistic, benefit from consistent surroundings and sequences, with each tool in its expected place and sessions following a familiar format. Some patients may require additional sensory stimulation with tactile or proprioceptive input to sharpen their body schema in preparation for movement. Cognitive abilities may require simplification of directions that are short, simple, clear, and concrete. Special tools or adaptations may be beneficial to assist with physical limitations. The occupational therapist must be careful about setting up contrived methods of performing the activity, however, because this diminishes the value of the selected activity in an adult patient and usually does not work at all with a child. Contrived methods require both the therapist and the patient to constantly focus attention directly on the movement rather than on the end result of the activity. This diminishes satisfaction and enjoyment and may well interfere with developing coordinated, smooth, voluntary motion. The best activity is one that intrinsically demands the exact movement that the client needs to improve.

Bruner (1966) focuses on intrinsic, not extrinsic, rewards in learning. The intrinsic motives include curiosity, desire to achieve competence, aspiration to emulate a model, and reciprocity with others toward an objective. In occupational therapy, the doing becomes the reward. Bruner's rules for learning activities suggest that (1) activity needs sustained sequence, is habitual, and is routine; (2) an activity needs a beginning and an end that allows a determination of success; (3) an activity needs to be approved for age, class, and gender and to require skill a little beyond that presently possessed; (4) a teacher is required who is a working model to *interact* with the learner; and (5) situations have demand value in that one behaves in specific ways in church, at a baseball game, or in the supermarket.

To teach an activity, the occupational therapist must first analyze the component parts of the activity as well as the processes and steps to complete the task. This breaks down the activity into units and can justify amounts to be accomplished during each treatment session. The work area, tools, and supplies need to be prepared, and the occupational therapist should allow sufficient time for these preparation activities. The following are the four basic steps involved in the instruction of the client (Hopkins & Tiffany, 1988, p. 100):

Step 1: Preparation of the Client

- Establish rapport with the client to allay fear and encourage participation.
- Find out how much the client knows about the activity so that instruction may be geared accordingly.
- Involve the client in the activity to ensure interest in it. Be sure the client understands the purpose and value of performance of the activity.
- Place the client in a comfortable and correct position for performance of the activity. When demonstrating, work at the side of the client so that the process may easily be seen. In most cases, do *not* work opposite the client because this may create a reverse mental image. When teaching a client who has hand dominance opposite that of the therapist, however, it may be appropriate to instruct while sitting opposite the client. Better yet, it may be advisable for the therapist to demonstrate using the hand dominance of the client.

Step 2: Presentation of the Activity

- Give oral directions and demonstrate the process. Written directions and diagrams may be helpful, depending on the complexity of the activity and the learning ability and preferences of the client.
- Present the instruction slowly and patiently. Allow for lag time in the client's understanding since this is likely to be new or confusing information.
- Teach the process step by step, stressing key points.
- Teach no more than can be mastered at one time.

Step 3: Try-out Performance

- The client should perform the activity either step by step with the therapist or immediately after being shown.
- Correct errors as they occur. If possible, they should have been anticipated so they can be avoided.
- Have the client explain the process.
- Have the client repeat the activity several times to be sure he or she can perform it correctly.

Step 4: Follow-up

- Put the client on his or her own to work independently.
- Designate a person who can help if difficulties arise.
- Check progress frequently to correct errors and to ensure success in performance. Less frequent checks are sufficient as competence increases.

More than ever before, occupational therapists treat patients who are in acute rather than medically stable conditions. Therapeutic intervention may take place in special care units where many precautions must be observed. The occupational therapist in an acute care setting must put life-threatening issues first and restoration of function second (Dutton, 1989). Activities and learning for patients in this setting need to be adjusted for their vital capacity, medical status, pain, fear, sensory deprivation, medication, memory, and communication capabilities. Small increments of time, perhaps only 5 or 10 minutes, may be available to attend to a specific task. Even this may be interrupted by coughing, nausea, or medical procedures. Selection and teaching of tasks may need to be revised with regard to materials used, focus of activity, time allotted, and expectations to avoid frustration and further debilitation. Knowledgeable use of activity analysis, activity synthesis, and teaching and learning techniques can enhance occupational therapy intervention.

Summary

Activities are the core of the occupational therapy process. The therapeutic value of crafts and other life activities is determined by careful analysis of their intrinsic and extrinsic characteristics in combination with the growth potential those qualities can provide for the client. Active participation by the client in understanding the purpose of, selecting, and engaging in the activity is essential and motivating. The knowledge base of the occupational therapist supports the activity synthesis appropriate for specific patient needs through activity analysis, use of activity for evaluation and treatment, ability to provide suitable instructions, and ability to adapt the activity and the instructions to suit the circumstances.

References

Bing, R. B. (1981). Eleanor Clarke Slagle Lecture—Occupational therapy revisited: A paraphrastic journey. *American Journal of Occupational Therapy, 35,* 499–518.

Bruner, J. (1966). *Toward a theory of instruction.* Cambridge, MA: Belknap Press of Harvard University Press.

Csikszentmihalyi, M. (1975). *Beyond boredom and anxiety: The experience of play in work and games.* San Francisco: Jossey-Bass.

Cynkin, S. (1979). *Occupational therapy: Toward health through activities.* Boston: Little, Brown.

Dutton, R. (1989). Guidelines for using both activity and exercise. *American Journal of Occupational Therapy, 43,* 573–580.

Hopkins, H. L., & Tiffany, E. G. (1988). Occupational therapy—Base in activity. In H. L. Hopkins & H. D. Smith (Eds.), *Willard and Spackman's occupational therapy* (7th ed.) (pp. 93–101). Philadelphia: J. B. Lippincott.

Llorens, L. (1973). Activity analysis for cognitive-perceptual-motor dysfunction. *American Journal of Occupational Therapy, 27,* 453.

Meyer, A. (1922). The philosophy of occupational therapy. *Archives of Occupational Therapy, 1*, 1–10.

Miller, V., & Fox, J. (1988). Creativity: The forgotten link in occupational therapy. In *Occupational therapy: national Perspectives*. Proceedings of the 15th Federal Conference of the Australian Association of Occupational Therapists, August 17–20, 1988, Sydney, Australia.

Mosey, A. C. (1985). *Psychosocial components of occupational therapy*. New York: Raven Press.

Norristown State Hospital (1977). *Activity analysis*. Norristown, PA: Occupational Therapy Department.

Reed, K. L. (1986). 1986 Eleanor Clarke Slagle Lecture—Tools of practice: Heritage or baggage? *American Journal of Occupational Therapy, 40*, 597–605.

Representative Assembly (1979a). Resolution 531–79: Philosophical base of occupational therapy. *American Journal of Occupational Therapy, 33*, 785.

Representative Assembly (1979b). Resolution 532–79. *American Journal of Occupational Therapy, 33*, 785.

Schnebly, M. E., Prendergast, N. D. (Ed.), Pasch, M., & Evans, K. A. (1974). *A curriculum guide for occupational therapy educators*. Rockville, MD: American Occupational Therapy Association.

Swift, R. (1981). Images reflect: Letter to the editor. *American Journal of Occupational Therapy, 35*, 107.

West, W. L. (1984). A reaffirmed philosophy and practice of occupational therapy for the 1980s. *American Journal of Occupational Therapy, 38*, 15–23.

SECTION 4

Problem solving

HELEN L. HOPKINS

KEY TERMS

Assessment of Results   Problem Identification

Implementation of Plan   Solution Development

Plan of Action   Treatment Termination

LEARNING OBJECTIVES

Upon completion of this section the reader will be able to:

1. *Describe the five steps in generic problem solving.*

2. *Identify the sixth step in problem solving that is required in the treatment process.*

3. *Identify the basic ingredients needed for setting long- and short-term goals for treatment.*

The occupational therapy process seeks to help people who are ill or disabled and to provide conditions that will promote their optimal health and functioning. Occupational therapists work within a number of structures to achieve those purposes. In addition to providing treatment, therapists must be prepared to deal with issues such as scheduling, budget, staff supervision, and interdisciplinary relationships. At each level of functioning, the therapist needs to be prepared to carry out measures to effect change, to nurture growth, and to establish systems that will promote and support health. Skill in problem solving is basic to success.

Generic approach to problem solving

A generic approach to problem solving may prove useful to the therapist at all levels: administrative, supervisory, and clinical. This approach consists of five critical steps: problem identification, solution development, development of a plan of action, implementation of the plan, and assessment of the results (May & Newman, 1980). In the initial step, ***problem identification***, an effort is made to identify, specify, and clarify the nature of the problem and to analyze its elements and components. ***Solution development*** involves scrutiny of the information collected in the first step. On the basis of this scrutiny, alternatives are explored, and broad goals and objectives are set. From among the possible alternatives and goals, one choice is made at a time. The problem-solver next undertakes the development of a ***plan of action***, a realistic and sometimes detailed description of the activities that will be used to accomplish the goal selected. In the ***implementation of the plan***, those activities are carried out. The final step listed, ***assessment of results***, is in fact undertaken during, as well as at the end of, implementation. Often a fine-tuning of the plan or a second exploration of alternatives or choice of a different goal may be indicated.

Examples of administrative, supervisory, or interdisciplinary team problems for which the problem-solving steps would prove useful are providing wheelchair accessibility in an old building, enabling a reticent student to overcome difficulty in giving oral reports in staff meetings, and communicating the importance of proper positioning to a teacher of a cerebral palsied child. Many such problems are solved intuitively and smoothly, but occasionally, if one of the five steps is omitted, problems are magnified rather than diminished.

Adapting problem solving to clinical treatment

In the clinical treatment situation, the problem-solving steps become translated into the whole process of intervention. To provide valid and effective treatment for the disabled client, the occupational therapist must address a number of questions: On what basis do I understand this person? How do I conceptualize human personality, human behavior, physical function, and the ways in which human beings learn, grow, and change? How do I understand pathology or the disease process? What about its etiologic factors and its prognosis? What do I know about the external factors that impinge on this person? What about the social and work worlds in which this person must function now and in the future? What do I know about the methods of treatment and frames of reference for treatment being used with this person? How can I best communicate with this person so that we build a mutual understanding of reality that is as clear as possible?

In addressing these questions, the therapist is laying the groundwork for the problem-solving process to follow, a process that can be organized as a series of logical steps that parallel the steps of the generic approach to problem solving: initial assessment, setting treatment objectives, development of a treatment plan, implementation of the plan, and periodic or continual evaluation. A sixth step is added to the treatment process: treatment termination.

The initial assessment step requires collection of data that describe the client objectively. These data should include information about the existing pathology or disability and its effects on the client's life. They should also include information about the client's existing skills and strengths and educational and vocational background. They may include information about the client's personal history, developmental level, social and cultural world, and value systems.

Setting treatment objectives is the step in which reasonable predicted outcomes of the occupational therapy process are explored and named and in which realistic and objectively identifiable long- and short-term goals are stated. When the initial evaluation has been concluded, the therapist should have a clear picture of the client, of the client's assets and limitations, and of realistic expectations for future performance. In the evaluation, certain basic ingredients should have contributed to setting both long- and short-term goals for treatment:

- *The client's needs and goals.* However obliquely they may be communicated, the wishes and needs of the client are there. Unless the goals of treatment are mutually understood by therapist and client on some level, they probably cannot be achieved.
- *The treatment goals, the treatment approach, and the frame of reference for treatment used by the total team.* Coherence between the client's own goals and those of the team is important. The goals of occupational therapy must fit with both.
- *Knowledge of the client's disease process and the possible residual physical or psychological limitations.*
- *Knowledge of the treatment methods and approaches being used.* What medication is the client receiving?
- *Knowledge about the world in which the client is expected to live.* What skills are needed to cope with the demands of life at home, in the community, at work, at play, or in the institution?
- *Knowledge about the client's value system and what is important to the client.*

The therapist analyzes the evaluation data in light of the potential situation for occupational therapy. What does the therapist know about the prognosis for recovery or maintenance of function for people having a specific disease? Who are the other members of the treatment team, and what is the potential for collaborative efforts among them? Can the therapist expect professional and community support for efforts made in occupational therapy setting? To what extent will it be possible to manipulate objects and the environment to provide the best opportunities for the patient to grow and function to maximal capabilities? In what ways can we measure the success of the plan? These are hard but vital questions that must be faced in setting objectives and planning treatment.

Long-term objectives in occupational therapy usually represent a part of the long-term treatment objectives of the team. A long-term objective may be stated as follows: The patient will be able to function well enough to go back to his job. A long-term objective related to this in occupational therapy might be stated as follows: The patient will be able to organize his thoughts and actions to carry out a task from beginning to end. Short-term objectives contribute to the achievement of long-term objectives. A short-term objective related to the above example might be stated: The patient will be able to maintain attention to a given task for 15 minutes. Short-term objectives, then, represent the steps of achievement that will facilitate the attainment of the long-term objective.

Depending on the treatment situation and the pathology of the client, there may be either multiple or single sets of objectives. The results of the evaluation may also indicate that occupational therapy is not needed or relevant for a client at a given time. If attainable treatment objectives for occupational therapy cannot be determined, it is probably not appropriate for the client to be referred to occupational therapy.

It is on the basis of selected objectives that a treatment plan is developed. A description of the methods to be used to meet the treatment objectives constitutes the treatment plan. Just as the objectives represent an action-oriented summary of the client's evaluation, the plan represents a synthesis of the therapist's knowledge of the potential of activities and relationships as facilitators of growth and performance. It is a nuts-and-bolts statement of such things as the tools, materials, and equipment; the kinds of direction or guidance; the structure of the activity; the times and places in which the activity will take place; whether treatment will be accomplished individually or in a group; and the extent to which the family or the community is to be involved. A treatment plan is first stated in reference to each short-term objective, and it needs to be flexible enough to permit changes if reevaluation suggests that the plan is not working.

It is probably in the development of a treatment plan that the therapist is most often faced with the responsibility for sound professional judgment. The plan needs to be reasonable and possible, and should show a clear relation to the objectives of treatment.

The implementation of the treatment plan connects action and the performance of activities with the goals of treatment and acts on the implicit contract that has been developed between the therapist and the client. Implementation consists of three distinct phases: (1) the orientation phase, when the therapist and client define the parameters and expectations of the activities that will be used and when the therapist may describe or demonstrate the procedures that are involved; (2) the development phase, during which the therapist guides the client through exploration or practice in doing the activities; and (3) the termination phase, when the client has completed the plan, reevaluation takes place, and the need for setting further objectives is considered.

During the development phase, there should be continual evaluation to check the effectiveness of the plan and the relevance of the objectives. At this time, it is likely that new objectives and new treatment plans will evolve. Indeed, periodic or continual evaluation is essential in all three phases of treatment to assess the validity of the objectives and the efficacy of the treatment plan and process, to identify the need for changes in approach, and to determine when treatment can be terminated.

It is most satisfying when **treatment termination** takes place with a final assessment and clear indications for the future performance of the client. Termination can be an affirmation of the success of the plan and the process. For this reason, termination is a critical step in the occupational therapy process and deserves thoughtful planning. In reality, the termination phase is not always achieved. Clients may be discharged before objectives are met. In some situations, particularly with chronically ill patients, the treatment goal is maintenance of function, and therefore, short-term objectives are so numerous that the occupational therapy process may continue for a long time.

The use of the problem-solving process in occupational therapy requires creativity and imagination on the part of the therapist. The therapist must use knowledge, skills, and good professional judgment to find the best possible solution for each client (Marshall, 1965; Parnes, 1967).

It is important for the client to be involved in the process of problem identification so that the assets as well as liabilities of the situation may be determined. The goals established, the alternative chosen, and the plan of action must reflect what is desired by and acceptable to the client. To be successful, moreover, the plan of action and the approach must be compatible with those of other professionals working with the client. The values and lifestyle of the client's family should also be taken into consideration.

Each plan of action must be examined for its probable value and the potential outcomes of treatment or intervention. If the plan appears feasible, and if it offers a promising solution, it can be implemented. Short-term goals with manageable elements contribute to the achievement of long-term goals. The therapist needs to be clear about the relation between the long-term and short-term goals and their sequencing. There must be periodic reevaluation to determine progress—what goals have been reached and what problems have been solved. It may be necessary to make modifications or to adapt goals and plans as changes occur. There are occasions when abandonment of an unsuccessful plan is necessary, requiring a determination of another course of action. As new knowledge develops and as new viewpoints evolve, new alternatives arise that provide different approaches for intervention in occupational therapy.

Approaches to intervention

The selection of the issues and data that will be given attention in the problem-solving process and the choices among treatment plan alternatives are determined by the frame of reference within which the therapist is working. In occupational therapy today, there are several alternative approaches to intervention that may be chosen, depending on the therapist's orientation and rationale for treatment. Each approach has a specific knowledge base, each is built on stated concepts, and each uses a rationale that constrains the occupational therapy program by specifying the type of appropriate activities (see Chapter 4). These approaches overlap in some areas. Their importance lies in the fact that they provide the therapist with specific guidelines within which to apply knowledge and skills. The experience, values, sociocultural assumptions, points of view, and concept of reality inherent in an agency's philosophy promote the choice of a

specific frame of reference (Conte & Conte, 1977). For example, within the developmental approach, one occupational therapist, a group of therapists, or an agency may favor a neurodevelopmental perspective for treatment of children with cerebral palsy and may use the Bobath frame of reference, whereas others may favor a neurophysiologic perspective and may use a Rood frame of reference. Some agencies use more than one approach to intervention, depending on the type of client as well as on the preferences, biases, and expertise of the therapists. This increases the number and variety of frames of reference that may be used. The rationale and basis for choosing an approach and frame of reference, as well as the knowledge base and concepts inherent in that approach, must be understood by the therapist.

The occupational therapy intervention process differs according to the approach and frame of reference chosen, but the overall goals of the process can be described as prevention of conditions causing or resulting in loss of function; remediation, treatment, or rehabilitation for restoration of function and performance; and promotion and maintenance of health and optimal functioning.

Summary

Problem solving consists of five critical steps: problem identification, solution development, development of a plan of action, implementation of the plan, and assessment of results. In adapting generic problem solving to clinical treatment in occupational therapy, a sixth step must be added to the treatment process, that of treatment termination. Problem solving in occupational therapy requires creativity and imagination. It also requires that the therapist use knowledge, skills, and good professional judgment to find the best solution for each client.

The author thanks Elizabeth G. Tiffany for use of portions of her material from the 7th edition of this book.

References

Conte, J. R., & Conte, W. R. (1977). The use of conceptual models in occupational therapy. *American Journal of Occupational Therapy, 31*, 262.

Marshall, E. (1965). A problem solving method of learning, measured against a rote memory method. *American Journal of Occupational Therapy, 19*, 60.

May, B. J., & Newman, J. (1980). Developing competence in problem-solving: A behavioral model. *Physical Therapy, 60*, 1140.

Parnes, S. J. (1967). *Creative behavior guidebook*. New York: Charles Scribner's Sons.

SECTION 5

Therapeutic adaptations

SECTION 5A
Upper-extremity splinting

ELAINE EWING FESS and JUDITH H. KIEL

LEARNING OBJECTIVES

Upon completion of this section the reader will be able to:
1. *Identify the purposes and rational for splinting upper-extremity dysfunction.*
2. *Begin to apply splinting nomenclature and terminology appropriately.*
3. *Begin to define the relation of splinting to the scientific bodies of knowledge of anatomy, physiology, kinesiology, and biomechanics.*
4. *Differentiate between functional position and safe position and give appropriate applications of each.*
5. *Identify the principles of mechanics, design, construction, and fit as they apply to splinting.*
6. *Explain basic methods of splint pattern construction.*
7. *Recognize basic splinting material characteristics and their importance to therapists and patients.*
8. *Relate the effects of splinting and exercise as they are incorporated in treatment programs.*
9. *Explain therapist and patient responsibilities related to splint-wearing schedules, assessment, instructions, compliance, and precautions.*
10. *Recognize the psychological effect of hand disabilities, splinting, and rehabilitation programs.*
11. *Identify therapist management responsibilities regarding written documentation and pricing as they relate to upper-extremity splinting.*

History and philosophy

Although *orthotics*, the use of preventative or corrective appliances (Taber, 1989), has been employed for centuries (Fess, Gettle, & Strickland, 1981, pp. x–xi), upper-extremity splinting as it is now used by occupational therapists has emerged only over the past 30 years (Barr & Swan, 1988; Cannon et al., 1985; Colditz, 1990; Fess et al., 1981; Fess & Philips, 1987; Kiel, 1983; Malick, 1978, 1979; Moberg, 1984; Tenney & Lisak, 1986; Ziegler, 1984). These changes are the result of better understanding of biomechanics (Brand, 1985, 1990; Fess et al., 1981; Fess & Philips, 1987; Flatt, 1983; Malick, 1978) and of physiologic response of soft tissue to stress (Brand, 1985, 1990; Madden & Arem, 1981; Peacock, 1984; Weeks & Wray, 1978) and the development of specialized user-friendly splinting materials. Splinting is one of the most effective tools used in the conservative management of upper-extremity problems, yet it is only one of many techniques at the disposal of therapists involved in rehabilitation of the upper extremities (Hunter, Schneider, Mackin, & Callahan, 1990; Wynn Parry, 1981).

In preparing splints, it is important to begin "with a thorough understanding of the underlying anatomic alterations and realistic therapeutic considerations" (Fess et al., 1981, pp. ix), including pertinent medical, surgical, and rehabilitative factors. Additionally, for successful treatment of hand injuries or diseases, close communication must exist between the physician, therapist, and patient to create an interactive and effective rehabilitation team (Fess et al., 1981; Fess & Philips, 1987; Hunter et al., 1990; Wynn Parry, 1981; Ziegler, 1984).

Because it is both impossible and inappropriate to prescribe a single splint design for a particular diagnosis, occupational therapists create splints by adapting to individual patient variables. This generates a wide variety of splint configurations that are specifically designed to accomplish distinct therapeutic goals. It is therefore critical that therapists "thoroughly understand the exact purpose for the splint being prepared, the necessary mechanics to achieve it, and the available design options" (Fess et al., 1981, pp. xii).

Purpose

Made from a variety of materials, splints are external devices that are applied to treat upper-extremity problems resulting from injury, disease, birth defects, or the aging process. Splints serve one or more of four basic functions. They may be used to support, immobilize, or restrict a body part to allow healing after inflammation or injury to tendon, vascular, nerve, joint, or soft tissue structures. Correcting or preventing deformity is another function performed by splints. To achieve the "full potential of active joint motion of the hand, the remodeling of joint and tendon adhesions often requires the prolonged slow, gentle, passive traction that can best be provided by splinting" (Fess & Philips, 1987, pp. 72). Splints may also be used to artificially provide or assist motion to supple hands (normal passive range of motion) that are incapacitated due to muscle weakness or paralysis. By placing joints in better positions, or through use of assistive splint components, hands are often able to achieve functional motion more effectively. Finally, splints may serve as bases for attachment of self-help devices. Ranging from simple to complex, splints may be prefabricated or custom-designed and fitted.

Classification, nomenclature, and components

Many ways of classifying splints have been used, including external configuration, mechanical characteristics, source of power, materials, and anatomic part, to name a few (Fess et al., 1981; Long & Schutt, 1986; Malick, 1978, 1979). Although each of these methods has advantages and disadvantages, none exhibits the level of sophistication required by those currently involved in modern high-technology splinting endeavors.

Taking a major step toward eliminating confusion and redundancy in existing nomenclature, the American Society of Hand Therapists (1991) recently adopted a ***Splint Classification System*** (SCS). Created by a specially appointed committee of nationally and internationally recognized splinting experts, this system categorizes splints in an organized, logical, and practical manner, replacing more colloquial terminology that often described properties of splints themselves without regard for purpose or intent. Splints in this classification system are *not* categorized according to presence of dynamic or static components.

The SCS defines splints according to a series of four descriptors: anatomic focus, kinematic direction, primary purpose, and inclusion of secondary joints (Figure 9-3). Anatomic focus defines the primary joint(s) or segment(s) affected by the splint (eg, metacarpal phalangeal (MP), interphalangeal (IP), wrist, thumb, finger). Kinematic direction designates which way the primary joint(s) or segment(s) is moved (eg, flexion, extension, rotation). The primary purpose of a splint is described as one of three options: mobilization, immobilization, or restriction. Primary purpose mobilization splints enhance or encourage motion; primary purpose immobilization splints stop motion; and primary purpose restriction splints allow motion only in a partial, predetermined range. The fourth descriptor indicates the number of joints in a longitudinal pattern that are included in the splint but are not considered the primary focus joint(s). These joints are defined as secondary joints. If no secondary joint is included in a splint, it is designated as type 0; one secondary joint is type 1; two secondary joints are type 2, and so forth. The combination of the four descriptors accurately defines a splint without becoming lost in a multitude of specific design options. For example, a "cock-up splint" is considered to be a wrist extension immobilization splint, type 0 and an "MP arthroplasty splint" is categorized as an index through little MP extension–radial deviation splint, type 1.

The SCS enhances communication between medical personnel by defining the important aspects of splints while leaving decisions about design options to those who actually fabricate splints. This allows therapists greater flexibility and use of their knowledge bases.

Although a finished splint presents a unified and solid configuration, it is, in reality, an assemblage of integrated and interdependent components, each with a specific function and name designation (Bradley, 1968; Bradley, Fess, & Kiel, 1972; Fess et al., 1981; Fess & Philips, 1987; Kiel, 1978, 1983). Component terminology is usually based on function of the part or on its anatomic location.

When designing a splint, the therapist decides what the splint is to accomplish and what approach will provide optimal results. Experienced therapists often think in terms of components rather than final splint configurations, mentally putting together selected splint parts to build a splint whose final shape may be familiar or, as is often the case, completely original. Above all, it is important that a creative flexibility be maintained, allowing the therapist to draw from what is available to design and prepare a splint that best suits the needs of a specific hand problem. Understanding splint components, their potential combinations, and their capabilities provides this flexibility.

Evaluation and exercise

Evaluation provides the guidelines for treatment. Splinting and exercise programs cannot be established or carried out without careful assessment and reassessment of extremity volume, range of motion, sensibility,* strength, dexterity, physical daily living skills, and job requirements (see Chapter 18, Section 4 for further details).

Treating patients with upper-extremity problems requires continual evaluation and problem solving. Additionally, splinting must be combined with a carefully supervised exercise program. While splinting increases passive range of motion, active exercise provides critical gliding of musculotendinous units and pericapsular structures.

Fundamental concepts

Anatomy, kinesiology, biomechanics

The occupational therapist must first understand the complex and intricate interrelations of normal anatomic structures, their kinesiologic functions, and their biomechanical and physiologic ramifications before attempting to interpret, define, and treat the abnormalities that accompany upper-extremity problems. Many excellent books and articles are available regarding upper-extremity anatomy, kinesiology, and biomechanics. The reader is encouraged to independently pursue these subjects in greater detail. More harm than good may be accomplished when understanding of normal upper-extremity structure and function is superficial or incomplete. A careful review will provide a solid foundation from which therapeutic intervention may be directed.

---

* Sensibility is the "capacity to receive and respond to stimuli," while sensation is "a feeling or awareness . . . resulting from the stimulation of sensory receptors" (Taber, 1989, p. 525). In testing situations, patients are asked to receive and respond to stimuli, not just to receive.

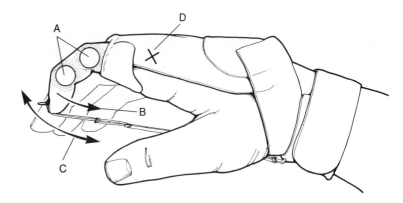

FIGURE 9-3. *Splints are grouped in the following manner: A: anatomic focus (IP joints); B: kinematic direction (flexion); C: primary purpose (mobilization); and D: number of secondary joints (one). According to the SCS, this is an IP flexion mobilization splint, type 1.*

Physiology

Living tissue responds in a predictable manner in its efforts to achieve homeostasis and healing. The normal physiologic response to injury results in an alteration and replacement of normal structures with scar tissue. It is therefore important to understand the **wound healing process** for surgical and therapeutic intervention to be effective (Madden & Arem, 1981; Peacock, 1984; Strickland, 1987). Tissue healing follows a normal sequence that includes inflammation, fibroplasia, scar maturation, and wound contracture. Scar in specialized tissues of the hand, such as tendon, bone, and joint, may lead to severe impairment of function. Scar results not only from accidental injury but also from surgical intervention and improperly applied therapeutic techniques (Brand, 1985; Fess & Philips, 1987; Strickland, 1987). Factors that cause increased scar formation include greater wound size, contamination, additional injury, and persistent edema. Although edema is part of the normal inflammatory response, if it is allowed to persist in the hand with its compact and mobile structures, the result will be marked tissue scarring and fibrosis (Bunnell, 1944; Hunter et al., 1990; Strickland, 1987).

Rest or stress

Scar remodeling is the foundation on which hand therapy treatment is based, and the fundamental question of rest or stress of living tissue is dependent on physiologic timing (Brand, 1985; Strickland, 1987). The inflammatory phase is characterized by transient vasoconstriction followed by vasodilatation of local small blood vessels and migration of white blood cells. Allowing the removal of dead tissue and foreign bodies by phagocytic cells, the acute inflammatory response generally subsides within several days. During this time, the injured part is usually immobilized to promote healing (Figure 9-4). In special instances where control of scar is critical, as with tendon gliding, early motion programs may be initiated (Figure 9-5) (Duran, Coleman, Nappi, & Klerekoper 1990; Kleinert, Kutz, & Cohen 1975; Evans, 1990).

Fibroplasia begins on the fourth or fifth day and continues for 2 to 4 weeks. This stage involves the synthesis of scar tissue by fibroblasts. As collagen fibers increase, the tensile strength (resistance to rupture) of the wound increases. During this stage, active motion may be initiated, and splints may be used to protect healing structures or to control unbalanced forces of uninjured musculature (Figure 9-6).

Changes in the architecture of the collagen fibers occurs during the scar maturation phase. Collagen becomes more orga-

nized, and tensile strength continues to increase (Madden & Arem, 1981). Carefully graded resistive activities may be added to existing active motion exercises, and gentle corrective splinting may be initiated (Figure 9-7).

As wounds age their edges contract and the area of scar becomes smaller. Remodeling of scar is a normal process that continues throughout life. Although a scar may not totally disappear, the deposition of new collagen and resorption of old collagen is a constant, ongoing process within the scarred area as well as in normal uninjured tissue. This remodeling process may be altered even in longstanding soft tissue contractures. Application of prolonged gentle traction is the key to influencing the remodeling process, and this is best done through a carefully supervised splinting program (Brand, 1985, 1990; Fess & Philips, 1987).

Timing for splinting programs must take into consideration all the above information while treating specific abnormalities on an individualized basis. Although diagnoses may be similar, no two patients respond in exactly the same manner to injury and subsequent therapeutic intervention.

Splints may be used to immobilize healing tissues, or they may permit controlled motion to influence adhesion formation

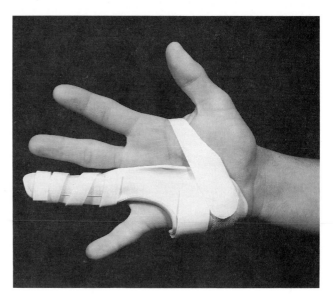

FIGURE 9-4. *To promote healing, this ring-finger immobilization splint, type 0, stops motion at all three joints. (From* Hand splinting: Principles and methods *[2nd ed.] by E. E. Fess and C. A. Philips, 1987, St. Louis: C. V. Mosby.)*

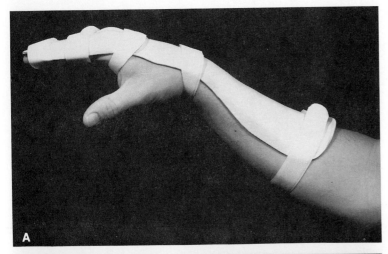

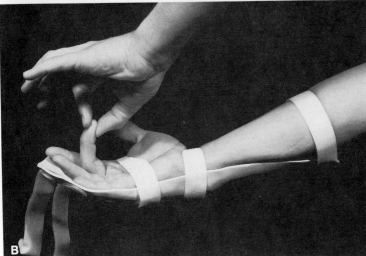

FIGURE 9-5. *Early passive motion of repaired superficialis and profundus tendons of the long finger is permitted in this wrist–finger immobilization splint, type 0.* (*From* Hand splinting: Principles and methods [*2nd ed.*] *by E. E. Fess and C. A. Philips, 1987, St. Louis: C. V. Mosby.*)

and enhance tensile strength of repaired structures. They may be used to correct existing joint deformity by providing constant gentle tension to remodel existent contracted, adherent, or scarred soft tissue structures. In the presence of supple joints and good tendon glide, splints may be used to maintain normal joint motion, and when muscle function is impaired, they may substitute for weak or absent muscle function. The timing is different for each of the above situations. It is therefore imperative that the physiologic implications be thoroughly understood before embarking on a method of treatment. Too much force applied to

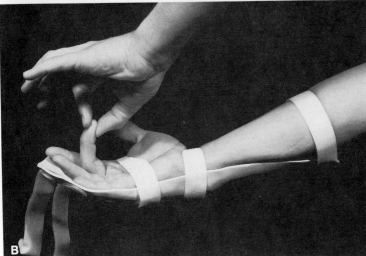

FIGURE 9-6. *Full PIP flexion is allowed, but extension beyond 25 degrees is blocked in this PIP extension restriction splint, type 0.*

healing tissue causes tearing and rupture, while too little force directed to stiffened joints or adherent soft tissue structures may result in little to no alteration of offending scar (Brand, 1985, 1990; Fess & Philips, 1987; Strickland, 1987).

Position of deformity

The presence of dorsal edema encourages a predictable ***position of deformity*** with the wrist flexed, MPs in hyperextension, IPs in flexion, and the thumb adducted (Figure 9-8) (Bunnell, 1944; Flatt, 1983; Strickland, 1987; Weeks & Wray, 1978). Acting as a biologic "glue," the protein-rich edema fluid fills the interstices[†] of the collateral ligaments and the soft tissues surrounding tendons and joints. Injured tissues, those immediately adjacent to the injury, and those in general proximity may all become involved as the fluid is replaced by collagen, forming scar and limiting both active and passive motion (Bunnell, 1944). Maintaining collateral ligament length by means of antideformity positioning is a fundamental concept to effective hand rehabilitation (Flatt, 1983; Hunter et al., 1990; Strickland, 1987; Weeks & Wray, 1978). It is important to understand the anatomy of each

[†] "A space that intervenes between one thing and another: a space between things" (Webster, 1981, p. 1183).

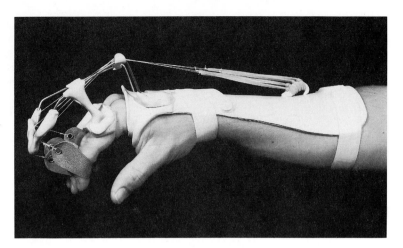

FIGURE 9-7. *Gentle tension is applied to remodel extrinsic flexor tendon adhesions and tight PIP pericapsular structures in this PIP extension mobilization splint, type 2. (From Hand splinting: Principles and methods [2nd ed.] by E. E. Fess and C. A. Philips, 1987, St. Louis: C. V. Mosby.)*

joint and the involvement of surrounding structures because the splinting position of choice differs significantly between the MP and IP joints.

Wrist position is the key to the posture of more distal digital joints (Flatt, 1983). Injury often results in adoption of a protective posture of wrist flexion. Additionally, the presence of dorsal edema places distention pressure on the extrinsic extensor tendons. This edema, coupled with a posture of wrist flexion, pulls the MP joints into extension or hyperextension, which in turn causes the IP joints to flex in a compensatory manner (Strickland, 1987). This zigzag collapse of the **longitudinal arch** is both predictable and preventable and may be averted by eliminating the instigating posture of wrist flexion. Providing there are no extenuating circumstances that would be contraindicated, the antideformity position for the wrist is neutral or dorsal extension.

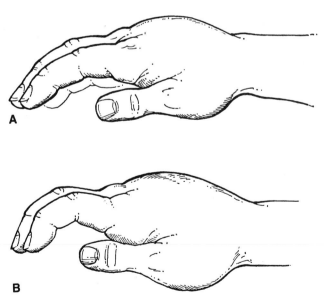

FIGURE 9-8. *In the position of deformity, ligamental shortening from uncontrolled edema and incorrect immobilization positioning prevents passive and active MP flexion and PIP extension of the fingers as well as abduction and extension of the thumb CMC joint. (A) Early stages of edema. (B) Later stage with increased deformity.*

Because of the cam configuration of the metacarpal head, the collateral ligaments are lax with the MP joint in extension (Bunnell, 1944; Flatt, 1983; Strickland, 1987). Injury or chronic edema around the joint can result in deposition of new collagen around the slackened ligaments, allowing them to shorten. Flexion is limited according to the degree of ligament shortening (Figure 9-9).

The IP joints are hinge articulations permitting motion in only one plane. Often the result of poor positioning after injury, IP flexion contractures usually involve shortening of the palmar plate and collateral ligaments (Strickland, 1987). Additionally, adhesion of the palmar skin, flexor tendons, or flexor tendon sheaths may be associated.

Functionally devastating, thumb web space contractures may involve skin, fascia, or musculature of the first web space (Flatt, 1983; Strickland, 1987; Weeks & Wray, 1978). Resulting from direct injury, ischemia, or chronic edema, secondary stiffening of the carpal metacarpal (CMC) joint may occur. Distention pressure on the extensor pollicis longus from dorsal edema also contributes to a posture of thumb adduction.

Functional position versus safe position

For many decades, the **functional position** (wrist, 20- to 30-degrees extension; MPs 45-degrees flexion; proximal interphalangeal (PIPs), 30-degrees flexion; distal interphalangeal (DIPs), 20-degrees flexion; and thumb abducted) for the hand was considered the posture of choice in hand splinting (Figure 9-10) (Bunnell, 1944; Malick, 1979; Wynn Parry, 1981). When an entire hand required immobilization, it was placed in a functional position unless special circumstances dictated otherwise. In the 1960s, hand specialists began to reevaluate this traditional approach, initially with specific diagnoses such as burns (Evans, Larson, & Yates, 1968; Koepke, Feallock, & Felle, 1963; Von Prince & Yeakel, 1974). This led to better understanding of the anatomic configuration of the joints of the hand and of the role that collateral ligaments play in producing a predictable pattern of deformity. "The position desired is not necessarily a functional position, but rather one which will prevent the deformity caused by contracture" (Von Prince & Yeakel, 1974, p. 30). As a result, a **safe position** was developed that maintained collateral ligament length, considerably diminishing chances of development of MP extension, IP flexion, and thumb CMC adduction contrac-

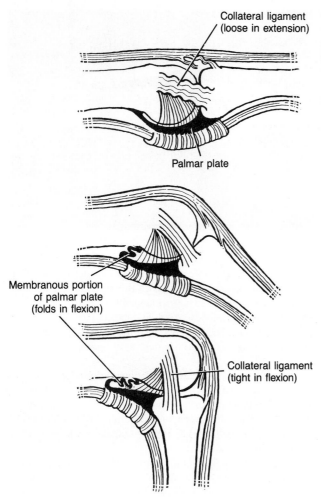

FIGURE 9-9. *A slight palmar projection (cam) of the metacarpal head causes inconsistent tension on the collateral ligaments as the proximal phalanx moves from extension (slack) to flexion (tight). (Modified from Hand splinting: Principles and methods [2nd ed.] by E. E. Fess and C. A. Philips, 1987, St. Louis: C. V. Mosby.)*

tures with immobilization. It is now thought that this antideformity position should be used as a preventive measure whenever a hand that has a tendency to develop stiffness requires immobilization for a period of time. This, of course, excludes instances when other postures are prescribed to promote healing of specialized tissues, as with flexor tendon repairs or fractures, or when functional needs dictate alternate measures, as with the development of a tenodesis hand.

In light of better knowledge, the functional position now may be viewed as that hand posture from which function is most easily initiated. To attain a functional position, soft tissue length, especially that of the collateral ligaments of the small joints of the hand, must be present. Maintenance of collateral ligament length requires that the wrist be positioned in neutral to slight extension, the MPs flexed 70 to 90 degrees, the IPs held in full extension, and the thumb CMC joint positioned in full abduction or extension, otherwise known as the safe position (Figure 9-11).

Mobilizing splints: how much force

Splinting, the method of choice for increasing passive range of motion, provides prolonged gentle stress that positively influences collagen remodeling and tissue growth. Too much force too quickly causes microscopic tearing of tissue, and the cycle of scar production begins anew (Brand, 1985, 1990; Fess & Philips, 1987; Strickland, 1987). *Stretch* is a temporary elongation of tissue that is not sustained for a sufficient length of time to promote collagen remodeling (Brand, 1985). Forceful passive stretch increases scar formation by disrupting tissue and reinitiating the inflammatory response and collagen synthesis.

As with other therapeutic techniques, splinting forces must be carefully controlled or they too may be of sufficient magnitude to cause harm. Force applied to prevent contracture should be just enough to properly position the involved segment. Because the hand is already supple, measurement of the force used is not necessary so long as care is taken not to overcorrect by applying more force than is required to place the hand in the desired position (Figure 9-12) (Fess & Philips, 1987). Forces used to correct joint deformity must be carefully monitored. Depending on structures involved and physiologic timing, experienced therapists use forces between 100 and 300 grams (Brand, 1978, 1985; Fess et al., 1981; Fess, 1984; Fess & Philips, 1987; Malick, 1978; Pearson, 1978). Caution must be exercised when using commercial splints because studies (Fess, 1988; Bledsoe, 1991) have shown that certain designs create forces that greatly exceed safe parameters (Figure 9-13).

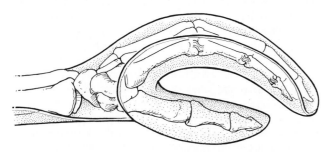

FIGURE 9-10. *With the MPs in 45 degrees of flexion and the IPs in 20 to 30 degrees of flexion, in the traditional functional position the collateral ligaments are lax.*

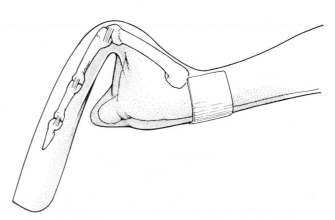

FIGURE 9-11. *In the safe position, with MPs flexed 70 to 90 degrees and IPs in extension, the collateral ligaments are at maximal length.*

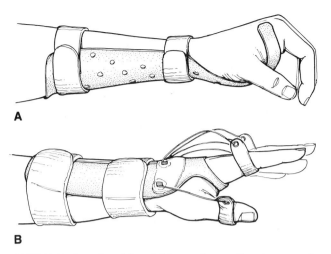

FIGURE 9-12. *In a hand in which passive motion is normal but active motion is limited, as with a radial nerve palsy, splints may be used to position the wrist (A), or to position the wrist and MP joints (B).*

Elastic or inelastic traction

Traditionally, elastic traction has been the method of choice for splinting directed at correction of joint deformity. In addition to rubber bands and elastic thread, springs are now available in differing strengths (Roberson, Breger, Buford, & Freeman, 1988).

As a result of the work of Brand (1952) and Bell (1987, 1990), the value of inelastic traction for correcting joint deformity is better understood. Minimal force applied by a series of splints that are refitted every 2 to 3 days has been shown to be an effective method for increasing passive motion of stiffened joints, especially those of a chronic nature (Figure 9-14).

Principles of splinting

The use of splints in rehabilitation programs is a serious undertaking and should not be regarded lightly. When employed appropriately, splinting is very effective; however, misuse of a

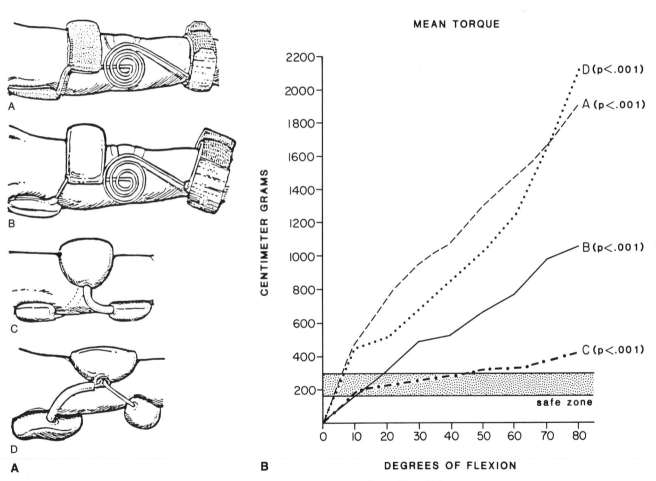

FIGURE 9-13. *Four commercial spring and spring-wire PIP joint extension splints (A) were tested to determine how much force (B, vertical axis) they exerted on the PIP joint with progressively increasing degrees of joint flexion (B, horizontal axis). All four splints applied far too much corrective force, exceeding the recommended force magnitude of 100 to 300 g (B, safe zone) by as much as 2000 g. Note that torque magnitude increases as the amount of joint flexion increases. (From Fess, E. E. [1988]. Force magnitude of commercial spring-coil and spring-wire splints designed to extend the proximal interphalangeal joint. Journal of Hand Therapy 2:1.)*

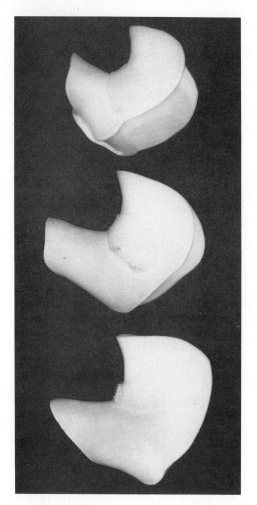

FIGURE 9-14. *These thumb CMC abduction mobilization splints, type 0, demonstrate how increased passive range of motion of a joint, in this case the CMC joint, may be achieved through progressive serial splinting.* (From **Hand splinting: Principles and methods** [*2nd ed.*] *by E. E. Fess and C. A. Philips, 1987, St. Louis: C. V. Mosby.*)

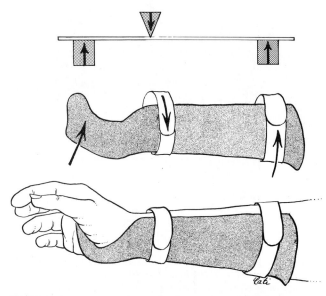

FIGURE 9-15. *Arrows indicate the three points of pressure applied by this wrist immobilization splint, type 0.* (From **Basic hand splinting: A pattern designing approach** *by J. H. Kiel, 1983, Boston: Little, Brown.*)

splint through ignorance or haste can lead to dire consequences, resulting in needless additional injury to an already debilitated extremity. To provide a splint that meets individual patient requirements, fits comfortably, and functions efficiently, certain basic criteria must be achieved. These criteria are relevant to the creation of all splints regardless of intent of application, final configuration, or material from which they are constructed. Integration of the principles of mechanics, design, construction, and fit will generate splints that are appropriate, wearable, and functional.

Mechanical principles

Because splinting involves direct application and manipulation of external forces to the extremity, it is important to understand basic ***principles of mechanics*** (Brand, 1978, 1985; Fess et al., 1981; Fess & Philips, 1987; Malick, 1978). Use of mechanical principles helps make splints comfortable, durable, and effective

and diminishes chances of additional injury secondary to splint application.

Mechanically, splints may be grouped into two categories: those that apply three-point pressure (Brand, 1985, 1990; Fess et al., 1981; Fess & Philips, 1987; Malick, 1978), and those that pull adjacent articulated bony segments together through circumferential pressure (P. Van Lede, personal communication, February 1991). Most splints employ three-point pressure; however, a few frequently used splints fall into the circumferential-pressure category. Three-point–pressure splints function through a series of reciprocal forces, with the middle force directed opposite to the two end forces (Figure 9-15). In the circumferential-pressure splint, the middle reciprocal force is absent (Figure 9-16). Those engaged in designing and fitting splints must understand the fundamental differences between these two types of splints to use them correctly and to anticipate potential problems arising from their application. For example, pressure necrosis is most likely to occur at the point of application of the middle reciprocal force in a three-point–pressure splint (Figure 9-17); whereas the forces in a circumferential splint are equally dissipated over two or more opposing surfaces. The latter are more apt to precipitate edema problems due to their inherent circumferential design.

Pressure and ***shear***[‡] may be reduced by increasing the surface area of the splint and by ensuring ***contiguous fit*** on the extremity. Short, narrow splints or components are often problematic because they apply forces to a small area, creating pressure necrosis of underlying soft tissue. Longer splint designs increase mechanical advantage and make splints less susceptible to causing pressure problems (Figure 9-18). Rolling or flanging splint edges, especially those at the proximal or distal ends, also

‡ "A strain resulting from applied forces that cause or tend to cause contiguous parts of a body to slide relative to each other in a direction parallel to their plane of contact" (Webster, 1981, p. 2090).

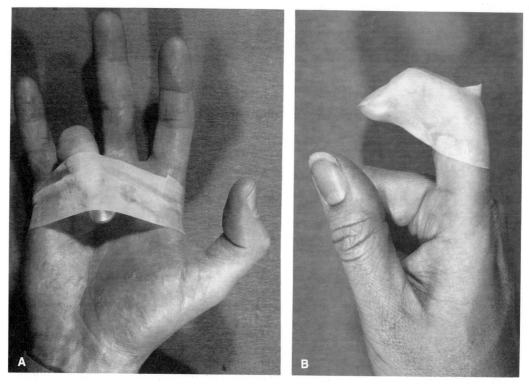

FIGURE 9-16. *The finger flexion mobilization splint, type 0* (A) *and IP flexion mobilization splint, type 0* (B) *are examples of circumferential pressure splints. The middle reciprocal force is absent in both splints.* (*From* Hand splinting: Principles and methods [*2nd ed.*] *by E. E. Fess and C. A. Philips, 1987, St. Louis: C. V. Mosby.*)

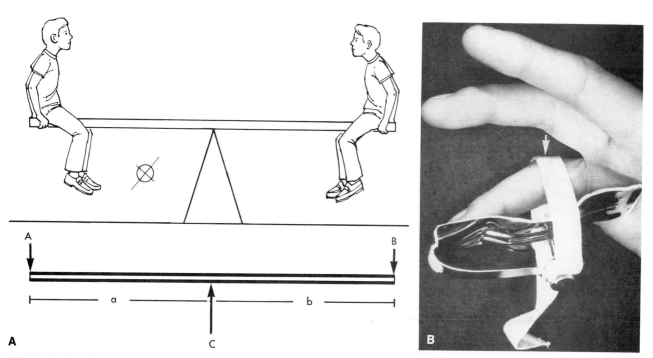

FIGURE 9-17. (A) *Pressure is greatest at the point of the middle reciprocal force in a splint, just as it is in this scale drawing. The combined proximal* (A) *and distal* (B) *forces equal the middle force* (C): A + B = C. (B) *For this splint, the greatest amount of pressure occurs on the dorsal aspect of the PIP joint* (arrow), *the point of application of the middle reciprocal force.* (*From* Hand splinting: Principles and methods [*2nd ed.*] *by E. E. Fess and C. A. Philips, 1987, St. Louis: C. V. Mosby.*)

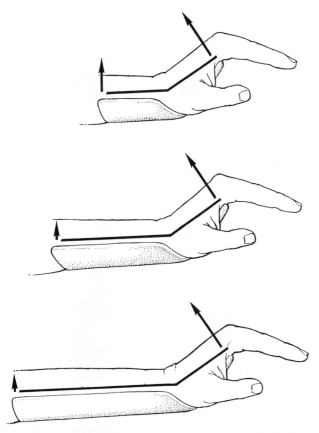

FIGURE 9-18. *The amount of proximal force required to support the weight of the hand in a splint is diminished by increasing the length of the forearm bar.* (*From* Hand splinting: Principles and methods [*2nd ed.*] *by E. E. Fess and C. A. Philips, 1987, St. Louis: C. V. Mosby.*)

diminishes shear and pressure forces (Figure 9-19). Additionally, dangerous shear forces may be diminished by attaching the splint snug to the extremity and by aligning articulated splint components with their respective anatomic joint axes, eliminating friction between splint and soft tissue surface as the extremity is moved. Splint strength and durability is also enhanced through the use of wider and longer components and through providing material contour.

Understanding the effects of proximal or distal joints within the longitudinal ray is another critical concept. Corrective forces

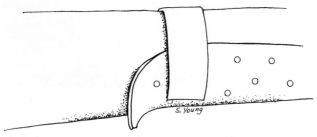

FIGURE 9-19. *To reduce pressure, it is often helpful to flange splint edges.* (*From* Basic hand splinting: A pattern designing approach by J. H. Kiel, 1983, Boston: Little, Brown.*)

may be abated or rendered ineffective if normal or relatively less stiff joints are not controlled when fabricating splints to mobilize stiff joints (Figure 9-20).

When splints are used to effect joint motion, a ***90-degree angle of approach*** of the mobilizing force must be used to avoid compression or distraction of articular surfaces (Figure 9-21). If the splint has been fitted to increase motion of a stiffened joint, a 90-degree angle of approach must be maintained as the joint motion changes through adjustments to the outrigger length. This mobilizing force must also be perpendicular to the joint axis of rotation (Figure 9-22). Additionally, components that provide immobilizing or stabilizing forces, such as straps or dorsal phalangeal bars, should have a 90-degree angle of approach to the joint or segment being immobilized or stabilized.

Design principles

Principles of design may be divided into two categories: general and specific (Fess et al., 1981; Fess & Philips, 1987). General principles incorporate broad concepts that help generate a splint that is practical for both the patient and the therapist, while more specific principles focus the splint design on individual patient requirements.

Patient factors, such as age, intelligence, motivation, body size, activity level, socioeconomic status, and proximity to the clinic, must be considered in addition to how long the splint will be used and the exercise program that will be incorporated. Splints should be as simple as possible, allowing optimal function and sensation of the extremity. Generally, they also should provide ease of application and removal. For children or for patients who cannot or will not accept responsibility for their treatment, however, splints may need to be designed to discourage voluntary removal. Acknowledging that splints are inherently strange-looking devices at best, care should be taken to make them aesthetically pleasing through attention to detail and neatness. The design should also allow efficient construction and fit, thereby controlling time and economic factors. These general principles are taken into consideration by the therapist during the early stages of design. They are approached not in lock-step, 1-2-3 fashion but rather as a simultaneous mental balancing of multiple factors.

Specific principles of design provide substance and detail to the emerging splint configuration. Decisions made at this point are based on specific personal, technical, and medical considerations, leading to substantially different splint configurations for seemingly similar diagnoses or therapeutic needs. Key primary joints are identified, and the purpose of the splint is reviewed. It should be determined whether the splint is intended to immobilize structures, partially restrict motion, increase passive motion, substitute for active motion, or serve as a base for attachment of self-help devices. The surface of the extremity on which the splint will be based is determined, and secondary joints that need to be controlled or positioned are noted. Areas of diminished sensibility are identified, as are anatomic variations, soft tissue defects, suture lines, and the presence of external or internal hardware, such as pins, plates, and screws, or external fixators. Because application of a splint often alters internal and external forces to proximal or distal joints, the kinetic effects of the splint must also be considered, including what will be the forces on unsplinted joints and what will be the ramifications to extrinsic and intrinsic musculotendinous structures (Fig-

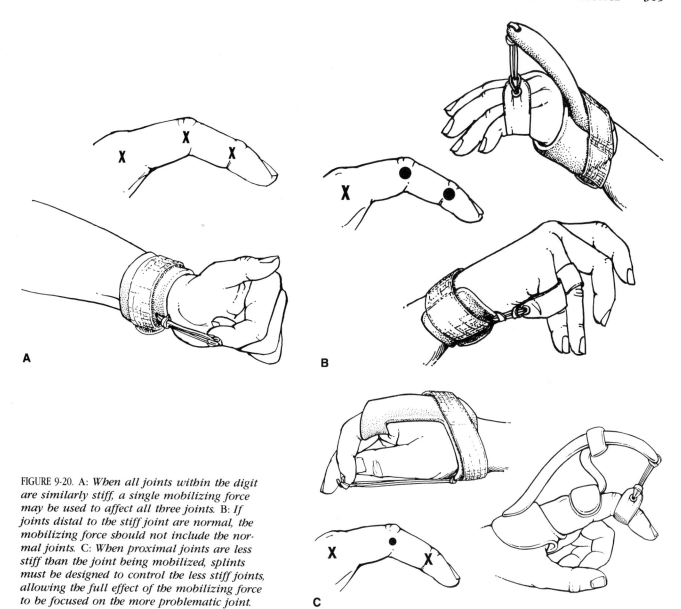

FIGURE 9-20. A: *When all joints within the digit are similarly stiff, a single mobilizing force may be used to affect all three joints.* B: *If joints distal to the stiff joint are normal, the mobilizing force should not include the normal joints.* C: *When proximal joints are less stiff than the joint being mobilized, splints must be designed to control the less stiff joints, allowing the full effect of the mobilizing force to be focused on the more problematic joint.*

ure 9-23). Mechanical principles directly influence splint structure and shape. Splint designs must also be reflective of the inherent properties of the splinting materials to be used.

All these factors and many more have considerable influence on the final splint configuration. It is easy to understand, in light of the above information, why "cookbook" approaches to splinting are potentially dangerous. With such a plethora of individual variables requiring attention, no single splint design is always appropriate for a given diagnosis or circumstance.

Construction principles

Principles of construction (Bradley, 1968; Bradley et al., 1972; Fess et al., 1981; Fess & Philips, 1987; Kiel, 1978, 1983) encompass concepts related to splint ***durability***, ***aesthetics***, and ***comfort***. Careful adherence to these principles provides a well-finished, wearable product that will withstand the rigors of daily use. Because splinting materials vary considerably in their respective physical properties, the type of heat, temperature, and the equipment employed to fabricate splints should be matched appropriately with the materials used. For the protection of both patient and therapist, safety precautions should be observed during all stages of construction. To achieve a good aesthetic effect, splint edges should be carefully smoothed, and both internal and external corners of all components, including straps, should be rounded appropriately (Figure 9-24). The hook portion of hook-and-loop fastening systems should be completely covered; joined components should be secure; and rivets or fastening devices should be finished, eliminating points or surfaces that might inadvertently cause injury or catch on clothing. Ventilation may be provided as necessary, and padding should be secured without surface overlap or wrinkling. Straps also need to be secured on one end to prevent loss or confusion with adjacent straps.

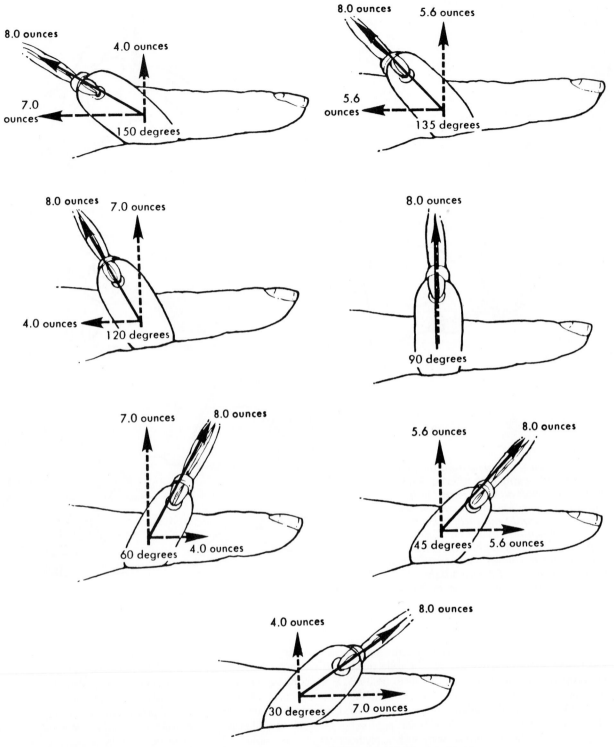

FIGURE 9-21. *Force used to correct joint deformity must be applied at a 90-degree angle of approach to the segment being mobilized. If this is not accomplished, the amount of rotatory force to the joint is diminished and the joint surfaces are pushed together or pulled apart, causing additional injury.* (*From* Hand splinting: Principles and methods [*2nd ed.*] *by E. E. Fess and C. A. Philips, 1987, St. Louis: C. V. Mosby.*)

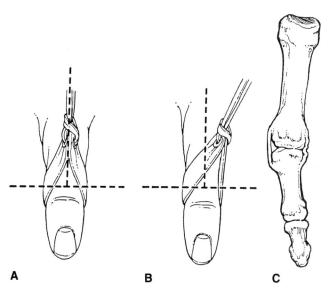

A   **B**   **C**

FIGURE 9-22. *The mobilizing force also must be perpendicular to the joint axis of rotation. If it is not, unequal stress is placed on the joint, and attenuation of the greater stressed collateral ligament may occur. (From* Hand splinting: Principles and methods [*2nd ed.*] *by E. E. Fess and C. A. Philips, 1987, St. Louis: C. V. Mosby.)*

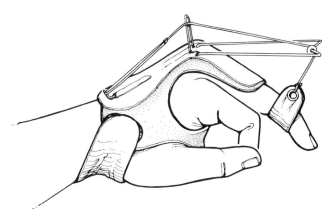

FIGURE 9-24. *Splint corners should be rounded. Internal or external corners that are not rounded create potential for weakness in the splint or pressure for the patient as well as poor aesthetic quality.*

Fit principles

The best design concepts and fabrication techniques may be rendered useless if a splint is not well fitted. The ***principles of fit*** (Bradley, 1968; Bradley et al., 1972; Fess et al., 1981; Fess & Philips, 1987; Kiel, 1978, 1983; Malick, 1978, 1979) serve as guidelines to this technically demanding final phase. It is at this point that the previously discussed principles come together to provide a well-functioning splint.

Mechanical principles play an important role during the fitting of a splint. Contiguous fit of the splint to the extremity reduces pressure on bony prominences as well as soft tissue (Figure 9-25). Optimal, 90-degree rotational forces prevent mi-

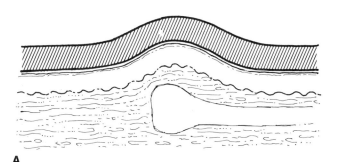

A

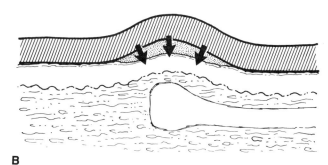

B

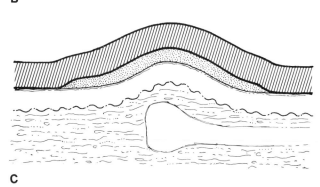

C

FIGURE 9-25. (A) *Contiguous fit reduces pressure. If padding is used, allowance must be made for its thickness. If this is not done, pressure is increased.* (B) *Incorrect.* (C) *Correct. (From* Hand splinting: Principles and methods [*2nd ed.*] *by E. E. Fess and C. A. Philips, 1987, St. Louis: C. V. Mosby.)*

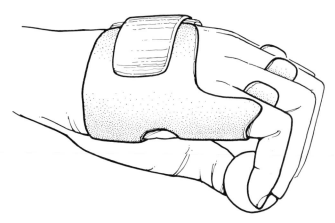

FIGURE 9-23. *When splints are applied, forces to unsplinted joints may be altered. It is important to carefully evaluate these changes to ensure that unsplinted joints are not damaged when the hand is used.*

gration of the splint and associated components, such as finger cuffs (Figure 9-26). Careful alignment of splint articulations with anatomic joint axes eliminates friction, and use of optimal leverage increases comfort and durability.

Anatomic considerations are also critical during fitting. **Skin creases** serve as anatomic guidelines to articular motion. If motion is desired at a given joint, the splint should be fitted so that it does not impinge on skin creases corresponding to the joint. Frequently impaired by poorly fitted splints or casts that inadvertently limit MP motion, the distal palmar crease should be free of splint material if the MP joints are to be permitted full range of motion. The same is true of the thenar crease. If full CMC joint motion of the thumb is required, the splint must not cross to the radial side of the palmar thenar skin crease. Bony prominences should be identified and the splint contoured to provide a smooth, close fit. In some cases, such as the radial styloid process at the wrist, the splint material may be molded to avoid contact, or padding may be employed to reduce forces

under a narrow component, such as a dorsal phalangeal bar (Brand, 1990). Splints that incorporate the second through fifth metacarpals should exhibit the **dual oblique angles** resulting from the combination of progressive radial to ulnar metacarpal shortening and from the relative mobility of the fourth and fifth metacarpals (Capener, 1956). Both **transverse** and **longitudinal arches** (Figure 9-27) should be supported. Careful attention should be directed toward digital joints on which corrective traction is applied. Rotational force applied in a direction that is not perpendicular to the axis of joint rotation results in unequal stress to pericapsular structures, causing irrevocable attenuation or lengthening of one of the two supporting collateral ligaments.

When fitting a splint, it is important to remember that the configuration of the hand and extremity change with movement. For example, as the fingers flex, the relative length of the dorsum of the hand elongates, while the palmar surface undergoes a relative shortening. The converse is true but to a lesser extent as

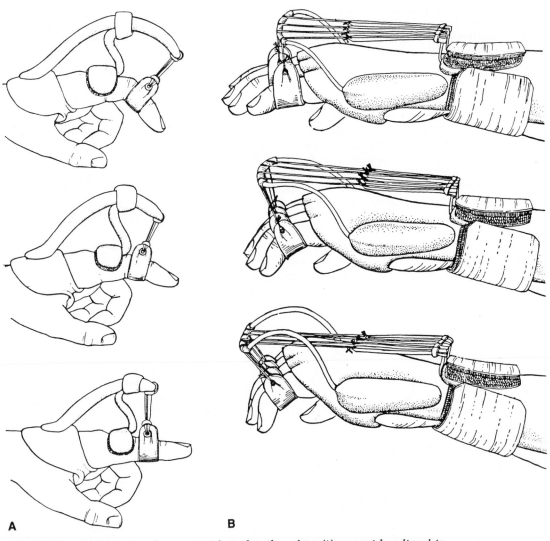

A   **B**

FIGURE 9-26. *As joint motion changes, outrigger length and position must be altered to maintain a 90-degree angle of approach of the mobilizing force.* (*From* Hand splinting: Principles and methods [*2nd ed.*] *by E. E. Fess and C. A. Philips, 1987, St. Louis: C. V. Mosby.*)

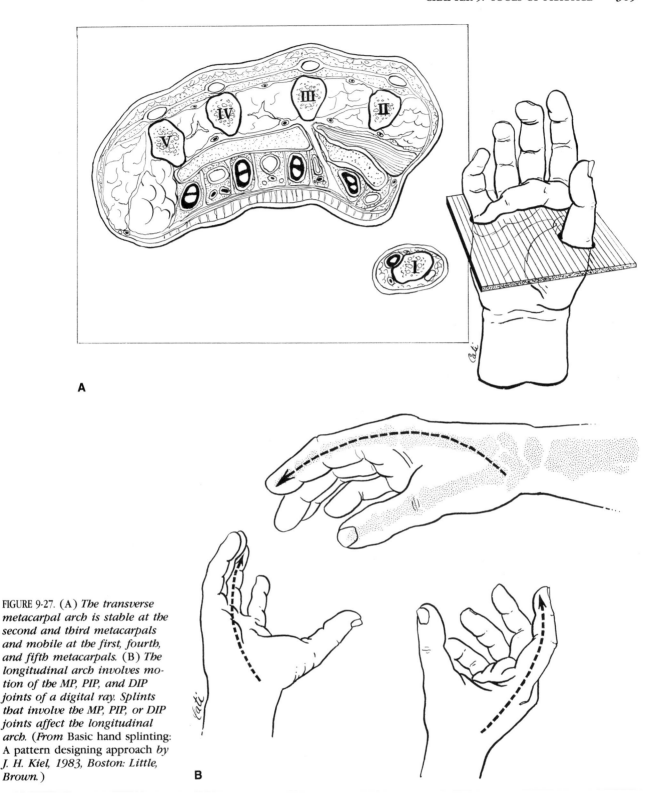

FIGURE 9-27. (A) *The transverse metacarpal arch is stable at the second and third metacarpals and mobile at the first, fourth, and fifth metacarpals. (B) The longitudinal arch involves motion of the MP, PIP, and DIP joints of a digital ray. Splints that involve the MP, PIP, or DIP joints affect the longitudinal arch. (From* Basic hand splinting: A pattern designing approach *by J. H. Kiel, 1983, Boston: Little, Brown.)*

the fingers are extended to neutral position. Opposition of the thumb results in similar changes, but it is the relative width of the hand that is altered, with dorsal width increasing and palmar width shortening as the thumb is moved in an ulnar direction. Any splint that allows motion must be fitted to adapt to these kinematic changes.

In addition to assessing component parts as they are constructed and fitted, it is important to mentally evaluate and reevaluate the entire splint as a whole, including those portions already completed. If one aspect of a splint is poorly constructed or fitted, it may cause other components or portions of the splint to be incorrect.

Application

Pattern construction

Once a design has been created mentally, it usually progresses through a pattern stage before becoming reality. Many methods have been published for constructing patterns (Fess & Philips, 1987; Kiel, 1983; Malick, 1978, 1979; Tenney & Lisak, 1986; Ziegler, 1984), each with merits and drawbacks. Ultimately, pattern fabrication seems to be dependent on the personal preference and style of the individual therapist. Experienced therapists often use entirely different methods of pattern construction, with end results being very similar. Additionally, it is not uncommon to find experienced therapists who adapt commercially available, precut splint blanks or who opt to fit a splint without the use of patterns. Newer materials whose inherent physical properties facilitate stretching, draping, and molding are more forgiving. Therapists with limited splinting experience, however, should be cautioned that attempts to make splints without patterns can lead to expensive, frustrating, and time-consuming errors.

An effective method of pattern construction is taping individual paper splint components to form the whole of a splint (Bradley, 1968; Bradley et al., 1972; Fess et al., 1981; Fess & Philips, 1987; Kiel, 1978, 1983). This is particularly useful for novices or in circumstances requiring unusually complicated designs.

Materials

The number of companies that provide materials for the construction of splints can be overwhelming. Most of these companies provide several types of materials along with aids to facilitate the splint construction process (AliMed, 1991; North Coast Medical, 1991; Smith & Nephew Rolyan, Inc., 1991; Sammons, 1991; WFR/Aquaplast, 1991). A skilled therapist not only must understand splinting theory and technique, but also is responsible for keeping current with new splinting products—adding, replacing, or rejecting as clinic requirements dictate (Cailliet, 1976). Although not all splinting needs may be purchased commercially, it is important to investigate and identify those that facilitate the fabrication process.

Excluding plaster of Paris and those materials from which specialized components are constructed, most basic splinting materials used today are **low-temperature thermoplastics**. With heat, these materials become soft and pliable, and when cooled, they retain the shapes to which they were conformed. Although thermoplastic materials differ in chemical content and physical properties, they may be grouped into two categories. The more plastic group has a polycaprolactone base, and the more rubber group has a polyisoprene base (Shafer, 1989; Breger-Lee & Buford, 1991). This provides a wide array of materials that may be matched selectively to individual patient problems and therapist preferences.

Qualities that influence the degree of material moldability include **stretchability**, **drapability**, **rebound**, and **elastic memory** (J. Hobbs, personal communication, October 1991). These characteristics are present in varying degrees in most thermoplastic materials and directly affect therapist effort required for forming splints.

Highly moldable materials require little therapist effort to conform. Once heated and cut to shape, these materials drape and stretch easily, allowing close, contiguous fit with minimal therapist intervention. These highly drapable materials are often easier to control by using gravity-assisted positions during fitting. This is especially helpful when working with splints designed for large surface areas. It is also possible to roll these materials into balls or tubes with no visible seams. Most highly moldable materials require close monitoring of applied heat levels since too-high temperatures result in excessive material softening and flow.

Rebound and elastic memory refer to the degree to which heated, stretched, or molded materials tend to return to their original sizes and shapes. Materials with large amounts of rebound or elastic memory require more therapist intervention to fabricate splints. Since these materials are inherently less drapable, they must be gently pushed or pulled into place; and once fitted, they must be carefully held in place until cool to prevent inadvertent loss of shape. Although materials possessing rebound properties attempt to return to their original manufactured shape to some degree when heated, they are altered somewhat by stretching and molding and are unable to achieve completely their premolded flat, smooth configurations. On the other hand, high elastic memory materials return to their original flat manufactured shape with little or no alteration when heated and left unattended.

The thermoplastic and memory qualities of splinting materials require constant awareness of the importance of completely cooling finished splints or sections of splints during fabrication. Splints or portions of splints that remain warm are susceptible to loss of shape, conforming to surfaces on which they have been placed or simply returning to their original flat shape. Without proper caution, it is also possible to accidentally direct heat to completed areas while working on adjacent spots, thereby requiring reforming of previously finished areas. The properties of thermoplasticity and elastic memory also require that patients be cautioned to clean splints in cool water and to store splints away from heat sources when they are not being worn.

Hot air and hot water most frequently are used to heat thermoplastic materials so that they may be cut, assembled, and fitted. Usually, heat guns are chosen for application of dry heat, although dry electric skillets may be employed with specific materials. Hair driers may be used for materials with relatively low heat thresholds, and in some cases, an electric burner may suffice. With a burner, however, it is difficult to direct the heat to individual splint parts. It is important to note that gas burners should be avoided because some materials are flammable. Wet heat may be obtained by heating water in electric skillets, large cooking pans, hydroculators, specialized splinting pans, or commercial restaurant steam tables. Hot water has the advantage of heating materials evenly. Although specific portions of splints may be heated in hot water by dipping, there may be areas that cannot be accessed without affecting adjacent finished parts. To avoid accidental burns to the patient or therapist when using hot water, it is critical to thoroughly dry materials before fitting.

Care must be used with all materials when tracing patterns to avoid leaving unsightly and undesirable residual marks on completed splints. Finding implements that make marks that are visible during transfer and cutting stages but that dissolve or erase after these stages have been completed is a continual challenge for therapists. Maintaining clean work areas is also important to fabricating splints because it is easy for dirt or scraps of material to become embedded in warm splint surfaces.

Therapists involved in splinting must thoroughly read information sheets provided with thermoplastic materials to identify the best and most efficient methods for working with each material. Techniques for cutting, heating, smoothing edges, and bonding with or without solvent often differ considerably from material to material.

Plaster of Paris–impregnated bandage, an often overlooked, older splinting material, continues to be used by experienced hand rehabilitation specialists. Although it has a tendency to absorb moisture and wound exudates and is not as durable as plastic, plaster is inexpensive, has superior capacity to conform, and allows skin to breathe. Plaster bandage is especially useful when correcting joint deformity through serial casting (Bell, 1987; Bell-Krotoski, 1990) (Figure 9-28). Because plaster tends to soften when exposed to moisture, patients must be cautioned to keep their plaster splints dry.

Trouble-shooting and assessment

As therapists make splints, supervise the construction of splints, or examine splints that have been brought back to the clinic by patients, there are guidelines that may be followed to ensure that these splints are designed, fabricated, and fitted appropriately. Since therapists often need to assess splints extemporaneously, it is helpful to be familiar with these guidelines. A list of **splint evaluation criteria** (Table 9-8) provides an organized approach to evaluating splints (Fess & Philips, 1987; Kiel, 1983). During this process, it is important to remember to assess the splint as a whole as well as its individual components.

Exercise

Splints and exercise must be carefully integrated to allow patients to achieve their full rehabilitation potential (Fess & Philips, 1987, pp. 325–369). Unfortunately, in practice, splinting has sometimes been viewed incorrectly as an isolated treatment technique. Splints are used to improve passive motion, substitute for weakened or lack of active motion, or infrequently are fabricated to provide resistive exercise. The effect of splinting on active range of motion is a secondary benefit that *may* occur after the attainment of these goals. Involving voluntary use of extrinsic and intrinsic upper-extremity musculature with adhesion-free tendinous excursions, active motion is the key factor to establishing and maintaining hand function.

Before active range of motion may be realized, corresponding passive joint motion must be present. For this reason, splinting is often used early in rehabilitation programs when exercise alone is insufficient to achieve or maintain motion. There are many instances when exercise alone is appropriate, but there are very few times, if any, when splinting may be used as an isolated entity.

Additionally, the occupational therapist must remember that use of a corrective splint to improve passive motion involves application of forces to effect tissue remodeling. This application of resistance must be appropriate to the level of physiologic timing of the problem. If resistive exercises are not appropriate, corrective splinting may also be inappropriate.

Evaluation measurements provide the guidelines from which coordinated splinting and exercise programs are orchestrated (Fess, 1990; Fess & Philips, 1987, pp. 103–121). Without these measurements treatment intervention is directionless and limited in effectiveness, potentially causing more harm than good. Assessment, splinting, and exercise are intricately intertwined in hand rehabilitation.

Creation of splint-wearing schedules is dependent on individual patient circumstances and physiologic timing. When splints are applied to influence tissue healing or remodeling, they must be worn for long periods of time to affect collagen realignment and tissue growth. Concomitantly, it is important to maintain or improve normal gliding capacity of adjacent struc-

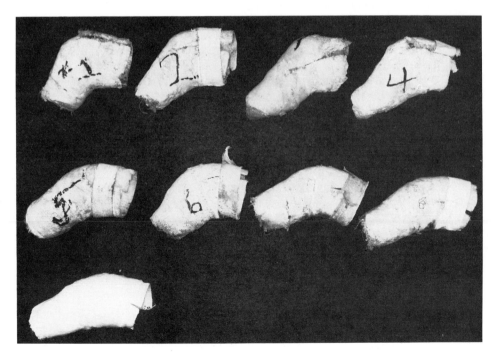

FIGURE 9-28. *Plaster of Paris– impregnated bandage is an excellent material for fabricating serial casts that are used to improve passive motion of stiff joints.* (*From* Hand splinting: Principles and methods [*2nd ed.*] *by E. E. Fess and C. A. Philips, 1987, St. Louis: C. V. Mosby.*)

TABLE 9-8.   *Splint Evaluation Criteria**

Need

1. Is application of splint necessary on initial examination?
2. Does it continue to be necessary on reevaluation?

Design

Given the diagnostic requirements, does the splint meet *general* design concepts, including adaptation for:

1. Individual patient factors (age, motivation, intelligence, clinic proximity, etc.)
2. Duration of time splint is to be used (temporary, semipermanent, permanent)
3. Simplicity (no irrelevant parts; splint is applicable and pertinent to the need)
4. Optimal function (splint allows usage and performance without unnecessary reduction of motion)
5. Optimal sensation (splint permits as much sensory input as possible)
6. Efficient fabrication (no extraneous parts or procedures, such as the use of reinforcement parts instead of curving contour, bonding instead of uninterrupted coalescing of components, straps instead of contiguous fit, inappropriate use of padding)
7. Application and removal (appropriate to individual patient factors)
8. Patient suggestions (requested adaptation that would not alter or jeopardize splint function)

Given the diagnostic requirements, does the splint meet *specific* design concepts, including adaptation for:

9. Influencing primary and secondary joints (motion allowed or restricted appropriately; components accomplish intended functions)
10. Attaining purpose (support, immobilize, or restrict motion; prevent or correct deformity; provide or assist motion; or provide attachment base for devices)
11. Affect on joints not included in splint; kinetic effects (avoids application of contraindicated forces to nonsplinted joints)
12. Anatomic variables (surface of application appropriate, healing structures protected as necessary, external hardware considered)
13. Exercise regimen (permits efficient execution of prescribed therapeutic exercises)

Mechanics

Given the diagnostic requirements, does the splint meet mechanical criteria, including adaptation for:

1. Reduction of pressure and shear (length and width of components appropriate; edges flanged as required; contiguous fit of components present)
2. Immobilization or stabilization forces (90-degree angle of approach to involved segment or joint)
3. Mobilization forces (90-degree angle of approach to segments mobilized, perpendicular to joint axes)
4. Magnitude of mobilization forces (supple joint: force sufficient to position segment; stiff joint: force does not exceed safe limits)
5. Difference of passive mobility of successive joints (relative stiffness of joints considered; mobilizing force is not abated at less stiff or normal joints)
6. Material strength (properties of material correlate to strength requirements; curving contour present at potential weak areas)
7. Elimination of friction and shear (joint axes aligned with splint articulations; contiguous fit present)

Construction

Given the diagnostic requirements, does splint fabrication and workmanship provide:

1. Good overall aesthetic appearance
2. Corners rounded, edges and surfaces smooth
3. Joined surfaces stable and finished (bonds solid, securing devices of sufficient number and correctly applied, internal edges smoothed, securing devices finished)
4. Ventilation (appropriately placed, splint strength not jeopardized)
5. Padding and straps secured

Fit

Given the diagnostic requirements, has the splint been fitted appropriately to adapt to:

1. Anatomic structure (bony prominences, arches, dual obliquity, skin creases)
2. Ligamentous stress (mobilization or immobilization forces correctly applied to avoid damage or attenuation)
3. Joint alignment (anatomic axes aligned with splint articulation; splint does not shift inappropriately on extremity)
4. Kinematic changes (splint does not inappropriately inhibit motion of unrestricted or partially restricted joints)
5. Contiguous fit of components on extremity

(continued)

TABLE 9-8. *Splint Evaluation Criteria* (continued)*

Patient Education

Given the diagnostic requirements, does the splinting program include consideration of and instructions for:

1. Wearing times and exercise regimen (reflects physiologic timing; is adapted to patient routine; is understood by patient)
2. Donning and doffing (process explained and demonstrated, understood by patient)
3. Wearability (patient gadget tolerance not exceeded; interfaces such as stockinette or powder used appropriately; acceptable to age and personality characteristics)
4. Precautions (written and verbal instructions provided, understood by patient)

* Although an attempt has been made to provide a complete listing, these criteria should not be considered all-inclusive.

tures. This requires delicate balancing between splint and exercise routines. Because patients with identical diagnoses may respond differently to therapeutic intervention, it is insufficient and often detrimental to adhere to rigid, predetermined protocols. Dictated by specific assessment data and physiologic parameters, treatment programs are tailored to individual patient needs. Some programs are relatively straightforward and uncomplicated, whereas others require constant alteration to keep pace with changing requirements. For example, a patient who needs to improve passive range of motion of a PIP joint may be instructed to repeat a splint-wearing and exercise routine every 2 hours throughout the day that involves wearing the PIP extension splint for 1 hour and 45 minutes, then removing the splint and exercising for 15 minutes, and then repeating the routine. Other programs may be more complicated. For example, it is not unusual for patients to have limitation of both flexion and extension, requiring that extension and flexion splints be alternated. Using the previously described splint-wearing and exercise cycle, a patient may be instructed to do three cycles with the extension splint, and on the forth cycle, to substitute the flexion splint. This repetition of a 3 : 1 splint extension/flexion ratio with exercise is used throughout the day. If a patient does not seem to have problems with developing stiffness in adjacent digits or joints, it may be appropriate to decrease the frequency of exercise. Conversely, if stiffness is a problem, exercises may be prescribed more often (eg, every 45 minutes). The key to effective splint-wearing and exercise regimens is to reassess frequently and to alter programs according to these measurements.

Special circumstances may also influence splint-wearing and exercise routines, and the astute therapist realizes that occasionally more creative approaches may be helpful in reminding patients to exercise on a regular basis. Television buffs readily adapt to exercising during commercials, whereas people working on an assembly line may be able to exercise only during breaks. Teachers and family members may need to be included when a child is wearing a splint. *Written instructions for splint wearing and exercise times should always be used to augment verbal instructions.*

Eliminating the exercise portion of a program, night splints may be the same as those used during the day, or they may have an entirely different, often more simple, design. Splints designed to correct joint deformity usually are coupled with night splints that maintain the advances made during the day. This requires careful monitoring and alteration of both day and night splints as changes occur.

Psychological effect and compliance

Because hands are constantly in use and visible, application of a splint often has psychological and socioeconomic ramifications. Therapists must be aware of the impact these factors may have on patient **compliance**. In reality, no splint may be considered beautiful, no matter how well designed and fabricated. Those patients who have greater physical limitations seem to be more accepting of splints, whereas the elderly often have difficulty adjusting lifetime habits and teenagers often are unwilling to accept anything that makes them different from their peers (Hopkins, 1966). Other patient conditions possibly causing noncompliance (eg, chemical dependence, lack of motivation, mental retardation) need to be identified as soon as possible. An unwillingness or inability to carry out instructions reliably may result in further damage or injury to the patient.

In general, a patient's **gadget tolerance** (Anderson, 1965; Feinberg & Brandt, 1981; Herman, 1984; Hopkins, 1966) may be enhanced if the benefits of wearing the splint are readily apparent. Patient education is critical to achievement of optimal functional results. It is important that patients be well informed about all aspects of their injury or illness and treatment program so they become integral members of the rehabilitation team. Indeed, the patient is the most important member of the team, and should be treated as such.

Precautions

Because splints are foreign bodies applied to living tissue surfaces, patients must be taught to monitor the status of their splinted extremities. The presence of pain, reddened areas, blisters, swelling, rashes, or other problems associated with wearing a splint must be reported to the therapist immediately, and use of the splint should be discontinued until the situation is assessed (Cannon et al., 1985). Self-examination instructions should be given to patients in writing, including telephone numbers for reporting problems.

Splint care should also be provided in writing. Patients should be cautioned about exposing their splints to warm or hot temperatures, such as hot water, heaters, or stoves. Additionally, they need to be reminded not to leave splints in hot car interiors. Thermoplastic splints may lose or alter their configurations in conditions such as these.

Management

Written documentation

"When writing a note in a patient's medical record about a splint, the same rules that apply to all professional writing should be used. In regard to the splint itself, the following . . . must be included" (Kiel, 1983, pp. 136–142): Patient name, identification number, age, sex, hand dominance, race, and ambulatory status provide basic information. Although the name and number usually appear on every page, the remaining data may be noted only once. The date, diagnosis, reason for referral, and referring physician are important in confirming the referral and application of the splint and in establishing third-party reimbursement procedures.

Initial baseline measurements of volume, range of motion, sensibility, strength, and dexterity define extremity condition before splint application. Results from other tests are included as needed. Documentation of passive and active range of motion is especially important if a splint is designed to improve joint motion. In the initial note, the splint is described, and the extremity to which it is fitted and the date of fitting are recorded. The purpose of the splint is briefly explained and its effect on the extremity confirmed, verifying that the splint does what it was designed to do. Wearing and exercise instructions are noted, and precautions are defined. Any unusual splint components or functions should also be included in the chart at this time. Additionally, documentation of explanations to the patient, nursing personnel, and family members should be delineated and, if possible, their level of understanding noted.

Notes from reevaluation sessions should include date and pertinent assessment measurements, with emphasis on identification of specific changes noted in the splinted extremity. Modifications made in the splint or in the splint-wearing and exercise program should be described in detail. Notation that these modifications were explained to the patient and pertinent others and that new instructions were provided in writing also should be recorded.

In practices in which many splints are fabricated, the use of standard forms may simplify and shorten the documentation process. In some cases, these forms are designed to meet the dual needs of patient education and medical-legal documentation.

Although clinics may differ slightly in their approaches, the above criteria are fundamental to documentation of splinting endeavors. With litigation procedures on the rise, no splint should be fitted to a patient without careful and thorough explanation in the medical record.

Cost and pricing

Most clinics develop a standard price list for frequently made splints that reflects material cost, therapist time, and overhead expenses per individual splint (Kiel, 1983, pp. 136–137). These prices are based on average fitting times and average-sized hands or extremities. Although extremes may occur, over time they are incorporated into the general patient population and a mean cost of materials and time is attained per splint design.

Material expense includes the cost per inch, or per square inch, of the amount of splint, strap, and padding materials used in each splint. Nonusable scraps are included as part of the cost of the splint. The individual cost of prefabricated components, fasteners, rivets, and so forth is also added to establish a basic price. Use of specialized products such as bonding solution and cooling spray must also be considered and usually is included on a general per application cost.

Therapist time involved in fabrication, fit, and explanation of the splint is added to the material expense. Therapist time is often figured at the same rate per hour used for other clinic treatments. To be representative of an average-experienced therapist, times for novice or highly specialized therapists are not used for determining splint prices. Therapist time involved in reassessing and altering finished splints on subsequent visits to the clinic may be included in the initial price of the splint or may be assessed on a time per alteration basis. Unfortunately, complicated splints often involve time-consuming alterations that considerably increase the price of the splint. Cost economy to the patient is another reason for opting for a simple splint design.

Summary

Many factors must be considered when splinting the upper extremity. The shear number of these variables makes it readily apparent that "cookbook" approaches must be avoided. Splints should be direct reflections of the individual patients for whom they are made. Factors that must be considered when creating splints include anatomic structures involved; type of surgical repair; physiologic timing; individual patient variables; kinetic and kinesiologic variables involving splinted and unsplinted joints; and the philosophic orientation of the physician and the therapist. Application of mechanical concepts enhances splint function, comfort, and durability, and adherence to construction principles results in aesthetically pleasing, well-fabricated final products. Additionally, implementation of the principles of fit ensures splint wearability and also influences splint function. When used appropriately, splints are an important and integral aspect of upper-extremity rehabilitation.

References

AliMed (1991). *Orthopedic rehabilitation products catalogue*. Dedham, MA: AliMed, Inc.

American Society of Hand Therapists, Splint Nomenclature Task Force (in press). *Splint classification system*. Garner, NC: The Society.

Anderson, M. H. (1965). *Upper extremities orthotics* (pp. 421). Springfield, IL: Charles C. Thomas.

Barr, N. R., & Swan, D. (1988). *The hand: Principles and techniques of splintmaking*. Boston: Butterworths.

Bell, J. A. (1987). Plaster casting for the remodeling of soft tissue (pp. 449–466). In E. E. Fess, & C. A. Philips, *Hand splinting: Principles and methods*. St. Louis: C. V. Mosby.

Bell-Krotoski, J. A. (1990). Plaster cylinder casting for contractures of the interphalangeal joints (pp. 1128–1133). In J. M. Hunter, L. H. Schneider, E. J. Mackin, & A. D. Callahan (Eds.), *Rehabilitation of the hand* (3rd ed.). St. Louis: C. V. Mosby.

Bledsoe, S. (1991). Comparison of the force magnitude of PIP flexion and extension commercial spring coil and springy wire splints to a commercial accordion spring configuration. Proceedings of the American Society of Hand Therapists. *Journal of Hand Therapy, 4*(1), 27–28.

Bradley, K. (1968). *Basic splinting manual*. (Unpublished handout, Indiana University Medical Center, Occupational Therapy Program, Indianapolis, IN.)

Bradley, K., Fess, E. E., & Kiel, J. H. (1972). *Basic splinting manual, revised.* (Unpublished handout, Indiana University Medical Center, Occupational Therapy Program, Indianapolis, IN.)

Brand, P. W. (1952). Reconstruction of the hand in leprosy. *Annals of the Royal College of Surgeons of England, 11,* 350–356.

Brand, P. W. (1978). The forces of dynamic splinting: Ten questions before applying a dynamic splint to the hand (pp. 591–598). In J. M. Hunter, L. H. Schneider, E. J. Mackin, & J. A. Bell (Eds.), *Rehabilitation of the hand.* St. Louis: C. V. Mosby.

Brand, P. W. (1985). *Clinical mechanics of the hand.* St. Louis: C. V. Mosby.

Brand, P. W. (1990). The forces of dynamic splinting: Ten questions before applying a dynamic splint to the hand (pp. 1095–1100). In J. M. Hunter, L. H. Schneider, E. J. Mackin, & A. D. Callahan (Eds.), *Rehabilitation of the hand* (3rd ed.). St. Louis: C. V. Mosby.

Breger-Lee, D. E., & Buford, W. L. (1991). Update in splinting materials and methods. In E. J. Mackin, & A. D. Callahan (Eds.), *Hand clinics* (pp. 569–585). Philadelphia: W. B. Saunders.

Bunnell, S. (1944). *Surgery of the hand* (pp. 198–203). Philadelphia: J. B. Lippincott.

Cailliet, R. (1976). *Hand pain and impairment* (2nd ed., pp. 150). Philadelphia: F. A. Davis.

Cannon, N. M., Foltz, R. W., Koepfer, J. M., Lauck, M. F., Simpson, D. M., & Bromley, R. S. (1985). *Manual of hand splinting.* New York: Churchill Livingstone.

Capener, N. (1956). The hand in surgery. *Journal of Bone and Joint Surgery, 38B*(1), 132.

Colditz, J. C. (1990). Dynamic splinting of the stiff hand (pp. 342–352). In J. M. Hunter, L. H. Schneider, E. J. Mackin, & A. D. Callahan (Eds.), *Rehabilitation of the hand* (3rd ed.). St. Louis: C. V. Mosby.

Duran, R. J., Coleman, C. R., Nappi, J. F., & Klerekoper, L. A. (1990). Management of flexor tendon lacerations in zone two using controlled passive motion postoperatively (pp. 410–413). In J. M. Hunter, L. H. Schneider, E. J. Mackin, & A. D. Callahan (Eds.), *Rehabilitation of the hand* (3rd ed.). St. Louis: C. V. Mosby.

Evans, B. E., Larson, D. L., & Yates, S. (1968). Preservation and restoration of joint function in patients with severe burns. *Journal of the American Medical Association, 204*(10), 91–96.

Evans, R. B. (1990). Therapeutic management of extensor tendon injuries (pp. 492–511). In J. M. Hunter, L. H. Schneider, E. J. Mackin, & A. D. Callahan (Eds.), *Rehabilitation of the hand* (3rd ed.). St. Louis: C. V. Mosby.

Feinberg, J., & Brandt, K. D. (1981): Use of resting splints by patients with rheumatoid arthritis. *American Journal of Occupational Therapy, 35*(3), 173–178.

Fess, E. E. (1984). Rubber band traction: Physical properties, splint design, and identification of force magnitude. *Journal of Hand Surgery, 9A,* 610. (From the Proceedings of the American Society of Hand Therapists.)

Fess, E. E. (1988). Force magnitude of commercial spring-coil and spring-wire splints designed to extend the proximal interphalangeal joint. *Journal of Hand Therapy, 1*(3), 86–90.

Fess, E. E. (1990). Documentation: Essential elements of an upper extremity assessment battery (pp. 53–81). In J. M. Hunter, L. H. Schneider, E. J. Mackin, & A. D. Callahan (Eds.), *Rehabilitation of the hand* (3rd ed.). St. Louis: C. V. Mosby.

Fess, E. E., Gettle, K. S., & Strickland, J. W. (1981). *Hand splinting: Principles and methods.* St. Louis: C. V. Mosby.

Fess, E. E., & Philips, C. A. (1987). *Hand splinting: Principles and methods* (2nd ed.). St. Louis: C. V. Mosby.

Flatt, A. E. (1983). *Care of the arthritic hand* (4th ed., pp. 15–35). St. Louis: C. V. Mosby.

Herman, H. (1984). Compliance with splint wearing schedule on a burn unit. *Journal of Hand Surgery, 9A,* 610. (From the Proceedings of the American Society of Hand Therapists.)

Hopkins, H. (1966). Self-help aides (pp. 647). In S. Licht (Ed.), *Orthotics etcetera* (9th ed.). New Haven, CT: Elizabeth Licht.

Hunter, J. M., Schneider, L. H., Mackin, E. J., & Callahan, A. D. (Eds.). (1990). *Rehabilitation of the hand* (3rd ed.). St. Louis: C. V. Mosby.

Kiel, J. H. (1978). *Basic splinting techniques.* (Unpublished handout, Indiana University Medical Center, Occupational Therapy Program, Indianapolis, IN.)

Kiel, J. H. (1983). *Basic hand splinting: A pattern designing approach.* Boston: Little, Brown.

Kleinert, H. E., Kutz, J. E., & Cohen, M. J. (1975). Primary repair of zone two flexor tendon lacerations (pp. 91–104). In American Academy of Orthopaedic Surgeons, *Symposium on tendon surgery in the hand.* St. Louis: C. V. Mosby.

Koepke, G. H., Feallock, B., & Felle, I. (1963). Splinting the severely burned hand. *American Journal of Occupational Therapy, 17*(4), 147–150.

Long, C., & Schutt, A. H. (1986). Upper limb orthotics (pp. 198–277). In J. B. Redford (Ed.), *Orthotics etcetera* (3rd ed.). Baltimore: Williams & Wilkins.

Madden, J. W., & Arem, A. (1981). Wound healing: Biologic and clinical features. In J. Sabiston (Ed.), *Davis-Christopher textbook of surgery* (12th ed.) (pp. 265–286). Philadelphia: W. B. Saunders.

Malick, M. H. (1978). *Manual on dynamic hand splinting with thermoplastic materials* (2nd ed.). Pittsburgh: Harmarville Rehabilitation Center.

Malick, M. H. (1979). *Manual on static hand splinting* (3rd ed.). Pittsburgh: Harmarville Rehabilitation Center.

Moberg, E. (1984). *Splinting in hand therapy.* New York: Thieme-Stratton.

North Coast Medical (1991). *Hand therapy catalog, 1991.* San Jose, CA: North Coast Medical.

Peacock, E. E. (1984). *Wound repair* (3rd ed.). Philadelphia: W. B. Saunders.

Pearson, S. O. (1978). Dynamic splinting. In J. M. Hunter, L. H. Schneider, E. J. Mackin, & J. A. Bell (Eds.), *Rehabilitation of the hand.* St. Louis: C. V. Mosby.

Roberson, L., Breger, D., Buford, W. L., & Freeman, M. (1988). Analysis of the physical properties of SCOMAC springs and their potential use in dynamic splinting. *Journal of Hand Therapy. 1*(3), 110–114.

Sammons, F. (1991). *Sammons catalog 1991.* Brookfield, IL: Fred Sammons.

Shafer, A. (1989). Demystifying splinting materials. In *O.T. product news 1.* Dedham, MA: AliMed, Inc.

Smith & Nephew Rolyan, Inc. (1991). *Splinting and rehabilitation products for occupational therapists and physical therapists, 1991 catalog.* Menomonee Falls, WI: Smith & Nephew Rolyan.

Strickland, J. W. (1987). Biologic basis for hand splinting. In E. E. Fess, & C. A. Philips (Eds.), *Hand splinting: Principles and methods* (2nd ed., pp. 43–70). St. Louis: C. V. Mosby.

Taber, C. W. (1989). *Taber's cyclopedic medical dictionary* (16th ed.). Philadelphia: F. A. Davis.

Tenney, C., & Lisak, J. (1986). *Atlas of hand splinting.* Boston: Little, Brown.

Von Prince, K. M., & Yeakel, M. H. (1974). *The splinting of burn patients.* Springfield, IL: Charles C. Thomas.

Webster's third new international dictionary of the English language, unabridged (1981). Springfield, MA: Merriam-Webster.

Weeks, P. M., & Wray, R. C. (1978). *Management of acute hand injuries: A biological approach* (2nd ed.). St. Louis: C. V. Mosby.

WFR/Aquaplast Corporation (1991). *1991 catalog.* Wyckoff, NJ: WFR/Aquaplast.

Wynn Parry, C. B. (1981). *Rehabilitation of the hand* (4th ed.). Boston: Butterworths.

Ziegler, E. M. (1984). *Current concepts in orthotics.* Menomonee Falls, WI: Rolyan Medical Products.

SECTION 5B

Assistive and adaptive equipment

KIRSTEN M. KOHLMEYER

KEY TERMS

Adaptive Equipment   Assistive Equipment

LEARNING OBJECTIVES

Upon completion of this section the reader will be able to:

1. *Define assistive and adaptive equipment.*
2. *Describe assistive and adaptive equipment options for a variety of deficits and applications toward personal care, communication, leisure, and home management activities.*
3. *Identify three to five considerations for evaluating the appropriateness of assistive and adaptive equipment.*

Definition

The American Occupational Therapy Association (1983) defines *therapeutic adaptation* as:

> the design and restructuring of the physical environment to assist self-care, work and play/leisure performance. This includes selecting, obtaining, fitting and fabricating equipment, and instructing the client, family and staff in proper use and care of equipment. Categories of therapeutic adaptation consist of: orthotics, prosthetics, and assistive and adaptive equipment (1983, p. 804).

By definition, a piece of **assistive equipment** gives "support or aid," while **adaptive equipment** is "made fit or suitable," often by modification (Webster, 1990).

Assistive and adaptive equipment can help patients maximize independence in activities of daily living such as self-care, home, work, school, and leisure activities. Assistive devices can also enhance health maintenance, deformity prevention, and energy conservation (Malik, 1988; Pedretti, 1985; Trombley & Scott, 1983).

Some devices are commercially available. Often, occupational therapists design or fabricate adaptive equipment in conjunction with their patients or other rehabilitation professionals, such as rehabilitation engineers or physical therapists.

TABLE 9-9. *Assistive and Adaptive Equipment Options for Various Activities of Daily Living*

Deficit Areas	Eating	Oral Facial Hygiene	Dressing	Toileting and Bathing
Range of motion	Universal cuff Elongated handles Built-up handles Cup holder Long straw and straw clip Plate guard Scoop dish	Sunbeam dental care system Electric toothbrush Water pik Extended handles Extended comb and brush Hand-held shower Extended faucet handles Shampoo basin (for caregiver)	Front-opening garments Large buttons Zipper pull Velcro fasteners Button hook Long shoe horn Reacher Sock aid donner Dressing stick Elastic shoelaces	Reacher Spray deodorant Long-handled sponge/toilet aid Long-handled skin inspection mirror Hand-held shower Terry cloth robe (for drying) Raised toilet and tub seat Safety rails
Strength and arm placement	Balanced forearm orthosis Swedish sling Lightweight utensils Serrated knife Water bottle Quad feeder Long straw and straw clip	Balanced forearm orthosis Swedish sling Hand-held shower Extended faucet handles Lightweight comb and brush Razor holder Soap on a rope	Large buttons Velcro fasteners Dressing stick Leg lifters and loops Sock aid and donner Bed and dressing ladder	Hand-held shower Long-handled sponge Soap on a rope Lever soap dispenser

Personal Care

Options for maximizing function

Although a multitude of equipment options exist for physical deficits, the occupational therapist can follow some basic principles in attempting to maximize patient function. Patients with range of motion limitations must compensate for lack of reach and joint excursion. Extended handles, reachers, and elastic or Velcro closures are several options. Compensation principles for decreased strength are to use gravity-assisted, lightweight, or electrical devices and to change body mechanics by using leverage. Incoordination in the form of tremors, ataxia, athetoid, or choreiform movements can cause difficulty in completing activities of daily living. Stabilizing proximal limb segments, weighting distal segments, and providing a safe environment help compensate for lack of balance and fine-motor skill. Patients with decreased hand function may use orthoses, universal cuffs, or straps to perform activities of daily living. The major compensatory technique for patients with hemiplegia is stabilization to substitute for the role normally assumed by the affected side. Secured objects, Dycem, and adaptive techniques are common options. Patients with low endurance should use energy conservation and work simplification techniques, such as prioritization, organization, pacing, and utilization of equipment that improves efficiency (Malik, 1988; Pedretti, 1985; Trombley & Scott, 1983). Table 9-9 lists assistive and adaptive equipment options for various activities of daily living.

Evaluation of fit

The occupational therapist considers numerous factors when deciding to introduce, loan, or issue assistive equipment. Patients need to understand the purpose of the device. Sufficient patient and caregiver education facilitates carry-over and use of proper techniques. Values related to effort level required, performance abilities with or without the equipment, caregiver needs, motivation, and sociocultural considerations should also be examined (Chiou & Burnett, 1985; Malik, 1988; Moy, 1987).

The therapist must consider clinical necessity. Little or no adaptive equipment should be used unless it is absolutely necessary. Often, adaptive techniques suffice over adaptive equipment for task performance. The therapist should determine whether the device has functional utility that facilitates performance outcomes, increases safety, or decreases energy or time expenditure and whether the equipment is reliable. Temporary devices may be appropriate during a transitional, functional stage of rehabilitation. Sufficient time should be allocated for adequate training before a definitive decision regarding equipment is made (Garber & Gregorio, 1990).

Economic factors, such as cost and reimbursement, should be considered. Level of technologic sophistication may impact cost and reimbursement, as may future acquisition and repair needs. Patients should be able to use their equipment in desired

(*Text continues on page 320*)

	Communication			Leisure	Home Management		
Reading	*Writing/Typing*	*Telephone Use*	*Games, Hobbies, Arts and Crafts, and Sports*	*Meal Preparation and Clean-up*	*Cleaning and Laundry*	*Environmental Control*
Electric page turner Mouthstick Book holder	Built-up pens and pencils Electric typewriter Word processor Typing sticks	Speaker phone Environmental control unit Push button Clip receiver holder	Mouthstick activities Bowling ball ramp Embroidery hoop Built-up handles	Reacher Nonslip mats Lightweight utensils Sponge cloth mitt Counter-top appliances	Extended handles for dustpans and mops Self-ringing mop lever Long-handled feather duster	Electric scissors Key holder Lever doorknob extension Reacher Environmental control unit
Electric page turner Mouthstick Book holder Balanced forearm orthosis Swedish sling Head wand	Inverted pencil in universal cuff Typing sticks Built-up pens and felt-tip pens Stabilized clipboard Electric typewriter with self-correcting ribbon Mouthstick with interchangeable tips	Speaker phone Head set Mouthstick Gooseneck phone holder Environmental control unit	Mouthstick activities Pneumatic control camera W/C camera tripod holder Trigger-release archery Built-up handles for pencil and brush grips Raised gardening Bowling ball ramp	Pan stabilizer Mirror over stove (if sitting) Push/pull oven rack piece Counter-top appliances	Reacher Front-loading machines Extended handles for dustpans and mops Long-handled feather duster	Environmental control unit Automatic door opener Pad or rocker switch Light-touch controls

(continued)

TABLE 9-9. *Assistive and Adaptive Equipment Options for Various Activities of Daily Living (continued)*

		Personal Care		
Deficit Areas	**Eating**	**Oral Facial Hygiene**	**Dressing**	**Toileting and Bathing**
Coordination and balance	Dycem Weighted utensils Weighted forearm cuffs Swivel utensils Long straw and straw guard Covered glass and sipping spout Rocker knife Scoop dish Friction mobile arm support	Wash mitt Soap stabilizer Soap on a rope Lever faucets Suction brush for nail and denture care Electric toothbrush Electric razor Shaving cream dispenser handle Shampoo dispenser Gooseneck-adapted hairdryer	Front-opening garments Large buttons Velcro closures Built-up button hook Elastic waists Zipper pull Elastic shoelaces	Roll-on deodorant Bath mitt Nonskid bath mat Bath seat and tub bench Hand-held shower Soap on a rope Safety rails Leg separator
Hand function	Dycem Adapted utensils (built-up handle, swivel, bent) Universal cuff Quad grip knife Sandwich holder Wrist/hand orthosis (WHO) Hand orthosis (HO)	Built-up handles Universal cuff Denture brush Floss holder Shaving cream dispenser handle Shampoo dispenser Make-up basket Soap on a rope	Velcro closures Loops and rings Zipper-pull cuff Thumb loop Button hook Elastic shoelaces W/C gloves (for friction)	Terry-cloth robe (for drying) Towel with loops Bath mitt Soap on a rope Skin inspection mirror Adapted catheter clamp Pneumatic or electric leg bag clamp Digital stimulator Suppository inserter
One-handed activities	Rocker knife Plate guard Dycem	Wash mitt Suction nail or denture brush Soap on a rope	Large, front-opening garments Velcro closures Button hook Reacher Dressing stick Long shoe horn	Wash mitt Long-handled sponge Soap on a rope Spray deodorant
Endurance	Flat-based utensils Lightweight utensils Balanced forearm orthosis	Electric toothbrush Lightweight comb and brush Balanced forearm orthosis	Reacher Dressing stick Long shoe horn Elastic shoelaces	Bath seat and tub bench Safety rail Hand-held shower

Communication			Leisure	Home Management		
			Games, Hobbies, Arts and Crafts, and Sports	*Meal Preparation and Clean-up*		
Reading	*Writing/Typing*	*Telephone Use*			*Cleaning and Laundry*	*Environmental Control*
Dycem Book holder	Typewriter holder Keyguard Weighted and enlarged pencil or pen Felt-tip pen Stabilized clipboard	Gooseneck phone holder Shoulder rest Large push buttons	Magnetic playing cards and board Enlarged and weighted game pieces Card holder Automatic card shuffler W/C bowling ball holder and ramp Chest strap and body harness Easy kneeler and seat	Pots with bilateral handles Dycem and nonskid mat Cutting board with rails, suction cup feet, and corner stabilizer Pot stabilizer Wall-mounted jar opener Heavy utensils and bowls Electrical appliances Counter-top appliances Long oven mitts	Suction bottle brush Dust mitts Wheeled cart Heavy, upright vacuum	Lever door handle Friction tape or rubber-covered door handle Key holder Pad or rocker switch Environmental control unit
Page turner Universal cuff with pencil inverted Pen holder with inverted pencil attached to orthosis Rubber finger Book holder	Wanchik writer Writing frame The Arthwriter Figure-8 writing splint Universal cuff with pencil inverted Pen holder	Large push buttons Phone holder (shoulder or gooseneck) Speaker phone Universal cuff with pencil inverted Clip receiver holder	Spring-loaded cue stick Quad grip frisbee Universal cuff Velcro straps and grip Enlarged game pieces Spring-loaded bowling ball Orthosis with utensil slot and vertical holder with inverted pencil Clamp frames	Wrist loop or strap Modified handles with high-temperature plastic Rocker knife Electric can opener Box topper Carton holder	Wash mitt Liquid soap dispenser Automatic faucet Faucet-mounted spray attachment Built-up or cuff handles on duster	Loop scissors Quick-clip scissors Key holder Pad or rocker switch Light-touch controls Lever handles Environmental control unit
Book holder	Stabilized clipboard Paper weight	Receiver holder (stand or shoulder)	Embroidery hoop Knitting needle holder Card holder Recreation Belt Electric retrieve fishing reel W/C bowling ball holder Bowling ball ramp	Dycem Suction devices Stabilized jar opener One-handed can opener One-handed rolling pin One-handed beater Cutting board with rails, suction cup feet, corner stabilizer	Standard equipment	Standard equipment Environmental control unit
Book holder Electric page turner	Built-up pens and pencils	Portable cordless phone Phone holder	Built-up handles Camera holder Embroidery hoop Clamp frames Easy kneeler and seat Bowling ball ramp	Pull-out shelves Lazy susans Vertical storage Lightweight utensils Electrical appliances Wheeled utility cart	Self-propelled vacuum Wheeled service cart Permanent-press clothing Dishwasher	Standard equipment Environmental control unit

environments. If equipment proves useless to the consumer, financial loss includes the cost of the equipment as well as the time spent in training sessions (Shaperman, 1984).

The most important basis for evaluating an assistive device is whether it satisfies the needs of the disabled consumer from the consumer's point of view. In a preliminary study of long-term users of assistive devices, Batavia and Hammer (1990) identified four key evaluation and selection criteria: effectiveness (the extent to which the function of the device improves one's living situation, functional capability, or independence), affordability (the extent to which the purchase, maintenance, or repair of the device causes financial difficulty), operability (the extent to which the device is easy to operate and responds adequately to commands), and dependability (the extent to which the device operates with repeatable and predictable levels of accuracy under conditions of reasonable use). Clinical implications from this consumer feedback are numerous. The consumer–provider relationship in equipment selection should be a partnership, not a teacher–student relationship. Therapists should use a systematic method of approaching the evaluation, usage, and prescription of adaptive devices so that important issues are not overlooked. Consumers should be educated in the variety of options available, with pros and cons of selections presented candidly. Finally, enhanced follow-up services by both prescribers and providers are necessary to meet consumers' changing needs.

References

American Occupational Therapy Association (1983). Standards of practice for occupational therapy. *American Journal of Occupational Therapy, 37,* 802–814.

Batavia, A. I., & Hammer, G. S. (1990). Toward the development of consumer-based criteria for the evaluation of assistive devices. *Journal of Rehabilitation Research and Development, 27*(4), 425–436.

Chiou, L., & Burnett, C. (1985). Values of activities of daily living. *Physical Therapy, 65,* 901–906.

Garber, S. L., & Gregorio, T. L. (1990). Upper extremity assistive devices: Assessment of use by spinal cord-injury patients with quadriplegia. *American Journal of Occupational Therapy, 44*(2), 126–131.

Malik, M. (1988). Activities of daily living. In H. Hopkins, & H. Smith (Eds.), *Willard and Spackman's occupational therapy* (7th ed.). Philadelphia: J. B. Lippincott.

Moy, A. (1987). Which aid? In E. Bumphrey (Ed.), *Occupational therapy in the community* (pp. 74–89). Maryland: Aspen Publishers.

Pedretti, L. W. (1985). *Occupational therapy: Practice skills for physical dysfunction* (2nd ed.). St. Louis: C.V. Mosby.

Shaperman, J. (1984). From another perspective: A clinician's view of the theme. *Occupational Therapy in Healthcare, 1,* 5–7.

Trombley, C. A., & Scott, A. D. (1983). *Occupational Therapy for Physical Dysfunction.* Baltimore: Williams & Wilkins.

Webster's ninth new collegiate dictionary (1990). Springfield, MA: Miriam-Webster.

Bibliography

Abrams, A., & Abrams, M. (1990). *The first whole rehab catalog.* White Hall, VA: Betterway.

ADL Catalog (1991). San Jose, CA: North Coast Medical.

Hale, G. (Ed.). (1979). *The source book for the disabled.* New York: Paddington Press.

McCluer, S., Conroy, E. E., Gephardt, S. L., Rice, W., & Wilke, R. (1971). *Assistive devices and equipment for rehabilitation.* Hot Springs, AR: Hot Springs Rehabilitation Center.

Professional healthcare catalog (1991). Burr Ridge, IL: Fred Sammons.

SECTION 5C
Environmental adaptation

KIRSTEN M. KOHLMEYER and
JEANNE ERICSSON LEWIN

KEY TERMS

Accessibility

Americans with Disabilities Act

Environmental Adaptations

LEARNING OBJECTIVES

Upon completion of this section the reader will be able to:

1. *Define environmental adaptation.*
2. *Identify the historical progression of legislation that has had the greatest impact on environmental adaptation.*
3. *Describe the two main components that guide the clinician's thinking when evaluating the environment for accessibility.*
4. *Discuss three available options for adapting the environment.*

This section focuses on physical barriers in the environment that interfere with a person's optimal performance of a desired task. Environmental barriers occur in both private (eg, home) and public (eg, workplaces, schools, restaurants) places.

Definitions

Environmental adaptations relate to changes in the physical space or environment that facilitate easy access and mobility to those who are physically challenged. Whether a person's disability involves mobility needs, requiring wheelchair use, a sensory-system deficit, as in the case of an aging person, or a visual or hearing impairment, evaluating the need for environmental adaptations is a primary concern of the occupational therapist.

An environmental assessment is performed by measurement of physical properties (Figure 9-29), naturalistic observations, self-reports, and interpretive analysis (Spencer, 1978; Davidson, 1991). This assessment is performed by occupational therapists, often in conjunction with other rehabilitation professionals, such as rehabilitation engineers, physical therapists, case

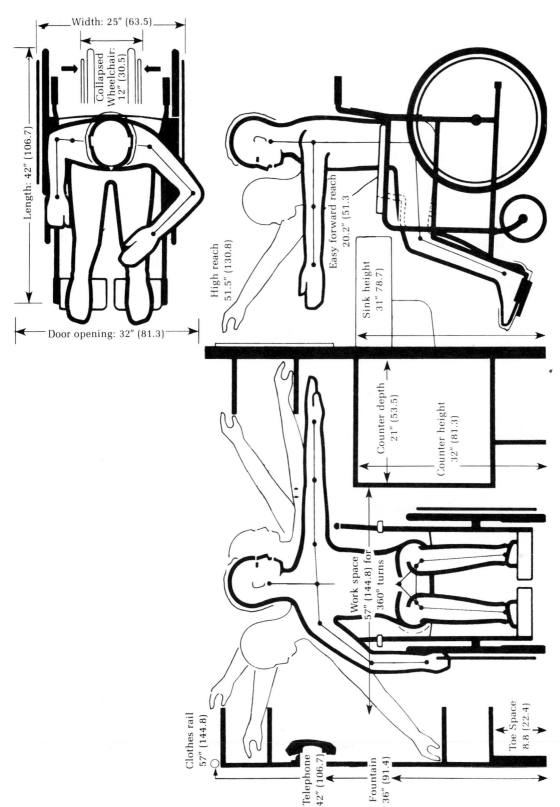

FIGURE 9-29. *Basic measurements and proportions can be used when planning home modifications. Measurements are given in inches and centimeters. (Adapted from "Humanscale 1/2/3" by N. Diffrient, A. R. Tilley, and J. Bardagey, 1974, Cambridge, MA: MIT Press, Designer: Henry Dreyfuss Associates.)*

managers, or tradespeople (eg, electricians, plumbers, computer experts). The primary goal of environmental adaptations is to match the needs of the disabled person with demands of the intended tasks (eg, self-care, home management, work).

Laws impacting *accessibility* include the Architectural Barriers Act of 1968, Federal Rehabilitation Act of 1973, Comprehensive Rehabilitation Services Amendment of 1978, Fair Housing Amendment Act of 1988, and *Americans with Disabilities Act* (ADA) of 1990.

The Architectural Barriers Act of 1969 was the first federal legislation in the United States to require certain federal and federally funded building projects to be accessible to people with physical disabilities (Federal Register, 1984; U. S. Department of Education, 1987). The Federal Rehabilitation Act of 1973 further mandated that any institution receiving federal funds could not discriminate against people with disabilities because of existing institutional architectural barriers (Nugent, 1978). The Architectural and Transportation Barriers Compliance Board was created to enforce provisions of the Rehabilitation Act. Because of inadequate compliance with the Rehabilitation Act, the federal legislatures passed the Comprehensive Rehabilitation Services Amendment in 1978.

Uniform Federal Accessibility Standards were then developed to be consistent with the Standards of the American National Standards Institute (ANSI) to establish accessibility guidelines (ANSI, 1986; Federal Register, 1984). The Fair Housing Amendment Act of 1988 extended the coverage of Title VIII of the Civil Rights Act of 1968 to prohibit discriminatory housing (Federal Register, 1988).

The ADA is one of the most important pieces of legislation for people with disabilities in the United States' history. President George Bush signed the ADA into Public Law 101-336 on July 26, 1990. The ADA is based on the Civil Rights Act of 1964 and significantly expands rights created by Title V of the Rehabilitation Act of 1973 in the areas of employment, public services and transportation, public accommodations, and telecommunications (ADA, 1990; Antone & Falk, 1991; Baker & McKenzie, 1991; Batavia, Dejong, Eckenhoff, & Materson, 1990; Ellek, 1991; Federal Register, 1991; Verville, 1990).

Environment-behavior principles

When evaluating the environment for potential adaptations, the occupational therapist must consider the client's psychosocial status for such changes as well as those modifications that are feasible within the specified physical environment.

Client-related considerations

When the therapist promotes opportunities for the client to make choices and control events that will have an impact on the home or work environment, the likelihood of the client's accepting the adaptations is enhanced. Therefore, whenever the client is mentally capable, the environmental adaptations should be designed by the occupational therapist with the consultation of the client. When the client is unable to consult with the therapist because of cognitive limitations, the client's family or primary caregiver should be consulted. When the occupational therapist provides a rationale for suggesting certain environmental adaptations, the client and the family or caregiver develops an under-

TABLE 9-10. *Recommendations for Environmental Adaptation Strategies*

Deficit	Suggestions for Modifications
Hearing	Use teletypewriters and teletype-displays to increase communication between hearing-impaired people and hearing peers. Use amplifiers in handsets of telephone; audible warning signals accompanied by visual or vibratory device to ensure safety. Carpet floor and install drapes on windows to reduce sharp noises and distracting background noise or echoes. Explore purchase of vibrating alarm clocks, amplified television set, flashing lights hooked up to the doorbell.
Vision	Use white or reflecting tape to clearly mark changes in floor levels. Position furniture away from high-traffic areas. Use higher wattage lightbulbs to increase illumination and distribute the light evenly. Keep a consistent light level in bedrooms and hallways and install night lights. Minimize glare by avoiding the use of shiny surfaces. Be aware that yellow-oranges and reds are most easily distinguished by people with low vision. Use contrasting colors between doorways and walls, dishes and tablecloths, and risers and flat surfaces of stairs.
Hand limitations	Use large, lever-type controls on faucets, door latches, and appliance knobs. Consider this rule of thumb when determining whether a person with dexterity limitations can use a control: if an able-bodied person can operate the control with the fist closed, then the person with hand limitations will be able to operate the control.
Frailty, disorientation, poor judgment	Avoid unstable, easy-to-knock-over furnishings and those with sharp corners to minimize the injury if one does fall. Remove scatter rugs and clutter. Consider placing barriers at potentially dangerous locations, such as at the top of a stairway, to prevent inadvertent falls.
Mobility impairments (includes restricted mobility due to heart disorders and other physiologic limitations)	Relocate bedrooms or living spaces onto one level. Provide convenient storage areas to minimize bending, reaching, lifting, and carrying. Keep paths free of clutter between commonly used rooms in the environment. Eliminate loose rugs and electric cords.

standing of why the recommendations have been made and are likely to follow through on the suggestions.

The functional needs of the client must be considered because the environment has the greatest effect on the person with the least capability. The occupational therapist should consider the status of the client's ability to process sensory information as well as the client's mobility status.

The occupational therapist should have a thorough understanding of the client's perceptual motor competencies when developing strategies for environmental adaptations. For example, for the client with a hearing impairment, sound reverberation caused by a lack of acoustic materials such as carpeting or draperies could interfere with the client's ability to function optimally within that environment. Considerations for the client with visual impairments include evaluating the lighting throughout the home or work environment, determining whether glare-reducing window and lighting treatments are an option, increasing the size of lettering on signs and written instructions wherever feasible, and using contrasting landmarks, such as wall hangings, to assist the client in negotiating through the environment. The floor surface (eg, vinyl flooring; carpeting) can influence the client's ability to move through space safely. The client with a diminished sense of proprioceptive and vestibular perception (as is often the case with elderly people) may perceive a reflective surface as having wet spots. In an attempt to step around the shiny or wet spots, the client compromises safety and risks falling.

Other considerations in designing an adaptive environment include whether the client lives alone or with other family members who might perceive the changes as an intrusion or inconvenience and the client's financial and physical resource capabilities to implement the modifications. Tables 9-10 and 9-11 provide specific recommendations for environmental adaptations.

TABLE 9-11.   *Special Adaptations for a Barrier-free Environment*

Adaptation	Considerations for Adaptability and Accessibility
Ramps	Consider the incline (12 inches of length for each inch of vertical rise) and surface material for safety; use nonslip surfaces. Portable ramps are available but take time to assemble and dissemble and are cumbersome for peoples with upper-body weakness.
Landings	5-foot-long landings should be located at top and bottom of ramp; intermediate landings should be used where a ramp changes direction or rises beyond 3 feet. Edge protections prevent falling off.
Materials	Wooden ramps are relatively inexpensive and easier to construct than concrete ramps but are a potential fire hazard. Ramp surface should be fireproof. Broom-finished concrete, in which broom strokes are perpendicular to the slope of the ramp, provides a nonslip surface. Avoid using carpeting, waxed linoleum, or glossy, painted surfaces.
Cover or roof	Consider building a protective roof in case of inclement weather.
Handrails	Handrails are necessary on both sides of the ramp.
Bathrooms	Consider increasing access by removing the doors and replacing the cabinet beneath the sink with a curtain (for under-sink storage). Cover the hot water supply and insulate pipes to protect against burns.
Vanity top	Usually 30 to 34 inches high provides easy access for a wheelchair.
Faucets	Single-level faucets provide an easy visual display of the water temperature; gross movements may be used to operate them.
Toilets	18-inch-high seat is recommended for easy access on and off.
Grab bars	Grab bar should be screwed directly into wall studs and reinforced for maximal strength and safety. *Pivoting grab bars* can be moved out of the way when not needed; *wall-mounted grab bars* offer the most stability; *sheltering arm grab bars* offer greater support than wall-mounted bars because they have legs that are supported on the ground and bolted to the toilet. They allow use of both the arm and leg muscles to lower oneself onto the toilet.
Tub seats	Built-in tub seats are more stable and safer than removable ones; the tub seat must be designed for drainage back into the tub.
Shower and tub controls	Single-lever controls are best; antiscald temperature controls are available so that the maximal water temperature can be preset.
Shower curtains and doors	Shower curtains are recommended over sliding doors with tracks, which provide a barrier and often have sharp edges.
Portable, hand-held shower head	Hand-held showers may be attached to the lavatory; with a floor drain installed, one may shower in a bath chair without extensive modifications to the bathroom.
Telephone	Install a telephone line or an emergency call system in the bathroom in the event of an emergency.
Ground-fault-interrupted circuits	All electrical circuits should be ground-fault-interrupted for safety in the event a hair dryer, electric shaver, or other electrical device falls into a tub or sink of water. Install circuits within wheelchair reach.

Environmental considerations

Environmental considerations relate to the potential adaptability of the environmental space that is considered for modification. How flexible is the environment to support changes to fit personal needs? Is the environment accessible to the client with specialized mobility needs? Are the modifications aesthetically pleasing? Have all safety and security issues been addressed? Table 9-12 provides decision-making strategies for planning a barrier-free space.

Strategies for decision making

By developing an understanding of the multiple ways in which the environment mediates the client's functioning, health care providers can be attuned to the clients' daily routines (Rogers, 1989). In making recommendations for environmental adaptations, the occupational therapist should consider a number of factors in addition to the previously described environment-behavior principles. The therapist should define the level of the accommodations by answering the following questions: Can the

TABLE 9-12.   *Decision-Making Strategies for a Barrier-free Environment*

Barrier	Considerations for Adaptability and Accessibility
Doors	Is there easy access through at least one entry (preferably two)? Are all doors along the accessible path between bedroom, kitchen, and bathroom easily accessed? Consider what type of door is most suitable for individual mobility needs if door modifications or placements are planned. Consider that (1) *swinging doors* require landings on both sides; (2) *sliding doors* require one to have strength to manage the weight and lateral movement to manipulate; the floor track may be a tripping hazard; (3) *folding doors* are lighter in weight, but the hardware may not withstand constant use; and, (4) *pocket doors* may be inexpensively mounted on the surface of an existing wall if the person has occasional needs for privacy.
Width	A standard-width 32-inch doorway cannot accommodate a wheelchair, whose standard width is 24 to 27 inches. Add 1½ inches on both sides of chair to allow for finger and knuckle clearance plus 1 or 2 inches to allow for inaccurate maneuvering and the usual oblique approach to doors.
Landing	Does the space on either side of the door allow a person who uses a wheelchair or other mobility-assisting device to approach and open the door?
Hardware	Can the latch or lock be reached and operated from a seated position? Is the person's hand dexterity sufficient to operate the hardware? Slide bolts with a lever arm welded or attached to an existing turn may provide an easier grip than standard slide bolts. Consider magnetic card readers, remote control locks, and push-button-activated locks. Avoid spring and hydraulic mechanisms.
Weight	Can the person manage the weight or spring pressure of the door?
Threshold	Can the threshold be ramped or removed? Abrupt changes in levels greater than ½ inch can create tripping hazards for people with mobility and vision impairments.
Doormats	Can the doormat be fastened in place with tacks, stables, or double-sided carpet tape? Loose mats create tripping hazards.
Kick plates	Is the doorway narrow, or does the person push the door open with the wheelchair foot rest? Consider a *thin* kickplate that extends from the floor up to a height of 16 inches to reduce wear on the door surface.
Vision panels	If there are interior passage doors that are normally left closed, the installation of a vision panel will help prevent a slowly moving person from being knocked over by others coming through the door. For security, one-way vision panels or peepholes on entrance doors allow one to survey any visitor before opening the door. For a person using a wheelchair, the peephole should be between 36 and 45 inches above the floor.
Stairs	
Handrails	Are there handrails on both sides of the stairway? If the stairway is wide, can a single handrail be installed in the center of the stairway? Can the user grip the rail between the thumb and fingers for safe use? Is the handrail mounted at least 1½ inches away from the wall to allow grasping space? Will it support up to 250 lb at any point? Extend the handrail beyond the top and bottom of the stairs to allow the support necessary to get on and off the last step.
Treads and risers	Risers higher than 6 to 7 inches provide tripping hazards; outside risers should be no more than 4 inches high. Tread width can be extended for safety, but the nosing should be beveled to avoid a tripping hazard. Open risers should be closed with pieces of wood. Use a nonslip surface.

task be performed in more than one way? Can the environment be rearranged, structurally modified, or relocated? Are commercially available products appropriate, or must a custom device be designed and fabricated? Other determinants of intervention options include self-image, cultural, and family concerns as well as the actual environmental characteristics. Whether the client rents or owns the space to be modified dictates the level of the modifications possible.

The therapist should be aware of the client's economic constraints when evaluating the home or work space for modifications. Inexpensive changes may include the use of adaptive devices and rearranging the environment, while more moderate changes may involve the installation of a hand-held shower or grab bar, and costly modifications may include a major building renovation with computerized environmental control systems (Barnes, 1991).

The client should try the suggested modification or simulated set-up before the therapist implements an intervention strategy that employs the modification. Other considerations in developing an intervention program are the length of time the client will need the modifications and the potential for change in the client's condition. The client's preferences and desire to be independent should impact the selection of the intervention strategies. The goal of an environmental adaptation is to assist the client to live as independently as possible (Barnes, 1991).

References

American National Standards Institute, Inc. (1986). *American National Standard for Buildings and Facilities providing accessibility and usability for physically handicapped people.* New York: American National Standards Institute.

Americans with Disabilities Act of 1990. (Public Law 101-336). 42 USC 12101.

Antone, T. M., & Falk, R. N. (1991, March/April). Physical access. *Team Rehabilitation Report,* 27–30.

Baker & McKinzie United States Employment Law Update Legislative Bulletin. (1991, July). Chicago: Baker & McKenzie United States Employment Law Practice Group.

Barnes, K. (1991). Modification of the physical environment. In C. Baum, & C. Christiansen (Eds.), *Occupational therapy—Overcoming human performance deficits.* Thorofare, NJ: Slack.

Batavia, A., DeJong, C., Eckenhoff, E., & Materson, R. (1990). After the Americans with Disabilities Act: The role of the rehabilitation community. *Archives of Physical Medicine and Rehabilitation, 71,* 1014–1015.

Davidson, H. (1991). Assessing environmental factors. In C. Baum, & C. Christiansen (Eds.), *Occupational therapy—Overcoming human performance deficits.* Thorofare, NJ: Slack.

Ellek, D. (1991). The Americans with Disabilities Act of 1990. *American Journal of Occupational Therapy, 45*(2), 177–179.

Federal register (Vol. 49, No. 153). (1984). Washington, DC: General Services Administration, Department of Defense, Department of Housing and Urban Development, U. S. Postal Service, and the Architectural and Transportation Barriers Compliance Board.

Federal register (Vol. 53, No. 215). (1988). Washington, DC: Department of Housing and Urban Development.

Federal register (Vol. 56, No. 144). (1991). Washington, DC: Department of Housing and Urban Development.

Nugent, T. (1978). *The problem of accessibility to building for the physically handicapped.* Framington, CT: The Stanley Works.

Rogers, J. (1989). The occupational therapy home assessment: The home as a therapeutic environment. *Journal of Home Health Care Practitioners, 2*(1), 73–81.

Spencer, J. (1987). Environmental assessment strategies. *Topics in Geriatric Rehabilitation. 3*(1), 35–41.

U. S. Department of Education Clearinghouse on the Handicapped (1987). *Pocket guide to federal help for individuals with disabilities.* Washington, DC: U. S. Department of Education.

Verville, R. (1990). The Americans with Disabilities Act: An analysis. *Archives of Physical Medicine and Rehabilitation, 71,* 1010–1013.

SECTION 6

Technology

SECTION 6A
Assistive technology

BEVERLY K. BAIN

KEY TERMS

Assistive Technology	*Control Interface*
Augmentative Communication	*Environmental Control Unit*
Biofeedback	*Powered Wheelchair*
Communication Aids	*Switch*

LEARNING OBJECTIVES

Upon completion of this section the reader will be able to:

1. *Discuss the significant contribution the occupational therapist can make to the interdisciplinary rehabilitation technology team.*

2. *Discuss the theoretical foundation of occupational therapy that relates to the application of assistive technology.*

3. *Describe a technology model and the interdependence of each component.*

4. *Describe the assessment, selection, and application of various technologic assistive devices with a variety of clients.*

5. *List major suppliers of technologic devices and key resource centers.*

For most people technology makes things easier. For people with disabilities, however, technology makes things possible.

MARY PAT RADABOUGH

As society moves into the technologic age, so too does the profession of occupational therapy. Historically, occupational therapists have used adaptive equipment to enhance the functional abilities of their clients in self-care, work, and leisure. With advances in technology have come new assistive devices that can increase functional abilities and foster independence of clients of all ages at various functional levels. Technologic devices, such as motorized wheelchairs and remote **environmental control units** (ECUs), are used by physically and sensory impaired clients to perform activities of daily living not possible a decade ago; specially adapted computers and augmentative communication aids now make it possible for severely disabled, nonverbal children to participate in classrooms, for adults with impaired hand function to become gainfully employed, and for people with physical, sensory, or psychosocial disabilities to enjoy leisure-time activities in the community.

The Technology-Related Assistance for Individuals with Disabilities Act (1988) defines an **assistive technology** device as: "any item, piece of equipment, or product system, whether acquired commercially off-the-shelf, modified, or customized, that is used to increase, maintain, or improve functional capabilities of individuals with disabilities." This broad definition includes low-technology devices that can be purchased from electronic or specialty stores, such as a simple attachment to a standard lamp that allows a person in the dark to turn the lamp on with the touch of any part of the hand rather than fumbling with a hard-to-find, small switch. The definition also includes complex, high-technology devices, such as a powered, computerized wheelchair that enables a person to control the chair, turn on and off lights and appliances, use the phone, and operate a computer through one integrated system.

The knowledgeable occupational therapist can use these advanced devices to increase, maintain, and improve the functional capabilities of many clients. The competent therapist must be able to: (1) assess the client, the technologic device, and the environments in which the device will be used; (2) select with other interdisciplinary team members the most effective and cost-efficient devices to meet the client's needs and abilities; (3) train the client in the use and maintenance of the device; (4) reevaluate the client, all devices, and environments periodically; (5) contribute to the development and field testing of new devices; and (6) serve as a consultant to other professionals, clients, and caregivers.

New technologic devices are being developed daily; therefore, it is prudent for the occupational therapist to know the therapeutic concepts and principles that are built on the profession's body of knowledge because these remain constant. This section presents these concepts and principles as they apply to the treatment of various clients who use technologic devices as a part of the total habilitation or rehabilitation process.

Commercial names of specific technologic devices are not mentioned in this section because the most appropriate selection of a specific device can be made only after a thorough assessment of the client and all possible environments in which the device will be used. Usually, use of both a standard or manual aid plus an electronic or technologic device is advisable.

Examples of occupational therapy clients who can benefit from high and low technology are multiply disabled infants who can be taught to press switches, thereby learning cause and effect and how to interact with their environment; learning-disabled, school-aged children, who can be taught to use computers to enhance their verbal and written communication skills; young adults with lower-extremity paralysis, who can be taught to become independently mobile with **powered wheelchairs** and adapted vans; and elderly clients, who can be taught energy conservation and safety with the use of low-technology ECUs.

Others in the occupational therapy rehabilitation process who can benefit from technology are caregivers of people with disabilities, who can use energy-saving technologic devices such as powered wheelchairs and ECUs and who can better communicate with their clients through the use of augmentative **communication aids**. Furthermore, occupational therapists can enhance their administrative responsibilities by using computers to keep records and for scheduling. For technologic assistive devices (TADs) to become effective tools of the profession, however, their application must be based on a sound theoretical foundation and assessment methods.

Assistive technology can be viewed as a system of three integrated and interdependent components: the client; the TAD; and the environment (Figure 9-30). Each component must be evaluated in the context of the others, selected on the basis of how it interfaces with the others, and applied as it interacts with the others. Because devices are being developed so rapidly and because some are extremely expensive, the professional can no longer simply match the device to the client without consideration of the various environments in which the client may need to use the device (eg, from a bed, at school, in the workplace, or in the community). Nor can the occupational therapist think of each new device on the market as the best for all clients. Each client must be evaluated and trained from a holistic perspective, each device must be evaluated and selected by an interdisciplinary team, and both the immediate and the future environments must be considered.

The TADs addressed in this section are powered mobility, including motorized wheelchairs, scooters, and adapted vehicles; written and verbal communication aids; ECUs; and adaptations to facilitate computer access.

Therapeutic foundation

In the area of occupational therapy technology practice, the therapeutic foundation is based mainly on the following frames of reference: *biomechanical*, specifically, the work simplification and energy conservation principle; *acquisitional*, specifically

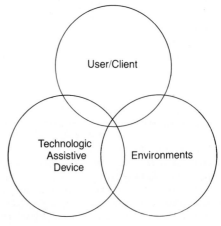

FIGURE 9-30. *The technology model.*

learning and maturation theories; and *rehabilitation*, specifically adaptations.

The biomechanical principle of work simplification and energy conservation is the therapeutic basis for teaching an accountant who has severe arthritis, for example, to reduce the stress and long hours of grasping accounting pens by using a personal computer's numeric key pad and accounting software. Word processing on the computer also simplifies the writing of reports.

The acquisitional frame of reference "provides a structure for linking learning theories, the reality aspect of purposeful activities, and the process of acquiring specific skills needed for successful interaction in the environment" (Mosey, 1986, p. 433). For example, clients with lower-extremity impairments can learn to interact successfully in their environments by learning to use powered wheelchairs and adapted vans to solve their mobility problems.

The major learning theories relevant to the occupational therapy process include classical conditioning, operant conditioning, and social or imitational conditioning. When teaching a client to use a TAD, the therapist may use one learning theory or a combination. For example, an augmentative communication aid is prescribed for a nonverbal person who might randomly press various keys on the aid. If that person accidentally strikes a certain key and hears the communication aid speak the word *food*, and if the person strikes the key again and the response is repeated, the person has learned through classical Pavlovian conditioning that pressing a designated key gives a definite response. That person can further learn, through operant conditioning, that to strike a series of keys (receiving positive reinforcement each time) expresses the desire to have lunch because the synthesized voice says, "I want to eat lunch now." Furthermore, this person may learn through social imitation that the preferred way to ask for lunch is to use the augmentative communication device rather than pounding on the table or making grunting noises.

The rehabilitation frame of reference is closely associated with the therapeutic application of adaptive equipment and adaptations of the environment to compensate for physical and sensory impairments or deficits. TADs are a new dimension of adaptive equipment, and through the application of devices such as computers, power wheelchairs, and ECUs, many environments require fewer adaptations. Technology is congruent with the philosophic assumption that "rehabilitation must be dynamic and keep in step with both scientific advances and changes in society" (Hopkins & Smith, 1983, p. 135). Another principle of the rehabilitative approach is the commitment "to the restoration of the disabled to a life that is purposeful and satisfying, one that allows each individual the opportunity to function . . . as a member of society with the capabilities to meet the responsibilities of that society" (Licht, 1983, p. 135).

Based on these assumptions, an occupational therapy treatment program for a severely involved client with a C4 quadriplegia, for example, would be to teach the person to use an ECU to compensate for the lack of hand manipulative skills; a power wheelchair to foster independent mobility; and a computer to increase possible educational, avocational, and vocational activities, enabling the client to be involved in a community. In addition, the treatment process may include technologic adaptations of the home, school, and workplace environments to help the client to live a more purposeful and satisfying life.

These are only a few examples of how technology and the basic occupational therapy therapeutic foundations relate to each other. The domain of concern for the profession—the occupational performances of activities of daily living, school, work, and play, leisure, and recreation activities—can be enhanced through the application of assistive technology. As has been previously stated, ECUs, powered wheelchairs, computers, and augmentative communication devices can increase a client's function. In addition, the client's motor, sensory, cognitive, psychological, and social abilities must be carefully evaluated before the therapist selects or uses any technologic device. For example, each TAD must be activated, which requires some form of motor function (this can be in the form of pressing a switch, blinking an eye, or saying a command); each device has some form of feedback, which is usually visual or auditory, requiring sensory integration; and each device requires a certain amount of cognitive ability, such as learning sequencing in word processing on the computer. In addition, the client must be motivated to use the equipment for any device to be effective. If successfully employed, however, technologic devices can help clients with disabilities to become participating members of society, with the ability to speak, be mobile, participate in school, seek employment, and be content and safe in their homes and in the community.

Further substantiating the therapeutic foundation of technology in the practice of occupational therapy, the definition of *occupational therapy* provided by the American Occupational Therapy Association (1981) is as follows: "Occupational therapy is the use of purposeful activity . . . in order to maximize independence, prevent disability and maintain health" (1981, p. 798). The purpose of assistive technology is to direct clients and make it possible for them to participate in many more purposeful tasks, which in turn can lead to restoration and improvement of their functional abilities.

Occupational therapy's fundamental concern is ensuring the client's capacity throughout the lifespan to perform with satisfaction those tasks and roles essential to productive living and to the mastery of self and environment. TADs can be used throughout the lifespan; for example, infants at risk can operate toys that allow them to interact and learn from the environment, and the elderly can use powered scooters and ECUs to increase their independence in performing tasks safely. Technology, however, is one tool of the profession and should not be considered the only solution. Rather, technology provides an extension of the abilities of selected clients treated by a reflective therapist who has thoroughly assessed the various TADs and the environments in which the individuals will use them.

Assessment of clients, TADs, and environments

A holistic assessment of the client, various TADs, and possible environments in which the devices will be used is a primary responsibility of the occupational therapist. A structured assessment is necessary in view of the number of available devices, the increasing number of clients being referred to occupational therapy for these aids, and the price range of different devices. Today's professional can no longer randomly match the latest device on the market with every client but must systemically evaluate each client's functional need for each device and all possible environments in which the client will use the device.

A valid technologic assessment should be a collaborative team effort that includes the client, physician, occupational therapist, physical therapist, rehabilitation engineer, speech pathologist, social worker, teacher, vendor, and caregiver. The trained occupational therapist contributes valuable and unique professional skills to the assessment team: the ability to assess clients with disabilities in all performance components and the ability to analyze tasks required to successfully use a TAD. Most devices are activated by switches; therefore, the optimal *control sites*, which are the anatomic parts of the body that are used to activate the switches, can best be determined by a therapist who evaluates a client's motor abilities. For example, a client who has a deficit in motor coordination of the upper and lower extremities may use as the control site the head or neck or eye motion to activate the switches that propel the powered wheelchair. In addition, the therapist must evaluate the client's spatial and depth perception abilities as well as cognitive ability. Furthermore, an experienced therapist is cognizant of the psychological implications that adaptive equipment may have on a client and can determine when to best introduce TADs into the treatment program. For severely involved clients who require complex technology systems, the primary occupational therapist (1) gathers data about the client's background and needs, (2) evaluates the client's abilities, and (3) relates this information to a occupational therapy technology specialist. The specialist should (1) have knowledge of and experience with various devices, (2) evaluate the client with several devices before recommending the appropriate TAD, (3) continue to evaluate both the client and TAD system during the training process, (4) teach the client all applications and maintenance of the TAD, and (5) be responsible for the integration of all technologic and standard equipment that the client requires.

In settings in which off-the-shelf technologic devices are used, the certified occupational therapy assistant, consulting with a specialist, is able to follow through with the application of the TAD and report when reevaluation of the client or TAD or when maintenance of the TAD is required.

A structured assessment instrument has been developed and field tested with various populations, including severely physically disabled adults and children, sensory-impaired adults, and clients with developmental disabilities (for a complete description and a copy of the form, see Bain, 1989). The primary areas to consider in the problem-solving approach to the assessment of clients for TADs by the entry-level therapist are presented in this section, with specific guidelines for switches, powered wheelchairs, augmentative communication aids, ECUs, and adapted computers.

The four major areas of assessment of clients for TADs are (1) data collection of the client's background and needs, (2) evaluation of client's abilities, (3) planning with the client, caregivers, and rehabilitation team members, and (4) selection of appropriate TADs that will enhance the client's functional abilities throughout the day and in a variety of environments. As with all assessments for any assistive or adaptive equipment, a problem-solving approach is essential. The following guidelines have proved to be effective:

- What are the client's needs and goals?
- What are the client's abilities?
- What TAD(s) would be appropriate based on the client's needs, goals, and abilities, considering: (1) the input, throughput, output, and display characteristics; (2) the commercial availability of a TAD or the adaptability of a commer-

cial TAD; (3) safety and reliability; (4) practicality; and (5) affordability.
- Where will the TAD be used? (Consider all present and possible future environments.)
- Based on the evaluation of the client, the TAD, and the environments in which the TADs will be used, various TADs should be tried with the client. (Most vendors and manufacturers of TADs will lend therapists equipment on a trial basis).
- Where can the TAD be ordered, and will it need to be adapted?
- Who will train the client to use the device, and how many treatment sessions will be required?
- Who will document the assessment, and where?
- Who and when should the client, TAD, and environment be reevaluated? (See Table 9-13 for details.)

These guidelines may be modified to meet the clinical setting and the qualifications of the rehabilitation technology team members. Many sites will not have all members of the desired team, and frequently the occupational therapist will be responsible for the coordination of the team assessment.

In summary, a few words of caution should be noted: Technologic devices are usually ordered only once, some are expensive, and many times they are discarded or underused. Therefore, a precise, structured assessment of each part of the system is worthy of professional time and effort, often requiring two or more sessions. Also, the clinical judgment of the therapist and members of the rehabilitation team should take precedence over the salesmanship of vendors or manufacturers, who may try to influence the selection of devices. The best assistive device is the one that best facilitates the client's functional abilities. It may be an expensive, high-technology, integrated system, or it may be an affordable, low-technology, single piece of equipment. In either case, the decision must be based on clinical knowledge of the entire team, which includes the client and caregiver.

Switches, control interfaces, and input devices

Each TAD system has four parts: (1) the input, known as the **switch** or **control interface**, which activates the device, (2) the throughput, which is the processing unit of the device, (3) the output, which is the result of a successful operation, and (4) the display, which is the visual, auditory, or tactile feedback that informs the operator that the system is activated. When one turns on a light by pushing or twisting a switch (input), the electric current in the building is the throughput and the light turning on is the output and also the visual display. When operating a flashlight, the battery is the throughput and the red light indicating the on button is the display.

Switches enable people with disabilities to interact with their environment, to increase functional activities, and to extend their capabilities. The purpose of switches is to control devices, therefore, in the technology literature, they are usually referred to as control interfaces. It has often been said that the most magnificent technologic device or the simplest toy is underused or useless if the person cannot efficiently operate it; it can also be the most frustrating experience for the client, caregiver,

TABLE 9-13. *Steps in a Problem-Solving Approach to the Assessment of Clients for Technological Assistive Devices (TADs)*

Steps	Part of System	Problem	Action
1.	Client	Identify needs and goals Communication Mobility Environmental controls Computer adaptation Switch or control interface	Review records Interview clients, caregivers, and family Observation
2.	Client	Identify abilities in lying, sitting, and standing positions	Formal testing Motor Manual muscle test, reflexes, range of motion Coordination Endurance Sensory Psychosocial Cognitive Social Interview Observation
3.	TAD	Based on 1 & 2, identify possible devices	Characteristics Input, processing, output, display Commercial availability Safety and reliability Practicality Affordability
4.	Environment	Present and future Bed Home Institution Community	Interview Observation On-site visits
5.	All	Trial period	Try various devices in a variety of environments
6.	TAD	Selection	Order, adapt, or fabricate
7.	Client	Application	Train in use and maintenance
8.	All	Documentation	Record in departmental and institutional records
9.	All	Reevaluation	Periodically reevaluate client, TAD, and environment

and therapist. Thus, the therapist must be certain that the client can readily and efficiently activate the switch or control interface.

Because the switch selection and mounting system of TADs are usually the responsibility of the occupational therapist, the therapist should first evaluate several control sites to determine the most accurate, reliable, and efficient movement that the client can make (Wright & Nomura, 1990). Next, the therapist determines the proper mounting system for the switch, which depends on both *where* the switch will be used and *what* devices it will interface with. For example, an ECU or augmentative communication aid needs to be controlled when the user is in bed as well as when the user is in a wheelchair. The trend toward integrated technology systems warrants the use of one switch to control many TADs.

The technology specialist should be able to select several possible control sites where the client demonstrates purposeful movement by reviewing the physical abilities assessment, by interviewing the client, and by observing the client's voluntary motion in various environments. Almost any part of the body can be used as the optimal control site; for severely involved clients, this may be the head, eyes, tongue, chin, toes, breath, or voice as well as the leg or foot.

A wide variety of switches and control interfaces are available commercially, and some can be readily fabricated by the therapist, other clients, family members, or caregivers. The most commonly used switches include (1) mechanical switches, such as joysticks, cushions, treadles, rockers, and pneumatic switches, such as sip and puff switches; (2) electromagnetic switches, such as light-beam infrared switches, LED detectors, and optical head-pointers; (3) electromyographic switches, such as those used to control myoelectric prostheses; and (4) sonic switches, such as ultrasound and voice switches that convert sound levels to switch closure. Different disabilities require different types of switches. A client with a spinal cord injury who has limited motion and muscle power requires a sensitive switch (sip and puff), whereas a client with poor gross motor control may require a strong pressure switch with individual slots to restrict inadvertent selections.

Single, dual, and multiple switches are used to operate technical aids: for a simple on/off toy, a single cushion switch may be used; for an ECU that requires scanning and then selection, a dual pneumatic switch may be needed; for a power wheelchair that moves in many directions, a multiple joystick may be required (Table 9-14).

Switches operate in momentary or latching modes. A momentary switch activates the device only as long as pressure or contact is being applied—for example, a car horn, an electric bed switch, or a power wheelchair switch. A latching switch requires one motion to turn on the device, which remains on until the switch is reactivated, disengaging the latch to the off position—for example, a wall light switch or the on/off switch of a computer.

Switches act as the interface between the person and the device; they activate or deactivate the device and also control the device by direct selection, scanning, or certain encoding techniques. Direct selection is the most frequently used and efficient selection technique. It can require more motor control than scanning, which requires higher cognitive and visual tracking skills. The two types of scanning are linear scanning, whereby each element is sequentially pointed to, and row or column scanning, whereby the row or column is selected first, followed by linear scanning of each element in the selected row or column. The latter technique reduces time and effort. Encoding can be used with both direct selection and scanning techniques and usually requires multiple selections, such as Morse code. Encoding is an abbreviated or accelerated selection technique. When recommending a switch or control interface, the therapist should take into consideration which selection technique will be used for each device to integrate the total assistive technology system. For example, many ECUs and augmentative communication aids require scanning techniques, but some powered wheelchairs do not; therefore, whenever possible, all devices should be integrated to use the same switches or control interfaces with a compatible selection technique.

TABLE 9-14.   *Switch or Control Interface Comparison Chart*

Number of Switches or Control Interfaces Name	Single Treadle	Dual Pneumatic	Multiple Joystick
Operational Features			
Activation	Light-to heavy pressure	Blowing and puffing	touch
Force required	Can be graded	Breath minimal	Can be graded
Feedback: T, tactile; A, auditory; V, visual	T/A		T/A
Momentary	✔		✔
Latching		✔	
Size of contact surface	1/4 to 3 inches	Straw	1 to 2 1/2 inches
Connecter type	1/8 inch mini phone	Stereo mini phone	9-pin DIN
Selection Technique			
Direct selection	✔		✔
Scanning		✔	✔
Encoding		✔	✔
Mounting			
Flexible (gooseneck)	✔	✔	
On body	✔		✔
Universal	✔		✔
Other	Head band	Caterpillar	Chin
Interface with			
Augmentative communication	✔	✔	✔
Computer	✔	✔	✔
ECU/telephone	✔	✔	✔
Powered wheelchair	✔	✔	✔
Cars and vans			✔
Other (eg, toy)	✔		✔

In communication, speed is an important factor and should be taken into account when choosing the appropriate technical aid. For instance, a client using a picture communication board who wishes to convey the desire for a glass of water can indicate that desire by pointing directly to the appropriate picture on the board. If the client is using a more complex communication board that has letters of the alphabet in rows of eight letters per row, however, the client may point first to the third row, where the letter *w* appears, then to each letter in that row until *w* is selected. When the message sender can reduce the effort and time it takes to make a selection, the communication becomes more effective. An example of the increased communication speed of high technology might be a computerized communication aid that has been programmed so that when a nonverbal client points to two or three icons, the computerized voice says, "I want a drink of water, please." This communication aid has switch encoding selection ability, whereby one or more symbols, letters, or words can be coded to convey a complete phrase or sentence.

Most switches require some form of mounting to keep the switch within reach and to allow for effective operation. Some switches can be kept in place on table tops, wheelchair trays, or bed rails using Velcro with adhesive backing or clamps. Other switches may require a switch clamp, a single or multiple joint mounting arm, and a mounting clamp. There are rigid, stainless steel, tubular mounting arms or flexible gooseneck or caterpillar arms. Switches can also be mounted directly on the client's head or chin or worn on the client's chest. A rehabilitation engineer may assist the therapist if a customized mounting system is necessary.

The variety of available interface systems and the range in prices warrant that a therapist check various suppliers' catalogs, carefully evaluate the client's abilities and all the environments where the switch will be used, and integrate the switch and mounting system with other equipment that the client may use. A primary consideration when selecting a control interface always should be the client's position in lying or sitting so as not to elicit reflexes or poor posture. If a complex system is used, the occupational therapist should draw a diagram or take pictures of the system so that all caregivers mount the switch correctly.

Because switches that control interfaces are critical to the operation of most TADs, the guidelines presented in the display are suggested to facilitate the therapist selection. In summary, it should be noted that (1) the selection of the switch or control interface is crucial to the operation of all assistive devices, (2) the occupational therapist is primarily responsible for selecting the switch and mounting system, but collaboration with other team members is essential, and (3) one switch or control interface system should be selected to integrate all the clients assistive devices.

Augmentative communication

The two basic areas of communication are verbal or conversational and written. Historically, the occupational therapist and the classroom teacher screened, evaluated, and trained children in the area of written communication. Today, there is an increasing use of the computer as a writing and drawing aid for the physically impaired. This section focuses on verbal communication and the vital role of the occupational therapist in collaborating with the speech pathologist, who is usually the technology coordinator of augmentative communication aids. The term ***augmentative communication*** is defined as "some way of communicating that does not require speech" (Trace Reprint #7, 1990); this may be through gesturing, facial expressions, body or sign language, or use of picture-letter-word boards, commonly known as communication boards. When a physically impaired client lacks the motor ability to convey a message, an adaptive or augmentative communication system is required. An effective speech system includes both standard nonelectronic and electronic aids. The most frequently used nonelectronic communication system requires the user or communication partner to point to choices to convey messages. Pointing by the user may be done with the hand, a head pointer, a light beam pointer, or with the eyes. An electronic augmentative communication system uses a form of electronic technology as the throughput. The input can be a single pressure switch, a dual rocker-lever switch, a joystick, an optical pointer, a keyboard, an eye-blinking switch, or any other control interface that is properly mounted and readily

GUIDELINES FOR SWITCH OR CONTROL INTERFACE SELECTION

1. Establish the optimal position for the client, noting all other functions, especially activities of daily living.
2. Determine with what TADs the client needs the switch to interface (toy, wheelchair, ECU, communication aid, computer, or others).
3. Evaluate the client's abilities, considering the senorimotor, cognitive, and psychosocial components (voluntary control, action, range of motion, endurance, speed of response, vision, etc.).
4. Note all precautions (seizures, respiration, fatigue, other).
5. Discuss with the client and/or significant others their thoughts, opinions, and desires.
6. Test the client for two or three possible control sites by observing, formal testing, interviewing, and reviewing the initial assessment (if client cannot communicate, be sure to observe all voluntary motions that are accurate, reliable, and efficient).
7. Evaluate the switch operational features: activation, force requirements, distance switch must travel, size of the control surface, durability, feedback, connector type, and momentary or latching mode (see comparison chart).
8. Analyze the selection technique required by the TAD (direct selection, scanning, or encoding).
9. Determine where the switch will be used (in bed, on wheelchair, at a workstation, or other).
10. Mount the switch temporarily. *Do not hold the switch.*
11. Try the switch with a temporary mounting; if this is not successful, try another switch or change the mounting; if successful, mount the switch permanently and note the position in writing (draw a picture) so all caregivers will be informed.
12. Reevaluate periodically.

delivery of electronic communication, the four substantial contributions of the occupational therapist are (1) the holistic evaluation of the clients, including physical abilities (eg, seating and positioning, range of motion, coordination, reflexes) and cognitive and perceptual abilities; (2) evaluating and recommending the most effective control interface and selection technique; (3) training the client to access the aid; and (4) collaborating with other team members (Angelo & Smith, 1989; Fishman, 1987). The speech therapist usually determines the client's communication needs, assesses the client's language ability, collaborates in the selection of an aid, and trains the client and major communication partners. Other professional members of the team may include a physician, who is required to sign orders for equipment; a social worker, who may counsel the client and family; a rehabilitation engineer, who may modify the control interface and mounting system; the vendor or manufacturer, who designs and produces the electronic aid; and the special education teacher, who is responsible for language development and implementation of the aid in the school setting. To be effective, this professional team must work closely with the nonverbal client and the client's communication partners.

As with all TADs, the optimal approach to augmentative communication aids includes the following: (1) the aid meets the client's needs, (2) the client, various aids, and all environments in which the aids will be used are carefully evaluated, (3) the selection is a result of the collaboration of the rehabilitation technology team members, (4) a back-up, standard nonelectronic aid is also available to the client, and (5) the augmentative communication aid can be integrated with all other assistive devices. The occupational therapy technology specialist needs to be aware of various aids. A comprehensive list of commercially available aids is found in the *Rehab Education ResourceBook I*, which contains descriptions and photographs (Brandenburg & Vanderheiden, 1987). In addition, speech pathologists, manufacturers, and vendors are available for in-services, workshops, and training institutes where the therapist can access knowledge in this area. The occupational therapist needs to know what equipment is available and what are the control interfaces. The speech pathologist is responsible for evaluating the client's language communication ability.

Powered mobility

For most people, mobility is the function that enhances their independence and quality of life; for the physically impaired, individual powered mobility is the assistive device that liberates the person to move about the home environment and into the community. Various powered mobility aids are available; the most frequently used are the three-wheeled, battery-powered scooters, adapted vehicles, and powered wheelchairs.

A scooter requires the user to have good sitting balance, good eye–hand coordination, adequate spatial and figure-ground perception, and good judgment. Therefore, the user must be carefully evaluated (Warren, 1990). Scooters can be used in conjunction with walkers, canes, or standard wheelchairs in the home, workplace, or when traveling in the community by people who have limited stamina.

Adapted cars and vans are another source of powered mobility for the physically impaired, including those with limited function of both lower and upper extremities, one arm and one

accessible to the user. The output can be synthesized speech, visual display, printed copy, or a combination of these.

The key characteristics of any communication system are (1) the rate or speed that a message can be conveyed, (2) portability of the aid, (3) its accessibility to the user in various positions, (4) dependability of both manual and electronic power sources, (5) quality of the output, (6) durability, (7) independence of the user, (8) vocabulary flexibility (programmable or fixed), and (9) the time required for repairs and maintenance of the aid (Fishman, 1987; Vanderheiden, 1984; Webster, Cook, Tompkins, & Vanderheiden, 1985). All these characteristics should be considered by the rehabilitation technology team when screening and evaluating the client, selecting the appropriate aid so that it can be interfaced with other equipment, training the client to maximize the application of the aid, and evaluating the system as the client's needs change (Angelo & Smith, 1989; Fishman, 1987).

To deliver the appropriate augmentative communication services to a client requires team cooperation. In the service

leg, restricted joint motion, or absence of lower extremities. Scrupulous evaluation must be done by the occupational therapist and the driving specialist before the client is trained and issued a license. In most clinics, the primary occupational therapist evaluates the client's strength, range of motion, eye–hand coordination, and cognitive and perceptual abilities; the driving specialist performs both simulated and on-the-road training. Driving standards for people with disabilities have been established by the Veterans Administration and most state motor vehicle agencies. Driver training is a specialty area that requires additional training, certification, and experience and is beyond the scope of this section.

The entry-level therapist should be aware of various vehicle adaptations, including proportional steering and hand controls, braking systems and safety back-up systems, auxiliary control boxes, and hydraulic lifts. Vans with lifts are the preferred means of transportation because powered wheelchairs with batteries can weigh between 225 and 250 lb and can carry people who weigh up to 250 lb. Lifts can conserve energy and the time required to transfer a person into a car and push or disassemble the powered wheelchair before placing it into a car. The independence and opportunities gained by a person who is able to drive to attend school, work, and recreational activities must be considered in perspective with the safety of the client and others on the road.

The occupational therapist is a valuable member of the rehabilitation technology team that selects and then trains severely impaired clients who need powered wheelchairs. The clients most frequently referred for powered wheelchairs are high-level spinal cord injury clients with C4 and above involvement; clients with advanced muscle weakness due to such diseases as amyotrophic lateral sclerosis, multiple sclerosis, or muscular dystrophy; and clients with poor coordination in all extremities, such as those with cerebral palsy. Clients of all ages who have to travel long distances and tire readily usually need a powered wheelchair; however, they will also need a standard wheelchair as a back-up when their powered chair is being repaired and for those times when a powered chair cannot be transported. Since 1980, an increasing number of young children have been referred for powered mobility, but always with two main concerns: safety for the user and others and the potential adverse effects on the child's physical development. There is limited research on the effects of power mobility on the child, but specialists agree that a comprehensive evaluation of each child's proper positioning and cognitive and perceptual development and of all possible environments where the chair will be used is crucial (Barnes, 1991; Jaffe, 1987; Warren, 1990).

Members of the rehabilitation technology team most responsible for determining the optimal powered wheelchair system are the occupational therapist, physical therapist, rehabilitation engineer, manufacturer or vendor, family members or caregivers, and social service professionals. The occupational therapist has a vital role in evaluating the client holistically, collaborating on the selection of a powered wheelchair system, verifying the wheelchair prescription with the user, training the user and caregivers, and following up periodically, especially as children grow and as adults' physical conditions change. The user's primary therapist and the occupational therapy technology specialist can collaborate on the holistic evaluation of the client; positioning; physical abilities to access the control interface; cognitive ability to follow instructions and use judgment;

perceptual skills, especially spatial relations and figure-ground perception; and user motivation. Proper positioning is the key to successful use of any TAD. It is therefore necessary for the occupational therapist to collaborate with the physical therapist, seating specialist, and caregivers. The technology specialist must also assess the user's optimal control site because power mobility, more than any other TAD, necessitates accuracy, reliability, and efficiency. In addition, the technology specialist is usually responsible for trying and recommending the switch and mounting system and for collaborating on a detailed wheelchair prescription.

Most wheelchair vendors have worksheets or prescription forms that are completed at a wheelchair clinic or by the coordinator in conjunction with other team members. It is imperative that the rehabilitation technology team work with a reliable, reputable, dependable vendor who will service the powered chair after it is purchased. Once the chair has been delivered, the therapist should carefully check each part against the prescription before training the user. Depending on the age, cognitive ability, and physical function of the user, training sessions may vary. Some powered wheelchairs are equipped with augmentative communication aids, ECUs, and computer interfaces; therefore, an integrated control system is advisable. This requires additional training by the therapist or other team members. In addition to training the user with the controls, the therapist should train the user in various environments, including on rough and smooth surfaces, indoors and outdoors, on inclines and declines, in large and small spaces (most powered wheelchairs have a turning radius of 30 inches), and in different climatic conditions.

The occupational therapist is qualified to assess architectural barriers in the user's home, school, work, and community. With the passage of the Americans with Disabilities Act (ADA) (1990), there should be an increase in public accommodations, public transportation, and employment opportunities for people with disabilities.

In addition to evaluating the user and the environments, the occupational therapy technology specialist should carefully assess the numerous powered wheelchairs available. Some have power that allows the user to stand, some allow the user to stand and move about, and one can climb stairs. The power base is the first portion of the chair that is selected, with special consideration given to types of battery (led or gel); safety brakes; any additional powered equipment, such as communication aids or powered recliners; ventilation; and phrenic nerve stimulator platforms. Next, the therapist needs to select the control method: proportional or nonproportional, momentary or latching systems. The control interfaces most frequently used are proportional joysticks, with fingertip, chin, lip, or tongue control; pneumatic (sip and puff control); and scanning, with four single switches attached to a headrest. Almost any part of the body can be used to control a wheelchair. Recently, microprocessors have been integrated into wheelchair control systems, which allows the rate and degree of control to be programmed according to the users motor abilities. Microprocessors also allow the client to operate the ECU through the same control system; therefore, it is necessary to select the ECU that is compatible with the powered chair by checking with the manufacturer and reading the literature carefully.

In conclusion, powered mobility can enhance the opportunity for severely and not so severely impaired clients to become self-reliant, to pursue employment, and to participate in the community. Usually, a standard wheelchair is also required.

Environmental controls

The ECU is the TAD for which the occupational therapist is mainly responsible; the occupational therapist undertakes the evaluation, selection, client training, and application of the ECU. An ECU is defined as:

> a means to purposefully manipulate and interact with the environment by alternately accessing one or more electrical devices via switches, voice activation, remote control, computer interface, and other technologic adaptations. The purpose of an ECU is to maximize functional ability and independence in the home, school, work, and leisure environment. (Bain, DiSalvi, Gold, Kollodge, & Schein, 1991, p. 55)

In the past 5 years, there has been a technology explosion in commercially available, convenient, remote controls for television, lights, telephones, emergency calls, door locks and openers, temperature regulators, and other appliances in the home and workplace. Currently, there are over 30 ECU systems: some are simple systems that control two or three appliances; others are more complex and control over 200 appliances; some can be integrated with augmentative communication aids, wheelchairs, computers, and telephones. For the person with poor hand manipulation skills, ECUs can be operated by switches; for the person with low physical stamina, tasks can be completed with greater speed and less energy; for the person with pulmonary and cardiac complications who needs constant monitoring, an ECU can be a safety device; and for the caregiver, an ECU saves time and energy by increasing client self-reliance, self-confidence, and independence. ECUs can be used by clients of all ages with various levels of function. Some require limited cognitive ability, while others require problem-solving, sequencing, memory, and concept formation abilities. Most ECUs have auditory, visual, or tactile feedback and therefore enable successful application for clients with sensory or motor impairment.

Each ECU consists of the four standard TAD parts: input, which can include buttons on the device, various switches, computer command, or voice activation; throughput, which can be operated by means of batteries, household current, or household current plus a module, radio waves, or infrared; feedback, which can include the response of the device; and output, which is sometimes referred to as the action of the appliances or peripheral.

The assessment of a client for an ECU begins with an evaluation of the client's needs and functional abilities; next, all environments where the ECU will be used must be considered, especially to determine if a portable system is required. Assessment of the ECU should include the access method, feedback requirements, integration with other equipment; expandability for future use; flexibility (eg, adjustable rate and method of scanning); installation; and cost (see the display on pages 334 to 348).

Because ECUs are rarely covered by funding agencies, another responsibility for the occupational therapist working in conjunction with the social worker and family is to find funding for the ECU system that best meets the clients needs. Sometimes this may mean beginning with an affordable ($50 to $100), off-the-shelf unit purchased by the family or friends and then pro-

gressing to a more comprehensive system as funding becomes available.

When requesting funding for ECUs, rehabilitation technology team members need to include in their calculations the hours and cost of attendant care that will be saved when the client can be independent because of the ECU. At present, there is not sufficient data to validate this savings, and therapists must research this area. The occupational therapist can wisely spend time by searching electrical specialty shops and trade magazines and by attending workshops on affordable off-the-shelf ECUs.

Other important factors to consider when prescribing an ECU are its safety features, its durability, and the reliability of the manufacturer. It is frustrating to the client, caregivers, and therapist when the system needs constant repairs or when the manufacturer is not reliable. A classification system was developed to help the occupational therapist and client select the appropriate ECU (see the display on page 339).

Telephones

Telephones mean safety as well as convenience and leisure for people with disabilities. Numerous technologic telephone advances have been made that benefit people with hearing, speaking, visual, and motor impairments. These include the following. For the visually impaired, there are telephones with enlarged numbers as well as enlarged stick-on numbers that can be applied to any phone. In addition, telephone bills can be printed in braille. Another useful aid for the visually impaired and for people with motor impairments is to dial the operator, who will then assist by dialing the complete number. For people who need assistance dialing 0, there is an overlay that fits over the buttons and requires only a gross motion to push down the 0 button. Other telephone aids for people with motor impairment include telephones that can be controlled by switches or interfaced with an ECU; portable, lightweight headset telephones; telephones with four-button emergency attachments; memory storage; battery back-up; conference calls; and redial capabilities. For people with weak voice quality, there are telephones that amplify the voice; and for those with poor voice volume, there are electronic artificial larynxes.

Great advances have been made in technology to increase the telephone capabilities of people with hearing impairments and those who are deaf. The hearing impaired can attach small amplifiers to any handsets or purchase a handset with adjustable amplification built-in. Deaf or speech-impaired people can call person-to-person to another deaf person or to anyone, anytime of the day, any day of the year, through the use of a telecommunications device for the deaf and the telephone company dual relay system (check your local telephone directory for details). Section IV of the ADA ensures that interstate and intrastate telecommunications relay services will be available to hearing- and speech-impaired people within 1 year of enactment of the law.

Monitoring systems

Personal response systems are technologic devices that are worn or carried by people who wish to live alone or who are left alone, such as the frail elderly, physically disabled people, or children who are old enough to care for themselves after school but who need help if there is an emergency. These devices can be acti-

(*Text continues on page 338*)

ENVIRONMENTAL CONTROL SYSTEMS NEEDS ASSESSMENT

CLIENT NAME: _____ **AGE:** _____ **SEX:** _____

DIAGNOSIS/DATE OF ONSET: _____

REASON FOR REFERRAL: _____

1. DEVICES TO BE CONTROLLED:

DEVICES	QUANTITY	LOCATION/COMMENTS
Call Bell		
Emergency Call System		
Telephone		
Intercom		
Bed		
Television		
VCR		
Stereo		
Radio		
Tape Recorder		
Light		
Fan		
Temperature		
Computer		
Page Turner		
Door Opener		
Door Lock		

COMMENTS:

(continued)

ENVIRONMENTAL CONTROL SYSTEMS NEEDS ASSESSMENT (*continued*)

2. ENVIRONMENTS AND LOCATIONS WHERE ECU WILL BE UTILIZED:

	WHEELCHAIR	BED	WORK STATION	OTHER:
Home				
Institution				
School				
Work				
Other				

LOCATIONS (column group header over WHEELCHAIR, BED, WORK STATION, OTHER)

COMMENTS:

3. ACCESS METHOD:

ACCESS METHOD	CLIENT POSITIONING		COMMENTS:
	SUPINE	SITTING	
Direction Selection			
Scanning			
Encoding			

4. DOES THE CLIENT REQUIRE FEEDBACK?   [ ] Yes [ ] No

TYPE OF FEEDBACK	SWITCH	ECU SYSTEM	COMMENTS:
Auditory			
Visual			
Tactile		N/A	

5. DOES THE SYSTEM NEED TO BE INTEGRATED WITH OTHER EQUIPMENT?

[ ] Yes [ ] No   If yes, with what other devices?

EQUIPMENT	MANUFACTURER/MODEL
Wheelchair	
Computer	
Communication Aid	
Other:	

COMMENTS:

(*continued*)

ENVIRONMENTAL CONTROL SYSTEMS NEEDS ASSESSMENT (*continued*)

6. **EXPANDABILITY FOR FUTURE USE:**

A. **WHAT ARE THE CLIENT'S GOALS**

Vocationally:

Avocationally:

Educationally:

B. **MEDICAL STATUS: (PROGNOSIS/POTENTIAL FOR IMPROVEMENT)**

7. **FUNDING:**

ADDITIONAL COMMENTS:

ENVIRONMENTAL CONTROL SYSTEMS LEVEL COMPARISON CHART

CONTROL SYSTEMS	LEVEL			
OPERATIONAL FEATURES:				
Numbers of Inputs				
Type of Access: Direct Selection				
Scanning				
Encoding				
Feedback: Visual				
Auditory				
FUNCTIONAL CAPABILITIES:				
# of 110 V AC on/off line receptables on base unit				
# of low V control circuits				
# of plug-in modules (ie, X–10, ultrasound)				
Momentary				
Latching				
Low V peripheral control (examples): Nurse call				
Intercom				
Electric bed				
TV channel selector				
Radio channel changer				
Page turner				
Other				
Telephone Control: Direct dial				
Operator assist				
Redial				
# of Memory locations				
Battery back-up				
Other				
FLEXIBILITY:				
Adjustable rate of scan				
Adjustable method of scan				
Interface with various switches				

(*continued*)

ENVIRONMENTAL CONTROL SYSTEMS LEVEL COMPARISON CHART (*continued*)

Access by caretaker				
User programmable				
Integrate with: Augmentative/Alternative Communication				
Wheelchair				
Computer				
Remote control transmission				
INSTALLATION:				
Hard wiring required				
Mounting hardware available				
COST: (1991)				

Adapted from Environmental Control Systems: Assessment, Selection, and Training *by B. K. Bain, M. DiSalvi, J. Gold, B. Kollodge, & R. Schein, 1991. Paper presented at 1991 AOTA Annual Conference, Cincinnati.*

vated by various switches; for severely impaired people, sip and puff, light pressure, or eyebrow switches are usually used. The switch sends a signal to a monitoring center, which then puts the user in touch with a relative, friend, neighbor, or an emergency service. Most users are linked directly to hospital monitoring centers. This device can be cost-effective in reducing nursing home or hospital stay while granting safe independence to the user and comfort to relatives who are unable to offer constant care (Joe, 1990). There are several systems throughout the United States and in many European countries; the client, therapist, and family need to evaluate each system in view of the user's needs.

Another means of monitoring people in the same house is an inexpensive (less than $50) baby monitor, which is sensitive enough to hear breathing anywhere in the house.

To summarize, historically, occupational therapists have used adaptive equipment to increase the functional capabilities of their clients; today, TADs add a new dimension to this area of practice when used in a holistic approach. The therapist must be cognizant of the client's tolerance to equipment and the psychological factor of being dependent on aids. Every effort should be made to prescribe only the ECU that will enhance the client's functional abilities and improve or maintain the client's independence. Often, the most efficient solution is for the therapist to suggest architectural changes in the environment (see Chapter 9, Section 5C).

Biofeedback

In the past 20 years, biofeedback has been used by occupational therapists in conjunction with other traditional treatment procedures for clients with physical and psychosocial dysfunction. Currently, it is being used, with special computer programs, for muscle reeducation, to reduce spasticity, for stress reduction, for

cardiovascular exercise, and to control body temperature and blood pressure. **Biofeedback** was defined by a leader in the field as "the technique of using equipment (usually electronic) to reveal to human beings some of their internal physiologic events, normal and abnormal, in the form of visual and auditory signals in order to teach them to manipulate these otherwise involuntary or unfelt events by manipulating the displayed signals" (Basmajian, 1983, p. 1).

Because the safe application of biofeedback machines requires special training, it is strongly recommended that the occupational therapist seek additional education resources, such as the American Occupational Therapy Association strategies training package. Some clients who may benefit from biofeedback are those with hand injuries, spinal cord injuries, arthritis, cerebral vascular accident, cerebral palsy, peripheral nerve injuries, cardiac arrhythmias, Raynaud's disease, and bronchial asthma. In addition to clients with these physical conditions, biofeedback may be effective for stress reduction, weight control, preventing substance abuse, and pain control. The nature of biofeedback is congruent with the philosophy of occupational therapy because the client is in control of the treatment and the therapist's role is that of a facilitator. When using biofeedback as an adjunct to therapy, the therapist must be aware of the whole client because the psychological effect of relaxation has a definite effect on the physical performance of the client (Abildness, 1988; Brown & Nahai 1983; Eakin, 1989).

Several advantages of electronic feedback are: (1) it is a natural extension of the use of verbal feedback generally given by therapists to motivate clients; (2) the feedback information is objective and can be monitored by the client, and (3) the results of each session can be used for accountable documentation of the client's treatment progress and validates reports. More specific advantages of biofeedback are: (1) electromyography feedback units are designed to detect low-functioning motor units not possible for the therapist to detect, (2) with psychiatric

CLASSIFICATIONS OF ECUs

Level I

- Devices are available off the shelf
- Devices do not require an adaptive switch
- Devices use direct selection and may be used with adaptations such as mouthstick, typing pegs, hand splints, and so forth.
- Devices offer primarily latching control, but very limited momentary control
- Devices allow control of on/off functions of appliances and lights (which can also be brightened and dimmed); includes telephones, multiple stand-alone devices, or small units that will control more than one appliance
- Devices may use infrared and radio frequency remote controls

Level II

- Devices are available through specialty equipment manufacturers
- Devices are controlled by an adaptive switch
- Devices use direct selection or scanning
- Devices offer primarily latching control
- Devices allow control of on/off functions of appliances, lights (including brightening and dimming), television, VCR, and adapted access to telephone functions
- Devices may use remote control through infrared, radio frequency, and ultrasound transmissions

Level III

- Devices are available through specialty equipment manufacturers
- Devices are controlled by an adaptive switch
- Devices use scanning, with the exception of voice activation
- Devices offer both latching and momentary control
- One system allows control of all functions of multiple devices, including full telephone and bed control
- Devices may use remote control through infrared, radio frequency, ultrasound, and telephone telemetry transmissions

Level IV

- Devices are available through specialty equipment manufacturers
- Devices are controlled by adaptive switch
- Devices use scanning
- Devices offer both latching and momentary control
- One system allows control of all functions of multiple devices, including full telephone and bed control
- Devices incorporate integration with other electrical devices such as augmentative or alternative communication aids, power wheelchair electronics, and computers using the same switch to access all functions

Level V

- Future developments integrating technology into the community

Adapted from Environmental Control Systems: Assessment, Selection, and Training *by B. K. Bain, M. DiSalvi, J. Gold, B. Kollodge, & R. Schein, 1991. Paper presented at 1991 AOTA Annual Conference, Cincinnati.*

patients, galvanic skin response can be monitored during various activities or in different situations, (3) cardiac clients can be monitored during exercise as they receive feedback alert signals and if they are exerting themselves, and (4) in pain management treatment programs, the use of drugs can be decreased as the client gains awareness of muscle and vascular tension levels (Abildness 1988; Basmajian, 1983; Brown & Nahai, 1983; Peffer, 1983; Trombly 1989).

Another area where occupational therapists are using biofeedback is with electrokinesiologic devices, such as electrogoniometers for shoulder, elbow, wrist, finger, and hip joints. These wearable biofeedback goniometers are used to monitor clients while they are performing activities in the clinic and throughout the day. The devices are calibrated to definite thresholds and are useful for evaluating range of motion, strength changes and alerting clients if they are exceeding their limits.

This is most beneficial in preventing further injury and maintaining proper joint alignment (Abildness 1988; Brown & Nahai 1983; Eakin 1989). These biofeedback goniometers have been developed and found effective with different clients in Massachusetts, Georgia, California, and Texas.

Biofeedback as an adjunct occupational therapy treatment modality has several limitations, some of which are the few trained and qualified professionals, the limited number of clinical sites that have this expensive equipment, the sparse research results, and the limited number of clients who will accept the modality and are capable of following through. The literature review shows that biofeedback was a popular treatment modality in the late 1970s and early 1980s; with the advent of its use in conjunction with the computer, a new interest may occur.

Summary

In the past 10 years, occupational therapists have learned to use assistive technology to extend the abilities of clients of all ages and with varying degrees of function. It is the intent of this section to encourage the entry-level occupational therapist and certified occupational therapy assistant to seek additional information, knowledge, skills, and competency by attending workshops, enrolling in technology courses, and networking with other professional groups.

In 1991, the American Occupational Therapy Association formed a special interest group in technology, and additional information can be obtained by contacting the Division on Practice. Another informative professional group is RESNA, the Association for the Advancement of Rehabilitation Technology. RESNA has excellent resources in the book *Assistive Technology Sourcebook* (Enders & Hall, 1990) and holds national and regional meetings once a year; in addition, some states have local groups that meet bimonthly.

As with any specialty area, assistive technology builds on the body of professional occupational therapy knowledge. It is advisable to first learn about switches and control interfaces and then to progress to an area for which your occupational therapy department or clinical site is responsible, such as toys, wheelchairs, ECUs, or computers. At first, it may seem impossible to keep up-to-date on the rapid advances in technology, but networking with occupational therapists, other professionals, and consumers is beneficial. Remember that assistive technology is one of many tools of the occupational therapy profession, and attempts should be made to avoid inappropriate application of high technologies when they are not needed and to use them only when their application is beneficial.

Assistive technology can make many tasks possible for many clients when it is based on occupational therapy therapeutic foundations, an on-going comprehensive assessment of all parts of the system, an interdisciplinary team making decisions on the selection of TADs, and the individual client's needs.

References

Abildness, A. (1988). Biofeedback. In H. L. Hopkins & H. D. Smith (Eds.), *Willard and Spackman's occupational therapy* (7th ed., pp. 346–353). Philadelphia: J. B. Lippincott.

American Occupational Therapy Association (1981). Occupational therapy definition: Representative assembly minutes. *American Journal of Occupational Therapy, 35,* 798.

Americans with Disabilities Act. (1988). (Public Law 100-366), 42, USC 12101.

Angelo, J., & Smith, R. O. (1989). The critical role of occupational therapy in augmentative communication services. In American Occupational Therapy Association, *Technology review '89: Perspectives on occupational therapy practice* (pp. 49–54) Rockville, MD: AOTA.

Bain, B. K. (1989). Assessment of clients for technological assistive devices. In American Occupational Therapy Association, *Technology review '89: Perspectives on occupational therapy practice* (pp. 55–59). Rockville, MD: AOTA.

Bain, B. K., DiSalvi, M., Gold, J., Kollodge, B., & Schein, R. (1991, June 1). *Environmental control systems: Assessment, selection, and training.* Paper presented at the 1991 AOTA Annual Conference, Cincinnati.

Barnes, K. H. (1991). Training young children for powered mobility. *Developmental Disabilities Special Interest Section Newsletter, 14,* 1–2.

Basmajian, J. V. (1983). Biofeedback treatment of foot drop after stroke compared with standard rehabilitation technique: Effects on voluntary control and strength. *Archives of Physical Medicine and Rehabilitation, 56,* 231.

Brandenburg, S. A., & Vanderheiden, G. C. (Eds.). (1987). *Rehab/education technology resourcebook series: Resourcebook 1: Communication aids.* Boston, MA: College-Hill Press.

Brown, D. M., & Nahai, F. (1983). Biofeedback strategies of the occupational therapist in total hand rehabilitation. In J. V. Basmajian (Ed.), *Biofeedback principles and practices for clinicians* (2nd. ed., pp. 90–106). Baltimore: Williams & Wilkins.

Eakin, V. S. (1989). The use of the biofeedback goniometer device in hip rehabilitation. In American Occupational Therapy Association, *Technology review '89: Perspectives on occupational therapy practice* (pp. 73–74) Rockville, MD: AOTA.

Enders, A., & Hall, M. (1990). *Assistive technology sourcebook.* Washington, DC: RESNA Press.

Fishman, I. (1987). *Electronic communication aids.* Boston, MA: College-Hill Press.

Hopkins, H. L., & Smith, H. D. (Eds.). (1983). *Willard and Spackman's occupational therapy* (6th ed.). Philadelphia: J. B. Lippincott.

If someone has a severe physical disability and can't communicate by speaking, what techniques or aids are available? (Trace Reprint #7). Madison, WI: University of Wisconsin Press.

Jaffe, K. (Ed.). (1987). *Childhood powered mobility: Developmental, technical, and clinical perspectives.* Washington, DC: RESNA.

Joe, B. E. (1990). International symposium focuses on emergency response devices. *Occupational Therapy Week, 4,* 4–5.

Licht, S. (1983). In Hopkins, S., & Smith, H. (Eds.), *Willard and Spackman's occupational therapy* (6th ed.). Philadelphia: J. B. Lippincott.

Mosey, A. C. (1986). *Psychosocial components of occupation therapy.* New York: Raven Press.

Peffer, K. E. (1983). Equipment needs for the psychotherapist. In J. V. Basmajian (Ed.), *Biofeedback principles and practice for clinicians.* (2nd ed., pp. 330–340). Baltimore: Williams & Wilkins.

Radabough, M. P. (1990). Speech given at the RESNA Conference, Washington, D.C., June 1990.

Technology-Related Assistance for Individuals with Disabilities Act (ACT). (1988). (Public Law 100-407), 29 USC 2202.

Trombly, C. A. (1989). Biofeedback as an adjunct therapy. In C. A. Trombly (Ed.), *Occupational therapy for physical dysfunction.* (3rd ed., pp. 316–327). Baltimore: Williams & Wilkins.

Vanderheiden, G. C. (1984). High and low technology approaches in the development of communication systems for severely physically handicapped persons. *Exceptional Education Quarterly, 4.4,* 40–56.

Warren, C. G. (1990). Powered mobility and its implications. In S. P. Todd (Ed.), *Choosing a wheelchair system* (pp. 74–85). Washington DC: Veterans Health Services and Research Administration.

Webster, J. G., Cook, A. M., Tompkins, W. J., & Vanderheiden, G. C. (Eds.).

(1985). *Electronic devices for rehabilitation.* New York: John Wiley & Sons.

Wright, C., & Nomura, M. (1990). *From toys to computers: Access for the physically disabled child* (2nd ed.). San Jose, CA: Wright.

SECTION 6B
Computer applications in occupational therapy

RENEE OKOYE

KEY TERMS

Administrative Support Functions	Multitasking
Analog Events	Research Functions
Communication Functions	Shell
Criteria-Referenced Guide	Software Analysis
Data	Spreadsheet
Database	Task Analysis
Data Management	Teaching Functions
Fields	Technologic Tools
Interface Devices	Treatment Documentation
Management Functions	User-Friendly
Merge Function	Word Processor

LEARNING OBJECTIVES

Upon completion of this section the reader will be able to:

1. *Define conceptual frameworks involved in the integration of computer applications.*
2. *Identify common strands of computer applications in occupational therapy.*
3. *Describe the function of a database used in clinical practice.*
4. *Design a merged document for treatment documentation.*
5. *List several common clinical problems for which computer applications can be a viable solution.*
6. *Identify key limitations to computer applications in clinical practice.*
7. *Identify domains of treatment in which computer applications can be implemented.*
8. *Describe strategies and methods for clinical implementation of computer technology in various domains of treatment.*
9. *Explain the purposes of software analysis and criteria-referenced guides for software selection.*

The purpose of this section is to provide a better understanding of how and when computer applications are indicated for use in occupational therapy. The application of computer technology to assist both administrative and clinical areas of practice is rapidly expanding. Computer technology is being applied successfully in many of our more multifaceted problem areas, such as administrative paper work, time utilization, and treatment documentation. The ability to effectively discharge all the responsibilities incorporated within the job description of the occupational therapist may well lie in an increased appreciation of how and when computer applications should be used. Many of the software programs, their modalities, and their accompanying peripheral devices offer reasonable and efficient alternatives for dealing with issues related to time and methodology that are routinely encountered in practice. The electronic marvels of computer applications are not without their pitfalls, however. It is not unusual for the therapist to become so overwhelmed by the *means* (DOS commands, database design, positioning of switches, workstation modifications, CD ROM disks, merge variables, video discs, and so forth) that the *end*—the task and its desired functional objectives—is lost.

Successful implementation of computer technology in clinical practice requires the ability to analyze and integrate three different conceptual frameworks. The first conceptual framework relates to a mechanical approach to the hardware and biomechanical aspects of access. The therapist must match the technologic equipment to the physical abilities of the end user, the patient. The second conceptual framework relates to software analysis. This framework includes not only the logical operations formatted to the screen but also the cognitive, sensory-integrative, and motor functions inherent to clinical use of the program, a therapeutic objective. The third conceptual framework is the traditional biopsychosocial orientation, from which much of our perspective of activity is derived. It is necessary to be able to integrate these conceptual frameworks and use the results as a structural matrix from which to compare the task demands of a given computer application with the abilities and needs of a specific patient. The ability to interdigitate these three conceptual frameworks in a semiautomatic manner can be likened to **multitasking**, an aspect of performance that is characteristic of a truly integrated computer system. Multitasking refers to the ability of a system to either perform different operations simultaneously or to run several different programs concurrently.

To some extent, development of multitasking abilities stemming from the rapid interdigitation of different bases used for task analysis is a natural product of occupational therapy education. The ability to apply this skill, however, to the logical problem-solving world of computer technology within the clinical theater of operations requires real-time practice. Real-time practice is needed to allow the therapist to become desensitized to the mechanics of the **technologic tools** and the logical operations of the programs involved. These technologic tools simply offer alternative means by which certain clinical objectives may be accomplished. Once desensitization to the technologic tools has occurred, generalization of previously acquired skills of task analysis can be more readily applied, and smooth transitions that incorporate computer applications as media in clinical practice can be accomplished more easily.

Computer technology offers an alternative, totally flexible, nonstructured medium with a uniquely different set of tools by which certain types of treatment objectives can be accomplished. Unlike other equipment used in occupational therapy, the computer can serve as tool, medium, and source of information management. A wide array of alternative means by which widely divergent clinical objectives may be accomplished are readily available through computer applications.

Computer applications in occupational therapy are divergent and consist of many strands. Most of these strands have evolved from differences in function and areas of practice among therapists. There are functions in occupational therapy that are similar to those of other professions, and in these functions, similarities in computer applications can be found. Administrative, teaching, and research functions are shared among many professional groups. Computer applications in these functions have little differentiation, apart from content, to distinguish them as particular to the occupational therapy profession. However, in specific areas of clinical implementation—such as in the remediation of cognitive functions, integration of sensorimotor skills, prevocational exploration, training in activities of daily living, use of the nonhuman environment, and therapeutic use of self—the distinctive factors of occupational therapy may be seen.

Although the parameters of computer technology in occupational therapy are broad, they can be seen as supporting two major strands of function. These are administrative support functions and clinical implementation functions. Other strands of function that commonly are shared by both administrative and clinical practice are functions such as management, research, and instructional applications. This section profiles strands of computer applications that support administrative, research, and clinical functions (Table 9-15).

Administrative support functions

In most instances, *administrative support functions* are no longer relegated to a computer room located deep in the bowels of the institutions where therapists work. Instead, at least one personal computer sits on a desk in the occupational therapy

---

TABLE 9-15.   *Computer Applications in Occupational Therapy*

Administrative Support Functions

Communication Functions

Treatment documentation
  Progress notes
  Treatment logs
  Evaluation summaries
Word processing
  Merged documents
  Tabulated reports
Desk-top publishing
  Articles
  Brochures
  Signs
  Floor plans
  Slide presentations
Management functions
  Scheduling
  Time management
  Databases
  Budgeting

Research Functions

Data collection
Statistical analysis
Data tabulation
  Sorting functions
  Searching functions
  Categorization of data
Spreadsheets
Graphic representation
  Circle graphs
  Bar graphs
  Line graphs
  Three-dimensional graphs

Teaching Functions

Clinical instruction
  Programmed instruction
  Basic clinical procedures
  Interactive video disks

Access libraries via modem
  Review articles and abstracts
  Perform indexed library searches
  Scan indexed bibliographies
Continuing education
  Applied sciences update
  Instruction in use of new equipment

Clinical Applications

Assessment Functions

EMG
Goniometry
Ergonometry
Cognitive functions
Application of orthotics
Seating
Work tolerance
Neuropsychological deficits
Disorders of ocular motility
Prevocational skills inventory
Access to environmental devices

Use of the Computer as a Tool or Modality for Treatment

Biofeedback
Cognitive remediation
Prevocational training
Work samples
Keyboarding
Work simulations
Behavior modification
Therapeutic exercise
Motor skills training
Event simulations
  Interviews
  Group interactions
  Family visits

office, and often at least one other is available for ***treatment documentation*** or treatment implementation in the main clinic area. The presence of computers in our offices and clinics has placed the responsibility for computer literacy, staff training, and program implementation squarely on the therapist as an administrative function.

Administrative support functions that can be appropriately and efficiently accomplished through computer applications include: (1) ***communication functions***, such as electronic mail, access to bulletin boards and databases, merge mail, treatment documentation, monthly statistics, and desk-top publishing applications; (2) ***research functions***, such as use of the computer as a tool for data collection, storage, organization, and statistical analysis as well as for computer-generated reports, charts, and graphs; (3) ***teaching functions***, such as integrated media presentations, interactive programmed instruction, rehearsal of clinical skills, library searches, and a vehicle for accessing new skills and new areas of knowledge; and (4) ***management functions***, such as scheduling and time management, budgeting, billing, departmental statistics of personnel, and patient records. All these administrative functions can be supported through appropriate use of software designed to aid communication functions.

Communication functions

Many types of communicative functions that assist in the administration of occupational therapy services can be appropriately and efficiently handled by a computer. Examples of these communicative functions include the following:

- Repetitive formats with few variables that are set up as merge letters, such as some forms of treatment documentation, progress reports and evaluation summaries, and billing procedures
- Presentation of repetitive numeric functions that are set forth in tables, such as monthly departmental statistics, categorized lists, tabulated reports, and accounting functions
- Text formats that require basic editing functions that are easily handled by a word processor, such as using search, find and replace, move, copy, delete, spell checker, and thesaurus functions
- Text that requires manipulation of fonts, text effects, or

formats as well as use of graphics, graphic tools, and the ability to manipulate layout or design, such as for desk-top publication of professional reports, proposals, departmental forms, and articles

Two basic types of computerized tools are necessary to the communicative functions of the administrator: the database and the word processor. Ideally, both should be ***user-friendly***, that is, easy to use, even for the novice. A ***database*** is a compilation of computer-generated forms that are used to store information relating to generic categories, such as people, items, transactions, events, or situations. The structure of a database (also known as a *file*) is generally composed of one basic form (also known as a *record*) that contains several fields. The database itself contains many filled-out forms. A single database generally stores information relating to only one generic category at a time. Several databases may be required to store information about all the categories necessary to the communication functions of an occupational therapy department. Use of a database helps to organize the way in which information is stored so that it can be efficiently retrieved and analyzed. A database is designed in much the same way as any other form, but the blanks to be filled in are called ***fields*** and the written prompts that let the filer know what type of information to place in each field are called *field labels*. The information filled out in each field is called ***data***. Once the form is filled out and saved, it is referred to as a record and is added to the file (Figure 9-31).

When properly designed, a database can be used to assist administrative functions by being able to retrieve quantitative data that answers questions regarding how much or how many. For example, how many patients with cerebral vascular accident are being treated? During which months are the greatest number of patient treatments provided? What proportion of the patient population is composed of young adults? A database can be used to locate selected items of interest. For example, where can I get this piece of equipment? In which periodical was the article about sensory integration and math skills located? From which specific geographic area do most of our patients come? A database can be used to show relations between fields of data. For example, are there relations between age or gender and diagnosis? demographics and diagnosis? equipment use and diagnosis? therapists and types of treatment interventions?

A user-friendly database has a built-in capacity for change without destroying data that has been previously entered. This

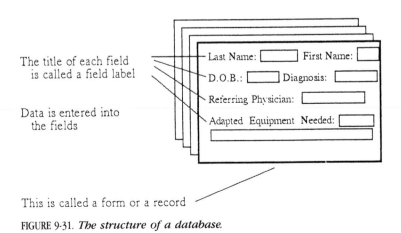

FIGURE 9-31. *The structure of a database.*

feature allows for adaptation and growth of the database through alteration of the design as administrative task demands change over time.

The second basic type of computerized tool used in administrative communicative functions is a **word processor**. The word processor, with its **merge function**, serves to alleviate the expenditure of costly human hours set aside for repetitive types of mandatory paper work, such as daily or weekly documentation of progress. The merge function allows a document that has been created by the word processor to be merged with specific fields of data contained within a database. Use of a computer for these repetitive but necessary communicative tasks allows the therapist to retain executive decision making through use of sort, retrieve, and other programming commands of the database. By merging the functions of the word processor with those of the database, however, the burden of output is shifted from the therapist to computer peripherals, such as printers, modems, and disks. Computerized outlines that have blank spaces that are filled in by a word processor as it reads the data contained in the fields of the database are called **shells** or *templates*. The computerized outline is merged with the data from specific fields of the database to produce completed progress notes, evaluation reports, bills, and so forth. (Figure 9-32).

Treatment documentation, monthly departmental statistics, and billing procedures are common examples of repetitive record-keeping procedures whose costs in terms of human hours can be significantly diminished through appropriate use of a computer as a tool. Although favorites in terms of database programs and word processors can be set up to perform merge functions, an integrated package that provides database, word processor, report generator, and utilities all in one program (such as *Q & A* by Semantec or *Appleworks* by Apple) is strongly recommended as the mainstay of administrative functions. Although this type of program is more costly, it tends to offer the kind of built-in variability that is essential for program survival, given the wide variety of administrative functions demanded of an occupational therapy department. Integrated packages are generally designed to be user-friendly. They are designed to be used by administrators or executives who have only basic computer literacy skills. They are designed so that maintenance functions, such as changes in database design, report, and print specifications, can be accomplished by the administrator without the additional assistance of a programmer.

Flexibility and the ability to make changes easily are vital aspects of computer applications in administrative support functions. As administrative tasks vary, so do the programs and formats used to accomplish those tasks. Flexibility provides a measure of longevity to the basic mechanisms of departmental record keeping since simple changes can be made to accommodate new governmental regulations and institutional and departmental policies without totally overhauling the structure of the database and its reports or documents.

Research functions

Flexibility in **data management** is a major aspect of computer applications in research functions, where it is often necessary to organize data into widely differing formats. Although a database can be used in some instances to organize data collected during different phases of research, the primary tool of computer applications in the area of research functions is the **spreadsheet**. A spreadsheet differs from a database both in structure and design.

A database is generally designed to look like an index card within a card file and is structured to sort quickly through the entire file of cards. A spreadsheet is generally designed to look like one gigantic table of values that is organized into rows and columns. It is designed to perform arithmetic operations, and its basic structural unit is the *cell* rather than the field. The data, or contents of each cell, can be either fixed as a value assigned by the researcher or variably derived from a formula based on the contents of cells located elsewhere within the spreadsheet. For example, a cell could hold a pretest score that 1 patient out of 20 who participated in group therapy achieved on a particular rating scale. Each row could be assigned to a specific patient, and each cell in that row would then represent either a pretest or posttest score from a different assessment scale. The contents of the cell at the end of each row could be derived from a formula based on the sum of all the patient's pretest scores divided by the number of pretest scores, or the patient's average score. The contents of the cells at the bottom of each column could be derived from the average of all group members' scores on a specific scale. The contents of a cell can be derived from a formula based on the mean, the standard deviation, the standard error, or whatever arithmetic relation was expressed in a formula that met the criteria of the researcher.

A spreadsheet is used to organize categories of numbers in much the same way that a database is used to organize categories of things. The product of a spreadsheet is generally some form of graphic representation of the data. Tables, charts, and graphs are used to translate the formulas and findings derived from the spreadsheet into the more commonly understood language of graphics.

Although computer programs are helpful in storing and organizing research data, certain computer applications can be used to collect research data as well. Software used in areas of cognitive remediation, prevocational assessment, and behavior modification commonly provide both the modality for treatment and an opportunity for data collection. This type of software is programmed to count the frequency of errors made on specific levels or branches of the program while it is being run. After completion of the exercise set, the program provides a numeric score, a ratio, and at times even a simple graph to represent the accuracy of performance in the area of competency tested. "Diagnostic" or "error analysis" claims of programs used in clinical applications refer to those counting functions of the program that have been designed to count the frequency of errors made in particular branches of the program and match them with specific behavioral objectives. The data collected can then be used to document improvement through quantitative analysis. Storing and then retrieving this type of data for comparison among different patient populations can provide an excellent vehicle by which to provide normative or standardized measures of instrumentation within a department.

Another application of computer technology that makes more sophisticated research available to the practicing clinician is the use of peripheral **interface devices** to convert **analog events** (changes that occur in the physical environment) into numeric or digital measures. These devices provide the clinician with access to events occurring on the microscopic rather than macroscopic level, where subtle changes that could not otherwise be seen can be registered and documented. Sophisticated measures of internal events, such as joint movement, changes in the electrical potential of muscle groups as they contract, and changes in chemical reactions of skin surfaces due to stress or

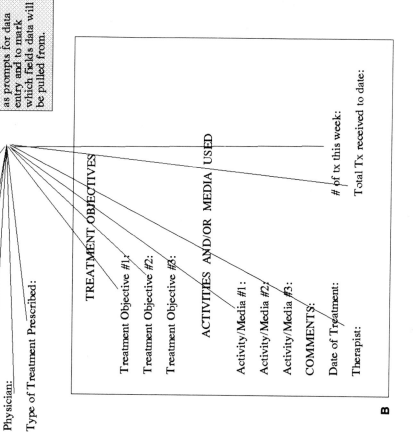

OCCUPATIONAL THERAPY TREATMENT LOG

These are field labels. They serve as prompts for data entry and to mark which fields data will be pulled from.

Last Name: First Name:

D.O.B: Diagnosis:

Physician:

Type of Treatment Prescribed:

TREATMENT OBJECTIVES

Treatment Objective #1:

Treatment Objective #2:

Treatment Objective #3:

ACTIVITIES AND/OR MEDIA USED

Activity/Media #1:

Activity/Media #2:

Activity/Media #3:

COMMENTS:

Date of Treatment: # of tx this week:

Therapist: Total Tx received to date:

B

WEEKLY PROGRESS REPORT

Occupational Therapy Department

Date: *Date of Tx*

First Name *Last Name* received *Type of Treatment Prescribed* this week.

# of tx this week this week.

Activity/Media #1, *Activity/Media #2*, and *Activity/Media #3* were used to accomplish the following clinical objectives:

Treatment Objective #1

Treatment Objective #2

Treatment Objective #3

First Name *Last Name* *Comment*

Therapist, OTR

These "merge variables", match the field labels of the database. The program will use data from these fields and merge it with the text of this shell of a report to create a weekly progress report.

A

The computerized merged document reads as:

WEEKLY PROGRESS REPORT

Occupational Therapy Department

Date: October 10, 1993

Timothy Jones received Functional Occupational Therapy three times this week.

Bilateral sanding activities on an inclined plane, bilateral shoulder ladder activities, and weighted skateboard activities were used to accomplish the following treatment objectives: to increase muscle power in the right shoulder flexors, to increase active range of motion in the right elbow, and to increase passive range of motion in the right wrist.

Timothy Jones's muscle power in the right shoulder flexors is now Fair + , a.r.o.m. in the right elbow is now 25 degrees of flexion and extension, p.r.o.m. in the right wrist remains severely limited.

Suze Smoothey, OTR

C

FIGURE 9-32. (A) The shell of a progress report. (B) A form from a database used for treatment documentation. (C) The computerized merged document.

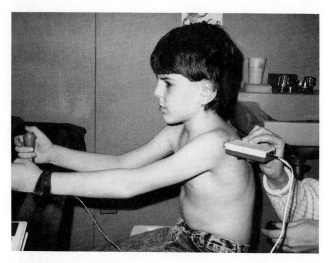

FIGURE 9-33. *Use of a interface device to record electromyogram changes.*

anxiety, are available for clinical application. The data collected by these interface devices gives the clinician an opportunity to view changes occurring on the biochemical or biomechanical level that precedes clinical manifestation of behavioral change. Data collected in this manner can be used to verify the effectiveness of techniques, materials, and equipment used in clinical practice and affords a different level of sophistication to clinical implementation of treatment procedures.

For example, one method of intervention that is becoming more widespread in developmental disabilities is the use of cerebral electrical stimulation to improve motor and sensori-integrative functions (Logan, 1988). One group of clinicians used a computerized electromyography (EMG) program with an interface that allowed for surface scanning of muscle surfaces to quantify the electrophysiologic changes that occurred within groups of muscle fibers during active contraction (Cram, 1986). A

spreadsheet was used to aid in comparison of the data that was collected. Graphic representation of the data was accomplished through use of a program (Harvard Graphics) designed to convert numeric values into charts that allowed for ease of comparison. The results of the study served to verify clinical observations of improved motor and sensory-integrative functions after cerebral electrical stimulation applications (Okoye, Malden, & Abramson, in press). Computer applications not only allowed for statistical analysis of the data but also afforded comparison of the variables in a number of quantifiable objective formats. Use of the computer as a tool eased the processes of collection, storage, and organization of the data within a clinical arena and also allowed for presentation of the findings in a professional manner (Figures 9-33 and 9-34).

Another study questioned whether or not motor skills were improved during use of joystick-controlled computer games. In this study, 23 neurologically impaired children were matched and placed into two groups. Children in the cognitive group continued with their regular therapy program and also used computer games that had been selected to provide rehearsal of cognitive skills surrounding motor functions (such as spatial relations and motor planning); however, they used keyboard entry rather than a joystick controller to play the games. Children in the executive motor group also continued with their regular therapy program, but in addition, they used joystick-controlled computer games that had been selected to provide rehearsal of motor executive skills (such as visual motor control, regulation of force, speed, and direction of motor output). These children were required to hold the joystick with both hands rather than rest the joystick base on the table for support. Surface EMGs and other adapted tests were used as extrinsic pretest and posttest measures. The duration of the intervention strategy was 6 weeks or six 30-minute computer treatment sessions.

The results indicated that children in the cognitive group performed better at tasks requiring size discrimination, while children in the executive motor group performed better at tasks of spatial orientation and shape discrimination. Children in the

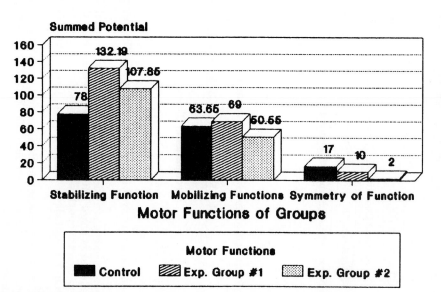

FIGURE 9-34. *Assessment of motor functions in dominant extremities.*

executive motor group showed significant difference in their motor skills at posttest. They showed better organization of motor control in terms of proximal stabilization with distal mobilization. The results of this research project were shared at the 1991 Annual Closing the Gap Conference (Okoye, Malden, Latourrette, Dapice, & Okoye, 1991) (Figure 9-35).

Research functions represent a domain of function that is shared by both administrative and clinical applications. Skilled use of computer applications as a tool in research can contribute to administrative and management functions, such as treatment documentation, cost effectiveness of intervention methods, budgeting, allocation of funds, and justification for staffing patterns. Research functions also serve to assist clinical implementation processes by helping to identify those procedures, practices, methods, tools, and media that are most effective in producing clinical change.

Use of the computer as a tool in clinical implementation

Computer applications exist for almost every stage and type of treatment implementation process in occupational therapy; however, underlying assumptions need to be considered that tend to establish guidelines for tenable application of computer technology in clinical practice. For example, use of a computer as a tool in clinical applications is based on the assumption that there is a job to be performed, a task to be accomplished, or a problem to be solved that requires technologic assistance. In a similar fashion, use of a computer as a tool in clinical practice is based on the assumption that the software, program, and peripheral devices used can be adjusted to meet the developmental,

psychological, emotional, physical, and cognitive needs of the patient in addition to meeting the treatment objective. Furthermore, use of a computer as a tool in clinical applications is based on the assumption that this tool allows the necessary task to be performed in a manner that is at least equally efficient in terms of time and equipment as use of other, more conventional media.

Guidelines

The following list contains common clinical problems for which computer applications can be a viable solution. It is by no means exhaustive but is offered as a set of guidelines by which to consider the feasibility and suitability of computer applications in given instances of clinical practice.

The use of a computer as a tool in clinical practice should be considered when the particular application can be used to meet the treatment objectives as well as to:

- perform the task in a manner that is more efficient and less time-consuming than other media (eg, keyboarding rather than typewriting in prevocational training)
- provide documentation that is otherwise unobtainable (eg, biomechanical assessment procedures of the hand, assessment of ocular motility or fields of vision)
- provide otherwise unavailable opportunity for multitasking (eg, use of CD ROM formats to facilitate simultaneity in integration of visual, auditory, and motor stimuli)
- provide opportunities for uniform, consistent repetition of skill without the element of interpersonal frustration (eg, motor training with the physically disabled, rehearsal of cognitive and academic skills with the brain injured)
- present the therapeutic activity in an engaging medium when the activity at face value would otherwise be avoided

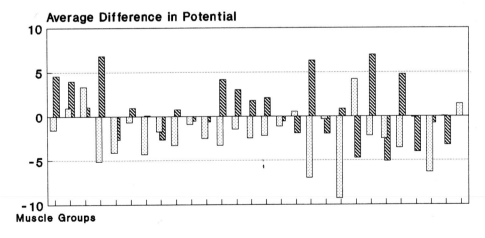

FIGURE 9-35. *Improvement of motor skills among 23 neurologically impaired children during use of joystick-controlled computer games.*

(eg, remediation of visual–associative and psycholinguistic skills with a learning-disabled child)

- provide opportunities for mastery and support of ego functions through use of controlled environmental experiences (eg, use of a word processor or graphics program with patients who have progressive degenerative neurologic disorders, use of a architectural planning program in group therapy with a group of men, use of programming options for an environmental control device with a quadriplegic patient)
- allow for parallel moves in treatment by providing for rehearsal of the same, sometimes boring, treatment objectives through an alternate medium (eg, therapeutic exercise routines)
- facilitate integrative and adapted responses to real-time events in physical, perceptual motor, cognitive, or affective domains (eg, intruding on processing time delays with attention-disordered patient)
- provide for collection of necessary data within the knowledge base but beyond the in-depth skill level of the therapist (eg, use of computerized, prevocational work samples or computerized personality, neuropsychological, or academic inventories)
- provide psychosocial modifiers through use of a medium that is of value to the patient (eg, fulfilling the needs for either consistency or randomization of reward based on predetermined behavioral contingencies)
- provide opportunities for development of relations with the nonhuman environment (eg, modifying social skills of a paranoid patient within a prevocational program)
- provide an environment that cannot be easily manipulated (eg, behavior training for behavior-disordered teen-agers)

Beyond these guidelines and examples for implementing computer technology within clinical settings, computer applications have broadened to incorporate a wide scope of physical settings, treatment milieus, and patient populations over the past several years. Clearly definable areas of specialization have emerged that incorporate distinctions such as types of software used, specialized adaptations and peripheral devices, and use of selected instructional methods. These specialized areas include augmented communication, hand therapy, orthotics and prosthetic fabrication and training, cognitive rehabilitation, prevocational training, pediatric psychiatry, early intervention, school-based occupational therapy, adult physical disabilities, environmental control, and biofeedback.

One key limitation to computer applications in clinical practice that is frequently overlooked is the inability of the program to interpret quality of performance on a multidimensional scale. A key process inherent in the science of occupational therapy is *task analysis*. This is the ongoing evaluation process of data compilation that occurs as the therapist observes and interprets the patient's physical, psychological, emotional, and cognitive reactions to treatment. The feedback (data) gained from this process contributes to a database of information for the therapist from which successive treatment plans will emerge. Although computer programs can provide documentation regarding frequency of errors and details of where and when they occur, by themselves they cannot provide the behavioral descriptors of patient performance so necessary to the field of occupational therapy.

In the final analysis, effective use of a computer as a tool in clinical practice is generally limited to those instances when the treatment objectives cannot be readily or effectively accomplished by use of conventional means. Computer applications are commonly used for assessment procedures when the needed degree of accuracy or other referenced criteria simply cannot be obtained through use of conventional media. In treatment implementation, computerized methods are commonly used when the necessary therapeutic intervention cannot be effectively administered or efficiently documented through use of alternate methods.

Task analysis: A common area of difficulty

There are common elements that frequently serve to block effective use of computer applications in clinical practice regardless of the setting. They tend to center around the difficulties inherent in performing a task analysis with technologic media. One aspect of this difficulty involves the need to plan meaningful therapeutic activity sequences that incorporate computer applications in an integrated fashion. Several stages of task analysis are necessary before computer applications can be incorporated successfully into clinical practice. These stages include careful selection of software, planning for the physical setup and accessibility of the hardware, making the necessary program adaptations so that the software meets the needs of the patient, and planning for complementary preparatory and follow-up activity sequences.

Generally speaking, computerized activities are like any others in that the purpose and manner in which they are used define the nature of the intervention as occupational therapy. The content and purpose of the therapeutic processes that surround computerized activity tend to determine whether or not the intervention qualifies as occupational therapy.

Another obstacle to the use of software as a medium for activity is related to the difficulty in deciding which treatment objectives can be met through the use of a particular program. As therapists, we tend to become more confident in our ability to perform task analyses when tangible media whose physical form serves to prompt our attention are used. With people or groups, the structure and content of psychosocial interactions often serve as cues to prompt and focus our analytic skills. A disk, on the other hand, apart from its label, offers no cues as to its contents or what physical or cognitive requirements its contents will demand of the user. With a disk, we are dependent either on our powers of observation or the claims of the publisher for such cues. If the program is to be used for occupational therapy domains of treatment, the therapist must provide the necessary cues before treatment implementation can begin. Often, these cues are obtained through use of *software analysis* or a *criteria-referenced guide* to software selection.

Software selection

Many forms for software analysis are available to the occupational therapist (eg, AOTA's Computer Information Packet). Some have been borrowed from other professions that share similar domains of treatment, whereas others have been designed by therapists in specific areas of clinical practice. It is more cost effective to modify an existing format for software analysis than to muddle about without an organized approach for clinical implementation of computer applications.

One of the first steps in selecting a program for a software library is to determine whether or not its inherent skills are appropriate for the area of clinical practice for which it is intended. Key elements in software selection include the physical, cognitive, and affective skills required to use the program, the developmental levels represented by those skills, the multiplicity of required skills, and the speed required for integrating or processing those skills. Use of a good format for software analysis provides these key elements.

Another method for ensuring that software used for occupational therapy implementation is appropriate for a particular clinical setting is through development of a criteria-referenced guide for software selection. As with any other format that requires development, the initial processes of constructing a criteria-referenced guide for software selection is time-consuming. Once common objectives of treatment within a specific clinical facility have been identified, however, one of the major elements that frequently serves to block successful use of computer applications in clinical practice will have been ameliorated.

The purpose of the criteria-referenced guide to software selection is threefold: (1) to screen software for suitability, (2) to indicate which subskills can be addressed through use of the program, and (3) to categorize the software according to domain of treatment. Programs can then be easily identified and retrieved for use in remediation of specific treatment objectives. The criteria-referenced guide should contain a grid or matrix that lists domains of treatment that lie within the scope of practice for the clinical setting and can also be remediated through use of computer applications (eg, cognitive, motor, psychosocial, and activities of daily living skills). The matrix for the criteria-referenced guide should also identify subskills within each domain of treatment that are most commonly addressed within the clinical setting. For purposes of comparison, only an equal number of subskills within each domain should be included in the matrix. After the matrix is completed, it is used to score familiar software first. Subskills that are inherent to success in the program can be scored as 1.0, while those that are only somewhat necessary can receive a score of 0.5. A score for each domain can be determined for purposes of comparison. The purpose is not to make an exhaustive list of subskills presented by a particular piece of software but rather to make a general determination as to whether or not the program can be of benefit to the patient population served by the clinic. If so, then the domains in which the program is likely to offer the broadest application already will have been identified. Software is then selected for clinical application based on the extent to which its content offers rehearsal, remediation, and instruction or assessment of subskills within domains of treatment addressed by the clinical practice. Figure 9-36 shows a criteria-referenced guide to software selection developed for a community-based, private pediatric practice (Okoye, 1986).

Ideally, as the matrix for the criteria-referenced guide is filled out on each program used in clinical applications, the data should be entered into a database. Reports can then be generated to provide the practicing clinician with a printout of software holdings, complete with physical cues about the domains, subskills, and developmental levels represented in the contents of each program. This aids not only in software selection but also in designing complementary activity sequences.

Strategies and methods of clinical implementation

General methods of implementing computer applications can be grouped according to domains of treatment. The domains of treatment for which computer applications are available include motor, sensory, cognitive, academic, and affective domains as well as activities of daily living. Each domain of treatment tends to have its own particular strategies for clinical implementation and can be identified according to types of device and common methods of approach.

Motor domains of treatment

Computer applications in the domain of motor functions are characterized by use of technologic means by which the motor output of the patient is recorded and measured. Sometimes peripheral devices, such as cuffs and interface devices, are applied to the patient to obtain the necessary physiologic data and convert it into digital form that can be manipulated by a software program. For example, *The Body Log* (by Body Link) is a computerized exercise program that uses cuffs placed around muscle bellies to obtain readings of potential, resulting from their activity to move objects on the screen. *The Cram Scan* (Cram, 1986), a computerized program for performing surface EMGs, uses an interface device with surface electrodes to obtain readings of potential being generated during muscle activity. Other low-technology means include switches and lever arms. For example, *Motor Training Games* (Cooper, 1989) is a collection of simple games of motor skill that use single-switch input to improve motor skills, such as timing, force, and sequencing skills. The *UBE* (by Cybex) is an upper-back and upper-extremity exerciser that requires the patient to perform measurable work by manipulating lever arms to engage the program. While the patient manipulates the levers, the program counts the frequency of movements and calculates the work completed by multiplying the frequency by the resistance being applied. Computer applications in the motor domain have been heavily influenced by trends in sports medicine, health, and fitness. Computer applications for assessment and treatment of motor functions typically require the user to choose training options from a simple menu and then to select criteria for measuring the amount of resistance or load to be applied, frequency of work, levels for reinforcement, and duration of the exercise. This type of computer application is able to provide realistic multisensory feedback for the patient during exercise segments. Stimulating visual, proprioceptive, tactile, and auditory feedback are often built into the programs. Another characteristic of this kind of equipment is that it usually has been designed to provide feedback for the therapist by means of a hard-copy printout or screen graphic representation of the type and degree of work performed. Simple graphs, statistical measures, and ratios of performance are often provided for descriptive documentation that can be added to the patient's chart.

Sensory domains of treatment

Many of the computer applications that are used for assessment and treatment of sensory domains of function are dedicated to the development of compensatory strategies for those with low vision. Computerized tactile, proprioceptive, vibratory, and auditory mechanisms have been developed to provide alternative

Title:

Publisher:

Code:

Program Characteristics:

Attentive Functions

☐ Selective Attention

☐ Selective Inhibition

☐ Ordering & Sequencing

☐ Simultaneity

☐ Focus-Shift-Refocus

☐ Total Attentive Skill Score:

_____ Developmental Level

Visual Functions

☐ Figure Ground Discrimination

☐ Visual Pursuit

☐ Shape and Form Discrimination

☐ Pattern Recognition

☐ Visuo-spatial Orientation

☐ Total Visual Skill Score

_____ Developmental Level

Motor Functions

☐ Motor Planning

☐ Bilateral Motor Control

☐ Fine Motor Control

☐ Kinesthetic Awareness

☐ Regulation of Force, Speed, Movement

☐ Total Motor Skill Score

_____ Developmental Level

Language Functions

☐ Decoding

☐ Encoding

☐ Sequencing

☐ Object Recognition

☐ Spatial Language

☐ Total Language Skill Score

_____ Developmental Level

Sensori Integrative Functions

☐ Visual Association

☐ Eye-hand Coordination

☐ Logical Problem Solving

☐ Kinetic Memory

☐ Self-cuing Memory

☐ Total Integrative Skill Score

_____ Developmental Level

© Okoye, 1987

Program Description:

Comments:

FIGURE 9-36. *Criteria-referenced guide to software selection developed for a community-based private pediatric practice.*

sensory channels to aid the visually impaired in all aspects of daily living. One of the primary functions of a computer is conversion of one type of energy into another (eg, conversion of input into a binary code; conversion of binary into alternate forms of output, such as screen, printer, disk, modem). Perhaps this is why a computer can readily be designed to convert print that is based on human response to light energy into almost any other sensory channel. The use of a computer as a tool to aid in compensatory strategies for the visually impaired include screen adaptations that format extremely large print to the screen, braille input devices that convert text to braille, braille keyboard overlays (by the American Printing House for the Blind) for different keyboard configurations, and page scanners (computerized devices that convert braille to speech or text to speech). For example, the *Large Print Display Processor* (by TeleSensory) is an optical character recognition device that provides for large print display (as large as 5-inch letters) of a computer screen so that word processors and other programs using text formats can be used by the visually impaired. *Braille 'n Speak* (by Blazie Engineering) is a talking device that transcribes braille to speech or braille to print and can be used for instructional purposes. *DocuRead* (by Adhoc Reading Systems) is a computerized page scanning device that converts text to speech so that a book may be "read" by passing a hand-held scanner over its pages. This allows the visually impaired access to the same printed documents as the normally sighted. Evaluation of the ability of the multihandicapped user to access compensatory devices and training the multihandicapped user in use of these devices are important categories of application that lie within the scope of practice of the occupational therapist.

Another common computer application within the sensory domain is the implementation of computer technology in the area of vision training. This is an area of occupational therapy that is often shared with optometry and neuropsychological services. Methods of application often incorporate use of computer-generated light sources and patterns of movement with visual targets to be scanned and responded to by the patient. Strategies of implementation in this domain of treatment typically involve either software with screen presentations of graphics, letters, and words or oversized devices with programmable moving sources of light. Although certain aspects of vision training can be more easily accomplished with traditional media, such as beads on a string, flashlights, and index cards on a wall, training of smooth scanning patterns, simultaneous visual attention to multiple stimuli, and integration of peripheral with central vision is more effectively accomplished with use of computer applications. Computerized devices for vision training and programs designed specifically to improve visual attentive behaviors have been shown to be more effective than traditional means in remediating disorders of ocular motility and visual attention. For example, the *Visual Perceptual Diagnostic, Testing and Training Program* (by Computability Corp.) is a computerized tool designed by an occupational therapist that is used to assess visual field deficits and to train various patterns of ocular motor control. Computerized packages offering visual training exercises, including visual pursuit, and visual attentive behaviors have been successfully incorporated into several areas of clinical practice. Training in visual functions, in postural stabilization of the head, and in basic optic–kinetic skills heavily impacts success in many daily living skills. The sensory domain is one in which clinical

implementation of computer applications has become prominent in occupational therapy.

Domains of daily living skills

The area of daily living skills encompasses a wide array of treatment domains, each with its own set of subskills that can be accomplished more readily with computer applications. For example, the disabled homemaker has benefited greatly from technology applied to homemaking. Given meal preparation using a microwave, food storage using computerized refrigeration, computerized communications using word processors and electronic bulletin boards, hands-free speaker phones and telephones with memory dialing features, computerized shopping and banking using a modem, and a measure of environmental control using remote-controlled devices (by X-10 USA), even a severely disabled homemaker can be fairly independent. Key objectives for the occupational therapist in training disabled homemakers in use of these computerized applications include access, attention, and cognitive levels of function. These three objectives are also key functions of computer applications in the area of prevocational training.

Since so many office settings require some level of computer literacy, prevocational training involves the occupational therapist in assessment of a computer system as a workstation for the disabled worker. Details of access that become prominent in this area of clinical practice include height, reach, type of hand function and muscle power required, and accessibility of disk drives, printers, keyboard, and switches. Seating modifications, postural stability, and motor control also have an impact on access. For the severely physically challenged worker, computer applications typically substitute the use of peripheral devices for direct keyboard access. For example, the *Headmaster* (by Prentke Romich) is a mouse emulator and puff-and-sip unit that translates head rotation into cursor movement for keyboard control. Miniature keyboards and microswitches offer other alternatives to direct keyboarding for the severely physically disabled. Most of these peripheral devices are designed to be fully compatible with MS-DOS applications so that the programs used in the workplace can be reviewed in the clinic, where any access problems can be worked out before the worker returns to the office.

Software programs for prevocational instruction as well as computerized assessment programs are readily available. Programs for prevocational application tend to be characterized either by paper-and-pencil tasks or by sorting and coding tasks that have been formatted to a screen. A unique feature of prevocational applications for the occupational therapist is the availability of an extremely broad range of job samples at the click of a button. The accuracy with which the job samples have been portrayed and the ability of the program to determine which academic skills and level of cognitive functions are necessary to each vocational sample (*The Vocational Resource* by Conover) add to the appeal of the programs. Software for prevocational applications range from interest inventories, vocational aptitude tests, and worker personality profiles to work simulations and actual job samples for a variety of vocations. The prospective worker can actually try out a job to some extent before going for training in a specific area of interest.

Computer applications are also used in restorative functions for the disabled laborer. In work hardening applications, computerized workstations such as the B.T.E. (by the Baltimore Therapeutic Equipment Co.) are used to replicate the lifting, pushing, pulling, gripping, turning, hammering, and so forth of physical activities. These types of computerized workstations assess patient preparedness for physical labor, train for multitasks, and provide printed documentation of patient status.

Cognitive domains of treatment

One domain of practice that relies heavily on computer applications in both pediatric and adult physical disability and psychiatric clinics is the domain of cognitive functions. Dedicated software can assist with treatment objectives in the following cognitive domains: attentive functions, psycholinguistic functions, visual–perceptual functions, sensorimotor functions, virtually all academic areas of competency, and problem-solving skills. Computer applications used in occupational therapy that support cognitive domains of treatment usually involve software with few peripheral devices beyond a mouse or joystick. At times, options for the *TouchWindow* (Edmark), *PowerPad* (Dunamis), graphic tablet, or peripheral keyboard may be available. Another characteristic of this type of application has been the development of increasingly sophisticated graphic presentations with a preponderance of attention to visual detail. Multisensory formats, such as videodisks and CD-ROM technology, have resulted in striking presentations that can be used to combine both cognitive and sensory processing functions. The cognitive domain of clinical implementation requires greater skill on the part of the therapist in terms of use of guidelines for software selection, selection of criteria-referenced software, and sequenced incorporation of the computerized activity into the overall occupational therapy treatment plan. Several sources of software for remediation of cognitive functions are available. A partial listing of sources with software conducive to occupational therapy intervention is included at the end of this section.

Affective domains of treatment

Software applications are available for assessment and treatment of some subskills within the affective domain. Within the domain of affective functions, it is the method of implementation rather than the software per se that differs. In addition to the methods of clinical implementation already mentioned, therapists who use computer applications in this area of practice tend to specialize in use of a computer as an object. The values and status our culture ascribes to a computer, its use, and people who use computers can be capitalized on to influence patients with affective disorders, behavioral disorders, and psychosocial dysfunction. This orientation opens a panoramic spectrum of computer applications in areas of object relations, ego functions, behavioral contingencies, the nonhuman environment, social relations, group interactions, and simulations. Methods of implementation in this domain need to be highly interactive, highly structured, or deliberately nonstructured.

Summary

Computer applications in the field of occupational therapy represent a broadly expanding sphere of influence. Computer technology impinges on almost every aspect of practice, including the communicative functions of administrative support, the use of research applications to document effectiveness of various treatment methods, and the implementation of computer technology in general areas of clinical practice.

Many positive influences of computer applications have been observed. These include: (1) increased efficiency in administrative functions, which provides more time for administrators and clinicians to be involved with patient care rather than paper work; (2) increased professional visibility and credibility; and (3) expansion of the scope of occupational therapy practice through use of computer applications to offer a broader spectrum of services to the disabled.

References

Cooper, R. J. (1989). *Motor Training Games* [Computer program]. Available from Don Johnston Developmental Equipment, 100 N. Rand Rd., Bldg. 115, P. O. Box 639, Wauconda IL 60084

Cram, J. R. (1986). *Clinical EMG, Muscle Scanning for Surface Recordings* [Computer program]. Available from Clinical Resources, 901 Boren Ave., Ste. 1020, Seattle WA.

Logan, M. (1988, October). *Improved mechanical efficiency in cerebral palsy patients treated with cerebral electric stimulator (CES)*. Paper presented at the annual meeting of the American Academy for Cerebral Palsy and Developmental Medicine, Toronto.

Okoye, R. (1986). *Software selection guide for sensorimotor education*. (Privately published).

Okoye, R., Malden, J., & Abramson, D. (in press). Technological tools within a neurobiological framework: Agents in perceptual motor integration. *Journal of Occupational Therapy in Health Care*.

Okoye, R., Malden, J., Latourrette, D., Dapice, S., & Okoye, A. (1991, October). *Use of criteria-referenced software to teach motor skills*. Paper presented at the annual meeting of Closing the Gap Computer Conference, Minneapolis.

Additional resources

Adhoc Reading Systems, Inc., 28 Brunswick Woods Dr., E. Brunswick, NJ 08816 (produces *DocuRead*)

American Occupational Therapy Association, 1383 Piccard Dr., Rockville, MD 20850 (distributes the 1990 *Computer Information Packet*)

Appleworks is produced by Apple Corp. and is available from any authorized Apple dealer or from Apple Computers, Inc., 20525 Marian Avenue, MS 36AS, Cupertino, CA 95041, (408) 974-7910.

Blazie Engineering, 3660 Mill Green Rd., Street, MD 21154 (produces *Braille 'n Speak*)

Body Link, Mt. Kisco, NY (distributes *The Body Log*)

Brain Train, Inc., 1915 Huguenot Rd., Richmond VA 23235

Computability Corp., 40000 Grand River, St. 109, Novi, MI 48375 (distributes *Visual Perceptual Diagnostic, Training and Testing Program*)

Conover Co., P. O. Box 155, Omro, WI 54963 (produces *Reasoning Skills on the Job, Microcomputer Evaluation of Career Areas*, and *Career Planning System, The Vocational Resource.*)

CREATE, P. O. Box 28, Hales Corners, WI 53130

Cybex Corp., 2100 Smithtown Ave., P. O. Box 9003, Ronkonkama, NY 11779 (produces *UBE*)

Dunamis Inc., 3620 Hwy 317, Suwanee, GA 30174 (produces the *Power Pad*)

Edmark, P. O. Box 3903, Bellevue, WA 98009 (produces the *Touch Window*)

Software Publishing Corp. (produces *Harvard Graphics* [1989])

Prentke Romich Co., 1022 Keyl Rd., Wooster, OH 44691 (produces *Headmaster*)

Psychological Software Services, Inc., 6555 Carrollton Ave., Indianapolis, IN 46220

Sunburst, 101 Castleton St., Pleasantville, NY 10570 (produces *Right Job*)

Symantec Corp., 10201 Torre Ave., Cupertino, CA 95014 (publishes *Q & A* [1988])

TeleSensory, 455 N. Bernardo Ave., Mountain View, CA 94039 (produces *DP-10 Large Print Display Processor*)

Vocational Resource, 2017 Cedar St., Berkeley, CA 94709 (produces *Realistic Assessment of Vocational Experiences* [RAVE])

Unicorn Engineering, 5221 Central Ave., Ste. 205, Richmond, CA 94804 (produces the *Smart Keyboard*)

X-10 USA, 185A LeGrand Ave., Northvale, NJ 07647 (produces *X-10 Home Automation Interface* and *X-10 Powerhouse Wireless Remote Control*)

UNIT III

The health care system

CHAPTER 10

Occupational therapy's place in the health care system

SECTION 1

The health care delivery system today

LINDA L. LEVY

LEARNING OBJECTIVES

Upon completion of this section the reader will be able to:

1. *Identify the function and structure of the health care delivery system.*
2. *Describe the evolution of the health care delivery system in the United States.*
3. *Discuss the changes in the health problems of the population during this century.*
4. *Explain how health care systems are financed.*
5. *Discuss problems of access to the health care delivery system.*
6. *Explain how financial issues affect quality of care.*
7. *Explain the reasons for the current crisis in health care as well as efforts to reform the current delivery system.*

KEY TERMS

Alternative Practice Models	*Hospice Care*
Commercial Insurance	*Independent Practice*
Comprehensive Continuous	*Associations*
Care	*Medicaid*
Cost Plus Fee-for-Service	*Medicare*
Crisis in Health Care	*Non-Profit Hospital*
Diagnostic-Related Group	*Nursing Home Care*
For-Profit Hospital	*Preferred Provider*
Fragmented Care	*Organizations*
Geographic Maldistribution	*Private Division*
Health Maintenance	*Private Funds*
Organizations	*Prospective Payment System*
Health Promotion/Disease	*Public Division*
Prevention	*Public Funds*
Home Health Care	*Risk Factors*

A revolution is occurring in our health care delivery system. Within the past two decades, economic, social, and political pressures have been added to those of science and technology, producing a demand for a new concept of health care, a new ethic of responsibility for both consumers and providers, and a new structuring of health care institutions to deliver broader, better, and more cost-effective care. As a result, the health care delivery system has not become a changed system, but rather a perpetually changing one. In light of the rapid changes that are occurring, the practice of occupational therapy a few years hence will likely be significantly different from what it is today.

To understand some of these changes, it is necessary to have a basic understanding of the system's function and structure. At the outset, it should be acknowledged that the term *system* is a misnomer. In reality, the United States does not have a single comprehensible system for delivering health care. Instead, the system is a conglomeration of many, often-independent components that overlap and interact in a variety of ways.

Function of the health care delivery system

The *function* of the health care delivery system is to deliver *equitable*, *efficient*, and *effective* services to the population. The services are derived from the veritable explosion in medical research and technology in the last decade, which has produced profound effects on the state of medicine and what it is capable of doing. And yet, paradoxically perhaps, there are serious concerns about health care and its delivery in the United States. The system by which these magnificent medical advances are made available to the public has been described as a "no-system system," or "push-cart vending in the age of supermarkets." That is, for all its technologic sophistication, it does not provide the health care the population needs; and the health care it does provide is delivered inefficiently.

These views are gaining credibility. Our research and technology are unequalled by any other nation, yet the United States is hardly a leader in the delivery of health care. Indicators of *health status*, such as infant mortality, maternal mortality, life expectancy, and death rates for middle-aged citizens, reveal that the United States lags far behind almost every nation in Western Europe. To make matters worse, few countries in the world spend as much money as the United States on health care, either in absolute terms or as a percentage of the *gross national product*. And, as is reflected in indicators of health status, the benefits do not appear to be justifying the costs. Furthermore, health costs are rising faster than practically any other segment of the nation's economy and have reached what many leaders consider intolerable levels. Health costs are draining resources from equally essential sectors, such as housing, education, and national defense, and are contributing significantly to the national deficit.

There are also mounting concerns about the *availability*, *accessibility*, and *quality* of health care services. It has become apparent that good health care is simply not available to many Americans. People seeking health care face many *geographic* and *economic barriers*. Wide geographic variations exist in the distribution of physicians and other health care workers. As a result, in many rural areas and in the poor parts of large cities, it is difficult, if not impossible, for many people to obtain proper health care. Also, more and more Americans are denied access to health care because they cannot afford insurance or have health problems that, by current standards, make them uninsurable. In fact, very few are covered against the costs of catastrophic illness or long-term care. To complicate the issue further, the quality of care varies greatly, particularly when one's eligibility for care is determined by the vagaries of one's insurance coverage rather than by one's need. Moreover, even when citizens have adequate insurance coverage, there are still vast differences in the quality of care available in different geographic regions and even in different sections of the same city.

Increasingly, critics contend that we have all but ignored the delivery of health care in our preoccupation with developing technology to treat diseases. They further question how such inequities can be tolerated in a society with so much know-how. One conclusion, however, is little disputed: in the United States, there is a ***crisis in health care***.

Origins of the problem

The health care crisis in America affects all people financially and in terms of the availability and quality of care they receive. Simply stated, the crisis is due to the fact that our knowledge of health care (ie, technology) has evolved at a much greater rate than our ability to deliver that care. This has created a large discrepancy between the demand for health care and the supply of services, which—true to market principles—results in sharply increasing costs. To understand how this situation came about, some historical background is necessary.

At the turn of this century, all health care was provided by general fee-for-service family physicians engaged in solo practice. It was a time when medicine had few effective remedies, and, as historians note, patients who went to physicians had only a 50-50 chance of benefitting from the encounter (Henderson, 1941). In 1910, as a result of the Flexner report, medical education became a university undertaking, and health care began to be firmly rooted in medical science. Thereafter, knowledge

about the workings of the human body and the causes of disease developed rapidly, which led to a need for highly trained specialists who were better equipped to handle the new technologies. General family physicians were gradually replaced on medical school faculties with full-time specialist physicians; thus, medical students had little contact with those who were practicing general medicine, and specialists became their only role models. This trend away from the general physician toward the more narrowly oriented specialist was further reinforced in World War II, when specialists were rewarded with higher rank and pay in the armed forces than general physicians.

Thus, by the late 1940s, general physicians began to disappear, replaced by an ever-increasing variety of specialists with more prestige and higher incomes. The problem for the health care delivery system was that no resources were developed to take the place of the family doctor, who heretofore had been central to health care delivery, providing the general medical care needed by most of the population. Furthermore, family doctors could coordinate the diverse services of the emerging specialities and were willing to provide continuing care. Now the more expensive specialists dominated the health care system. At times, internists, pediatricians, and obstetrician–gynecologists would assume responsibility for the general medical care that was most needed by the population. More often, however, Americans had to forgo general medical care or had to depend on hospital emergency rooms and clinics for diagnostic assistance and care. In either case, general medical care became increasingly unavailable (ie, the supply decreased). Concurrently, the costs began to rise.

The now-predominant specialists adopted the same solo practice model for the delivery of health care used by the general physician at a time when illness could be managed by a single family doctor. They continued to operate relatively independently, notwithstanding consultation agreements with other physicians, laboratories, and hospitals. This was another unfortunate development for the health care system because no mechanisms were designed to coordinate their specialized services. The links among specialists were informal and difficult to maintain and became inefficient and inconvenient to consumers. It was not unusual for patients to go to a number of different specialists and hospitals for one disease episode, and there were few general physicians available to provide the requisite continuing care. To this day, most patients receive ***fragmented care*** without a general family physician to provide continuity of care. This situation has become especially problematic given the changing nature of the diseases that the health system currently confronts—diseases that are more chronic, complicated, and difficult to defeat and that require ***comprehensive continuous care***. Thus, with the rise in specialist technology, health care became fragmented as well as more costly.

The specialization of physicians was accompanied by an increasing variety and number of allied health practitioners. In addition, an increasing complexity developed in the services provided by hospitals, the essential "workshops" of many of the new specialists (Freymann, 1977). A technologic gap developed between the care that could be provided in physicians' offices and the care provided in hospitals by highly specialized medical personnel using complex equipment. Consequently, hospitals were elevated to the central position in health care delivery. Note that before this century, hospitals were places to avoid because they were notorious for filth and overcrowding as well as for high rates of mortality. The postoperative infection rate, for instance, was 100%, and the postoperative mortality rate was 80% (Crichton, 1970). Wealthier patients were treated at home by their family physician. Now the role and function of the hospital in health care delivery was completely reversed.

The central position of hospitals in the health care delivery system became reinforced and solidified in the Depression era by the development of health insurance. The providers of care, first hospitals and then physicians, were concerned about the increasing inability of many consumers to pay their rising health care bills. Health insurance (eg, Blue Cross and Blue Shield) was created to spread the risk of health costs among consumers and to ensure that the hospitals themselves would be paid. It became an enormously popular benefit for American employees after World War II because the premiums were tax deductible for the employer and not taxable to the employee. As unions found it increasingly difficult to obtain wage increases, health insurance became a desirable benefit to bargain for during negotiations. Today, health insurance is one of the benefits employers are expected to offer employees.

Although health insurance did help provide for the consumer's need for protection, at the same time it produced untoward effects on the delivery of health services. The plan that the hospitals and physicians created largely served their interests and was inevitably inflationary. It clearly favored inpatient acute hospital care and specifically excluded equally important and less expensive nonhospital-based services. There were no cost-control measures built into the plan that would restrain the use of high-cost facilities and procedures. In fact, the plan was based on a ***cost plus fee-for-service*** system, which rewarded hospitals and physicians for providing more services rather than fewer. In addition, it became economically favorable for both patients and physicians to use hospitals, since hospital services were covered, whereas less expensive alternatives were not. We know that increased demand results in increased costs. In this case, it is important to recognize that health insurance increased the demand for the most expensive of medical services (ie, hospital services) rather than for the less expensive alternatives. As a result, insurance served to increase overall health care costs rather than to offset them.

To complicate matters further, the federal government replicated this hospital-based, cost plus fee-for-service model of health insurance in 1965 with the introduction of ***Medicare*** for the elderly and ***Medicaid*** for the poor. These entitlement programs were enacted in the era of the *Great Society* to address the critical problems of lack of access to health care for the elderly and the poor. Heretofore, health care services had been limited to the middle class worker with health insurance or the well-to-do. Subsequently, millions of people, many with serious health problems, were provided access to health care, and the demands on the health care system increased dramatically. No cost-control measures had been introduced into the system, so that billions of federal dollars were spent—virtually without control—on hospital services. Hospitals flourished and became the heart of the health care system. As a result, high-technology, high-cost, hospital-based services became the primary focus of the health care delivery system. This rapid expansion of acute care hospital services occurred at the unfortunate expense of the general medical, long-term care, rehabilitation, and preventive services that are needed to serve the dominant health problems of our population.

Some final points about health insurance are important. Not only did it promote the rapid growth of hospitals, its taken-for-granted nature led to the development of a political philosophy that considered health care an entitlement in this country, that is, a right rather than a privilege and a part of the good life that all should share. This philosophical change produced even more powerful demands on the health care delivery system. Insurance provided unlimited access to health care, and the costs of that care were no longer checked by one's ability to pay; nor was anyone really concerned about excessive use of services or rising costs when everyone knew the bill would be paid. Costs and demand, then, rose sharply. Moreover, with the increase in use of health services, the system has become crowded. As a result, health care has become not only more costly but harder to get (ie, the demand has far surpassed the supply.)

We are only beginning to realize the unfortunate effects of both this shift in political philosophy and our inflationary model of health insurance. The costs of health insurance have risen dramatically, which has made it inaccessible to the near poor (those ineligible for Medicaid) and to a growing number of middle-income families. Also, unions and industry are beginning to recognize that making private health insurance coverage universal and passing health insurance costs on to consumers have made it difficult for the United States to compete with other countries. For example, General Motors Corporation spends more for health insurance benefits for its employees and their families than it pays for steel to manufacture its automobiles. In 1989, the Chrysler Corporation was paying annually for health care more than $5300 per employee (Himmelstein & Woolhandler, 1989). These costs clearly have a serious impact on the nation's economy.

There was another consequence of specialist technology that, for all practical purposes, decreased the supply of health services: the ***geographic maldistribution*** of physicians. The distribution of physicians in this country is weighted heavily toward metropolitan areas, yet poverty-stricken areas of the cities are unable to attract the services of private physicians. Specialists, in particular, tend to cluster around hospitals in big cities, partly to keep up with their specialties, partly to have the sophisticated equipment and hospital support services they need, and partly to have access to a population large enough to provide sufficient incidence of the diseases for which their services are needed. They also tend to practice in those communities that can best afford their services. The geographic maldistribution has become worse, not better, in the last decade, and it contributes to the lack of availability of health care in many sections of the country (ie, the supply) and, consequently, to the increased costs of health care.

The costs of health care as well as its quality are also affected by the distinctive nature of the medical marketplace. With the purchase of health care services, a great deal of information is hidden from the consumer. Most consumers are not knowledgeable about what services are available, what costs are involved, and what alternatives are available. They are not in a position to evaluate the quality of care they receive, nor are they able—especially in times of emergency—to shop around for the best service at the best price. This, too, translates into large variations in quality and into higher and higher costs.

There is a final factor that contributes substantially to the crisis in health care. We have witnessed medical miracles, such as organ transplants and open heart surgery, and expect that these sophisticated methods will be available for all people and for all diseases. Ironically, these increased expectations about what medicine ought to be able to accomplish are contributing to the health care crisis because people have come to expect more from the health care system than it can provide. As was mentioned earlier, there is profound national concern that despite massive health expenditures, the nation's health has improved less than expected. There is a critical assumption underlying this expectation: that health care makes people healthy. The problem for the health care system is that, contrary to this popular belief, health care will *not* make people healthy. A brief overview of the leading causes of death and disability in this country may shed light on this issue.

Before this century, the major causes of illness and death were infectious diseases, such as pneumonia, influenza, tuberculosis, diphtheria, cholera, and smallpox. Cures such as antibiotics and immunizations were not available, and unsophisticated public health standards, such as the lack of safe water and milk and inadequate sewage disposal, contributed to widespread infection of the population. Today, improvements in sanitation, breakthroughs in antibiotic therapy, and immunization have greatly reduced the role of infectious diseases as causes of deaths, and other disease categories are taking their place. Specifically, diseases of the heart and circulation now account for more than half of all deaths and disability. Cancers account for about half of the remainder, with the other primary causes of death being cirrhosis of the liver, diabetes, and accidents. These diseases, plus arthritis and musculoskeletal impairments, are also the primary causes of disability.

Ironically, the prevalence of these more chronic diseases is testimony to our success in eliminating infectious diseases. (Accidents, the one nondisease cited, have become a major cause of death in this century because of the use of the automobile.) Survival from the diseases that used to kill early in life dramatically increased life expectancy and thereby allowed the illnesses that occur later in life to increase in frequency. Consequently, the present-day health care system is faced with an older, more illness-prone population, whose disabilities are much more difficult and costly to treat. Concomitantly, this age shift in the population has dramatically increased the demand for health services. The key questions to be asked are the following:

- For how many of today's diseases do we now have an effective technology for cure or prevention, comparable to antibiotics for the treatment of pneumonia?
- Are we failing to treat these diseases effectively because of deficiencies in the health care delivery system?
- Or, do present mortality and disability rates from these diseases merely reflect the absence of any known technology that works?

The unfortunate reality is that with the present state of our knowledge, there is no medical treatment that will prevent heart disease, stroke, diabetes, cirrhosis, arthritis, or injuries, nor do we possess any effective technology for cure of these diseases. The medical treatment that we do possess will relieve pain, stabilize the patient's condition, arrest deterioration, provide support, and reduce disability to some degree, yet there is little evidence that our technology has contributed substantially to improved health or longevity. In other words, even if we had the best health care delivery system in the world, there are very real limits to the impact it could have on the major health problems that Americans face today.

This is not to say that nothing can be done to increase the health of the American people. There may well be little hope for prevention or cure of these diseases through medical intervention, yet there is much to suggest that these diseases occur prematurely, that many have significantly more damaging effects than are necessary, and, in some cases, that they are avoidable through control of unhealthy lifestyles and behaviors. In fact, the whole ***health promotion and disease prevention*** (HP/DP) movement is based on the recognition that the most useful solutions to the most prominent health problems of our time are prevention and control of the progress of these diseases. To illustrate:

- Heart disease is the most common cause of disability of Americans over the age of 40, yet it has been estimated that 80% of all deaths from heart disease occur prematurely and are facilitated by unhealthy habits, primarily cigarette smoking, overweight, and sedentary lifestyle.
- Lung cancer is our most common lethal malignancy, yet it is estimated that 80% of all lung cancer deaths are directly caused by cigarette smoking. Other types of cancer are also related to, and worsened by, smoking (oral and bladder cancer), the ingestion of food additives and certain drugs, and the inhaling of a wide variety of noxious agents.
- Cirrhosis is directly related to, and worsened by, excessive ingestion of alcohol together with poor nutrition.
- Accident fatalities are directly related to alcohol ingestion, excessive speed, and refusal to use seat belts (Knowles, 1977).
- Anywhere from 4% to 100% of patients with diabetes, hypertension, ulcers, rheumatic fever, or tuberculosis fail to comply with medical and rehabilitative recommendations designed to lessen the effects of their diseases (Marston, 1970).

A recurring theme in these examples is that the diseases that most threaten the health of the American public have a number of well-established ***risk factors***. By removing the risk factors associated with the progress of these diseases, one can postpone their occurrence, lessen their debilitating effects, and, in some cases, even prevent them from occurring at all. To a large extent, control of present major health problems entails modification of individual behaviors and lifestyles.

In light of these observations, convincing arguments have been made that the next major advances in the health of the American people will be made, not by what the health care system is able to provide, but rather by what people are willing to do for themselves. More attention is being paid to studies that reveal that good health and longevity are as much related to a self-enforced regimen of sufficient sleep, regular well-balanced meals, moderate exercise and weight, no smoking, and little or no drinking as they are to professionally delivered services (Breslow, 1973). If people were willing to do these things, the impact on the nation's health would be enormous, and billions of health care dollars would be saved. Otherwise, we probably should stop complaining about the steadily rising costs of health care and the lack of expected results (Knowles, 1977). We must realize that more medical care will not, in itself, result in better health.

The tragedy is, however, that this insight is little promoted by the health care system. In addition, it requires a rejection of an assumption that is widely accepted (ie, that health care makes people healthy) as well as modifications of behaviors that are notoriously difficult to change. Although reorganization of our health care system is undoubtedly needed to improve accessibility and quality and to contain costs, the fact is that improving the health care system is not necessarily the most effective way of improving health. This is not to say that the health care system is good for nothing; rather, it is not good for everything.

In summary, we have inherited our present health care delivery system from nearly a century of haphazard growth. It was derived from a family doctor-centered health care system that worked reasonably well at a time when medical science and education were less sophisticated, health problems were more straightforward, delivery of health care was simpler, and society, correctly doubting the benefits anyway, was less demanding. The system is now proving inadequate in the face of new demographic, epidemiologic, and social problems that are largely the result of medicine's technologic success (Freymann, 1977).

The most striking characteristic of the health care system, as Freymann (1977) notes, is *imbalance*. We have gone from no science to little but science, from no specialists to practically all specialists, from widespread fear of hospitals to widespread veneration of them, from insufficient funding to financing that overloaded the system, from life familiar with death to a long lifespan that is almost guaranteed, from lavish support of one fragment of the system (acute care) to neglect of the others (chronic, psychiatric, and preventive services), from an abundance of inadequate doctors to a maldistribution of good ones, from no faith in medicine to unrealistic faith in it. Yet it is the imbalance that has developed between the *supply* of health services and the *demand* for health services that has created the most devastating impact on the delivery of health services. There are a number of forces that have contributed to this imbalance. These include changes in research and technology, which fostered specialization; the status of hospitals; the methods of financing care; the role played by government; public values and expectations; the nature of disease; and the age composition of the population. All these forces have caused demand to increase faster than supply can increase. The result has been continuing rapid rises in health care costs.

Reform of the health care system: Past, present, and future

The frequent frustration of unmet demands and concern about costs have created increasing political pressure for major changes in the health care delivery system. Notable examples of efforts at reform include the following:

National health insurance proposals, which attempt to ensure that all Americans are covered by a more comprehensive (less hospital-based) model of health insurance and which would also protect them in the event of catastrophic illness. The United States is the only developed nation in the Western world that does not have a universal program of health insurance.

Social Security Amendments of 1972 (P.L. 92-603), which provided for the establishment of Professional Standard Review Organizations to ensure that federally funded programs, such as Medicare and Medicaid, were used in an efficient and effective manner. These organizations were succeeded by the Professional Review Organizations, which continue to be Medicare's quality assurance program today.

Health Maintenance Organization Act of 1973 (P.L. 93-222), which provided for the planning and development of **health maintenance organizations** (HMOs) to encourage less costly ambulatory care outside the hospital, including preventive, diagnostic, therapeutic, and rehabilitative services

National Health Planning and Resources Development Act of 1974 (P.L. 93-641), which established regional health systems agencies to assume responsibility for health care planning for community needs and for cost containment. The Act required hospitals that wished to engage in major construction or to change service programs to be reviewed.

The National Consumer Health Information and Health Promotion Act of 1976, which attempted to set rational goals for health information and education

Health Professions Educational Assistance Act (P.L. 94-484), which provided incentives for medical schools to increase the number of family practice physicians to half of their graduates and also attempts to attract physicians to underserved areas by subsidizing their medical education

Omnibus Budget Reconciliation Act of 1981 (PL 97-35), which reduced federal spending for the provision of direct health services by one quarter and which encouraged the expansion of HMOs and **preferred provider organizations** (PPOs).

Tax Equity and Fiscal Responsibility Act of 1982 (PL 97-246), which set up the Professional Review Organizations, an external audit system, to ensure that health care services paid for with public funds are of high quality.

Title VII of the Medicare Prospective Payment Legislation (P.L. 98-21) in 1983, which provided incentives for cost containment and better management of resources by a reimbursement structure based on a patient's diagnosis rather than the direct costs of care

Any proposals for reform of the health care system—in the past, present, or the future—bring with them hopes to contain costs, to provide accessibility of services for all, and to improve the quality and continuity of health care. They also hope to encourage more effective and rational use of services by both provider and consumers by modifying the demand for the most expensive health services and by structural reform of the delivery system. Their goal is to make our acute care, hospital-dominated system more comprehensive and continuous. It is, however, fair to suggest that in the present environment of sluggish economic growth, low productivity growth, and inflation, it is the *cost of health care* that is moving politicians to basic reform of the health care delivery system rather than any concerns they have about the performance, structure, and efficiency of that system. As we have seen, basic market principles dictate that any proposal aimed at containing costs will have to increase supply more than demand.

Structure of the health care system

The *structure* of the health care system is based on the historic precedents and economic incentives discussed above. It is composed of many independent components affiliated in a variety of ways and of many smaller systems serving specific groups of people. We will begin to explore its structural components by looking at its two major divisions.

The two basic divisions for delivering health care in the United States are the **public division** and the **private division**. The public system is operated by federal, state, and local governments and has two major concerns. The first is primary prevention services provided at the public health level to prevent disease. Examples include sanitation systems, water purification and fluoridation, and immunization programs for children of low-income families. The second major concern of the public system is the operation of a series of smaller subsystems to provide health care to specific groups of entitled citizens. For example, the military operates its own health care system for people in the armed services, the Veterans Administration provides ongoing care for veterans with service-connected illnesses and injuries, and the Indian Health Service is responsible for caring for Native Americans on reservations. In addition, there has been a long tradition that care of the developmentally disabled child and the severely or chronically mentally ill adult is provided by a public system developed at the state level.

The private health system consists of a loose association of independent health professionals who provide personal health care services on a fee-for-service basis. Most health care expenditures—more than 90%—occur within the private system (National Center for Health Statistics, 1989). Because of its predominance, the rest of this discussion will focus on the private health system.

The major components of the private health care system include financing, payment mechanisms, health care personnel, institutions for delivering care, and system regulation. A brief description of each component follows.

Financing

The health care system accounts for more than $733 billion in national expenditures (Castro, 1991). Of these funds, about 42% is spent on hospital care, 19% on physician services, 6% on dentist services, 7% on drugs, 8% on nursing home care, and the remainder on a wide variety of other activities, including research and prevention (National Center for Health Statistics, 1989). Health care costs are increasing faster than practically any other aspect of the nation's economy. The percentage of the gross national product (all economic activity) spent on health care in the United States has increased from about 5% in the 1960s to 12% now (Castro, 1991).

This more than doubling of the resources devoted to health care is of great concern to those who finance it, from two perspectives. The first is reflected in questions about whether the economy can afford such large expenditures for health care when there are so many other needs to be met from the same funds. As we spend more for medicine, there is necessarily less available for other critical sectors of the economy, including education, housing, nutrition, transportation, income supplementation, and defense. As will be seen, these economic limits have already imposed de facto rationing in health care. At this rate of growth, Americans will be spending a third of all resources on health care within 20 years. The second perspective is reflected in questions about what we are getting for our health care dollar. Critics note that for all our increased expenditures, there has been no statistically significant change in the health of the American population (Eisenberg, 1977). Thus, valid arguments are being raised that we would be healthier if we spent the money on education, better public housing, or better highways.

Another important trend in financing health care is the increasing share of the health care bill that is paid by federal or state governments (ie, the taxpayer). In the early 1960s, governments paid for 25% of all health care; now governments pay more than 40% of the nation's health care bill (National Center for Health Statistics, 1989). The two publicly financed national entitlement programs, Medicaid and Medicare, account for most of these funds. The costs of these programs have increased so dramatically that taxpayers and governments are beginning to reassess their abilities to provide access to services for the poor and the elderly.

Ultimately, the people pay all health care costs; however, there are two sources of income for the health care system. The first is individuals and families. They pay directly for services (eg, dental services, pharmaceuticals, ambulatory care) and also pay indirectly through their own health insurance premiums; through federal, state, and local taxes; and through the purchase of goods and services (a portion of domestic consumer prices reflects the costs of the workers' health insurance premiums). The other income source is the employer. Employers pay an equal share of Social Security taxes as well as health insurance premiums and corporate income taxes. Funds from these two sources, individuals and employers, are transferred to private insurers and governments, who purchase health services. Private and public insurance have become the major forms of financing medical care, accounting for 75% of expenditures for all personal health care and 90% of all hospital care expenditures (National Center for Health Statistics, 1989).

Payment mechanisms

As noted above, both **public funds** (about 40%) and **private funds** pay for the health care received in the United States. Within each sector, there are a variety of spending sources. Public funds, for example, come through such diverse programs as temporary disability insurance, workmen's compensation, public assistance, Veteran's Administration, Office of Economic Opportunity, Defense Department, public health services, maternal and child health services, school health, and vocational rehabilitation. As indicated earlier, however, the major sources of public funding of health care are Medicare and Medicaid. Private health expenditures consist of direct payments by consumers for health care and, more commonly, insurance payments made on their behalf. Private insurance is sold largely through employers. There are three major types: Blue Cross, **commercial insurance**, and **alternative practice models**, such as HMOs, **independent practice associations** (IPAs), and PPOs.

In the United States, access to health care is dependent on the availability of insurance, and 85% of the population has some form of health insurance protection, either public or private (Swartz, 1984). This means that 15% of all Americans have no insurance protection, a problem that has become worse in the last decade.

The principal insurance plans are presented below.

Medicare

Medicare consists of a basic program of hospitalization insurance under which most people aged 65 years and over are protected against the major costs of hospital and related care (Part A); and a supplementary insurance program through which people aged

65 years and over are aided in paying physician, home health care, and other health care bills (Part B). Coverage under Part A is automatically available to all those covered by the Social Security system. Part B requires a premium payment from the beneficiary to cover part of the costs. Medicare is a single federal program funded by workers' payroll taxes and administered by the Social Security Administration.

Health care costs under Medicare have skyrocketed from $5 billion at the inception of the program to $110 billion today. Since the 12% of the U. S. population that is over 65 years of age currently accounts for 36% of all health care expenditures, there are serious concerns about the precipitous escalation in expenditures when this population figure swells to 20% of the population, as predicted for the year 2000 (Mathiessen, 1989). The major proportion of Medicare expenditures, nearly 70%, is for acute inpatient hospital services. Until recently, all attempts to control costs had been directed at regulating the use of health care services. More recently, however, attempts to control Medicare costs have been directed at reimbursement. The most dramatic change was the introduction in 1983 of the ***prospective payment system*** for Medicare hospitalization, which limits the amount of reimbursement for physicians and hospitals on the basis of the patient's particular medical problem, or ***diagnostic-related group*** (DRG). Before the introduction of this legislation, physicians and hospitals had little incentive to increase efficiency or to control costs because they were reimbursed for whatever services were provided. Now a fixed payment is made for each DRG. This encourages both the physicians and hospital to restrain their expenditures to the amount that they expect to receive. There is, however, allowance made for the fact that medical problems are unpredictable by permitting some increase in payment if there are either complications or coexisting medical problems. Medicare is also beginning to reimburse HMOs and hospice services (to be discussed more fully later) on a prospective basis.

Many people incorrectly assume that at age 65, all medical expenses will be covered by Medicare. Currently, Medicare payments cover only 49% of the total medical costs of the elderly (U. S. Senate Special Committee on Aging, 1989). This is due, in part, to medical needs of the elderly, including preventive care, care of chronic conditions on an outpatient basis, long-term care, and supportive care, which are not covered by Medicare.

Medicaid

Medicaid provides federal assistance to states to cover certain medical expenses of specified groups of low-income people (eg, the needy aged, the blind, the disabled) and welfare recipients. Revenues for the Medicaid program come from general tax revenues at the federal, state, and local levels. The size and the scope of the program is determined by the individual states, but participating states are required to cover the following basic services for the welfare population: inpatient hospital services, outpatient hospital services, skilled nursing home services, physician services, and limited home health services. In addition, a number of services can be supplied at state option, including, for example, clinic services, dental care, occupational and physical therapy services, drugs, vision care, prosthetic devices, and skilled nursing home services. As a result, Medicaid provides widely varying coverage and might best be conceptualized as a series of 50 separate programs, each administered by individual

state welfare departments. Medicaid is the fastest growing spending program in the United States (Castro, 1991). It pays, for example, for half of all nursing home patients (at an annual cost of $37,000 per person), severely impaired crack infants, AIDS victims, poor single mothers, and pregnant teenagers. As with Medicare, the rapid escalation in costs has led to cutbacks in eligibility, benefits, and payments for providers. Although Medicaid is supposed to insure those who cannot pay for coverage, it can barely afford to help 40% of the poor (Castro, 1991). And, in some states, Medicaid pays as little as 40% of physician charges. Consequently, providers are becoming more reluctant to treat Medicaid patients. Accessibility to health care for the poor and the elderly may decline as the government finds it increasingly difficult to pay the bills.

Blue cross

Blue Cross is the largest private financier of hospital care in the United States. Even though there are actually 75 independent Blue Cross plans, these plans are linked by the National Blue Cross Association, which represents them in national affairs and provides services in marketing, education, research, and public relations. Blue Cross plans are primarily nonprofit voluntary organizations that operate under enabling legislation specifically enacted to cover nonprofit prepayment plans. Therefore, they are often subject to state regulation of their rates and benefits, usually by the insurance department of the state in which the plan operates.

In general, Blue Cross coverage is designed to provide reasonably full payment of the total bill for most hospitalizations. Other than that, there is no standard plan. Employers can buy any package of benefits and other plan characteristics that they want, and the insurer "costs out" the benefit package that is selected to determine the premiums. Individual policies may also cover, for example, outpatient physician services, prescription drugs, or services provided by psychologists, chiropractors, podiatrists, and nurse practitioners.

It is important to recognize that the predominance of Blue Cross plans for private insurance coverage was reinforced by the federal government with the passage of Medicare and Medicaid legislation because Blue Cross was designated as the fiscal intermediary between hospitals and Medicare.

Commercial insurance

From the consumer's point of view, commercial insurance is not noticeably different from Blue Cross. However, insurance contracts in this area are indemnity contracts, offered by for-profit insurance companies through employers. Under indemnity insurance, when the enrollee uses health care services that are covered by the benefits of a specific plan, the insurance company pays the person a certain amount of money, and the person is responsible for paying the provider. Hence, this method of insurance involves more administrative paper work than Blue Cross because the enrollee must file claims for benefits.

In contrast to Blue Cross, commercial insurance companies are profit-making businesses that can provide similar benefits to people in different states. This is advantageous for large employers, who are able to obtain uniform benefits for employees in different states by access to only one company. In addition, health insurance is usually only one of the many types of insurance offered by commercial insurance companies.

Health maintenance organizations

In the early 1970s, the federal government promoted prepaid group practice through HMOs. A prepaid group practice is an organization that agrees to provide most or all the care that enrollees need in return for an established monthly or annual fee. The organization, in turn, hires or contracts with physicians and hospitals for enrollees' care. The HMO thus has an incentive to contain health care costs since its income is fixed regardless of how much care is provided. The HMO also assumes a significant portion of the financial risk of providing health care services that were previously borne by the reimbursers. HMOs often provide a wider range of services at less cost than traditional insurance programs. They also provide more preventive care since it is in their interests for enrollees to stay healthy. Indeed, HMOs achieve their savings through lower rates of hospitalization despite higher rates of ambulatory care.

There is considerable national interest in HMOs because they are 10% to 40% less expensive than the conventional system for delivering health care (Arnould, 1984). There are estimates that by the year 2000, about half the U. S. population will receive their health care through some form of an HMO. HMOs are also being tested as a mechanism to administer Medicare funds.

A variant of an HMO is the IPA. In this model, the HMO or insurance company contracts with a number of individual physicians who operate out of their private offices. Patients are enrolled in these private practices, and the HMO or insurance company pays the independent practitioner an established fee per patient to provide services to the enrollees. Physicians are free to derive additional income through their traditional fee-for-service practices.

Preferred provider organizations

Since 1986, PPOs have become an additional alternative practice model. Service is provided to members for a set fee that is lower than the usual market price. The goal of a PPO is to sign up a large number of physicians (the preferred providers) who will accept a predetermined fee that is lower than the market price. PPOs are somewhat of a hybrid of a fee-for-service system and a prepaid group health plan. Once a physician provides a service, the insurance company pays the prearranged fee. In this sense, the PPO operates as a fee-for-service system, while the prospective payment concept is derived from the fact that the fees-for-service are predetermined.

Who is excluded?

Although insurance coverage provided by both the private and the public sectors for health care is extensive, there are still many Americans who have no coverage. These include the unemployed, the independently employed (health insurance is very costly for people who cannot obtain group coverage), those employed in transient jobs, those who change jobs frequently or changed jobs recently, those with "bad" diagnoses, and the chronically sick. Most of the *uninsured* are the families of low-income workers in small firms that offer either no insurance

plans or plans that cover workers but not their dependents. Current federal administration policies have shifted the emphasis from access to health care to issues having to do with the control of costs. As a result, health care cutbacks have worsened access to health care for large parts of the population.

As of this writing, legislation has been introduced in Congress to require all employers to provide medical insurance to their employees. Reaction to this proposed legislation is mixed. Businesses and other groups, wary of federal mandates, are suggesting alternative approaches. There is no easy solution to covering the nation's uninsured.

Health care personnel

Almost ten million people are employed directly or indirectly in the health care delivery system (National Center for Health Statistics, 1989), making health care the second largest employer in the United States, exceeded only by the construction industry. Health care is also one of the fastest growing industries: between 1970 and 1980, the number of people employed increased by 70% (National Center for Health Statistics, 1989). This rapid growth of manpower is mainly the result of the rapid advances in technology and the need for more specialized personnel. Health care personnel were rarely scrutinized in the past for the efficiency, efficacy, or cost effectiveness of their services because of the open-ended flow (until recently) of third-party payments for many services. Times are changing rapidly, however, and health care rationing has become a major concern. This will undoubtedly affect the health care workforce.

The number of physicians has also increased dramatically. In 1970, there were about 255,000 physicians providing patient care in the United States. By 1986, this number had risen by 70%, to 436,877 (National Center for Health Statistics, 1989). Although in the 1960s there was fear about a doctor shortage, there now are questions about a doctor surplus. While debate continues about how many physicians and what types are actually needed, we know that an increase in the supply of doctors means more medical care and, ultimately, higher costs because physicians create their own demand for services by ordering tests, hospitalizations, and referrals. This is also the case with other types of health professionals. An increase in the supply of health providers will increase the supply and, often, the demand for their services. That is, more occupational therapists means more services, which tends to increase the demand for their services. Again, this translates into higher costs.

In terms of practice type, about 85% of physicians in the United States are specialists (National Center for Health Statistics, 1989), and the need for more general practitioners is well recognized. As indicated earlier, one of the key provisions of the Health Professions Educational Assistance Act of 1976 was to require medical schools with teaching hospitals to provide a greater proportion of their medical residencies in family practice medicine. The rewards of specialty practice in terms of prestige, income, and lifestyle, however, continue to outweigh those of general medical practice. For example, specialists can earn over $300,000 per year compared with the average family practitioner's income of $96,000 (Castro, 1991). Another major problem with our supply of physicians has also been mentioned; that is, most physicians want to practice in metropolitan areas, where the potential for peer interaction, for working in the best hospitals, and for higher incomes has been the greatest. As a result, many inner-city and rural areas have shortages of physicians, while other parts of the country have surpluses. Federal programs have attempted to attract physicians to shortage areas, such as through the National Health Corps (P.L. 94-484), which subsidizes medical education in return for a commitment to practice in medically underserved areas. Just as we cannot force physicians to choose family practice instead of a specialty, however, there is no way to force physicians to practice where they are most needed. Similar maldistribution occurs for all other health professionals, including occupational therapists.

Physicians exert the most powerful influence over the health care industry because they control hospital use, drug prescriptions, and referral for services reimbursed by Medicare, Medicaid, and other insurance plans. In fact, this dominance is guaranteed by law. Hence, the ability of other health care professionals to influence the health care system is limited. And yet physicians represent only a minority (9%) of professionals involved in the delivery of health care; nurses represent the majority of health care professionals, nearly 55% (U. S. Bureau of the Census, 1986). With 40,000 practitioners, occupational therapists represent about 0.5% of the people employed in health-related activities.

Health care institutions

Hospitals

The hospital is the center of our health care delivery system, accounting for the highest percentage of health care expenditures. Of the approximately 7000 hospitals in the country, nearly 6000 are community hospitals (American Hospital Association, 1984), most of which focus on the provision of short-term acute care. This total, however, includes hospitals with specialized missions, such as children's rehabilitation as well as hospitals owned and operated by the federal government (eg, Veterans Administration or military hospitals). Most private hospitals in this country are owned by nonprofit corporations, such as religious groups and city or county corporations, although private hospitals increasingly are being bought by chains, most of which are for-profit companies.

There are large geographic disparities in hospital distribution. The number of hospital beds per 1000 population is, on average, 60% greater in the industrial New England and Mid-Atlantic states than in the Rocky Mountain states (National Center for Health Statistics, 1989). This reflects too many beds in metropolitan areas as well as too few in rural areas.

The most significant trends in the hospital industry over the past decade have been the development of multihospital systems and the proliferation of *for-profit hospitals*. Multihospital systems are being organized largely by for-profit corporations, although **nonprofit hospitals** are beginning to affiliate with each other as well. Hospitals are attempting to coordinate and consolidate services to allow them to compete more aggressively, increase efficiency, and remain financially viable. As a result, it is likely that independent nonprofit community hospitals will be forced out of business in the near future.

In addition to the growth of multihospital systems, there has been rapid growth in the number of for-profit (proprietary) hospitals. Today, proprietary hospitals are owned and operated by large national or international corporations that can buy supplies and equipment in bulk and that employ a wide range of experts in financing, marketing, and planning to manage the hospital.

Some trends bear watching. As indicated earlier, in 1983, Medicare Prospective Payment legislation was enacted that changed the way acute care hospitals are reimbursed for Medicare bills. (Currently, psychiatric hospitals, rehabilitation hospitals, children's hospitals, and long-term care hospitals are exempted from prospective payment.) Under the new system, diagnoses are divided into DRGs, and the government has set a fixed price for treatment of each diagnosis, regardless of what services are provided. If hospitals spend less, they make money; if they spend more, they lose money. Clearly, this offers a financial incentive to limit treatment and discharge patients as early as possible. And, as one might predict, the average length of hospital stay has declined continuously since 1983. The DRG reimbursement policy also encourages hospitals to change the mix of services they provide in favor of those that are most profitable. Consequently, there is concern that low-profit but essential services—such as head trauma and burn care—may be eliminated by hospitals seeking to maximize their overall reimbursement.

Another ominous trend is the closing and relocation of hospitals that have traditionally served the poor and minorities in the inner-city. Hospitals faced with the economic burdens of providing free or underreimbursed care tend to relocate to the more affluent suburbs. Thus, hospital care has become increasingly inaccessible for poor inner-city residents. Closing and relocation is particularly common among for-profit hospitals (Rice, 1987).

Nursing homes

The fastest growing category of health care spending in the United States is **nursing home care**. There are about 22,000 nursing homes in the United States, a total that by all estimates falls far short of the national need. Moreover, it is estimated that an additional 1.2 million nursing home beds will be needed by the year 2000 just to maintain present levels of service (U. S. Bureau of Census, 1978). Nursing homes provide both inpatient care that is less intense than that provided in hospitals and care for the permanently dependent, such as the severely affected Alzheimer disease victim. Most nursing homes are small proprietary institutions with fewer than 100 beds. Less than 20% are nonprofit or owned by the government (U. S. Bureau of Census, 1978). Increasingly, however, nursing homes are being bought or built by large health care corporations.

Nursing home care is subject to severe financial restrictions that affect the availability of nursing homes as well as the quality and scope of services they can provide. There are two tests that must be met for nursing home care to be covered by Medicare: (1) care must be skilled, not merely custodial; and (2) care must be rehabilitative, that is, based on some chance of recuperation. Medicare provides minimal assistance in paying for nursing home care: in fact, only 1% of Medicare's budget is expended on nursing home care (U. S. Senate Special Committee on Aging, 1988). Reimbursement is available under Medicaid, but patients must exhaust both Medicare benefits and their personal financial resources to become eligible for Medicaid reimbursement. Even then, as mentioned earlier, levels of reimbursement under Medicaid are typically low. If sufficient political pressure were exerted to increase funding for nursing home care, the quantity, quality, and range of services offered would undoubtedly improve (see Chapter 27).

Home health care and hospice care

Two additional institutions for the delivery of health care that have grown rapidly within the last decade are home health care and hospice care.

Home health care has been called the sleeping giant of the health care industry (Balinsky, 1985). Although it is still in its infancy, compared to hospitals and nursing homes, it is rapidly expanding as a result of pressure from an aging population, skyrocketing Medicare and Medicaid expenditures, a hospital and provider industry experiencing financial stress, and a business community searching for more cost-effective health care benefits for its employees. Home health care services have also become a preferred method of providing health care to a large segment of the population. Bringing services to people in their own homes is seen as a realistic and more humane approach for all but the most complex of health care services. The major goals of home health care have been to prevent hospitalization and to delay or avoid residential health care placement. However, home health care, a less costly method of service delivery, has become especially attractive to institutions attempting to make the DRG system profitable by sending patients home quicker and sicker (Coleman & Smith, 1984).

Home health care is generally considered to include the provision of skilled nursing services; occupational, physical, and speech therapy; medical social services; dietary services; homemaker services; home health aide services; respiratory therapy; and medical supplies, drugs, and appliances. These services are provided through public agencies; nonprofit agencies, such as visiting nurses associations; agencies operated by hospitals, skilled nursing facilities, or rehabilitation facilities; and proprietary organizations. Many hospitals are responding to the advent of DRGs by establishing their own agencies to replenish revenues lost under prospective payment. Reimbursements for services vary but are derived most commonly from Medicare and Medicaid as well as from the Veterans Administration, the Civilian Health and Medical Program of the Uniformed Services, Title III of the Older Americans Act, Social Services Block Grants to states (formerly Title XX), private health insurance, and private payment by patients (see Chapter 28).

Hospice care is both a philosophy and an organized program of care designed for terminally ill patients and their families. It has only recently become a significant component of the health care delivery system. The overall goal is to minimize suffering and heroic intervention while offering palliative care to the patient and support to the patient and family during the process of dying. As such, it is viewed as an organized reaction to a significant social problem: the depersonalization of care for the terminally ill and the failure of the existing medical care system to meet the needs of the dying (Paradis, 1985). Hospice is also being seen as a cost-saving alternative in health care delivery.

A variety of organizational structures deliver hospice care, including free-standing or independent programs, hospital-based programs, home health agency–based programs, and community-based (or volunteer) programs. Hospices provide or arrange for the following services: nursing, physician services, social work, pastoral care, bereavement counseling, nutrition, physical and occupational therapy, psychological services, pharmacy services, medical supplies, laboratory services, home health aide services, personal care, housekeeping and homemaker services, and short-term inpatient services.

Reimbursement for hospice care has increased dramatically in the past few years. In 1981, Blue Cross initiated coverage for hospice care. Shortly thereafter, a number of commercial insurers followed their lead. Medicare reimbursement was established in 1983 within the Tax Equity and Fiscal Responsibility Act, and in 1986, the Omnibus Budget Reconciliation Act sanctioned the addition of a hospice benefit to the list of services that states may choose to add to their Medicaid plans. With these reimbursement mechanisms, hospice care has been placed in the mainstream of the health care delivery system (see Chapter 30).

System regulation

The private health care system functions under a complex set of rules and regulations. The law has assumed a steadily increasing role in health care, given its interests in protecting the public health, safety, and welfare and in protecting the rights of providers and patients in the health care process.

Traditionally, the primary responsibility for formulating *health care policy* has rested within individual states. For example, licensing of health personnel; accreditation of hospitals, nursing homes, and other health facilities; protection of patients' rights; statutes that define criteria for pronouncing death; and the negligence, liability, and malpractice systems are operated primarily by the states. The federal government, however, is assuming more of a role over health care issues to protect its increased stake in the system, primarily through regulations that are attached to the use of Medicare and Medicaid funds. Further, the federal courts have become significantly involved in bioethical questions, especially those bearing on abortion, the definition of death, human subject research, informed consent, right to treatment, and right to refuse treatment.

In addition, the private health care system functions under a set of professional regulations. The involvement of individual professions in the regulatory process acknowledges that specific professional competence is needed to evaluate the quality of care given by health providers. Consequently, accreditation of medical, dental, and allied health professional schools; requirements for certification examinations; certification of the qualifications of health providers; and malpractice criteria have become the responsibility of professional associations.

Health promotion and disease prevention

Within the last decade, there has been a growing trend toward wellness-oriented health care, disease prevention, and health promotion. A number of the social and demographic factors discussed previously have sparked this interest, including the change in focus from acute infectious diseases to chronic degenerative diseases, the recognition of lifestyle and individual behaviors as significant factors in the disease process, the increasing shortcomings of traditional medicine, the age shifts in our population, and the unbearable economic prospect of maintaining an ailing elder population (Dychtwald, 1986). In 1974, the government cited "the promotion of activities for the prevention of disease" as one of the 10 national health priorities (P.L. 93-641, Section 1502). This law acknowledged the importance of taking action either to avoid illness or to reduce the premature occurrence of disabilities attending the chronic diseases that medicine today is unable to cure as a way of reducing the cost of treatment. Beyond this acknowledgment, however, lie more important issues, chief among them being the actual resources we are willing to commit to this effort. Of the $733 billion spent annually on health care in the United States, only about 3% is spent on prevention services.

Notwithstanding, in 1979, the federal government began a 10-year public policy initiative for HP/DP. The 1979 report, *Healthy People: The Surgeon General's Report on Health Promotion and Disease Prevention* (Public Health Service, 1979) cautioned that improvements in the health of Americans would not come from advances in medical care and increases in health expenditures alone but rather could best be accomplished through efforts designed to *prevent* disease and *promote* health. The report set goals to reduce death and disability rates for 1990 for different age groups, and it set strategic targets for 1990 that included 15 topics divided into the following three areas:

1. Preventive health services, designed to increase health through medical care, specifically, high blood pressure control, family planning, pregnancy and infant health, immunization, and sexually transmitted diseases
2. Health protection for population groups, aimed at modifying environmental risks, specifically toxic agent and radiation control, occupational safety and health, accident prevention and injury control, fluoridation and dental health, and control of infectious diseases
3. Health promotion for population groups, aimed at modifying lifestyle risk factors to good health, specifically smoking cessation, drug and alcohol abuse treatment, nutrition, physical fitness and exercise, and control of stress and violent behavior

A later report gave priority to the *1990 Health Objectives* for the Nation in terms of a specialized focus for each of five age groups (Public Health Service, 1986).

For infants younger than 1 year old, the national goal was to reduce deaths by 35% by focusing on low birth weight and birth defects. For children aged 1 to 4 years, the goal was to reduce deaths by 20% by focusing on growth, development, and injuries. For adolescents and young adults, the goal was to reduce deaths by 20% by focusing on motor vehicle injuries, alcohol, and drugs. For adults aged 25 to 64 years, the goal was 25% fewer deaths by focusing on heart attacks, strokes, and cancers. And for older adults, the goal was 20% fewer sick days by focusing on influenza, pneumonia, and functional independence.

The 1990 Objectives introduced into health care policy a major emphasis on functional independence and the value of health care in facilitating functional ability, which has been further underscored in the *Year 2000 Health Objectives for the Nation* (U.S. Department of Health and Human Services, 1990). This new emphasis represents a subtle yet significant shift from earlier health care policies, which emphasized cost factors rather than outcomes, in the provision of health care. In the 1990s, health care policy is looking more and more to functional ability as a critical health care outcome. This trend bodes well for the profession of occupational therapy (see Chapter 29).

In addition to, and in support of, governmental policy and planning initiatives, a number of hospitals are beginning to establish their own HP/DP programs, in large part to make money and also to improve their images in the community. The American Hospital Association's Center for Health Promotion has been a major stimulus and guide for hospitals in developing these programs (Jonas and Rosenberg, 1986). The HD/DP programs include one or more elements of primary prevention (the prevention of disease before any symptoms are present), secondary prevention (screening, early detection, and early treatment of clinically inapparent disease in a person who has been defined as at risk), and tertiary prevention (the treatment of acquired disease in a manner designed to minimize the development of complications). The recommended core HP/DP programs include:

In primary prevention, the "basic seven" personal preventive interventions:
Exercise promotion
Smoking cessation
Weight loss
Stress management
Nutrition counseling
Substance abuse control
Personal accident prevention
In secondary prevention, screening and early detection of:
Cancer
Hypertension
Diabetes
Heart Disease
Glaucoma
In tertiary prevention:
Cardiac rehabilitation
Pulmonary rehabilitation
Musculoskeletal rehabilitation

Final comments

The health care system of the United States has been described as a nonsystem. Clearly, it is not a unified system; rather, it is a loose network of a number of components within which health care services are provided. Services are somewhat interdependent since each component serves a specific function and depends on the others for referrals, although each component still functions relatively independently in policy and decision making. It is little wonder that it is considered an "underpreventive, overspecialized, poorly coordinated, unaccountable, and inaccessible" health care system (Weiner et al., 1987, p. 426).

All components of the health care system are faced with the formidable challenge of meeting public demands for universal access and high quality, comprehensive, and continuous care while at the same time controlling costs. Although previous attempts at major reform have run into a gridlock of conflicting interests among physicians, hospitals, and insurers, public opinion now holds promise for breaking the impasse. A recent survey revealed that 91% of the American public believes that the health care system needs fundamental change, and 70% stated that they would be willing to pay higher taxes to ensure that all Americans have insurance coverage (Castro, 1991). For the first time in history, political candidates in the 1992 presidential campaign placed universal health care at the top of their agendas.

Yet as available resources shrink in relation to health care needs, we are all facing the difficult task of reconciling the *Hippocratic Oath*, which requires that we do all we can to sustain life, with *allocative justice*, which requires that we use resources where they can save the most lives. When a single procedure designed to save one life may involve enough money to save the lives of hundreds, this dilemma raises profound and troubling choices that force us to move beyond the needs and rights of individuals, as poignant as these are, to a broader social perspective. These choices will severely test our national will and wisdom as we *all* are faced with the challenges that accompany our successes in living longer.

References

American Hospital Association. (1984). *Hospital statistics, 1984* (Appendix I [A 10]). Chicago: American Hospital Association.

Arnould, R. (1984). Do HMOs produce services more efficiently? *Inquiry, 21*, 3–6.

Balinsky, W. (1985). Home care: Current trends and future prospects. *New York Business Group Health Newsletter, 5.*

Breslow, L. (1973). Research in a strategy for health improvement. *International Journal of Health Services, 3*, 7–16.

Castro, J. (1991, November 25). Condition: Critical. *Time,* 34–42.

Coleman, J., & Smith, D. (1984). DRGs and the growth of home health care. *Nursing Economics, 2*, 391–396.

Crichton, M. (1970). *Five patients: The hospital explained.* New York: Alfred E. Knopf.

Dychtwald, K. (1986). *Wellness and health promotion for the elderly.* Rockville, MD: Aspen.

Eisenberg, L. (1977, Winter). The search for care. *Daedalus,* 235–246.

Freymann, J. G. (1977). *The American health care system: Its genesis and trajectory* (pp. 96–97). Huntington, NY: Robert Krieger.

Henderson, L. J. (1941). *The study of man.* Philadelphia: University of Pennsylvania Press.

Himmelstein, D., & Woolhandler, S. (1989). A national health program for the United States: A physician's proposal. *New England Journal of Medicine, 320*(2), 102–108.

Jonas, S., & Rosenberg, S. (1986). Health, manpower, and ambulatory care. In S. Jonas (Ed.), *Health care delivery in the United States.* New York: Springer.

Knowles, J. H. (1977, Winter). The responsibility of the individual. *Daedalus,* 57–80.

Marston, M. V. (1970). Compliance with medical regimens: A review of the literature. *Nursing Research, 19*, 312–318.

Mathiessen, C. (1989). Unsurance. *Hippocrates, 3*, 36–46.

National Center for Health Statistics (1989). *Health, United States, 1988.* DHHS Pub. No. (PHS) 89-1232. Public Health Service. Washington DC: U. S. Government Printing Office.

Paradis, L. F. (1985). *Hospice handbook.* Germantown, MD: Aspen.

Public Health Service. (1986). *The 1990 health objectives for the nation: A midcourse review.* Washington DC: DHHS.

Public Health Service. (1979). *Healthy people: The surgeon general's report on health promotion and disease prevention.* Washington DC: DHHS

Rice, M. F. (1987). Inner city hospital closures/relocations: Race, income status, and legal issues. *Social Science and Medicine, 24*(11), 889–896.

Swartz, K. (1986). Testimony Before the Subcommittee on Health of the Committee on Finance, U. S. Senate, April 27, 1984. Washington, DC: U. S. Government Printing Office.

U. S. Bureau of Census (1986). *Statistical abstract of the United States: 1985* (Table 156). Washington, DC: U. S. Government Printing Office.

U. S. Bureau of Census (1978). *1976 survey of institutionalized persons: A study of persons receiving long-term care.* Current Population Reports, Series P-23, No. 69. Washington, DC: U. S. Government Printing Office.

U.S. Department of Health and Human Services. (1990). *Healthy people 2000: National health promotion and disease prevention objectives.* Washington, DC: U.S. Government Printing Office.

U. S. Senate Special Committee on Aging. (1989). *Aging America: Trends and projections.* Washington DC: AARP Publications.

Weiner, J., Maxwell, J., Sapolsky, H., Dunn, D., & Hsiao, W. (1987). Economic incentives and organizational realities: Managing hospitals under DRG's. *The Millbank Memorial Fund Quarterly, 65*(4), 463–487.

SECTION 2

Occupational therapy practice in the health care system

JUDITH M. PERINCHIEF

KEY TERMS

Ambulatory Care	*Home Care*
Community-Based Services	*Hospital-Based Services*
Competition	*School-Based Services*
Cost Containment	*Service Delivery Models*

LEARNING OBJECTIVES

Upon completion of this section the reader will be able to:

1. *Identify the major environmental and societal issues confronting occupational therapy practice.*

2. *Describe the major impacts of the health care system on the occupational therapy profession, personnel, education, and practice.*

3. *Identify how efforts toward cost containment and competition for health care dollars may affect the practicing occupational therapist.*

4. *Discuss the implications of the changing health care system on a variety of practice areas in occupational therapy.*

5. *Discuss methods that the practitioner and the profession as a whole should employ to prepare for occupational therapy practice in the 21st century.*

The intent of health care in the United States is to provide equitable, efficient, and effective care to the population. This care should be available and accessible to all and of assured quality. As a provider within the health care system, the occupational therapist is confronted with numerous issues and dilemmas.

Issues

Environment and society

Traditionally, the occupational therapist practiced in institutionally based service areas, and coverage for service was of little concern. The cost of service was frequently incorporated in the per diem charge for hospitalization and was occasionally covered by selling projects made by patients. Philanthropic gifts and funds from volunteer organizations were often used to augment the budget.

In the 1960s, with the expansion of national health insurance programs on a private and federal government basis, financial support from these sources greatly diminished, and occupational therapy managers were suddenly involved in extensive budgeting for their departments. Previously, providers had been shielded from **competition**. Now all allied health practitioners were competing for a controlled if not shrinking health care dollar. The practitioner was confronted with situations that limited occupational therapy services or made them inaccessible under a given insurance program. In the past, occupational therapists had not had to consider the importance of their services in relation to others; suddenly, reimbursement sources were determining the provision of care, and occupational therapy was not necessarily among the services recognized for coverage. For the most part, occupational therapy had not been represented in the political arena when the determination regarding coverage was made on a national level. The practitioner now had to justify service and validate practice previously taken for granted by the system at large. The consumer, who had acquired power in demanding care, had little knowledge or understanding of the services of the occupational therapist because, previously, the consumer had relied on the physician to determine which services were required. The physicians had become occupied with protecting their own practice and had little concern for the plight of other health care professionals. The power began to shift from the provider to the consumer.

Profession

For the occupational therapist to provide service, methods had to be instituted to educate consumers, legislators, reimbursement agencies, and other practitioners. The occupational therapy profession was confronted with significant public relations issues and was placed in the position of having to explain, defend, and validate services. The American Occupational Therapy Association (AOTA) began to take steps in the national office at the direction of the Representative Assembly. Public relations efforts increased, position papers were drafted and published, and the Government and Legal Affairs Division was instituted. To facilitate occupational therapists' negotiations with commercial insurance companies for coverage of service, a handbook on third-party reimbursement was prepared in 1976 by the Government and Legal Affairs Division.

Twenty years ago, public discussion of the quality of occupational therapy services barely existed, but within a decade, quality assurance became a major issue for the profession. The AOTA Division of Practice launched workshops and initiated publications to disperse information and knowledge to the practitioner within hospital-based programs requiring quality assurance and peer review. Increasingly, materials became available on utilization review, quality assurance, program evaluation, and performance appraisal of employees. By 1982, the government had instituted a massive effort to develop a nationwide quality assurance system. In the future, it is expected that the quality assurance system will encompass nonhospital institutional care, ***ambulatory care***, and care reimbursed by private health insurers.

Education

Educational programs in occupational therapy continued to prepare generalists for practice, while the health care system shifted emphasis to the specialist in practice. The occupational therapist became a specialist through experience in practice, and this is still the method open to most practicing therapists. Contrary to former employment habits, the occupational therapist today does not move from one area of practice to another but rather refines skills and knowledge in a specific area of practice; for example, hand therapy, drug and alcohol programs, head injury, burn treatment, and early intervention programs. These choices, unintentional though they may be, tend to favor programs recognized as necessary and reimbursable by funding sources. The profession made a commitment to high-quality educational programs at the entry level, but the needs of practitioners to be prepared for the marketplace were largely ignored.

In answer to this problem, continuing education training programs were developed by the AOTA to provide competence in special areas of practice, such as TOTEMS, PIVOT, ROTE, and SCOPE. In addition, position papers describing the role and function of occupational therapy in specialty areas of practice were developed, and free packets of literature in specialty areas were made available to AOTA members.

Personnel

Occupational therapy has been identified by the U. S. Bureau of Health Manpower (1984) as having significant manpower shortages. This statistic is noted in spite of a 230% growth in occupational therapy between 1966 and 1978 (Bezold, 1982). The growth of the profession can be traced to the overall expansion of the health care system and to an increased awareness of the value of rehabilitation services. A manpower study by the profession in 1985 also indicated a geographic maldistribution of occupational therapists, which was related to location of other health care providers, of delivery systems, and of educational programs (Ad Hoc Commission, 1985).

In 1984, 18% of surveyed hospitals indicated that they would be adding or expanding occupational therapy departments over the next 2 years (Freeland & Schendler, 1984). This is an interesting fact in light of the institution of the Medicare prospective payment system that was then facing the health care industry. With the development of new and alternative health care programs, the demand for occupational therapy services should increase proportionally. Although there have been efforts to encourage migration of occupational therapists to less professionally populated areas, there is no way to force occupational therapists to choose a specific practice area or geographic location.

Practice

With the onset of the Medicare prospective payment system and diagnostic-related groups (DRGs), the decreased length of stay and limitations on treatment for cost and profit purposes, occupational therapists began to look for alternative ways to provide service. Occupational therapy service was limited when lengths of stay were shortened, and therapists were heard to comment that patients were discharged too soon or sicker at the next level of care under the new system. This was particularly evident in moves from acute care to rehabilitation or home care settings. Therapists practicing in nursing homes talked about an increase in the number of patients referred who required intensive intervention within that setting. The economics of the system, rather than the need or condition of the patient, dictated the amount and level of occupational therapy service. Now the therapist must examine alternatives for the well-being of the patient. Occupational therapy was frequently not covered at the next level of care to which the patient would be transferred, or the coverage was time-limited for a patient who actually needed a greater length of service as a result of shortened service at the previous level of care.

As a result, occupational therapy services provided within the hospital have been streamlined to maintain quality yet provide vital services in a shorter time. The evaluation process has become more efficient to allow more time for intervention. The occupational therapist prioritizes goals and treatment in accordance with the estimated length of stay and anticipated intervention at succeeding levels of care. This increases the demand for effective communication between the occupational therapists practicing at various levels within the health care system, not only to avoid duplication of effort but also to allow for cost-effective service to meet the needs of the patient.

The occupational therapist today must be acutely aware of and extremely knowledgeable about health care reimbursement as the therapist plans and implements treatment programs for the individual patient. It is not sufficient to know that a given patient has private insurance coverage; the therapist must be aware of the limitations of that coverage and of the alternatives for coverage should the need arise. This frequently becomes part of patient education during the treatment process.

Over the last 10 years, occupational therapists have witnessed an increase in independent practice opportunities. There has been a redistribution of jobs toward outpatient facilities, home health agencies, and nontraditional settings. The allied health personnel as a group have been striving for professional status and thus have become very competitive in the health care marketplace. The occupational therapist as a member of this group has sought recognition as an independent practitioner. **Home care** has become a major area of practice for increasing numbers of occupational therapists. Despite the fact that reimbursement has been difficult, until the passage of recent legislation (Reconciliation Act of 1986), the profession recognized the need for and potential growth of service in home care. This is also true of the therapist who practices in a nursing home.

Maintenance of health, prevention of further disabling conditions, and promotion of independence within the community are major issues for the population receiving service through home health agencies. In providing service at this level, the occupational therapist helps the patient avoid a more costly level of care, that is, in a hospital or skilled nursing facility.

Implications for the future

The ways in which occupational therapy services are delivered has begun to change from traditional models of **hospital-based service** to **community-based** and **school-based services**, and the profession must continue to change with changing times. Target components of the health care system include multihospital systems, health maintenance organizations (HMOs), home health providers, and integrated health service systems.

Throughout the late 1980s and into the 1990s, legislators have discussed and proposed national health programs for children, mothers, the elderly, the chronically ill, and the disabled. None of these programs have come to fruition, however, and it can only be assumed that attempts will be made to achieve more equitable and affordable health care for all people in the United States through legislative efforts. As practitioners, occupational therapists can expect regulation to continue to effect the provision of treatment, documentation, quality assurance, and reimbursement.

Practice arenas

A number of clinical areas to be considered should include the following examples. The occupational therapist possesses the tools for practice in each of these practice arenas but will need to anticipate, influence, and shape the changes in health care in the coming years.

Acute care

Health care industry experts predict that 40% of all U. S. hospitals will close by the year 2000. Hospital costs have continued to grow faster than the gross national product in the last 10 years. Hospitals have begun to aggressively search for alternative services and markets. This is evidenced in the number of new hospital-based programs that are aligned with assured reimbursement patterns in health care. Reimbursement on a prospective and cost-minus basis is projected to continue as a means of **cost containment** in Medicare and Medicaid programs. The private insurance industry has begun to adopt prospective methods of reimbursement and will continue to do so in the future. Hospital-based services will be constrained, and a shift to ambulatory and chronic care settings will prevail. Occupational therapists are well positioned to provide care at these levels but must remain competitive in their services.

Chronic and long-term care

Between 1980 and 2050, the 85-year and older age group is projected to increase to over 500% (U. S. Bureau of the Census, 1984). Given the needs of the older adult population today, one can predict the intensity of chronic care needs the elderly will require as we move into the 21st century. Since occupational therapists are primary providers of long-term care, even more dramatic shortages can be anticipated. Services such as diagnosis and treatment of the chronically ill will continue to be provided in acute care settings, but the increase in the demand for services will shift to the community level of care, either in ambulatory care or long-term care facilities. With efforts toward more cost-effective health care delivery, improvements in community-based ambulatory and chronic care services will be necessary. The focus for practice in these settings will be functional and environmental assessments—skills that form the basis of the occupational therapy profession.

Pediatrics and developmental disabilities

Over 18% of occupational therapists practice in school-based programs according to the AOTA Member Data Survey (1990), and this number will continue to grow because of the federal mandate for the provision of occupational therapy services within school systems. Practice in the school system is framed within the educational model. Occupational therapists who have traditionally been trained within the medical model must develop knowledge and skills to practice within the school setting. Many of the skills that the occupational therapist has learned within the medical model can be transferred to the educational setting through modification of those skills, such as documenting functional goals using individual educational plans (IEPs) instead of the problem-oriented medical record and consulting with educators and parents rather than physicians and other allied health professionals.

Another 18% to 20% of occupational therapists practice in pediatric settings, such as early intervention, hospital-based, and community-based programs. Federal legislation under discussion will mandate health care for children through a national health program. Any resemblance of this legislation will have a large impact on the practice of occupational therapy. Given that about one third of the occupational therapists in practice today are in pediatric arenas, with an increase in the demand for service that this legislation could produce, one can only surmise the number of occupational therapists that will be required. The occupational therapist practicing in these arenas must have keen consultation skills and effective methods for the provision of service (see Chapter 25).

Home care

The Health Care Financing Administration (1986) has projected that the cost of home care will grow to over $460 billion by the year 2000. Consumers continue to express preferences for insurance programs that include home health care benefits. The number of older people demanding home care services is projected to triple by the year 2030. Occupational therapists hold a large market share in home care and are well positioned to respond to these needs and preferences. Therapists practicing in this area must become involved in the political arena and advocate with the insurance industry to ensure that occupational therapy is included in health care coverage (see Chapter 28).

Industrial rehabilitation and health promotion

Work hardening and vocational rehabilitation have long been a specialty area for occupational therapists. Occupational therapists are highly qualified to provide work analysis, work assessments, and back-to-work programs. The Americans with Disabilities Act (1990) will have an impact on this area of practice since it will affect how occupational therapists work. These programs have the potential to grow into prevention of illness and work injury as growth in federal interest parallels the overall growth in wellness and self-help movements (see Chapter 8, Section 2B).

Mental health and addiction programs

Practice in mental health has shown an increasing shortage of occupational therapy practitioners. Programs in drug abuse and addiction demonstrate a need for occupational therapy services that are currently limited. These positions are being filled by other professionals whom administrators believe can perform the same functions as the occupational therapist. Regulators of these programs have specified that occupational therapy services must be available, and these services are reimbursable through most major medical policies. As patients seeking these services move from inpatient to community care settings, occupational therapists must be prepared to practice in those settings. Community-based programs with strong functional living skills can be provided by occupational therapists (see Chapter 17).

Individual practitioner and the profession

Occupational therapists have demonstrated strengths in home care, designing living space and adapting environments, adapting toys, working in prisons, designing programs for the homeless, and teaching life skills to young, unwed mothers. These represent some of the emerging nontraditional settings for practice. It is important that the profession be prepared to change rapidly, to adapt or modify ***service delivery models*** in accordance with the health care system demands, and to educate personnel to practice in these emerging settings.

With the advent of certification in specialty areas of practice (hand therapy and pediatric certification have been initiated and sensory integration treatment certification already exists), certification may well become the rule rather than the exception.

The total impact of the prospective payment system (P.L. 98-21, 1983) is still emerging. There is strong evidence, however, of increased demands for productivity, cost effectiveness, and new sites of delivery of service. Current trends can be interpreted for future areas of programming based on societal emphasis on health promotion. These include survival of people with previously life-threatening disabilities or disease processes as the result of improved technology, increases in health maintenance programs in the workplace and among the older population, and the mainstreaming of mental health patients into the community. The occupational therapist has the expertise to offer programs for each of these areas; the profession must be prepared to meet the need, or others will fill the positions.

The profession has identified several goals as the result of the manpower study. These include promotion of new educational programs in underserved states; development of nontraditional educational and recruitment programs to meet the demand for qualified professionals; expansion of continuing education programs to increase the skills of the practicing therapist; examination of the opportunities available in occupational therapy educational programs to expand exposure to nontraditional practice settings; ensuring that future therapists are equipped with knowledge and skills in management, systems behavior, health economics, and marketing; development of promotional materials for use in marketing services; and increasing research and promotional activities to meet the needs of unserved or underserved populations.

As a result of the changes in the health care delivery system over the last few years, AOTA Directions for the Future and the strategic integrated management system approach have been adopted to identify changes that will impact on the profession and to enable the profession to adapt to these changes.

Each occupational therapist must become a self-confident, assertive, risk-taking, and critically thinking person (Labovitz, 1986) because the therapist is a participant in the provision of health care in a time of increased competition for status, recognition, and reimbursement. Occupational therapy must be developed as a scientific discipline to gain a stronger position with a strong professional identity. There must be increased dialogue between educators and clinicians to define common goals.

Finally, the occupational therapist must assist people to gain control of their health through advocacy, new programming, technologic advances, and expanded educational programs. By marketing services to corporations and to the insurance industry, through political activity, through research and collaboration with researchers in other fields, and through consultation and collaboration with multidisciplinary health care providers, consumers, caregivers, and advocates, the occupational therapist will be equipped to meet the challenges of the future in health care.

References

Ad Hoc Commission on Occupational Therapy Manpower (1985). *Occupational therapy manpower: A plan for progress*. Rockville, MD: American Occupational Therapy Association.

American Occupational Therapy Association. (1990). *Member data survey*. Rockville, MD: author.

Bezold, C. (1982). Health care in the U. S.: Four alternative futures. *The Futurist, 16*(4):14.

Freeland, M.S., & Schendler, C.E. (1984). Health spending in the 1980's: Integration of clinical practice patterns of management. *Health Care Financing Review, 5*(3):1.

Health Care Financing Administration (1986). National health care expenditures estimates for 1986. *Health Care Financing Review, 8*(4), 1–36.

Labovitz, D. (1986, October). *Meeting the challenge: Occupational therapy survival, 2000 and beyond*. Keynote address, New York State Occupational Therapy Association Annual Conference.

U. S. Bureau of Census (1984). *Demographic and socio-economic aspects of aging in the United States: Current population reports*. Washington, DC: U. S. Government Printing Office, 84, 23.

U. S. Bureau of Health Manpower, Health Resources Administration (1984). *Report on allied health personnel*. Washington, DC: U. S. Government Printing Office, Dept. of Health, Education and Welfare Pub. HRA 80–28.

Bibliography

American Occupational Therapy Association. (1989). *Directions for the future*. Rockville, MD: American Occupational Therapy Association.

Capra, F. (1982). *The turning point: Science, Society and the rising culture*. New York: Simon and Schuster.

Child health: Lessons from developed nations. (1990). Washington, DC: House Select Committee on Children, Youth and Families.

Ginzberg, E. (1987). Sounding board: A hard look at cost containment. *New England Journal of Medicine, 316*(18), 1151.

Johnson, E. A., & Johnson, R. L. (1986). *Hospitals under fire: Strategies for survival*. Rockville, MD: Aspen.

Scott, S. J., & Acquaviva, J. D. (1985). *Lobbying for health care*. Rockville, MD: American Occupational Therapy Association.

The state of U. S. hospitals in the next decade. (1989). Washington, DC: National Association for Hospital Development.

UNIT IV

Management

CHAPTER 11

Service management

JUDITH M. PERINCHIEF

SECTION 1

Management functions and strategies

LEARNING OBJECTIVES

Upon completion of this section, the reader will be able to:

1. *Identify management theories and techniques as they apply to the delivery of occupational therapy services.*
2. *Identify and describe management styles.*
3. *Describe the application of leadership principles in occupational therapy.*
4. *Recognize the role of planning in relation to occupational therapy management.*
5. *Describe the application of supervision principles in occupational therapy.*
6. *Recognize the role of policies, procedures, and productivity in relation to management of an occupational therapy service.*

Historically, the emphasis in occupational therapy has been on the treatment aspects of service. In the first few years of professional experience, the occupational therapist concentrated on acquiring expertise in clinical skills through continuing education courses, workshops, and professional journals. Knowledge and skill in management, organization, and administrative areas were learned through daily experience and by a trial-and-error process. Since its beginning, the occupational therapy profession has been struggling for proper recognition among the medical professions. This struggle has been based largely on the fact that many occupational therapists do not use proper administrative techniques. This is substantiated by Johnson (1973) in her statement that the success of occupational therapy may well depend on the ability to clearly identify the product and services, to determine the best environment to provide the services, and to obtain adequate sources of support. These characteristics clearly define the functions of the occupational therapist in management. An understanding of the principles of management and administration and the ability to implement them are fundamental to successful practice in occupational therapy.

Until the early 1980s, administrative knowledge and practice were little valued or emphasized within the profession. Thus, those practitioners at administrative levels were not compelled to develop knowledge and skill beyond the opportunities provided on the job or through life experiences in community work and the raising of a family. In the early 1980s, the profession began to recognize that education and resources had to be supplied from within the professional structure as a means of providing qualified administrators. During this era, the American Occupational Therapy Association (AOTA) took the initiative by providing resource materials, a special interest section for management and administration, and continuing education workshops and seminars for administrators.

For the purpose of this section, ***administration*** is defined as the management of institutional affairs. The importance of administration in a large institution can easily be seen, but it is becoming increasingly important in all levels of health care delivery because of the increasing interaction between the health care facility and the community. For the purpose of this section, *organization* is defined as a body of people organized for the attainment of a specific goal. The organizational environment must be conducive to assisting people to reach and maintain their maximal potentials.

The key to effective management is understanding what organizational behavior is all about, understanding styles and philosophies of management, and selecting those with which one feels most comfortable. Historically, the functions of management have been designated as *organizing, planning, directing*, and *controlling*. All administrative aspects of the manager's job fall into one of these categories.

Organizing

The manager's role as an organizer encompasses activities aimed at creating and maintaining a formal structure for accomplishing tasks within a system, with designated roles and responsibilities. Professional management was developed early in the 1900s. As society expanded, the increasing use of technology required more organizational structure. Between 1935 and 1955, the "science" of management began to develop. In health care, integrated hospital care grew, and practitioners focused their activities in the hospital setting. Things began to be measured and counted. During this period, the impact of World War II was influential on medical organization and delivery of care. The Systems Movement of the period from 1955 to 1970 evidenced the expectation that the health care system would deliver limitless quality care. Organizational structures stressing accountability and planning processes became formalized during this period. In the 1970s, networking took on greater importance as regulation took a firmer hold on the health care industry. It was during this period that for-profit health care systems began to develop. During the 1980s, high technology, high costs, and high expectations were drivers for change in the health care industry. Managers began to downsize operations and build management teams to contend with the demand for more rapid decision making. Conflict within organizations increased in an attempt to determine managerial direction—to increase bureaucratic control or liberalize the decision-making process. This caused stress on the managers and tested the organization's ability to implement change. In the 1990s, economic competition will continue to affect managerial styles. Focused management teams will replace more traditional management structures. Managers who are willing to take risks and are visionary will replace the types of manager seen in the past.

Management styles and principles

A variety of principles and styles of management have evolved as organizations and managers have been studied and researched. Studies have identified that no one style or theory is the definitive answer to management; nor is there one correct way to manage. A manager works with the style that is most comfortable and protective for the manager in the given environment. Different environments and situations call for different approaches on the part of a manager. It is therefore important for managers to recognize their own capabilities.

The factors that affect **management styles** include the environment in which the manager works, the beliefs and value system of the manager, the personality of the manager, and an element of chance. Management styles are not fixed. These are subject to modification through formal education or self-training.

The Managerial Grid (Blake & Mouton, 1964) is a theory of managerial behavior based on degrees of concern for people and concern for production. Characteristics that evidence concern for people include accountability, self-esteem, personal commitment to completing a job, ability to establish and maintain working conditions, recognition of the importance of equitable salary structure and benefits, and ability to conduct positive social relations with associates. Characteristics that evidence concern for production include attention to the quality of policy decisions, procedures or processes; creative thinking; concern for the quality of services staff provide; and awareness of the workload and efficiency of individual workers.

The Managerial Grid theory proposes that when acting as a manager, one makes assumptions about how to solve problems of achieving purpose through people. The manner in which a manager views the linkage of concern for people and concern for product defines how the manager uses the hierarchy of the grid. The character of concern differs at different grids, even though the degree may be the same. Through the clustering of various qualities of managers, managerial styles have emerged. These styles change in popularity and situation, but most of the styles discussed below can be seen in managers today.

Country-club style

The main assumption of the country-club style is that production requirements are contrary to people's needs. A manager who uses this style feels that attitudes and feelings of people are important. The manager plans, directs, and controls activities of subordinates but does not push. This type of manager demonstrates and supports staff and may even pitch in to assist staff. This manager expects devoted loyalty from supervised staff.

Laissez-faire style

The main assumption of the laissez-faire style is that there is a basic incompatibility between production requirements and the needs of people. This type of manager has low involvement with people and contributes minimally toward organizational purpose. This style may create a failure situation for the manager and the organization since minimal exertion of effort is required to get work done. This style is most common in bureaucratic, noncompetitive organizations with routine operations and repetitive actions.

Authoritarian style

The main assumption of the authoritarian style is that goals are quotas for the people who work to achieve them. Human relationships are at a low point in this style of management. Efficiency in the operation results because of the arrangement of work conditions so that human elements will interfere minimally.

Participatory style

The main assumption of the participatory style is that people want to work and assume responsibility. It is further believed that if treated properly, people can be trusted and will put forth their best effort. Participatory managers motivate workers by use of internal factors, such as satisfaction with assigned tasks, self-esteem, and recognition for a job well done. Delegation is an important factor in this managerial style.

Rules-oriented style

The main assumption of the rules-oriented style is that people require reinforcement from the manager to function. This type of manager believes that things must be done by the book; enforcing policies, rules, and procedures with employees ensures motivation and achievement. These managers tend to be police-like and bureaucratic.

Motivation theories

It is essential that a manager understand theories of motivation and behavior and be able to apply these to the management situation. A comprehensive discussion of organizational psychology is beyond the scope of this section; however, purposes can be served with a summary of the tenets of three of the major contributors to the literature: Abraham Maslow, Frederick Herzberg, and Douglas McGregor.

Theory X and Theory Y

McGregor (1960) described the traditional assumptions about human motivation and a contrasting set of assumptions about human nature as applied to the workplace. Theory X assumes that economic incentives primarily motivate employees and that since these incentives are controlled by the organization, employees are passive agents to be controlled by the organization. This theory further assumes that people are basically lazy, irrational, and incapable of self-discipline in relation to the workplace. In contrast, the Theory Y tenets are that people can and will control their own work, that economic incentives are only one reason people work, and that most employees enjoy some parts of their work and will accept responsibility in numerous work situations.

Hierarchy of needs

Maslow (1943) saw people as creatures of unending wants or needs that are organized into a series of levels, forming a **hierarchy**. Those needs at the lowest level are the physiologic needs of food, shelter, and so forth. Subsequent levels include safety needs, social needs, esteem needs, self-fulfillment needs, and self-actualization needs. Maslow demonstrated that a significant portion of motivation comes from having an internal need that drives the person to take action. A satisfied need is never a motivator; therefore, management action should be directed toward unmet needs of an employee.

Two-factor theory

Herzberg (1966) studied the importance of work and job conditions on the lives of the average worker. Herzberg determined that the good feelings workers had about their jobs were linked to job content, and he labeled these *motivator factors*. He determined that the bad feelings workers had about their jobs related mostly to job surroundings and labeled these *hygiene factors*. Herzberg felt that hygiene factors were prerequisite to effective motivation but did not motivate workers to do a better job.

Managerial systems

Management by Objectives (MBO) is a system of management that emphasizes a goal-oriented philosophy and attitude (Ordiorne, 1965). Goal-oriented management emphasizes the result rather than the method used to achieve a goal; this is a contrast to traditional American management systems that emphasize methods and techniques. The major reason for an organization to adopt the MBO approach is to improve productivity of everyone concerned with the product and to improve overall organizational productivity. This system places a great deal of emphasis on effective communication between levels within the organization. Two important ingredients in setting objectives under MBO are: (1) the objectives must be quantified, and (2) there must be a specified time frame in which the objectives will be accomplished. It should be kept in mind that MBO is a complete system of management rather than a management technique. Its purpose is to make managers more effective.

An overview of the MBO system is outlined below, followed by a case study to enhance understanding of the application of this system.

MBO System Overview

1. State mission and goals.
2. Identify people who are to participate.
3. Set measurable objectives and determine approach for each objective.
4. Develop events as they are to occur in relation to each other with specific time frames for initiation and completion.
5. Determine training needs and deterrents of progress.
6. Measure progress and take corrective action as needed.

MBO CASE STUDY

The multidisciplinary treatment team on the spinal cord injury service has determined that an educational manual for staff training and patient and family education is needed. The team meets and develops the following plan of action. Each member contributes to the development of the plan and assumes responsibility for a designated activity.

Mission: Develop an educational manual for care of spinal cord–injured patients

Goals: (1) develop standardized information that will be presented to staff for care of spinal cord–injured patients; (2) train personnel; (3) train patients and families; (4) complete manual by December 20; (5) implement manual by February 20

Participants: Physician, social worker, nurse, occupational therapist, physical therapist, psychologist

Objectives and approach: (1) social worker to chair committee; (2) physician to provide medical information in written form by November 18; (3) nurse, occupational therapist, physical therapist, psychologist, and social worker to provide written procedures for care, equipment, and teaching responsibilities for respective services by November 18; (4) committee to critique all information for clarity and level of presentation by December 5; (5) committee to provide final approval of all material by December 15; (6) materials to be sent to printer by December 20; (7) training sessions to be scheduled by each team member for their respective departments during the 2 weeks of February 5 to 17

Training needs: Staff of each department who is responsible for care and treatment of spinal cord-injured patient

Deterrents: Members absent from meetings; members not meeting time lines; difficulty obtaining resources for typing and illustrations; difficulty obtaining funding for printing manual

The team instituted the plan as outlined above. The chair of the committee was assigned the responsibility of discussing resources and funding with the unit administrator in addition to other duties as a member of the team.

Planning

Planning is the process of making decisions in the present to bring about an outcome in the future. It is the most fundamental management action and precedes all other management functions. Planning is characterized by a cyclic process in which some goals and specific objectives are recycled.

Participants in planning

Top-level managers set the basic tone for planning. They determine the overall goals for the organization and give direction on content of policies and planning documents. The board of trustees or managers of a given institution are considered to be the top-level managers. Chief executive officers or presidents of an institution are also considered top-level managers within the overall organization. At a departmental level, directors or chiefs of service are considered top-level management. These latter managers are responsible for the planning processes in their areas; they identify goals and set policies for their departments. As a result of federal legislation, specifically the Rehabilitation Act of 1973 and subsequent legislation in 1974, consumers also participate in planning, particularly in federally funded programs. Within an individual institution or department, others may participate in planning as delegated by top-level management. Staff planners or planning consultants have been used in the past to develop plans and then give them to top management for implementation. This strategy has become more or less obsolete, and staff or consultants in this capacity are now more effectively used when they act as facilitators of a planning process that seeks to establish organizational direction. Staff or consultant planners assist the planning process by facilitating group interaction and by stimulating creativity.

Organization goals

The goals of an organization originate in the mission embodied in the statement of purpose or philosophy of the organization. Goals are the ends toward which activity is directed. In a sense, a goal is never completely achieved but rather is in a continuing ideal state. Organizational goals may be found in the charter of the institution, articles of incorporation, the mission statement, or official bylaws of the organization.

Organizational planning

Planning takes many forms within an organization. Planning may be formulated around a program, as in a new service or an extension of an existing service. Planning may be formulated on the physical arrangement, either new or renovated space. In any event, planning is based on the philosophy, goals, and objectives of the organization, and these must be reviewed in the initial considerations of planning for new or expanding programs. Regardless of the program to be developed and the setting, certain principles are involved in devising the plan of action. In approaching organizational planning, the following three major elements should be considered:

Survey: A survey is used to identify the need for the program. The population to be served, the source of referrals, the needs of the staff, the treatment methods, and the anticipated case-load all must be identified.

Interviews: Interviews with top level administrators should be conducted to determine the nature and extent of the program desired. The philosophy of the institution must be kept in mind during this phase of planning. Fiscal considerations and administrative restrictions must be accommodated. Interviews should be conducted with potential consumers to determine the appropriateness of the scope of the program.

Evaluation: This phase of planning is the translation of all the information gathered into a workable plan. At this stage, personnel and facilities are matched with the needs of the organization and the program.

The following case study illustrates the three phases of planning.

PLANNING CASE STUDY

A large, university-based teaching hospital is considering expanding rehabilitation services to include special programs in traumatic head injury. The *survey* conducted by planning leadership included review of the number of inpatient days for patients with head injuries during the last 5 years and the sources of referral of these patients. A significant increase was found in the number of patient days and referrals within the last 3 years. Further study of demographics revealed that the geographic area for referrals had increased to include six contiguous counties, only three of which had previously referred patients. The study also revealed that four community hospitals in the geographic area had discontinued all but emergency care of patients with these types of injuries and that these four institutions referred all patients with these types of injuries to the university hospital. The survey also revealed that the neurology and neurosurgery services had recently expanded their residency programs and were prepared to develop specialized programs in head injury. The expertise for these programs exists within the current medical staff. The survey indicated that from 100 to 175 new head injury cases could be anticipated each year as the result of motor vehicle, sports, and domestic accidents. Further investigation identified a model program in another part of the country that integrated the care of head injury patients through coordination of emergency care, neurosurgery, and physical medicine services.

Interviews were conducted with top administrators within the university hospital and with the chairpersons of the neurology, neurosurgery, orthopedic, and physical medicine departments. In addition, interviews were conducted with administrators and emergency room coordinators at local hospitals in the area, particularly the four community hospitals identified in the survey phase of planning. Department managers who supplied staff across program lines within the emergency room, neurology, neurosurgery, orthopedics, and physical medicine services were interviewed to determine increased resource demands that would result from program expansion. Selected planning leaders visited the model program identified in the survey and interviewed the key administrators for the various services and departments involved in the program. At each level in the interview process, fiscal implications were enumerated and health insurance coverage issues were identified.

During the *evaluation* phase of planning, the data collected during the survey, the reports generated from the interviews, and the cost and accounting implications were studied. A marketing plan was discussed, and outreach educational programs were proposed as a result of the information gathered in the first two phases of planning. A final report was generated incorporating all the data and information collected and a carefully detailed plan for implementation of the new program. This report was forwarded to the chief executive officer of the institution and subsequently to the board of trustees for approval.

Planning for growth

As health care organizations intensify their competitive strategies and move into new markets, planning for organizational growth becomes more important. Understanding the strengths and weaknesses of the organization is a necessary first step in planning for growth. Despite the competition and cost-constraint pressures, continued growth, upgrading, and expansion of health care facilities is projected into the 21st century. Existing health care facilities will continue to be replaced to comply with codes, to maintain accreditation, and to gain competitive advantage. The demand for medical care programs is increasing in the outpatient and new technology sectors. In the 1990s, major facility development issues will involve the retrofitting of inpatient facilities as well as the development of free-standing alternative health care centers. Generally speaking, these delivery centers will be designed for ambulatory, non–life-threatening conditions that need not be treated in a hospital. Careful, cost-effective planning will need to take place to meet the projected needs of the health care consumer. All members of the health care profession will need to be prepared to participate in meeting these planning demands.

Planning in an occupational therapy department

Occupational therapy managers are involved in planning both within the department and across program lines on a continual basis. At this level, managers need to be intimately aware of the resources necessary for various programs and the financial implications of providing these resources. The department manager must analyze the costs and benefits of programs, including

comparing expenses with projected revenues. The manager must also identify the probability of securing the staff necessary for expanding or new programs. An analysis of space and equipment needs must also be conducted by the manager to identify provision of resources in a cost-effective manner. The occupational therapy manager should be well versed in the various provisions of coverage of occupational therapy service by third-party payers. Since coverage varies dramatically depending on the services rendered, this information is paramount in planning. The occupational therapy manager should be involved in initial planning meetings and should submit a report to top-level management based on data and revenue and expense projections for resources that are necessary for expanding or new programs within the institution.

Planning takes many forms within an occupational therapy department, such as planning for programs, for physical arrangement of space and equipment, or for development of services within an existing agency. Regardless of the purpose of planning, certain factors should be considered, including the type of institution, agency, or service needed; the principal diagnoses to be treated; the bed capacity devoted to the service; the projected average monthly census and rate of turnover; and the eligibility of patients by payer mix. In addition, personnel requirements must be determined, such as the number of registered occupational therapists, certified occupational therapist assistants, and support staff that will be needed and the ratio of patients per therapist. The number of professional and support staff needed to operate a department is difficult to ascertain and may be misleading. Many variables should be considered, including patient diagnosis, complexity of problems presented by patients, size of institution or service, referral rates, and average length of stay. Little reliable data is available to assist a manager in planning for staffing. A general guideline for a patient/staff ratio is 8 : 1 for individual treatment caseload and 15 : 1 for group treatments. A manager can base planning for program expansion on current staff patterns and use of space.

In determining space allocation, the basic areas to be considered are primary treatment areas for assessment, work stations, and specialized treatment rooms; support areas for reception and waiting; storerooms and dressing rooms; and administrative areas for management and staff offices, rooms for clerical staff, conference rooms, and classrooms. Factors that influence space requirements include the patient load at any one time, the number of personnel using the area at one time, the work flow, and equipment and storage needs. Specific consideration should be given to location of office and waiting room space so that they are adjacent to treatment areas. Safety features should also be considered in planning space, including panic bars on doors, sprinkler systems, fire extinguishers, emergency alarm systems in secluded treatment areas, storage for flammable materials, and proper receptacles for disposal of materials. Accessibility of communication systems, whether they are telephones, intercoms, or paging systems, should also be included in space planning. Plumbing considerations should include grease or plaster traps in sinks and accessibility of sinks, toilets, or water fountains for the proposed patient population.

The following are some examples of departmental planning:

- The Occupational Therapy Department in the Department of Physical Medicine in a large metropolitan 320-bed hospital is developing an outpatient service for patients with upper-extremity disabilities primarily caused by traumatic accidents. The Physical Medicine Department has allocated a room that measures 20 feet × 18 feet for this program. The Director of Occupational Therapy must develop a plan for the use of physical space and the equipment that will be necessary for this program. There are no additional staffing needs because the program will be covered by existing staff.

- The 30-bed Psychiatry Department of a large teaching hospital has determined that to meet accreditation standards, occupational therapy services are needed in addition to activity programming currently provided for all inpatients. The Chief of Occupational Therapy in the Physical Medicine Department has been asked to plan for the staff and resources that will be required for this program expansion.
- The Chief of Occupational Therapy in a children's hospital will be involved in planning for the expansion of services and relocation of the Occupational Therapy Department into a proposed new physical facility. The new facility will include 42 new beds, which will be divided between neonatology, orthopedics, and neurology services. The Chief of Occupational Therapy has been asked to plan for increased staffing and to determine the cost of new equipment and of moving the Occupational Therapy Department to the new facility.

Strategic planning

Regardless of the purpose of planning, a systematic approach to planning is strongly recommended. Systems for planning have been developed by various professions, and business has developed a strategic model for those in management positions that is referred to as **strategic planning**. Strategic planning relates to goals that are essential, basic, or critical to the continuation of an institution or organization. Strategic planning involves the allocation of resources to achieve an organization's long-range goals. It deals with three basic questions: where are we; where do we want to be; and how do we get there?

Strategic planning should be one of the routine daily activities of top-level managers. Based on daily contact with the reality in which the organization operates, top-level managers determine strategy for the organization. This suggests that top-level managers have to incorporate more long-range thinking into their daily activities. Planning tests managers. Strategic planning involves the expenditure of effort to define the organization's mission, collect data to identify trends, and then project this into the future. Countless meetings among those involved in the planning process are required. Good strategic planning suggests the need for close interrelationships between the planners and executives.

Strategic planning is a five-step process that involves participation from all levels in the organization.

1. *Assessment* involves a thorough appraisal of the current and future states of the organization. Environmental assessments lend themselves to development by groups of people. At this stage, there is the opportunity to involve many managers and employees with special expertise. Involving groups of employees in the development of assessments provides those employees with a sense of ownership of the strategic plan. Through the assessment phase, issues are identified and ranked in order of priority.
2. *Analysis* is the first step in developing a focus. Issues are selected from the assessment that could influence the organization's response. A literature review is essential at this point in the process. Trends should be analyzed, and implications for the future should be considered.
3. During the *decision-making* phase, advantages and disadvantages are discussed regarding each of the issues that were analyzed. At this stage, preferred options are determined and ranked; these become the strategic plan.
4. Once the strategic plan has been determined, methods to *implement* the plan must be developed. Since this is the stage at which failure commonly occurs, it is advantageous to determine action steps, set time tables, and allocate resources for each step.
5. The final step involves *evaluation* of outcomes. The usual way is to measure the actual outcomes against a standard. Questions should be asked to determine when an issue is resolved and how this can be measured. If the plan is not working within a particular parameter, then the people involved in planning should return to the decision-making phase to consider ways of improving or eliminating the action plans or to develop new plans.

A successful strategic planning process results in values and themes that guide and strengthen an organization's ability to succeed in changing environments. The process, however, has been criticized for requiring too much time, fostering loss of focus on the purpose of strategic planning, and using inadequate inputs to planning. Steiner (1979) listed the following pitfalls to avoid in the strategic planning process:

1. Assuming that planning can be completely delegated to a planner
2. Top-level managers spending insufficient time on strategic planning
3. Using unsuitable goals as the basis for planning
4. Involving major personnel inappropriately
5. Not using a manager's contribution to achieving the plan as the basis for evaluating the manager's performance
6. Failing to develop a climate congenial to strategic planning
7. Failing to integrate planning into the entire management process
8. Injecting such formality into the system that it becomes inflexible and restrains creativity
9. Top-level managers failing to review middle managers' plans
10. Managers making intuitive decisions that run counter to formal plans

Directing

A basic responsibility of a manager is to shape and modify employee behavior through directing so that an employee can acquire the necessary knowledge and skills to perform assignments in compliance with policies and procedures of the institution.

Leadership

Leadership is a managerial function that links the organization's policy makers and those delivering service. Leaders must focus on the emotions, values, degrees of commitment, and aspirations for success of employees as well as the organization as a whole. Leaders set organizational direction. In contrast, managers focus on the physical, human, financial, and material resources of an organization. Merging the functions of leadership and management can be accomplished by adapting styles and strategies to the organizational environment. An effective leader is flexible, honest in dealing with those being led, and aware of forces within himself or herself, the group, and the environment. An effective leader makes certain that necessary decisions are made and does not try to avoid responsibility.

A great deal has been written in behavioral science about leadership. Leadership is not easily acquired, nor is it bestowed on a person. It is the process of influence that occurs between one who leads and those who follow. Leadership may be formal or informal. Formal leadership is defined as legitimate authority. Informal leadership is defined as influence through the strength of personality. An understanding of the concepts of power, influence, and formal authority leads to a better understanding of leaders and leadership. The *concept of power* denotes the authority that is legitimized by virtue of a person's formal role in an organization. The *concept of influence* differs from that of power in the manner in which compliance is evoked. Influence is accepted voluntarily; power is coercive in nature. Through the use of influence, a leader may elicit compliance without relying on formal action, rules, or force. The *concept of formal authority* is that which carries a mandate and is reinforced by organizational charts, job descriptions, procedure manuals, and work rules. Formal authority differs from influence in that it is clearly vested.

Leaders give orders and directives. Orders should have an autocratic tone. Giving orders is a major function of a manager's daily role. It is often taken for granted that every manager knows how to give orders. Issuing effective orders requires attention to timing and language. Leaders must prepare employees in many ways so that when orders are actually given, they are both acceptable and effective in terms of essential communication. Leaders must also be prepared to discipline. Disciplining is more likely to address behavior than to address work results. Discipline may have a connotation of punishment but should be used by a leader to improve employee behavior and to motivate employees to display self-discipline and effective job performance. A manager can discipline by calling attention to correct behavior in an effective manner and by calling attention to responsibilities and making suggestions. An employee should be treated as a person with a problem, not as a problem employee. Regardless of circumstances, all disciplinary action should be handled as a private matter between the manager and the employee. Good leaders have objectives in leading, but these objectives may or may not be obvious to those being led. They include raising the level of member motivation, improving quality of all decisions, developing teamwork and morale, furthering individual development of members, and increasing readiness to accept change.

Supervision

Leaders in an occupational therapy department frequently are responsible for the **supervision** of employees. A supervisor can be defined as any person having authority in the interests of the employer to hire, transfer, lay off, recall, promote, assign, reward, or discipline other employees. The primary duties of a supervisor consist of the management of a unit and the direction of two or more employees to promote the growth of the employee. Contact between a supervisor and employee may vary from close daily interaction to only monthly contact. A line staff member in an occupational therapy department may have daily contact with a supervisor; on the other hand, the unit supervisor in the occupational therapy department may have only weekly or biweekly contact with the department manager. Supervisors are defined by the Fair Labor Standards Act of 1972 as those who do not devote more than 20% of work hours to activities that are not supervisory in nature. Supervisors are the middle managers who represent the administration to employees and employees to the administration. Supervisors must master the art and science of consultation. Two-way communication with a feedback loop is the key to successful supervision. Almost every technique of supervision can be learned, and the basic principles can be transferred from one workplace to another.

There are two types of supervisor, and one type is not preferable to another, although one type may be more effective in one situation than another. The *traditional* supervisor sets goals for subordinates and defines standards and the results expected. This type of supervisor sets examples, trains and checks subordinates, and disciplines people to keep them in line. A traditional supervisor is knowledgeable and develops and installs new methods. This supervisor develops subordinates for promotions and recognizes achievements, but does not hesitate to point out failures. The *emerging concept* supervisor participates with staff in problem solving and goal setting and enables people to check their own performance. This type of supervisor creates an environment for learning and provides opportunity for improving methods. The emerging concept supervisor recognizes achievements and helps people learn from failure.

The best clinicians do not always make the best supervisors, nor do the best workers always make the best supervisors. There are a number of reasons why supervisors fail, but the primary reason is the person's inability to adjust to new and changing conditions. Other reasons include poor general relations with workers or other managers, lack of initiative and unwillingness to spend the necessary time and effort to improve, and lack of understanding of the management point of view.

A supervisor should be a facilitator and coach, not a friend. Those characteristics that are valued in a friend are usually not those that a person seeks in a role model. Both the supervisor and employee are responsible for the relationship and for keeping communication lines open. The relationship should involve mutual respect between both parties.

Learning styles

Supervisors facilitate learning and are trainers; therefore, they should understand that people learn differently. Different learning styles should be taken into account when designing learning experiences for employees. Employees' feelings of success are related to their level of participation in the learning experience. A number of learning style inventories are available to supervisors. Research has been conducted by occupational therapists regarding the learning styles of students in classrooms and clinical settings (Katz 1988, 1990; Cunningham & Trickey 1983; Rogers & Hill, 1980).

Decision making

Regardless of the management position, the process of making decisions is a key component of managing. There are two elements to decision making: the quality of the decision and the acceptance of the decision by those it affects. Decisions that are made at the top level of management are considered centralized. Many daily decisions that managers face must be made on the spot. Most decisions are based on intuition as well as logic and experience. When time and style permit, a manager may involve employees in the decision-making process and may involve others through group consensus. This is a common practice in decentralized decision making when the process is moved from the top level of management to incorporate participation by those at lower levels of the hierarchy. The brainstorming technique used in the team approach to problem solving is often helpful in the decision making process. Regardless of the style of decision making, the traditional approach to problem solving is (1) analysis of the issue, (2) definition of objectives, (3) interpretation of the facts, (4) evaluation of proposed solutions and alternatives, (5) selection of the best solution, (6) development of an action plan with attention to time sequencing and use of resources, and (7) implementation with follow-up.

Controlling

Hierarchy in organizations

Management takes place within an organization. Organizations have several characteristics that are universal—that is, regardless of the product or setting, they are present to some degree. By effectively managing these universal characteristics, efficient production and, thus, a sound organization result. The three universal characteristics of organizations are *purpose, people,* and *hierarchy.* For example, the purpose of an industrial organization is to make a product, and the purpose of a health care organization is to supply quality health care at a cost-effective level. Purpose cannot be achieved without people. The process of achieving purpose through the efforts of several people results in some people attaining authority to supervise, plan, control, and direct others through a hierarchic arrangement.

Relationships in formal organizations are highly structured in terms of authority and responsibility. The flow of authority and responsibility that can be observed in a hierarchy constitutes a chain of command. *Chain of command* is defined as an organizational pattern that results from using the scalar principle to link the highest manager in the hierarchy to the lowest in an unbroken chain of authority, responsibility, and accountability. *Unity of command* is the uninterrupted line of authority from superior to subordinate so that each person reports to only one superior. A clear chain of command shows who reports to whom, who is responsible for the actions of an employee, and who has authority over the employee. According to classic organization principles, a supervisor can only direct a limited number of subordinates; this is referred to as *span of control.* No exact number of employees who can be supervised effectively is ever prescribed, and the span of control may differ given the supervisor's level within the organization. Generally, organizational theories hold that the more efficient organizations have a smaller span of control. To further clarify these concepts, a discussion of organizational patterns is provided next.

Organizational patterns

Organizational patterns are schematic representations that arrange positions in the organization in a hierarchic pattern. These patterns illustrate the chain of command within the orga-

nization or department. They are schemes of planned interaction and indicate responsibilities of employees working within a structure. The patterns may be *vertical, horizontal, pyramidal,* or *matrical.*

In a vertical pattern, the chain of command proceeds from top to bottom in a straight chain. The horizontal pattern proceeds from left to right. The pyramidal pattern proceeds from top to bottom, becoming more diversified as it proceeds down the chain. This pattern is viewed as the typical medical model. The matrical pattern is a combination of the vertical and horizontal patterns. As a model organizational pattern, it allows for the simultaneous existence of both the hierarchic (vertical) association through departmental organization and the lateral (horizontal) association across departments. The horizontal associations are typically called *programs* and are illustrated in patient care teams. Within this pattern, the program manager is responsible for overall management of the program group and, therefore, for results. The department manager retains responsibility for the functional department and is therefore responsible for providing resources to attain results.

Tables of organization

From the schematics described above, an organization or manager depicts a table of organization or organizational chart. The structure of any organization is a device that has been designed to assist management in achieving various objectives of a given organization. A table of organization or organizational chart depicts major functions, specific relationships, lines of communication, formal authority, and positions by title. No table of organization or organizational chart is static; each changes as the organization grows and changes. Organizational charts depict organizational relationships in a diagrammatic form (Figure 11-1). Usually, only major functions are shown, except at a departmental level, where greater detail of relationships may be depicted (Figure 11-2). Only formal lines of authority and communication are shown. Tables of organization or organizational charts cannot be properly interpreted without reference to support information such as that found in policy manuals or job descriptions.

Job description

A **job description** is defined as a written statement of a single position. The purpose of a job description is to identify, define, and describe the position that, by virtue of its definition, becomes a tool for controlling. A job description should cover every aspect of the job. It should be reviewed with prospective candidates for the position and reviewed annually with the person who holds the position. Since a job description enumerates all aspects of a job, the employee is ensured that significant elements of the job are known to both parties and that the job is correctly described. A job description ensures employees that the jobs of greater difficulty and value receive greater remuneration or pay. A job description also provides a means of performance appraisal as an ongoing part of self-evaluation and supervisory evaluation. Each organization or institution has its own method of writing job descriptions, but the following elements are common to all job descriptions:

- Job title
- Department or service work area or unit

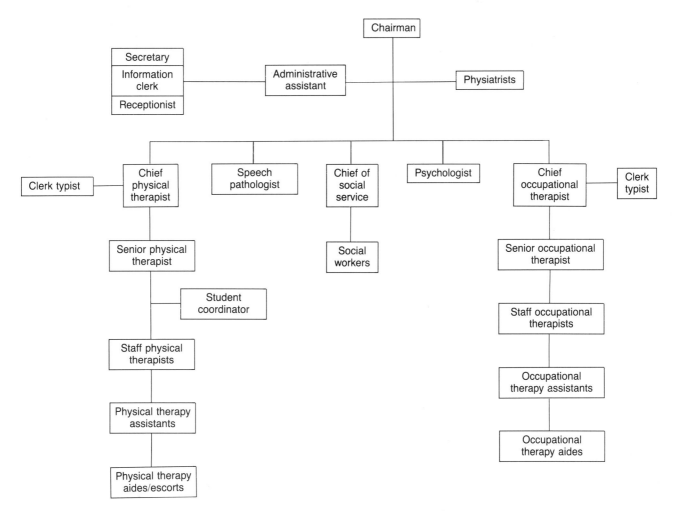

FIGURE 11-1. *Sample table of organization for physical medicine department in a large urban teaching hospital.*

- Supervision received and given
- Qualifications, including education, experience, certification, license, and physical demands
- Basic functions and duties recorded in a concise statement that summarizes the position's purpose
- Specific duties, including a description of tasks and responsibilities in relation to the patients, students, the department, and the institution

  See the display on page 384 for a sample job description.

Job specification

Once a job description has been completed and administrative approval for hiring has been received, a *job specification* is prepared based on the job description. A job specification delineates the minimal acceptable qualifications for the specific position, including education, experience, and physical abilities for the specific job. The format for a job specification usually is stipulated by the institution through the Human Resources Department. The job specification form is forwarded to the Human Resources Department to initiate the hiring process. See the display on page 385 for a sample job specification.

Policies and procedures

Policies and procedures are necessary to effectively control administrative management of a service, department, or organization. The extent of policies or procedures required is dictated by the size and complexity of the organization. Policies and procedures exist to greater or lesser degrees depending on the level of bureaucracy within the organization. Policies that apply in one organization may not be necessary for another. Under usual circumstances, policies and procedures are not transferable from one organization to another.

Policies

Policies are controlling in that they set forth regulations. They are a set of criteria of what is to be done, and they explain what activities are carried out within the organization, department, service, or program. Policies are never established on a verbal basis; they should be written and approved at top administrative levels. They should be reviewed regularly and updated or revised according to changing conditions or new regulations. There is no universal guide that applies to the development of policies. In writing specific policies at a departmental level, the

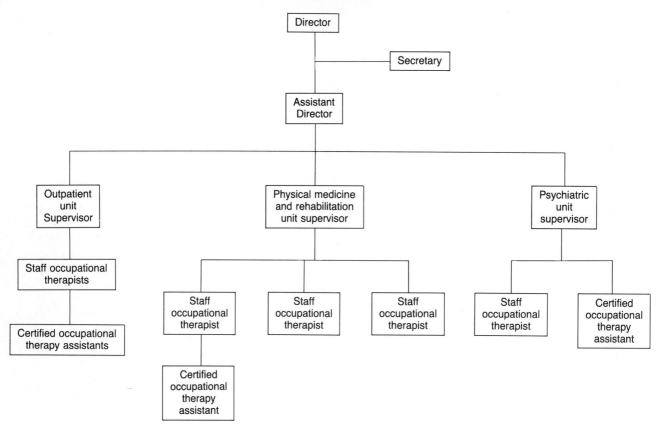

FIGURE 11-2. *Organization of an occupational therapy department.*

SAMPLE JOB DESCRIPTION

Department: Occupational Therapy
Job Title: Staff Therapist
Reports to: Unit Supervisor
Supervises: Unit Technician
Qualifications:
Education: Graduate of an accredited program in Occupational Therapy with a minimum of baccalaureate degree. Certified by the American Occupational Therapy Certification Board. Licensed by the State of New York.
Experience: Entry-level position, no experience required.
Physical: Good general health with no physical restrictions that would compromise patient care.
Basic Functions and Duties: Responsible for planning and implementing specific treatment programs for both individual and groups of patients according to the principles and practices of occupational therapy. Responsible for contributing to the clinical education program for students as assigned. Functions in a collaborative manner with the coordinating staff therapists.
Specific Duties:
With patients: Evaluates assigned patients. Develops treatment plans for assigned patients. Collaborates with patients in goal setting, including family when possible. Documents individualized evaluations, treatment plans, and summaries in accordance with departmental standards. Implements treatment with assigned patients in a timely manner.
Within department: Promotes and maintains open communication with departmental and other staff. Promotes and maintains safety standards within the department. Provides guidance and supervision to certified occupational therapy assistants, technicians, students, and volunteers. Provides clinical education to students as assigned. Represents the department at professional and related meetings and conferences as assigned. Contributes to quality assurance program of the department and the institution. Performs other duties as assigned by department director or immediate supervisor.

SAMPLE JOB SPECIFICATION

Box #5049
Date of Request: 5/14/93
Department: Occupational Therapy
Requested by: Jane Stevens
Job Title: Staff Occupational Therapist
Replacement for: David Fleurhart
Vacancy due to:
   New position: _____
   Promotion: _____
   Resignation: __X__
   Termination: _____
Explanation: Current employee took more prestigious
   position elsewhere.
Working hours: 8:00 AM to 4:00 PM
Work week: Monday through Friday
FT: __X__ PT: _____
Salary range: $28,000 to 31,000 per year
Date needed: 6/1/93
Name of supervisor: Mary Castle/Jane Stevens
Education required: B.S. in Occupational Therapy
Special skills required: Evaluation and treatment of
   hand disabilities
Organizational relationships: Collaboration with other
   occupational therapists, physical therapists, nurses,
   social workers, and physicians.
Duties: Evaluation and treatment of patients; participate
   in teaching and clinical research; function as a team
   member.
Promotional possibilities: Unit Supervisor
Interviewer: Jane Stevens
Department location: 3rd floor, East
Name of Candidate Hired: _____
Starting date: _____
Starting salary: _____

first consideration should be the way in which the departmental policy will blend or relate to those of the institution. The second consideration should be that the policy reflect the philosophy of the department.

Policies should provide the user with information about action to be taken, action to be avoided, and when and how to respond. They must be flexible; thus, policy statements often use phrases such as "whenever possible" or "as circumstances permit." Once policies are written and reviewed by top management, they should be distributed at all staff levels to which they apply and permanently filed in a policy manual.

The following list represents the types of policy typically found in an institution.

Personnel policies (eg, salary administration, work schedules, vacation allowances, sick leave, personal time off, probationary periods, employee separation, benefits, transfers, and promotions)

Institutional policies (eg, interview of applicants, preemployment and annual physical examinations, performance appraisal, fire and safety, medical records, and quality assurance)

Departmental policies (eg, treatment, referral, equipment maintenance, fees and charges, documentation, safety, and dress code)

See the display below for a sample administrative policy.

Procedures

Procedures are criteria for how things are to be done—a course of action or way of doing something. Procedures are more detailed than policies; they should state precisely how and in what specific order an activity is to be carried out. Generally, a procedure is developed for each regulating policy if the policy requires certain activities for fulfillment. Once procedures have been written, authorized, and implemented, they are assembled in manageable form—usually in a manual. Procedure manuals are required by accrediting bodies such as the Joint Commission on Accreditation of Healthcare Organizations (JCAHO) and the Commission on the Accreditation of Rehabilitation Facilities (CARF).

Institutional procedures are developed by the service with specific responsibility for a given activity; for example, fire and safety procedures would be written by the manager responsible for risk management in the institution. Examples of institutional procedures include fire, evacuation, disaster, accident, communication, and accounting.

Departmental procedures are developed within a specific department by those responsible for the service or their designee; for example, an occupational therapy documentation procedure would be written by the director of occupational therapy. Examples of departmental procedures include record keeping, equipment and supplies, maintenance and repair of equipment, quality assurance, staff orientation, referral, scheduling, patient evaluation or assessment, tests and measurements, treatment modalities, reporting, and charting. See the display on page 386 for a sample procedure.

Productivity

Productivity is viewed as a controlling mechanism for top-level management. Productivity is defined as the ratio between the output and the resources expended to obtain the desired output. A given level of quality is always implied for any output. The importance of obtaining productivity data relates to the cost effectiveness of a program. It is not unusual for administrators to set goals for productivity and strive for a minimal goal of 5% to 15% improvement annually. It is highly unlikely that 100% pro-

SAMPLE ADMINISTRATIVE POLICY

Newcombe Community Hospital Administrative Policy

All new employees will receive training in and demonstrate proper procedures to be followed in the event of fire or disaster within the institution. Training is to be scheduled by immediate supervisor and completed within 3 weeks of employment.
Effective: 9/1/90
Reviewed: 10/91, 10/92

SAMPLE PROCEDURE STATEMENT

Newcombe Community Hospital Procedure for Fire and Disaster Training Policy

1. Supervisor will provide new employee with written procedures for fire and disaster within 2 days of employment.
2. Supervisor will schedule training session with Plant and Risk Management Supervisor.
3. Supervisor will note date and time of training in writing and provide the employee with written schedule. Schedule for training will be noted in employee's departmental record.
4. Upon successful completion of training, the Plant and Risk Management Supervisor will notify employee's supervisor and forward completed training certificate to the Human Resources Department.
5. Human Resources Department will file certificate in employee's personnel record.

Effective: 9/1/90
Reviewed: 10/91, 10/92

---

ductivity would ever be achieved, and administrators do not strive for percentages beyond 80% to 90%. The information gathered in productivity studies can assist in planning new programs, making personnel projections, balancing work loads, improving staff effectiveness, and reducing or containing costs.

If an occupational therapy program is not cost effective, the service will not be competitive in the health care industry of the future. By evaluating productivity data, a manager can evaluate how much time is spent in direct and indirect service. The data may be reported by the individual therapist, by diagnosis, by modality, or by treatment outcomes. Productivity data can assist the occupational therapy manager improve efficiency by integrating planning information to ensure fiscally viable products and services without sacrificing quality care. It is important that an occupational therapy manager inform the staff about the purposes of productivity studies. This is a sensitive topic, and staff tend to react negatively to this type of study if they are not informed of its purpose. The involvement of staff in data collection and analysis can help to alleviate fears of loss of position or major changes occurring within the department. If handled well by the manager, productivity studies can be extremely beneficial to the department and may even result in increased staff, space, support personnel, or financial resources.

Summary

The issues of organizing, planning, directing, and controlling have been discussed and illustrated in their application to health care delivery and occupational therapy. The entry-level therapist should be aware of administrative and management functions and their effects on the setting in which the therapist is employed. The occupational therapy manager provides an image of the profession among peers in the health care delivery system and thus must be highly qualified as an administrator. The future

growth of the occupational therapy profession requires qualified, effective managers. In a time when occupational therapy is regarded as an expanding field, the profession must be prepared to meet these needs through education and professional standards.

References

Blake, R. R., & Mouton, J. S. (1964). *The managerial grid*. Houston, TX: Gulf Publishing.

Cunningham M. J., & Trickey, B. A. (1983). The correlation of learning styles with student performance in academic and clinical course work. *Occupational Therapy Journal of Research, 3*, 54–55.

Herzberg, F. (1966). *Work and the nature of man*. New York: Thomas Y. Crowell.

Johnson, J. A. (1973). Occupational therapy: a model for the future. *American Journal of Occupational Therapy, 27*, 1.

Katz, N. (1988). Individual learning style: Israeli norms and cross cultural equivalence of Kolb's learning style inventory. *Journal of Cross-Cultural Psychology, 19*, 361–379.

Katz, N. (1990). Problem solving and time: Functions of learning style and teaching methods. *Occupational Therapy Journal of Research, 10*(4), 221–235.

Maslow, A. H. (1943). A theory of human motivation. *Psychological Review, 50*(6), 370–396.

McGregor, D. (1960). *The human side of enterprise*. New York: McGraw-Hill.

Ordiorne, G. S. (1965). *Management by objectives*. New York: Putnam.

Rogers, J. C., & Hill, D. J. (1980). Learning style preferences of bachelor's and master's students in occupational therapy. *American Journal of Occupational Therapy, 34*, 789–793.

Steiner, G. A. (1979). *Strategic planning: What every manager must know*. New York: Free Press.

Bibliography

Bair, J., & Gray, M. (Eds.). (1992). *The occupational therapy manager*. (2nd ed.). Rockville, MD: American Occupational Therapy Association.

Bair, J., & Gwin, C. (Eds.). (1985). *Productivity systems guide for occupational therapy*. Rockville, MD: American Occupational Therapy Association.

Barris, R., Kielhofner, G., & Bauer, D. (1985). Learning preferences, values and student satisfaction. *Journal of Allied Health, 14*, 13–23.

Baum, C. M., & Luebben, A. J. (1986). *Prospective payment systems: A handbook for health care clinicians*. Thorofare, NJ: Slack.

Bryson, J. M. (1988). *Strategic planning for public and nonprofit organizations*. San Francisco: Jossey-Bass.

Desatnick, R. L. (1970). *A concise guide to management development*, New York: American Management Association.

Drucker, P. F. (1954). *The practice of management*. New York: Harper and Row.

Drucker, P. F. (1973). *Management, tasks, responsibilities, practices*. New York: Harper and Row.

English, C. (1984). *Management and supervision techniques for physical and occupational therapists*. Campbell, CA: North Coast Medical.

Hayes, R. H. (1985, November/December). Strategic planning—Forward in reverse? *Harvard Business Review*, –.

Kirk, R. (1988). *Healthcare quality and productivity*. Rockville, MD: Aspen.

Lewin, K. (1948). *Resolving social conflicts*. New York: Harper and Row.

Liebler, J., Levine, R. E., & Dervitz, H. L. (1984). *Management principles for health professionals*. Rockville, MD: Aspen.

Litman, T., & Robbins, L. (1984). *Health politics and policy*. New York: John Wiley and Sons.

Office of the Federal Register, National Archives and Records Administration. *Federal register*. Washington, DC: U. S. Government Printing Office.

Ordiorne, G. S. (1965). *Management by objectives*. New York: Putnam.

Thompson, A. M., & Wood, M. D. (1980). *Management strategies for women, or Now that I'm boss how do I run this place?* New York: Simon and Schuster.

Winston, S. (1983). *The organized executive*. New York: W. W. Norton.

SECTION 2

Documentation

KEY TERMS

Communication Barriers

Internal Classification of Impairment, Disabilities and Handicaps

Problem-Oriented Medical Record

Regulators

RUMBA Test

SOAP Note

Uniform Terminology

LEARNING OBJECTIVES

Upon completion of this section the reader will be able to:

1. *Identify the major purposes of documentation.*
2. *Describe the RUMBA test and its application to documentation.*
3. *Identify the components of a SOAP note.*
4. *Discuss the purposes and uses of uniform terminology in occupational therapy practice.*
5. *Identify the uses of ICIDH codes.*
6. *Identify the implications of accrediting bodies and reimbursement agencies for documentation in a variety of practice settings.*
7. *Discuss the implications for computerized documentation.*

Documentation is one of the most important functions performed by occupational therapists to support their intervention with patients. In other words, next to treatment, documentation accounts for a major part of time in the daily schedule of a practicing therapist. Documentation is the key to communicating the services of the occupational therapist to others on the professional team, to the patient, and to the reimbursement agency. In addition, documentation is the basis for measuring quality assur-

ance throughout the organization or system. Records and reports generated at various levels in a department or institution reflect the quality of activity taking place.

Issues of communication

Whether the method of communication is verbal or written, certain considerations should be taken into account. It is important for the therapist practicing in the health care system to understand issues that surround communication. True communication results in comprehension and understanding. Verbal communication has the advantage of continual feedback from the receiver of the message to the sender through facial expression or gestures. In written communication, the words stand alone without feedback to the communicator. Therefore, no adjustment can be made to the statements, and further clarification is not possible. For these reasons, written communication skills are important for occupational therapists.

Communication barriers should be understood to avoid some of the pitfalls common within an organization. There may be a lack of common meaning in language among participants, such as in the use of jargon, slang, or technical language. Unconscious motives fostered by inner thoughts, ideas, or emotions may cloud a person's ability to perceive or interpret events. Psychological factors, such as mistrust, fear, anger, or indifference, may shape the perceptions of a participant in communication. People develop preconceived notions about others and act on their preconceptions instead of reality. Logistic factors, such as lack of time, place, or space to communicate clearly, may produce negative results in communication. The organizational structure and the size of the organization may block communication channels simply because of the number of layers through which a communication must go. These factors should be kept in mind when communicating within the health care organization or system.

Purposes of documentation

The documentation of facts is the only evidence of professional decision making. It is the only method that ensures reimbursement agencies and accrediting bodies that something has taken place. Many therapists will use the saying, "if it isn't documented, it didn't happen" as a guideline for documentation considerations.

Documentation has four major purposes: (1) it facilitates effective treatment, (2) it justifies reimbursement, (3) it stands as a legal document, and (4) it provides communication among the patient, the treatment team, and the family (AOTA, 1986; Tiffany, 1983; Baum, 1983). Therefore, documentation has legal, ethical, and financial ramifications.

Guidelines for documentation

In considering the diversity of documentation requirements mandated by the variety of populations treated by an occupational therapist, it is a small wonder that documentation is frequently considered a chore or an overwhelming task by practicing therapists. The following suggestions may assist in organizing one's thinking process in approaching documentation and in reducing the negative connotation of documentation.

First, the therapist should consider the audience for which documentation is intended. It is important to consider who will read this documentation and who will benefit from it. Answers to these questions depend on the setting, the consumer, the payer, and other providers. That is to say, the rules for documentation in any work setting must be built on an understanding of: (1) the needs of the consumer (the patient, the family, or significant others), (2) the other team members (nurses, physical therapists, physicians, social workers, teachers), (3) the requirements of reimbursers (Blue Cross/Blue Shield, Medicare, Medicaid, commercial insurance companies, United Way), and (4) accreditation and governmental regulations (JCAHO, CARF, federal, state, and local government agencies).

RUMBA

The **RUMBA test** was originated by AOTA in the 1970s as a method used in quality assurance. RUMBA has developed further to be used as a method of self-assessment not only in quality assurance but also in documentation, intervention, and research. The RUMBA test can be applied to documentation by asking the following questions:

R = Is it RELEVANT?
U = Is it UNDERSTANDABLE?
M = Is it MEASURABLE?
B = Is it BEHAVIORAL?
A = Is it ACHIEVABLE?

Is it RELEVANT? Reports should reflect functional goals and achievements because these indicate the true relevance of an intervention. For example, the reporting of measurements taken on a weekly basis does not reflect meaningfully to members of the audience who will read the report. An increase in grip strength of 5 lb or an increase of 15 degrees of range of motion in the elbow with a muscle grade of 3 (good) in the triceps is meaningless, other than to demonstrate that the patient has greater strength or range of motion than last week. These facts standing alone are not relevant to function. However, when accompanied by statements that reflect that the patient is able to feed him- or herself a full meal independently as a result of improved grip strength or to transfer safely using a transfer board as a result of improved strength and increased range of motion in the elbows, the reader has a more complete understanding of the relevance of the documentation.

Is it UNDERSTANDABLE? There are several universal do's and don't's when it comes to documentation. First, the documentation must be readable, and therefore the writing must be legible. Jargon should be avoided. Other professionals, patients, and families do not understand the jargon of occupational therapy. Sentences should be concise, succinct, and constructed using proper grammar and spelling. Contrary to early professional standards in documentation, it is becoming more acceptable to use the first person in sentence structure; that is, "this therapist applied" or "I have determined." It is no longer acceptable to use noncommittal language; that is, "it seems" or "it appears that." A patient does not *appear* depressed; the patient either *is* or *is not* depressed as evidenced by the patient's behavior and the professional observations of the therapist. A patient

does not *seem to be* independent in donning a shirt; the patient either *does* or *does not* require assistance.

Is it MEASURABLE? Goals and statements should be written in measurable terms. Once these have been documented, other professionals can understand the measures being used. Measurements should be reported in terms of frequency and duration, that is, how long something occurred or how many times something was done. For example: Millie is able to write legibly her first name five times on wide-lined paper and then must refrain from any fine motor activity for 3 to 5 minutes; or, John is able to feed himself breakfast, lunch, and dinner independently after setup. Readers have a common understanding of how long it takes to write the word Millie or to eat a meal.

Is it BEHAVIORAL? Occupational therapists are trained to be fine observers of behavior. Behaviors are those occurrences that are seen and can be measured. One can count how many times a child loses balance to the right, how many times a patient loses control during a group activity, whether a patient cries, or whether a patient reaches for an object. The words *friendly*, *depressed*, *appropriate*, and *unmotivated* do not describe behaviors, nor can they be measured; therefore, they should be avoided.

Is it ACHIEVABLE? At this step, the occupational therapist should try to step outside the situation and look at the goal statements from the perspective of the reimburser or accreditor. The question is: Is this plan or goal achievable for this person, given the time constraints imposed by reimbursement or regulatory standards? If the answer is no, then the goal is not realistic, given the treatment setting and constraints, and the documentation should be reworked.

Problem-oriented medical record

The **Problem-Oriented Medical Record** (POMR) was developed by Weed (1971) as a means of providing structure for progress note writing. The system is based on a list of problems that is generated as a result of assessing the patient's abilities and limitations. These problems are numbered, and each subsequent progress note is written with reference to the problem list. The SOAP method for writing progress notes is commonly used in medical institutions. The structure of a **SOAP note** is as follows:

S = *Subjective:* the therapist records information as reported by the patient, the family, or significant other. This information might include what a patient says that cannot be measured.
O = *Objective:* the therapist records measurable, observable data, usually obtained through formal assessment or evaluation tools. Specific medical information and history are included here.
A = *Assessment:* the therapist records his or her professional judgment or opinion as to functional expectations or limitations based on the objective data noted in the previous section.
P = *Plan:* the therapist records a specific plan of action to be followed to resolve problems. This section may include short- or long-term goals, how long treatment should be provided, and how often the patient should receive treatment.

The SOAP format may be used for initial notes, interim or progress notes, and discharge notes. Determination to use the

POMR is made by the institution. The problem list is a master list developed by the treatment team collectively, and each SOAP note written in the medical chart must refer to a problem on the list. Thus, any reader tracking a particular problem can readily see progress from all treatment areas. Under the POMR system, service notes are not written; instead, members of the treatment team write SOAP notes to address those problems that are appropriate to their interventions.

Uniform terminology

In 1977, the Secretary of Health and Human Services was required by legislation (P.L. 95-142) to establish regulations for uniform reporting systems in hospitals. The AOTA developed a uniform reporting system in 1979 for use throughout the profession. Despite the fact that the Department of Health and Human Services never adopted the system due to concerns about price fixing and antitrust issues, the AOTA Uniform Terminology for Occupational Therapy Services (AOTA, 1989b; see Appendix C) is widely used by occupational therapists.

Since all occupational therapy services collect data on attendance, intervention, and treatment results, it is beneficial that the information collected can be compared and contrasted from one setting to another. The use of standardized **uniform terminology** can assist in avoiding disparity in the types of coverage from one region to another. The use of uniform terminology in reporting services facilitates review for reimbursement in that reviewers are accustomed to the terminology. The benefits of using uniform terminology can impact on standards, reimbursement, management, and research.

Classification codes

Within the last few years, reimbursers have shifted from approving therapy claims based on impairments to approving those based on functional limitations. This change has implications for occupational therapy documentation. The AOTA recommends that the World Health Organization's **International Classification of Impairments, Disabilities and Handicaps** (ICIDH) be used in documentation of occupational therapy outcomes. The classification system provides a uniform language for documentation of services and assists in tracking outcomes.

Arenas for communication

Hospitals

Within a hospital organization, the occupational therapist is guided in documentation by departmental policies and procedures and by requirements of accrediting bodies such as the Joint Commission of Accreditation of Healthcare Organizations (JCAHO) and the Commission of Accreditation of Rehabilitation Facilities (CARF). In addition, the requirements of reimbursers must be taken into consideration. Institutions generally tailor their documentation techniques to comply with JCAHO monitoring standards. Despite this fact, there continues to be a question of accountability for determining quality of medical care and good documentation. Since JCAHO defines occupational therapy services, the provision of services should be retained within the scope of practice described. If services provided are outside the scope of practice prescribed or if documentation is incomplete, the accreditation can be jeopardized. Likewise, noncompliance can jeopardize reimbursement. JCAHO publishes an *Accreditation Manual for Hospitals* (1990) from which occupational therapists may obtain the most current guidelines and requirements for documentation. Most institutions have copies of this manual in the medical library, the Health Information Management department (Medical Records), and administrative offices. For those institutions or units that are accredited by CARF, their documentation standards should be reviewed and followed to avoid loss of accreditation or reimbursement.

Community agencies

Documentation is governed by policies and procedures within the community agency and by various **regulators** of the agency, usually at local, state, and federal levels. The types of practice considered here are home health agencies, public health agencies, outpatient clinics, and private practice. Reimbursement for services rendered in these agencies may include commercial insurance providers, Medicaid, health maintenance organizations (HMOs), Easter Seals, public schools, or the Division of Services for Crippled Children. With such diversity in reimbursers and in regulations governing documentation, the therapist practicing in these settings must review the guidelines for each reimburser to document properly. For example, Medicaid guidelines are state-specific within the federal guidelines but cannot be generalized from one state to another; and, in some instances, occupational therapy services are not covered by Medicaid.

Residential agencies

Within residential agencies, documentation is regulated by federal and state laws. Medicaid guidelines have the greatest influence on documentation in residential settings as a result of the Department of Health and Human Services Health Care Financing Administration Rulings (U. S. Government Health Care Financing Administration, 1988). Therapists working in mental health facilities should be informed about current local and state regulations but should also keep in mind that these facilities may also be accredited by JCAHO and must therefore meet JCAHO regulations governing documentation.

Schools

Within the school system, documentation is guided by local educational agencies to comply with state and federal regulations. The Education of the Handicapped Act (U. S. Government, 1975 and 1986) is the definitive guide for documentation procedures in the school system. In addition, the U. S. Department of Education regulations for implementation are a valuable resource regarding the influence of legislation on documentation. The AOTA incorporated the federal guidelines in the Guidelines for Occupational Therapy Services in School Systems (AOTA, 1989). An individual education program (IEP) must be completed for any child to receive special services within the school setting (U. S. Government, 1981). The IEP is a collaborative plan put in writing as a commitment of resources and services and serves as the evaluation device for determining a child's progress toward meeting proposed outcomes. Current performance levels, annual goals and short-term objectives, special education and related services involvement, amount of regular class placement, projected dates for initiation and anticipated duration of services, and evaluation criteria and schedules for measurement must all be included on an annual basis in each IEP.

Computerized documentation

Computerized medical records are standard in many health service organizations. The POMR lends itself to computerization because it is a standardized system. Computerization requires standardization, and standardization can improve reliability. Computerized systems for reporting statistical data have been a part of the health care industry since the mid-1970s. These systems are constantly being updated to meet the demands of administrators, payers, and governing bodies. In consideration of documentation requirements and the professional time spent to meet these requirements, computerization has the potential to become a cost–benefit measure within the health care organization.

Summary

Documentation is not a simple skill that can be acquired in one setting and transferred to another. Although skill in documentation may be acquired in terms of use of terminology, legibility, structure, and phraseology, additional knowledge must be updated continually in terms of regulations set forth by regulators and accreditors. The AOTA has published numerous reference sources for the documentation process for practicing therapists. These are listed in the bibliography (see also Appendix E).

References

American Occupational Therapy Association (1986). Guidelines for occupational therapy documentation. *American Journal of Occupational Therapy, 40*, 830–832.

American Occupational Therapy Association (1989a). *Guidelines for occupational therapy services in the school systems.* Rockville, MD: AOTA.

American Occupational Therapy Association (1989b). *Uniform Terminology for Occupational Therapy Services* (2nd ed.). Rockville, MD: AOTA.

Baum, C. M. (1983). Management of finances, communication, personnel with resources and documentation. In H. L. Hopkins, & H. D. Smith (Eds.), *Willard and Spackman's occupational therapy* (6th ed.) (pp. 815–826). Philadelphia: J. B. Lippincott Co.

Joint Commission for Accreditation of Healthcare Organizations (1990). *Accreditation manual for hospitals.* Chicago: JCAHO.

Tiffany, E. G. (1983). Psychiatry and mental health. In H. L. Hopkins, & H. D. Smith (Eds.), *Willard and Spackman's occupational therapy* (6th ed.) (pp. 267–334). Philadelphia: J. B. Lippincott.

U. S. Government (1975 and 1986). *Education for All Handicapped Children Act and Amendments.* (Public Law 94-142 and Public Law 99-457). Washington, DC: U. S. Government Printing Office.

U. S. Government (1981). Assistance to states for education of handicapped children; Interpretation of the individualized education program. *Federal Register, 46*(12), 5462.

U. S. Government Health Care Financing Administration (1988). *Conditions of participation for long term care facilities.* Part 483 of Department of Health and Human Services Medicaid Program Conditions for Intermediate Care Facilities for the Mentally Retarded. Washington, DC: U. S. Government Printing Office.

Weed, L. L. (1971). *Medical records, medical evaluation and patient care.* Chicago: Yearbook Medical Publishers.

World Health Organization (1980). *International classification of impairments, diseases and handicaps: A manual of classification relating to consequences of disease.* Geneva, Switzerland: WHO.

Bibliography

American Occupational Therapy Association (1986). *Guidelines for occupational therapy documentation.* Rockville, MD: AOTA. (Appendix F)

American Occupational Therapy Association (1987). *Guidelines for occupational therapy services in hospice.* Rockville, MD: AOTA.

American Occupational Therapy Association (1987). *Guidelines for occupational therapy services in home health.* Rockville, MD: AOTA.

American Occupational Therapy Association (1989). *Guidelines for occupational Therapy services in early intervention and preschool services.* Rockville, MD: AOTA.

American Occupational Therapy Association (1989). *Family centered care: An early intervention resource manual.* Rockville, MD: AOTA.

American Occupational Therapy Association (1989). *Guidelines for occupational therapy services in school systems* (2nd ed.). Rockville, MD: AOTA.

American Occupational Therapy Association (1989). *Occupational therapy product output reporting system and uniform terminology for reporting occupational therapy services.* Rockville, MD: AOTA. (Appendix C)

American Occupational Therapy Association (1989). *A user's guide to the occupational performance history interview.* Rockville, MD: AOTA.

American Occupational Therapy Association (1990). *Resident assessment system.* Rockville, MD: AOTA.

American Occupational Therapy Association (1990). *OT FACT: A software system for functional performance profile.* Rockville, MD: AOTA.

Bair, J. (Ed.). (1987). *Occupational therapy in acute care settings: A manual.* Rockville, MD: AOTA.

Berni, R., & Readey, H. (1978). Problem oriented medical record implementation. *Allied health peer review.* St. Louis: C. V. Mosby.

Kettenbach, G. (1990). *Writing S.O.A.P. notes.* Philadelphia: F. A. Davis.

Mahoney, F., & Barthel, D. (1965). Functional evaluation: The Barthel index. *Maryland Medical Journal, 14*, 61–65.

Montgomery County Association for Retarded Citizens (1978). *IEP: Individualized educational program. What is it/how does it work?* Silver Springs, MD: author.

Scott, S. J., & Dennis D. C. (Eds.). *Payment for occupational therapy services.* Rockville, MD: AOTA.

SECTION 3

Quality assurance

LEARNING OBJECTIVES

Upon completion of this section the reader will be able to:

1. *Discuss quality assurance as a method for evaluating program delivery and outcomes.*
2. *Define the major components of a quality assurance program.*
3. *Identify three aspects of quality assurance.*
4. *Describe a method for monitoring quality.*
5. *Describe the implications of utilization review for occupational therapy practice.*
6. *Apply the steps of program evaluation to occupational therapy services.*

Quality assurance lies at the heart of the basic purpose of health care. Consumers demand assurance that the health care that they receive is provided at quality levels. Quality assurance is a process of assessing and improving health care outcomes. Quality assurance deals with aggregates, not individual patients. From the perspective of a manager, quality assurance is an evaluating method for program delivery and outcomes, personnel performance, and staff productivity and, as such, assures the highest possible level of care and quality of service.

Historical perspective of quality assurance

Historically, the hospital was the primary focus for quality control of the practice of medicine. The board of trustees or governing body of the medical institution had the ultimate responsibility to assure quality of care. In 1918, the American Congress of Surgeons inaugurated the accreditation effort in health care to assure quality in service. In 1951, the Joint Commission for the Accreditation of Hospitals (JCAH) was formed, and by 1955, JCAH had initiated the use of monitors in medical records for problem resolution. Over the years, the right to quality medical services has changed from a luxury to a utilitarian necessity, and society has been given a role in determining when, where, and what services should be delivered. Health care costs spiraled upward, and quality of care came under greater scrutiny. As a result, federal legislation was imposed to improve quality and reduce costs. The legislation mandated quality assurance and utilization review to measure the necessity for service. The JCAHO now mandates quality assurance, utilization review, and program evaluation within its quality assurance program regulations for accreditation.

Quality assurance programs defined

Quality assurance involves defining quality by continuously measuring outcomes against standards and then taking corrective action when problems are identified. A quality assurance program includes the following components:

Quality assurance, which identifies problems in health care service delivery and remedies them. Those benefits considered achievable that are not achieved are the focus of quality assurance.

Utilization review, which monitors the use of facilities and services. This assures that patients receive no more and no less care than is needed, that the care is medically necessary and delivered in the most economical way.

Program evaluation, which defines and reviews the results achieved after provision of service. This assures that monitoring of outcomes of intervention is taking place.

Donabedian (1982) classified the elements of quality care by defining three aspects. Assurance of quality begins with inquiry into these three aspects:

Structure: the way in which the institution is organized and the resources used to provide care (ie, personnel and equipment)

Process: the totality of interaction between the consumer and the provider of care, including what is and what is not done

Outcome: the results of intervention and interaction with the system, that is, the status of the patient after care is provided.

Quality assurance may be measured in two ways: concurrently as the care is being delivered and retrospectively after the care has been delivered.

Quality assurance monitoring

Quality assurance starts by asking and answering questions. These questions might include: What would I see if my department were providing quality care? Do all the patients return home? Do patients participate in setting their own goals for treatment? Are patients able to participate and perform certain tasks? How many patients? How many hours a day? What are the costs? These questions can be answered through quality assurance monitoring by continually measuring outcomes against standards that have been set within the department, the institution, or the profession. When a problem is identified, corrective action is taken by changing a procedure, retraining a person who performs a procedure, or changing the program altogether.

The JCAHO requires a continuous monitoring system of quality assurance. The following illustrates one method for meeting the JCAHO standard. There are five stages in quality assurance monitoring. In stage 1, the indicators of quality care are identified. The indicators should be those aspects of care that have high priority, high risk, and high volume and that are perceived as solvable should a problem occur. In stage 2, data are collected that are measurable, that is, functional scales and standardized performance measures that reflect the indicators. In stage 3, cause is determined, and if a problem is found, remedial action is indicated. In stage 4, the remedy is implemented. This is a crucial step that is sometimes overlooked. The remedy should be short and simple and should not be too costly to implement. In stage 5, the measurement process is performed again to determine if the problem has been solved. If the problem has not been solved, the process reverts to stage 3, and the cause is reinvestigated. If the problem is solved, it should be monitored periodically with lengthened measurement intervals to determine that no further complications have occurred.

Within the occupational therapy department, quality assurance monitoring may be carried out by an individual or a committee, depending on the size of the department. Regardless of how the monitoring is managed, the study must be documented and reported to top-level management and ultimately to the governing body.

QUALITY ASSURANCE MONITORING CASE STUDY

A manager in an acute care occupational therapy unit and her staff have identified several standards of treatment outcomes for patients with hip fracture. One of these standards is that 80% of the patients with a diagnosis of hip fracture will achieve independence in upper- and lower-extremity dressing within 5 days of referral to occupational therapy. In collaboration with staff, the manager sets up a monitoring system to determine if the standard is being met. The format takes the following form:

Indicator: Outcome of activities of daily living treatment for patients with hip fractures.
Data source: Occupational therapists' documentation in patients' charts.
Criteria: 80% of patients achieve independence in dressing. The maximal acceptable standard of nonachievement is 20%. All nonachievement records are reviewed.
Sample size: 20 patients
Sample method: Next 20 patients referred to occupational therapy
Time frame of study: Next 4 weeks.

The monitoring takes place, and the results indicate that 30% of the records were in the nonachievement category. The study indicated that one of the patients developed additional medical problems and received further surgery. The remaining five patients were not issued the necessary equipment, nor were they treated after the assessment session. All were assessed by the same occupational therapist and were to be treated by the same certified occupational therapy assistant.

The problem has been refined further to indicate that the five patients did not receive necessary treatment. The cause of this problem was that the occupational therapist did not communicate the need for treatment to the certified occupational therapy assistant.

The staff collaborates in designing a form to be used for intradepartmental referral information so that the certified occupational therapy assistant member of the treatment team is advised in writing of assessment outcome and necessary intervention. The new form procedure will be monitored for the next 2 weeks. The original indicator (activities of daily living treatment outcomes in patients with hip fractures) will be remeasured at the end of 3 weeks to determine if remediation has affected outcomes.

In this case study, a quality assurance study has been conducted, a problem has been identified, remediation has been implemented, and as a result, another study has been generated. In addition, remeasurement of the initial study has been assured to identify any further problems with outcomes of this particular indicator. The cyclical nature of monitoring is seen in the example, and the generation of problem-based studies is illustrated. Monitoring is shown to be systematic, continuous, and comprehensive. It involves clinicians and is part of everyday treatment functions.

A discussion of the quality assurance monitoring would not be complete without discussion of other important elements of the process. JCAHO requires that studies be documented and reported through the chain of command to the board of trustees. Since the ultimate responsibility for quality assurance rests with the board of trustees, all services should be involved in monitoring studies, even contract services, such as joint ventures for the supply of equipment to patients. Written documentation of monitoring studies should be forwarded through the department head to the quality assurance committee or similar committee or department with review authority, to the chief executive officer, and to the board of trustees in a report format, usually drafted by the chief executive officer.

Utilization review

Utilization review is a hospital- or facility-wide function. It is a program that monitors the use of facilities and services. As noted previously, utilization review assures that the patient receives only those services that are medically necessary. In addition, utilization review assures the payer that the care is medically necessary, delivered economically, and conforms to criteria determined by peers within the facility.

Utilization review programs are coordinated by a person who has extensive knowledge of all aspects of patient care. These coordinators are often nurses or health information managers. Utilization review coordinators are responsible for certifying admission, reviewing for length of stay, and notifying the attending physician of any problem that occurs or issues that might warrant the discharge of a patient. The implications for the occupational therapist are that documentation must be accurate, timely, and understandable in terms of goals and progress since it is the record that is reviewed for utilization of facilities and services. It is important for the occupational therapist to be aware of the admission certification date and approved length of stay because this may have an impact on the projected treatment program and goals.

Program evaluation

Accrediting agencies, such as JCAHO and CARF, require that each institution has a system for evaluating the program of care delivered. Program evaluation defines and reviews the results achieved after the provision of care; it is an outcome-monitoring system that reflects the impact of services on consumers. The actual method of evaluation varies from one program to another and from one department to another.

The methodology for program evaluation generally is conducted by diagnosis or service rendered (eg, patients with myocardial infarction, or neurosurgical intervention in patients with parietal lobe trauma). As in other quality assurance programs, program evaluation studies involve the identification of goals, purpose, indication for treatment, recommended services, patient status at discharge, and need for follow-up or community-level services. Data on outcomes are related to those consumers who achieved the goals or have demonstrated change as a result of receipt of service. A committee reviews data collected retrospectively and determines the strengths, weaknesses, and shortcomings of the program being evaluated. The results of the study are shared with those involved with the program, and plans are made for implementing any changes to improve the program or service.

Another method for evaluating a program is to conduct a patient satisfaction survey. This is a common practice in evaluating specially funded programs, such as those financed by a grant.

Either of the above methods may be used to evaluate an occupational therapy program. The studies should be conducted within the department by management-level staff or designees. Examples of program evaluation studies in an occupational therapy department include achievement of functional goals for head trauma patients; levels of self-care skills among patients with left-sided hemiplegia as measured by the Barthel Index; parallel group participation of patients performing on an Allen Cognitive Level 4; and patient and family satisfaction with training programs in occupational therapy. Program evaluation in an occupational therapy department may be used to communicate to third-party payers, meet accreditation standards, assist in marketing, plan new programs, and improve benefits to consumers.

Summary

Quality assurance programs, including utilization review and program evaluation, are evaluating and monitoring tools for measuring the outcomes of services provided. These programs are the result of the need for health care providers to be accountable to consumers and third-party payers. The methods described assist the occupational therapy manager in determining the extent to which programs are meeting the established goals and objectives.

Reference

Donabedian, A. (1982). *Exploration of quality assessment and monitoring. Vol. 2: The criteria and standards of quality.* Ann Arbor, MI: Health Administration Press.

Bibliography

American Medical Association (1974). *PSRO program manual.* Chicago: American Medical Association.

Commission on Accreditation of Rehabilitation Facilities (1982). *Pro-gram evaluation: A guide to utilization.* Tuscon, AZ: Commission on Accreditation of Rehabilitation Facilities.

Graham N. (1982). Historical perspective and regulations. In N. Graham (Ed.), *Quality assurance in hospitals.* Rockville, MD: Aspen.

Joe, B. E. (1985). Quality assurance. In J. Bair, & M. Gray (Eds.), *The occupational therapy manager.* Rockville, MD: AOTA.

Joint Commission of Accreditation of Healthcare Organizations. (1990). *The accreditation manual for hospitals.* Chicago: JCAHO.

Joint Commission of Accreditation of Hospitals. (1980). *The quality assurance guide.* Chicago: JCAH.

Ostrow, P. C. (1983). Historical precedents for quality assurance in health care. *American Journal of Occupational Therapy, 37*(1), 23–26.

Ostrow, P. C., & Kuntavanish, A. K. (1983). Improving the utilization of occupational therapy: A quality assurance study. *American Journal of Occupational Therapy, 37*(6), 388–391.

Ostrow, P. C., Williamson, J. W., & Joe, B. E. (1983). *Quality assurance primer.* Rockville, MD: AOTA.

Shimeld, A. (1983). A clinical demonstration program in quality assurance. *American Journal of Occupational Therapy, 37*(1), 31–34.

SECTION 4

Fiscal management

KEY TERMS

Balance Sheet	*Indirect Costs*
Chart of Accounts	*Master Budget*
Cost Accounting	*Operating Budget*
Cost Centers	*Revenue and Expense*
Direct Costs	*Budget*

LEARNING OBJECTIVES

Upon completion of this section the reader will be able to:

1. *Discuss the importance of fiscal management in relation to an occupational therapy manager's role.*

2. *Identify and discuss the impact of key legislation for reimbursement in health care.*

3. *Define the basic terminology used in financial management.*

4. *Describe the budgeting process for an occupational therapy manager.*

Fiscal management is the method of controlling the economics of problems at hand. It is an activity concerned with discovering, developing, defining, and evaluating the financial goals of the department. This activity is usually the responsibility of administrators or managers; however, the success of fiscal management is often dependent on combined efforts by staff at all levels. If sound financial management is in its proper perspective, it can do much to augment the quality, quantity, and effectiveness of health care by providing a system that makes service available and accessible at a reasonable cost.

Reimbursement

Any discussion of fiscal management must include issues surrounding coverage for services. It is crucial that an occupational therapy manager be knowledgeable about reimbursement issues in relation to the programs that are being administered. This knowledge should include existing coverage for occupational therapy services, the terminology used by third-party payers, current federal legislation regarding services and reimbursement for given populations, denials for reimbursement within the institution or organization in which occupational therapy services are provided, reasons for rejections of reimbursement, and appeal mechanisms. An overview of reimbursement legislation is included in the display to provide guidelines for the basis of acquiring this knowledge.

Financial management terminology

A basic discussion of terms used in accounting practices in health care is necessary to facilitate an understanding of fiscal management. *Cost accounting* includes theories, methods, and procedures for identifying, measuring, and reporting the cost of obtaining or providing services. The principle objective of cost accounting is to measure the resources used to produce a service. There are a number of formulas for cost accounting, and the processes of cost accounting are too involved for extensive discussion here. Occupational therapy managers usually consult with accountants or financial officers of the institution to determine the formulas to be used in their services.

The *tax exempt status* of an organization is determined by the ownership and control classification of the organization. Health care organizations are classified as nonprofit, for-profit, or government-controlled. *Nonprofit organizations* are usually determined to be tax exempt by government standards. *For-profit organizations* are owned by a group or individual for the care of their own consumers. These include investor-owned facilities that provide services with the anticipation that a profit will be made and distributed to investors.

MAJOR U. S. LEGISLATION AFFECTING REIMBURSEMENT

1935 **Social Security Act** (P. L. 74-241) **and Amendments**. Provided financial support for disabled workers and retirement income for the elderly, including medical benefits.

1956 **Disability Insurance Benefit Program**. Provided benefits to qualified disabled individuals with work experience.

1965 **Title XVIII** (P. L. 89-97, Medicare) **and Title XIX** (P. L. 89-97, Medicaid) **of the Social Security Act**. Established reimbursement based on reasonable cost for medical services for the elderly and through state grants to the poor.

1972 **Social Security Amendments** (P. L. 92-223). Authorized Intermediate Care Facilities under Medicaid for residents in active treatment.

1974 **Rehabilitation Act** (P. L. 93-112) **and Amendments** (P. L. 93-516). Provided vocational rehabilitation of the handicapped, particularly the severely disabled.

1975 **Education of All Handicapped Children Act** (P. L. 94-142). Provided for free appropriate education for handicapped children and funding for related services.

1981 **Omnibus Reconciliation Act** (P. L. 97-35). Provided financing through Medicaid for community-based services for people with developmental disabilities when services were demonstrated to be less expensive than institutional care.

1982 **Tax Equity and Fiscal Responsibility Act** (TEFRA). Placed limits on inpatient hospital costs, eliminated nursing salary differential, and reduced reimbursement for other charges for Medicare and Medicaid patients. Occupational therapy was among those services on which limits were placed.

1983 **Omnibus Social Security Act** (P. L. 98-210). Established a prospective payment system based on a fixed price per diagnosis-related group (DRG) for inpatient services.

1984 **Developmental Disabilities Act Amendments** (P. L. 98-527). Ensured that developmentally disabled people received necessary services and established a monitoring system.

1984, 1985, 1986 **Deficit Reduction Legislation Acts** (P. L. 98-369, P. L. 99-272, and P. L. 99-509). Extended coverage for services through modification of Medicare legislation.

1986 **Education of All Handicapped Children Act Amendments** (P. L. 99-457). Provided funding for preschoolers and mandated early intervention programs for handicapped infants and toddlers.

Cost centers are the segments of activity for which costs are collected. The cost centers in each service are numbered for accounting purposes. Occupational therapy is a revenue-generating cost center since services are reimbursed.

A ***chart of accounts*** is a basic accounting method for organizing data in reference to costs. Most charts of accounts are number-coded for ease of identification and organization. These charts should allow for expansion and contraction to accommodate changes in goals, but they should maintain basic uniformity for recording and reporting information. These differ from one facility to another depending on the size and complexity of the organization.

A *budget period* is a time frame for budgeting purposes. The time frame may be 12 months, as in a calendar or fiscal year, or 3, 5, or 10 years, depending on the purpose of the budgeting function. A fiscal year is the usual accounting period for an annual or operating budget. The longer time frame is frequently used for depreciation or capital equipment budgets.

A ***balance sheet*** portrays the assets, liabilities, and fund balances at a particular time within the fiscal year. ***Direct costs*** are those that can be traced to a specific unit or activity. ***Indirect costs*** are those that cannot be traced to a particular service. Whether a cost is direct or indirect depends on the level of sophistication of the accounting system used in the institution. In general, a manager tries to make as many costs as possible direct since these are usually reimbursable.

Budgeting

Budgets ensure that program objectives are formulated with financial realities in mind. Budgeting is a planning and controlling tool. As a plan, a budget is a specific statement of anticipated results, expressed in numeric terms, covering a specific time period and is the basis of continuing and future plans in financial terms. When administered properly, a budget controls. The organizational structure based on department goals and functions is reflected in a budget. A budget is an educated estimate of future needs and is based on past records, personal experience, knowledge, and projected planning. Budgets are generally rigid but should be flexible enough to allow success with respect to established objectives and to allow for unforeseen demands on the organization or individual departments.

Types of budgeting

A variety of budgets are used within an organization. The ***master budget*** is the central, composite budget for the entire organization. This budget usually is provided to top-level management and the board of trustees of an organization. Individual units are reflected in the master budget but usually only in general terms as to revenues and expenses.

Departmental budgets become part of the master budget. These budgets are working, detailed budgets for each unit and are usually developed by the unit manager in collaboration with employees from the fiscal or financial department. Departmental budgets tend to be highly specific and permit identification of each item as well as close coordination and monitoring of revenues and expenses.

A *capital budget* is used to reflect anticipated expenses to be incurred for the purchase of major equipment or improvements to the facilities. A capital budget often covers more than the fiscal year—usually a budget period of 2–5 years. Items included in a capital budget are generally those items that have at least a 5-year life expectancy and cost more than $300. This budget may indicate amounts of money to be allocated to specific units that have submitted requests for capital expenditures, or the budget may reflect specific equipment that is to be purchased for specific units. The format of a capital budget varies from one organization to another.

The most common type of budget is the ***revenue and expense budget***, which reflects anticipated revenues from payment of services rendered, endowments, special funds, grants, and other special sources. Expenses are enumerated in terms of personnel, equipment, supplies, and benefits. This type of budget is often referred to as the ***operating budget*** and usually reflects the activity of a given fiscal year. Each department has an operating budget for a fiscal year, which is usually referred to as the *department budget*.

Other special types of budgets that may be used within a health care organization include *personnel budgets, student education budgets, special project budgets,* and *development budgets.* The use of these types of budgets varies from one institution to another depending on the size and complexity of the organization.

Budgeting process and methods

To establish a budget, specific information about direct and indirect costs must be gathered. A number of formulas are used for determining revenue and expenses. The manager should check with fiscal advisers within the organization to determine the formulas to be used for budgeting purposes.

The first step in the budgeting process is to identify the direct costs. Direct costs include salaries, payroll taxes, overtime, vacation relief, supplies, student programs, educational expenses, in-services, and reimbursable equipment. The expenses in each category are listed separately and then totaled.

The next step in the process is to determine the indirect costs. Indirect costs include administrative support for personnel, accounting, purchasing, cleaning and maintenance of department, laundry and plant operation costs, and utilities. The determination of indirect costs is based on the percentage of space used or allotted to the department in relation to the total facility space. The formula is as follows:

$$\frac{\text{departmental square footage}}{\text{total facility square footage}} = \% \text{ of usage}$$

For example, for an occupational therapy department that uses a space measuring 50 feet × 42 feet in a facility whose total square footage is 120,000 feet, the following would apply:

$$\frac{2100 \text{ square feet}}{120,000 \text{ square feet}} = 0.0175$$

Therefore, if the cost to the facility for utilities were $8000, the portion allocated to the occupational therapy department would be $140.

In the third step, the direct and indirect costs are then totaled for the total budget figure. If the organization includes a bad debt allowance in the operating budget, this figure would be added to the total.

The fourth step in the process is the determination of the fee-for-service once the total budget has been ascertained. The formula for this process is to divide the total budget by the number of projected treatment procedures for the budget period. For example:

$$\frac{\text{total budget}}{\text{projected number of treatment procedures}} = \frac{\$378{,}234}{24{,}750} = \$15.28 \text{ (cost per procedure)}$$

This figure would be determined in consultation with fiscal administrators.

In final form, the budget includes all the data gathered through methods outlined above. Once the budget has been developed, it is approved through administrative channels and becomes part of the master budget. Through review of the monthly cost center report generated by the financial department, ongoing monitoring of revenues and expenses is possible.

Summary

An important function for an occupational therapy manager is that of financial accountability. Without knowledge and skills in financial management, a manager cannot justify fees-for-service, staffing, or service costs. Occupational therapy managers have the greatest involvement in developing and monitoring their departmental budgets. The manager should involve staff in budget planning, particularly as a tool to assist staff in recognizing and supporting the financial management of the department and institution.

Bibliography

American Hospital Association (1976). *Chart of accounts for hospitals.* Chicago: American Hospital Association.

Baum, C. M., & Luebben, A. J. (1986). *Prospective payment systems: A handbook for health care clinicians.* Thorofare, NJ: Slack.

Berman, H. J., & Weeks, L. E. (1982). *The financial management of hospitals.* Ann Arbor, MI: Health Administration Press.

Laase, S. M. (1985). Financial management. In J. Bair, & M. Gray (Eds.), *The occupational therapy manager.* Rockville, MD: AOTA.

Neumann, B. R., Suver, J. D., & Zelman, W. N. (1984). *Financial management: Concepts and applications for health care providers.* Owings Mills, MD: National Health Publishing.

Roemer, M. I. (1986). *An introduction to the U. S. health care system* (2nd ed.). New York: Springer.

Scott, S. J. (1988). *Payment for occupational therapy services.* Rockville, MD: AOTA.

SECTION 5

Marketing

KEY TERMS

Consumer Research

Marketing

Marketing Plan

Marketing Segmentation

Market-Oriented Institution

LEARNING OBJECTIVES

Upon completion of this section the reader will be able to:

1. *Differentiate between advertising and marketing.*
2. *Describe the components of a marketing plan.*
3. *Apply marketing principles to an occupational therapy service.*
4. *Discuss the implications of marketing for occupational therapy staff.*

Health care marketing evolved in the mid-1970s when concerns arose about increased regulation of health care, decreased resources, increased competition for those limited resources, and changes in reimbursement practices for health care. Today, greater attention is given to alternative delivery systems and copayment by consumers as a means of reducing health care costs. This section is intended to provide an overview of a complex system for marketing in the health care industry.

Marketing defined

Marketing is a process that focuses the organization on the needs of the consumer. Marketing has meant advertising a product, but marketing professionals have long acknowledged that advertising alone does not produce large increases in demand. Marketing requires a vision of where the organization is going as well as a plan for getting there. Marketing begins by asking what are the needs and desires of consumers. This is in contrast to strategic planning, which asks what are the organization's mission and goals (Figure 11-3). Both processes proceed in similar ways until the methods of achieving the plan are questioned. Marketing then turns to public relations and sales methods, whereas strategic planning considers economic alternatives.

To understand what consumers want, an analysis of consumer desires and behaviors plays a large part of the marketing planning process. Techniques used by industry may assist in understanding the process. ***Marketing segmentation*** is a fundamental concept in marketing. It should be based on research rather than logic. Segments need to be determined for specific services since purchase behavior is being predicted. The market segment is a group of consumers who are distinguished

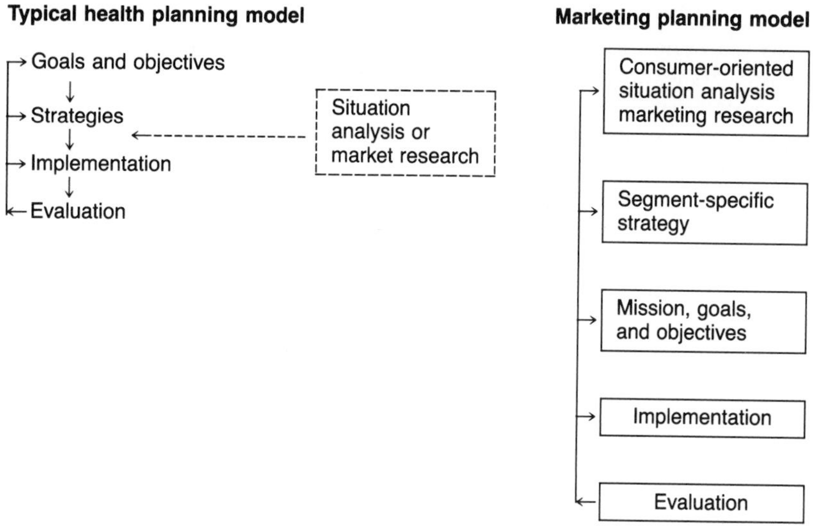

Typical health planning model

→ Goals and objectives
  ↓
→ Strategies ←------ → Situation analysis or market research
  ↓
→ Implementation
  ↓
←— Evaluation

FIGURE 11-3. *A traditional model and a marketing planning model.*

Marketing planning model

Consumer-oriented situation analysis marketing research
↓
Segment-specific strategy
↓
Mission, goals, and objectives
↓
Implementation
↓
Evaluation

by one or more characteristics believed to affect their purchasing behavior. **Consumer research** is conducted to determine how consumers behave and the attitudes, knowledge, and beliefs that affect their behavior. Surveys, by mail or personal interview, are a common method for this type of data gathering.

Marketing plan

Once the surveys have been completed, the goals must be established in the **marketing plan**. The goals state the broad purpose to be accomplished. They may emphasize growth or entry into new markets. Objectives are then delineated. These are the anticipated, measurable results that are defined in terms of quantity and time. For example, an objective may be to increase the number of referrals by 20% by 1993. The objectives should be realistic but challenge the services to meet them. Strategies or plans of action for each objective are developed next. Programs are the key components of strategies. These might include programs for promoting a particular facet of the service that is underused, visits to other services within the institution to identify potential consumers, in-service presentations within the institution, or special breakfast meetings sponsored by the organization to educate potential consumers in the insurance industry. The budget must be established so that the plan can be carried out with the necessary resources for the marketing plan. Throughout the budgeting phase, it should be kept in mind that good marketing is a sound investment in the future, but it is a long-range reward and quick results should not be anticipated.

Marketing strategies in health care

By refocusing the institution from a production orientation to a marketing orientation, federal legislation has played a role in developing marketing as a tool for health care institutions. A **market-oriented institution** sees its roles as identifying and serving the evolving needs of the consumers and the public. Marketing experts suggest that the health care professions have neglected market research and have overlooked the development of market strategies in the pursuit of methods to produce quick results.

Marketing in health care is a growing discipline that combines a knowledge of health care, its environment, and analytic design with a study of their interactions. Analysis of consumer behavior, attitudes, knowledge, and beliefs are changing the way some health care organizations are planning for new services. The number of new programs being offered that emphasize lifestyle change, disease detection, and alternatives to hospital care suggests that some organizations are changing their behavior.

Marketing implications for occupational therapy

Marketing follows a sequence of steps similar to that of treatment planning. The marketing strategist assesses the client's needs, develops the marketing plan, and then implements it. The occupational therapist can collect information by reviewing patient records or referrals; examining demographic trends, such as age, gender, income, location, and disability; and reviewing changes in paying methods. It is also important to monitor trends in society to determine the impact the service may have. Once the market analysis has been completed, the marketing position is written as part of the marketing plan.

A concise and precise position statement should be written that specifies the service in the way clients should perceive the program. Since most patients are referred by physicians in a hospital setting, the physician must be attracted to the program for the therapist to have access to the patient. In the school setting, the target would most likely be the teacher or school administrator who arranges for service rather than the parent of the potential client. Promotion of an occupational therapy service may be accomplished through brochures, advertising, newsletters, public relations events, or public speaking. Occupational therapists who volunteer in a speaker's bureau have the opportunity to promote their services to a variety of audiences.

Occupational therapy managers can successfully incorporate marketing into their administrative practices by combining proved marketing strategies with traditional practice methods. Such a combination can maintain professionalism, deliver high-quality care, and satisfy the needs of potential patients while ensuring the viability of the program. Marketing concepts can be used effectively within an organization in demonstrating the service to other providers or services. Methods of internal marketing strategies might include a departmental open house, inservices provided to the nursing or social service departments, and feature articles in employee newsletters. Progress notes, memorandums, and reports, as well as participation in case conferences, are other methods of demonstrating the benefits of service and therefore can be construed as marketing tools. Marketing also can be used externally to educate consumers to the need and availability of occupational therapy services, such as through a community newsletter, seminars and workshops for special disability groups, articles about staff accomplishments in local newspapers, and participation in health fairs within the community or region.

The occupational therapy manager must educate staff regarding the merits of marketing to ensure a commitment to marketing on all levels. Many staff members do not perceive themselves as having a role in marketing a service. Staff can be reminded that the impression they create with patients or visitors to the clinic is in fact a means of promoting the service. Staff also can be reminded that marketing is necessary to create public awareness of occupational therapy and to differentiate occupational therapists from competing health care providers.

Summary

The occupational therapy manager would be wise to include market research as a step in program evaluation to ensure maximal use of resources. It would not be practical for an occupational therapy manager to embark on a marketing research program independently unless the therapist is managing a private practice. Resources within the organization can be tapped for developing a marketing plan. Although marketing does not ensure success, a lack of marketing may curtail growth or even the life of the service. Yoder (1984) advocated aggressive marketing when he stated that consumer education has an important role in building acceptance and awareness of professionals who are marketing their services. The more the public knows the more they will seek our services. The more we can demonstrate our competency, the more the consumer will benefit from our services.

Reference

Yoder, D. (1984). Presidential Address to American Speech and Hearing Association.

Bibliography

Cooper, P. D. (Ed.). (1979). *Health care marketing: Issues and trends.* Rockville, MD: Aspen.

Berkowitz, E. N., & Flexner, W. A. (1978). The marketing audit: a tool for health service organizations. *Health Care Management Review, 3*(4), 52–53.

Gilkeson, G. E. (1985). Occupational therapy leadership potential can be developed through marketing techniques. In F. Cromwell (Ed.), *Work-related programs in occupational therapy.* New York: Haworth Press.

Gilkeson, G. E., Glenn, J. M., & Webb, R. S. (1988). Marketing: a reasonable administrative approach to decision making. In F. Cromwell, & C. Brollier (Eds.), *The occupational therapy manager's survival handbook.* New York: Haworth Press.

MacStravic, R. E. (1977). *Marketing health care.* Rockville, MD: Aspen.

UNIT V

Research in occupational therapy

CHAPTER 12

Research: A systematic process for answering questions

JEAN C. DEITZ

KEY TERMS

Control

Correlational Research

Dependent Variable

Descriptive Research

Experimental Research

External Validity

Group Research

Independent Variable

Internal Validity

Interobserver Agreement

Operational Definition

Population

Procedural Agreement

Qualitative Research

Quantitative Research

Reliability

Sample

Single system research

Triangulation

LEARNING OBJECTIVES

Upon completion of this chapter the reader will be able to:

1. *Define research and explain its importance to occupational therapy.*

2. *Describe quantitative group and single system research designs and demonstrate a basic understanding of concepts relevant to these types of research.*

3. *Describe and give an example of qualitative research.*

4. *Appreciate the variety of research types and designs and the value of each to occupational therapy.*

As a practicing therapist or as an educator, questions emerge. The clinician may wonder:

Will this splint prevent contractures?

Will more of my clients in the nursing home participate in the walking group if a new destination is planned for each walk rather than a familiar path each session?

At what age can typically developing children access a computer to play a simple cause-and-effect game involving switch control?

What are the activity patterns of parents with children who are multiply disabled?

What is the nature of occupational therapy practice in acute care psychiatry?

According to Cox and West, research is "a systematic approach to the discovery of knowledge" (1982, p. 5). It is a process involving a logical sequence leading from a question to an answer, which in turn may result in a new question. Inherent in this process is systematic observation.

Gilfoyle and Christiansen (1987) contend that research "is essential to the survival and continued development of occupational therapy" (p. 7). They further maintain that the "challenge that confronts our profession . . . concerns a commitment to inquiry, knowledge development, and responsible (scientifically based) clinical practice" (p. 7). Research is important to occupational therapy for three reasons. First, it develops and extends the knowledge base of the profession; second, it contributes to the development and validation of occupational therapy tests and measurements; and third, it documents the effectiveness of occupational therapy interventions. In the process, research plays an important role in theory testing and building.

Types of research

There are different types of research and each is relevant and appropriate for answering different types of questions. In some cases, however, the same question may be answered by two or more research approaches.

Although research approaches have been classified in a variety of ways, for purposes of this chapter, they are divided into two major types: quantitative research and qualitative research. The former will be further subdivided into quantitative group research design and quantitative single system design. The type of research used is influenced by (1) the nature of the research question; (2) the ability to control variables; and (3) the extent of the knowledge base related to the area of concern. Additionally, research ethics make an impact on choice of method. For example, although it may be ideal from a scientific perspective to withhold treatment from a no-treatment control group, this might not be justifiable from an ethical perspective. Therefore, the researcher may decide against the use of a research design that requires the withholding of treatment. Likewise, a researcher may decide against a qualitative research approach that requires the researcher to immerse himself or herself in the family life of a person with a disability because this approach might be perceived as an unacceptable invasion of privacy.

Quantitative research

The quantitative research process involves a series of logical steps:

1. Identifying a question that merits answering
2. Reviewing existing literature and knowledge related to the question
3. Clarifying the question based on the review just mentioned
4. Designing a study to answer the question
5. Carrying out the procedures of the study
6. Analyzing the data collected
7. Interpreting the data to determine the extent to which the identified question has been answered
8. Identifying new questions that emerge as a result of the research
9. Disseminating research findings

Vocabulary

Relating to quantitative research, the following terms are important:

Operational definition—"a definition based on the observable characteristics of that which is being defined" (Tuckman, 1978); method by which you quantify or measure a variable

Independent variable—treatment variable; a condition that is manipulated by the researcher

Dependent variable—the outcome or measured variable; the variable used to measure the effect of the independent variable

Reliability—the consistency or stability of measurement

Interobserver agreement—the extent to which two or more observers agree in assigning scores or ratings to the performance of a subject or a group of subjects

Procedural agreement—the extent to which the experimental procedures (independent variables) are applied in accordance with the delineated plan (Billingsley et al., 1980)

Internal validity—a condition that exists when the observed effect on the dependent variable can be attributed to the independent variable (ie, a condition that exists when you can attribute the outcome of the study—for the person or group studied—to the treatment)

External validity—a condition that exists when generalizations can be made from the sample to the population.

Quantitative group research

Quantitative **group research** design is characterized as being group-focused, reductionistic, and carefully controlled. The designs for this type of research can be categorized into descriptive, correlational, and experimental research designs. To some extent, these designs are sequential. According to Payton (1988), if little or nothing is known about a topic, the general sequence of research designs is from descriptive to correlational to experimental. In reality, however, some overlap is seen in these designs. For example, the design of a single study may include both descriptive and correlational design elements.

The three basic types of quantitative group research design differ relative to (1) the kind of question asked, (2) the degree to which the researcher manipulates the sample, (3) the statistical tools used to summarize or interpret the data, and (4) the types of statements the researcher makes on the basis of the data collected and analyzed (Payton, 1988).

Before addressing the three types of quantitative group research designs, it is important to discuss populations and samples. A **population** is a well-defined group of people or objects that meet the criteria set by the researcher. Such groups have some characteristics in common (Cox & West, 1982). For example, a population might be adults with multiple sclerosis or typically developing 4-year-old girls or people treated at the Helpful Hand Clinic in Florida in 1991.

In some instances, the subjects in a research study may include the entire population. For example, it might be possible to include the population of all people treated at the Helpful Hand Clinic in Florida in 1991 in one study. On the other hand, it would be almost impossible to include the 1991 population of all typically developing 4-year-old children in the United States in a study. Instead, the researcher selects a **sample** (small subset of the population) designed to be representative of the population. The researcher should carefully describe the sample selection process and the steps taken to ensure that the sample was representative of the population.

For example, if the researcher desires a sample reflecting the population of typically developing 4-year-old girls, the researcher should describe such factors as how it was determined that the subjects were typically developing and how he or she ensured that children were included from a variety of ethnic groups and diverse socioeconomic backgrounds. This is desirable because often when a sample is used, the researcher wants to obtain information that is generalizable to the population, in this case, typically developing 4-year-old girls. Therefore, it is important to know that the subjects in the sample are comparable to those in the population. One of the best ways to ensure this is through *random selection* of subjects. This is exemplified by listing all members of a specified population and using a random numbers table to select the desired number of subjects for the sample.

Descriptive research

The research question for quantitative **descriptive research** focuses on the characteristics of the world relative to the specific question. The purpose of such research is to gather data relevant to a clearly defined problem from either a specifically identified sample or population. For example, the researcher might ask, "How many people with C5-6 quadriplegia in Michigan, who were initially fitted with wrist-driven splints, continue to wear them 6 months following discharge?" After compiling a list of all facilities in Michigan where persons with C5-6 quadriplegia are treated, the researcher might randomly select six facilities from the list. Next, the researcher would find the names of all the people in these settings with C5-6 quadriplegia who were discharged between given dates and at the time of discharge were wearing wrist-driven splints. The researcher might then develop a carefully designed questionnaire regarding the respondent's use of wrist-driven splints and mail it to all persons identified as having wrist-driven splints at the time of discharge.

Data from this survey might be reported in terms of the number or percentage of persons answering each of the questions in a given way. If the research question had been phrased in terms of the number of hours that persons with C5-6 quadriplegia wear such splints, data would be reported using statistics reflecting the central tendency (mean, median, or mode) and the extent of score spread or dispersion (variance, standard deviation, range) of the responses to a specific item.

Survey and normative studies are examples of quantitative descriptive research. The preceding hypothetical study as well as a study by Kanny et al. (1991) exemplifies the former. The study by Kanny et al. (1991) had two purposes. The first was to document the status of technology training in entry-level curricula; the second was to "identify the factors that were barriers and those that would facilitate the development of technology training components in entry-level occupational therapy curricula" (Kanny et al., 1991, p. 313). The population was defined as the 67 schools offering entry-level occupational therapy programs. Therefore, surveys were mailed to these 67 institutions, 59 of which returned their questionnaires. Thus, the response rate was over 88%. The answers to the questions on these surveys were compiled and the final results were reported in a table and a graph. For other examples of survey research relevant to occupational therapy, refer to studies by Holcomb et al. (1989) on the scholarly productivity of occupational therapy faculty members; by Crowe and Kanny (1990) on occupational therapy practice in school systems; and by Stone and Mertens (1991) on educating entry-level occupational therapy students in gerontology.

An example of a normative study is that completed by Mathiowetz et al. (1986). They collected normative data on four

tests of hand strength, reporting findings for a sample of 231 males and 240 females. These subjects ranged in age from 6 to 19 years. The normative data for these subjects were reported descriptively in tables. See Table 12-1 for an example.

Normative information such as this is useful clinically in that it assists in interpreting evaluation results and setting realistic treatment goals. For additional examples of normative studies, refer to test manuals for the Miller Assessment for Preschoolers (Miller, 1982), the Sensory Integration and Praxis Tests (Ayres, 1989), and the Manual for Application of the Motor-Free Visual Perception Test to the Adult Population (Bouska & Kwatny, 1983).

Correlational research

The purpose of **_correlational research_** is to determine the extent to which two or more phenomena tend to occur together. For example, a researcher would use correlational research to find out the extent to which hyperactivity and scores on a test of sensory integration are related or to find out the extent to which two tests of hand function measure the same thing. To do this, the researcher uses correlational statistics to examine the degree of relationship between two or more variables. Note that correlation does not imply causation. For example, relative to the former question, if the researcher determines that hyperactivity and low scores on a test of sensory integration are related, the researcher should not say that poor sensory integration causes hyperactivity or that hyperactivity causes poor sensory integration. Instead, the researcher should say only that hyperactivity and poor sensory integration tend to occur together. Thus, the conclusions based on correlational research should be focused on degree of relationship, not on causation. Such research might lead to questions regarding cause and effect, which might then become the focus of future research using experimental research designs.

A study by Crowe et al. (1987) exemplifies a correlational study. This study was designed to examine the relationship among infants' scores on the Bayley Scales of Infant Development (BSID) (Bayley, 1969) during the first 2 years of life and their motor and cognitive performance at 4½ years. The sample consisted of children identified at birth as biologically at high risk for developmental problems. The 70 children in this study were evaluated at

TABLE 12-1. *Average Performance of Normal Subjects on Palmer Pinch (Pounds)*

Age	Hand	Males			Males		
		Mean	*SD*	*Range*	*Mean*	*SD*	*Range*
6–7	R	10.0	2.2	5–13	9.0	1.7	6–12
	L	9.2	2.0	5–13	8.4	1.4	6–11
8–9	R	11.6	2.3	7–17	10.7	2.1	8–17
	L	11.2	2.8	6–16	10.3	2.2	6–20
10–11	R	13.9	2.7	7–21	13.5	2.2	11–22
	L	13.2	2.9	8–23	12.6	2.0	10–17
12–13	R	15.5	3.6	8–26	15.4	2.6	11–23
	L	15.1	4.1	8–23	14.2	2.8	10–20
14–15	R	19.2	4.2	11–28	15.6	3.3	9–26
	L	18.8	5.0	10–33	14.7	3.4	8–25
16–17	R	22.2	5.0	17–39	17.8	3.9	12–27
	L	20.3	4.1	14–31	16.6	3.9	10–26
18–19	R	23.8	4.3	17–34	20.2	3.3	10–26
	L	23.4	4.5	16–34	19.0	3.0	14–25

(From Mathiowetz, V., et al. [1986]. Grip and pinch strength: Norms for 6- to 19-year olds. American Journal of Occupational Therapy, 40, 708.)

corrected ages of 4 months, 1 year, and 2 years on the BSID. These same children were evaluated at 4½ years (corrected age) on a measure of gross motor development and a cognitive measure, the Wechsler Preschool and Primary Scales of Intelligence (Wechsler, 1963). The latter has both a verbal and a performance scale. Findings from this study indicated that for this sample, scores on the BSID at 4 months did not relate to 4½-year-old motor and cognitive performance. As expected, however, the BSID motor scale scores at 12 months related significantly to the measure of gross motor performance when the BSID was administered at 4½ years. The BSID mental scale score at 12 months related significantly to both the measure of gross motor performance and the measure of cognitive performance at 4½ years. When administered at 24 months, the BSID mental scale score related significantly to later cognitive performance and the BSID motor scale score related significantly to later motor performance.

The information obtained on the BSID is important for occupational therapists involved in developmental assessment of infants and toddlers identified as high risk for biologic problems because it provides them with information about the validity of this commonly used test. It warns them to be cautious about predicting future performance of a 4½-month infant on the basis of scores on the BSID. It also warns them to be cautious about interpreting BSID mental scale scores of 12-month-old infants as cognitive measures because these scores relate to both cognitive and motor outcome measures. Therefore, it is possible that a child who is motor-impaired may be falsely identified as "cognitively impaired" on the BSID mental scale, when in fact the child's score may reflect a motor deficit.

The study by Crowe et al. (1987) has added to the understanding of the relation between BSID scores at three stages of infancy and later preschool performance. It exemplifies the types of questions answered by correlational research and the way such research can contribute to quality clinical practice.

For additional examples of correlational research, refer to journal articles by Edwards et al. (1991) on the contributions of constructional apraxia to functional loss in Alzheimer's disease; by Larson (1990) on activity patterns and life changes in persons with depression; and by Walker and Burris (1991) on the correlation of scores of normal children on the Sensory Integration and Praxis Tests (Ayres, 1989) and the scores of the same children on the Metropolitan Achievement Tests (Prescott et al., 1978).

Experimental research

Experimental research is used to establish cause-and-effect relationships among variables. With this type of research, the question is generally one of comparison:

For a particular group of subjects—Is treatment A better than treatment B relative to a specifically desired outcome?
For a particular group of subjects—Is treatment A better than no treatment relative to a specifically desired outcome?

Experimental research is interpreted in terms of probability. For example, the answer to a research question regarding whether treatment A or treatment B is more effective relative to a desired outcome may be that the chances are 5 in 100 of being wrong in saying that treatment B is better than treatment A. In other words, it might be stated that the results were significant at the 0.05 level, a commonly selected minimum standard.

Experimental research designs can be divided into true experimental designs, pre-experimental designs, and quasi-experimental designs (Campbell & Stanley, 1963). All are discussed and evaluated in terms of a series of factors that can jeopardize their internal or external validity. Internal validity (see definition earlier in chapter) is the "basic minimum without which any experiment is uninterpretable" (Campbell & Stanley, 1963, p. 5).

Consider a study designed to address the question regarding whether treatment A is better than treatment B. If that study has good internal validity and the results are significant in favor of treatment A, the researcher can say that treatment A was better than treatment B for the group of persons studied. If the study does not have good internal validity, the researcher cannot say that treatment A is better than treatment B, even if the results are significant in favor of treatment A.

Internal validity is a prerequisite for good external validity, but it does not ensure external validity (see definitions). To have good external validity, the results of the study must be generalizable to other situations. Although good external validity is desirable, external validation is usually possible only to a limited extent.

A critical concept to the discussion of experimental research is **control**. Experimental research involves the manipulation of the independent variable (treatment); the control or holding constant of all other variables; and the observation of the effect of the manipulation of the independent variable on the dependent variable (Cox & West, 1982). According to Cox and West (1982), control

> . . . refers to the attempt by the researcher to rule out the effects of any variables, other than the independent variable, on the dependent variable so that statements about the relationship between the independent and dependent variables will be accurate. (p. 34)

The concept of control relates directly to the validity of the study; it relates to the extent to which the therapist can have confidence in the results of the research. The following are examples of how control can be incorporated into the design of a research study. All examples relate to the internal validity of the described study. Imagine a study with two groups—an experimental group and a control group. An *experimental group* is the group that experiences the treatment (independent variable). The *control group* is a group of subjects "whose selection and experiences are identical in every way possible to the treatment or experimental group except that they do not receive the treatment" (Tuckman, 1978, p. 94). In the hypothetical study, the experimental group receives a treatment specifically designed to improve grip strength and the control group receives no treatment. To help rule out the possibility that the subjects in one group at the beginning of the study are stronger, the researcher could partially control for this threat to validity by randomly assigning subjects to the two groups. The validity of the same study also can be threatened by differences between data collectors.

For example, if two data collectors were administering grip strength measures for all subjects before the onset of treatment (pretest) and at the completion of the study (posttest), one data collector might be naturally more encouraging and the subjects that this data collector tests might perform better. This variable can be partially controlled by standardizing the interactions between the data collectors and the subjects and checking for procedural agreement. This standardization involves checking to see that the data collectors follow the same preset plan for data collection. This variable also can be controlled by counterbalancing the study so that each data collector tests 50% of the subjects in the control group and 50% of the subjects in the experimental group for both the pretest and the posttest.

A shorthand code is used for displaying research designs (Campbell & Stanley, 1963; Tuckman, 1978). According to this code, *X* designates a treatment; a *blank space* designates the absence of treatment; *O* designates an observation (a pretest or a posttest); *R* indicates random assignment; and a *dashed line* (- - -) indicates that intact groups have been used. Tuckman (1978) uses *R* to indicate either randomization or other techniques used to control factors other than the independent variable that could make an impact on the outcome of the study. This shorthand code was used in the following example.

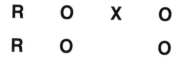

According to the design depicted, subjects were randomly divided into two groups. The first group experienced a pretest, a treatment, and a posttest; the second group experienced a pretest and a posttest and no treatment.

True experimental designs

With true experimental designs, it is possible to control for threats to internal validity. Two of the most common designs in this category that are appropriate for use in occupational therapy are the pretest–posttest control group design and the posttest–only control group design. The former was previously depicted. According to this design the subjects are randomly divided into two groups—a control group receiving no treatment and an experimental group receiving the treatment to be studied. Subjects in both groups are pretested before the institution of the treatment and are posttested after completion of the treatment. This study successfully controls for such threats to internal validity as history, maturation, and instrumentation.

History refers to events that occur between the first and the second measurement in addition to the experimental variable. In this case both groups should have similar histories because the subjects are randomly assigned. *Maturation* refers to processes within subjects that operate as a function of time, such as getting tired or hungry, growing older, or changing as a result of a disease process. For example, if the sample for the grip strength study included persons who had had cerebrovascular accidents resulting in hemiparesis, their grip strength scores might improve with the passage of time because of the normal course of recovery. If the researcher had only one group, the researcher, measuring the change in scores, might attribute that change to his or her treatment. *Instrumentation* refers to changes in the observers or scorers or changes in the calibration of the testing instruments. For example, in the grip strength study, the calibration of the dynamometer may change with use and it may become easier to obtain higher grip strength scores. Since this is true for both groups with a pretest–posttest control group design, it doesn't lead to the false conclusion that the subjects have improved because of the treatment, since the improvement would be observed in both the treatment and the control groups.

The second design, the posttest-only control group design, is depicted below.

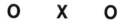

This design is exemplified in a study entitled "Added-Purpose Versus Rote Exercise in Female Nursing Home Residents" (Yoder et al., 1989). The authors of this study hypothesized that "the subjects engaged in the added-purpose, occupationally embedded exercise would engage in more exercise repetitions than would the subjects engaged in rote exercise" (p. 584). Thirty women residents in two nursing homes who met predetermined criteria on the Parachek Geriatric Rating Scale were randomly divided into two groups—a rote-exercise group and an added-purpose group. Therefore, 15 women were in each group. The rote-exercise group participated in an occupation designed to elicit rotary arm exercise; the added-purpose group participated in the same occupation except that they had the added-purpose of stirring cookie dough. The tested hypothesis was that "the subjects engaged in the added-purpose, occupationally embedded exercise would engage in more exercise repetitions than would the subjects engaged in the rote exercise" (Yoder, et al., 1989, p. 584).

This hypothesis was tested using inferential statistics and the results were significant ($P < 0.05$). The design of this study was strong with respect to threats to internal validity, but was not as strong relative to external validity because the subjects were drawn from only two nursing homes and only two examiners were used. This limits the generalizability of the results. When the results of this study are combined with those from similar studies, however, the external validity is improved and together they provide "support for the traditional occupational therapy idea of embedding exercise within occupation" (Yoder et al., 1989, p. 581).

Pre-experimental designs

Pre-experimental designs contain some elements of experimental designs, but they typically do not provide adequate control for threats to internal validity. Two of the more common pre-experimental designs seen in occupational therapy literature are the one-group pretest–posttest design and the intact-group comparison. The one-group pretest–posttest design is depicted as follows.

O   X   O

With this design, a group of subjects are administered a pretest followed by a treatment, then followed by a posttest. The treatment is considered to be effective if there is a significant difference between pretest and posttest scores. This design is exemplified in a study by Shillam et al. (1983) on the effect of occupational therapy intervention on bathing independence of persons with disabilities. The example for this study consisted of nineteen patients being treated in an inpatient rehabilitation facility. The pretest–posttest measure was the bathing section of the Klein-Bell Activities of Daily Living Scale. The treatment was specific to the person and involved bathing training, including provision and training in the use of adaptive equipment. Results of the study indicated that all subjects performed better on the posttest than on the pretest and as a group, mean scores were significantly higher ($P < 0.01$) on the posttest than on the pretest.

A one-group pretest–posttest design such as that used in the study by Shillam et al. (1983) is subject to threats to internal validity. For example, it is possible that something other than the treatment caused the change in scores from pretest to posttest, such as the subjects' experiencing spontaneous recovery between the pretest and posttest period. This was unlikely in this study, however, because patients with changing pathology were not included and because all patients were reported to have stable medical conditions. Nevertheless the study design did not rule out the potential effects of other concurrent therapies on the bathing skills of the subjects; therefore, caution is indicated in interpreting the results. This design was chosen by the authors because of ethical and practical concerns related to the withholding of treatment from a no-treatment control group.

The second pre-experimental design is the intact-group comparison depicted as follows.

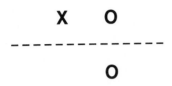

This design includes an experimental group and a control group, but subjects in the two groups are not selected or assigned randomly. For example, the subjects in one group might be all the patients in one rehabilitation facility and the subjects in the other group might be all the patients in another rehabilitation facility. With this design, one group experiences a treatment, after which both groups are tested. The posttest scores of the two groups are compared in an effort to ascertain whether the treatment was effective. This design is subject to threats to validity because steps are not taken to ensure comparability of the two groups. It is possible that differences in the outcome are related to inherent differences in the two different subject groups. Also, differences in outcome may be related to differences in the staff in the two facilities rather than to a specific treatment that is used. Therefore, findings from such studies should be viewed cautiously.

Quasi-experimental designs

Quasi-experimental designs typically are better than pre-experimental designs because they control for some but not all sources of internal invalidity. Two of the more common designs are the time–series design and the nonequivalent control group design. The former is depicted as follows.

O   O   O   X   O   O   O

The time–series design differs from the one-group pre-test–posttest design in that a series of pretests are given before the treatment is instituted. The treatment is then followed by a series of posttests. Effectiveness of the treatment is demonstrated if the change between the last test before the treatment and the first test after the treatment is significantly greater than the change between any of the adjacent pretests or posttests.

The nonequivalent control group design is similar to and an improvement over the intact-group comparison because a pretest is added for both groups. This makes it possible to compare the two groups on the dependent variable before implementing the treatment. Ideally, at the time of pretesting, the two groups should be very similar relative to this variable. Then, if posttest differences are revealed, the researcher can have more confidence that the posttest differences were not reflective of initial differences in the dependent variable between the two groups. The nonequivalent control group design is depicted as follows.

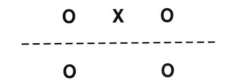

For additional examples of experimental research, refer to studies by Carlton (1987) on the effects of body mechanics instruction on work performance and by Sents and Marks (1989) on the effect of positioning on preschool children's I.Q. scores.

Quantitative single system research

Single system research, sometimes referred to as single subject research, differs from quantitative group research in that the focus is on a single person or system. The unit of study may be one person or a group that is considered collectively. With this type of research the subject serves as his or her own control and measurements of the same dependent variable or variables are repeated over time. Also, while other factors are held constant, there is the systematic application, withdrawal, and sometimes variation of the treatment (independent variable). Quantitative single system research methods are suggested for use in occupational therapy for several reasons. First, groups of subjects with similar disabilities and characteristics are not required. Therefore, single system research is applicable in the clinical setting, where often the therapist has one or, at most, a few clients with whom a particular treatment is used.

Using group research methods, the effects of the specific treatment on numerous clients from numerous settings would have to be evaluated to address a question regarding the merits of the treatment. By contrast, with single system research the effects of a specific treatment can be evaluated in a systematic way by studying one subject in a single setting. Hence, quantitative single system methods are highly appealing for answering specific questions in the clinical setting related to the effectiveness of treatment, especially for subjects with less common diagnoses and disabilities.

The second reason why single system research is recommended is that this type of experimental research does not require the withholding of treatment from a no-treatment control group. Because each subject serves as his or her own control, the treatment typically is withheld from the subject for one or more periods of time and then instituted or reinstituted. The third reason for recommending this type of research is that the financial and time demands are realistic for the clinical setting since data are maintained on only one or a small number of subjects. Also, because of the moderate financial and time demands, this research method is appropriate for pilot studies conducted before more costly group experimental studies involving numerous subjects and multiple sites.

Single system research to answer a clinical question

Example

An occupational therapist worked in a residential facility with adults with cerebral palsy who were dependent on outside help for eating (Einset et al., 1989). In this setting the people were fed by staff members. Because of cost factors and a desire to increase self-sufficiency, the use of feeding devices to help these people eat was explored. Based on her clinical experience with this client group, the therapist identified a specific feeder that she believed would be useful for her clients. She obtained two of these devices. Before recommending the purchase of more feeders, however, the therapist was interested in determining the extent to which these mechanical feeders were effective in relation to three dependent measures: (1) the amount of time needed to eat a meal; (2) the amount of staff time necessary for feeding a person who was physically dependent; and (3) the percentage of food ingested per meal by the client. She also was interested in determining her clients' impressions of the usefulness of the feeder.

Together with others (three faculty members with expertise in the areas of cerebral palsy, measurement, and single subject research), this occupational therapist designed a study to answer her questions. Next, she identified four subjects, all of whom (1) had a diagnosis of athetoid cerebral palsy; (2) were being fed by staff; (3) had functional communication skills as determined by a speech pathologist; and (4) were able to remove food from a spoon using their lips or teeth. Data systematically were collected for each of the first three dependent measures for each of the subjects individually. Each subject experienced a series of days of being fed (baseline phase), followed by training in the use of the mechanical feeder and a series of days of using the mechanical feeder (treatment phase). Finally, this was followed by a series of days of being fed (return to baseline). Throughout all phases of data collection, efforts were made to hold all factors constant that could have influenced the results of the study. All data collection meals were eaten in the same room and the same therapist provided feeding assistance and collected data.

Data were graphed and examined for each subject individually. For an example of graphed data for one variable for one subject, refer to Figure 12-1. Results for this study indicated that use of the feeder increased the length of the meal for some subjects, decreased the amount of staff time needed for feeding

for some subjects, and decreased the percentage of food eaten by all subjects. At the end of the study, only two of the four subjects indicated that they would choose to use the feeder on a regular basis. On the basis of these results, the therapist questioned the advisability of using the feeder in her setting on a regular basis, primarily because of the decrease in percentage of food ingested by all subjects. This was of particular importance since each subject was thin and had a diagnosis of athetoid cerebral palsy. If this therapist hadn't systematically collected data in both baseline and treatment conditions, she might not have been aware of this difficulty when using the feeder.

Studies such as the one just described assist the therapist in effective decision making and, when shared through professional journals, assist others in the clinical decision-making process. For additional examples of single system research studies designed to answer clinical questions in occupational therapy, refer to studies by Case-Smith (1988) on the effects of daily occupational therapy on the nutritive and nonnutritive sucking of three high-risk infants; by Ray et al. (1983) on the effects of techniques to facilitate mouth closure on the drooling of a child with cerebral palsy; and by Ottenbacher (1982) on the effects of a program of sensory integration therapy on the duration of postrotary nystagmus in three children with learning disabilities.

Presentation of data

Typically, with single system research, data for each variable for each subject or system are graphed individually on either equal interval graph paper or the standard behavior chart (sometimes referred to as six-cycle graph paper). The primary benefit of the former is that it is easily understood. Benefits of the standard behavior chart are that behaviors with extremely high or low rates can be recorded on the chart and that the graph progresses in semilog units, thus facilitating the estimation of linear trends in the data. Carr and Williams (1982) clearly describe the rationale for and use of the standard behavior chart.

Demonstration of change

With single subject research, effectiveness of treatment is demonstrated by a change in level, trend, or variability between phases when treatment is instituted or withdrawn (Wolery & Harris, 1982; Ottenbacher & York, 1984). For potential patterns of data reflecting change and no change, refer to Figure 12-2.

Common single system designs

A simple notation system is used for single system designs, where A represents baseline; B represents the intervention or treatment phase; and C and all other letters represent additional treatments or conditions. The design on which all others are built is the *A–B design,* which can be exemplified by looking at both the first baseline phase (*A*) and the treatment phase (*B*) on Figure 12-1 for the electric feeder study. This displays the data for one subject for percentage of food ingested. The vertical axis of the graph indicates the percentage of the meal eaten and the horizontal axis indicates the days. During the first baseline phase (*A*), this subject experienced 12 days of being fed as usual and data were systematically kept on percentage of food ingested. Note that the subject consistently ingested more than 90% of the food served. On the 17th day, phase *B* (intervention) was started. The intervention consisted of use of the feeder and assistance with meal-

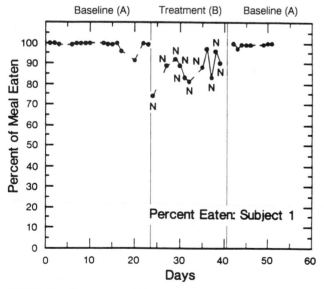

FIGURE 12-1. *Percentage of food intake for subject 1 during three phases: baseline, treatment, and baseline.* (*From Einset, K., et al. [1989]. The electric feeder: An efficacy study.* Occupational Therapy of Research, 9, *46.*)

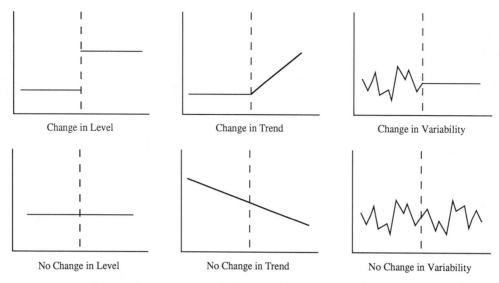

FIGURE 12-2. *Potential patterns of data reflecting change and no change.*

time tasks as needed. Note that the percentage of the meal eaten dropped substantially during the treatment phase. If the study had stopped after data were collected for only a baseline phase and an intervention phase, this would have been an *A–B* design.

A common variation of the *A–B* design is the *A–B–C* successive intervention design, in which a second treatment is introduced in the *C* phase. For example, the therapist studying the effects of the electric feeder might have chosen to introduce one feeder in the *B* phase and a totally different feeder in the *C* phase to see whether one feeder was more effective for the client than the other. Another variation of the *A–B* design is the *A–B–C* changing criterion design, in which the criterion for success changes with each successive treatment phase (Hartmann & Hall, 1976). For example, in the *B* phase, a therapist, working on scissor cutting with a child with fine motor deficits might count how many times the child goes outside 2-inch boundaries when cutting a 10-inch strip of paper. After the child achieves success with this criterion, the *C* phase would be entered, and the criterion for success would change to staying within a 1-inch boundary.

With both the *A–B* and the *A–B–C* designs, no causal statements can be made. In the electric feeder study, if data had only been collected for an initial baseline phase and a treatment phase (see Figure 12-1), the therapist wouldn't have known if some factor other than the introduction of the electric feeder resulted in the drop in percentage of food ingested. For example, the subject might have become ill on the 17th day or there might have been a change in cooks in the residential facility in which the subject was eating meals. Therefore, this design is subject to threats to internal validity.

Because of this, the *A–B–A* or *withdrawal design* was developed. This design consists of a minimum of three phases: baseline, treatment, and baseline. It is exemplified by the electric feeder study in which the feeder was removed after the treatment phase and data were again collected under baseline conditions (see Figure 12-1). Because this design involves a return to baseline, it is most appropriate for behaviors that are reversible (likely to return to the original baseline levels when intervention is withdrawn). This is a true experimental design in the sense that causal inferences can be made relative to the subject studied.

For example, in the electric feeder study, because the percentage of food ingested decreased during the intervention phase and then returned to the original baseline levels during the second baseline phase, it is possible to say that the use of the electric feeder by subject 1 is likely to have resulted in a decrease in the percentage of food ingested.

If the treatment (use of the electric feeder) resulted in a desirable change, the advisability of ending on a baseline phase would be questionable. The *A–B–A–B* design was developed for such situations in which treatments are expected to be effective. With this design the treatment is reinstated after the second baseline phase.

The next category of designs is the *multiple baseline designs*. These designs require repeated measures of at least three baseline conditions that typically are implemented concurrently, with each successive baseline being longer than the previous one. Multiple baseline designs can be (1) across behaviors, (2) across subjects, or (3) across settings.

In a multiple baseline design across behaviors, the same treatment variable is applied sequentially to separate behaviors in a single subject. Consider the hypothetical example of a child in a mental health setting who, when in the presence of other children, frequently displays three aggressive, antisocial behaviors: biting, hitting, and kicking. The therapist is interested in knowing whether or not her intervention (a 5-minute time-out) is successful in reducing or eliminating the incidence of these behaviors.

For 5 days, during a 2-hour peer socialization group the researcher collects baseline data on these aggressive behaviors in the natural situation, making no change in treatment (Figure 12-3). On the sixth day, the researcher introduces the intervention, thus starting the treatment phase (*B*) for the first behavior (biting). This involves consequating episodes of biting with a 5-minute time-out. The researcher makes no change in the treatment program for hitting and kicking. These two behaviors remain in baseline phase (*A*). After 10 days the researcher initiates the time-out treatment for hitting and, after 15 days, the same treatment for kicking. If the researcher can demonstrate a change in behavior across all three behaviors following the institution of the treatment, this provides support for the effec-

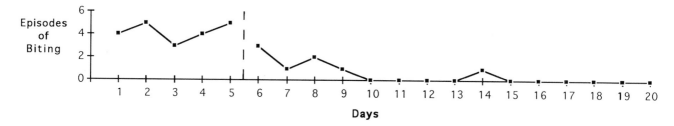

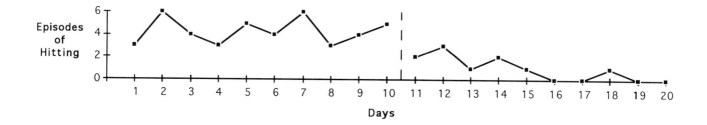

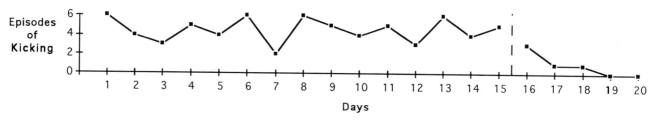

FIGURE 12-3. *Graphed data for a hypothetical study using a multiple baseline design across behaviors.*

tiveness of time-out in decreasing aggressive, antisocial behaviors in the child studied. This exemplifies a multiple baseline study across behaviors.

With a multiple baseline design across subjects, one behavior is treated sequentially across matched subjects. For example, if three subjects had limited wrist extension, you might institute treatment for the first subject on the fourth day, for the second subject on the seventh day, and for the third subject on the tenth day. Figure 12-4 displays hypothetical data for such a study.

The last type of multiple baseline design is that which is across settings. With this design the same behavior or behaviors are studied in several independent settings. Consider the client with dementia who is in a nursing home. This person repeatedly interrupts by singing inappropriately. She does this in the dining room during mealtimes, in the dayroom during movies, and on recreational outings in the van. First, the therapist collects baseline data in all three settings for 4 days. Then she tries an intervention in the dining room (the first setting) while simultaneously continuing to collect baseline data in the other two settings. After 3 more days, she introduces the intervention in the second setting (the dayroom during movies) while continuing to collect baseline data in the third setting. Last, after 2 more days, she introduces the treatment in the third setting (the van during recreational outings). For a graphic display of hypothetical data for such a study, refer to Figure 12-5.

With all these multiple baseline designs, effectiveness of treatment is demonstrated if a desired change in level, trend, or variability occurs only when treatment is introduced. In addition,

the change in performance should be maintained during the treatment phase or improvement should continue as long as treatment is maintained.

Multiple baseline designs have three major strengths. First, they require no reversal or withdrawal of intervention. This makes them appealing and practical for clinical research where continued therapy is sometimes indicated to maintain the client's performance at the optimal level; therefore, the discontinuation of therapy to collect data for a second baseline is contraindicated.

The second strength of multiple baseline designs is that they are useful when behaviors are not likely to be reversible. Typically, in occupational therapy, therapists hope that the treatment will cause a difference that will be maintained even when the treatment is withdrawn. For example, after a therapist has taught a client with a stroke to eat independently using only the nondominant hand, the therapist expects the client to be able to eat independently even when therapy is withdrawn. The therapist expects the effects of therapy to be long-lasting. This makes it difficult to use the withdrawal design discussed earlier, because traditionally with a withdrawal design, treatment effectiveness is demonstrated by having the behavior return to the original baseline level when treatment is withdrawn.

The third strength of a multiple baseline design is that results of research based on it provide some support for the demonstration of causal relationships because the therapist is showing that change can be effected in multiple situations.

The weakness of multiple baseline designs is the requirement of more data collection time because of the staggered

Subject #1

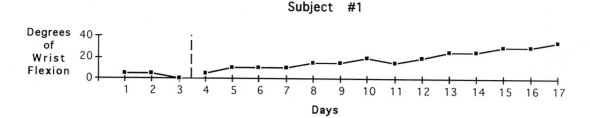

Subject #2

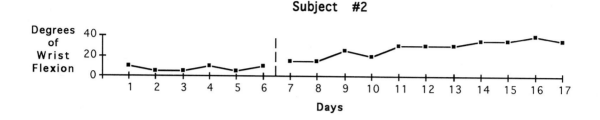

Subject #3

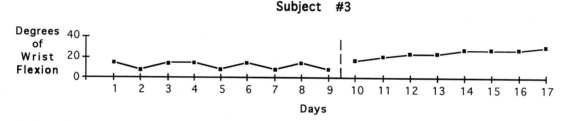

FIGURE 12-4. *Graphed data for a hypothetical study using a multiple baseline design across subjects.*

starting times for the intervention phases. Also, because of this, some behaviors or subjects are required to remain in the baseline phase for longer periods of time. Sometimes in clinical settings, these long baseline requirements can be problematic. For example, in the first hypothetical study involving a child in a mental health setting, the last behavior (kicking) was allowed to continue for 15 days before the institution of treatment. This would be contraindicated for others in the setting because of the potential for injury.

The last type of single subject design is the *alternating treatments design* (Barlow & Hayes, 1979). This design and minor variations of it have also been termed multi-element baseline designs, randomization designs, multiple schedule designs, and simultaneous treatments designs. These designs can be used to compare the effects of treatment and no treatment, or they can be used to compare the effects of two or more distinct treatments. In all cases, these designs involve the fast alternation of two or more different treatments or conditions. They usually have a baseline phase and require interventions that will produce immediate and distinct changes in behavior.

Harris and Riffle (1986) used an alternating treatments design when studying the effects of inhibitive ankle–foot orthoses on standing balance in a 4-year-old boy with cerebral palsy who was not walking independently. The researchers wanted to know whether orthoses would improve the child's ability to main-

tain two-foot standing balance. The independent variable was ankle–foot orthoses and the dependent variable was duration of two-foot independent standing. See Figure 12-6 for a graph of the data.

During the first phase of the study, baseline data on independent standing were collected for five sessions. The child did not wear ankle–foot orthoses during this phase. Phase 2 began after the subject had been wearing a new set of orthoses for 1 week. The subject's standing balance was measured both with and without orthoses during each session. The order of the two conditions (with and without orthoses) was counterbalanced by random assignment. Therefore, for three of the five sessions in phase 2, duration of standing balance was measured first with orthoses. For the other two sessions, duration of standing balance was measured first without orthoses. As depicted in the graph, the child's ability to maintain independent standing rapidly improved, thereby providing support for the use of orthoses with this child with cerebral palsy. This study exemplifies use of a single subject alternating treatments design to answer a clinical question.

The alternating treatments design has three primary strengths. First, it does not require a lengthy withdrawal of the treatment, which may result in a reversal of therapeutic gain. Second, it often requires less time for a comparison to be made because a second baseline is not required. Third, with this design

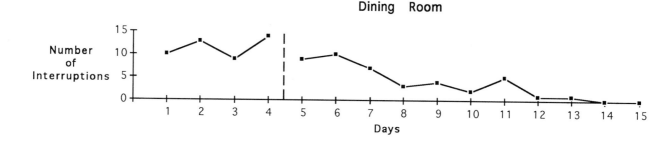

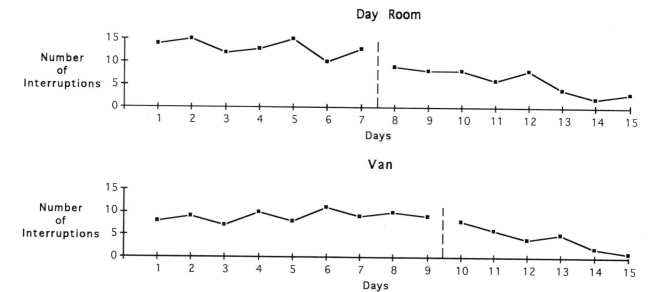

FIGURE 12-5. *Graphed data for a hypothetical study using a multiple baseline design across settings.*

it is possible to proceed without a formal baseline phase. This is useful in clinical situations in which ethically it is difficult to justify baseline data collection.

The primary weakness of the alternating treatments design stems from its vulnerability to an internal validity threat relating to the influence of one treatment on the adjacent treatment. As a partial control for this threat, all variables that could potentially influence the results of the study should be counterbalanced. For example, in the study by Harris and Riffle (1986), the conditions (with orthoses and without orthoses) for measuring duration of two-foot standing balance were counterbalanced by random assignment. Instead, if the child always had stood first without orthoses and second with orthoses, it is possible that the improved performance might be a function of the practice in the "without orthoses" condition.

For additional readings related to single subject research, refer to the Bibliography.

Qualitative research

According to Yerxa (1991), qualitative research,

> . . . is a generic term encompassing many research approaches. In general, it is descriptive, uses the natural setting as the direct source of data, is concerned with the process as well as the outcome,

analyzes data inductively (so theory is built from the ground up), and has an essential interest in meaning from the participant's perspective. (p. 200)

This type of research "seeks to understand and portray the social life of a particular group within its own physical, social, and cultural context" (Kielhofner, 1982a). For example, Krefting (1989) used a qualitative approach to study the experience of head injury from the insider's perspective. Her desire was "to uncover new variables, rather than testing existing ones" (Krefting, 1989, p. 68).

Qualitative research methods have their historical roots in anthropology, sociology, history, and political science (Miles & Huberman, 1984; Kielhofner, 1982a). These research methods, rather than starting with operational definitions, isolate and define categories during the research process. As a result they have impressive complexity-capturing capabilities and are useful for studying the content, pattern, and meaning of experiences. With qualitative research, an area of interest is identified and broad questions are asked. As data collection proceeds, the questions may change or become more focused and the research question continues to unfold (Lincoln & Guba, 1985).

Qualitative research is appropriate in a variety of situations. It is particularly useful in the exploratory stages of inquiry and also in situations in which the focus of concern is the study of

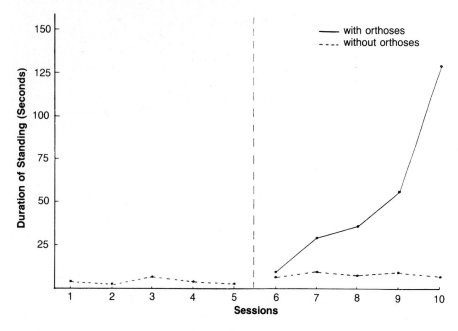

FIGURE 12-6. *Graphed data for a hypothetical study using an alternating treatments design: Duration of independent standing in seconds with and without orthoses* (*From Harris, S. R., & Riffle, K. [1986]. Effects of inhibitive ankle-foot orthoses on standing balance in a child with cerebral palsy. Physical Therapy, 66, 665.*)

persons in their environmental contexts. Largely because qualitative research is contextualized, its methods are compatible with occupational therapy's humanistic values and its focus on occupational performance (Yerxa, 1991; Kielhofner, 1982b). As Kielhofner (1982b) maintains,

> There is a special harmony between the concerns of occupational therapy and the paradigm and methods of qualitative research. Both focus on the realities of everyday life. Both appreciate the richness of mundane affairs. (p. 162)

Data collection and analysis

With qualitative research the data typically are extensive and in the form of words rather than numbers. Such data are a source of "well-grounded, rich descriptions and explanations of processes occurring in local contexts" (Miles & Huberman, 1984, p. 15).

The data collection process for qualitative research is more loosely structured, inductively grounded, and emergent than that used for quantitative research. This process is labor-intensive and may last for months or years. Data are collected using observation, interviews, extracts from documents, and tape recordings. For example, Krefting (1989), in her study of persons with moderate head injuries, used four approaches in an attempt to "experience life" from the perspective of a person with a head injury (p. 69). The first approach involved over 80 hours of nonstructured interviews with persons with head injuries, their families, and their friends. Each interview ranged from 1 to 4 hours. The second approach involved participant observations and the recording of the researcher's own actions, the behavior of others, and aspects of the the sociocultural situation. To do this, the researcher attended meetings, social events, and treatment sessions, and accompanied the persons with head injuries and their families on a variety of outings. The third approach was to review documents such as a diary that had been kept by a person with a head injury, human interest stories from newspapers, and newsletters from organizations concerned with head injury. The last approach involved maintaining a field log in which Krefting noted her thoughts, feelings, ideas, and hypoth-

eses generated by her contact with persons with head injuries and their families and friends.

With qualitative research, data from sources such as interviews and participant observations are organized into extended texts, the most common form of which is narrative text. For example, the data from Krefting's study (1989) were transcribed into almost 1000 pages of text. Special techniques are used for reducing the data and for sorting and organizing it to identify themes and patterns. In contrast to most quantitative methods, the methods used in a qualitative study can be changed in response to emergent findings.

Research design

Qualitative research designs range from being loose and emergent to relatively prestructured. The former is exemplified by the work of Goodall, who immersed herself over a period of years in the environment of chimpanzees in Tanzania, even going so far as imitating some of their behaviors and sampling their foods (Moritz, 1967). The relatively prestructured research design is exemplified by the long interview method, which is a "sharply focused, rapid, highly intensive interview process," calling for "special kinds of preparation and structure, including the use of an open-ended questionnaire" (McCracken, 1988, p. 7). In reality, most of the qualitative research currently being done falls between the two extremes (Miles & Huberman, 1984).

Numerous factors merit consideration when a researcher chooses the extent to which a qualitative research design should be structured. Some of these are the extent of knowledge related to the phenomena of concern, the amount of time available for the research, the type of analysis to be used, the instruments available (Miles & Huberman, 1984), and the extent to which privacy of subjects is an issue. For example, because of privacy issues, a researcher might choose a more prestructured and less time-consuming approach to studying the meaning of having a child with a disability in the home. It is understandable that families may not be open to having a researcher be included within their family routines over a long period of time (similar to the approach taken by Goodall when she studied chimpanzees in Tanzania).

Selection of subjects

Samples for qualitative research studies tend to be small. The emphasis is on working longer and with more depth with a few subjects. The selection of subjects is determined by a desire to gain access to cultural categories. For example, the sample for Hinojosa and Anderson's (1991) study regarding mothers' perceptions of home treatment programs for their preschool children with cerebral palsy consisted of eight mothers of preschool children with cerebral palsy who had experienced a home program for their children. These mothers varied in ethnicity and economic level.

Investigator

In qualitative research, the investigator assumes the role of participant-observer. In addition, the researcher initiates and monitors methods for and quality control of data collection and documents methods used in collecting, analyzing, and interpreting data (Kielhofner, 1982a).

Rigor in qualitative research

With qualitative research, as with other methods, rigor and the related issues of validity and reliability are important (Kielhofner, 1982a). These relate to the credibility and dependability of the findings. According to Kielhofner (1982a), the issue of validity centers on taking observations of social actions and the underlying common sense structures and transforming these into theoretical constructs that are accurate reflections of everyday life, including the related meanings and organizational structures.

Numerous approaches have been advocated to help ensure the credibility or internal validity of findings. One approach relates to the researcher's effectiveness in developing the participant-observer role such that he or she has access to the "everyday meanings, rationales, and actions employed by subjects" (Kielhofner, 1982a, p. 73). Prolonged engagement allows the informants to become accustomed to the investigator and for the investigator to develop rapport with the informants. If this is not achieved, validity is compromised because the investigator may not have access to aspects of the social system known only to the participants. Therefore, the researcher may have a restricted view of reality for that social group. This involvement, although increasing the validity of the study, may also be a source of invalidity. An investigator may become overinvolved and lose the ability to interpret findings. In other words, there are two primary threats to validity related to the participant-observer role.

First, the researcher may have an effect on the site; conversely, the site may have an effect on the researcher. Miles and Huberman (1984) provide suggestions for countering such bias. Relative to countering researcher effects on the site, suggestions include using unobtrusive measures; having an informant at the site attend to and comment on the researcher's influence on the site and the people involved; and doing some interviewing off-site. Relative to countering the effects of the site on the researcher, suggestions include spreading out site visits and spending some time away from the site; concentrating on conceptual

thinking such that personal feelings are translated into theoretical thoughts; and using ***triangulation***. The latter involves gathering data from more than one source (persons with head injuries, their parents, and documents), using more than one method (interview and participant/observation), and using different researchers. Ideally, information from all sources should agree with and not contradict the emerging theory. This information should converge and be mutually supportive, and should provide a more complete view of the subject of study.

If the investigator intends to make generalizations based on his or her qualitative research study, then strategies are needed to enhance transferability (Krefting, 1991). Also, the investigator has the responsibility to provide rich descriptive information about the people or groups that he or she is studying. The research consumer is then better able to evaluate the extent to which those studied are comparable to the people or groups with whom the consumer is concerned. In many cases, such comparisons are inappropriate because the group studied is unique.

Dependability, or reliability, of findings from a qualitative research study also is of concern. Triangulation is one method that has been used to enhance the dependability of findings (Miles & Huberman, 1984). For example, two researchers may take parallel information at the same time. This makes it possible to double-check findings to make sure that there is agreement. Another method is to divide the data in half and have two separate research teams deal separately with the two halves.

Achieving rigor in qualitative research is a complex and time-consuming process. The above information provides examples of strategies for ensuring the trustworthiness of qualitative research only. More detailed information can be found in the work of Miles and Huberman (1984), Krefting (1991), and Lincoln and Guba (1985).

Example of a qualitative research study

Niehues et al. (1991) conducted a comparatively small qualitative study to explore the "nature of occupational therapy practice in public schools" (p. 195). Five expert school system practitioners were interviewed using an open-ended, in-depth format. All were asked to "narrate a situation from their practice when they felt their interventions had made significant differences for students and in students' abilities to learn in school" (Niehues et al., 1991, p. 195). These interviews were conducted by the principal investigator and lasted from 1 to 2 hours. All interviews were audiotaped and transcribed in their entirety. Data were analyzed for thematic content in a three-stage process.

First, the narratives from each interview were analyzed individually for the purpose of identifying the central themes of each. Second, the narratives were "compared with one another, successively, until basic commonalities and discrepancies across all five narratives were identified and categorized" (Niehues et al., 1991, p. 200). Last, the data were interpreted in light of the theoretical perspectives identified in relevant literature and the practical perspectives of the researchers, which were developed during their practice in public school systems. The results were presented as themes.

For example, the first theme dealt with the therapist helping other team members change their view of a student, which in turn enabled the other team members "to develop more effective strategies for teaching or parenting the student" (Niehues et al., 1991, p. 201). The researchers titled this theme "reframing." They discussed it in depth, sharing parts of therapists' practice stories, including direct quotations from some of the therapists. In addition, two other themes were identified and discussed. This study expanded understanding of occupational therapy practice in school settings.

Strengths and weaknesses of quantitative and qualitative research

The possibility of getting a distorted view of reality exists with both quantitative and qualitative research. The primary benefits of quantitative research are that (1) it is possible to obtain precise, objective information about subjects; (2) it is possible with group designs to obtain extensive information about numerous subjects in a parsimonious manner; and (3) it is possible to control for factors that could jeopardize either the internal or the external validity of a study. If well designed and well conducted, quantitative research is objective and reproducible. Also, because decisions regarding the design of the study (the operational definitions of independent and dependent variables, the methods by which data will be collected, the ways in which reliability in data collection will be ensured) are made a priori, the effect of researcher or examiner bias on the results of the study is minimized.

According to Philips and Pierson (1982), qualitative methods are vulnerable to factors that influence objectivity, especially as related to the investigator's assuming two roles, participant and observer. They express concern about the "relative lack of scientific rigor" in qualitative research "to protect against the undue influence of the researcher's beliefs on the findings" (Philips & Pierson, 1982, p. 167). However, authors such as Miles and Huberman (1984), Lincoln and Guba (1985), and Krefting (1991) offer methods for evaluating the trustworthiness of qualitative research.

The primary strengths of qualitative research stem from its groundedness in everyday life and its complexity-capturing capabilities. Consequently, qualitative research is a valuable approach relative to the identification of emerging theory. It is appropriate for the study of the gestalt and of complex relationships and meanings. On the other hand, quantitative research has been criticized because of its potential for oversimplifying findings and distorting reality when data are reduced to graphs and statistics. Also, experimental research designs have been criticized because their need to control all variables except the independent variable can result in the creation of an artificial situation that doesn't relate to typical life situations.

Qualitative and quantitative research: Joint contributors to the knowledge base in occupational therapy

Studies using qualitative research methods and studies using quantitative research methods have contributed to the knowledge base of occupational therapy. Both are suited to answering important questions and to expanding knowledge related to occupational performance and the components of function. Sometimes one method is more suited to a particular question than another. When the answer to a question requires precision, quantitative methods are preferred; when the answer to a question involves capturing the complexity in a situation, qualitative methods are preferred. At other times, the question can be answered using either quantitative or qualitative methods. In such cases, research with one method can be used to confirm or expand on the findings demonstrated by the other method.

Consider the situation in which the desire is to understand more about children's mobility when using power mobility devices as opposed to manual wheelchairs. Using qualitative methods, a researcher observes four children, all of whom use power mobility devices. The researcher unobtrusively observes these children in the home and school environments. After weeks of intensive observation, followed by transcription of notes, and so on, the researcher identifies several themes. One theme relates to distances traveled. The researcher notes that the children in the power mobility devices move continuously on the playground, offer to go on errands, and frequently move around the classroom. Are these children exceptionally outgoing and not typical of most children who use power mobility devices? Is this reality only for these four children, or is it a general theme related to the use of power mobility devices?

From this research, a hypothesis may be generated, which may be confirmed by further investigation with quantitative methods. Such a study might be designed and conducted using 30 children with motor impairments requiring the use of wheelchairs. All would be capable of using either manual chairs or power mobility devices. For 1 week, 50% of the subjects would use a power mobility device and 50% would use a manual chair. The following week the conditions would be reversed. All chairs would be equipped with odometers so that distances traveled could be measured objectively. The distances traveled by all children when using manual chairs would be compared with the distances traveled by the same group when using power mobility devices. Imagine that the findings were significant in favor of greater distances traveled by the children when using the power mobility devices. These findings would complement those from the qualitative study and improve the generalizability of the findings related to distances traveled. Conversely, the findings from the qualitative study would add depth to the quantitative study and provide insight into what "increased distances traveled" might mean to the child in his or her school environment. Thus, findings from qualitative and quantitative research can be complementary.

The issue is not whether one type of research is better than the other; the issue is how to use the two types of research to complement one another for the benefit of knowledge development in occupational therapy. These two types of research cannot be substituted for one another because they facilitate the observation of different aspects of the same reality. This is highlighted by McCracken (1988), who contends that qualitative research offers the opportunity to glimpse the complicated character, organization, and logic of culture, and that the extent to which what is discovered exists in the rest of the world can best be decided by quantitative methods.

Research ethics

Important considerations when designing and conducting both quantitative and qualitative research are ethics as they relate to the researcher and the research process. The researcher has the responsibility to adhere to high scientific standards in designing and conducting research studies and in analyzing and reporting research findings. Scientific misconduct includes such acts as fabrication, falsification, and plagiarism. In addition, ethical implications are related to the researcher's decisions and actions concerning the rights of subjects. Researchers need to check with the human subjects' review boards in all the institutions in which subjects will be approached. They need to consider whether participation in the study could be contraindicated for the subject. This consideration should focus not only on physical issues, but also on issues related to such factors as stress and invasion of privacy. Subjects or subject advocates must give informed consent before participation in a study, and they must be informed of their right to withdraw from participation at any point while still maintaining the services to which they are otherwise entitled.

Research skills of occupational therapists

All occupational therapists have the responsibility to become knowledgeable consumers of research so that they can evaluate the research literature relevant to their practice arenas. It is the professional responsibility of therapists to be able to read, understand, and critically review the research literature in journal articles, newsletters, and test manuals. To do this, therapists must have a basic understanding of statistics and the different types of research, including their respective strengths and weaknesses.

Most professional journals in occupational therapy have a peer review process whereby each manuscript is reviewed and critiqued by a minimum of two or three colleagues with expertise in the area of the research before the manuscript is accepted for publication. Even so, there is great variability in the quality of the articles published. Thus, the last step in the review process is that taken by the informed consumer.

Some therapists extend beyond the role of research consumer to that of researcher. Such therapists may contribute through formulation of research questions, systematic data collection, or the design, implementation, and dissemination of research studies. Often research is the product of many persons (clinicians and academicians) working collaboratively using a systematic process to find answers to questions of mutual concern.

References

Ayres, A. J. (1989). *Sensory integration and praxis tests manual.* Los Angeles: Western Psychological Services.

Barlow, D. H., & Hayes, S. C. (1979). Alternating treatments design: One strategy for comparing the effects of two treatments in a single subject. *Journal of Applied Behavior Analysis, 12,* 199–210.

Bayley, N. (1969). *Manual for the Bayley Scales of Infant Development.* New York: Psychological Corp.

Billingsley, F. F., White, O. R., & Munson, R. (1980). Procedural reliability: A rationale and an example. *Behavioral Assessment, 2,* 229–241.

Bouska, M. J., & Kwatny, E. (1983). *Manual for application of the Motor-Free Visual Perception Test to the adult population.* Philadelphia: P.O. Box 12246.

Campbell, D., & Stanley, J. C. (1963). *Experimental and quasiexperimental designs for research.* Chicago: Rand McNally.

Carlton, R. S. (1987). The effects of body mechanics instruction on work performance. *American Journal of Occupational Therapy, 41,* 16–20.

Carr, B. S., & Williams, M. (1982). Analysis of therapeutic techniques through use of the standard behavior chart. *Physical Therapy, 52,* 177–183.

Case-Smith, J. (1988). An efficacy study of occupational therapy with high-risk neonates. *American Journal of Occupational Therapy, 42,* 499–506.

Cox, R. C., & West, W. L. (1982). *Fundamentals of research for the health professional.* Laurel, MD: RAMSCO Publishing Company.

Crowe, T. K., Deitz, J. C., & Bennett, F. C. (1987). The relationship between Bayley Scales of Infant Development and preschool gross motor and cognitive performance. *American Journal of Occupational Therapy, 41,* 374–378.

Crowe, T. K., & Kanny, E. (1990). Occupational therapy practice in school systems: A survey of northwest therapists. *Physical and Occupational Therapy in Pediatrics, 10,* 69–83.

Edwards, D. F., Baum, C. M., & Deuel, R. K. (1991). Constructional apraxia in Alzheimer's disease: Contributions to functional loss. *Physical and Occupational Therapy in Geriatrics, 9*(3/4), 53–68.

Einset, K., Deitz, J., Billingsley, F., & Harris, S. (1989). The electric feeder: An efficacy study. *Occupational Therapy Journal of Research, 9,* 38–52.

Gilfoyle, E., & Christiansen, C. (1987). Research: The quest for truth and the key to excellence. *American Journal of Occupational Therapy, 41,* 7–8.

Harris, S. R., & Riffle K. (1986). Effects of inhibitive ankle-foot orthoses on standing balance in a child with cerebral palsy. *Physical Therapy, 66,* 643–667.

Hartmann, D. P., & Hall, R. V. (1976). The changing criterion design. *Journal of Applied Behavior Analysis, 9,* 527–532.

Hinojosa, J., & Anderson, J. (1991). Mothers' perceptions of home treatment programs for their preschool children with cerebral palsy. *American Journal of Occupational Therapy, 45,* 273–279.

Holcomb, J. D., Christiansen, C. H., & Roush, R. E. (1989). The scholarly productivity of occupational therapy faculty members: Results of a regional study. *American Journal of Occupational Therapy, 43,* 37–43.

Kanny, E., Anson, D., & Smith, R. O. (1991). A survey of technology education in entry-level curricula: Quantity, quality, and barriers. *Occupational Therapy Journal of Research, 11,* 311–319.

Kielhofner, G. (1982a). Qualitative research: Part one—paradigmatic grounds and issues of reliability and validity. *Occupational Therapy Journal of Research, 2,* 67–79.

Kielhofner, G. (1982b). Qualitative research: Part two—methodological approaches and relevance to occupational therapy. *Occupational Therapy Journal of Research, 2,* 150–164.

Krefting, L. (1989). Reintegration into the community after head injury: The results of an ethnographic study. *Occupational Therapy Journal of Research, 9,* 67–83.

Krefting, L. (1991). Rigor in qualitative research: The assessment of trustworthiness. *American Journal of Occupational Therapy, 45,* 214–222.

Larson, K. B. (1990). Activity patterns and life changes in people with depression. *American Journal of Occupational Therapy, 44,* 902–906.

Lincoln, Y., & Guba, E. (1985). *Naturalistic inquiry.* Beverly Hills, CA: Sage Publications.

Mathiowetz, V., Wiemer, D., & Federman, S. M. (1986). Grip and pinch strength: Norms for 6- to 19-year olds. *American Journal of Occupational Therapy, 40,* 705–711.

McCracken, G. (1988). *The long interview* (Qualitative Research Methods Series, Vol. 13). Newbury Park, CA: SAGE Publications.

Miles, M. B., & Huberman, A. M. (1984). *Qualitative data analysis: A sourcebook of new methods.* Newbury Park, CA: Sage Publications.

Miller, L. J. (1982). *Miller assessment for preschoolers.* Littleton, CO: The Foundation for Knowledge in Development.

Moritz, C. (Ed.). (1967). *Current biography yearbook.* New York: H. W. Wilson Company.

Niehues, A. N., Bundy, A. C., Mattingly, C. F., & Lawlor, M. C. (1991). Making a difference: Occupational therapy in the public school. *American Journal of Occupational Therapy, 11,* 195–211.

Ottenbacher, K. (1982). Patterns of postrotary nystagmus in three learning-disabled children. *American Journal of Occupational Therapy, 36*, 657–663.

Ottenbacher, K., & York, J. (1984). Strategies for evaluating clinical change: Implications for practice and research. *American Journal of Occupational Therapy, 38*, 647–659.

Payton, O. (1988). *Research: The validation of clinical practice.* Philadelphia: F. A. Davis.

Philips, B. U., & Pierson, W. P. (1982). Commentary: Qualitative research in occupational therapy. *Occupational Therapy Journal of Research, 2*, 165–170.

Prescott, G. A., Balow, I. H., Hogan, T. P., & Farr, R. C. (1978). *Metropolitan Achievement Tests.* New York: Psychological Corporation.

Ray, S., Bundy, A., & Nelson, D. (1983). Decreasing drooling through techniques to facilitate mouth closure. *American Journal of Occupational Therapy, 37*, 749–753.

Sents, B. E., & Marks, H. E. (1989). Changes in preschool children's IQ scores as a function of positioning. *American Journal of Occupational Therapy, 43*, 685–687.

Shillam, L. L., Beeman, C., & Loshin, P. M. (1983). Effect of occupational therapy intervention on bathing independence of disabled persons. *American Journal of Occupational Therapy, 37*, 744–748.

Stone, R. G., & Mertens, K. B. (1991). Educating entry-level occupational therapy students in gerontology. *American Journal of Occupational Therapy, 45*, 643–650.

Tuckman, B. (1978). *Conducting educational research.* New York: Harcourt Brace Jovanovich.

Walker, K. F., & Burris, B. (1991). Correlation of Sensory Integration and Praxis Test scores with Metropolitan Achievement Test scores in normal children. *Occupational Therapy Journal of Research, 11*, 307–310.

Wechsler, D. (1963). *Manual for the Wechsler preschool and primary scale of intelligence.* New York: Psychological Corporation.

Wolery, M., & Harris, S. (1982). Interpreting results of single-subject research designs. *Physical Therapy, 62*, 445–452.

Yerxa, E. J. (1991). Seeking a relevant, ethical, and realistic way of knowing for occupational therapy. *American Journal of Occupational Therapy, 45*, 199–204.

Yoder, R. M., Nelson, D. L., & Smith, D. A. (1989). Added-purpose versus rote exercise in female nursing home residents. *American Journal of Occupational Therapy, 43*, 581–586.

Bibliography

Babbie, E. R. (1973). *Survey research methods.* Belmont, CA: Wadsworth.

Barlow, D. H., & Hersen, M. (1984). *Single case experimental designs: Strategies for studying behavior change* (2nd ed.). New York: Pergamon Press.

Bogdan, R., & Taylor, S. (1984). *Introduction to qualitative research methods.* New York: John Wiley & Sons.

Campbell, P. H. (1988). Using a single-subject research design to evaluate the effectiveness of treatment. *American Journal of Occupational Therapy, 44*, 732–738.

Dillman, D. A. (1978). *Mail and telephone surveys: The total design method.* New York: John Wiley & Sons.

Elzey, F. F. (1974). *A first reader in statistics.* Belmont, CA: Wadsworth.

Kazdin, A. E. (1982). *Single-case research designs: Methods for clinical and applied settings.* New York: Oxford University Press.

Ottenbacher, K. (1986). *Evaluating clinical change: Strategies for occupational and physical therapists.* Baltimore: Williams & Wilkins.

## PART II

Practice issues: Occupational therapy intervention across the life span

Implementation of occupational therapy in pediatrics

CHAPTER 13

Developmental disabilities

SECTION 1

Mental retardation

RUTH HUMPHRY and KAAREN JEWELL

LEARNING OBJECTIVES

Upon completion of this section the reader will be able to:

1. *Define mental retardation and describe how it is diagnosed.*

2. *Know the terms used to describe persons with mental retardation and the implications of the level of severity for occupational performance.*

3. *Differentiate between causes of mental retardation and the importance of a biopsychosocial approach in understanding some sources of intellectual deficits.*

4. *Relate philosophical concepts about services for persons with mental retardation to the role of occupational therapy.*

5. *Compare different treatment approaches used to serve children and adolescents with mental retardation.*

6. *Discuss key issues related to selecting occupational therapy goals, treatment planning, and practice when a young person has mental retardation.*

7. *Discuss the role of occupational therapy in collaboration with the family and as a source of family support.*

8. *Recall the different residential and work alternatives for older adolescents and adults with mental retardation and the importance of transition planning.*

9. *Associate the importance of the young person's age and the severity of mental retardation to goal planning and selecting between the different treatment approaches.*

10. *Describe the importance of a multidisciplinary team approach in services for people with mental retardation.*

Definition and measurement issues

Mental retardation is a general term used to describe a condition marked by intellectual and functional ability deficits. The person with mental retardation is identified during childhood to demonstrate subaverage mental abilities as reflected by learning at a slower rate and problems in the cognitive performance component. Mental retardation occurs in 3 or 4 per 1000 people (McLaren & Bryson, 1987). The presence of an intellectual deficit is a chronic condition, but improved occupational performance does occur, especially with family and program support.

Intelligence tests are administered by a psychologist and result in an intelligence quotient (IQ) that usually has an average of 100 with a standard deviation of 15 points (Shae et al., 1987). The possibility of mental retardation is suggested if the person scores more than 2 standard deviations below the mean (IQ of 70). There are several different forms of intelligence tests (Shae et al., 1987), and the occupational therapist or certified occupational therapy assistant who serve persons with mental retardation should become familiar with the strengths and weaknesses of various tests.

Although some infant tests report a mental or cognitive score, assessment of the cognitive component before the child is 3 years old has not proven to be a reliable measure of future intellectual skills (McCall, 1979). Mental retardation is usually not identified during infancy although children with some syndromes or medical conditions may be considered at risk for mental retardation.

Intellectual abilities are difficult to define and accurately assess. As a result, subaverage intelligence is only one criteria in identifying mental retardation. The presence of limitation in functional areas or adaptive skills such as self-direction, social interaction, community use, and performance at school or work are included in a definition (Luckasson et al., 1992). Many instruments are used to document adaptive skills. Two common assessments are the American Association on Mental Retardation (AAMR) Adaptive Behavior Scale (Lambert & Windmiller, 1981) and the Vineland Adaptive Behavior Scale (Sparrow et al., 1984). By interviewing family members, teachers, or residential staff about the person's abilities in areas such as self-care, social skills, and maladaptive behaviors, data can be collected in a systematic way.

To be considered valid, assessment of intellectual deficits and functional problems must be made within the context of the person's cultural and social context (Luckasson et al., 1992). The importance of assessments within the environment is revealed by Koegel and Edgerton's (1984) term "the 6 hour retarded child." These authors discuss the situation in which a child appears mildly retarded in an academic setting but at home neither the family nor peers feel that the child is retarded. The prevalence of minorities who do not do well on standardized IQ tests warns to use caution in using only one measure to identify the presence of mental retardation (Broman et al., 1987).

Classification

There are several ways to group persons with mental retardation to discuss common characteristics among subgroups. One approach is to categorize based on the cause of the subnormal intellectual development. This approach is used in the following text to discuss etiology and characteristics of some diagnostic groups. Another approach advocated by service providers in social and educational programs is to discuss the person based on IQ scores and functional abilities (Goodman, 1990). Table 13-1 gives commonly used educational terms and descriptions of abilities at adulthood.

Associated problems, such as cerebral palsy and mental health problems, occur in 30% of persons with mental retarda-

TABLE 13-1. *Expected Academic Outcome for Different Levels of Mental Retardation*

Severity	I.Q.	Education	Adult Academic Abilities
Mild	70 to 55–50	Educatable	Elementary grade skills
Moderate	55–50 to 40–35	Trainable	Early elementary grade skills
Severe/profound	less than 35		Emphasis on self care skills, basic tasks

(Adapted from Kirk, S., & Gallagher, J. J. [1989]. Children with mental retardation. In Educating exceptional children [p. 00]. Boston: Houghton Mifflin.)

tion. The severity of the associated problem tends to increase with the amount of intellectual deficit (McLaren & Bryson, 1987). In providing services it is important not to allow the presence of mental retardation to overshadow other problems that warrant treatment. **Dual diagnosis** is a term used to indicate that mental health problems and mental retardation are both present in a person. In one study, about 10% of the people had a diagnosis for mental retardation and a psychiatric diagnosis (Borthwick-Duffy & Eyman, 1990). Another study found that 39% of the sample of those with mental retardation had problem behaviors such as impulsiveness, inability to get along with peers, attention seeking and oversensitivity; this suggests that persons with mental retardation may be more vulnerable to personality problems (Reiss, 1990).

Multiply handicapped describes persons with mental retardation who have physical disabilities. Those with mental retardation may also have problems such as cerebral palsy and visual impairment. Epilepsy is another common problem associated with mental retardation. Multiple handicapping conditions present considerable challenge. For example, if the person is physically challenged and lacks speech, an accurate assessment of the level of retardation is difficult. Psychologists and educators may look to occupational therapy to identify the best position for function or the best motor response to use as a communication signal.

Causes of mental retardation

During normal development the acquisition of new skills is influenced by a wide range of internal and environmental factors. In trying to understand why a person has mental retardation, the reader must remember that development is a result of transactions among the person's genetic potential, current biologic and psychological abilities, and characteristics of the environment (Sameroff, 1990). Problems within the person or environmental deficits each can result in lower than normal intelligence.

Genetic and metabolic causes

Of the known syndromes linked with abnormal genes, 503 have mental retardation listed as an associated problem (Wahlstrom, 1990). Fragile X syndrome is the most common inherited cause of mental retardation and affects up to 1 in 1000 boys (Rogers & Simensen, 1987). Girls with fragile X syndrome may experience learning problems but usually are not mentally retarded. Down syndrome is due to a deficit in the 21st chromosomes and occurs in both boys and girls. In both conditions the defective gene is present during embryonic and fetal development and usually affects physical features of the person as well as intellectual abilities.

Congenital problems may not directly affect brain development during the fetal period. Phenylketonuria (PKU) is a condition in which the amino acid phenylalanine is not metabolized correctly. Infants are usually tested for this problem at birth. Those with the condition must follow a special diet that eliminates phenylalanine; otherwise, severe mental retardation may result. Even with early treatment of PKU, research suggests that there may be differences in how the child performs during problems (Welsh et al., 1990).

Prenatal causes

A wide range of events or conditions can affect the development of the central nervous system during embryonic and fetal development. Malformations of the brain can occur, often for unknown reasons. About 8% of birth defects in infants are associated with identifiable teratogens or environmental agents (Schor, 1984). Brain development appears to occur during critical periods so that the implication of a teratogen for intellectual abilities of the person depends on when it occurs and whether the condition persists. Congenital infections such as rubella (German measles) and cytomegalic inclusion disease (CMV) result from transmission of a virus through the placenta (Blackman, 1984). The developing brain and other structures such as the eyes may be affected.

Maternal lifestyle during pregnancy can influence embryonic and fetal brain development. Poor maternal nutrition has been linked to a reduced number of brain cells and fewer synaptic connections. Maternal use of drugs or consumption of alcohol can also affect the developing brain. Fetal alcohol syndrome (FAS) is the leading known cause of mental retardation (Abel & Sokol, 1987). Adolescents and adults with FAS do not appear to have the same distinctive physical features seen during childhood but they continue to have impaired intellectual function and severe maladaptive behaviors such as poor concentration, dependency, social withdrawal, and periods of high anxiety (Streissguth et al., 1991).

Birth complications such as hypoxia are thought to account for 11% of severe/profound mental retardation (McLaren & Bryson, 1987). It is difficult, however, to distinguish prenatal causes that may affect the fetus's ability to withstand the stress associated with birth.

Postnatal causes

Postnatal mental retardation occurs after birth and before 18 years of age and reflects inadequate acquisition of cognitive ability (Luckasson et al., 1992). Several potential causes of mental retardation after the baby is born result from trauma or disease that affects the central nervous system. Meningitis is an example of an illness that can leave the child with mental retardation. Lead poisoning is described as the most common environmental disease of children and can also lead to mental retardation (Needleman, 1991).

Nonorganic mental retardation

Many persons with mental retardation have no identified medical cause for below-normal intellectual abilities (Weisz, 1990). The severity of the mental retardation for this group tends to fall in the mild-to-moderate range; frequently no physical features or associated physical handicaps are present, and a significant percentage of persons with nonorganic mental retardation come from families who are minorities and who live in poverty (Broman et al., 1987). The term *familial* or *environmental retardation* has been used to describe the condition of persons whose general environment appears to play a significant role in the etiology.

To fully appreciate factors contributing to nonorganic mental retardation, the reader should consider the biopsychosocial nature of development. More than one factor may play a role in the subsequent mental retardation of a child. For example, 55% of African American children who live in poverty have blood levels of lead that exceed the recommended minimum (Needleman, 1991). Potential effects of lead poisoning may be one in a series of risk factors such as poor prenatal care, which have a negative accumulated effect on intellectual abilities. Home environmental factors such as overcrowded living situations and the lack of learning opportunities during the preschool years can also have a cumulative effect on intellectual abilities, which are revealed when the child starts academic programs.

Cause of retardation and treatment planning

Does the cause of mental retardation make a difference in treatment planning? The effects of habilitation and educational programs vary according to the cause of mental retardation. Intervention services with all levels of retardation are important but expected outcome may vary. For those with mild familial retardation, sustained intervention programs may raise the intelligence quotient so that the children are no longer retarded (Garber, 1988). If moderate or severe/profound mental retardation has an organic basis, it may be more appropriate to discuss outcome in terms of preventing secondary problems and maximizing the person's adaptive skills. Successful intervention could be defined as reaching the family's goals for their member and helping the person achieve a degree of independence rather than measuring the efficacy of intervention by changes in intellectual performance.

Developmental psychology and medical sciences are expanding our understanding of neurobehavior and cognitive abilities to the extent to which some authors argue that the term mental retardation is too broad to be useful (Landesman & Ramey, 1989). Diagnostic group differences in information processing, behavior, personality, and life span prognosis exist. After potential differences due to cause are recognized, the pattern of strengths and needs of the person who is mentally retarded and is served in occupational therapy should be assessed.

Guiding philosophical concepts in programs

Caring for children and adults with mental retardation has been part of our society for over a century (Zigler et al., 1990). With an understanding of current issues, occupational therapists and occupational therapy assistants will be able to identify how our profession plays many important roles in programs for people with mental retardation.

Our society's approach to helping persons with mental retardation has changed with time and reflects political, economic, and social forces (Zigler et al., 1990). At a time when segregated educational systems and the deplorable conditions in large institutions were a point of social concern, the concept of **normalization** was embraced. The philosophy of normalization suggests that persons with mental retardation are best served when they experience everyday (normal) life. Thus, children and adults who are retarded participate in household routines, leave for school or work in the morning, and have time off for vacations. Quality programming for persons with mental retardation has aimed at emphasizing a normal way of living and participation in the community.

Part of normalization of lifestyle is to assist the person with meaningful, **age-appropriate activities**. An activity is age-appropriate when it is consistent with the activities engaged in or materials used by normal agemates in the same culture. Because persons with mental retardation appear superficially to behave at a younger age than they are, it may seem appropriate to engage them in activities consistent with their mental age. However, use of immature activities makes the person with mental retardation seem even more different than his or her agemates and contributes to social isolation. Occupational therapy, which emphasizes adaptation of activities, can suggest ways to simplify age-appropriate activities so that they are consistent with limited cognitive abilities.

Under the philosophy of normalization, an argument has been made that services should be those that are available in the "normal" community (Zigler et al., 1990). This led education services to promote the practice of mainstreaming children with mental retardation into the regular classroom. **Mainstreaming**, or placing the child with special needs among his or her agemates, permits social interaction and unique learning opportunities. At the same time, service providers, such as occupational therapists and educators, need to be committed to making mainstreaming work. One way is to structure activities that encourage interaction with normal peers. In addition, occupational therapy can play an important role in maximizing occupational behaviors expected of school-age children such as independence in personal care, toileting, and self-feeding.

Any program philosophy that is taken as dogma misses the range of individual differences among those with mental retardation. The best practice includes options for specialized or segregated services if they best meet the person's needs and may ultimately lead to greater community participation (Zigler et al., 1990).

In defining goals for persons with mental retardation, a general direction is to ensure a high **quality of life**. Engaging in meaningful activities that lead to developing new skills and pleasurable interaction with the social and inanimate environment can be seen as leading to an enhanced quality of life. Occupational therapy can play an important role in enabling those with mental retardation to reach this goal through emphasis on the occupation that is meaningful as defined by that person and by the family.

General issues

This section focuses specifically on occupational therapy services for children and teenagers. The reader should remember, however, that mental retardation is a chronic condition and occupational therapy can address the needs of persons with mental retardation throughout their lifespan. For example, a new area is occupational therapy for the geriatric person with mental retardation. Persons with mental retardation also may acquire disabilities such as spinal cord injury. Rehabilitation needs are best met in the hospital and rehabilitation center and occupational therapy procedures need to be adapted to meet the patient's learning abilities.

With our emphasis on occupational performance areas, it may seem that occupational therapy should address all performance areas and components of performance that are delayed. Occupational therapy is usually one of many professional services sharing the common goals of enhancing development of functional skills and the quality of life of those with mental retardation. Following are some general considerations that may help narrow the focus of occupational therapy services as we collaborate with other team members.

First, although the person with mental retardation may show delays in many areas of function, the occupational therapist needs to consider the **profile of strengths and needs** within the context of the person's cognitive abilities. Peaks and valleys of abilities exist even when all areas of function are retarded. For example, children with mental retardation may have strengths in their social skills but may be more delayed in self-help skills. Service providers who consider the whole person will regard performance areas that are more mature than others as assets or strengths, even when the stronger abilities are retarded compared with those of average persons. *Occupational therapy services may be indicated if the problems in performance areas cannot be explained by the level of the intellectual deficits.*

A second point is to set realistic expectations for therapy. Remember that the child with mental retardation can and does learn new things. The *rate of learning* is slower and varies according to the severity of retardation. A child with severe retardation may take 2 years to acquire the same skills it took a child with moderate level of mental retardation skills 6 months to master. Treatment objectives with times for the behavioral outcomes are based on the past rate of change. Previous assessments and information provided by the family help to establish how rapidly changes have occurred in the past. Through activity analysis, goals related to more immediate changes in a general area can help everyone adjust their expectations to be consistent with the child's rate of learning. For example, when dressing is a goal, progress can be defined as pulling on clothes rather than complete independence in dressing. Specifically targeted objectives that reflect anticipated incremental changes can be used to support the efficacy of occupational therapy services.

Another important issue in planning services is **generalization of learning**. With basic abilities in abstract thinking, most children recognize familiar elements in new situations. Past experiences and skills are generalized to fit a new setting so that most children do not have to be taught the same skills for each new situation. The child or teenager with mental retardation may not perceive similarities between situations. As a result of a more concrete and situational learning style, therapy services are most effective when provided in the context of real life situations. Practicing to dress oneself as part of getting ready for swimming or to leave for the bus are intervention strategies that compensate for reduced ability to generalize. If occupational therapy services need to take place out of the context of the home or classroom, practice in real life situations should be coordinated with parents, teachers, and other caregivers. An occupational therapist who develops and monitors a program carried out by others must be sure that the suggestions work toward goals shared by the person responsible for implementation.

Therapists may identify times when it is important to work on an isolated or splinter skill. **Splinter skills** occur when one activity is learned by rote. When developmental progress in the performance component is slow, occupational therapy may train the person with mental retardation through repetition to perform an activity. However, there are limitations to teaching one skill at a time. Splinter skills do not generalize to other situations and may be forgotten if they are not practiced regularly. For example, the therapist may teach a teenager how to sign his name so he can cash a check from his part-time job. At the same time,

TABLE 13-2. *Strategies to Encourage Participation in Activities*

Check Your Style

Make your communication consistent with the developmental level of the receptive language skills of the child.

Try to sound animated, excited, or surprised.

Provide natural and specific reinforcers when an effort is made such as "Good try at coloring in the lines," or, "You climbed half the way up, great!"

If the child is getting stuck, offer to take turns doing a task, before frustration sets in.

Structure the Environment and the Session

Use the social environment to enhance motivation and include another child who can model the activity.

Eliminate distractions that tend to overwhelm the child causing him or her to become a spectator rather than a participant.

Use a picture chart to "tell" the child what to expect during each session.

Give the child a choice between two activities that would meet your treatment objectives.

Pace each activity so challenges are followed by desired or easier activities so the child is rewarded and experiences success often.

---

the therapist, recognizing this as a splinter skill, does not expect the adolescent to be able to write other words.

An important issue in occupational therapy services for persons with mental retardation may be *motivation*. The inner drive or motivation to engage in purposeful activities is usually a key concept in treatment planning. A person who is mentally retarded may not think of alternative activities or see a need to try something new. Thus, he or she may develop a learned helplessness characterized by passivity and lack of initiation (Weisz, 1990). Table 13-2 provides a list of suggestions on ways to elicit participation in activities. Use of a behavioral approach is discussed later in this section.

Treatment approach alternatives

Occupational therapy services may use several different treatment approaches to meet the complex, individual needs of a child or teenager with mental retardation. Different treatment approaches should not be mixed without reflection on their underlying assumptions (Parham, 1987). The discussion that follows reflects suggestions from the authors regarding when a specific treatment approach *might* be used. The ideas should not be viewed as formulas but as options. Decisions regarding which approach to follow should be based on each child's strengths and needs, on family priorities, on associated handicapping conditions, on the therapist's specialty skills, treatment objectives, and on other services.

Developmental approach

In general, it is assumed that people with mental retardation follow a developmental sequence similar to normally developing children (Hodapp et al., 1990). A comprehensive understanding of the developmental flow of different components of function acts as a model for occupational therapy intervention. A developmental approach simulates learning experiences that result in skill acquisition during normal development. A key assumption of the developmental approach is that skills are hierarchical and that later ability is built on earlier skills. Occupational therapy

services emphasize enhancing developing competence in components of skills such as manual dexterity or body scheme, on the assumption that they are needed for success in later occupational performance areas. With a knowledge of emerging performance components, the therapist can identify the "zone of proximal development" or that ability the child or teenager can do almost independently but needs a little assistance for success (Lyons, 1984). Practicing emerging skills also offers opportunities to further consolidate abilities lower on the developmental continuum (Gilfoyle et al., 1990).

In occupational therapy, technology can be an important medium to promote development related to performance areas such as communication and play. Computers and adapted toys can be used to help the physically challenged child engage in activities that develop concepts such as cause and effect practice and a consistent motor signal needed for communication. Coordination of basic skills training with communication activities often results in naturally motivating activities that may speed learning (Musselwhite, 1988). Computers and high-interest electronic toys can also be excellent motivators to enhance both cognitive development and play skills for children with retardation who do not have physical handicaps.

Sensorimotor treatment approach

Motor problems are frequently identified in children with mental retardation. Although sensorimotor treatment approaches are a variation of the developmental approach, their frequent use warrants consideration. A sensorimotor approach uses sensory input to promote motor development by eliciting an adaptive motor response. The sensorimotor approach proposed by the Bobaths (Bobath, 1971; Semans, 1967) has been the foundation for the neurodevelopmental treatment (NDT). The NDT view of motor behavior and postural mechanisms has become widely accepted in occupational therapy for children with cerebral palsy (Carrasco, 1989). If the child has multiple handicaps due to cerebral palsy, incorporation of an NDT approach may be important (see Chapter 13, Section 2). Concepts from an NDT approach may be applied when abnormal motor tone is present due to other causes. For example, hypotonia is a characteristic of children with genetic syndromes such as Down or fragile X.

Among children with moderate-to-severe mental retardation, delayed motor development is not unusual. NDT literature can be a resource for understanding basic gross motor development, especially in infancy (Bly, 1983). Other sensorimotor approaches may be used to develop intervention programs for general motor delays (Farber, 1982; Gilfoyle et al., 1990; Connolly & Montgomery, 1987).

Sensory stimulation approach

Performance component areas addressed in occupational therapy services include consideration of the various sensory systems that provide each person with information about the environment. Variations in preferences for and tolerance of sensory stimulation are present in everyone, including those with mental retardation. Occupational therapy services can play an important role by helping other professionals recognize individual differences in sensory processing among young people with mental retardation. Reframing perceived inappropriate behavior as sensory defensiveness or a need to seek out intensive sensory stimulation may help other professionals or the family to understand the behavior in a new light.

The concept of a meaningful sensory diet has been applied to young babies but can be expanded to occupational therapy services for persons with mental retardation (Wilbarger, 1984). Sensory stimulation is an important part of day-to-day life at all ages. Persons with severe mental retardation may need assistance obtaining varied sensory input due to impaired understanding on how to become involved in an activity or limited mobility due to multiple handicaps. The appropriate level of stimulation becomes an important issue and occupational therapy services play a role in environmental adaptation to avoid overstimulation or understimulation.

Stereotyped behaviors are apparently purposeless, habitual motor acts, which the person with mental retardation engages in repeatedly. The behaviors may be so severe that interaction with the environment and learning cannot occur. Sensory stimulation may be used to help change the person's level of arousal and to focus attention (Farber, 1982). Although some evidence exists that sensory stimulation may reduce stereotyped behavior (Bonadonna, 1981; Bright et al., 1981), a controlled study did not show sensory stimulation to be more effective than talking and touching (Iwasaki & Holm, 1990). Activities providing meaningful sensory stimulation may interrupt stereotyped behavior but should not be expected to eliminate the underlying cause of the behavior.

Environmental adaptation to provide appropriate sensory stimulation should not be confused with a sensory integration approach. Sensory integration dysfunction reflecting sensory modulation problems and developmental dyspraxia may coexist with mental retardation but could be difficult to isolate. Many of the clinical observations used to identify sensory integrative problems can be observed in persons with mental retardation. There may be alternative explanations to behaviors suggesting sensory integration dysfunction; however, because mental retardation can be associated with damage in other parts of the nervous system clinicians should avoid overidentification of these problems (Fisher & Murray, 1991). Sensory integrative dysfunction may be identified appropriately, especially when mental retardation is mild (Murray & Anzalone, 1991). An important clue is the clinical observations of sensory integration dysfunction, which cannot be explained by the degree of retardation.

Behavioral approach

The behavioral approach uses the principles of learning and behavior management to teach functional skills. This approach may include training in specific skills combined with work toward eliminating other behaviors (Whitman et al., 1983). For example, self-feeding, because it requires holding a spoon, is incompatible with constant throwing behavior. **Reinforcers**, which include any desired object or activity that is rewarding to a person, are used to increase desired behaviors.

When skills are already present, reinforcement methods can be used effectively to motivate the child to use them functionally. If skills have not yet been learned, behavioral techniques, including prompting and shaping, may be used in teaching. Prompts include social or verbal cues and visual aids such as picture cues. Physical guidance through a task may be necessary when other prompts are not effective. Prompts are gradually reduced to shape behavior as the child does more on his or her own. For example, when teaching a child to eat with a spoon, initially hand-over-hand physical guidance may be necessary.

Later the physical help may be reduced to guidance at the forearm and finally eliminated (Whitman et al., 1983). Similarly verbal cues might be gradually eliminated as a child learns a skill.

Behavioral techniques of forward or backward chaining can be applied to teach sequential steps of a functional task. In *forward chaining*, if the skill is putting on a shirt, the child is first rewarded for picking up the shirt and receives assistance in completing the other steps. Next, he or she is expected to complete the first two steps (picking up the shirt and orienting it correctly) before receiving a reward. Successive steps are reinforced until the skill is mastered. *Backward chaining* reverses the procedure.

A behavioral approach can also be applied to behaviors that interfere with learning or limit integration into the community. Eliminating the cause of behavioral problems should be the first option examined. Excessive demands or overstimulation may lead to acting out behavior. In these situations, program adaptation—not a behavioral program—should be considered. If a behavioral program to eliminate maladaptive behaviors is needed, services will be most effective if problems are addressed early with a team effort. When behaviors interfere with functional performance, procedures to prevent reinforcement, called *extinction techniques*, may be used. Punishment, in the form of a "time-out" procedure might be used in extreme cases. For example, if the child throws a spoon during feeding, he or she may be removed from the table for several minutes for a time-out.

Compensatory approach

Assisting the person with mental retardation to function at maximum level is an important part of occupational therapy services. Assistive devices, wheelchairs, and computers help the person to participate in activities such as communication, mobility, self-care, and play. Planning compensation begins by considering the child's relative needs and the social and physical environments where the person will function. An interdisciplinary team evaluation is often used to integrate insight into physical (including hand skill) and cognitive abilities, motivation to use the device, and the demands that use of the device places on caregivers who have to help the person with mental retardation.

For those with mental retardation and speech problems, augmentative communication techniques can be used to stimulate development of skills and to provide a means of communication. As persons with retardation make a transition to work and living environments outside the home, communication with unfamiliar people becomes increasingly necessary. Effective communication affects a person's ability to participate in the community. Voice output devices are an ideal means to interact with both peers and unfamiliar adults.

Specific treatment issues

Assessment and treatment issues introduced in the following text vary greatly based on chronologic age and the severity of mental retardation. The implications of different levels of retardation for occupational performance of children and teenagers are presented in Tables 13-3 and 13-4, respectively. These suggested abilities reflect generalization to help the reader. In reality each person with mental retardation may achieve more or less, depending on programming and the presence of associated handicapping conditions.

TABLE 13-3. *Occupational Performance of 5-Year-Old Children with Different Levels of Mental Retardation*

Level	Activities of Daily Living	Study	Play
Mild	Toilet: independent Feeding: feeds self Dressing: needs help with fasteners	Pre-academics: draws shapes, matching, counting, colors, etc.	Seeks contact with younger peers Imitation, playground, plays simple games
Moderate	Toilet: time trained, may signal needs Feeding: independent Dressing: needs prompts, assistance with garment once started	Attending, learn class routines; Recognizes shapes, construction	Parallel and interactive play; functional use of toy
Severe/profound	Toilet: dependent Feeding: may fingerfeed, messy use of spoon if any Dressing: dependent, cooperates with activity	Basic sensorimotor skills; reach, manipulation	Enjoys social contacts, exploration of objects

Assessment issues

The occupational therapist may serve as a program consultant or receive referrals to see persons with mental retardation for a variety of reasons. An initial screening may be necessary to establish the occupational performance area or component that the therapist wants to assess. Before assessment begins, information is needed about the general level of the severity of retardation and the presence of associated conditions such as cerebral palsy or hearing loss, which would affect testing.

Two types of standardized tests, norm-referenced or criterion-referenced evaluations, are typically available in pediatric practice (Rogers & Simensen, 1987). If the therapist wishes to compare the child's motor abilities with other children of the same age, evaluation tools such as the Peabody Developmental Motor Scales (Folio & Dubose, 1983) and the Bruininks-Oseretsky Test of Motor Proficiency (Bruininks, 1978) are examples of norm-referenced tests. *Norm-referenced tests* are most appropriately used when the child being tested is similar to those children used to establish the norms. Frequently children with mental retardation are excluded during test development. When the child has mental retardation, limited language and attention may then affect how he or she responds to standardized test situations. If the therapist adapts the testing procedures (ie, gives the child demonstrations and uses different materials) the reliability of a norm-referenced test may be compromised. *In reporting test results, the therapist must note whether adapta-tions to standard procedures were made to accommodate for special needs of the child.*

The other type of test, the ***criterion-referenced test***, consists of descriptions of abilities used to compare with those of the child. This leads to an understanding of what that child can and cannot do. Programs may choose to use criterion-referenced instruments because changes in the child's ability are easily tracked and progress is documented in a positive manner. A checklist, for example, of feeding skills arranged in developmental order may serve as a criterion tool to chart progress. The therapist can say that last year the child may have had only 50% of the skills on the list, whereas now the child has 98% of the skills.

The Erhardt Developmental Prehension Assessment (Erhardt, 1982) provides a description of fine motor skills organized in a developmental sequence. The child's reflexive arm and hand positions, control of voluntary reach and grasp, and prewriting skills can be noted. Although this instrument does not meet psychometric criteria, it does offer an effective means to observe and document progress (Dunn, 1983). Another criterion-referenced assessment is the Sensorimotor Performance Analysis (Richter & Montgomery, 1989). This screening tool offers an easy way to document qualitative changes in gross and fine motor skills of school-age children.

Clinical observations form an important evaluation tool for the occupational therapist working with people with mental retardation. In *ecologically based observations,* the person is observed in his or her natural environment (class or workshop);

TABLE 13-4. *Occupational Performance of 15-Year-Old Adolescents With Different Levels of Mental Retardation*

Level	Activities of Daily Living	Work/Study	Play/Leisure
Mild	Independent in grooming Community mobility developing Aware of context, tries to fit in Uses phone, can write simple notes	Simple home management Shops, uses money Expresses job interests Demonstrates functional reading/writing	Interest in peer groups Opposite-sex friends Agemates for leisure activities Knows TV and popular movies
Moderate	Independent in self-care Can follow learned routes in neighborhoods	With supervision participates in cooking and housekeeping routines Prevocational classes to learn basic job skills	Spectator activities Peer and family outings
Severe/profound	May be independent in feeding, dressing with supervision Not independent in community travel Social skills best with familiar people	Needs help with home management Sheltered workshop tasks	Enjoys repetitive social games; outings

these observations are important for collecting information about occupational performance areas. The young person with mental retardation may have functional skills within the context of his or her home or school but may not demonstrate the abilities when given unfamiliar material in occupational therapy. The occupational therapist uses a clinical reasoning approach to develop hypotheses regarding abilities and disabilities (Rogers, 1983). Modification of hypotheses is based on repeated observation, interactions with the child, and input from the primary caregivers.

Occupational therapy services

Occupational therapy services may address such diverse issues as developing components of performance areas, specific skills in occupational behaviors, compensation for disabilities, and prevention of further handicapping conditions. Direct service is provided but other models are also important parts of occupational therapy for children and adolescents with mental retardation. Due to the gradual nature of changes and the need to provide learning opportunities in the context of daily routines, monitoring programs developed in occupational therapy may be identified as the way to provide the highest quality of service. Consultation with family members, teachers, and other program staff is therefore a frequent part of occupational therapy services. Other persons working with the child or teenager may need assistance in problem solving around a daily activity and suggestions from an occupational therapy perspective lends new insight. Selection of the correct model of service is influenced by the occupational therapy goals, the chronologic age of the person with mental retardation, the rate developmental change are anticipated, and the presence of other handicapping conditions.

CASE STUDY 1

Lisa is a 10-year-old girl with a diagnosis of mosaic Down syndrome. Psychological testing when she entered school suggested that Lisa was severely mentally retarded, functioning at a level between 1 and 2 years of age. At school Lisa is placed in a life skills class with children who are moderately to severely retarded. As part of her school program, an occupational therapist consults with her teacher about activities to promote fine motor and self-care skills development.

Lisa was brought to a private occupational therapist by her mother, who hoped Lisa would achieve more independence in self-help skills at home. Her mother reported that Lisa needed assistance with dressing and feeding. From her mother's perspective, Lisa did not play with toys appropriately and "acted out" in waiting rooms or when shopping. Occupational therapy evaluation revealed low muscle tone with hyperextensible joints. During the assessment Lisa pulled away from physical guidance. She refused to explore materials with texture, such as clay, and was distracted with trying to rub this material off her hands. Items from the fine motor section of the Peabody Developmental Motor Scale were used to structure observations (Folio & Dubose, 1983). Based on her performance the therapist thought that Lisa's fine motor skills were at a level under 24 months. Throughout the evaluation noncompliant behavior was a problem. Lisa would push away materials or the table itself.

A period of weekly occupational therapy was recommended to begin working on building occupational performance skills. Fine motor skills were targeted if they were linked to self-help skills addressed in therapy. Lisa's mother identified dressing, use of toilet paper, drinking from a straw, and independent play as goals. The school occupational therapist was contacted so services and behavior management would be coordinated.

Lisa's preferences during activities were noted to identify possible reinforcers. Instruction and practice with targeted skills were presented as parts of desired activities. For example, practice dressing was achieved by having Lisa put on a special "jumping shirt" in preparation for a reinforcing activity, jumping on a small trampoline. Repetitions of selected fine motor skills were built into the session. Lisa practiced manipulation skills by opening and closing jars in the context of getting motivating activities or putting things away.

Desired activities that offered experience with different textures were followed in the same treatment session by a functional activity that had a tactile element Lisa seemed to avoid. Her tolerance for different textures increased as Lisa became familiar with activities. She continued to be noncompliant when new activities were introduced. Discussion with her mother enabled the family to see that some of Lisa's noncompliant behavior was due to a need to build familiarity with the novel tactile aspects of new activities.

Repeated sessions were needed to identify which aspects of the behavioral approach would be effective in helping Lisa learn new skills. Repetition and physical prompts were used to elicit participation and to shape behavior. To address noncompliant behavior, a regular routine for the therapy session was established. Lisa's mother observed treatment sessions and provided suggestions such as withdrawal of adult attention and waiting for participation.

Since generalization of skills learned in therapy to home and school environments was important, Lisa's mother brought in items that were part of her daughter's routine. Lisa learned to manipulate a zipper when desired items were in the backpack that she took to school. Therapy also focused on using existing play skills more independently by practicing short functional activity sequences. For example, to teach independent coloring, materials were presented in a box. Lisa was guided to open the box, use the materials appropriately, then put them away. As skills became more independent in therapy, her mother presented the activity in the same container at home.

After weekly private therapy and coordinated effort at home and school, Lisa is slowly developing new functional skills. She drinks from a straw, puts on a shirt, and wipes off the table. With minimal supervision she can entertain herself by coloring pictures for short periods of time.

Discussion

Important aspects of occupational therapy are illustrated with Lisa's treatment. Her mother played an active role in identifying her daughter's treatment goals, which ensured that therapy addressed relevant skills. Lisa's mother was also an important resource in understanding how to best work with Lisa and deal with noncompliant behaviors. Although she had significant pervasive fine motor delays, in consideration of her chronologic age, individual therapy emphasized using a behavioral approach to enhance self-help skills rather than addressing overall sensory and motor performance components. Direct therapy for a period has been useful in bringing out new skills that were needed at home. A consultation model will be implemented when Lisa's family feels she has reached their goals.

CASE STUDY 2

Mark was referred for occupational therapy at the suggestion of his speech/language pathologist when he was 3¹/₂ years old. He had received speech therapy since the age of 30 months because of language delays related to oral dyspraxia. Mark's parents expressed concern about his clumsiness, difficulty playing with toys, and his social skills. Mark attended a regular day care center but staff reported behavior problems. Mark was described as overly active and was reported to hit other children and grab their toys.

An interview with his parents revealed that Mark started sitting at 9 months and walked when he was 17 months old. They reported that he was an irritable baby. Occupational therapy assessment revealed that Mark was delayed in gross and fine motor development. His cooperation for standardized testing procedures could not be obtained because he was active and had difficulty paying attention to structured activities. Observed skills suggested scattered abilities at levels between 18 and 29 months. Clinical observations included low muscle tone and immature ability to do gross motor skills requiring balance, such as navigating steps without reverting to crawling.

Attentional difficulty with fleeting eye contact was observed. Mark became engrossed with a toy clock, would not attend to other activities, and had a tantrum when the clock was put away. Mark's parents reported similar difficulties with activity changes at home. Mark seemed to enjoy a variety of sensory activities (eg, playing in a sandbox) but often rejected manipulative materials after briefly attempting to use them.

Individual weekly occupational therapy sessions were initiated using a sensorimotor developmental approach to enhance Mark's ability to manipulate toys. Fine motor activities incorporated the use of large toys for manipulation such as oversized beads strung on plastic tubing to reduce frustration. In the context of play, Mark could be motivated to try manipulative activities such as stringing beads to make a necklace for a toy animal. A consistent routine in therapy sessions was established and attending behavior improved so that Mark would sit at a table for 8 to 10 minutes.

After 2 months of occupational therapy, Mark did not make anticipated progress in learning activities, even with repetition and structure. Unusual obsession with some activities continued, drawing elicited intense, overfocused interest and subsequent difficulty shifting to another activity. The therapist's observations and Mark's limited progress were discussed with his parents. They agreed that Mark should be referred for an interdisciplinary evaluation to better understand his strengths and needs.

The team evaluation included professionals from audiology, psychology, speech/language pathology, medicine, and social work. Medical evaluation identified characteristics sug-

gestive of fragile X syndrome including autistic-like behaviors such as poor eye contact. The pediatrician also noted attention problems, perseveration, and delayed development. The doctor noted physical features such as joint hyperextensibility and prominent forehead. The audiologist tested hearing, which was found to be normal. On a psychological test appropriate for a nonverbal child, Mark scored in the mild range of mental retardation. The language assessment revealed that he had concrete speech but did not seem to understand abstract references. The social worker administered the Vineland Adaptive Behavior Scale, which showed mild deficits in all areas of function. In addition, the social work interview revealed that Mark's parents wondered about his future, felt guilty that they had not done more to help him earlier, and were concerned about their plans for more children.

With an improved understanding of the range of Mark's problems, a comprehensive intervention plan was established by his parents and the team. He was placed in a developmental day care center where he could get an individualized educational program with related services including occupational therapy and speech/language therapy. Further medical testing and genetic counseling were planned to explore the diagnosis and address Mark's parents' concerns. The family was also told about a parent-to-parent support group in which a volunteer parent of an older child with mental retardation could meet with them to discuss the future from a parent's perspective.

Weekly occupational therapy services continued to address fine motor development, which the parents selected as a priority. Activities to improve hand dexterity and manipulation of objects were first practiced at the table with structure and then incorporated into play. For example, work with plastic blocks that fit together was introduced with hand-over-hand guidance. Physical help was gradually reduced until Mark could pull apart and stack the blocks himself. The blocks were then introduced during free play on the floor. Once a month the occupational therapy treatment session consisted of the therapist working with Mark in the classroom. The therapist worked with Mark's teacher to provide opportunities for Mark to practice activities like the blocks in play with other children.

Discussion

The case report on Mark illustrates how important multidisciplinary assessments are to the identification and programming for children with mental retardation. Mark's problem originally was identified as a language delay and he appeared to have problems with planning and executing movements. With insight into his intellectual abilities, Mark became eligible for a more comprehensive program. Mark's motor skills were more delayed than his general cognitive level, and occupational therapy sessions were continued but expanded to provide repetition and practice across all environments for maximum generalization of skills. Treatment sessions in Mark's classroom ensured continuity of experience and helped Mark apply new play skills in social situations. Since Mark was a young child, a developmental approach was used to select activities to promote the fine motor component of function rather than a behavioral approach to teach specific skills.

Occupational therapy and families

Families of children and teenagers with mental retardation are important participants in the habilitation process. Intervention, education, and support programs change as children get older but families are a continual and powerful force in the lives of people with mental retardation. Our philosophy of family participation is changing. Research has demonstrated that there are many sources of stress for families with a child who is mentally retarded (Singer & Irvin, 1989). At one time, parents were viewed as assistants to carry out home programs developed in occupational therapy (Bazyk, 1989). Emphasis on a deficit view of the child with mental retardation (as suggested by a list of problems parents should work on) may only add to family stress. Rather than ask caregivers to take on the role of therapist as well as that of parent, families are encouraged to decide their own level of participation. An appreciation of a family's expertise regarding the member with special needs and the importance of family support lead to a collaborative relationship between occupational therapy personnel and families (Bazyk, 1989).

Many of the occupational performance skills that therapists address are acquired in the context of family life. Thus, occupational therapy services that respond to family priorities in activity of daily living training are important. Professionals need to be sensitive to potential barriers to parent participation in programs. Logistical problems of meeting at a time convenient for program personnel, unfamiliarity with school systems (especially among parents with minority backgrounds), a sense of inferiority combined with the attitude that professionals must know what is best, and uncertainty about the child's problems may make parents hesitant to become involved (Turnbull & Turnbull, 1986). Occupational therapists who help parents bridge communication gaps and increase their participation in planning services provide the most effective services possible for young people with mental retardation.

Addressing family stress

The amount and nature of family stress associated with a member who has mental retardation will change over the life span of the family. There are anticipated periods of stress in which professionals can be an important part of the family support system (Turnbull & Turnbull, 1986). For example, although a family knows that an infant has delayed development, diagnosis of mental retardation may not come until the child is in the preschool years. The process of learning about and adjusting to the diagnosis of retardation takes time. Families frequently have questions after they leave the doctor's office or the diagnostic session with the psychologist. They want to know where to learn more about the identified problems and the implications for the future, and they need clarification of terms. Occupational therapy personnel should be ready to help families find resources to answer questions as they arise.

Special events, such as seeing a younger sibling achieve developmental milestones that the child with mental retardation has not reached, may trigger new feelings of loss of an "ideal" child. At the same time, families should not be seen as if they were in constant mourning. Many parents can point to positive things that they have learned and skills acquired as the family learns to live with the extra needs of a child with mental retardation.

Normal periods of family stress can have new meaning when the child has mental retardation. When families deal with starting new programs, transition periods between programs, and making the right placement decisions, tension is created, especially when the child has special needs. Occupational therapy services for the parents to plan for program changes, explore alternatives, and identify skills the child or teenager will need in the next program will help families deal with anxiety about changes. Transition planning should be a routine part of long-term treatment goals of each program and not introduced only when decisions need to be made.

Families of adults with mental retardation

A natural period of family development is when children become young adults. One problem is that parents and professionals may continue to view the person with special needs as a child, thus not allowing the young person the opportunity to grow up (Turnbull & Turnbull, 1986). Two major aspects of growing up are living away from home and engaging in daily activities that are meaningful. Knowledge about future programming options ensure that occupational therapy services participate in preparing the older child and later the adolescent for transition into adulthood. Discussion of how skills learned in occupational therapy relate to the future can help families shift toward viewing their "child" as someone who will assume some parts of adult roles.

The guiding principles of the least restrictive and most normal environments are factors in decisions that determine where an adult with mental retardation will live. Public and private institutions and specialized nursing homes offer close supervision and care, especially for those with severe/profound mental retardation. The advantages of services concentrated in one site must be weighed against the potential isolation from community involvement. Over the last two decades there has been a decline in the number of large state institutions (Braddock et al., 1991). Foster homes, group residences, and semi-independent living arrangements offer alternatives for adults with mental retardation to live in neighborhoods. Adults with severe/profound mental retardation can be successful residents of a group home if they are given proper support. Occupational therapy services and program consultation are frequently provided to enhance independence in activities of daily living and home maintenance skills.

A range of work alternatives is important to meet the varied needs of adults with mental retardation (Haney et al., 1988). Vocational alternatives may be an *adult activity center,* where basic concepts, functional activities, and leisure time interests are addressed. *Sheltered workshops* help the person master basic work skills. Activities may include simple assembly or the sorting of objects to be packaged. Supervision of the activities is ongoing and pay is less than minimum wage if the sheltered workshop is involved in contract work. *Supported employment* takes place if the adult with mental retardation is engaged in an actual job. The work may be a position adapted for that person but it usually fulfills a need in a place of business. Training and supervision are provided as needed by a job coach.

Occupational therapy services are often part of activity centers, sheltered workshops, and supported employment. Training in activity analysis is especially valuable in planning how to help the person with mental retardation perform skills necessary for specific work-related tasks. Although sheltered workshops continue to be the most common form of adult programming, there are philosophical and economic arguments to expand opportunities for supported employment (Schuster, 1990).

An important part of being an adult is the ability to decide what one wants to do. Conversely, asking a person about goals and activities communicates a respect for the rights of adulthood. In preparing for adulthood, teenagers with mental retardation should be given increased opportunities to make choices about program and leisure time alternatives.

Summary

Mental retardation indicates limitation in the cognitive component of performance that occurs during the developmental period. The range of intellectual problems can vary from mild to severe; multiple handicapping conditions may further limit occupational performance. Heterogeneity of characteristics of people who are mentally retarded should be expected due to individual differences and varied causes of intellectual and adaptive skill deficits.

Occupational therapy services use a considerable variety of treatment approaches and models of service. With children, the emphasis in occupational therapy services may be to assist family and other caregivers in helping the child develop a foundation for self-help and academic skills. Therapy may address problems in performance components such as sensorimotor skills if developmental delays in the components appear to be more significant than the intellectual limitations. In later childhood and adolescence, occupational therapy is often part of multidisciplinary teams that work to develop functional self-care, home maintenance, and prevocational skills. With persons of all ages occupational therapy techniques are important intervention strategies when there are associated handicapping conditions. Throughout the life span of the person with mental retardation, occupational therapy service has a role in maximizing independence and a high quality of life.

References

Abel, E. L., & Sokol, R. J. (1987). Incidence of fetal alcohol syndrome and economic impact of FAS related anomalies. *Drug Alcohol Dependency, 19*, 51–70.

American Journal on Mental Retardation, 95, 1–12.

Bazyk, S. (1989). Changes in attitudes and beliefs regarding parent participation and home programs: An update. *American Journal of Occupational Therapy, 43*, 723–730.

Blackman, J. A. (1984). Congenital infections. In J. A. Blackman (Ed.), *Medical aspects of developmental disabilities in children birth to three* (pp. 71–76). Rockville, MD: Aspen Publications.

Bly, L. (1983). *The components of normal movement during the first year of life and abnormal motor development*. Chicago: NeuroDevelopmental Treatment Association.

Bobath, K. (1971). The normal postural reflex mechanism and its deviation in children with cerebral palsy. *Physiotherapy, 57*, 515–525.

Bonadonna, P. (1981). Effects of a vestibular stimulation program on stereotype rocking behavior. *American Journal of Occupational Therapy, 35*, 775–781.

Borthwick-Duffy, S. A., & Eyman, R. K. (1990). Who are the dually diagnosed? *American Journal on Mental Retardation, 94*, 586–595.

Braddock, D., Fujiura, G., Hemp, R., Mitchell, D., & Bachelder, L. (1991). Current and future trends in state-operated mental retardation institutions in the United States. *American Journal on Mental Retardation, 95*, 451–462.

Bright, T., Bittick, K., & Fleeman, B. (1981). Reduction of self-injurious behavior using sensory integrative techniques. *American Journal of Occupational Therapy, 35*, 167–172.

Broman, S., Nichols, P. L., Shaughnessy, P., & Kennedy, W. (1987). *Retardation in young children*. Hillsdale, NJ: Erlbaum.

Bruininks, R. H. (1978). *Bruininks-Oseretsky Test of Motor Proficiency*. Circle Pines, MN: American Guidance Service.

Carrasco, R. C. (1989). Children with cerebral palsy. In P. N. Pratt & A. S. Allen (Eds.), *Occupational therapy for children* (pp. 396–421). St. Louis: C. V. Mosby.

Connolly, B., & Montgomery, P. (1987). *Therapeutic exercise in developmental disabilities*. Chattanooga, TN: Chattanooga Corporation.

Dunn, W. (1983). Critique of the Erhardt developmental prehension assessment. *Physical and Occupational Therapy in Pediatrics, 3*(4), 59–68.

Erhardt, R. P. (1982). *Developmental hand dysfunction: Theory-assessment-treatment*. Laurel, MD: Ramsco.

Farber, S. D. (1982). *Neurorehabilitation: A multisensory approach*. Philadelphia: W. B. Saunders.

Fisher, A. G., & Murray, E. A. (1991). Introduction to sensory integration theory. In A. G. Fisher, E. A. Murray & A. C. Bundy (Eds.), *Sensory integration: Theory and practice* (pp. 3–26). Philadelphia: F. A. Davis.

Folio, R., & Dubose, R. F. (1983). *Peabody Developmental Motor Scales*. Allen TX: DLM Teaching Resources.

Garber, H. L. (1988). *The Milwaukee Project: Preventing mental retardation in children at risk*. Washington, DC: American Association on Mental Retardation.

Gilfoyle, E. M., Grady, A. P., & Moore, J. C. (1990). *Children adapt* (2nd ed.). Thorofare, NJ: Slack.

Goodman, J. F. (1990). Technical note: Problems in etiological classification of mental retardation. *Journal of Child Psychology and Psychiatry, 31*, 465–469.

Haney, J. I., Wilson, J. W., & Halle, J. (1988). Adults with mental retardation: Who they are, where they are and how their communicative needs can be met. In S. N. Calculator, & J. L. Bedrosian (Eds.), *Communication assessment and intervention for adults with mental retardation* (pp. 67–94). Boston: Little, Brown & Co.

Hodapp, R. M., Burack, J. A., & Zigler, E. (1990). The developmental perspective in the field of mental retardation. In R. M. Hodapp, J. A. Burack & E. Zigler (Eds.), *Issues in the developmental approach to mental retardation* (pp. 3–26). New York: Cambridge University Press.

Iwasaki, K., & Holm, M. B. (1990). Sensory treatment for the reduction of stereotype behaviors in persons with severe multiple disabilities. *Occupational Therapy Journal of Research, 9*, 170–183.

Kirk, S., & Gallagher, J. J. (1989). Children with mental retardation. In Kirk, S., Ed. *Educating exceptional children* (pp. 130–177). Boston: Houghton Mifflin.

Koegel, P., & Edgerton, R. B. (1984). Black "six-hour" retarded children" as young adults. In R. B. Edgerton (Ed.), *Lives in process: Mildly retarded adults in a large city* (pp. 145–171). Washington, DC: American Association on Mental Deficiency.

Lambert, N. M., & Windmiller, M. (1981). *AAMD Adaptive Behavior Scale, School Edition*. East Aurora, NY: Slosson Educational Publications.

Landesman, S., & Ramey, C. (1989). Developmental psychology and mental retardation. *American Psychologist, 44*, 409–415.

Luckasson, R., Coulter, D., Polloway, E., Reiss, S., Schalock, R., Snell, M., Spitalnik, D., & Stark, J., Eds. (1992). *Definition and classification in mental retardation*. Washington, DC: AAMR publishers, 1992.

Lyons, B. G. (1984). Defining a child's zone of proximal development: Evaluation process for treatment planning. *American Journal of Occupational Therapy, 38*, 446–451.

McCall, R. B. (1979). The development of intellectual functioning in infancy and the prediction of later I.Q. In J. Osofsky (Ed.), *Handbook of infant development* (pp. 707–741). New York: John Wiley & Sons.

McLaren, J., & Bryson, S. E. (1987). Review of recent epidemiological studies of mental retardation: Prevalence, associated disorders, and etiology. *American Journal of Mental Retardation, 92*, 243–254.

Murray, E. A., & Anzalone, M. E. (1991). Integrating sensory integration theory and practice with other intervention approaches. In A. G. Fisher, E. A. Murray & A. C. Bundy (Eds.), *Sensory integration: Theory and practice* (pp. 354–383). Philadelphia: F. A. Davis.

Musselwhite, C., & St. Louis, K. (1988). *Communication programming for persons with severe handicaps*. Boston: College Hill Press.

Needleman, H. L. (1991). Lead exposure: The commonest environmental disease of childhood. *Zero to Three, 11*(5), 1–6.

Parham, D. (1987). Toward professionalism: The reflective therapist. *American Journal of Occupational Therapy, 41*, 555–561.

Reiss, S. (1990). Prevalence of dual diagnosis in community-based day programs in the Chicago metropolitan area. *American Journal on Mental Retardation, 94*, 578–585.

Richter, E., & Montgomery, P. (1989). *The sensorimotor performance analysis*. Hugo, MN: PDP Products Press.

Rogers, J. C. (1983). Selection of evaluation instruments. In L. King-Thomas & B. J. Hacker (Eds.), *A therapist's guide to pediatric assessment* (pp. 19–34). Boston: Little, Brown & Co.

Rogers, R. C., & Simensen, R. J. (1987). Fragile X syndrome: A common etiology of mental retardation. *American Journal of Mental Deficiency, 91*, 445–449.

Sameroff, A. J. (1990). Neo-environmental perspectives on developmental theory. In R. M. Hodapp, J. A. Burack & E. Zigler (Eds.), *Issues in the developmental approach to mental retardation* (pp. 93–113). New York: Cambridge University Press.

Schor, D. P. (1984). Teratogens. In J. A. Blackman (Ed.), *Medical aspects of developmental disabilities in children birth to three* (pp. 223–226). Rockville, MD: Aspen Publications.

Schuster, J. W. (1990). Sheltered workshops: Financial and philosophical liabilities. *Mental Retardation, 28*, 233–239.

Semans, M. A. (1967). The Bobath concept in treatment of neurological disorders. *American Journal of Physical Medicine, 46*, 732–785.

Shae, V., Towle, P. O., & Gordon, B. (1987). Psychological and cognitive tests. In L. King-Thomas & B. J. Hacker (Eds.), *A therapist's guide to pediatric assessment* (pp. 287–332). Boston: Little, Brown & Co.

Singer, G. H. S., & Irvin, L. K. (1989). Family caregiving, stress, and support. In G. H. S. Singer & L. K. Irvin (Eds.), *Support for caregiving families* (pp. 3–26). Baltimore: Paul Brooks.

Sparrow, S., Balla, D., & Cicchetti, E. (1984). *Vineland Adaptive Behavior Scales*. Circle Pines, MN: American Guidance Services.

Streissguth, A. P., Aase, J. M. Clarren, S. K., Randels, S. P., LaDue, R. A., & Smith. D. F. (1991). Fetal alcohol syndrome in adolescents and adults. *Journal of the American Medical Association, 265*, 1961–1967.

Turnbull, A. P., & Turnbull, H. R. (1986). *Families, professionals and exceptionality: A special partnership*. Columbus, OH: Merrill Publishing.

Wahlstrom, J. (1990). Gene map of mental retardation. *Journal of Mental Deficiency Research, 34*, 11–27.

Weisz, J. R. (1990). Cultural-familial mental retardation: A developmental perspective on cognitive performance and helplessness behavior. In R. M. Hodapp, J. A. Burack & E. Zigler (Eds.), *Issues in the developmental approach to mental retardation* (pp. 137–168). New York: Cambridge University Press.

Welsh, M. C., Pennington, B. F., Ozonoff, S., Rouse, B., & McCabe, E. R. B. (1990). Neuropsychology of early-treated phenylketonuria: Specific executive function deficits. *Child Development, 61*, 1697–1713.

Wilbarger, P. (1984). Planning an adequate sensory diet: Application of sensory processing theory during the first year of life. *Zero to Three, 5*, 1–3.

Whitman, T., Scibak, J., & Reid, D. (1983). *Behavior modification with the severely and profoundly retarded* (pp. 25–59; 117–145). New York: Academic Press.

Zigler, E., Hodapp, R. M., & Edison, M. R. (1990). From theory to practice in the care and education of mentally retarded individuals.

SECTION 2

Cerebral palsy

RHODA P. ERHARDT

KEY TERMS

Classification of Cerebral
Palsy

Myofascial Release

Neurodevelopmental
Treatment

Orthotics

Positioning

Seizures

Sensory Integration

Spasticity

LEARNING OBJECTIVES

Upon completion of this section the reader will be able to:

1. *Define cerebral palsy, its scope, and classification types.*

2. *Compare normal and atypical development and its effects on upper extremity function.*

3. *Describe the consequences of atypical neurologic development in terms of primitive reflexes, abnormal muscle tone, sensory deficits, compensations, and effects on function.*

4. *List disorders associated with cerebral palsy.*

5. *Identify assessments and intervention models appropriate for people with cerebral palsy.*

6. *Be knowledgeable in the general treatment methods of occupational therapy and in the relationship of occupational therapy to other treatments.*

Historical perspective

It was not until 1843 that William John Little, an English orthopedist, recognized that various deformities in children were associated with what he called "infantile spastic paralysis." His definitive paper in 1861 documented correlations between abnormality of pregnancy, labor, delivery, and subsequent developmental deficits (Little, 1862).

Although interest in "Little's disease" spread to other medical disciplines, emphasis was on identification and cause. Specific approaches to treatment were slow in developing until orthopedic surgery to correct specific deformities became popular after the turn of the century. Initial surgical benefit was frequently followed by disappointing long-term results, however, as deformities returned or new ones developed.

Another orthopedist, Winthrop M. Phelps, expanded the work of Bronson Crothers, a pediatric neurologist, who recognized the need for a broader approach that included developmental, neurologic, and psychological considerations as well as surgery. Phelps emphasized the need for exercise and bracing. He began his interest in handicapped children during the period before World War II and coined the term *cerebral palsy* to distinguish the condition from mental retardation (Phelps, 1940).

The postwar years brought renewed interest in children with handicaps by a variety of community groups, including the Easter Seal Society for Crippled Children and Adults, which formed a Cerebral Palsy Division in 1946 to create a forum for sharing ideas and interdisciplinary information. Soon after, a United Cerebral Palsy Association developed chapters throughout the United States.

Almost simultaneously the American Academy for Cerebral Palsy was established in 1947 as a multidisciplinary professional organization to stimulate research and training in the field. The founders included Phelps (the first president), Crothers (neurologist), Meyer Perlstein (pediatrician), Temple Fay (neurophysiologist), George Deaver (physiatrist), and Earl Carlson (internist who also had cerebral palsy). This small group gained momentum, and by 1977 recognized the broad area of developmental disabilities to become the American Academy for Cerebral Palsy and Developmental Medicine (AACPDM) (Scherzer & Tscharnuter, 1990). In 1991, membership had grown to about 1500 professionals from almost 40 countries, including those in the major medical disciplines, with related therapy, educational, and psychological services (AACPDM, personal communication, October 14, 1991).

Treatment for cerebral palsy has moved from a rehabilitative to a habilitative approach, with early intervention essential to help each child reach a maximum level of potential in all areas of development to achieve functional independence. Technologic developments in prenatal, perinatal, and postnatal care in the last 50 years have reduced infant mortality. With more at-risk infants surviving, however, morbidity from neurologic and developmental deficits presents significant challenges to all members of transdisciplinary teams. These critically ill newborns, supported by advanced medical technology, have longer lifespans and require occupational therapy services throughout their entire lifespans (Neistadt, 1986). Adaptation to cerebral palsy and satisfaction with one's level of independence involves a process that begins early in life and continues through adulthood. It requires the establishment of satisfying routines, reliance on functional techniques and equipment, and dependence on a set of social supports. Thus, enhancement of function requires consideration of the person in daily life contexts (McCuaig & Frank, 1991).

In summation, the perception and concept of cerebral palsy have undergone a dramatic change in the 150 years since William Little first became concerned about children with deformities. Originally perceived as an orthopedic disorder with a neurologic basis, cerebral palsy has been recognized as a multihandicapping condition, a major disorder in development, and a disability emerging as the child grows. It requires early identification and management by many specialties and services (Scherzer & Tscharnuter, 1990).

Scope of cerebral palsy

Definition

The term *cerebral palsy* refers to a number of disorders of movement and posture that are due to a nonprogressive abnormality of the immature brain (Batshaw & Perret, 1986). It is a static motor impairment, occurring during the prenatal, perinatal, or postnatal period, with associated handicaps that may include vision and auditory deficits, seizures, mental retardation, learning disabilities, and feeding, speech, and behavior problems. Impairment, disability, and handicap are defined according to the *World Health Organisation Manual*. *Impairment* represents disturbance at the organ level; *disability*, the consequence of impairment for function and activity; and *handicap*, the disadvantage experienced by the person as a result of impairment and disability, thus reflecting the person's interaction with and adaptation to the environment (Wiklund & Uvebrant, 1991).

Because cerebral palsy influences the way children develop, it is known as a developmental disability. Because the disability is primarily *motor* in nature, it is distinguished from conditions such as organic brain deficits, autism, emotional disorders, or mental retardation syndromes (Gersh, 1991a; Scherzer & Tscharnuter, 1991).

Incidence and etiology

Cerebral palsy occurs in about 1 of every 500 live births (Torfs et al., 1990) with only 60% having an identifiable cause according to Hagberg's 1979 study (Batshaw & Perret, 1986). Causative factors during the first trimester may be exposure to teratogenic drugs or intrauterine infection. In later pregnancy, fetal–placental function may place the child at risk. Complications during labor, delivery, and the neonatal period are asphyxia, sepsis, and prematurity (noted in at least one third of cases). Maternal infection is a major source of fetal central nervous system pathology and includes rubella, toxoplasmosis, cytomegalovirus, herpes, and, most recently, acquired immunodeficiency syndrome (AIDS). Early childhood disorders affecting the developing brain are meningitis, toxins, and head injury (Scherzer & Tscharnuter, 1990; Batshaw & Perret, 1986). Even more recent studies have stated that about 10% of cerebral palsy is caused by *perinatal* events, 10% by *postnatal* events, and more than 75% is thought to be secondary to underlying *prenatal* influences such as central nervous system malformations, chromosomal aberrations, and congenital infections. However, definite etiologies have not been established for the majority of cerebral palsy cases believed to be of prenatal origin (Coorssen et al., 1991). Recent public health studies confirm that the strongest predictors of cerebral palsy are congenital anomalies and low birth weight that are related to prenatal factors, not to perinatal asphyxia (Torfs et al., 1990).

Comparison of normal and atypical development

Basic concepts of normal brain function

The normal developmental sequence reflects the neurophysiologic basis of an ascending development of brain center control. Initially, newborn infant behavior is largely reflexive, mediated primarily through the brain stem. However, some degree of voluntary movement is present even in the neonate. Maturation then proceeds toward higher centers, ultimately reaching independence in full voluntary control, with individualized responses replacing mass behaviors (from total motor synergies to differentiated motor patterns). Motor maturation also proceeds in a cephalo-caudal direction as well as a proximal to distal direction.

Postural control

Postural control against gravity is gained through the automatic responses of righting and equilibrium responses in a sequence relative to the three body planes: (1) sagittal, using extension and flexion against gravity; (2) frontal, using lateral flexion; and (3) transverse, using rotation within the body axis. The sequence is repeated in different positional levels: prone and supine, sitting, crawling, standing, and walking; it can be correlated to a similar sequence of vertical, horizontal, and diagonal movements in oculomotor skills, perception, and eye–hand coordination, especially in drawings.

In atypical development, important components of posture and movement are missing. Insult to the central nervous system of the neonate initially affects brain stem function, with alteration in the expression of primitive reflex behavior and delayed development of postural reactions. Muscle tone is altered—either increased or decreased. Developmental milestones are also delayed, affected by the nature and degree of the central nervous system pathology. Instead of variable and adaptive responses, stereotyped behaviors predominate. Atypical development also proceeds in a cephalo-caudal and proximal–distal direction. Postural control may be arrested at the initial stage of extension/flexion (sagittal plane), with delayed lateral righting (frontal plane) and no rotation (transverse plane). Central nervous system dysfunction is demonstrated by a lack of inhibition, resulting in total (synergic) motor patterns instead of selective, differentiated movements (Scherzer & Tscharnuter, 1990). According to Bobath (1985), the central nervous system uses lower centers (brain stem, cerebellum, midbrain, basal ganglia) to maintain posture and equilibrium. When the restraining influence of the cortex is absent, abnormal postural reflex activity is released, resulting in abnormal coordination of muscle action.

Functional skills such as self-feeding, dressing, and writing require very complex and selective patterns of muscular coordination, which depend on an intact central nervous system and a foundation of basic motor patterns acquired during early life. All movements require constant changes of posture and adjustment to the changes in the center of gravity. These automatic, unconscious shifts of postural tone are dynamic and variable, preceding movement as well as accompanying it (Bobath & Bobath, 1972). The normally developing child also finds appropriate points of stability from which he or she achieves smooth and comfortable mobility. Without these automatic postural adjustments, the child with cerebral palsy "fixes" in various parts of the body.

Table 13-5 shows a comparison of developmental postures in prone and sitting positions of a normal 3-month-old and a child with cerebral palsy whose postural patterns at the age of 10 months are delayed but fairly normal. By the time the child reaches 3 years of age, the emergence of abnormal patterns reflects this delay plus the effects of primitive reflexes and poorly regulated muscle tone. Finally, when the child reaches 11 years of age, the current functional compensatory patterns are illustrated while he operates an electronic keyboard in a prone positioner and while communicating with a lighted head pointer in his adaptive seating system.

Upper-extremity function

Upper-extremity function, such as reaching, controlled arm movements in space, and manipulative skills, requires dynamic postural stability of the shoulder girdle on a stable trunk and dissociation of movement between the head and shoulders and between the shoulders and arms. These skills develop initially during activities in weight bearing (Scherzer & Tscharnuter, 1990). Skilled arm and hand function also requires a dynamically stable sitting base, which allows weight shift during arm mobility such as reaching. Thus, all parts of the body are connected, with the pelvis as the central point. Muscle activity between the upper trunk and the pelvis and between the pelvis and the legs makes a significant impact on upper extremity function (Hypes, 1988). Poor spinal stability can result in excessive flexion or extension of trunk or legs. Asymmetry is another factor affecting postural alignment and balance throughout the body. Without good sitting balance, the hands are not free for manipulation.

Weight bearing

Efficient patterns of upper extremity weight bearing in the prone position are based on the gradually developing ability to shift weight through the trunk and pelvis in lateral as well as posterior directions. This developmental progression affects positions of the head, shoulders, arms, and hands in prone position during rest, head raising, and approach (Table 13-6). If primitive patterns are retained, arms may be posterior to the shoulders and internally rotated, and hands may be fisted with thumbs inside palms. Consequently, head control cannot develop and the arms don't begin to move separately from the shoulder girdle. Accurate reaching and fine-graded manipulative skills are impeded (Scherzer & Tscharnuter, 1990).

Reflexive patterns

Primitive reflexes and postures provide many basic sensorimotor experiences precluding volitional movements. For example, the asymmetrical tonic neck reflex (ATNR) results in the infant's first visual awareness of his or her own hand as head rotation causes extension of the arm on the face side. If the child does not achieve voluntary control, however, he or she may rely on the ATNR for stability and not develop symmetry and bilateral eye and hand function. Specific reflexes affecting prehension also prepare the infant for important developmental components of voluntary skills. For example, the grasp reflex is responsible for sustaining early grasp, allowing a toy to be brought to the mouth

TABLE 13-5.   *Normal, Delayed, and Abnormal Development and Compensatory Functional Patterns*

Position	Normal (3 months)	Delayed (10 months)	Abnormal (3 years)	Function (11 years)
Prone	Beginning head control and symmetry, elevated shoulders, arms internally rotated, hands fisted or partly open, eyes straight	Incomplete head control and symmetry, elevated shoulders, arms internally rotated, hands fisted, eyes not straight	Inadequate head control, asymmetry, elevated shoulders, wrists and hands fisted, eyes not straight (strabismus)	Independent use of electronic keyboard
Sitting	Beginning head control, sitting with trunk support, hands partly open, arms and legs abducted, general low muscle tone	Incomplete head control, sitting with trunk support, hands fisted, arms and legs adducted, low proximal muscle tone, high distal tone	Inadequate head control, sitting with trunk support, athetoid hand posturing, low proximal muscle tone, high distal tone (feet)	External head support needed for control of lighted head pointer with communication system

for exploration. The avoiding response, which causes the fingers and wrist to extend in response to light touch, helps modify the grasp reflex and allow release of an object (Twitchell, 1965, 1970). Persistence of these automatic grasping responses after 6 months, however, can prevent the development of skilled voluntary prehension. The grasp reflex interferes with release and delicate manipulation; the avoiding response interferes with sustained grasp.

Voluntary movements

Components of voluntary fine motor function described in developmental scales include items such as visual regard or inspection, approach or reach, grasp, manipulation or manual dexterity, release, and eye–hand interaction or coordination. For example, voluntary movements in the Erhardt Developmental Prehension Assessment (EDPA) are organized into sequential clusters that illustrate development from birth to 15 months. They are approach (supine, prone, sitting), grasp and release (dowel, cube, pellet), and manipulation. The 15-month level, when essential pattern components are functional, can be considered the maturity of prehension. Further refinement, in-

creased skill, and the use of tools develop through learned experiences.

Atypical development is characterized by both delays and abnormal patterns, which may be the result of gaps in sequences and combinations of pattern components from different developmental levels. For example, a common abnormal posture of cube grasp (flexed wrist and hyperextended metacarpophalangeal joints) is a combination of certain components of normal 3-month and 9-month patterns (Erhardt, 1982). Figure 13-10 (see page 448) presents some examples of these developmental sequences and typical abnormal patterns seen in children with cerebral palsy.

In-hand manipulation, which generally develops between the ages of 1 and 7 years, refers to movement of an object within a person's hand such as getting coins out of a coin purse, moving them from fingers to palm, and from palm to fingers to insert into a machine slot one at a time (Exner, 1989). The mastery of buttons, zippers, shoelaces, scissors, and other tools requires the most complex distal movement patterns of manipulation. These fine motor blends are a combination of simple patterns, performed sequentially and concurrently to complete a functional task (Boehme, 1988).

TABLE 13-6. *Developmental Progression of Upper Extremity Weight Bearing in Prone Position*

Age	At Rest and During Head-Raising	Approach
7 Months		
6 Months		
5 Months		
4 Months		
3 Months		
2 Months		
1 Month		
Natal		

(*From Erbardt, R. P. [1982]. Developmental hand dysfunction: Theory assessment, and treatment (pp. 51, 57). Tucson, AZ: Therapy Skill Builders.*)

Eye–hand coordination

Eye movements generally precede hand movements to visual targets, providing both quantitative and qualitative visual information to guide the hand accurately to the target. At the same time, coordinated hand movements influence the eyes, as both systems exchange information needed for adaptation to rapidly changing environmental conditions (Erhardt, 1992). Visual–motor function, or oculomotor control, develops rapidly during the first 6 months of life, as primitive ocular reflexes become integrated and voluntary eye movements reach a stage of maturity nearly identical with that of the adult. Eye–hand interaction occurs not only during visual localization and reaching toward an object, but also during fixation upon grasp and tracking during manipulation (Erhardt, 1990). The coordination of hand and eye depends first on the control of the head, enabling the eyes to monitor the task of the hands. A stable shoulder girdle then dictates the effectiveness of the arm in transporting the hand to its task and maintaining it during manipulation (Penso, 1990). The functional role of the hand, accomplished through combined movements of the forearm, wrist, and the dynamic palmar arches, is to shape itself around the viewed object (Boehme, 1988). Atypical motor development can dramatically affect function of the eyes and hands and their interactions.

Grasp of the pencil and other utensils

During the early use of writing implements, only the crayon tip touches the page, while the arm and hand move unanchored through space to produce exploratory scribbles. The trunk and shoulder provide internal stability for crude arm mobility. Later, the forearm glides on the surface (external stabilization) as more definitive strokes are made. Next, the wrist and forearm stabilize on the surface, and the hand's movement creates recognizable drawings. Finally, with maturity, the hand itself stabilizes, allowing finger movement dissociated from the metacarpophalangeal (MCP) joints for precise, small productions of drawings, letters, and numbers. This progression of the stabilizing point of external control from proximal to distal joints has been correlated with the developmental progression of crayon or pencil grasp in the Erhardt Developmental Prehension Assessment (EDPA) (Erhardt, 1982). Table 13-7 illustrates this sequence from 1 to 6 years and a common atypical grasp in children with cerebral palsy.

The relationships between external/internal and proximal/distal stability have important clinical implications. Although all prehension components, normally acquired by 15 months, are present and functional, demands for high-level manipulation skills and writing still require adequate external support in normal children. Children with cerebral palsy, who lack some of these developmental components, regulate muscle tone poorly and don't use automatic points of stability such as the other arm on the surface or the feet on the floor and revert to more primitive patterns due to stress (Erhardt, 1982; Hirschel et al., 1990).

Types and classifications of cerebral palsy

Uniformity of diagnostic description of cerebral palsy has been controversial, since many different professionals attempted to provide an understanding of cerebral palsy and give direction to treatment and management. In 1956, the American Academy for

TABLE 13-7. *Normal and Abnormal Development of Crayon or Pencil Grasp*

Dynamic Tripod Posture
4½–6 Years

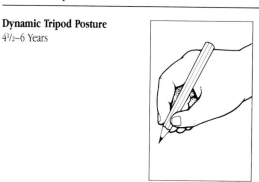

Static Tripod Posture
3½–4 Years

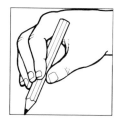

Digital–Pronate Grasp
2–3 Years

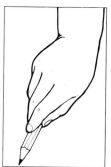

Palmar–Supinate Grasp
1–1½ Years

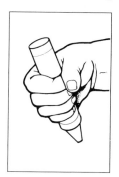

Abnormal Pattern

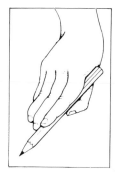

(From Erhardt, R. P. [1982]. Developmental hand dysfunction: Theory, assessment, and treatment (pp. 43, 65). Tucson, AZ: Therapy Skill Builders.)

Cerebral Palsy accepted a classification prepared by Minear, which included not only eight motor types, but also, for the first time, distribution and degree of involvement (mild, moderate, severe). Categories according to muscle tone were (1) spasticity, (2) athetosis, (3) rigidity, (4) ataxia, (5) tremor, (6) atonia, (7) mixed, and (8) unclassified (Scherzer & Tscharnuter, 1990). Categories according to distribution and location of involvement in the body included:

Monoplegia—one extremity (arm or leg)
Hemiplegia—upper and lower extremity on one side
Paraplegia—both lower extremities
Diplegia—both upper and lower extremities, with mild upper involvement (Gersh, 1991a; Scherzer & Tscharnuter, 1990).
Quadriplegia—equal involvement of both upper and lower extremities

Because Minear's classification was published 35 years ago, when cerebral palsy was diagnosed late on the basis of a fixed motor deficit, some recent efforts have been made to consider early signs of development and emerging motor characteristics in more flexible classification systems. A diagnosis of cerebral palsy in the very young child is formulated on the basis of developmental history, abnormal tone, and reflex behavior. In the older child (beyond 1 year), the diagnosis can indicate a specific motor type, which is emerging but also changing. As the child grows, the extent and degree of involvement can be specified (Scherzer & Tscharnuter, 1990). As indicated in Table 13-5, the younger child demonstrates developmental delay with fairly normal patterns, which become more abnormal as the child gets older and develops compensatory patterns for function.

Many physicians, however, still use the classification in Hagberg's 1979 study as a basis for diagnosis (Batshaw & Perret, 1986). It groups cerebral palsy into three broad types, according to the location of brain damage:

Pyramidal type. About 50% of all children with cerebral palsy have spasticity caused by damage to either the motor cortex, which controls voluntary movement, or the pyramidal tracts, which link the cortex with nerves in the spinal cord that relay signals to the muscles. Hypertonia (high muscle tone) is often accompanied by persistent primitive reflexes, an exaggerated stretch reflex, and clonus (rapid and rhythmic involuntary muscle contractions, usually in the ankles).
Extrapyramidal type. About 25% of all children with cerebral palsy have involuntary movements caused by damage to the cerebellum or basal ganglia, which process signals from the motor cortex to achieve smooth, coordinated movements and to maintain posture. Fluctuating muscle tone and purposeless movements interfere with skills requiring coordination such as feeding, talking, reaching, grasping, and manipulation. Different types of involuntary extrapyramidal movements have been further classified as (1) chorea (abrupt, jerky), (2) athetosis (slow, writhing), (3) dystonia (slow, rhythmic), (4) ataxia (incoordination, imbalance), and (5) rigidity ("lead-pipe").
Mixed type. Mixed type cerebral palsy is present in about 25% of the children, who have both high muscle tone and involuntary movements due to lesions in both pyramidal and extrapyramidal areas of the brain (Batshaw & Perret, 1986; Gersh, 1991a).

Consequences of atypical neurologic development

For children with cerebral palsy, *quality of development* is just as important or even more important as the *rate of development*, which depends on the type and severity of their impairments (Blacklin, 1991). Factors interfering with quality of posture and movement are primitive reflex activity, abnormal muscle tone, and sensory deficits, which lead to compensations and deformities.

Primitive reflex activity

The persistence of reflexes, which influence muscle tone and limb movements, is one of the chief diagnostic signs of cerebral palsy. Instead of being gradually integrated into voluntary movement as the infant matures, these primitive patterns are stronger and longer-lasting. They cause stereotyped, obligatory postures and movements, which are incompatible with higher level automatic balance reactions and eventually complex motor skills (Batshaw & Perret, 1986). It is difficult, however, to isolate the various reflexes in children with cerebral palsy, since their volitional efforts to move complicate the total picture. For that reason, Bobath (1985, May) stated that she no longer tested for reflexes, but preferred to examine the individual patterns of hypertonus and its interference with normal activity.

Abnormal muscle tone

Spasticity, or hypertonia, affects movement because the increase in tone creates an imbalance between muscle groups. The spastic child has difficulty with transitions (moving from one position to another). Gross and fine motor movements are slow and require excessive effort. Restricted range of motion and limited manipulation delays the development of play and self-care skills.

Flaccidity, or hypotonia, affects movement because the decreased tone and lack of joint integrity do not provide a balance of stability and mobility for almost all postures and motor control, especially those against gravity. Many flaccid infants develop spasticity later as they recruit excessive tone in their attempts to move or maintain postures.

Athetosis is characterized by fluctuating muscle tone and poor midrange control. Co-contraction is lacking in proximal joints; thus, distal control is difficult such as fixation of head and trunk for activities requiring eye–hand coordination.

Muscle tone abnormalities are determined by observation of body posture and movement. Hypertonia is characterized by too much resistance to movement, hypotonia by too little resistance, and fluctuating tone shifts between both.

Children may also have combinations of muscle tone and movement disorders, requiring the occupational therapist to be aware of the type and distribution in different parts of the body. For example, when planning treatment, it should be noted that mobility is needed for areas with hypertonia, and stability is needed for areas with fluctuating tone (Powell, 1985; Fraser et al., 1990).

Sensory deficits

Interpreting and using information from the senses may be impaired. The most common problems are with touch, position, movement, and balance. Tactile hypersensitivity or defensiveness can cause withdrawal or agitation to normal touch and can cause intolerance to restricted positioning. Hyposensitivity can result in delayed or diminished responses to the tactile stimulation of touch, temperature, and pain as well as an inability to process sensory stimuli (Fraser et al., 1990; Foltz et al., 1991). In a study of tactile preferences for hard or soft objects, children with cerebral palsy and normal children were compared. The apparent preference of children with cerebral palsy for hard objects suggested that they needed greater proprioceptive input because of decreased tactile awareness (Curry & Exner, 1988).

Compensations and effects on function

Persons with multiple handicaps develop habitual patterns of flexion or extension synergies, which limit isolated, selective movements. Sustained postural abnormalities lead to soft tissue imbalances, eventually resulting in contractures and skeletal deformities.

"Tailbone sitting," a common pattern in spastic diplegia, originates with the lack of automatic balance reactions and postural control in this higher-gravity position. Limited range of motion between the legs and hips also interferes with upright sitting. Compensatory kyphosis (rounding of the back) and increased tightness in anterior flexors (neck, trunk, extremities) become secondary problems. Figures 13-1 and 13-2 compare the sitting positions of a normal 3-year-old and her twin sister who has spastic diplegia.

Figure 13-3 illustrates arm and hand patterns in a child with athetosis and spasticity; asymmetry is demonstrated during reaching with retraction of the opposite arm and shoulder. During bilateral manipulation (Figure 13-4), the child's flexor

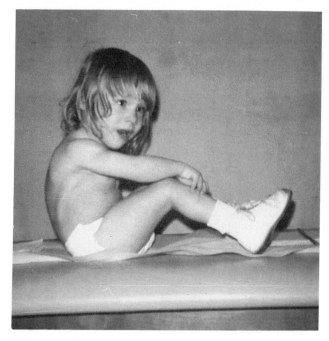

FIGURE 13-2. *The "tailbone" sitting position, common in spastic diplegia.*

synergies are expressed in elevated shoulders, rounded spine, internal rotation of arms and legs, and flexion of elbow and wrist joints. Because his flexed wrist prevents him from resting his right arm and hand on the table surface, he finds stability instead with his fingers, hyperextended at the MCP joints. The subluxed proximal joint of his right thumb is further evidence of this instability and underlying low muscle tone. Figure 13-5 shows the use of a commercial corner seat to provide trunk

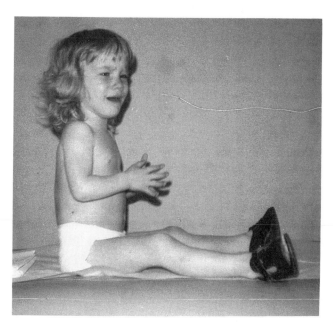

FIGURE 13-1. *A normal sitting position.*

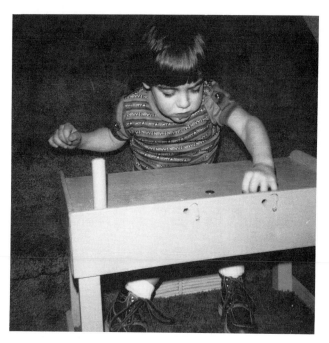

FIGURE 13-3. *Retraction of opposite arm and shoulder during reaching. (Courtesy of Therapy Skill Builders.)*

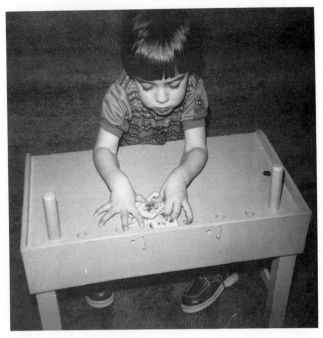

FIGURE 13-4. *Atypical patterns during manipulation.* (*Courtesy of Therapy Skill Builders.*)

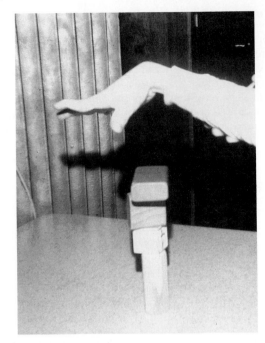

FIGURE 13-6. *Compensatory hand posture used for function.*

support, a low bench to keep legs apart, and dowels to normalize hand patterns during grasp for stabilization (right hand) and release (left hand).

Figure 13-6 shows the flexed wrist used for stability during approach, necessitating hyperextension of the MCP and proximal interphalangeal (PIP) joints to open the hand and prepare for grasp with the flexed distal phalangeal (DP) joints. Table 13-8 illustrates the effects of different types of cerebral palsy on

muscle tone, movement, and personality as well as general needs of these children.

Disorders associated with cerebral palsy

Feeding problems

Difficulties with feeding are often one of the first signs of cerebral palsy, because the young baby is unable to coordinate sucking and swallowing, to tolerate solid food textures, and to successfully bite and chew a variety of foods (Blacklin, 1991). Primitive oral and general reflexes such as rooting, biting, and the ATNR are not integrated; thus, involuntary movements predominate over voluntary ones. Oral–motor function is also affected by problems with sensory integration and muscle tone, not only in the mouth area, but also throughout the trunk because of the respiratory support needed for feeding as well as speech (Foltz et al., 1991).

Gastroesophageal reflux (GER) is a condition in which food and stomach acid juices back up from the stomach after meals. It may cause pain, vomiting, or aspiration into the lungs. Contributing factors to constipation, another major digestive problem, are inactivity, inadequate fluid and fiber intake, and poor rectal sphincter control (Batshaw & Perret, 1986).

Visual problems

Visual impairments can result from problems with any part of the visual system, including the eyes, eye muscles, optic nerve, and areas of the cerebral cortex that process visual information (Gersh, 1991b). Optic nerve damage, visual field losses, and cataracts are common in premature infants with retinopathy of prematurity (ROP). Children with cerebral palsy exhibit a variety of problems with acuity and focusing, ocular motor performance, and visual perception (Duckman, 1984).

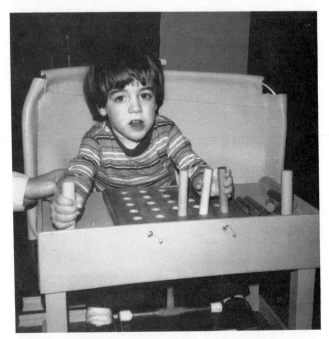

FIGURE 13-5. *External supports to normalize hand patterns during grasp and release.*

TABLE 13-8. *Effects of Cerebral Palsy*

Type	Muscle Tone	Movement	Personality	Needs
Spastic (hypertonic)	Ranging from normal to very high, depending on stimulation	Small, labored, limited, in midrange only, not selective, abnormally learned	Fearful, stereotyped responses, difficulty adapting to change, perseveration	Assistance to achieve movement, strong but graded stimulation, time to adjust, avoid excessive effort
Flaccid (hypotonic)	Very low tone with intermittent extensor tone, sinks into gravity in all positions	No co-contraction, full range but not used, hypermobile joints	Happy and comfortable, high pain threshold, slow response time, not motivated to move, limited interaction with environment	Head control, stimulate to increase muscle tone and initiate effort, slow and steady handling, wait for reaction, developmental sequences
Athetoid	Fluctuating from low to normal or low to high	Extreme ranges, no midrange grading, no fixation, large jerky movements, uses asymmetry for stability	Unstable, immature, happy, friendly, fearless, sudden mood swings	Stability, control of entire body, symmetry, reduce movement, avoid overstimulation
Athetoid with spasticity	Moderately high, ranging from normal to high	Poor control in midrange, poor selective movements	Similar to Spastic, but more fearless and adaptable	Balance, symmetry, midrange control of head, shoulders, and arms
Ataxic	Low or ranging from low to normal	No sustained postural control or fixation, normal but primitive coordination	Same as Athetoid	Sustained posture

(From Bobath, B. [1977, October/November]. NDT 8-week certification course. London. Unpublished material.)

Acuity

Almost 75% of children with cerebral palsy have refractive errors including nearsightedness or farsightedness and astigmatism. Cortical visual impairment, especially common in infants with ROP, is defined as partial or total blindness due to injury in the visual pathways or visual cortex of the brain, rather than in the eye itself (Erhardt, 1990; Gersh, 1991a, 1991b).

Ocular motor control

Parents of children with cerebral palsy and other movement disorders have often been aware, even during the first year, that "something was wrong" with their child's eyes. Some of the comments parents tell therapists later are, "His eyes weren't always straight, especially when he was tired"; "She didn't always notice me when I was across the room"; "He wasn't interested in books and pictures"; "She seemed to ignore everything on one side of her body"; "He never watched his hands." Yet, they are told by eye doctors that their child is too young to test, or, if tested, that the eyes are fine with normal acuity.

New techniques do allow more precise testing of infants and young children. Visual acuity, which relies on the accommodative system to bring objects at specified distances into focus, is only part of the vision process, however. The six eye muscles, which are constantly locating, watching, and following objects, are part of the body's neuromuscular system. Thus, cerebral palsy may cause eye muscles to be stiff and slow-moving (spastic) or constantly in motion (athetoid). Visual development may be delayed with visual reflexes still active and voluntary movement patterns still primitive.

Table 13-9 shows examples of normal visual–motor levels and warning signs of delays. By 6 months, the normal infant's visual–motor control is almost identical with that of an adult. Visual reflexes are integrated; that is, they do not interfere with voluntary eye movements. Localization, fixation, ocular pursuit, and gaze shift are accurate, efficient, and effortless. There is

always cause for concern if these 6-month milestones have not been achieved by 1 year.

Coordination of eye muscles is usually related to neuromuscular function in the entire body. Thus, children with delayed integration of general primitive reflexes such as the ATNR may also show delayed integration of visual reflexes. For example, a child with severe cerebral palsy may use the ATNR position for stability to look at and reach for an object. A child with spasticity may use a total flexor synergy for a functional task such as writing, and has slow, difficult eye movements within a limited range. Even an older child with mild cerebral palsy and imperfect head control may use primitive patterns such as asymmetrical neck extension to gain stability for a high-level motor and cognitive task such as reading, which requires eye movements dissociated from head movements. These oculomotor problems, related to muscle imbalance, are manifested by conditions such as strabismus (misalignment), amblyopia (lazy eye), and nystagmus (involuntary movements) (Erhardt, 1990).

Visual perception

The process of obtaining information from the environment is defined as visual perception, which includes discrimination, memory, spatial relationships, form constancy, sequential memory, figure–ground, and closure. Occupational therapists are frequently the professionals designated to assess and treat children with visual–perceptual problems. Children with cerebral palsy and normal intelligence have been found to score significantly lower than normal children on motor-free tests of visual–perceptual skills (Menken et al., 1987).

Auditory problems

Two types of hearing impairments, sensorineural and conductive, reduce the level of a child's sound perception; these impairments range from mild to profound. Sensorineural loss is due to

TABLE 13-9. *Guidelines for Visual-Motor Development and Signs of Delay*

Between Birth and 6 Months	By 6 Months to 1 Year	Signs of Delays
Localization of Faces		
Not consistent	Consistent	Looks at parent's face briefly or not at all
Binocular Fixation		
Not consistent	Consistent	One eye turns in or out
Eyes Follow Moving Target While Head Remains Still		
Eyes and head move together	Eyes move separately from head	Eyes and head always move together
Eyes Watch Hands		
Eyes watch only one hand	Eyes watch both hands	Eyes do not watch hands or watch only one hand; eyes and hands cannot come to midline
Downward Gaze		
Asymmetrical neck extension	Neck elongation and controlled chin tuck in midline	Cannot use downward gaze in prone and sitting

(Adapted from Erhardt, Winter 1991–1992.)

damage in the inner ear, the auditory nerve, or both. It may be hereditary or congenital (present at birth) or acquired later in childhood from meningitis, high fever, or medications. Conductive loss is due to middle ear conditions (anatomic malformations or infections). Middle ear fluid, which accompanies colds or allergies, can cause temporary hearing loss at a critical time during early speech and language development in the first 3 years of life (Gersh, 1991b).

Speech problems

Muscle tone problems in the entire body influence oral–motor control, movements of jaw, lips, tongue, and facial muscles used in speaking. Trunk muscles of respiration are often inadequate, interfering with breath control for volume and articulation. These children show early feeding problems, since the same muscles are involved (Gersh, 1991a). The development of a progressive interaction between stability and mobility, characteristic of all sensorimotor behavior, is also reflected in the oral–pharyngeal system through development in the first 3 years. Positional or external stability is provided, as one body part is steadied against another body part or external source. Postural or internal stability is more dynamic, achieved through control of paired muscles and possible during movement. For example, the normal infant stabilizes the mouth on a toy as the tongue and lips explore it. The older child stabilizes with jaw muscles while the lips and tongue articulate words. The child with cerebral palsy lacks midrange jaw control and dissociated movements of the lips and tongue needed for feeding and speech (Morris, 1982).

Mental retardation

Most people define intelligence as the ability to reason, think, and solve problems. However, it also reflects the ability to take care of oneself in the world and behave in socially appropriate ways. Standardized tests are used to measure intelligence (IQ score), with scores between 70 and 130 considered normal. In the United States, about 3% of all children and 25% of children with cerebral palsy are said to have mental retardation, or scores below 70. Estimates vary because testing is often done with tests that are inappropriate for children who cannot talk or control their hands to respond correctly. The wide range of retardation means that the ability to learn varies greatly, although generally children with mental retardation learn new skills more slowly than other children, may not be as motivated, and do not generalize new skills to similar but not identical situations (Gersh, 1991a). See Chapter 13, Section 1 for a more detailed discussion of mental retardation.

Seizure disorders

About 50% of children with cerebral palsy have **seizures**, involuntary movements or changes in consciousness or behavior caused by abnormal electrical activity in the brain. Seizures may be *partial* or *generalized*, and can affect the motor, sensory, and autonomic systems. For example, motor symptoms include jerking of muscle groups or an extremity. Sensory seizures cause visual or auditory hallucinations or disturbances of taste or smell. The autonomic system reacts with rapid heartbeat, sweating, pallor, flushing, or anxiety.

New terminology for generalized seizures (with previous terms in parentheses) includes the following:

Absence (petit mal)—brief, abrupt loss of consciousness for a few seconds, associated with staring or eye blinking, followed by rapid, complete recovery

Infantile myoclonic (infantile)—sudden, brief, involuntary muscle contractions, producing head drops and flexion of extremities (jackknife)

Tonic-clonic (grand mal)—muscle stiffening and falling into unconsciousness (tonic phase), followed by rhythmic jerking (clonic phase), breathing problems, drooling, and loss of bladder control, and finally confusion and sleepiness. A tonic-clonic seizure brought on by fever is called a *febrile seizure*, common in young children (Gersh, 1991b).

See Chapter 13, Section 7 for a more detailed discussion of seizure disorders.

Health-related procedures for medically fragile children

Schools are experiencing an increase in the number of students with multiple and severe handicaps who require medical and health-related procedures during the school day. Because of federal legislation in 1978, which inaugurated policies of mainstreaming and inclusion, these medically fragile children are remaining at home in their own communities instead of in institutions, and often attend neighborhood schools. Therapists and teachers are dealing with issues that have been relegated exclusively to nurses and physicians in the past. For example, a survey revealed that in more than 80% of these classrooms, procedures related to seizure problems, such as administration of medication, seizure monitoring, and emergency measures, were the responsibility of teachers and other classroom staff. Other health-related procedures, with school nurses also involved, were postural drainage, shunt care, nasogastric tube and gastrostomy feeding, prosthesis care, catheterization, machine and syringe suctioning, and tracheostomy care. As policies evolve that define the roles of professionals in these new situations, occupational therapists must become knowledgeable about these serious medical conditions and aware of their effects on function (Mulligan-Ault et al., 1988).

Assessment

Comprehensive assessment of the child with cerebral palsy requires consideration of both the child and the environment as a single unit. This ecologic assessment process places equal importance on information gathered from interviews, checklists, and observations of the child functioning within his or her environment, as well as from tests. Observations, when used properly, are a nonbiased reporting method of the child's interaction with the environment, either animate (people) or inanimate (objects) (Huber & King-Thomas, 1987).

Developmental skills have always been the most important aspect in assessment of young children. In the 1950s, early developmental scales addressed gross motor, fine motor, communication, adaptive, and social skills, emphasizing developmental milestones. In the last 40 years, with the technologic advances of modern medicine, younger infants with more severe handicaps have survived, and therapists have had to consider the quality as well as the quantity of milestones achieved. The biologic and social sciences foundation of occupational therapists allows for expansion of the developmental scales to include both motor and sensory components of movement, play, and self-help skills, and thus a broader perspective on the child's function within his or her environment (Mather & Weinstein, 1988).

Evaluations must not only describe the neurologic deficits, but also the functional consequences of those deficits. Management of the young child in particular should be analyzed in terms of handling, positioning, bathing, dressing, and feeding. As the child matures, evaluation procedures need to expand to include function in the school and community (Scherzer & Tscharnuter, 1990). Assessment is most useful if it leads directly to treatment, and "treatment is ongoing assessment," according to Barbro Salek (Mather & Weinstein, 1988, p. 5).

Tests and evaluation instruments

Observable quantified behaviors can be measured by standardized instruments such as the Bayley Scales of Infant Development (Bayley, 1969) and the Peabody Developmental Motor Scales (Folio & Fewell, 1983). These scales measure gross motor abilities such as balance and strength, and skills such as sitting and walking; fine motor abilities measured include manual dexterity and eye–hand coordination, and skills such as stacking blocks and drawing (Stewart et al., 1988). Although the use of standardized tests prevents unreliability in judgment, relatively few pediatric therapists use them in clinical practice because the goals of developmental therapy are to make qualitative improvements in movement patterns, or to accomplish specific functional objectives. Such outcome measures are not reflected on standardized motor tests, which do not always assess quality of movement, identify improvement in children who change slowly, and measure functional skills (Harris, 1988; Campbell, 1990). Also, most of these tests rely on the child's ability to execute verbal and/or motor responses and are not appropriate for those who are nonverbal or physically handicapped, or both. Modification of standardized tests, however, renders the standardization meaningless (Hacker & Porter, 1987).

Thus, many therapists rely on a variety of detailed nonstandardized evaluations of muscle tone, reflex patterns, motor development, and sensory status, as well as their observations of spontaneous behaviors (Cook, 1991). For example, Mary Fiorentino's pioneering work has helped therapists identify specific reflexes and expectations for emergence and integration (Fiorentino, 1973). Sarah Semans developed a cerebral palsy assessment chart, which scored the child's ability to be placed, sustain, and assume different postures against gravity (Semans, 1965a, 1965b). The Gesell Developmental Scales have been used by many therapists to assess adaptive, language, and personal–social areas as well as gross and fine motor levels (Knobloch et al., 1980). The Erhardt Developmental Prehension Assessment measures involuntary (positional reflexive) and voluntary (cognitively directed) arm–hand patterns from the prenatal period to 15 months, and pencil grasp/prewriting skills from 1 to 6 years (Erhardt, 1982). Prefeeding skills and oral–motor function can be assessed within the framework of therapeutic feeding programs developed by professionals such as physical therapists, nurses, physicians, dietitians, and nutritionists as well as occupational therapists (Smith et al., 1982; Morris, 1982; Morris & Klein, 1987; Fee et al., 1988; Jelm, 1990).

Age-appropriate functional skills also need to be assessed. For example, the Pediatric Assessment of Self-Care Activities scores the child's degree of independence according to defined developmental sequences of feeding, toileting, hygiene, and dressing, including the use of fasteners (Coley, 1978). The Preschool Play Scale measures abilities such as exploration, imitation, participation, and management of materials and space (Knox, 1974).

Comprehensive evaluations are needed when equipment needs to be prescribed. For example, positioning for adaptive seating devices requires assessment of the following:

1. Medical and surgical history (for considerations of skin condition, allergies, continence, respiratory status)
2. Muscle tone, skeletal alignment, and postural control (levels of passive and active movement, effects of reflexes and external stimuli, contractures and deformities)
3. Functional skills (compensatory patterns, additional equipment to interface with wheelchair, transfers, propulsion)
4. Cognitive, behavioral, and communication status (safety awareness, perception, receptive and expressive interactions)
5. Goals of both the person and the team, and the current environment (therapy restrictions, accessibility, acceptance, maintenance, transportation; Bergen et al., 1990)

Finally, other transdisciplinary team members contribute important information about vision, hearing, speech, social/emotional adjustment, and cognition, which must be synthesized with that describing the child's physical condition and skill levels (Scherzer & Tscharnuter, 1990).

Assessment/intervention models

Practical models incorporating assessment and intervention can be useful in programs that address functional and environmental issues. For example, the Family Daily Routine model was developed in 1979 at the University of Wisconsin, Department of Rehabilitation Psychology and Special Education. Its purpose was to facilitate communication among parents, teachers, and therapists in collaborative home–school partnerships by providing a base of information for structuring an appropriate home program (Rainforth & Salisbury, 1988). Another model based on both developmental and functional approaches is presented in Table 13-10, which considers the child's intrinsic motivation in the context of cognitive and play developmental levels. Exploratory stages of visual and tactile behaviors lead to eye–hand interaction, and ultimately to purposeful, goal-directed activities. These eye–hand skills are achieved through developmentally targeted interventions and functionally appropriate adaptations (Erhardt, 1992). See Chapter 7 for a more detailed discussion of occupational therapy assessment.

Overview of treatment methods for cerebral palsy

Intervention approaches have been grouped in various categories. For example, Schmoll described four groups: *neuromotor*, emphasizing neurophysiologic and developmental sequences as the foundation for motor learning; *functional*, stressing the

TABLE 13-10. *An Operational Model for Eye–Hand Coordination Intervention*

System Components	Developmentally Targeted Interventions	Functionally Appropriate Adaptations
Cognitive motivation	Piaget's schemas, developmental play sequences	Adapted age-appropriate toys, switches, adapted positioning
Visual exploration	Environmental awareness (near, middle, and far space, central and peripheral fields), linkage with other stimuli (sound, movement)	Adapted materials, lighting, and positioning (trunk support for eye–head mobility, head support for eye mobility)
Tactile exploration	Developmental sequences of approach, grasp, manipulation, release; touching objects within reach, experiencing size, shape, texture, temperature	Adapted materials, equipment, and positioning (trunk support for arm mobility, table surface for hand/finger control)
Eye–hand interaction	Visually directed exploration, repetition, adaptation	Adapted seating and positioning to ensure both hand and object in visual field, appropriate proximal stability for distal mobility
Purposeful activity	Goal-directed, problem-solving manipulation, self-help activities, tool use, pre-writing developmental sequences	Adapted utensils, task analysis, graded work surfaces, low-tech aids, high-tech electronic equipment

(*From Erhardt, R. P. [1992]. Eye–hand coordination. In J. Case-Smith & C. Peboski (Eds.). Development of hand skills in the child (p. 23). Rockville, MD: American Occupational Therapy Association.*)

improvement of the person's functional skills within his or her own environment; *psychoeducational*, based on the theory that sensorimotor development is a necessary foundation for learning; and *orthopedic*, using orthoses, casting, and surgery to improve musculoskeletal structure and function (Fraser et al., 1990). These theoretical approaches are usually combined, with emphasis on a specific approach depending on the person's age, severity of condition, and cognitive level. Thus, the younger child with a mild handicap would benefit most from neuromotor and psychoeducational approaches, whereas the older more severely affected child with structural deformities would need functional and orthopedic approaches.

Historically, physicians such as Crothers, Phelps, and Deaver were proponents of orthopedic methods, especially surgery. Certain principles they developed continue to be a basic guide for current acceptable methods. For example, Crothers stressed the need for active movement and urged independence rather than overprotection. Phelps was the first to develop a systematic treatment approach, involving sensory as well as motor stimulation. Deaver emphasized function in activities of daily living. Fay, a neurophysiologist, postulated the concept of ontogeny recapitulating phylogeny, that is, motor development following the evolutionary process. Doman, a physical therapist, and his partner Delacato integrated these concepts into their method of "patterning," which became one of the more controversial treatment methods.

Kabat and Knott used "proprioceptive neuromuscular facilitation" to increase voluntary muscle contraction through central excitation. Exercises were designed to use large diagonal movements, required cooperation from the patient, and thus were not always as useful in pediatric practice (Scherzer & Tscharnuter, 1990).

Margaret Rood, an occupational therapist, encouraged developmental patterns of movement after activating muscles through sensory receptors, using heat or cold accompanied by stroking or brushing selected areas on specific muscle groups. Her work has been continued and expanded by Wilbarger (1984), who treats sensory processing problems by planning an adequate "sensory diet," especially during the first year of life. Shereen Farber (1982) also incorporated Rood's techniques in an eclectic sensorimotor approach based on the works of A. Jean Ayres; Karel and Berta Bobath; Signe Brunnstrom; Herman Kabat, Margaret Knott, and Dorothy Voss; A. Joy Huss; and others.

In clinical treatment situations, many therapists prefer an eclectic approach, choosing a variety of modalities from established theoretical bases and individualizing each program according to the child's changing needs as well as their own professional strengths. Although this approach is flexible and effective, it causes problems for efficacy research, which requires uniformity and systematic identification of procedures (Scherzer & Tscharnuter, 1990).

Current theoretical models

Neurodevelopmental treatment

The ***neurodevelopmental treatment*** (NDT) approach was originated in England in 1943 by Berta Bobath, a physiotherapist, in collaboration with her husband, Dr. Karel Bobath, who helped develop the knowledge base of normal and abnormal movement and the neurophysiologic rationale for the clinical results of the treatment. According to information distributed by the Neuro-Developmental Treatment Association (based in the United States), NDT is a form of therapy used with persons who have central nervous system disorders resulting in abnormal posture and movement. The treatment approach attempts to initiate or refine the normal stages and processes in the development of movement. Specific handling techniques as well as adaptive equipment are used to achieve inhibition of abnormal patterns, normalization of muscle tone, and facilitation of more normal movement. These techniques vary according to different therapists and the needs of different children, but the theory of NDT remains relatively constant. The following are its main principles:

1. The damaged central nervous system blocks normal movement.
2. Abnormal muscle tone results in abnormal patterns of posture and movement.
3. These abnormal patterns affect all function, including respiration, speech, feeding, perception, self-care, and walking.
4. Because the basis of movement is sensation, change requires the person to *feel* more normal movements.

5. Optimal gains are achieved only with an interdisciplinary effort that includes the patient, family, physician, therapists, and teachers.

During a symposium in Neuro-Developmental Treatment in the United States in 1985, Berta Bobath reviewed the changes in NDT during the past 40 years. She stressed that although the emphasis on various aspects has shifted and that much was learned from other professionals such as Kabat, Rood, and Peto, the basic concept remained the same. The most significant changes were related to the need for more direct transition of treatment into functional activities. This was best accomplished by observing the child during everyday activities to assess his or her abilities and disabilities and by treating the child in functional situations in home and school to ensure carryover (Bobath, 1985, May).

The concept that movements range from "least automatic" to "most automatic" has been useful in explaining the NDT approach to therapeutic handling, which attempts to obtain active, automatic movements from the child, leading to voluntary, purposeful movements. Although the child is responding automatically rather than volitionally, he or she is not passive. The child gains normal sensorimotor feedback from active movements, achieved without excessive effort. Through expert handling, normal patterns of movement are facilitated, and abnormal patterns are inhibited. For example, in Figure 13-7 the child responds to lateral movement of the carpeted barrel with automatic righting reactions of head and trunk while the therapist helps him achieve elongation of his weight-bearing side. The next step is active elongation through reaching forward and upward to bring in rotation as well.

The role of occupational therapy in NDT emphasizes upper body control and acquisition of hand skills for self-care, academics, leisure, and community activities, leading to as much independence as possible. Handling techniques are designed to normalize muscle tone and obtain postural alignment throughout the entire body and to prepare upper and lower extremities for weight bearing, weight shifting, and function (Foltz et al., 1991).

Neurodevelopmental treatment has also been combined with sensory integration treatment, since both approaches address adaptive responses of the person and use sensory input to produce the motor response. Main differences are that NDT focuses on the motor output, the production of motor control, whereas sensory integration focuses on the sensory processing aspect (Blanche & Burke, 1991).

Sensory integration therapy

Sensory integration (SI) therapy is a treatment approach developed by occupational therapist A. Jean Ayres. Sensory integration is the organization and processing of sensory information from the different sensory channels, and the ability to relate input from one channel to that of another to emit an adaptive response (Dunn, 1987). Information from three basic senses (touch, movement, position) is used to plan and sequence movements, to coordinate both sides of the body, to develop balance, to coordinate eye and hand movements, and to develop body awareness. Many children with cerebral palsy have problems receiving and processing sensory input, which results in (1) hypersensitivity or hyposensitivity to touch (tactile system), (2) gravitational insecurity (vestibular system), and (3) motor planning problems (dyspraxia) (Foltz et al., 1991).

Treatment principles for sensory integrative deficits include (1) to normalize sensory input, (2) to consider development in terms of the stability/mobility spiral process, (3) to determine effectiveness by the child's response, and (4) to require the child to be an active participant, responding appropriately as he or she achieves mastery over movement and the environment (Dunn, 1987).

Treatment techniques for *tactile problems* focus on providing a combination of exploratory and structured play experiences, which assist in sensory modulation for the child who is overreacting or underreacting to tactile stimulation. Activities may include firm, deep pressure through weight bearing on different parts of the body or rolling while wrapped in a blanket.

Vestibular problems in children with cerebral palsy respond well to a combination of SI and NDT approaches. For example, a child who needs and enjoys rough housing with a parent may become more spastic, with legs stiffening in extension and adduction. The therapist will recommend that this play be continued, but with the child's legs straddling the parent's leg or waist to keep them straight and apart.

Children with *dyspraxia* have trouble planning movements and putting them into complex sequences, which affects their ability to move from one position to another, to construct a drawing, and to manipulate buttons (Foltz et al., 1991).

Therapy aims to increase registration and integration of sensory input (especially tactile), to develop mature postural control and movement patterns, and to improve body scheme. This is achieved by providing constantly changing activities that require the child to be adaptive and goal-directed. Ideation and organization can be improved in a dressing activity, for example, if the child is asked to verbalize (talk his way through the movement sequences). The therapist can provide guidance and modeling when needed (Ellig, personal communication, December 16, 1991).

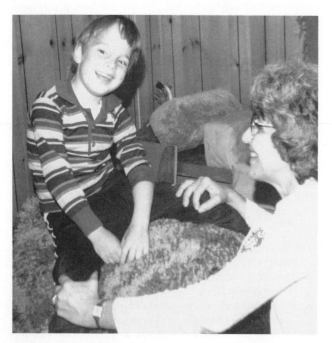

FIGURE 13-7. *Automatic righting reactions and elongation of the weight-bearing side.*

Relationship of occupational therapy to other treatment modalities

Medication

The use of drugs for problems associated with cerebral palsy has a relatively recent and not always successful history. Muscle relaxants and tranquilizers—oral, rectal, and injected—have shown some limited benefit in reducing muscle tone and involuntary movement but may also show certain side effects such as drowsiness, disorientation, weakness, nausea, headaches, and increased drooling (Albright et al., 1991; Armstrong et al., 1991). Seizure medication, of course, has played a significant and essential role in management. Drugs for attentional deficits, hyperactivity, and severe emotional disturbances have been useful, especially in preparing the child to obtain maximum participation and benefit from therapy and education (Scherzer & Tscharnuter, 1990; Batshaw & Perret, 1986). Team members need to be aware of drug side effects that influence behavior and function (Fraunfelder, 1976).

Myofascial release

The purpose of **myofascial release** (MFR) techniques is to release restrictions that are secondary to tonal dysfunction in children and adults. The lengthening of superficial and deep soft tissue is accomplished by changing the viscosity of the fascia ground substance and by gentle and sustained stretch of the muscular elastic components of fascia. Many occupational therapists have been combining MFR techniques with neurodevelopmental treatment to integrate the improved structural alignment into postural and movement patterns (Barnes, 1991; Boehme, 1991).

Orthotics

Early bracing, with metal and leather components, was used with orthopedic surgery as the main treatment modality for most children with cerebral palsy until the early 1960s. It was restrictive and passive, without active carryover. Currently, treatment with **orthotics** is well established to maintain postsurgical correction and to be used in combination with an active task-oriented therapy program. The new and wide variety of thermoplastic materials to fabricate customized orthotics provides many options for upper and lower extremities as well as for the trunk (Scherzer & Tscharnuter, 1990; Fraser et al., 1990) (see Chapter 9, Section 5A).

The least restrictive devices, soft splints, can be constructed from webbing, neoprene, hook-and-loop fastener material, and other substances. Soft splints do not limit dynamic mobility and sensory feedback as much as do thermoplastics. For example, the thumb abduction supinator splint (TASS) positions the forearm in supination and the thumb in abduction during upper extremity function (Casey & Kratz, 1988). Many types of orthoses for the hands are available. They are fitted to the arm and position the hand and wrist to maximize function.

For children with moderate degrees of spasticity, stronger molded thermoplastic materials are necessary to provide stability. They are lighter in weight than the original metal and leather braces and are easily cleaned; some of the low-temperature plastics can be altered as growth or changes occur. Ankle–foot orthoses (AFO) and shoe inserts can be fitted to the foot and leg, which are held in alignment during fabrication; they provide stability during standing, transitions, and walking. Multiple and severe handicaps may require spinal orthoses and seating orthoses for correction of curvatures such as scoliosis, kyphosis, and lordosis (Fraser et al., 1990).

Occupational therapists have also found that upper extremity casting, which provides prolonged, gentle stretch to spastic or contracted muscles, is an effective adjunct to therapeutic techniques. These casts are fabricated with plaster or fiberglass casting tape. The effects of upper extremity, short-arm casts, extending from below the elbow to the palm and maintaining the wrist in neutral or slight extension, have shown increased quality of movement and wrist extension in children with spasticity (Law et al., 1991). Serial casting protocols for certain children may begin with a rigid circular elbow cast, which is changed as frequently as necessary to accommodate increasing range of elbow motion as muscle length increases. Children with hemiplegia may benefit from a long-arm cast to improve forearm supination and extension as well as elbow extension. The long-arm cast can be bivalved and strapped for use as a night splint. A platform cast can be applied for a child with mild involvement of the long finger flexors to improve wrist and finger function.

Results of upper extremity casting have been significant, with increased strength, control, and spontaneous use of the impaired arm as well as bilateral hand use during play and transitional movements (Yasukawa & Hill, 1988; Yasukawa, 1990). Use of upper extremity inhibitive weight-bearing mitts during transitional movements such as crawling, can be used to reduce muscle tone in children with spastic hemiplegia, with carryover demonstrated by improved functional performance of the impaired upper extremity (Smelt, 1989). Results with older, more severely impaired children with fixed contractures may be less effective or inconsistent (Cruikshank & O'Neill, 1990). The casting program is always integrated into the overall therapy program, with the same functional goals (Yasukawa & Hill, 1988). See Chapter 9, Section 5A for a more detailed discussion of therapeutic adaptations including splinting.

Surgery

At one time, surgery aimed to eliminate all deformities. Changing priorities have led to more realistic goals and a different approach to the timing of surgical procedures. Today surgeons hope to achieve a straight spine and flexible hip and leg joints for postural alignment in adaptive seating or energy-efficient gait with or without assistive devices (canes, crutches, walkers). Instead of one operation at a time, one-session surgeries correct as many deformities as possible. Soft tissue procedures such as tendon or muscle lengthenings, tendon transfers, neurectomies, and myotomies (cutting nerve or muscle) have replaced late operations on bone such as osteotomies (removing and repositioning bone parts) and arthrodeses (fusion of bones) (Gersh, 1991b; Rang & Wright, 1989).

Most upper-extremity surgical procedures for children with cerebral palsy have been orthopedic, involving tendon transfers, small joint arthrodeses, and muscle releases or lengthenings. They have been most beneficial when deformities are mild, and neuromuscular reeducation is provided in follow-up therapy. Surgical goals for the population with multiple and severe deformities are related to function: (1) cosmetic, to achieve more normal arm/hand postures; (2) facilitative, to achieve manual communication board use, for example; and (3) hygienic, to open fisted hands for skin care (Fraser et al., 1990).

Recent increases in neurosurgical operations have involved cutting certain nerves in the spine to reduce muscle tone in upper or lower extremities or in the trunk. The most common of these surgeries, the selective posterior (dorsal) rhizotomy, has affected occupational therapists because postures are improved in many developmental positions, especially sitting, thus allowing improved upper-limb function. Gains in the ability to assume and maintain these positions result in more active participation in activities of daily living such as feeding, dressing, and bathing. Therapists who are part of rhizotomy teams have developed postsurgical protocols to improve upper- as well as lower-extremity function (Berman et al., 1990; Bretas & Dias, 1991; Gersh, 1991b).

Occupational therapy treatment for cerebral palsy

Effective treatment depends on the ability of the professional team members to integrate and synthesize all information gathered and shared during assessment. The child must be considered within the social context of family, school, and community as a unique, goal-oriented person, who influences the world as much as he or she is influenced by it and who is intrinsically motivated to seek stimulation and interaction. Occupational therapy programs for children with special needs are designed to promote adaptation and prevent secondary complications that would occur during development. Adaptation is facilitated through purposeful participation in meaningful and natural activities. By discussing assessment and intervention in terms of daily life experiences, the team can move away from the model of pathology toward everyday problems and solutions (Gilfoyle et al., 1990).

Holistic models that synthesize occupational therapy theory, evaluation, and treatment can be useful to achieve this task. Powell (1985) presented such a model, which contained neurologic, sociocultural, psychosocial, and orthopedic components. These frames of reference can be used separately or in combination, tailored to meet the individual needs of each child. Traditionally, neurologically based sensorimotor approaches, especially neurodevelopmental treatment, have been used most widely in the management of cerebral palsy, because motor behavior is recognized as the major problem.

Occupational therapy in neurodevelopmental treatment

Functional goals

Neurodevelopmental treatment (NDT) is an interdisciplinary therapy approach, which is used to enhance the quality of motor performance, teach new movement skills in preparation for greater function, and prevent disability resulting from abnormal movement patterns. Physical, occupational, and speech therapists all may work during treatment to increase head and trunk control. The physical therapist works to prepare the child for gross motor skills such as locomotion (rolling, crawling, walking). The speech therapist works to prepare the child for oral–motor skills such as feeding and speech. The occupational therapist works on head and trunk control to prepare the child for fine

motor skills such as reach, grasp, manipulation, and release. In other words, the occupational therapist uses NDT to develop the motor competence required for the performance of specific occupational behaviors. One goal of NDT, for example, is to provide foundational patterns for the learning of self-care skills such as feeding, dressing, and hygiene, which is particularly relevant to the field of occupational therapy (Lilly & Powell, 1990).

Current theory related to treatment techniques emphasizes the importance of developing postural organization as an objective to achieving functional goals. The focus is on kinesthetic perception and sensory cues preceding and surrounding motor patterns. Thus, priorities of treatment principles are the following:

1. The relationship between gravity and the base of support
2. The distribution and adaptability of muscle tone to provide postural stability for optimal mobility instead of inappropriate compensatory patterns
3. Control of movement in both end ranges as well as in midrange, modeled after normal developmental sequences
4. Global tactile, proprioceptive, and kinesthetic input provided to the child, who achieves postural organization by orienting to gravity and the base of support (Scherzer & Tscharnuter, 1990).

Moving efficiently against gravity requires muscle and joint range of motion, muscle strength and synergy, postural alignment, and the ability to react appropriately to shifts in the base of support. With true facilitation by the therapist, the child gains control of movement components and learns to use them to develop both gross and fine motor skills (Hypes, 1991).

General treatment strategies for upper-extremity function

After the therapist has determined which movements the child can do independently and which can be done with assistance, missing components can be identified and abnormal muscle tone that is interfering with execution of movement can be inhibited. The therapist can concurrently facilitate all or part of the movement pattern by (1) helping the child maintain proper alignment and relationship to the center of gravity, (2) guiding the speed and excursion of the movement, (3) inhibiting inefficient patterns, and (4) reinforcing the child's improved movement verbally and reducing support (Figure 13-8; (Boehme, 1988). The following are additional general guidelines for treatment:

1. Normalize muscle tone, either increasing or decreasing, in positions where inhibition works best, providing enough postural support but no more than necessary, so that the child is as active as possible. Teach new skills in positions where the child is most stable and tone is most normal.
2. Try to fill most developmental gaps in the young child, but only necessary ones in the older child (not enough time or socially inappropriate).
3. Strengthen present skill levels to prepare for easy sequential transitions but introduce higher developmental levels also, because normal children overlap by attempting new skills before perfecting previous ones.
4. Grade treatment by beginning with passive movement (placing and holding), then assistive movement (providing

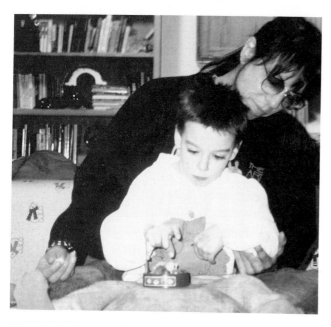

FIGURE 13-8. *Treatment for upper-extremity function. (Courtesy of Regi Boehme.)*

support), and finally active movement (independent). If abnormal patterns appear, return to lower levels, provide more postural support, or increase external control.

5. Be aware of visual components, such as the need for eye-pointing before initiation of hand movements and the maintaining of fixation during manipulation.

6. Remember that the child needs help in learning how and where to stabilize certain parts of the body to enable other parts to move efficiently.

7. Elicit more automatic movements (subcortical) performed without excessive effort, by directing child's attention to the task or to play, not to the way it is being done. If possible, reinforce correct movements and ignore incorrect ones, unless the child needs awareness to correct.

8. Generalize new skills, experimenting with wider ranges, variety of speed and directions, and different positions, as patterns stay fairly normal. Integrate skills into functional activities (self-help, play, educational tasks) and encourage problem solving and new ideas from the child as well as from parents and other caregivers.

Task analysis for specific treatment planning

Another model that integrates assessment and treatment arose from a theory of inappropriate prehension patterns relating to developmental hand dysfunction (Figure 13-9). Developmental sequences are used as a basis for analyzing abnormal hand patterns, determining missing components, and planning appropriate treatment. For example, Figure 13-10 illustrates a typical abnormal grasp of the cube, well-established in older children with cerebral palsy. The wrist is flexed, the thumb is adducted with excessive effort, and the fingers are accommodating to the object's shape in a maladaptive manner. Although many normal components are present at the 3-, 5-, and 9-month levels, a key element is missing—the 7-month radial–palmar grasp. This is normally one of the most stable of all grasps because of the large area of contact by palm and fingers. Treatment to facilitate the

FIGURE 13-9. *A theory of inappropriate prehension patterns relating to developmental hand dysfunction. (From Erhardt, R. P. [1982]. Developmental hand dysfunction: Theory, assessment, and treatment. Tucson, AZ: Therapy Skill Builders.)*

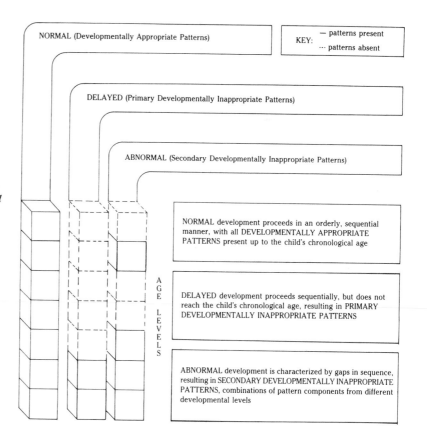

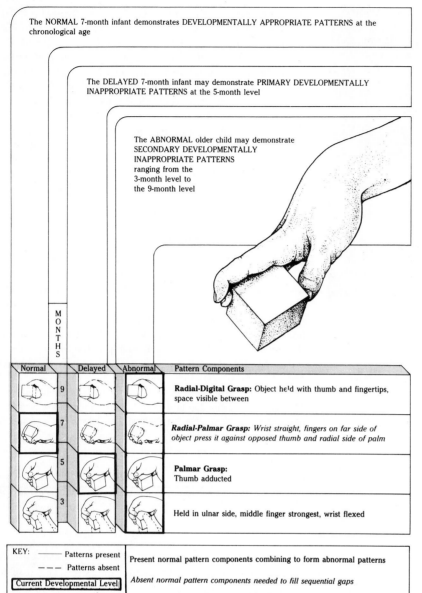

The NORMAL 7-month infant demonstrates DEVELOPMENTALLY APPROPRIATE PATTERNS at the chronological age

The DELAYED 7-month infant may demonstrate PRIMARY DEVELOPMENTALLY INAPPROPRIATE PATTERNS at the 5-month level

The ABNORMAL older child may demonstrate SECONDARY DEVELOPMENTALLY INAPPROPRIATE PATTERNS ranging from the 3-month level to the 9-month level

M O N T H S

Normal	Delayed	Abnormal	Pattern Components
9			**Radial-Digital Grasp:** Object held with thumb and fingertips, space visible between
7			**Radial-Palmar Grasp:** *Wrist straight, fingers on far side of object press it against opposed thumb and radial side of palm*
5			**Palmar Grasp:** Thumb adducted
3			Held in ulnar side, middle finger strongest, wrist flexed

KEY: ——— Patterns present
- - - Patterns absent
| Current Developmental Level |

Present normal pattern components combining to form abnormal patterns

Absent normal pattern components needed to fill sequential gaps

FIGURE 13-10. *A comparison of normal, delayed, and abnormal prehension development and a treatment model: grasp of the cube. (From Erhardt, R. P. [1982].* Developmental hand dysfunction: Theory, assessment, and treatment. *Tucson, AZ: Therapy Skill Builders.)*

radial–palmar grasp is planned by considering and adapting treatment variables such as (1) positioning, (2) points of stability, (3) direction and range of mobility, (4) type, position, shape, size, and weight of stimulus, and (5) amount and place of external support (Erhardt, 1982).

Home management

Self-care

Most children with cerebral palsy need some level of assistance with the self-care activities of feeding, dressing, toileting, bathing, grooming, and other hygiene tasks. Some remain totally dependent on caregivers for all basic needs. Others gain varying degrees of independence in activities of daily living (Fraser et al., 1990).

Feeding

Mealtime is a social occasion for nonhandicapped persons, a time to enjoy food and conversation. Physical problems such as abnormal muscle tone, retained primitive reflexes, and delayed oral–motor development make independent feeding difficult, time-consuming, and often unpleasant for many children and adults with handicaps. Without early intervention, these feeding problems may lead to long-term eating disorders, including rejection of some or all foods or textures, failure to thrive, and disturbed parent–child interaction. Nutritional inadequacy is a common problem in about two thirds of children with cerebral palsy, whose height and weight are under the 10th percentile. Malnutrition, which is associated with apathy, decreased energy, and increased susceptibility to infections, can be due to one or more causes such as inadequate calories offered or not consumed because of oral–motor dysfunction, dental problems, or food refusal, and inadequate calorie retention because of vomiting or GER.

The role of occupational therapy in the assessment and management of feeding problems varies according to the child's current environment. Thus, the therapist may be part of a team of nurses and other hospital staff in the Newborn Intensive Care Unit (NICU) or of an outpatient support group program for parents of NICU graduates (Chamberlain et al., 1991). In the home, occupational therapy may be in the form of consultation to all family members and respite caregivers who feed the child to facilitate appropriate methods as well as positive social interaction during the process (Erhardt, 1985, 1986). In the school environment, the therapist may provide direct service by being the designated feeder at lunchtime, or the therapist may monitor paraprofessional classroom staff.

Evaluation for a feeding program usually includes: (1) review of background information (medical considerations, gross and fine motor function, sensory impairments); (2) examination of the mouth and oral structures (lips, teeth, gums, palate, tongue); and (3) observation of the present feeding/eating process to assess positioning, developmental components, and responses to food textures, utensils, and presentation methods (Bergen & Colangelo, 1985; Fraser et al., 1990; Morris & Klein, 1987).

Some medical conditions that affect feeding are respiratory insufficiency and frequent respiratory infections leading to chronic gagging, coughing, and possible aspiration of food. Conservative management of GER involves dietary changes, medications, and inclined positioning. Surgery may be indicated in severe cases to avoid continued pain, regurgitation, and aspiration.

Primitive reflexes affecting feeding are the following:

1. ATNR, which interferes with hand-to-mouth movements (arm flexion causes the head to turn away)
2. Symmetrical tonic neck reflex (STNR), which interferes with head and trunk stability (neck flexion causes arm flexion and leg extension and vice versa)
3. Tonic labyrinthine reflex (TLR), which interferes with swallowing and hand-to-mouth movement (total synergies of flexion or extension)
4. Oral–motor reflexes (biting, rooting, gagging, suck–swallow), which interfere with the attainment of mature voluntary function

Other problems may be poor lip closure, jaw or tongue thrust, tonic bite, ineffective swallowing, and hypersensitivity to touch. Lack of automatic swallowing mechanisms also contribute to excessive drooling, with associated problems of hygiene, skin irritation, social concerns, and, in severe cases, risk of aspiration (Fraser et al., 1990). Major treatment approaches for drooling include oral-motor therapy, behavior modification, medication, and surgery. Various medications and surgeries to reduce drooling have produced partial or mixed results, with some unpleasant side effects (Siegel & Klingbeil, 1991). Behavioral programs using cuing, positive reinforcement, and overcorrection have been more successful because policies against aversive techniques and punishment have been accepted. Oral–motor stimulation methods of brushing, firm pressure, vibration, jaw control, and so on, before or during feeding have also been successful in reducing, but not eliminating, drooling in children with multiple disabilities (Domaracki & Sisson, 1990; Lammatteo et al., 1990).

Children who are unable to achieve adequate nutrition orally or who are in danger of aspiration may need a temporary nasogastric (NG) tube, or a gastrostomy (G-tube) for longer periods or permanently. The NG tube is inserted into the stomach through the nose, is invasive, and can be irritative. The G-tube is an opening between the stomach and the outside surface of the abdominal wall and can be used to supplement oral feedings or to be the sole source of nutrition (Fraser et al., 1990).

A variety of adaptive feeding equipment is commercially available for dependent feeders (those whose oral–motor dysfunction does not allow them to place food in their mouths) and assisting feeders (those who have upper-extremity control and oral–motor skills allowing them a degree of active participation in the feeding process) (Fraser et al., 1990). These devices include bottles, cups, and spoons for dependent feeders. Assisting feeders may use plates with food guards, suction cups, adapted utensils, special cups, and more sophisticated feeding systems. Figures 13-11 and 13-12 show a child with hypotonia learning to use a ball-bearing feeder, which eventually becomes unnecessary as strength and coordination improve (Figure 13-13). Updated product catalogues are an excellent resource for new therapists as well as for experienced ones who want to be apprised of new products. Frequently, however, utensils used by the normal population can be adapted to meet the needs of a specific child. For example, children with low muscle tone may have difficulty lifting a cup to the mouth for straw drinking. A tall sport cup, with an added saucer base for stability, promotes more normalized postures of head and trunk as well as more independence.

Dressing

Caregivers need encouragement and techniques to help children participate in the dressing process as much as possible. The NDT principle of providing proximal *stability* to foster distal *mobility* can be useful in assistive techniques. For example, support of the pelvis can facilitate reaching upward to place an

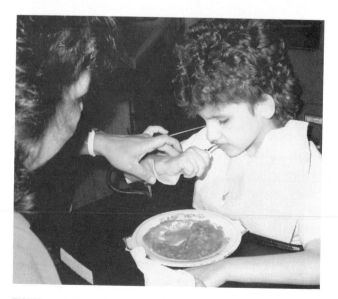

FIGURE 13-11. *An adapted ball-bearing feeder leading to independent feeding.*

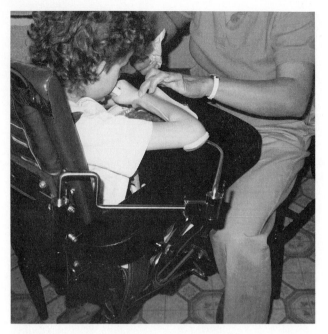

FIGURE 13-12. *An adapted ball-bearing feeder leading to independent feeding.*

arm into a sleeve or downward to pull on socks. Another important NDT concept is that automatic postural adjustments free higher cortical centers to plan intentional or voluntary movements. Self-care skills such as dressing are basically voluntary, but become more automatic through practice. To establish goals for complex functional tasks, the therapist must identify the movement components required (task analysis) and assess which of those the child possesses and what compensatory patterns are used instead. Preparation, treatment, and carryover are aimed at facilitating more automatic reactions and the subse-

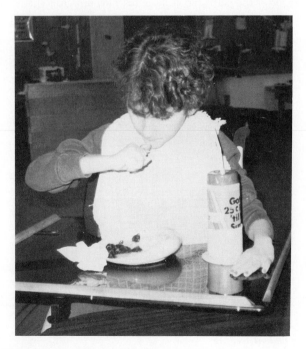

FIGURE 13-13. *Independent feeding.*

quent learning of efficient intentional movements through handling, play, and adapted materials. Adaptive clothing can make dressing easier for semi-independent dressers as well as for caregivers of totally dependent persons, who also need to learn good body mechanics to protect their own physical health (Boehme, 1985; Fraser et al., 1990).

Hygiene and grooming

Hygiene consists of toileting, bathing, and grooming. Many children with multiple handicaps are incontinent and remain so throughout their lives. Others either can participate in a scheduled toileting program or can eventually be independently trained. Adapted seats and chairs that provide stability and comfort can make this process easier and more effective. Bathing aids range from portable devices to bathtub or shower seats, chairs, or hydraulic lifts (Fraser et al., 1990). A lightweight portable bath chair provides head and trunk support has suction cups on its legs for stability in the tub or shower. Practical suggestions for bathing children with cerebral palsy can be individualized and taught to caregivers by therapists (Dunaway & Klein, 1988).

Play

A primary occupation of childhood, play is characterized by fun and spontaneity. It involves exploration, experimentation, imitation, and repetition (Florey, 1981). Play deprivation is common in children with physical disabilities because of many different forms of barriers. These barriers include: (1) limitations imposed by caregivers, who are overprotective and fear injury; (2) physical limitations of the child, whose lack of mobility has prevented exploratory play with household objects; (3) environmental barriers in homes, schools, and community; and (4) social barriers, due to limited interaction with nonhandicapped peers. Therapists can facilitate parents in establishing safe, enjoyable play routines (Missiuna & Pollack, 1991). Toys should possess the following four elements, if possible:

1. *Attention attraction*—interesting and age-appropriate
2. *Variety value*—capable of being used in different ways
3. *Teaching trait*—arousing curiosity and providing new information
4. *Family factor*—stimulating social interaction and fun

Simple activities stimulating visual control are appropriate for all infants, with or without disabilities, and can be done by parents at home during everyday positioning, handling, and play. The therapist can demonstrate specific play procedures for individualized functional goals, such as head control in prone position for downward gaze into a mirror (Figure 13-14) and eye–hand coordination and bilateral hand use in popping soap bubbles (Figure 13-15). Parents often ask therapists to recommend appropriate toys for birthday or Christmas presents. Figures 13-16 and 13-17 show how the skills learned from playing with a switch-adapted, battery-operated toy can serve as preliminary training for operation of a powered chair, as well as computers, augmentative communication devices, and environmental control systems (Williams & Matesi, 1988).

By integrating play within therapy sessions, therapists can promote interaction with the environment and mastery of new skills and develop risk-taking, problem-solving, and decision-making abilities (Reilly, 1974). Integrating play into NDT can be particularly effective because normal patterns of movement can

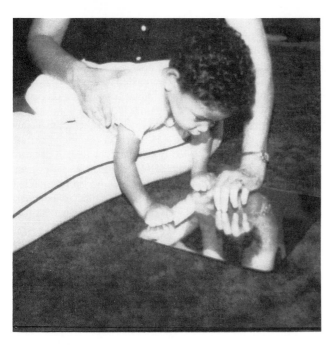

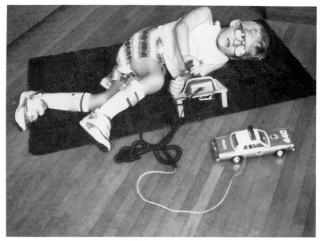

FIGURE 13-16. *A switch-adapted, battery-operated toy preparing for powered chair operation.*

FIGURE 13-14. *Developing head control during mirror play. (From Erhardt, R. P. [1987]. American Journal of Occupational Therapy, 41(1), 46.)*

be promoted and abnormal postural reactions can be prevented while the child is engaged in functional, purposeful activities. NDT aims to produce automatic movement patterns without placing conscious attention on the process and eliciting excessive effort. A child absorbed in play is not focused on the specific motor demands of the activity and can be stimulated to use therapeutically appropriate movements to improve control of head, trunk, and arms during manipulation of toys. The occupational therapist's task analysis skills are used to continually adapt:

(1) size, shape, and consistency of materials; (2) rules and procedures; (3) position of child or materials; and (4) nature and degree of personal interaction (Anderson et al., 1987).

The physical, social, emotional, language, and intellectual needs of children with disabilities are no different from those of normal children. Adapted playgrounds, which stimulate spontaneous play, can be valuable environments for meeting those needs by providing opportunities for peer interaction as well as public awareness, which facilitates the process of community mainstreaming. Occupational therapists are ideal professionals to help design playgrounds for young children with disabilities because therapists understand what modifications are needed to eliminate architectural barriers and to ensure safe environments

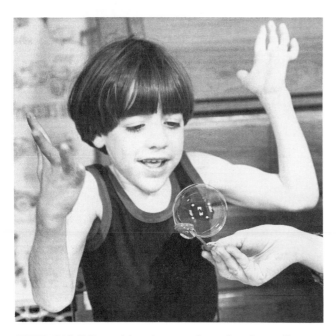

FIGURE 13-15. *Bilateral hand use and eye–hand coordination. (Courtesy of Therapy Skill Builders.)*

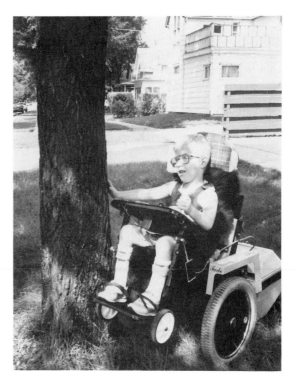

FIGURE 13-17. *Operation of a powered chair.*

despite cognitive, sensory, and physical limitations (Stout, 1988). See Chapter 8, Section 3 for a more detailed discussion of play/leisure in terms of occupational therapy performance areas.

Positioning and handling

Parents have many opportunities for therapeutic handling during feeding, dressing, and play. Therapists can help them and other caregivers to understand the difference between normal and abnormal movement patterns and to develop spontaneous and natural handling skills as part of their automatic physical interaction with their child (Stern & Gorga, 1988). Positioning is important for infants, who rapidly develop new movement patterns that become well-established habits. As they grow older, appropriate positioning is essential for increasing function. Children with severe and multiple handicaps are even more dependent on adaptive seating and positioning. Proper positioning not only minimizes the influence of pathologic forces on body posture but provides a stable base of support for performance and function; thus, it is the key to increased independence and improved self-esteem.

The positioning and handling program is always developed by members of the team, with the caregivers' participation, to ensure that recommended techniques are compatible with established home routines and schedules. As much as possible, even when optimal seating is gained in a specific adaptive seating system, several other positioning options should be available throughout each day, since normal children do not remain in one position for prolonged periods of time (Fraser et al., 1990).

Adaptive equipment for patients with cerebral palsy

Prescribing equipment that allows maximum function with minimum pathology is considered both a science and an art, with certain guidelines but no firm rules. Therefore, professional judgment, educated experimentation, and personal sensitivity are essential for the team of therapists, physicians, educators, and equipment providers working with the client and the family. Proper seating and positioning can potentially provide the following benefits (Bergen et al., 1990):

1. Decreases abnormal neurologic influences on the body
2. Increases active and passive range of movement, maintains skeletal alignment, and controls or prevents deformities or contractures
3. Manages pressure to prevent potential for decubitus ulcers
4. Provides stability to enhance function
5. Increases tolerance and comfort
6. Enhances autonomic nervous system function
7. Decreases fatigue
8. Facilitates components of normal movement in developmental sequences
9. Provides maximum function with minimum pathology

General principles for optimum seating are: (1) head maintained in the vertical plane; (2) hips, knees, and ankles maintained at 90 degrees unless pelvic thrust or posterior tilt require more hip flexion; and (3) feet supported. Most of the currently available equipment is designed to be extremely adaptable, but continual monitoring is always necessary, because simple repairs

may be necessary as the child grows or as changes in function occur (Bergen & Colangelo, 1985; Taylor & Trefler, 1984).

Although commercial equipment may be available for a specific type of problem, many therapists use their creative talents to invent or adapt devices needed for one or a group of their patients. For example, positional support for premature infants in newborn intensive care units (NICU) may include: (1) supine support pillow constructed from foam, which facilitates symmetrical flexion postures; (2) lambskin-covered water pillows constructed from sealed plastic bags for flexion in prone and sidelying; (3) preemie comfort bags filled with polystyrene beads (beanbags) for placing very small ventilator-dependent infants in supine or sidelying position (Updike et al., 1986). Numerous commercial products designed for neonatal positioning, especially in intensive care incubators, are available.

Custom-made adaptive seating devices (ASDs) have been found to improve sitting postures and eating skills of young children with multiple handicaps (Hulme et al., 1987). A variety of adjustable seating inserts, wheelchairs, and support systems are available, such as individualized foam and gel pack cushions in solid contoured seat and back bases. These individualized seating systems have knit covers and can be inserted into wheelchairs or powered mobility vehicles such as scooters (Figures 13-18 and 13-19).

Use of accepted therapeutic guidelines for wheelchair positioning have resulted in increased rate and accuracy in skills such as head-controlled typing in adults with cerebral palsy (Bay, 1991; Taylor & Trefler, 1984). Figures 13-20 and 13-21 illustrate custom-molded seating system fabricated for a person who has severe deformities of the spine and pelvis. The system provides postural support for access to augmentative communication and powered mobility.

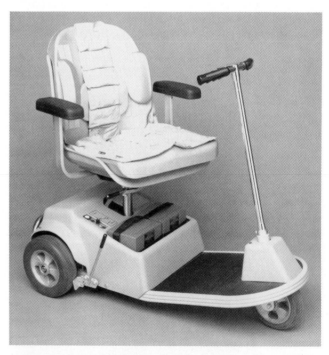

FIGURE 13-18. *Amigo three-wheeler with Jay seat and back, uncovered. (Courtesy of Health Care Accessories, Fargo, ND, Amigo Mobility, Inc., and Jay Medical Inc.)*

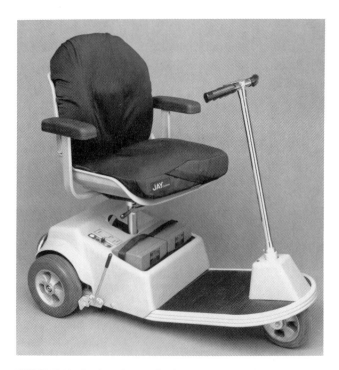

FIGURE 13-19. *Amigo three-wheeler with Jay seat and back, with knit covers. (Courtesy of Health Care Accessories, Fargo, ND, Amigo Mobility, Inc., and Jay Medical Inc.)*

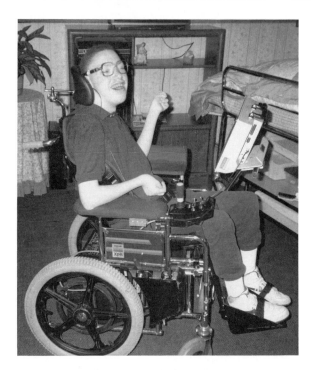

FIGURE 13-21. *Use of custom-molded seating system for augmentative communication and powered mobility. (Courtesy of Adaptive Equipment Services, Developmental Center, Grafton, ND.)*

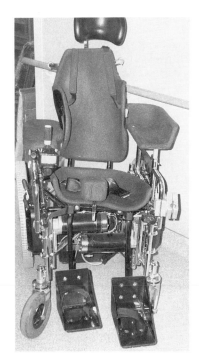

FIGURE 13-20. *Custom-molded seating system. (Courtesy of Adaptive Equipment Services, Developmental Center, Grafton, ND.)*

The challenge of evaluating older children and adults with severe motor disabilities for switch control can lead to rewarding successes, especially when cognitive and motivational levels are high. For such people innovative postures such as sidelying may be needed to access functional, isolated movements of an extremity (Einis & Bailey, 1990).

Figures 13-22 and 13-23 show the typical standing posture of children with spastic diplegia and show how an innovative, adjustable walker based on the Bobath use of vertical walking sticks facilitates extension, abduction, and external rotation in arms and legs as well as in spinal extension. Adjustable in height and width, the walker is used as an intermediate step between assistive and independent walking to promote better upper as well as lower extremity function and to prevent the persistence of abnormal patterns.

Educational considerations

Eye–hand coordination for function

After a child enters school, functional eye–hand skills are essential for writing and prevocational activities such as keyboard use. Scribbling, coloring, and drawing have provided the visual–motor experiences that are necessary for complex writing tasks. These tasks are learned by tracing (eyes direct hand to follow the visual representation), imitating (eyes watch and remember another's action to repeat the same action and production), and copying (eyes alternate glances between visual representation and own production in process). A person whose development has been delayed or compromised by damage to the central nervous system may demonstrate obvious hand dysfunction, but

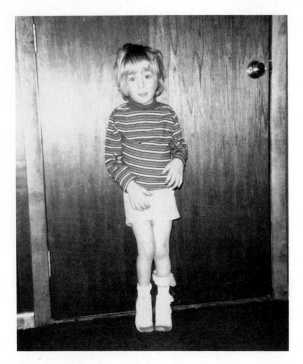

FIGURE 13-22. *Standing posture common in spastic diplegia.*

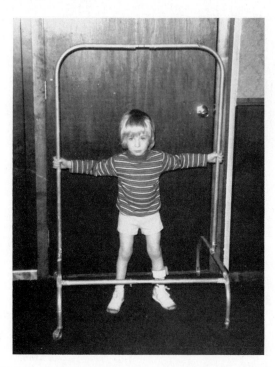

FIGURE 13-23. *Erhardt Abduction Walker used to normalize arm and leg postures. (Courtesy of Erhardt Developmental Products, Maplewood, MN.)*

visual problems involving motor control as well as acuity and perception may be more subtle and difficult to identify. Comprehensive evaluations are needed to analyze the disruption of the visual process as well as fine motor deficits, which interfere with eye–hand mechanisms (Erhardt, 1992).

Strategies for handwriting and keyboard use

The normal hand is usually held in a position of about 45 degrees supination, with the wrist in slight extension for handwriting and drawing, a task requiring static grasp of the pencil at the same time as dynamic movement of the arm. For operating a keyboard, the hands are usually held in a pronated position with wrists in slight extension. The hand postures of persons with cerebral palsy typically have limitations of wrist supination and extension, which interfere with these skills for written communication (Penso, 1990). Additionally, visual monitoring of the hands is often inconsistent, because of inadequate head control or the persistence of primitive reflexes.

Strategies to accommodate grasp and movement problems of the hand are: (1) positioning of the person in appropriate seating systems; (2) adjustment of the work surface with inclines or easels; and (3) the use of adaptations for crayons, pencils, pens, and markers, for example, grips of plastic, foam rubber, or thermoplastic material in triangular, cylindrical, ball, or customized shapes, which are also useful for other utensils and tools.

Augmentative and alternative communication

A major challenge for professionals and family members assisting the person with handicaps is identifying strategies to enable communication skills to develop. A person with limited or unin-

telligible speech requires an alternative method to communicate, and thus act upon and control events in his or her life. Technology has dramatically increased these opportunities in recent years, with a variety of commercial communication boards, voice output communication aides (VOCA), and accessibility switches. Transdisciplinary evaluations determine exactly which devices and which components of each device are appropriate for each person by identifying visual needs, the most effective body part movement, and the cognitive and language levels as well as projected potential. For example, visual needs may include symbols adapted for size and line thickness, specific placement of materials (eye level and focal length), and scanning skills. Activation of a single switch must consider placement for hand access and pressure required. Figure 13-24 demonstrates the use of a toggle treadle switch to operate a light-emitting diodes (LED) scanning system developed by local university engineering students, using large print materials.

Computer-assisted instruction (CAI) has also expanded within the educational system; new equipment may be accessed through keyboards, single or multiple switches, touch panels, touch windows, and voice input. The large variety of adapted software programs with graphics and voice feedback are highly motivating. They can be used with very young children for simple cause-and-effect activities and with older children who are reinforced by the interactive processes, allowing self-controlled learning. An individualized computer system for a person with severe handicaps may include a communication program, environmental control, and social–leisure activities (Fraser et al., 1990). See Chapter 9, Sections 5 and 6 for a more detailed discussion of assistive/adapted equipment and technology.

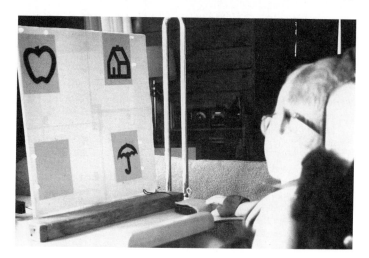

FIGURE 13-24. *Single-switch operation of an LED scanning system with large print symbols.*

Preparation for community integration and independence

Changing attitudes of society toward minority groups have benefited persons with disabilities. New federal, state, and local legislation, promoted by advocacy groups, has meant increased integration and more appropriate health care, accessibility, housing, and transportation. Lifestyles for children and adults with moderate and severe cerebral palsy have changed from total dependence in institutional settings to group homes, foster homes, and assisted independent living. Work opportunities have also changed from sheltered to supportive employment, with job coaches enabling the worker to function within more normal, competitive situations (Rang & Wright, 1989).

However, provision of lifelong special services, which fosters dependency, can significantly interfere with the child's acquiring of adult life skills. The developmental tasks of adolescence are achieving emotional independence from parents, preparing for close relationships with peers, learning socially responsible behavior, and beginning vocational exploration. These tasks are difficult when people are operating from a social position of passivity and helplessness, which is common in young adults with cerebral palsy, because of limited mobility, few opportunities to make decisions, and dependence on others for many activities of daily living. The occupational therapist who perceives young children with cerebral palsy in the context of their entire lifespan will recognize the importance of encouraging them at an early age to take responsibility, to be more self-reliant, and eventually to become more assertive in directing their own lives (Neistadt, 1987). Therapists working in school systems can address the self-esteem needs of children as they move toward adolescence and make sure they have opportunities to choose positive environments for their social interactions (Magill-Evans & Restall, 1991).

Summary

Children with cerebral palsy offer exciting challenges and opportunities for occupational therapists who can choose from many different settings with this population throughout their lives. Early intervention may begin in the hospital high-risk nursery or in screening programs for infants and toddlers. Preschool programs may be home-based or center-based, or a combination of both. Therapists may be employed as related service providers by school systems or hired by families to supplement insufficient school programs that are struggling with shortages of professional personnel. As part of these professional teams that are assisting adolescents with cerebral palsy to make transitions from high school to different levels of domestic and employment situations, occupational therapists' theoretical base of human occupation is invaluable. More people, handicapped as well as nonhandicapped, are gaining increased longevity. Thus, specialists in the area of developmental disabilities such as cerebral palsy are expanding their knowledge base from pediatrics through the adult continuum to geriatrics.

Appreciation is extended to the children, parents, and therapists who have graciously given permission for use of their photographs. In addition, Gary Baune's illustrations from some of my previous works have helped to clarify important points in this section (Erhardt, 1982, 1990).

References

Albright, A. L., Cervi, A., & Singletary, J. (1991). Intrathecal baclofen for spasticity in cerebral palsy. *Journal of the American Medical Association, 265,* 1418–1422.

Anderson, J., Hinojosa, J., Strauch, C. (1987). Integrating play in neurodevelopmental treatment. *American Journal of Occupational Therapy, 41,* 421–426.

Armstrong, R., Steinbok, P., Farrell, K., Cochrane, D., Kube, S., & Fife, S. (1991). Intrathecal baclofen for treatment of spasticity in children *Developmental Medicine and Child Neurology, 33,* Supplement No. 64 (Abstracts of Annual Meeting), 27.

Barnes, J. F. (1991). Pediatric myofascial release. *Occupational Therapy Forum,* July 19, 18–19.

Batshaw, M. L., & Perret, Y. M. (1986). *Children with handicaps* (2nd ed.). Baltimore: Paul H. Brookes.

Bay, J. L. (1991). Positioning for head control to access an augmentative communication machine. *American Journal of Occupational Therapy, 45,* 544–549.

Bayley, N. (1969). *Bayley Scales of Infant Development.* New York: Psychological Corporation.

Bergen, A. F., & Colangelo, C. (1985). *Positioning the client with central nervous system deficits: The wheelchair and other adapted equipment* (2nd ed.). Valhalla, NY: Valhalla Rehabilitation Publications.

Bergen, A. F., Presperin, J., & Tallman, T. (1990). *Positioning for function: Wheelchairs and other assistive technologies.* Valhalla, NY: Valhalla Rehabilitation Publications.

Berman, B., Vaughan, C. L., & Peacock, W. J. (1990). The effect of rhizotomy on movements in patients with cerebral palsy. *American Journal of Occupational Therapy, 44,* 511–516.

Blacklin, J. S. (1991). Your child's development. In E. Geralis (Ed.), *Children with cerebral palsy: A parents' guide* (pp. 175–208). Rockville, MD: Woodbine House.

Blanche, E. J., & Burke, J. P. (1991). Combining neurodevelopmental and sensory integration approaches in the treatment of the neurologically impaired child. Part I. *Sensory Integration Quarterly, 19,* 1–5.

Bobath, B. (1977, October/November). *NDT 8-week certification course.* London, England. Unpublished notes.

Bobath, B. (1985). *Abnormal postural reflex activity caused by brain lesions.* Rockville, MD: Aspen Publications.

Bobath, B. (1985, May). Changing Trends in NDT. In *Symposium on Neuro-Developmental Treatment.* Conducted at the meeting of the Neuro-Developmental Treatment Association (N. D. T. A.), Baltimore.

Bobath K., & Bobath, B. (1972). Cerebral palsy. In P. H. Pearson & C. E. Williams (Eds.), *Physical therapy services in the developmental disabilities* (pp. 31–185). Springfield, IL: Charles C. Thomas.

Boehme, R. (1985, November). Self-care assessment and treatment from an NDT perspective. *NDT Newsletter, 1,* 5.

Boehme, R. (1988). *Improving upper body control.* Tucson, AZ: Therapy Skill Builders.

Boehme, R. (1991). *Myofascial release and its application to neurodevelopmental treatment.* Milwaukee: Boehme Workshops.

Bretas, C., & Dias, L. (1991). Selective posterior rhizotomy. *Developmental medicine and child neurology, 33,* Supplement No. 64 (Abstracts of Annual Meeting), 26.

Campbell, S. K. (1990). Using standardized tests in clinical practice. In S. K. Campbell (Ed.), *Topics in pediatrics,* Lesson 11 (pp. 1–13). Alexandria, VA: American Physical Therapy Association.

Casey, C. A., & Kratz, E. K. (1988). Soft splinting with neoprene: The thumb abduction supinator splint. *American Journal of Occupational Therapy, 42,* 395–398.

Chamberlain, J. L., Henry, M. M., Roberts, J. D., Sapsford, A. L., & Courtney, S. E. (1991). An infant and toddler feeding group program. *American Journal of Occupational Therapy, 45,* 907–911.

Coley, I. L. (1978). *Pediatric assessment of self-care activities.* St. Louis: C. V. Mosby.

Cook, D. G. (1991). The assessment process. In W. Dunn (Ed.), *Pediatric occupational therapy: Facilitating effective service provision* (pp. 34–73). Thorofare, NJ: Slack.

Coorssen, E. A., Msall, M., & Duffy, L. C. (1991). Multiple minor malformations as a marker for prenatal etiology of cerebral palsy. *Developmental Medicine and Child Neurology, 33,* 730–736.

Cruikshank, D. A., & O'Neill, D. L. (1990). Upper extremity inhibitive casting in a boy with spastic quadriplegia. *American Journal of Occupational Therapy, 44,* 552–555.

Curry, J., & Exner, C. (1988). Comparison of tactile preferences in children with and without cerebral palsy. *American Journal of Occupational Therapy, 42,* 371–377.

Domaracki, L. S., & Sisson, L. A. (1990). Decreased drooling with oral motor stimulation in children with multiple disabilities. *American Journal of Occupational Therapy, 44,* 680–685.

Duckman, R. H. (1984). Effectiveness of optometric visual training in a population of severely involved cerebral palsied children utilizing profesional, non-optometric therapists. *Physical and Occupational Therapy in Pediatrics, 4,* 75–86.

Dunaway, A., & Klein, M. D. (1988). *Bathing techniques for children who have cerebral palsy.* Tucson, AZ: Therapy Skill Builders.

Dunn, W. (1987, May). Sensory integration. In *NDT OT Instructor Course.* Akron, Ohio.

Einis, L. P., & Bailey, D. M. (1990). The use of powered leisure and communication devices in a switch training program. *American Journal of Occupational Therapy, 44,* 931–934.

Ellig, D. D. (1991). Personal communication (December 16).

Erhardt, R. P. (1982). *Developmental hand dysfunction: Theory, assessment, and treatment.* Tucson, AZ: Therapy Skill Builders.

Erhardt, R. P. (1985). *Developmental prehension components of independent feeding (video).* Maplewood, MN: Erhardt Developmental Products.

Erhardt, R. P. (1986). *The consultant's role in evaluation and treatment of eating dysfunction (video).* Maplewood, MN: Erhardt Developmental Products.

Erhardt, R. P. (1990). *Developmental visual dysfunction: Models for assessment and management.* Tucson, AZ: Therapy Skill Builders.

Erhardt, R. P. (1991–1992, Winter). Improving visual control: Activities for parents and infants. *Teamtalk, 1,* 12–15. (Available from Teamtalk, PO Box 83165, Milwaukee, WI 53223).

Erhardt, R. P. (1992). Eye-hand coordination. In J. Case-Smith & C. Pehoski (Eds.), *Development of hand skills in the child* (pp. 13–33). Rockville, MD: American Occupational Therapy Association.

Exner, C. (1989). Development of hand functions. In P. N. Pratt & A. S. Allen (Eds.), *Occupational therapy for children* (pp. 235–259). St. Louis: C. V. Mosby.

Farber, S. (1982). *Neurorehabilitation: A neurosensory approach.* Philadelphia: W. B. Saunders.

Fee, M. A., Charney, E. B., & Robertson, W. W. (1988). Nutritional assessment of the young child with cerebral palsy. *Infants and Young Children, 1,* 33–40.

Fiorentino, M. R. (1973). *Reflex testing methods of evaluating C.N.S. development* (2nd ed.). Springfield, IL: Charles C Thomas.

Florey, L. L. (1981). Studies of play: Implications for growth, development, and for clinical practice. *American Journal of Occupational Therapy, 35,* 519–528.

Folio, R., & Fewell, R. R. (1983). *Peabody Developmental Motor Scales.* Hingham, MA: Teaching Resources.

Foltz, L. C., DeGangi, G., & Lewis, D. (1991). Physical therapy, occupational therapy, and speech and language therapy. In E. Geralis (Ed.), *Children with cerebral palsy: A parents' guide* (pp. 209–260). Rockville, MD: Woodbine House.

Fraser, B. A., Hensinger, R. N., & Phelps, J. A. (1990). *Physical management of multiple handicaps.* Baltimore: Paul H. Brookes.

Fraunfelder, F. T. (1976). *Drug-induced ocular side effects and drug interactions.* Philadelphia: Lea & Febiger.

Gersh, E. S. (1991a). What is cerebral palsy? In E. Geralis (Ed.), *Children with cerebral palsy: A parents' guide* (pp. 1–32). Rockville, MD: Woodbine House.

Gersh, E. S. (1991b). Medical concerns and treatment. In E. Geralis (Ed.), *Children with cerebral palsy: A parents' guide* (pp. 57–90). Rockville, MD: Woodbine House.

Gilfoyle, E. M., Grady, A. P., & Moore, J. C. (1990). *Children adapt: A theory of sensorimotor-sensory development* (2nd ed.). Thorofare, NJ: Slack.

Hacker, B. J., & Porter, P. B. (1987). Use of standardized tests with the physically handicapped. In L. King-Thomas & B. J. Hacker (Eds.), *A therapist's guide to pediatric assessment* (pp. 35–40). Boston: Little, Brown & Co.

Harris, S. R. (1988). Early intervention: Does developmental therapy make a difference? *Topics in Early Childhood Special Education, 7,* 20–32.

Hirschel, A., Pehoski, C., & Coryell, J. (1990). Environmental support and the development of grasp in infants. *American Journal of Occupational Therapy, 44,* 721–727.

Huber, C. J., & King-Thomas, K. (1987). The assessment process. In L. King-Thomas & B. J. Hacker (Eds.), *A therapist's guide to pediatric assessment* (pp. 3–10). Boston: Little, Brown & Co.

Hulme, J. B., Shaver, J., Acher, S., Mullette, L., & Eggert, C. (1987). Effects of adaptive seating devices on the eating and drinking of children with multiple handicaps. *American Journal of Occupational Therapy, 41*, 81–89.

Hypes, B. (1988). A kinesiological analysis of dynamic sitting. In R. Boehme (Ed.), *Improving upper body control* (pp. 189–209). Tucson, AZ: Therapy Skill Builders.

Hypes, B. (1991). *Facilitating development and sensorimotor function: Treatment with the ball*. Hugo, MN: PDP Press.

Jelm, J. M. (1990). *Oral-Motor/Feeding Rating Scale*. Tucson, AZ: Therapy Skill Builders.

Knobloch, H., Stevens, F., & Malone, A. (1980). *A manual of developmental diagnosis: The administration and interpretation of the revised Gesell and Amatruda Developmental and Neurological Examination*. New York: Harper & Row.

Knox, S. A. (1974). A play scale. In M. Reilly (Ed.), *Play as exploratory learning* (pp. 247–266). Beverly Hills: Sage Publications.

Lammatteo, P. A., Trombley, C., & Luecke, L. (1990). The effect of mouth closure on drooling and speech. *American Journal of Occupational Therapy, 44*, 686–691.

Law, M., Cadman, D., Rosenbaum, P., Walter, S., Russell, D., & DeMatteo, C. (1991). Neurodevelopmental therapy and upper-extremity inhibitive casting for children with cerebral palsy. *Developmental Medicine and Child Neurology, 33*, 379–387.

Lilly, L. A., & Powell, N. J. (1990). Measuring the effects of neurodevelopmental treatment on the daily living skills of 2 children with cerebral palsy. *American Journal of Occupational Therapy, 44*, 139–146.

Little, W. J. (1862). On the influence of abnormal parturition, difficult labours, premature birth and asphyxia neonatorum, on the mental and physical condition of the child, especially in relation to deformities. In *Transactions of the Obstetrical Society, Vol. III for the year 1861* (pp. 293–346). London: Longman, Green, Longman and Roberts.

Magill-Evans, J. E., & Restall, G. (1991). Self-esteem of persons with cerebral palsy: From adolescence to adulthood. *American Journal of Occupational Therapy, 45*, 819–825.

Mather, J., & Weinstein, E. (1988). Teachers and therapists: Evolution of a partnership in early intervention. *Topics in Early Childhood Special Education, 7*, 1–9.

McCuaig, M., & Frank, G. (1991). The able self: Adaptive patterns and choices in independent living for a person with cerebral palsy. *American Journal of Occupational Therapy, 45*, 224–234.

Menken, C., Cermak, S. A., & Fisher, A. (1987). Evaluating the visual-perceptual skills of children with cerebral palsy. *American Journal of Occupational Therapy, 41*, 646–651.

Missiuna, C., & Pollack, N. (1991). Play deprivation in children with physical disabilities: The role of the occupational therapist in preventing secondary disability. *American Journal of Occupational Therapy, 45*, 882–888.

Morris, S. E. (1982). *The normal acquisition of oral feeding skills: Implications for assessment and treatment*. New York: Therapeutic Media.

Morris, S. E., & Klein, M. D. (1987). *Pre-feeding skills: A comprehensive resource for feeding development*. Tucson, AZ: Therapy Skill Builders.

Mulligan-Ault, M., Guess, D., Struth, L., & Thompson, B. (1988). The implementation of health-related procedures in classrooms for students with severe multiple impairments. *Journal of the Association of Persons with Severe Handicaps, 13*, 87–99.

Neistadt, M. E. (1986). Occupational therapy treatment goals for adults with developmental disabilities. *American Journal of Occupational Therapy, 40*, 672–678.

Neistadt, M. E. (1987). An occupational therapy program for adults with developmental disabilities. *American Journal of Occupational Therapy, 41*, 433–438.

Penso, D. E. (1990). *Keyboard, graphic and handwriting skills: Helping people with motor disabilities*. London: Chapman & Hall.

Phelps, W. (1940). The treatment of cerebral palsies. *Journal of Bone and Joint Surgery, 22*, 1004.

Powell, N. J. (1985). Children with cerebral palsy. In P. N. Clark & A. S. Allen (Eds.), *Occupational therapy for children* (pp. 312–337). St. Louis: C. V. Mosby.

Rainforth, B., & Salisbury, C. L. (1988). Functional home programs: A model for therapists. *Topics in Early Childhood Special Education, 7*, 33–45.

Rang, M., & Wright, J. (1989). What have 30 years of medical progress done for cerebral palsy? *Clinical Orthopedics and Related Research, 247*, 55–60.

Reilly, M. (Ed.). (1974). *Play as exploratory learning*. Beverly Hills: Sage Publications.

Scherzer, A. L., & Tscharnuter, I. (1990). *Early diagnosis and therapy in cerebral palsy* (2nd ed.). New York: Dekker.

Semans, S. (1965a). Specific tests and evaluation tools for the child with central nervous system deficit. *Journal of the American Physical Therapy Association, 45*, 456–462.

Semans, S. (1965b). A cerebral palsy assessment chart. *Journal of the American Physical Therapy Association, 45*, 463.

Siegel, L. K., & Klingbeil, M. A. (1991). Control of drooling with transdermal scopolamine in a child with cerebral palsy. *Developmental Medicine and Child Neurology, 33*, 1013–1014.

Smelt, H. (1989). Effect of an inhibitive weight-bearing mitt on tone reduction and functional performance in a child with cerebral palsy. *Physical and Occupational Therapy in Pediatrics, 9*, 53–80.

Smith, M. A., Connolly, B., McFadden, S., Nicrosi, C. R., Nuckolls, L. J., Russell, F. F., & Wilson, W. M. (1982). *Feeding management of a child with a handicap: A guide for professionals*. Memphis: University of Tennessee.

Stern, F. M., & Gorga, D. (1988). Neurodevelopmental treatment (NDT): Therapeutic intervention and its efficacy. *Infants and Young Children, 1*, 22–32.

Stewart, K. B., Deitz, J. C., Crowe, T. K., Robinson, N., & Bennett, F. C. (1988). Transient neurologic signs in infancy and motor outcomes at 4½ years in children born biologically at risk. *Topics in Early Childhood Special Education, 7*, 71–83.

Stout, J. (1988). Planning playgrounds for children with disabilities. *American Journal of Occupational Therapy, 42*, 653–657.

Taylor, S., & Trefler, E. (1984). Decision making guidelines for seating and positioning children with cerebral palsy. In E. Trefler (Ed.), *Seating for children with cerebral palsy: A resource manual* (pp. 55–76) Memphis: University of Tennessee Center for Health Sciences, Rehabilitation Engineering Program.

Torfs, C. P., Van den Berg, B. J., Oechsli, F. W., Cummins, S. (1990). Prenatal and perinatal factors in the etiology of cerebral palsy. *Journal of Pediatrics, 116*, 615–619.

Twitchell, T. E. (1965). The automatic grasping responses of infants. *Neuropsychologia, 3*, 247–259.

Twitchell, T. E. (1970). Reflex mechanisms and the development of prehension. In K. Connolly (Ed.), *Mechanisms of motor skill development* (pp. 25–38). London: Academic Press.

Updike, C., Schmidt, R. E., Macke, C., Cahoon, J., & Miller, M. (1986). Positional support for premature infants. *American Journal of Occupational Therapy, 40*, 712–715.

Wiklund, L. M., & Uvebrant, P. (1991). Hemiplegic cerebral palsy: Correlation between CT morphology and clinical findings. *Developmental Medicine and Child Neurology, 33*, 512–523.

Wilbarger, P. (1984). Planning an adequate sensory diet: Application of sensory processing theory during the first year of life. *Zero to Three, 5*, 7–12.

Williams, S. E., & Matesi, D. V. (1988). Therapeutic intervention with an adapted toy. *American Journal of Occupational Therapy, 42*, 673–676.

World Health Organization (1980). *International Classification of impairments, disabilities, and handicap*. Geneva: WHO.

Yasukawa, A. (1990). Upper extremity casting: Adjunct treatment for a child with cerebral palsy. *American Journal of Occupational Therapy, 44,* 840–847.

Yasukawa, A., & Hill, J. (1988). Casting to improve upper extremity function. In R. Boehme (Ed.), *Improving upper body control* (pp. 165–188). Tucson, AZ: Therapy Skill Builders.

SECTION 3

Developmental delay: Early intervention

OLGA BALOUEFF

KEY TERMS

Assessment

Case Management

Center-Based

Developmental Delay

Early Intervention

Home-Based

Individualized Family
    Service Plan (IFSP)

Interdisciplinary Approach

Public Law 99–457,
    Part H

Multidisciplinary Approach

Team Approach

Transdisciplinary
    Approach

LEARNING OBJECTIVES

Upon completion of this section the reader will be able to:

1. *Identify various types of developmental delay.*

2. *Explain the meaning, rationale, and goals of early intervention.*

3. *Understand the effects of Public Law 99–457 on the development and delivery of early intervention services.*

4. *Explain the role of occupational therapy in early intervention.*

5. *Describe the various aspects of service delivery proper to early intervention, such as Individualized Family Service Plan and case management.*

6. *Select tests for assessment of infants and toddlers with developmental deviations and families' strengths and needs.*

7. *Identify ways to enhance parent–professional interaction.*

In the last 20 years, advances in biomedical technology, special education, and therapeutic services and a positive change in social attitudes toward persons with disabilities have created new opportunities for developmentally vulnerable infants and their families. Furthermore, beliefs and knowledge about the influence of a child's earliest years on later development have contributed to the establishment and expansion of early childhood intervention programs (Meisels, 1989). Parent advocacy and slow but steady recognition by health care professionals of the crucial role that families play in the care of their children have shifted the focus of services in pediatrics from children primarily to children *and* their families, creating a family-centered care approach (Shelton et al., 1987).

In 1986, with the passage of Public Law 99–457, early intervention programs for infants and toddlers with or at risk for developmental delay expanded in number throughout the United States. Occupational therapy is an integral part of these early intervention services.

Developmental delay

The term ***developmental delay*** refers to a wide range of childhood disorders and environmental situations (Clancy & Clark, 1990). Children are considered to have developmental delays when they are unable to accomplish the developmental tasks typical of their chronologic age (Clancy & Clark, 1990). They may be at risk or have developmental delays for a variety of reasons.

Tjossem (1976) identified three groups of children who have developmental delays or who are at risk for developmental deviations:

Infants with *established risk* are those manifesting early-appearing atypical development related to diagnosed medical disorders of known etiology (eg, Down syndrome, sensory impairments).

Infants at *biologic risk* are those who have an increased probability for delayed or atypical development from biologic insult(s) to the developing brain, acquired pre-, peri- or postnatally (eg, low birth weight, small-for-gestational age, fetal alcohol syndrome).

Infants at *environmental risk* are those who, although biologically sound, may develop developmental deviations due to depriving life experiences (eg, parental neglect, homelessness).

These three categories are not mutually exclusive, and many infants have a combination of risks for developmental deviations affecting them, their families, and society. For example, a child born early with a low birthweight to a mother who has an addiction to drugs and a chaotic lifestyle that limits her ability to properly care for her infant is at greater risk for developmental deviations than a child born prematurely in a stable, nurturing family.

Early intervention

Definition

The term ***early intervention*** has several meanings, depending on the context in which it is used. In this section it is defined as a comprehensive, coordinated, community-based system for developmentally vulnerable or delayed young children from birth to age 3 years and their families. Early intervention (EI) consists of multidisciplinary services designed to enhance child development, minimize potential delays, remediate existing problems, prevent further deterioration, limit the acquisition of additional handicapping conditions, and promote adaptive family functioning. The goals of EI are accomplished by providing developmental and therapeutic services for children, and support and instructions for their families (Meisels & Shonkoff, 1990). These services are *federally mandated, individualized,* and *family-focused*. For interventions to be meaningful and effective, they have to reflect the individual, cultural, and specific environmental characteristics and needs of the family.

Rationale for early intervention

EI services can be remedial or preventive in nature. Support for EI is drawn from neurophysiologic principles, studies of child development and families, and societal beliefs (Schaaf & Gitlin, 1989).

Early brain plasticity

During the prenatal and early childhood stages of life, the brain is experiencing rapid periods of development. Increased myelinization of the pathways and nuclei in the nervous system in the first year of life and rapid proliferation of synaptic connections ready the organism for environmental experiences (Anastasiow, 1990; Touwen, 1989). The immature brain of a young child is capable of adaptive recovery to a greater degree than the more differentiated and mature brain of an adult (Anastasiow, 1990). It is known to be highly plastic and to have more potential for neuronal restructuring following a lesion (Moore, 1969; Vohr, 1991).

Importance of early experience

Early experience is very important to children's development. Each person's development is formed by genetic processes but is also the unique product of experience. The final wiring of the brain occurs after birth and is governed by early experience (Aoki & Siekevitz, 1988). Environmental experiences cause the neurons to be activated. This neural activity stabilizes the synapses and makes persistent synaptic connections (Anastasiow, 1990). Early experience lays the foundation and affects later development.

Critical periods for experience

During particular or critical periods of brain growth, specific environmental stimulation is needed to promote normal development (Touwen, 1989). These critical periods for brain development extend from pregnancy to early childhood when the brain experiences rapid rates of development (Touwen, 1989). The synaptic stabilization is most sensitive and vulnerable to environmental experiences during the critical periods of development. Thus, before birth and during early childhood, the brain is not only highly receptive to environmental influence but is also highly vulnerable to it (Touwen, 1989; Vohr, 1991).

Importance of environment

The environmental context in which young children develop is crucial to their development. Sameroff and Fiese (1990) proposed that human development is a transactional process between the child and the significant "contexts or environment of life." The child's characteristics affect the environment and the child in turn is influenced by the environment that his or her behavior has in part produced. Development is seen as " . . . a product of continuous dynamic interactions of the child and the experience provided by his or her family" (Sameroff & Fiese, 1990, p. 122). Contributions from both members of the dyad have influenced development.

Caregiver's responses determine and are determined by the infant's behavior (Seligman, 1988). For example, infants with disabilities or poor sensory modulation may create problems for the parent and develop a mutually reinforcing style of ineffectuality, which could have profound negative consequences for both infant and parent (Greenspan, 1988; Seligman, 1989; Williamson, 1988). Prevention and remediation of such a disastrous chain of behaviors are crucial to the child's development (Greenspan, 1988; Resnik et al., 1988; Seligman, 1988; Williamson, 1988).

Interrelatedness of behavior across developmental areas

Areas of development (cognitive, language, motor, perceptual, emotional) are interdependent. Developmental gains or gaps in some areas affect development in other areas.

Sensory input by means of sight, sound, smell, and touch is important for a child's development. Failure to remediate a handicap can produce secondary deficits or lead to a cumulative developmental deficit. Accordingly, the earlier it is possible to intervene to improve impaired vision or hearing or to begin remedial sensory stimulation programs to compensate for these deficits, the better the child's developmental course will be (Adelson & Fraiberg, 1974; Klein & Schleifer, 1989).

Infants with poor sensory processing and organization, along with poor muscle tone and motor planning, may become limited in their ability to adapt to, explore, and learn from their environment (Greenspan, 1988; Williamson, 1988). Greenspan (1988) proposed that these children and their families require special assistance. The children need help in mastering emotional and cognitive milestones. Their parents have to learn ways to interpret their child's emotional development.

Economic expectations

Interventions in early childhood can help to reduce the educational costs to society by minimizing the need for special education and related services after infants and toddlers with special needs reach school age. Early intervention also maximizes the potential of these children for future independent living skills (Simeonsson, 1991).

Studies of early intervention with environmentally disadvantaged families have demonstrated positive effects on both parent and child (Barnett & Escobar, 1988, 1990; Seitz et al., 1985). Children demonstrated increased school success, measured by better school attendance records and lower special education costs. Likewise, it has been reported that infants born prematurely and weighing under 5.5 pounds who received early intervention services from birth had significantly better cognitive and behavioral organization at 2 and 3 years of age (Barrera et al., 1986; Bennett, 1990; Rauh et al., 1988; Richmond, 1990).

Legislation and its influence on services for children with developmental deviations

The last 25 years have produced several major pieces of legislation affecting the lives of children with handicaps and developmental disabilities (Dunn, 1989; Hanft, 1988; Hauser-Cram et al., 1988; Gilkerson et al., 1987; Klein & Schleifer, 1989; Meisels & Shonkoff, 1990):

In 1968, with the enactment of Public Law 90–538, the Handicapped Children's Early Education Assistance Act, funds were provided for the development, evaluation, and dissemination of model demonstration projects for children from birth to 8 years with handicaps and for their families.

In 1970, Public Law 91–230, the Education of the Handicapped Act, authorized funding for regional resource centers for blind and deaf children, experimental early childhood education programs, and personnel training.

In 1974, Public Law 93–380 mandated the provision of programs for unserved children with handicaps, including those of preschool age.

In 1975, a major federal legislation, Public Law 94–142, the Education of All Handicapped Children Act, was signed into law. This most extensive federal legislation affecting the education of children with disabilities is designed to ensure that states and localities provide free and appropriate education for all children with handicapping conditions. Under P. L. 94–142, the term "handicapped" refers to children who by reason of their special needs require special education and related services. School-age children (between 5 and 17 years) have a right to an education appropriate to their needs. States were also encouraged to identify children at risk for handicapping conditions from birth through a provision called *Child Find*. Additionally, this law encouraged the development of services for children with special needs from 3 to 5 years of age.

In 1986, Public Law 99–457, the Education of the Handicapped Act Amendments of 1986, became the most important legislation to affect the lives of young children with disabilities and their families. This legislation contains four main sections (titles), but Title I, Handicapped Infants and Toddlers, designated as the added part H of the Education of the Handicapped Act directly concerns early intervention services. This part of the law established a new discretionary program for states to facilitate the development of comprehensive systems of early intervention services necessary to meet the special needs of infants and toddlers with handicaps from birth to age 2 years inclusive.

Effects of P. L. 99–457 on early intervention services

P. L. 99–457 has been enacted to allow funding for individual states to plan, develop, and implement programs to provide for the needs of children with, or at risk for, developmental deviations (Hauser-Cram et al., 1989). Although the development of a service system beginning at birth is encouraged but not required

by this law, all of the states have elected to participate in *Public Law 99–457, part H* and to apply for funding.

How each state defines its policies and programs ultimately affects the nature of service delivery. The law mandated 14 minimum requirements for states seeking federal funding for their early intervention systems. States were given 5 to 6 years from the law enactment date to fulfill these requirements. Over the course of the implementation process, states must define "developmental delay," design an appropriate service delivery system, and provide a timetable for services availability. They must offer a comprehensive multidisciplinary evaluation of the needs of children and their families and provide an Individualized Family Service Plan (IFSP) that includes case management services. Public awareness focusing on early identification of children at risk for developmental deviations (Child Find), referral systems, interagency coordination, policies and procedures for personnel standards and personnel development, a system of program evaluation, procedural safeguards, and a single line of authority to a lead agency are part of the requirements dictated by law (Healy et al., 1989; Meisels, 1989).

Goals of early intervention according to P. L. 99–457, Part H

EI services are generally provided at no cost to the family and are designed to do the following:

a. Enhance child development and minimize potential for developmental delays or disabilities
b. Reduce the need for special education and related services . . . [when] school age [is reached]
c. Minimize the likelihood of institutionalization or other restrictive placements and maximize potential for independent functioning in society
d. Enhance the capacity of families to meet the special needs of their infants and toddlers with handicaps (Section 671, (a) 1 pp. 3, 4, P. L. 99–457)

According to this law early intervention services agencies must respond to the unique needs of infants and toddlers (by individualized programming) and their families (by a family-focused approach) and develop community collaboration (by an interagency system) (Hanft, 1988).

Role of occupational therapy

In early intervention, occupational therapists are members of an interdisciplinary team composed of health and education professionals and the child's parents (Gorga, 1989). The role of occupational therapy is to facilitate the independent functioning of infants and toddlers and their families (Case-Smith, 1989) (Figures 13-25 and 13-26).

Independent functioning of young children, according to their developmental age, is achieved through assessment and intervention efforts in the areas of motor control, sensory modulation, adaptive coping, sensorimotor development, social–emotional development, daily living skills, and play (Gorga, 1989).

In working with parents the major goals of occupational

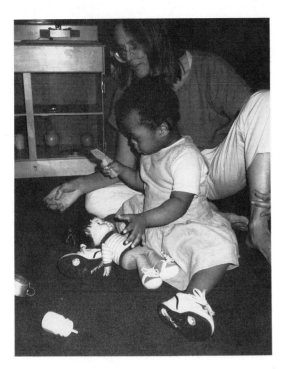

FIGURE 13-25. *Therapist is encouraging language and play skills.*

therapy are to support, enable, and empower them in creating a familial climate conducive to prevent or minimize development delays and to promote harmonious growth and development (Dunst et al., 1988). These goals can be achieved through identifying of *family needs, family strengths,* and resources; through facilitation of satisfying parent–child interactions; through supporting and educating parents to meet the special needs of their child and to enhance their child's competence and adaptation; through locating and linking families to informal and formal community resources to support parents' needs and goals; and through supporting and empowering parents to become advocates for their child's and their family's needs (Anderson & Hinojosa, 1984; Bazyk, 1989; Dunst et al., 1988).

In the case study later in this section, more specific and detailed goals and methods of occupational therapy assessment and intervention are presented.

Service delivery in early intervention programs

Team approaches

The complexity and interrelationships of very young children's developmental problems cannot be addressed by a single discipline and require services from various professionals. The *team approach* is used widely in early intervention. Depending on the setting and its staff composition, three types of teamwork are used: multidisciplinary, interdisciplinary, and transdisciplinary (Woodruff & Hanson, 1987). The interdisciplinary and transdisciplinary models are most often used in early intervention delivery systems. Professionals work together as a team to deliver the range of necessary services:

Multidisciplinary approach—in this approach, a group of professionals perform related tasks (evaluation or treatment) independently of one another and act as independent specialists. Professionals may consult or interact with each other, but there is not always a built-in coordination of services and communication mechanisms among them. This model is more frequently seen in medicine; when it is used in EI, a case manager is assigned to the family to provide coordination of services. Such may be the case of a child receiving additional services outside the main agency, such as evaluation or specialized treatment (Woodruff & Hanson, 1987).

Interdisciplinary approach—in this approach professionals of various disciplines, but in the same agency and location, assess and treat the child independently. However, there is a built-in mechanism for cooperation and communication. Decision making regarding the interpretation of the child's evaluation, diagnosis, goal setting, and treatment is shared and reflects the team consensus. Team members collaborate with each other. The interdisciplinary approach

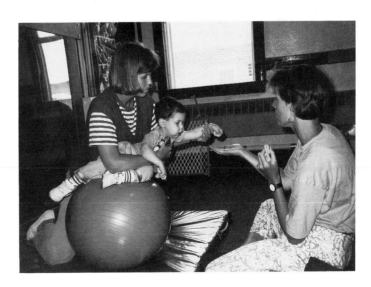

FIGURE 13-26. *Therapist is facilitating trunk elongation.*

takes into account the complexity of the child and the family needs and is built on the skills unique to each professional specialty (Woodruff & Hanson, 1987).

Transdisciplinary approach—in this approach professionals cross the lines of their own traditional professional limits and become more like generalists. They form a team that crosses and recrosses disciplinary boundaries to maximize communication, interaction, and cooperation among each other (Woodruff & Hanson, 1987). This approach gives the parents and the child access to one person who consistently works with them and limits the number of professionals coming in and out of their lives. Early intervention services provided by a single professional were generally reported as decreasing stress in mothers of children with developmental deviations (Shonkoff et al., 1990).

Whatever the setting and the model, occupational therapists in early intervention work as team members and always in partnership with the child's parents, who are acknowledged as full members of the team.

Location of service delivery

Although a number of components are common across all early intervention programs, other factors clearly distinguish one program from another (Filler, 1983). Services are community-based, and thus their location and structure vary with the characteristics of that community, such as geographic setting (rural, urban, and so on), the needs of the population served, the community resources, and the goals of the services (Zeitlin & Williamson, 1986). Services are provided either in the child's home or at the center. The setting in which services are delivered is usually a decision made according to the needs of the child, the family, and the resources and organization of the agency. A family may receive services at home (***home-based***) or at the center (***center-based***), or a combination of both. Advantages characteristic of each type of services are as follows:

I. Home-based (Filler, 1983, p. 378)
   A. Parent and child routines are preserved and more easily shared with the therapist.
   B. Family natural environment may be used and modified to facilitate developmental adaptations.
   C. Sessions are generally more regular because family does not have to travel to appointment.
   D. Interventions are relevant to family context.
   E. Child's health can be better protected.
   F. Parents may feel more in control because of being in their own territory.
   G. Young children may perform better in their own environment.
   H. Other members of the family can be more easily included in the intervention.
II. Center-based (Filler, 1983, p. 379)
   A. Opportunity for families to meet others in group setting (eg, parent-child groups; parent support group; father group) (Figures 13-27 and 13-28).
   B. Opportunity for child to socialize with other children (eg, play group; sibling group).
   C. Opportunity for child to learn new routines in preparation for preschool entry and transition from EI [early intervention] (eg, toddler group).

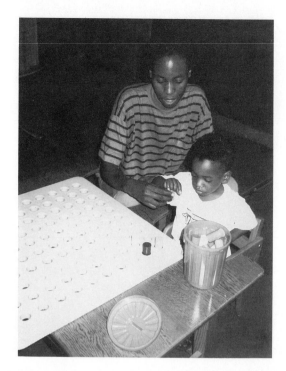

FIGURE 13-27. *Mother and child engaged in a fine-motor activity.*

   D. Opportunity for other EI staff participation (eg, interdisciplinary team).
   E. A special learning environment can be provided with access to larger diversity of toys and equipment.

Bronfenbrenner (1974) proposed that home-based or home-based plus center-based programs may be more effective than strictly center-based programs. Shonkoff et al. (1990), in their efficacy study on early intervention, reported that in their appraisal of their early intervention experience, parents (especially mothers) described home visits as the most helpful of all services received. The researchers also found that more frequent home visits were associated with significant decreases in the amount of parental stress or personal difficulty.

Frequency of services

At present, there are no reports in the EI literature regarding optimal scheduling of services for the various types of children with or at risk for developmental deviations. Schedule and frequency of services vary from program to program and from family to family (Shonkoff et al., 1990). Some children need more intensive intervention and may in infancy receive 1 hour per week of home visits plus 1 hour per week of parent–child group support at the EI center. Other infants need only developmental monitoring and may receive services once or twice per month for about 1 hour at home or at the center or at both. Toddlers may attend a *toddler group* twice per week for about 2.5 hours at the EI center. This prepares them for preschool placement when they reach 3 years of age.

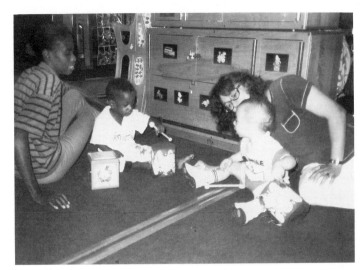

FIGURE 13-28. *Two mothers and their boys are enjoying play at the Parent-Child Playground.*

Services required by law

Three major types of services are required by law. These services occur in a team process: assessment, individualized family service plans, and case management.

Assessment

The family-focused P. L. 99–457 has specific guidelines regarding assessments (Dunst et al., 1988; P. L. 99–457, subpart D, Sec. 303.300–322). Assessment of children's strengths and weaknesses must take into account family factors as well. *Assessment* is an interactive process between the parents and the professionals. Guidelines for evaluations are as follows:

Screening and assessment should reflect several sources of information.

Screening and assessment procedures should be reliable and valid.

Parents are an integral part of that process, and are part of the assessment team.

Family assessments should be designed to determine the strengths and needs of the family related to enhancing the child's development.

Family needs and strengths should be assessed by the most natural and least intrusive methods.

Screening and assessment procedures and interpretation must be culturally sensitive.

Relevant and familiar tasks and settings enhance the results of the assessment.

Communication of assessment results to parents should be carried out in a sensitive, honest, caring, practical, and constructive manner.

Results of the evaluation should be written in a language understandable to the parents; they should stress the child's areas of competence and report areas of concerns with appropriate recommendations for remediation.

Screening and assessments should be made on recurrent, periodic bases.

Comprehensive training is needed for those who screen and

assess very young children (Bailey, 1991; Meisels & Provence, 1989, p. 24).

Procedures for assessments vary according to the organization of each EI program. For instance, in some programs a screening test is first administered by the professional who meets with the family during the intake interview. According to the needs of the child and the family, other appointments are scheduled later for a more in-depth assessment. The choice of instruments varies from program to program, depending on the professional staff preference and orientation. Tables 13-11 and 13-12 present several instruments that are commonly used in EI settings.

Meisels and Provence (1989) advised caution in the administration and interpretation of tests with young children: "Due to the dynamic nature of development, tests provide only an indication of a child's skills and abilities at a given time." (p. 50). Parents' perceptions of their child's strengths and problems are crucial to the evaluation process as they give a perspective on the child's daily functioning in the context of his or her environment.

The assessment is viewed as part of the therapeutic process. It seeks to enhance parents' understanding of their child and to improve the fit between the parents' caretaking style and the child's behaviors (Parker & Zuckerman, 1990). The evaluation of individual family needs, strengths, and supports is also viewed as part of the therapeutic process. It is a prerequisite for the planning and implementation of the family service plan.

Individualized family service plan

To ensure the parents' central role in the planning and administration of their child's program of services the law requires the development of a family-centered service plan. This plan, called the *Individualized Family Service Plan* (IFSP), is a written individualized plan of intervention developed by a multidisciplinary team, including the parent or the child's guardian.

The IFSP must include in writing the following information (P. L. 99–457, part H, Sec. 677. d.):

1. The child's present level of function in all developmental areas

TABLE 13-11. *Selected Assessment Tools for Birth to 3 Years*

Title and Source	Age Range	Norm-Referenced	Criterion-Referenced	Primary Purpose				
				Developmental	Motor	Sensory Integration	Play	Other
Battelle Developmental Inventory (DLM Teaching Resources, Allen, TX)	0–8 yr	Yes		Yes				
Battelle Developmental Screening Inventory Test (DLM Teaching Resources, Allen, TX)	0–8 yr	Yes		Yes				
Bayley Scales of Infant Development (Psychological Corporation, San Antonio, TX)	2–30 mo	Yes		Yes				
Callier Asuza Scales (University of Texas at Dallas, Callier Center for Communication Disorders, Dallas, TX)	0-5 yr		Yes					Yes
Denver Developmental Screening Test (Ladoca Publishing Foundation, University of Colorado, Denver, CO)	0–6 yr	Yes		Yes				
Denver II Developmental Screening Test (Ladoca Publishing Foundation, University of Colorado, Denver, CO)	0–6 yr	Yes		Yes				
Early Coping Inventory (Scholastic Testing Service, Bensenville, IL)	4–36 mo	Yes						Yes
Early Intervention Developmental Profile (University of Michigan, Ann Arbor, MI)	0–36 mo		Yes	Yes				
Early Learning Accomplishment Profile for Developmentally Delayed Young Children (Kaplan Press, P.O. Box 25408, Winston-Salem, NC)	0–36 mo		Yes	Yes				
Early Screening Profiles (American Guidance Service, Circle Pines, MN)	2–6 yr	Yes		Yes				
Erhardt Developmental Prehension Assessment (Therapy Skill Builders, Tucson, AZ)	0–15 mo			Yes	Yes			
Erhardt Developmental Vision Assessment (Therapy Skill Builders, Tucson, AZ)	0–6 mo			Yes				Yes
From Exploration to Play (Belsky, J. [1981]. *Developmental Psychology, 17*, 630–639)	7½–21 mo						Yes	
Hawaii Early Learning Profile (VORT Corporation, Palo Alto, CA)	0–3 yr		Yes	Yes				
Infant Monitoring Questionnaire (Bricker, Division of Special Education, College of Educations, University of Oregon, Eugene, OR)	0–3 yr	Yes		Yes				
Infant Mullen Scales of Early Learning (244 Deerfield Road, Cranston, RI)	0–38 mo	Yes		Yes				
Miller Assessment for Preschoolers (Harcourt Brace Jovanovich, San Antonio, TX)	2 yr, 9 mo–5 yr, 8 mo	Yes		Yes		Yes		
Movement Assessment of Infants (P.O. Box 4631, Rolling Bay, WA)	0–12 mo		Yes		Yes			
Neonatal Behavioral Assessment Scale (J. B. Lippincott, Philadelphia, PA)	0–1 mo	Yes		Yes		Yes		
Peabody Developmental Motor Scales (DLM Teaching Resources, Allen, TX)	0–83 mo	Yes			Yes			
Pediatric Evaluation of Disability Inventory (Haley, S., et al., Rehabilitation Medicine Dept., Tufts University School of Medicine, Boston, MA)	6 mo–7 yr	Yes						Yes

(*continued*)

TABLE 13-11. *Selected Assessment Tools for Birth to 3 Years (continued)*

Title and Source	Age Range	Norm-Referenced	Criterion-Referenced	Primary Purpose				
				Developmental	*Motor*	*Sensory Integration*	*Play*	*Other*
Preschool Play Scale (Bledsdoe & Shephard [1982]. *AJOT, 36*[12], 783–788)	0–6 yr		Yes				Yes	
Sensory Integration Observation Guide for Children (Jirgal & Bouma [1989]. *Sensory Integration Newsletter, 12*[2], 3)	0–3 yr					Yes		
Takata Play History (In Reilly [Ed.], *Play as Exploratory Learning.* Sage Publications, Beverly Hills, CA)	0–16 yr						Yes	
Test of Sensory Functions in Infants (Western Psychological Services, Los Angeles, CA)	4–18 mo	Yes				Yes		
Transdisciplinary Play-Based Assessment (Paul H. Brooks Publishing, Baltimore, MD)	6 mo–6 yr			Yes			Yes	
Vineland Social Maturity Scale (American Guidance Service, Circle Pines, MN)	0–26 yr	Yes		Yes				

2. The family's strengths and needs related to support of their child's development
3. The major outcomes to be achieved for the child and the family; the criteria, procedures, and timeline used to determine the degree to which progress toward achieving the outcomes is being made; whether modifications or revisions of the outcomes are necessary
4. The specific services needed to meet the unique needs of the child and the family, including the frequency, intensity, and the method of delivery services
5. The dates of services (initiation and anticipated duration)
6. The name of the family case manager (service coordinator)
7. The transition plan (when appropriate) to services provided under part B of the law (preschool services)

The main purpose of the IFSP is to identify and organize formal and informal resources to facilitate parents' goals for their child's optimal development and for their family. It acknowledges that (1) family strengths will be recognized and built on; (2) family needs will be met in a way that is respectful of their beliefs and values; and (3) parents' hopes and aspirations for their child will be encouraged and enabled (Deal et al., 1989).

The development of the IFSP goals occurs after the child and the family needs have been assessed. It involves a process of collaboration and mutual problem solving between parents and professionals to establish priorities in the intervention plan (McGonigel & Garland, 1988). It is written in a language understandable to parents and contains parents' own words in sections relative to parents' perception of needs and strengths.

The IFSP needs to be updated at regular intervals with a record of treatment activities and their effectiveness. An example of the IFSP is offered in the case study section at the end of this section.

Case management

Case management is central to the coordination of early intervention services. The law mandates that a case manager be named "... from the profession most immediately relevant to the child or the family's needs (P. L. 99–457, part H, Sec. 677). Occupational therapists are primary interventionists and are frequently designated as case managers" (Case-Smith, 1991).

Case management is an active and ongoing process throughout the duration of services (for some families, 3 years), which helps promote a coherent service system. The case manager (also called "service coordinator") is responsible for the following tasks (Case-Smith, 1990; P. L. 99–457, part H, Sec. 677):

To coordinate for the family all services in the EI agency as identified in the IFSP.

To assist parents in gaining access to other services as identified in the IFSP or as the need arises and to coordinate these services (for diagnosis, evaluation, and intervention purposes).

To ensure that the IFSP reflects the family's evolving needs and to continuously seek services reflecting those needs.

To facilitate program transition.

In providing services to the families, case managers engage in a variety of activities and roles, from specialist to service coordinator, advocate, teacher, helper, community liaison, partner, and so on (Bailey, 1989). First and foremost, case management has to be family-centered and to focus on the family's needs and strengths (Case-Smith, 1990). A successful partnership between the family and the case manager is crucial to the intervention program, reflecting the importance of harmonious parent–professional interactions.

TABLE 13-12. *Selected Assessment Tools for Evaluating Family Needs*

Test Name (Author)	Primary Purpose	Norm-Referenced	Source
Family environment scale (Moos & Moos)	Family social environment assessment	Yes	Consulting Psychologists Press Palo Alto, CA
Family functioning style scale (Dunst et al.)	Family functioning assessment		Brookline Books Cambridge, MA
Family needs scale (Dunst et al.)	Needs-based assessment		Brookline Books Cambridge, MA
Family resource scale (Dunst et al.)	Needs-based assessment		Brookline Books Cambridge, MA
Family strengths profile (Dunst et al.)	Family strengths assessment		Brookline Books Cambridge, MA
Family support plan (Dunst et al.)	Planning of family support		Brookline Books Cambridge, MA
Family support scale (Dunst et al.)	Sources of family support assessment		Brookline Books Cambridge, MA
Inventory of social support (Dunst et al.)	Person's social network assessment		Brookline Books Cambridge, MA
Parenting stress index (Abidin)	Assessment of parent stress in raising a child	Yes	Clinical Psychology Publishing Co. Brandon, VT
Perceived support network inventory (Dunst et al.)	Family members' personal network assessment		Brookline Books Cambridge, MA
Personal network matrix (Dunst et al.)	Person's social network assessment		Brookline Books Cambridge, MA
Profile of family needs and social support (Dunst et al.)	Family needs and social support assessment		Brookline Books Cambridge, MA
Questionnaire on resources and stress for families with chronically ill or handicapped members (Holroyd)	Assessment of stress in families who care for ill or disabled relative	Yes	Clinical Psychology Publishing Co. Brandon, VT
Resource scale for teenage mothers (Dunst et al.)	Needs-based assessment		Brookline Books Cambridge, MA
Support functions scale (Dunst et al.)	Needs-based assessment		Brookline Books Cambridge, MA

Parent–professional interactions

The birth of a child changes the life of a family forever. With few exceptions, the birth of a child with a disability or with a difficult perinatal course is not expected and thus brings emotional, organizational, and financial strains on the family. All parents in our modern society have to depend to some degree on the expertise and help from professionals in the care and education of their children. But for parents of children with special needs, this dependence is much stronger. The shape and quality of this dependence can influence the way families adapt to their temporarily or permanently altered lives (Featherstone, 1980; Healy et al., 1989).

For occupational therapists working in early intervention, the question is how best to contribute one's expertise and assistance in ways that will respect the family's integrity and promote competence and independence in both child and parents (Healy et al., 1989). Parents of children with special needs and professionals have made recommendations for ways to enhance this special relationship in several areas (Anderson & Hinojosa, 1984; Dunst et al., 1988; Featherstone, 1980; Hanft, 1988; Healy et al., 1989; Hobbs & Perrin, 1985; Provence, 1990; Redman-Bentley, 1982).

I. Communication
    A. Articulate information clearly and in a manner understandable to parents (no jargon).
    B. Share knowledge in parents' and family members' best learning style (pictures, hands-on approach, books, and so on).
    C. Deliver information according to parents' emotional and cognitive readiness.
    D. Give information regarding test results, changes in child's progress and program, and child's developmental needs.
    E. Emphasize child's and family's strengths.
    F. Teach parents and family members specific intervention techniques to promote child's development and parent–child interaction.

II. Attitudes
  A. Respect parents' and family's feelings, values, and priorities.
  B. Acknowledge child and family individuality.
  C. Listen to parents with respectful and sensitive attention.
  D. Demonstrate empathy.
  E. Be caring, honest, and truthful.
  F. Accept parents' emotional setbacks.
  G. Project optimistic feelings, positive attitude, and a sense of humor.
  H. Support and foster parents' efforts and competence in raising their children.
  I. Expect, encourage, and prepare parents to take an active role in their child's program.
  J. Offer support and help relevant to the family's culture.

III. Professional training
  A. Knowledge of typical and atypical infant development
  B. Knowledge of the parenting process and family life cycle
  C. Knowledge and skills in approaches, assessment, treatment planning, and intervention methods and practice for children with special needs and their families
  D. Knowledge of the effects on the whole family of having a child with special needs
  E. Knowledge of methods to support, enable, and empower families
  F. Knowledge of family advocacy practices
  G. Knowledge and skills in communication with parents, family members, and with other professionals
  H. Knowledge and skills in working in an interdisciplinary and transdisciplinary team
  I. Knowledge and application of decision-making and clinical reasoning skills
  J. Knowledge of social and cultural issues and practice (Figures 13-29 and 13-30)

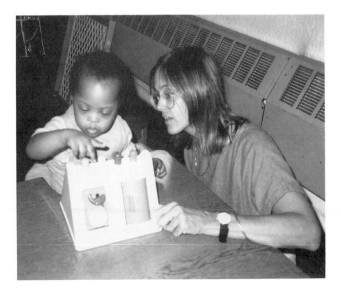

FIGURE 13-29. *Therapist and child engaged in fine-motor exploration.*

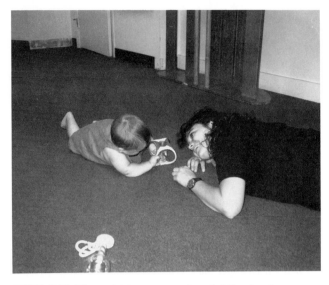

FIGURE 13-30. *Therapist is encouraging child's play in prone position.*

CASE STUDY

Steven, an infant with neurobehavioral problems, was referred to the EI program by his pediatrician.

Background History

Steven was born at 41 weeks of gestation, weighing 6 pounds, 12 ounces. Labor was induced when ultrasonography showed an insufficiency of amniotic fluid. Steven's mother was in labor for 30 hours but fetal monitors did not indicate any distress.

Steven's perinatal course was complicated by meconium aspiration, and a few hours after birth by a collapsed lung. He was transferred to the Neonatal Intensive Care Unit (NICU), where he stayed for 10 days, during which time he suffered three seizures (for which he is now on phenobarbital), was put on a respirator for 2 days, and was tube-fed for 9 days. A computed tomography (CT) scan indicated that he had suffered anoxic brain damage.

Steven is the third child in his family. He has two older sisters (10 and 6 years old). Three months before Steven's birth, the family moved because of the father's work. This has been particularly difficult on the family because they do not know anybody in their neighborhood. The girls have had a difficult adjustment to their new school, and Mr. and Mrs. P. have neither relatives nor friends in this area. The mother was working part-time in a bank before the move but is now home with Steven.

After the referral to EI, Steven (then 4 months) and his family were visited by the social worker. She met with them at their home and took a history of Steven's perinatal and early infancy as well as a family history. She inquired about family needs and concerns about Steven and themselves. This was done in a friendly and supportive interview format to establish contact and a basis for future assessment by an EI team.

Assessment of Case Study

Assessment was done at home by an EI interdisciplinary team of an occupational therapist and an educator. Instruments:

- EI Developmental Profile
- Neuromotor assessment
- Behavioral observations
- Interview with parent about Steven's sleep–wake patterns, mood, care, feeding, and daily routine
- Family support scale (Dunst et al., 1988)

Major Findings

I. Family strengths
   A. Family members are supportive of each other and Steven.
   B. Father and sisters participate in Steven's care.
   C. Home environment is conducive to children's growth and development (setting, furniture, toys, food).
   D. Family wants help from EI staff.
II. Steven's strengths
   A. Handsome baby who smiles when he is "happy"
   B. Enjoys family's attention most of the time
   C. Follows faces and toys with his eyes when presented in front of him
III. Family needs
   A. Mother needs socialization outside of home.
   B. Mother needs help in handling Steven at times, especially feeding.
   C. Father and sisters want to know why Steven is a cranky baby at times.
IV. Steven's needs
   A. Sensitive to noise and sudden changes of position
   B. Does not like baths and to be undressed
   C. Mild hypertonicity through trunk and extremities
   D. Minimal reciprocal movements in upper and lower extremities (UEs, LEs)
   E. Poor suck and "colicky" baby
   F. Strong Moro reflex
   G. Poor head control
   H. Sleep patterns poorly established

Individual Family Service Plan (IFSP)

After the evaluation, a case manager (service coordinator) was assigned to this family based on their major needs. These needs centered around Steven's hypersensitive neuromotor system and feeding needs. An occupational therapist was given the role. She met with the mother at home, and together they discussed Steven's assessment results and drew the IFSP for the first months of intervention. The schedule of services was as follows:

1 hour per week service provided for Steven at home by an occupational therapist (case manager in this instance)
1.5 hours for mother and child to *Baby Group* at the EI center provided by interdisciplinary team (social worker, occupational therapist, physical therapist, and educator)

The following are home-based intervention goals:

Decrease muscle tone in trunk, UEs, and LEs through proper positioning and relaxation methods (modeled from NeuroDevelopmental Treatment and Sensory-Motor approaches).

Instruct mother and the rest of the family on proper positioning of Steven during all activities and care (hands-on approach shown to mother and pictures of positioning with purpose left with her). (Baby Positioning stickers are available from Therapy Skill Builders, Tucson, AZ.)

Instruct mother on ways to calm Steven (swaddling, slow rocking, diminish noise, deep touch—no tickling—slow and firm stroking of extremities and hands, hold baby firmly).

Instruct mother on feeding position, nonnutritive sucking, and jaw control.

Increase Steven's tolerance to sensory input through individualized vestibular and tactile stimulation (modeled from sensory integration approach).

Help mother to bring some regularity to Steven's schedule.

Encourage visual exploration, grasping, babbling, soft auditory stimulation through developmental appropriate toys and activities.

Develop head and trunk control in prone, sitting positions.

Explain to family reasons for Steven's "crankiness," the meaning of hypersensitivity and avenues for controlling it and promoting positive interaction.

Inform mother about resources in the community of interest and assistance to her and family.

The following Baby Group intervention goals provide opportunities for:

Mother to socialize with six other mothers and to get out of her house,

Sharing common issues with other mothers,

Receiving support from the other mothers and EI professionals,

Exploring new toys and child care resources (books, pamphlets), and

Primary therapist (case manager) to ask for input from colleagues as they interact with Steven.

Goals were set in collaboration with the mother and should be reevaluated and recorded on the IFSP form periodically (at least every 6 months) or as often as the need arises.

See examples of several pages of Steven's IFSP in Figure 13-31.

Summary

Pediatric occupational therapy is a growing field in which areas of practice in the school system and in early intervention are mandated by law (eg, P. L. 94–142; P. L. 99–457).

Public Law 99–457 has opened more services for young children with developmental disabilities and those with or at risk for developmental deviations and for their families. It is a challenging concept of social, educational, and health care services focusing on prevention, habilitation, and remediation of children's developmental delays. Services are individualized, coordinated, and family-focused. Occupational therapists have an essential role in EI working in collaboration with parents and other professionals.

(*Text continues on page 473*)

INDIVIDUAL FAMILY SERVICE PLAN

Cambridge-Somerville Early Intervention Program—Preschool Unit
12 Maple Avenue
Cambridge, MA 02139

Child's Name: _Steven P._

Parent/Guardian: _Laurie P._

Parent/Guardian: _John P._

Address: _1233 Some Street, Some Town_

Initial Screening: _11/06/91_   Initial Assessment: _11/15/91_

Child's DOB: _7/14/91_

Relationship: _Mother_

Relationship: _Father_

Telephone: _(617) 555-2222_

Service Coordinator: _Sue M., MA, OTR/L_

Intervention Team:

	Role:
Laurie and John P.	Parents
Sue M.	Case Manager, MA, OTR/L
Ellen S.	MS, RiPT, baby group team
Ann R.	M. Ed., baby group team

I have had the opportunity to be as involved in the development of this plan as I would like and I agree with the plan and its provisions.

_____   _____
Signature of Parent/Guardian   Date

FIGURE 13-31. *Individual family service plans for Steven P.* (*Figure continues on next page*)

Child Profile: How would you describe your child?

Steven is our handsome baby boy.

He smiles when he is happy. He likes our attention.

He has had a hard time since his birth.

Child's Strengths:

Handsome and at times cheerful.

He enjoys our attention and playing with us.

Child's Needs:

He needs to suck better.

His muscles are not strong.

He is cranky at times and does not like to take baths, to be undressed, and to be moved suddenly.

Household/Family Members:

Mother and father

Susan (10 years old, sister)

Mary (6 years old, sister)

Family's Concerns, Priorities, and Resources:

We want help in feeding and taking care of Steven.

We want help with Steven's development.

We would like to meet other families with children like Steven.

We help each other, and the girls like to play with Steven.

Summary of Child Development Information

Fine motor perceptual:

Steven follows faces and toys with his eyes in all planes. He fingers his own hands in play at midline when lying supine. When trunk and head are supported he reaches for objects.

Cognition:

When supported he mouths objects and shakes rattles. He looks at faces and recognizes his family.

Language:

He exhibits differentiated crying. He turns his eyes and his head in direction of voices and sounds. He begins to vocalize when talked to.

Social emotional:

He smiles spontaneously and to familiar faces. He watches family walk across room. He likes to be with people.

Self-care:

He has a weak suck. He does not coordinate sucking, swallowing, and breathing well.

Gross motor:

He has:
a strong Moro reflex; moderate hypertonicity through trunk and extremities; minimal reciprocal movements in UEs and LEs; poor head control

Screening tool—Denver II Developmental Screening Test and Family Support Scale
Assessment tool—Early Intervention Developmental Profile; neurobehavioral observations

Comments:

Steven is also sensitive to noise and sudden changes of position. He is colicky, and his sleep patterns are poorly established.

FIGURE 13-31. (*Figure continues on next page*)

Child's Name Steven P.   Service Coordinator Sue M.   Date 11/25/91

INDIVIDUAL FAMILY SERVICE PLAN AND REVIEW

Child's Name: Steven P.

Evaluation Rating Scale:
1. No longer a need or goal.
2. Unchanged—still a goal.
3. Improved.
4. Resolved or attained.

Date	Goal/Need	Plan	Source of Support	Planned Achievement Date	Evaluation Dates
11/25/91	1. Decrease muscle tone in trunk and limbs	Position Steven according to pictures given by therapist. Therapist will use relaxation techniques.	Parents, Sue M.	6/25/91	
	2. Show ways to calm Steven	Therapist will show to the family techniques for calming Steven.	Sue M.		
	3. Increase sucking	Instruct parents on jaw control, feeding position, use of pacifier.	Parents, Sue M.		
	4. Increase socialization for mother	Parent–child playgroup and community resources.	Baby—group team		
	5. Increase motor development	Developmental activities	Parents, and Sue M., baby—group team		

Types of Service (Subject to the availability of resources)	Location	Personnel	Frequency	Total Hours/Week
Home visit: sensorimotor, developmental intervention	Home	Sue M.	1X/week	1.0/week
Baby group	Center	EI staff	1X/week	1.5/week
Consultation from other EI disciplines as needed.	TBA	TBA	As needed	As needed

I agree with this plan and its provisions.

_____ _____
Parent/Guardian   Date

FIGURE 13-31. (*Continued*)

472

References

Abidin, R. R. (1983). *Parenting stress index.* Charlottesville, MD: Pediatric Psychology Press.

Adelson, E., & Fraiberg, S. (1974). Gross motor development in infants blind from birth. *Child Development, 45,* 114–126.

Anastasiow, N. J. (1990). Implications of the neurobiological model for early intervention. In S. J. Meisels & J. P. Shonkoff (Eds.), *Handbook of early childhood intervention* (pp. 196–216). New York: Cambridge University Press.

Anderson, J., & Hinojosa, J. (1984). Parents and therapists in a professional partnership, *American Journal of Occupational Therapy, 38*(7), 452–461.

Aoki, C., & Siekevitz, P. (1988). Plasticity in brain development. *Scientific American,* December, 56–64.

Bailey, D. B. (1989). Case management in early intervention. *Journal of Early Intervention, 13*(2), 120–134.

Bailey, D. B. (1991). Issues and perspectives on family assessment. *Infants and Young Children, 4*(1), 26–32.

Barnett, W. S., & Escobar, C. M. (1988). The economics of early intervention for handicapped children: What do we really know? *Journal of Division for Early Childhood, 12,* 169–181.

Barnett, W. S., & Escobar, C. M. (1990). Economic costs and benefits of early intervention. In S. J. Meisels & J. P. Shonkoff (Eds.), *Handbook of early childhood intervention* (pp. 560–582). New York: Cambridge University Press.

Barrera, M. E., Rosenbaum, P. L., & Cunningham, C. E. (1986). Early home intervention with low birth weight infants and their parents. *Child Development, 57,* 20–33.

Bazyk, S. (1989). Changes in attitudes and beliefs regarding parent participation and home programs: an update. *American Journal of Occupational Therapy, 43*(11), 723–736.

Bennett, F. C. (1990). Recent advances in developmental intervention for biologically-vulnerable infants. *Infants and Young Children, 3*(1), 33–40.

Bronfenbrenner, U. (1974). Is early intervention effective? *Teachers College Record, 76,* 279–303.

Case-Smith, J. (1989). Working with families in early intervention: new strategies with traditional occupational therapy skills. *Developmental Disabilities Special Interest Section, 12*(1), 2–3.

Case-Smith, J. (1990). Case management in early intervention. *Developmental Disabilities Special Interest Section Newsletter, 13*(4), 5–7.

Case-Smith, J. (1991). Occupational and physical therapists as case managers in early intervention. *Physical & Occupational Therapy in Pediatrics, 11*(1), 53–69.

Clancy, H., & Clark, M. J. (1990). *Occupational therapy with children.* New York: Churchill Livingstone.

Deal, A. G., Dunst, C. J., & Trivette, C. H. (1989). A flexible and functional approach to developing individualized family support plans. *Infants & Young Children, 1*(4), 32–43.

Dunn, W. (1989). Occupational therapy in early intervention: new perspectives create greater possibilities. *American Journal of Occupational Therapy, 43*(11), 717–721.

Dunst, C., Trivette, C., & Deal, A. (1988). *Enabling and empowering families, principles and guidelines for practice.* Cambridge, MA: Brookline Books.

Education of the Handicapped Act Amendments of 1986 (Public Law 99–457), 20 U.S.C. 1400.

Featherstone, H. (1980). *A difference in the family life with a disabled child.* New York: Basic Books.

Filler, J. W. (1983). Service models for handicapped infants. In S. G. Garwood & R. R. Fewell (Eds.), *Educating handicapped infants, issues in developmental intervention.* Rockville, MD: Aspen Publications.

Gilkerson, L., Hilliard, A. G., Schrag, E. & Shonkoff, J. P. (1987). *Report accompanying the education of the handicapped act amendments of 1986 and commenting on P.L. 99–457,* Washington, DC: National Center for Clinical Infant Programs.

Gorga, D. (1989). Occupational therapy treatment practices with infants in early intervention. *American Journal of Occupational Therapy, 43*(11), 731–736.

Greenspan, S. (1988). Fostering emotional and social development in infants with disabilities. *Zero to Three, 9*(1), 8–18.

Hanft, B. (1988). The changing environment of early intervention services: Implications for practice. *American Journal of Occupational Therapy, 42*(11), 724–731.

Hauser-Cram, P., Upshur, C. C., Krauss, M. W., & Shonkoff, J. P. (1988). Implications of Public Law 99–457 for early intervention services for infants and toddlers with disabilities. *Social Policy Report, 3*(3), 1–16.

Healy, A., Keesee, P. D., & Smith, B. S. (1989). *Early services for children with special needs, transactions for family support.* Baltimore: Paul H. Brookes.

Hobbs, N., & Perrin, J. M. (1985). *Issues in the care of children with chronic illness.* San Francisco: Jossey-Bass.

Holroyd, J. (1974). The questionnaire on resource and stress: An instrument to measure family response to a handicapped member. *Journal of Community Psychology, 2,* 92–94.

Klein, S. D., & Schleifer, M. J. (1989). Early Intervention!! *Exceptional Parent,* Jan–Feb, 38–41.

McGonigel, M. J., & Garland, C. W. (1988). The individualized family service plan and the early intervention team: Team and family issues and recommended practices. *Infants and Young Children, 1*(1), 10–21.

Meisels, S. J. (1989). Meeting the mandate of Public Law 99–457: Early childhood intervention in the nineties. *American Journal of Orthopsychiatry, 59*(3), 451–460.

Meisels, S. J., & Provence, S. (1989). *Screening and assessment: Guidelines for identifying young disabled and developmentally vulnerable children and their families.* Washington, DC: National Center for Clinical Infant Programs.

Meisels, S. J., & Shonkoff, J. P. (Eds.). (1990). *Handbook of early childhood intervention.* New York: Cambridge University Press.

Moore, J. C. (1969). *Neuroanatomy simplified.* Dubuque, IA: Kendall Hunt.

Moos, R., & Moos, B. (1986). Family environment scale manual. Palo Alto, CA: Consulting Psychologists Press.

Parker, S. J., & Zuckerman, B. S. (1990). Therapeutic aspects of the assessment process. In Meisels, S. J. & J. P. Shonkoff (Eds.), *Handbook of early childhood intervention* (pp. 350–369). New York: Cambridge University Press.

Provence, S. (1990). Interactional issues: Infants, parents, professionals. *Infants and Young Children, 3*(1), 1–7.

Rauh, V. A., Achenbach, T. M., Nucombe, B., Howell, C. T., & Teti, D. M. (1988). Minimizing adverse effects of low birth weight: Four-year results of an early intervention program. *Child Development, 59,* 544–553.

Redman-Bentley, D. (1982). Parent expectations for professionals providing services to their handicapped children. *Physical and Occupational Therapy in Pediatrics, 2*(1), 13–27.

Resnik, M. B., Armstrong, S., & Carter, R. L. (1988). Developmental intervention program for high-risk premature infants: Effects on development and parent-infant interactions. *Journal of Developmental and Behavioral Pediatrics, 9,* 73–78.

Richmond, J. (1990). The infant health and development program: enhancing the outcome of low birth weight, premature infants: A multisite randomized trial. *Journal American Medical Association, 263*(22), 3069–3070.

Sameroff, A. J., & Fiese, B. H. (1990). Transactional regulation and early intervention. In S. J. Meisels & J. P. Shonkoff (Eds.), *Handbook of early childhood intervention* (pp. 119–149). New York: Cambridge University Press.

Schaaf, R., & Gitlin, L. N. (1989). Early intervention: new directions for occupational therapists. *Occupational Therapy in Health Care,* 6(2/3), 75–89.

Seitz, V., Rosenbaum, L. K., & Apfel, N. H. (1985). Effects of family support intervention: A ten-year follow-up. *Child Development, 56,* 376–391.

Seligman, S. (1988). Concepts in infant mental health: implications for work with developmentally disabled infants. *Infants and Young Children, 1*(1), 41–51.

Shelton, T. L., Jeppson, E. S., & Johnson, B. H. (1987). *Family-centered care for children with special health care needs.* Washington, DC: Association for the Care of Children's Health.

Shonkoff, J. P., Hauser-Cram, P., Krauss, M. W., & Upshur, C. C. (1990). *The early intervention collaborative study: Final report of phase one.* Worcester, MA: University of Massachusetts Medical School.

Simeonsson, R. J. (1991). Primary, secondary, and tertiary prevention in early intervention. *Journal of Early Intervention, 15*(2), 124–134.

Tjossem, T. D. (Ed.). (1976). *Intervention strategies for high risk infants and young children.* Baltimore: University Park Press.

Touwen, B. C. (1989). Critical periods of early brain development. *Infants and Young Children, 1*(3), vii–x.

Vohr, B. R. (1991). Preterm cognitive development: Biologic and environmental influences. *Infants and Young Children, 3*(3), 20–29.

Williamson, G. G. (1988). Motor control as a resource for adaptive coping. *Zero to Three, 9*(1), 1–7.

Woodruff, G., & Hanson, C. (1987). *Project KAI.* 77B Warren Street, Brighton, MA 02135.

Zeitlin, S., & Williamson, G. G. (1986). Early intervention for infants and toddlers. *Teaching Exceptional Children,* Fall, 57–59.

Bibliography

Carter, B., & McGoldrick, M. (Eds.). (1989). *The changing family life cycle.* Needham Heights, MA: Allyn & Bacon.

Crouthamel, C. (1988). Siblings of handicapped children: a group support program. *Early Child Development and Care, 37,* 119–131.

Dunst, C., Trivette, C., & Deal, A. (1988). *Enabling and empowering families.* Cambridge, MA: Brookline Books.

Fewell, R. R., & Vadasy, P. F. (Eds.). (1986). *Families of handicapped children, needs and supports across the life span.* Austin, TX: Pro-Ed.

Fisher, A. G., Murray, E. A., & Bundy, A. C. (1991). *Sensory integration theory and practice.* Philadelphia: F. A. Davis.

Greenspan, S., & Greenspan, N. T. (1985). *First feelings.* New York: Penguin Books.

Hanft, B. E. (Ed.). (1989). *Family centered care, an early intervention resource manual.* Rockville, MD: American Occupational Therapy Association.

Haynie, M., Porter, S. M., & Palfrey, J. S. (1989). *Children assisted by medical technology in educational settings: Guidelines for care.* Boston: Project School Care, Children's Hospital

Johnson, B. H., McGonigel, M. J., & Kaufman, R. K. (1989). *Guidelines for the individualized family service plan.* Washington, DC: Association for the Care of Children's Health.

Kochanek, T., & Friedman, D. (1988). *Incorporating family assessment and Individualized Family Service Plans into early intervention programs: A developmental decision making process.* Providence: Department of Special Education, Rhode Island College.

Meisels, S. J., & Provence, S. (1989). *Screening and assessment: Guidelines for identifying young disabled and developmentally vulnerable children and their families.* Washington, DC: National Center for Clinical Infant Programs.

Meisels, S. J., & Shonkoff, J. P. (1990). *Handbook of early childhood intervention.* New York: Cambridge University Press.

Meyer, D., Vadasy, P., & Fewell, R. (1985). *Living with a brother or sister with special needs.* Seattle, WA: University of Washington Press.

Nathanson, M. (1986). *Organizing and maintaining support groups for parents of children with chronic illness and handicapping conditions.* Washington, DC: Association for the Care of Children's Health.

Odom, S. L., & Karnes, M. B. (Eds.). (1989). *Early intervention for infants and children with handicaps: An empirical base.* Baltimore: Paul H. Brooks.

Pratt, P. N., & Allen, A. S. (1989). *Occupational therapy for children.* St. Louis: C. V. Mosby.

Schleifer, M. J., & Klein, S. D. (1985). *The disabled child and the family: An exceptional parent reader.* Boston: Exceptional Parent Press.

Shonkoff, J. P., Hauser-Cram, P. Krauss, M. W., & Upshur, C. C. (1990). *The early intervention collaborative study: Final report of phase one.* Worcester, MA: University of Massachusetts Medical School, Division of Developmental and Behavioral Pediatrics.

SECTION 4

Sensory integration/ learning disabilities

MOYA KINNEALEY and LUCY J. MILLER

KEY TERMS

A. Jean Ayres

Gravitational Insecurity

Praxis

"Research-Then-Theory"

"Theory-Then-Research"

Sensory Defensiveness

Sensory Integration and Praxis Tests

Sensory Integration Treatment

Sensory Integrative Equipment

Southern California Sensory Integration Test

LEARNING OBJECTIVES

Upon completion of this section the reader will be able to:

1. *Define sensory integration.*

2. *Summarize the theory of sensory integration.*

3. *Describe the development of sensory integration theory by A. J. Ayres.*

4. *Identify instruments that evaluate sensory integration dysfunction: The Southern California Test of Sensory Integration, the Sensory Integration and Praxis Tests, and other tests that permit observation and analysis of sensory integration.*

5. *Describe occupational therapy treatment using sensory integrative procedures including the conceptual model and the components of treatment.*

6. *Describe the clinical postulates underpinning the sensory integration approach.*

7. *Describe treatment strategies including writing goals and objectives, activity planning, and use of equipment.*
8. *Describe research of the effectiveness of sensory integration treatment including methods of studying sensory integration procedures.*
9. *Describe the importance of building an empirical consensus based on collective research.*
10. *Summarize the effectiveness of sensory integration intervention.*

Sensory integration theory

The theory of sensory integration was the life work of **Dr. A. Jean Ayres** (1920 to 1988) and continues to evolve and be modified by researchers and clinicians worldwide. The theory describes the way in which the brain works as a whole with the objective of improving functional ability. The development of the theory was originally based on work with learning-disabled children.

Sensory integration is defined as:

... the neurological process that organizes sensation from one's own body and from the environment and makes it possible to use the body effectively within the environment. The spatial and temporal aspects of inputs from different sensory modalities are interpreted, associated and unified. Sensory integration is information processing. (Ayres, 1989a, p. 11).

The theory is summarized by Ayres as:

Sensations from the body, especially during purposeful activity provide the means by which a neuronal model or precept of the body is established. ... An accurate body scheme is necessary for practic tasks, for a sense of directionality and for relating body to space. At the same time conceiving, planning, and executing adaptive action is a major means by which sensation is made meaningful and translated into a body precept. ... Praxis is a uniquely human aptitude that underlies conceptualization, planning and execution of skilled adaptive interaction with the physical world ... (and) is fundamental to purposeful activity. Praxis and perception are both end products of sensory integration. ... Somatosensory, vestibular, and visual input to sensory integration and praxis are essential to organism environmental interactions. (Ayres 1989b, pp. 11–12)

The purpose of theory in science is to provide a typology, a logical explanation, prediction and potential for control, and a sense of understanding (Reynolds, 1971). The two basic ways of developing a scientific body of knowledge are the "research-then-theory" approach and the "theory-then-research" approach (Reynolds, 1971).

Both approaches are useful for different purposes. The former is useful in the beginning stages of theory development. The **"research-then-theory"** process includes identifying a phenomenon, measuring the characteristics, analyzing the data to determine patterns, and making statements describing the outcome that contribute to developing the theory.

The **"theory-then-research"** strategy occurs more frequently when a theory has been developed and statements of theoretical relationships are being tested. If the statement from the theory does not correspond to the research results, appropriate changes are made in the theory or in the research design. In this way development of the theory is continuous through the interaction with empirical research.

The theory of sensory integration using both of the aforementioned approaches was developed in a methodical manner by Ayres over three decades until her death in 1988, first through factor analytic studies and later through predictive studies. Based on 15 years of clinical work, influences from the perceptual motor work of Newall Kephart and Marianne Frostig, and extensive reading of the neuroscience literature, Ayres determined that many of the behavioral and learning problems manifested by her clients had a biologic basis. Her hypothesis was that through therapeutic input designed to modify the neurobiologic basis of behavior, functional improvement could result.

Because there were no tests to evaluate these neurobiologic underpinnings, Ayres began to develop a variety of tests to quantify the phenomenon of interest, beginning with space visualization. She concomitantly continued to analyze and describe clinical phenomena.

Much of Ayres' early work is compiled in *The development of sensory integrative theory and practice: A collection of works of A. Jean Ayres* (Henderson et al., 1974). Ayres' work provided a unique perspective and constitutes one of the major theoretical frameworks of occupational therapy. The theory reflects her background in the neurosciences, psychology, and occupational therapy. She related neuropsychological processes to functional ability and behavior and developed postulates about the relationship between sensory input and brain development with the goal of changing the child's neuromotor efficiency and capacity.

After the development of testing tools, that is, the **Southern California Sensory Integration Tests** (Ayres, 1972a), the research-then-theory strategy was used to further refine and clarify components of the theory of sensory integration. A series of factor-analytic studies, which explored the relationships among perceptual and performance areas, and clinical observations were completed. The resulting theory was named "sensory integration."

Five basic assumptions underlie both the theory and the use of sensory integration treatment techniques (Ayres, 1972b):

1. There is *plasticity* within the central nervous system; thus, intervention procedures based on sensory integration theory can effect changes in the brain.
2. The sensory integrative process occurs in a *developmental sequence.*
3. The brain functions as an integrated whole but is composed of systems that are *hierarchically organized.*
4. Evincing an *adaptive response* promotes sensory integration, and the ability to produce an adaptive response is based on sensory integration.
5. An *inner drive* exists to develop sensory integration, which is manifested through participation in sensorimotor activities

In 1972, Ayres published her first book, *Sensory Integration and Learning Disabilities*, introducing the principles of brain function on which sensory integration theory was formulated. Six areas of dysfunction, related to learning-disabled children, were introduced and referred to as "syndromes":

- Auditory language disorder
- Bilateral integration
- Developmental apraxia

- Form and space perception
- Tactile defensiveness
- Unilateral disregard/right cerebral hemisphere dysfunction

In this volume, the six syndromes were described as well as methods for remediation of underlying disorders. The application of a child-directed therapeutic approach (guided exploration) and sensory integrative equipment (hammocks, balls, ramps, scooterboards) were detailed. Until that time the use of these techniques was not common in the profession of occupational therapy. In 1972, Ayres published her first test battery, the Southern California Sensory Integration Tests (SCSIT).

Experimental and predictive studies were necessary to determine the effectiveness of the approach and to further modify the theory. In a study sponsored by the Valentine Kline Foundation (1976), Ayres accomplished three objectives:

1. Exploring the relationship of academic, intellectual, language and sensory integrative functions
2. Determining the distribution of different types of disorders and the significance of those disorders to academic learning
3. Exploring the efficacy of therapeutic procedures

This study used The Post-Rotary Nystagmus Test (Ayres, 1975). For the first time in occupational therapy, the role of the vestibular system in learning disabilities was researched.

Another conceptual expansion of the theory occurred in 1985 as Ayres addressed the multiple aspects of developmental dyspraxia, with an emphasis on differentiating childhood-onset from adult-onset apraxia. For heuristic reasons she proposed three practic (motor planning) processes: ideation or conceptualization; planning or choosing a strategy for action; and motor execution.

At that time it was still unknown whether developmental dyspraxia was a unitary function. However, different functional areas manifesting apraxia and principles for intervention based on neurophysiologic literature were delineated. The functional areas included postural dyspraxia, motor sequencing deficits, dyspraxia on verbal command, oral dyspraxia, and constructional dyspraxia. About the relationship between praxis and language Ayres (1985) stated:

> Praxis is to the physical world what speech is to the social world, both enable interactions and transactions. Both are uniquely human; both are learned . . . some aspects of speech and language comprehension may be closely related—even dependent upon—the development of praxis. Both praxis and language require cognitive functions of ideation and concept formation, both require integration of sensory input and both require planning that enables motor expression. (p. 1)

In 1986, Rush University in Chicago and Western Psychological Services, the publisher of Ayres' tests, commenced a refinement and national restandardization of the existing test battery (SCSIT), eliminating some tests and adding five new tests to evaluate dyspraxia. The **Sensory Integration and Praxis Tests** (SIPT; Ayres, 1989a) were standardized on 1997 children in the United States and Canada.

The SIPT evaluates children ages 4 years, 0 months to 8 years, 11 months. The 17 subtests of the battery measure four domains of function: (1) form and space, (2) somatosensory and vestibular processing, (3) bilateral integration and sequencing, and (4) praxis.

With continued use of this relatively new test, the knowledge base in sensory integration will expand and the theory will grow and be modified in response to data accumulated from empirical research.

The fact that the theories and evaluative practices in sensory integration are evolving and changing is believed to be a strength by advanced clinicians (Clark, 1991), although the lack of stable "facts" may be frustrating to novice therapists. The changes are a result of new knowledge that impacts on theory and practice. Change can be threatening but, as Ayres stated,

> Knowledge—especially theoretical knowledge—is tentative, and constantly changing. . . . Theory is not fact but an organization of ideas, hopefully supported by some facts, which guides one in solving problems. . . . Observing the manner in which a body of knowledge grows step by step, each step providing a foundation for more advanced thinking, is helpful in maintaining a perspective. . . . The amount of change in thinking from early papers to later papers [in sensory integration] reminds one that even greater change in thought will occur in the years to come. . . . (Ayres, 1974 p. xi)

Ayres encouraged others to have the "courage . . . to think independently, and along unorthodox lines" (Ayres, 1974, p. xi). Students of Ayres were taught to have a questioning attitude and to conduct research to explore the many questions existing in the theory and evaluation of sensory integration. "Although A. J. Ayres is no longer among us, the theories and work she dedicated her life to developing are alive and changing" (Clark, 1991 p. ix).

The work that Dr. A. Jean Ayres began has stimulated research in occupational therapy for several decades. Numerous occupational therapists in clinical and academic settings have implemented research studies, as discussed in the text that follows. In addition, in 1972 an organization was founded to support and facilitate research in sensory integration. Originally called the Center for the Study of Sensory Integration Dysfunction (CSSID), this organization published a quarterly newsletter, publications, and films, and provided an opportunity for therapists to be trained in the original test (SCSIT). About 50 occupational and physical therapists were trained to be "Faculty" to teach SCSIT certification workshops. These persons have continued to expand sensory integration theory through lectures, research, and clinical practice, and are now known as "Faculty Emeritus."

As worldwide interest in sensory integration grew, in 1984 the mission of CSSID was expanded and the name was changed to Sensory Integration International (SII). SII purchased the Ayres Clinic, thus the expansion into areas of treatment, clinical education, and research could be accomplished.

Sensory Integration International participated in the update and standardization process for the new test, SIPT, and developed a new certification process for SIPT administration and interpretation. Currently, in addition to continuing education opportunities offered nationwide, a graduate level course in sensory integration is offered at the Ayres Clinic.*

Introduction to sensory integration evaluation

Tests yield numbers and numbers can do things that words or ideas cannot do. In occupational and physical therapy, measurement is central to differential diagnosis, gain or loss assessment, establish-

---

* For additional information on continuing education opportunities, contact Sensory Integration International, 1402 Cravens Ave., Torrance, CA 90501.

ing client status, predicting response to therapy, building and testing theory, and conveying information across fields. It is difficult to accomplish any of these goals without some form of measurement. (Ayres, 1989b)

Evaluation in sensory integration is a combination of science and art. The therapist must use a variety of quantitative and qualitative procedures to arrive at a final conclusion, so that appropriate treatment recommendations can be derived. Generally, the evaluation procedure is complex and involves the synthesis of numerous behavioral observations as well as test scores.

A variety of standardized and criterion-referenced evaluation techniques can be analyzed within the sensory integrative frame of reference. Data from these scales provide information about levels of functioning in the central nervous system, the sensory modalities, postural responses, and related functional abilities.

Dr. A. Jean Ayres was a pioneer in sensory integration theory and evaluation, and based test item development on a *neurobiologic model*, as already discussed. Her tests were designed to assess abilities to detect position and movement in space (vestibular processing), ability to sense body position (proprioceptive processing), tactile perception, ***praxis*** (motor planning skills), visual perception (eye–hand coordination and visual discrimination), and other abilities.

Because sensory integration evaluation and theory are relatively new, theory, evaluation, and treatment practices are still evolving, based on new research and clinical findings. Thus, the evaluation process in sensory integration has evolved, and the domains originally evaluated have been modified.

The evaluation emphasis has evolved as new knowledge has been gained. In the 1960s, Ayres' work focused on visual perception. In the 1970s, the SCSIT were published, and the interpretation of dysfunctional performance was grouped into the six syndromes just discussed (Ayres, 1972a; 1980). In the 1990s, the SIPT were published with an emphasis on practic (motor planning) abilities and sensory processing (Ayres, 1989b).

Specific sensory integration evaluations

Sensory integration and praxis tests

The primary instrument for identification of sensory integration dysfunction is the SIPT (Ayres, 1989a). The SIPT is a battery of 17 subtests that provides detailed information on the sensory integrative status of children ages 4 years, 0 months thorough 8 years, 11 months of age.

The SIPT can be administered in 90 to 120 minutes, depending on the age and ability of the child and the experience of the examiner. The SIPT is individually administered and computer-scored by the publisher, Western Psychological Services. This scoring system was chosen because it allows for "complex statistical comparisons between the tested child's pattern of SIPT scores and the typical score patterns observed in six different cluster groups" (Ayres & Marr, 1991).

Examiners who administer the SIPT must be carefully trained and must have extensive experience in pediatrics and at least one course in statistics and measurement. Examiners are required to complete three courses covering the theory, administration, and interpretation of the SIPT, and have successfully completed an observation session with a qualified observer before being eligible to take the SIPT Competency Examination.

These courses are offered by Sensory Integration International.

All 17 subtests require performance by the child; none is based on verbal responses, although one (Oral Praxis) is dependent on auditory processing and language comprehension. Although several of the subtests measure performance in more than one area, Ayres categorized the subtests into four groups (in following text).

Measures of tactile and vestibular–proprioceptive processing[†]

- Kinesthesia (Kin)*
- Finger identification (FI)
- Graphesthesia (Gra)*
- Localization of tactile stimuli (LTS)*
- Postrotary nystagmus (PRN)
- Standing and walking balance (SWB)

The somatosensory tests are Kin, FI, Gra, and LTS, and are administered with vision occluded. Aspects of vestibular–proprioceptive functioning are evaluated by PRN, SWB, and Kin.

Measures of form and space perception and visual–motor coordination

- Space visualization (SV)
- Figure–ground perception (FG)*
- Manual form perception (MFP)*
- Motor accuracy (MA)*
- Design copying (DC)*
- Constructional praxis (CPR)

Nonmotor visual perceptual abilities are measured by SV and FG, which can be compared with visual–motor coordination on MA and DC. The haptic (tactile) component of form and space is measured in MFP. Visual construction abilities, including elements of form and space perception, are measured by DC and CP.

Measures of praxis

- Design copying (DC)*
- Constructional praxis (CPR)
- Postural praxis (PPR)
- Praxis on verbal command (PVC)
- Sequencing praxis (SPR)
- Oral praxis (OPR)

Visual praxis abilities are evaluated through DC and CPR. Motor planning related to aptitude in assuming unusual body positions is evaluated with PPR. Motor planning based only on comprehension of verbalized directions is measured by PVC. Abilities to process and remember a specific order of positions following demonstration is measured in SPR. Ability to plan and execute oral motor movement patterns is measured in OPR.

Measures of bilateral integration and sequencing

- Oral praxis (OPR)
- Sequencing praxis (SPR)
- Graphesthesia (Gra)*
- Standing and walking balance (SWB)

† The subtests marked with an asterisk (*), were originally included in the SCSIT, although many of these include modified and improved versions of items in the SCSIT.

- Bilateral motor coordination (BMC)*
- Space visualization contralateral use (SVCU)
- Space visualization preferred hand use (PHU)

All these subtests assess the ability to integrate functioning on two sides of the body either in gross motor movements (SWB; BMC), fine motor movements (SPR; BMC), oral motor movements (OPR), and tactile perception (Gra). Two scores are derived from administration of SV; they measure ability of the child to cross the midline of the body (SVCU) and demonstration of preferred or dominant hand for writing (PHU).

The process of test development and national standardization has been well documented (Ayres & Marr, 1991; Ayres, 1989a). In addition, extensive reliability and validity information are reported in the literature and will continue to accumulate in future years (Ayres, 1989a; Ayres & Marr, 1991)

Southern California sensory integration test battery

The SCSIT was the precursor of the SIPT (Ayres 1972a; 1980). It included 17 subtests and was usually administered conjointly with the Southern California Postrotary Nystagmus Test (Ayres, 1975). The subtests above marked with an asterisk (*) originated with the SCSIT, although the SIPT includes modifications and improvements of some test items. In addition, the SCSIT also included the following subtests, which are not included in the SIPT because levels of reliability or validity were not acceptable: Crossing the Midline, Position in Space, Right Left Discrimination, and Double Tactile Stimuli Perception.

After the development and standardization of the SIPT, the publisher has ceased selling the SCSIT. Although normative information for the SCSIT is limited, some therapists originally certified in administration of the SCSIT use the subtests to supplement clinical observations of children's sensory integrative status.

Other tests that permit observation and analysis of sensory integration in children

Sensory integration, as defined in the preceding text, is a complex neurobiologic theory. It addresses the relationship among the sensory systems and between sensory processing and motor planning abilities. These sensory and motor processing abilities are considered essential to competent organization and appropriate functioning by the person within his or her environment. Thus, it can be seen that the evaluation of sensory integration is much broader than just the SIPT or SCSIT tests. Although these tests were milestone contributions to understanding sensory integration functioning in children ages 4 to 8 years, a variety of other measures exist that also provide insight into the sensory integrative status of people.

Sensory integration is a frame of reference. Sensory integration evaluation is not limited strictly to the subtests developed by Ayres. Thus, many assessments can be interpreted from a sensory integration frame of reference, although they were not initially intended as a specific measure of sensory integration status, as were the SIPT and the SCSIT.

For example, the Miller Assessment for Preschoolers (MAP; Miller, 1988a, 1982) was developed by an occupational therapist and describes in the theoretical chapter the underlying theoretical basis of that test as in part based on sensory integration theory. Although the MAP was originally intended as a screening test to provide information on preschool-aged children (2 years, 9 months to 5 years, 8 months) to assist in predicting children at risk for later developmental delays and learning difficulties, Miller (1988b) discusses the use of the scale to *assess* rather than *screen* sensory integrative aspects of functioning when the test is administered by a qualified therapist.

In particular on the MAP, items that measure what Ayres refers to as vestibular–proprioceptive sensory processing assess what Miller refers to as position and movement abilities. These items are Finger-Nose, Romberg, Stepping, and Vertical Writing. Two items specifically measure tactile abilities in preschoolers: Finger Localization and Stereognosis. A variety of items encompass the evaluation of motor planning skills, although Miller has labeled them "complex tasks": Draw-A-Person, Imitation of Postures, Block Designs, and Mazes.

Other tests that include items from which an understanding of the sensory integration abilities of children age 3 years through adulthood can be derived are the McCarron Assessment of Neuromuscular Development (MAND; McCarron, 1982) and the Haptic Visual Discrimination Test (HPVT: McCarron & Dial, 1979). McCarron is a neuropsychologist with a strong interest in psychoeducational testing and neurologic functioning.

Items on the MAND that provide information about sensory integrative functioning are Heel-Toe Walk and Stand One Foot in the Kinesthetic Integration subdomain, Beads on Rod and Nut and Bolt in the Bimanual Dexterity subdomain, Rod Slide and Finger-Nose in the Persistent Control subdomain, and Hand Strength and Jumping in the Muscle Power subdomain. Beads on Rod also provides interesting sensory integration information because vision is occluded during part of this item.

A frequently administered test, which is designed to measure gross and fine motor functioning in children ages 4 years, 6 months to 14 years, 6 months is the Bruininks-Oseretsky Test of Motor Proficiency (Bruininks, 1978). This assessment is designed to measure gross and fine motor proficiency of children. Although the author has a strong psychoeducational background, he does not come from a sensory integrative frame of reference. Thus, the descriptions in the test manual are from a physical education and motor learning point of view.

Nevertheless, many of the items administered can be interpreted from a sensory integrative frame of reference. For example, vestibular–proprioceptive processing can be inferred from performance in the Balance subtest and in Touching Nose with Index Fingers and Touching Thumb to Fingertips, eyes closed in the Upper-Limb Coordination subtest. Praxis can be observed throughout the assessment, but particularly in Bilateral Coordination, Upper-Limb Coordination, Visual-Motor Control, and Upper-Limb Speed and Dexterity subtests. Form and space perception and visual–motor coordination can be determined from results of the Visual-Motor Control, and the Upper-Limb Speed and Dexterity subtests. Bilateral Integration and Sequencing abilities can be detected through analysis of Bilateral Coordination, and Placing Pennies in Two Boxes with Both Hands, in Upper Limb Speed and Dexterity subtests.

Of primary importance in sensory integrative evaluations is differential diagnosis of motor-free visual perceptual dysfunction versus visual–motor integration disorders. Useful in this regard (supplementing or in place of the form and space perception subtests on the SIPT) is comparison of performance on a motor-free visual perception test such as the Test of Visual-Perceptual Skills, (Gardner, 1982) and the Motor-Free Test of Visual Perception (Colarusso, 1972) with performance on a test that requires the integration of visual and motor skills such as the Developmental Test of Visual-Motor Integration (Beery & Buktenica 1967), or the Test of Visual-Motor Skills (Gardner, 1986). A careful examination of the scores of items on these scales will show that some children have high scores on motor-free visual perceptual tasks and low scores on visual–motor coordination items, thus indicating that visual perceptual skills are intact, but either the motor component or the integration of motor and visual perceptual is causing the problem. In contrast, other children demonstrate low scores on both types of items, indicating a combination of both visual perceptual and motor problems.

A test useful in clinical interpretations of sensory integrative functioning is the DeGangi-Berk Test of Sensory Integration (TSI) (Berk & DeGangi, 1983). The TSI is a criterion-referenced test that hypothesizes three vestibular-based functions: postural control, bilateral motor integration, and reflex integration. The authors discuss that when used in the diagnosis of sensory motor dysfunction, the results should be incorporated with other relevant test results to reliably determine problem areas. Although the scoring system is subjective (particularly in the reflex integration subtest) and the test is not norm-referenced, the items are helpful in the clinical assessment of sensory integration functioning in this age group (3 to 5 years old). In particular, two areas can be supplemented by information from items in this scale: vestibular processing (by observation of the antigravity position items) and bilateral integration (by items such as Rolling Pin Activity, Jump and Turn, and Drumming).

A variety of other clinical assessments include items that tap into sensory integrative functioning. An inclusive review of all items from all assessments that measure sensory integration is beyond the purview of the material in this section. However, the concept has been presented that the domains of development identified by Ayres in over 30 years as an occupational therapist and scientist are measured by many items that are not necessarily labeled "sensory integration" by the test author. Thus, it becomes the responsibility of each clinician administering an evaluation or battery of tests to interpret those applicable parts within the sensory integration frame of reference.

Related areas in a sensory integration evaluation

A sensory integration evaluation should never be completed in the absence of the collection of other important data. An excellent description of additional components of a sensory integration evaluation and a detailed case study are presented by Fisher & Bundy (1991).

In general, the following components must be included before the results of a sensory integration evaluation can be interpreted.

Complete referral information

The therapist should ascertain exact symptoms that make the child a candidate for a sensory integration evaluation. This includes detailing the presenting problems and identifying possible areas of sensory integrative deficits as well as functional problems that may be related to sensory integrative deficits. In particular, the therapist should carefully explore the aspects of the child's *quality of life* on which sensory integrative disorders may have an impact. These aspects may include psychosocial functioning, learning difficulties, communicative disorders, and problems with activities of daily living. The therapist can then tie the evaluation results back to the presenting problem, and thus make interpretation and remediation suggestions that will be meaningful to the referring source.

Detailed developmental history

It is essential to obtain a complete developmental history on the child. This should include the mother's pregnancy and birth history information; infant behavior and functioning; milestone attainment of performance areas including motor, communication, cognitive, and social–emotional abilities; academic performance/problems; and factors that describe the family functioning including both protective and risk factors. Often a variety of factors in the history will help to confirm or rule out various aspects of sensory integration dysfunction that may not be evaluated during the test session.

Classroom observation

Whenever possible, observations of the child in the context of the classroom or home environment should be made. This provides an opportunity to observe the child in a natural environment and to demonstrate differences between functioning in the test session (one-to-one situation) and functioning in a group. A classroom observation may illuminate school-related problems and provides an excellent opportunity to interview the child's teacher. In addition, it affords an opportunity for evaluation and remediation suggestions to be directed to one of the child's main occupations, school.

Related clinical observations

Much of the understanding of sensory integrative functioning is based on observing the child in a variety of situations. Numerous areas of sensory integrative functioning have no standardized assessment. For example, muscle tone, reflex integration, co-contraction skills, crossing the midline, tactile defensiveness, and antigravity reactions must all be clinically observed rather than specifically measured using a test "score." In addition, clinical observations conducted (preferably) over several sessions and in a variety of circumstances (such as on the playground, in the clinic, or within the home) frequently allow the therapist an opportunity to confirm suspected areas of strength and dysfunction that may be hypothesized based on the standardized evaluation.

Interpretation of sensory integration evaluations

Interpretation of a person's sensory integration status is a difficult and complex process. When the SIPT is administered, the process is facilitated in some ways because standardized scores are derived in each of the component subdomains. However, good interpretation of the computerized SIPT results takes years of practice and necessitates completion of a professional training course.

The purpose of this section of Chapter 13 is to provide an overview of sensory integrative evaluation as a process, not detailed explanations of the interpretation of the SIPT (detailed descriptions available in Ayres, 1989a; Fisher et al., 1991); therefore, the following chart (Figure 13-32) has been compiled, which may apply to any evaluation that has sensory integration components. In using this chart the therapist should enter all information about the performance onto the chart, listing the child's strengths in the left column and limitations in the right column. An analysis of the chart will assist in an understanding of the child's sensory integrative status.

Occupational therapy using sensory integration procedures

Ayres developed a conceptual model of occupational therapy using sensory integration procedures, which is useful in identifying treatment priorities and planning treatment programs (Ayres, 1979) (Figure 13-33).

On the left side of this figure, the major sensory systems are depicted: auditory, vestibular, proprioceptive, tactile, and visual. Based on a person's development and experience, it is hypothesized that the input from these sensory systems is integrated and results in a variety of "end products," or adaptive functions.

Integrative tasks are demonstrated in a hypothesized hierarchy in levels 1, 2, and 3 in Figure 13-33 and include (for example):

Posture and balance abilities (level 1)
Efficient motor planning and coordination of two sides of the body (level 2)
Eye–hand coordination (level 3)

The end products (depicted on the right of Figure 13-33) include a variety of functional and adaptive abilities, such as self-esteem, self-control, and self-confidence. The capacity to demonstrate integrated and adaptive end products is based on efficient neurologic organization that includes competence in accurately perceiving sensory input, ability to process and integrate perceptions, and adaptive performance of the important occupations of life (such as learning, interacting, playing).

It is essential that occupational therapists focus on the end products when they use sensory integration techniques. Long-term objectives of treatment *must* reflect functional goals. The impact of using these techniques on the child's quality of life must always be the underlying motivation for normalization of his or her sensory perception and motor performance. A chart summarizing observable behaviors that may indicate sensory processing difficulties is provided by Dunn (1991).

Using the model in Figure 13-33 as a conceptual guide, occupational therapy using sensory integration treatment techniques can be planned and implemented after either a standardized or nonstandardized evaluation has been completed. The model provides an effective framework for assessing the full spectrum of ages from neonates to adults. In addition, it encompasses a variety of diagnostic categories including emotional disturbance, mental retardation, and physical handicaps.

It has been found that persons with a variety of diagnoses have sensory integrative deficits that impact negatively on treatment progress unless specifically addressed. This includes those with fragile X, substance-exposed or substance-affected children,

Subdomain of Development Assessed	Items Indicating Strengths in Subdomain Functioning	Items Indicating Limitations in Subdomain Functioning
Movement Perception		
Position In Space Perception		
Tactile Perception		
Visual Perception		
Visual–Motor Integration Abilities		
Fine Motor Abilities		
Gross Motor Abilities		
Postural Abilities		
Ocular Abilities		
Praxis Abilities		
Bilateral Integration Abilities		
Cognitive Abilities		
Auditory/Language Abilities		
Social/Emotional Abilities		

FIGURE 13-32. *Analysis of sensory and motor performance.*

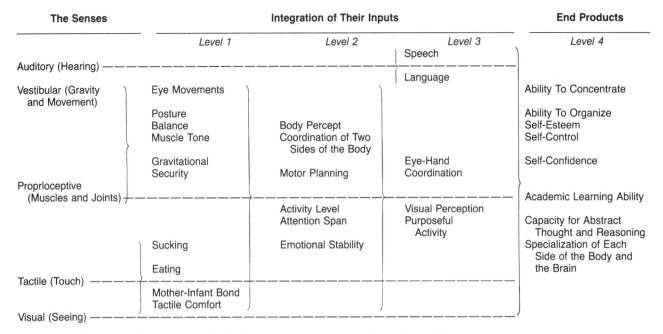

FIGURE 13-33. *The senses, integration of their inputs, and their end products. (From Western Psychological Services, 12031 Wilshire Blvd., Los Angeles, CA 90025.)*

abused children, and children with cerebral palsy, mental retardation, and autism. In these populations, although sensory integration or any therapy does not purport to change a child's medical condition, it can improve functional independence, motivation, self-esteem, and overall competence in performing the usual occupations of life.

Effective treatment planning is based on information gathered from standardized testing, clinical evaluations, and developmental and family history (as described in the preceding text), and can be effectively organized utilizing the framework presented by the model in Figure 13-33.

Sensory integration treatment is a complex treatment modality. Its complexity is due to the numerous variations all included under the title, "Sensory Integration Treatment." A good summary of characteristics of sensory integration treatment is provided by Kimball (1988). Included in her description are the following components:

Active participation by the person being treated
Client-directed activity
Individualized treatment based on the age, disorder, developmental status, and response of the client
Purposeful activities requiring an *adaptive response*
Sensory stimulation as a part of the activities
Improving underlying neurologic processing and organization
rather than focusing on the development of splinter skills
Treatment by a therapist with advanced training in specific sensory integration treatment techniques

Sensory integration treatment is neither predetermined nor fixed, but rather varies from one individual to the next, and changes in response to the individuals' response to therapy . . . [make] a concise description of the treatment difficult. (Kimball, 1988, p. 423)

Three clinical postulates form the foundation for the sensory integration approach to assessment and treatment planning:

1. A continuum exists between hyporesponsiveness and hyperresponsiveness in each sensory system, which affects the ability of the person to interact effectively and efficiently with the environment.
2. The symmetry (or asymmetry) of function between the two sides of the body and the two hemispheres affects efficiency of function.
3. The brain functions as a whole; however, a hierarchy within the central nervous system affects neurologic functioning, and thus affects behavioral manifestations of nervous system integrity.

Continuum of hyper- to hyporesponsivness

Over- and underresponsiveness to sensory stimuli including tactile, vestibular, auditory, gustatory and visual systems can affect the child's behavior and functioning. One of Ayres' earliest clinical observations was a cluster of behaviors that she studied extensively (Ayres, 1964) and labeled "tactile defensiveness." Tactually defensive behavior, or hyperresponsiveness of the tactile system, is characterized by an adversive (or defensive) reaction to nonnoxious, tactile stimuli. Behavioral manifestations include hyperactive and distractible behavior, withdrawn behavior, and aggressive responses to touch, sometimes called the "fight-or-flight reactions."

Techniques for normalizing overly sensitive tactile systems, called tactile defensiveness, have been developed by Ayres (1972b) and Wilbarger and Wilbarger (1991). Exploration of the neurologic mechanisms believed to be involved in remediation have been described by Fisher and Dunn (1983).

At the other end of the hypo- to-hyperreactive continuum in the tactile domain are children who have unusually high thresholds of sensory perception and registration. In these children, concomitant problems are often observed in tactile discrimination and haptic abilities. In addition, poor tactile discrimination (hyporeactivity) may be related to poor execution of motor skills that require a high degree of skill and planning.

Hypo- or hyperresponsiveness to vestibular stimulation may also be observed clinically. According to sensory integration theory, an underresponsive vestibular system may result in vestibular bilateral disorders or vestibular language disorders (Ayres, 1976, pp. 82–83). Evidence of an overreactive vestibular system may be demonstrated by either gravitational insecurity or intolerance to movement, depending on which part of the vestibular system is affected (Ayres, 1976).

Gravitational insecurity is manifested by fear, anxiety, and distress when the person assumes positions to which he or she is unaccustomed, particularly when moved by another person. A child with this condition feels safest with both feet on the floor, is cautious and fearful of falling, and avoids activities involving movement such as jumping, somersaulting, and the like. *Intolerance to movement*, in contrast, is manifested through a variety of autonomic reactions such as severe discomfort, nausea, and headache with rapid movement (Ayres, 1979).

Hyper- and hyporesponsiveness can also be observed in the other sensory systems but the reactions are less well documented in occupational therapy literature.

The concept of **sensory defensiveness** has been described by Wilbarger and Wilbarger (1991):

> Sensory defensiveness is a tendency to react negatively or with alarm to sensory input that is generally considered harmless or non-irritating . . . common symptoms may include oversensitivity to light or unexpected touch, sudden movement or over reaction to unstable surfaces, high frequency noises, excesses of noise or visual stimulation and certain smells. . . . Sensory defensiveness results in varying degrees of stress and anxiety although symptoms vary with each individual. (Wilbarger & Wilbarger, 1991, p. 3)

Abnormal reactions to sensory input may potentially have negative effects on every aspect of a person's life and may result in social and emotional problems.

The reactivity model demonstrated in Figure 13-34 formulated by Lorna Jean King is useful in understanding the behavioral parameters of hyper- and hyporeactivity. The relationship between the model presented by King in Figure 13-34 and the model presented by Ayres in Figure 13-33 is interesting. Both models relate the senses (including reactivity to sensation) to "end products" or quality of life. These theorists were interested in the effect of deficits in the perception and processing of sensory information on functional abilities, or the occupations of children's lives. As the neurophysiologic theories relating to sensory integration have become more advanced based on new knowledge, there is a tendency to forget the less technically sophisticated and more meaningful aspects of sensory integration treatment depicted in Figure 13-33 as "End Products," and in Figure 13-34 as "Defective Behaviors, and Impaired Learning."

Symmetry and asymmetry of function

There are some conditions in functioning in which symmetric abilities indicate strengths in abilities and other conditions in which more advanced performance on one side of the body indicates more mature responses. For example, in a normal person both sides of the body are expected to show similar balance reactions, similar reflex integration, and similar development of muscle tone. The presence of definite asymmetries in any of these areas (such as those seen in hemiplegia) would be evidence of dysfunction.

Although dysfunction due to hemiplegia is clinically obvious, subtle asymmetries in the perception of sensory information may also cause dysfunctional performance. For example, there is some evidence that vestibular-based asymmetry in muscle tone and balance responses may be associated with persistent inner ear infections (Denning & Mayberry, 1987; Schaaf, 1985). There is also evidence that children who demonstrate significantly different abilities to perceive tactile stimulation on the right and left sides of their bodies are more likely to demonstrate motor planning deficits and other functional problems associated with tasks of daily living (Ayres, 1972b).

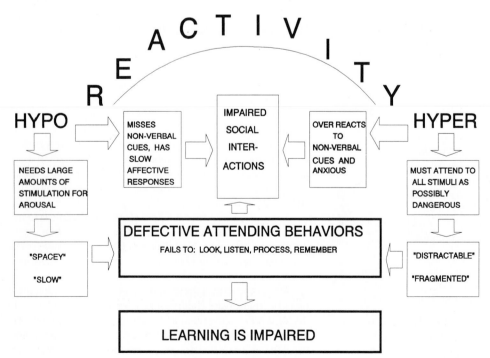

FIGURE 13-34. Schematic of hypo- and hyperactivity and their impact on attending and learning. (*From King, L. J.* [*1988*]. *Interpretation of social-emotional domain. In Miller assessment for preschoolers: Seminar administration and interpretation manual. San Antonio: The Psychological Corporation.*)

In other developmental tasks, however, it is appropriate to observe asymmetric functioning, that is, when one side of the body has developed particular skill in performance. One obvious example of this is in the establishment of hand dominance. It is anticipated that by a certain age children show particular skill and dexterity in performance of activities such as writing, eating, and other fine motor tasks. The lack of specialization (equal or symmetric performance by both hands) may be an indication of dysfunction if neither hand has established the skill needed to perform the activities expected at his or her age.

Clinical assessment of sensory and motor performance with particular emphasis on the presence of atypical asymmetry or on symmetric functioning when mature performance is based on one side demonstrating more advanced ability can be useful in indicating avenues of remediation.

Clinical testing of two sides of the body in the following areas can be useful in observing asymmetries:

- Muscle tone and strength
- Co-contraction
- Bilateral, smooth coordinated movements
- Diadochokinesis (rapid alternating movement patterns)
- Sequential fingertip opposition
- Tactile discrimination
- Crossing the midline of the body
- Tonic neck reflexes
- Fine motor skill and dexterity tasks

Levels of function

The central nervous system manifests a hierarchy anatomically and functionally. However, the brain functions as a whole and integration of the brain mechanisms including sensation occurs at many levels of the brain.

Occupational therapy using sensory integrative treatment techniques is founded on the belief that tactile, vestibular, and proprioceptive sensations that generate *purposeful movement and activity* provide a foundation for visual and auditory functions. A further postulate holds that efficient brainstem functions provide a foundation for higher level cortical functions (Seig, 1988).

Thus, the clinical symptoms for which a child may be referred to occupational therapy—poor handwriting and difficulties in motor performance—are often due to inefficient functioning at lower levels of the central nervous system. Thus, input directed at abilities mediated by lower central nervous system structures (such as reflex integration activities, tactile discrimination tasks, or activities which improve sense of position and movement) may affect other abilities mediated by higher central nervous system structures (such as cognitive, language, and integrative abilities). It is hypothesized that remediation focused on deficits in the lower levels of the central nervous system affect not only higher level central nervous system abilities, but also end products such as self-confidence, self-esteem, and academic performance.

CASE STUDY

José is referred for an occupational therapy evaluation by his teacher, who feels that he is demonstrating poor handwriting and immature motor abilities that are interfering with his schoolwork. After interviewing the teacher, the therapist finds out that José is extremely distractible, frequently fights in school, tends to play only with children younger than himself, and often displays "tantrums," particularly during self-care activities such as dressing, eating, and washing.

The therapist determines through observation, clinical assessment, and developmental history that the child is overreactive to sensory stimulation, particularly tactile. She concludes that the lowered threshold to sensory input (sensory defensiveness) is contributing significantly to José's distractibility in the classroom, and his difficulties completing self-care tasks.

On clinical assessment, José is found to have low muscle tone, which contributes to his difficulty sitting upright in a chair for an extended time without "wiggling." In addition, during writing and reading activities, José props his head on his hand (which, as the therapist observes, helps him to maintain an upright position and visually focus on the task in front of him).

Because José must use the nonpreferred hand to help him maintain balance, his alternate hand is not free to hold his paper when he is writing. In addition, his pencil grip is weak. Therefore, José demonstrates poor pencil control and illegible letter formation.

The therapist also clinically examines a variety of reactions and responses known to be related to efficient functioning of the vestibular system. José demonstrates low muscle tone, inability to hold the prone extension posture, inefficient balance responses, and difficulty with bilateral coordination. This set of observations suggests that his vestibular system may not be working efficiently and verifies the need for further standardized assessment.

Completed standardized testing confirms the presence of hyperresponsiveness in the tactile system, vestibular processing inefficiency, and bilateral integration difficulties.

Occupational therapy treatment is recommended to maximize José's potential in school. It is believed that by decreasing José's sensitivity to tactile stimulation, increasing his ability to efficiently process vestibular input, and normalizing his abilities to perform tasks requiring smooth integrated use of the two sides of the body, José will experience increased satisfaction at school in academic areas and in interpersonal relationships.

Long-term goals

  I. Academic and classroom performance
    A. Improve handwriting
    B. Decrease distractibility
  II. Social–emotional abilities at school
    A. Decrease aggressive behavior
    B. Increase interactions with children in his age group
 III. Self-care skills
    A. Improve abilities to dress independently
    B. Improve ability to take care of usual grooming skills for his age

Related therapeutic methods and modalities

For each of the above long-term goals, numerous therapeutic methods and modalities would be beneficial to use in a treatment plan. The development of a comprehensive treatment plan is an important and challenging part of the therapeutic process. Each child must have a comprehensive written treatment plan prior to initiating treatment.

Due to the complexity of developing treatment plans based on each child's diagnosis, strengths, and needs, it is difficult to synthesize the process in an introductory text as provided here. For each of the long-term goals, a variety of short-term goals and sensory and motor strategies (activities) can be used to achieve the goal. Examples of short-term goals are noted in the following text.

I. Improve handwriting[‡]
   A. Increase ability to copy shapes and forms
   B. Increase speed and dexterity of fine motor abilities
   C. Improve ability to organize writing on a page
   D. Improve pencil grasp
   E. Improve postural stability so that fine motor activities can be accomplished more easily
II. Decrease distractibility[§]
   A. Decrease hyperresponsiveness in the sensory systems, particularly reduce tactile defensiveness
   B. Raise threshold to distraction from outside, unrelated stimuli.
   C. Ensure that José's placement in the classroom is in the least distracting place in terms of outside environmental stimulation, peer distractions, and the like.

Goals and objectives of treatment

Goals of treatment and measurable objectives are required by school systems, hospitals, insurance companies, and others. However, the therapist must realize that the nature and wording of these objectives must be consistent with the intent of the organization through which the therapy is provided; the therapist also should take into account the purpose for which the goals and objectives are being written. For example, goals and objectives written for the family to take home and implement may well be different from those written for a referring physician.

Activity planning

Activities that address the short-term goals can be diverse. Many activities can be applicable to each goal. For example, above short-term goal A, "Increase ability to copy shapes and forms," the activities might include blackboard activities, tracing shapes in the sand, making finger-paintings with pudding, and so on. It is critical that the activities are specifically tied to the short-term and long-term goals for the child.

It must be realized that in occupational therapy using sensory integrative techniques, each goal and activity is designed based on an understanding of the neurobehavioral basis of the academic, social, or functional problem. Improvement in problems such as handwriting and distractibility is likely to result not only in improved handwriting, but in improved quality of life in terms of behavior, family relationships, peer interactions, and functional abilities. As a result, the end products (self-esteem, self-confidence, ability to organize, and so on) described in

Figure 13-33 will improve. After abilities such as focusing on tasks or maintaining an upright seated posture become automatic (instead of requiring cognitive effort), a child is much more able to put energy into other important activities such as cognitive skills (listening to the teacher, improvement in reading), social–emotional skills (relating to peers, following directions), and the like.

Sensory integrative equipment

A variety of **sensory integrative equipment** is commercially available to implement treatment based on sensory integration principles. This equipment may be categorized into four groups:

1. *Tactile equipment,* consisting of textured mats, brushes, vibrators, pillows, and a variety of therapist-developed activities
2. *Nonsuspended moving equipment,* consisting of balls of all sizes, rolls, barrels, tiltboards, ramps, scooter boards, trampolines, jumping boards, and sit-n-spins (Figure 13-35)
3. *Hanging equipment,* consisting of hammocks, bolsters, platform swings, suspended ladders, bars, gliders, and inner tubes (Figures 13-36 to 13-38)
4. *Motor planning equipment,* consisting of a variety of obstacle courses, jungle gyms, and other creative and innovative pieces of equipment that facilitate unique previously unexecuted activities (Figure 13-39)

Sensory input can be divided into two categories for each sensory system: (1) facilitory input and (2) inhibitory input. Generally, input that is expected, rhythmic, sustained, or slow tends to be inhibitory. Input that is unexpected, arrhythmic, uneven, or rapid tends to be excitatory.

The therapist must carefully assess the goals of the treatment to ascertain which type of equipment is useful in maximizing efficient and optimal functioning for the child. Duration, intensity, frequency, and careful monitoring of the child's response to the stimulation are required.

Occupational therapy using sensory integration techniques is complex, multifaceted, and process-oriented. A major component of treatment depends on the child's motivation, choice of

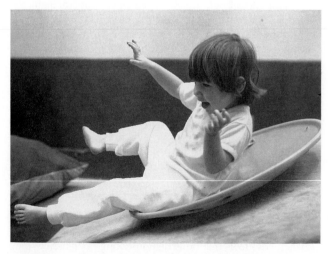

FIGURE 13-35. *Balance and righting responses are challenged when sliding on a nonlevel surface in the saucer.*

[‡] Many other examples of short-term goals related to improving handwriting could apply here.
[§] Many other examples of short-term goals related to improving distractibility could apply here.

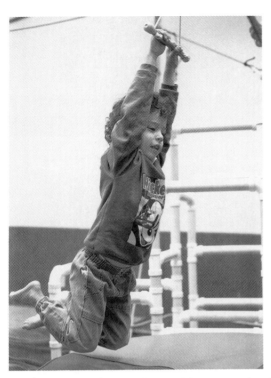

FIGURE 13-36. *Activities that require total body organization and movement help visual, spatial, and motor planning skills develop.*

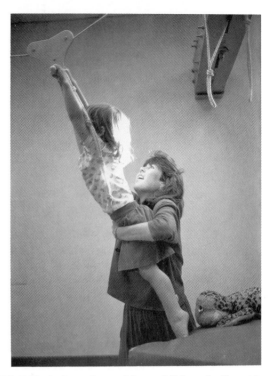

FIGURE 13-38. *A therapist enables a child to challenge herself on the flying trapese.*

equipment, and the type and degree of guided sensory input the therapist provides.

A discussion of the use of each of the types of available equipment is beyond the scope of the material presented here. A particular piece of equipment may be used in a multitude of ways

to provide the input appropriate to meet a child's needs. However, it was felt that by exploring the use of one common piece of equipment, for example, the large therapy ball, an understanding that pieces of equipment could be used for a variety of goals would be clear. Thus, the chart in Table 13-13 presents uses of the

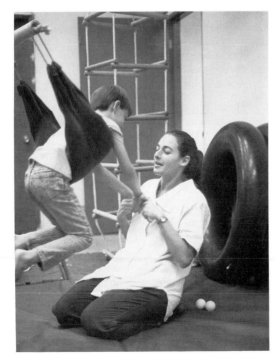

FIGURE 13-37. *A therapist and child use linear movement to develop vestibular proprioceptive responses in the neck, arms, and back.*

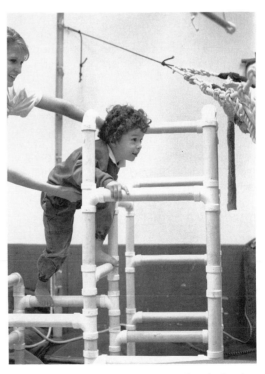

FIGURE 13-39. *A child's ability to motor plan is developed through challenging sensory motor experiences.*

TABLE 13-13. *Use of Therapy Ball in Sensory Integration Treatment*

Treatment Needs Addressed	Goal	Position of Child	Type of Sensorimotor Input
Hyperreactive tactile system	Reduce hypersensitivity	Child on floor; child lying prone on ball	Press ball on child, ventral pressure, slow rhythmic rock, head in inverted position
Hyporeactive tactile system	Increase tactile awareness	Sitting or lying on ball	Heavy bounce, bare skin on towel on ball, brisk movement, brisk rubbing
Hyperreactive vestibular system	Reduce hyperreactivity	Sitting or in prone	Slow predictable rhythmic movement tolerance, heavy bounce tactile input simultaneously all pressure
Hyporeactive vestibular system	Increase reactivity	Any/many positions	Quick movements in any position or direction, movement requiring body adjustments including protective extension and righting reaction
High tone	Reduce tone	Prone arms extended	Slow rhythmic rocking, weight bearing, weight shifting
Low tone	Increase tone	Prone	Heavy movement front to back, bouncing, sustained weight shift
Motor planning	Improve basic pattern on which motor planning is based	Prone; supine, rotational movements	Work on total body patterns of flexion, extension, and trunk rotation, activities on small balls in which the body controls the movement of the ball

large therapy ball in addressing a variety of treatment needs for a child.

Many occupational and physical therapists have expanded the application of sensory integration theory and the use of sensory integration treatment techniques to a broader population base than the learning-disabled children for which it was initially intended. This includes autistic children and adults (King, 1987), severely retarded and schizophrenic adults (Mailloux, 1987), chronically mentally ill patients in an institutional psychiatric setting (King, 1974) and applications relevant to preacademic, academic, and classroom skills (Knickerbocker, 1980). Other therapists have used this theory base in the development of testing tools, as previously discussed in the evaluation section.

Research on effectiveness of sensory integration treatment

The issues in analyzing research in all fields of occupational therapy are complex. For a more complete description of issues related to research, see Chapter 12.

Interpreting the results of sensory integration studies

Two aspects of interpretation are critical to discuss: the limitations of available instruments in occupational therapy and the importance and variety of outcome measures that are used.

Instrumentation was discussed already briefly in regard to sample selection. However, the importance of understanding the psychometric properties and intended purpose of scales that are used in a study cannot be overemphasized. Before undertaking research and even prior to finalizing the research questions, it is useful to explore the options available to measure the constructs

that are intended for study. Existing research is hampered by a serious lack in the profession of well-standardized, reliable, and valid measurement tools.

Cermak and Henderson (1989, 1990) documented the percentage of sensory integration efficacy studies that used each of the following outcome variables and found the following percentages:

Academic outcomes, 20%
Language outcomes, 45%
Motor outcomes, 45%
Postrotary nystagmus outcomes, 20%
Self-stimulation behaviors, 5%
Behavioral outcomes, 5%
Other outcomes, 10%¶

The choice of outcome measures is based on two factors: the research question and the validity of the measure. If the question relates to the effectiveness of sensory integration therapy in producing changes in school, academic measures might be of interest, for example. A review of the literature highlights the fact that in many instances the instrumentation is described, but the initial research hypothesis is not elaborated. It is not of particular interest, for example, whether children who receive sensory integrative treatment demonstrate changes in test scores unless documentation can be supplied that those test scores are indicative of changes in constructs that are under study.

Does a change in a test score on an intelligence scale mean that a child has become more intelligent? Probably not. Does the change mean that the child will be performing better in school? Not necessarily, although changes in the child that caused the child's test scores to improve may be related to changes that also affect school performance. Thus, it can be seen that researchers

¶ Some outcomes were used in more than one study; hence, the total is more than 100%.

need to clarify the choice of outcome measures and relate that choice back to the hypothesis of the study.

The psychometric properties and purpose of the outcome measures also need to be considered. Is a criterion-referenced scale appropriate for measuring change over time in a group of children? It may be valuable to provide descriptive documentation for a qualitative study, especially if the scores obtained represent small discriminating categories; however, if the purpose of the study is to document quantitative changes over time or compare the effectiveness of two treatment approaches, a scale with a reliable and valid final score must be used.

Unfortunately, few well-standardized scales in occupational therapy can be used for this purpose. Therefore, researchers are cautioned to modify the research question to those questions that can be answered using existing technologies and to use scales developed outside the profession, which are designed to measure related concepts. This does not mean that only standardized tests can be used in sensory integrative research, but that the choice of instrumentation in part determines the generalizability of results and the format of the research question. The obvious implications for the profession with regard to the importance of allocating resources to the development of standardized tests is emphasized once more by this discussion.

Cermak and Henderson (1989, 1990) include the following list of domains in which change in response to sensory integration therapy may be demonstrated: "organization, learning rate, attention, affect, exploratory behavior, biologic rhythm (sleep-wake cycle), sensory responsivity, play skills, self-esteem, peer interaction, and family adjustment" (p. 7). Although intriguing, these domains represent a challenge to the profession in terms of existing measurement technologies. With proper planning, implementation, and analysis, however, progress can be expected over the next decade in measuring these important aspects of the occupation of children.

Building an empirical consensus based on collective research

The concepts for building an empirical consensus are based on the thought-provoking and stimulating concluding chapter in the book by Fisher et al., *Sensory Integration: Theory and Practice*, to which all serious students of sensory integration are referred. In his chapter, Ottenbacher (1991) raises complex issues, including the importance of developing a consensual science that supports and documents the effective elements of sensory integration.

Because sensory integration is such a complex issue, Ottenbacher notes an "absence of a unifying research paradigm," and cautions that "research is only one component of science, and in fact, can produce little of lasting value unless it grows out of consensus supported by theory" (p. 398). Clark (1991) notes that Ayres in her more than 30-year career "discovered a new paradigm for explaining a variety of neurological disorders in children." Dr. Ayres was a proponent of change; it is a challenge for all students of sensory integration to follow her lead in asking questions and seeking answers. Our current challenge is to grow beyond the existing knowledge that she dedicated her life to developing and to continue to provide new knowledge that will help all potential clients to validate the new paradigm that Dr. Ayres constructed.

For a theory to become accepted as fact (or to represent a new paradigm), it must be carefully documented by a large body of well-implemented research. This research becomes meaningful only when discussed in terms of concepts that have pragmatic relevance to the field. Thus, the growth of theory is based on research, and the relevance of research is based on theory. Ottenbacher (1991) emphasizes the importance of a collective body of research in establishing empirical consensus that can be translated into professional agreement.

Cruickshank (1974) noted that Ayres

... has the unique role of not only having added much to the work of previous authors, but of having essentially turned a whole profession around. The writings of Jean Ayres, in large measure, have been instrumental in setting new directions for a total discipline, or at least have directed the profession of occupational therapy into areas that are historically and functionally different from that which characterized it prior to 1955. (p. viii)

Clark (1991) notes "how the work of scientists of lower standing is prone to resistance by scientists of higher standing" and cites as an example the criticism of von Nageli, who was in a position of authority over Mendel, who judged Mendel's groundbreaking work in genetics to be insignificant. This resistance may in part account for the slow acceptance of sensory integration into the main body of occupational therapy theory and practice.

Sensory integration therapy has been heavily criticized both from within occupational therapy and from the medical and educational professions. This may be partly due to the kind of resistance discussed by Clark (1991) and partly due to the lack of a well-researched or validated theory and research base (although despite methodologic problems, more research exists on sensory integration within the profession than on any other area of practice). Ottenbacher's statements regarding empirical consensus building in the context of collective research are critical for the profession of occupational therapy. Because not until professional agreement exists regarding the constructs of sensory integration based on empirical findings of research studies that are synthesized into a well-formulated theory base, will sensory integration make the transition from a set of ideas to a paradigm embraced by the profession.

Summary of the effectiveness of sensory integration therapy

A brief summary of the research that supports the efficacy of sensory integration procedures is provided by the American Occupational Therapy Association (Efficacy; Data brief, 1988). More detailed descriptions of studies are provided by Clark and Pierce (1988) and Cermak and Henderson (1989, 1990).

Cited in these reviews is the meta-analysis by Ottenbacher (1982), which examined 49 published research studies and included eight that met stringent criteria. Ottenbacher found that 78.8% of children who received sensory integration treatment demonstrated better performance than children who did not receive treatment. These advantages were found in motor performance, academic achievement, and language functioning.

The comprehensive review by Clark and Pierce (1988) provides the following conclusion: Positive treatment effects are documented in both single subject design studies (Madsen & Conte, 1980) and in group design studies (Ayres, 1972c), although there is not a consistent result among all studies (Carte et al., 1984).

An example of an experimental group design with a rigorously controlled design is provided by several studies completed by Ayres (1972c, 1976). In the 1972 study, Ayres found that in both the generalized sensory integration group and the auditory language problem group, children who received sensory integration treatment made greater academic gains in reading than the children who did not receive sensory integrative treatment. In the 1976 study, it was demonstrated that sensory integrative treatment ameliorates dysfunction identified by hyporeactive nystagmus and promotes efficiency of academic learning (as measured by scores on the Wide Range Achievement Test: Reading and Spelling).

Numerous other studies have been conducted using comparisons of groups. In summary, Clark and Pierce (1988) state:

> Results of these studies suggest that sensory integrative procedures seem to produce language or language-related gains in both learning disabled and mentally retarded children . . . that they may promote eye-hand coordination, and that their effects on nystagmus duration are unclear. (p. 4)

The review of research using single subject design highlights the usefulness of that technique in understanding the role of individual variation in response to sensory integration therapy. Single subject design studies serve as a useful tool for generating hypotheses for study in larger experimental approaches. In general, the findings of the case studies were "generally consistent with the findings of the studies on the effectiveness of sensory integrative treatment that utilized group designs" (Clark & Pierce, 1988, p. 5). Three of the four studies reviewed found positive effects of therapy on outcome measures.

Strong evidence exists in the literature that sensory integration may be effective; however, research evidence is not conclusive. Due to a variety of methodologic problems, many of the studies are open to criticism. *The lack of conclusive scientific evidence does not mean that the construct of sensory integration lacks validity, however.* Ottenbacher (1988), in reviewing efficacy studies in sensory integration, concludes that although there are design flaws in existing studies, *most sensory integration efficacy studies reveal that sensory integration treatment is effective.* Thus, he concludes that "an aggressive empirical effort [should be instituted] to establish the credibility of these initial findings" (p. 426).

As noted by Cermak and Henderson (1989, 1990), occupational therapists and professionals in education, medicine, and psychology are faced with similar dilemmas. It is important to believe in the efficacy of the treatment that you are undertaking. It is essential to feel that there is merit in the clinical approach that defines your profession and thus to respond to demands for service made upon the profession. Nevertheless, each discipline has an ethical obligation to question the efficacy of its treatment approaches and must be diligent in researching effects of various treatments. As new research results are reported, the field must be open to changes. Improvements in treatment modalities are only possible given the acceptance of data-based results of efficacy studies.

It is possible that the paradigm of sensory integration, as it continues to grow and change and is actualized into the profession in the future, may bare only partial resemblance to that envisioned by its originator, Dr. A. Jean Ayres. These changes, if based on collective research in the profession, will be positive and will support the importance of a questioning attitude and continued growth and expansion of knowledge, as exemplified by Ayres' statement, "Truth, like infinity, is to be forever approached, but never reached" (Ayres, 1972b, p. 4).

Where do we go from here?

It is hoped that this review of the methodologic problems inherent in sensory integration efficacy research has not dissuaded the serious student from completing research in this field. Obviously, the need for efficacy research with the concomitant theoretical leaps that can be made from a synthesis of new knowledge is immense.

It is apparent that a single person or even a few people are unlikely to produce the body of research needed to prove (or disprove) the efficacy of this paradigm of treatment. However, through multisite studies and collaborative research of other types, new knowledge can be gained that will shed light on which aspects of sensory integration treatment are valid and which must be modified.

Each person is well cautioned to take to heart some of the suggestions made by occupational therapists referenced in this section. Overly ambitious projects that attempt to answer unrealistic research questions will probably provide information that is so diffuse that it will not add to the body of knowledge in the field. However, studies that have carefully thought-out research questions, clearly delineated hypotheses, and detailed quantitative or qualitative research methodologies are likely to provide information that will have relevance for many decades and ultimately benefit many children. The profession of occupational therapy is responsible for valuing and supporting research in the profession, both financially and in terms of human resources. Only by integrating research into our clinical practice, can the necessary knowledge result in changes in treatment practices be actualized.

The photographs in this section were taken by Shay McAtee.

References

Ayres, A. J. (1964). Tactile functions: Their relation to hyperactive and perceptual motor behavior. *American Journal of Occupational Therapy, 18*(1), 6–11.

Ayres, A. J. (1972a). *Southern California Sensory Integration Tests: Manual.* Los Angeles: Western Psychological Services.

Ayres, A. J. (1972b). *Sensory integration and learning disorders.* Los Angeles: Western Psychological Services.

Ayres, A. J. (1972c). Improving academic scores through sensory integration. *Journal of Learning Disabilities, 5,* 24–28.

Ayres, A. J. (1974). *The development of sensory integrative theory and practice.* Dubuque, IA: Kendall/Hunt Publishing Co.

Ayres, A. J. (1975). *Southern California Postrotary Nystagmus Test: Manual.* Los Angeles: Western Psychological Services.

Ayres, A. J. (1976). *The effect of sensory integrative therapy on learning disabled children: Valentine–Kline Foundation Project.* Los Angeles: Center for the Study of Sensory Integration Dysfunction. Available from Sensory Integration International.

Ayres, A. J. (1979). *Sensory integration and the child.* Los Angeles: Western Psychological Services.

Ayres, A. J. (1980). *Southern California Sensory Integration Tests: Manual, revised.* Los Angeles: Western Psychological Services.

Ayres, A. J. (1985). *Developmental dyspraxia and adult onset dyspraxia*. Torrance, CA: Sensory Integration International.

Ayres, A. J. (1989a). *Sensory Integration and Praxis Tests*. Los Angeles: Western Psychological Services.

Ayres, A. J. (1989b). Forward. In L. J. Miller (Ed.), *Developing norm-referenced standardized tests*. New York: Haworth Press.

Ayres, A. J., & Marr, D. B. (1991). Sensory Integration and Praxis Tests. In A. G. Fisher, E. A. Murray & A. C. Bundy (Eds.), *Sensory integration: Theory and practice*. Philadelphia: F. A. Davis.

Beery, K. E., & Buktenica N. A. (1967). *Developmental Test of Visual-Motor Integration*. Chicago: Follett Publishing Co.

Berk, R. A., & DeGangi, G. A. (1983). *DeGangi-Berk Test of Sensory Integration: Manual*. Los Angeles: Western Psychological Services.

Bruininks, R. H. (1978). *Bruininks-Oseretsky Test of Motor Proficiency*. Circle Pines, MN: American Guidance Service.

Carte, E., Morrison, D., Sublett, J., Uemura, A., & Sektrakian, J. (1984). Sensory integration therapy: A trial of a specific neurodevelopmental therapy for the remediation of learning disabilities. *Journal of Developmental Behavior in Pediatrics, 5*, 189–194.

Cermak, S. A., & Henderson, A. (1989). The efficacy of sensory integration procedures. *Sensory Integration Quarterly Newsletter, XVII*(4), 1–4. Available from Sensory Integration International.

Cermak, S. A., & Henderson, A. (1990). The efficacy of sensory integration procedures. *Sensory Integration Quarterly Newsletter, XVIII*(1), 1–5. [Available from Sensory Integration International].

Clark, F. (1991). Foreword. In A. G. Fisher, E. A. Murray & A. C. Bundy (Eds.), *Sensory integration: Theory and practice*. Philadelphia: F. A. Davis.

Clark, F., & Pierce, D. (1988). Synopsis of pediatric occupational therapy effectiveness. *Sensory Integration News, 16*(2), 1–15.

Colarusso, R. P. (1972). *Motor-Free Visual Perception Test*. Novato, CA: Academic Therapy Publications.

Cruickshank, W. M. (1974). Foreword. In Henderson, A., Llorens, L. Gilfoyle, E., Myers, C., Prevel, S., Eds. *The development of sensory integrative theory and practice*. Dubuque, IA: Kendall/Hunt Publishing Company.

Denning, J., & Mayberry, W. (1987). Vestibular dysfunction in preschool children with a history of otitis media. *Occupational Therapy Journal of Research, 7*(6), 335–348.

Dunn, W. (1991). The sensorimotor systems: A framework for assessment and intervention. In F. P. Orelove & D. Sobsey (Eds.), *Educating children with multiple disabilities: A transdisciplinary approach* (2nd ed.). Baltimore: Paul H. Brooks.

Efficacy: Data brief: *Research supports efficacy of sensory integration procedures*. (1988). American Occupational Therapy Association, 5(3).

Fisher, A. G., & Bundy, A. C. (1991). The interpretation process. In A. G. Fisher, E. A. Murray & A. C. Bundy (Eds.), *Sensory integration: Theory and practice*. Philadelphia: F. A. Davis.

Fisher, A. G., & Dunn, W. (1983). Tactile defensiveness: Historical perspective, new research: A theory grows. *Sensory Integration Specialty Section Newsletter, 6*(2), 1–4.

Gardner M. F. (1982). *Test of Visual-Perceptual Skills*. Seattle, WA: Special Child Publications.

Gardner M. F. (1986). *Test of Visual-Motor Skills*. Seattle, WA: Special Child Publications.

Henderson, A., Llorens, L., Gilfoyle, E., Myers, C., & Prevel, S. (1974). *The development of sensory integrative theory and practice*. Dubuque, IA: Kendall/Hunt Publishing Company.

Kimball, J. (1988). The emphasis is on integration, not sensory. *American Journal on Mental Retardation, 92*(5), 423–424.

King, L. J. (1974). A Sensory integrative approach to schizophrenia. *American Journal of Occupational Therapy, 28*(9), 529–537.

King, L. J. (1982). Interpretation of social-emotional domain. Miller assessment of preschoolers: Seminar administration and interpretation manual; San Antonio: Psychological Corp.

King, L. J. (1987). A sensory integrative approach to the education of the autistic child. In Z. Mailloux (Ed.), *Sensory integrative approaches in occupational therapy*. New York: Haworth Press.

Knickerbocker, B. M. (1980). *A holistic approach to the treatment of learning disorders*. Thorofare, NJ.: Slack.

Madsen, P. S., & Conte, J. R. (1980). Single subject research in occupational therapy: A case illustration. *American Journal of Occupational Therapy, 34*, 263–267.

Mailloux, Z. (1987). *Sensory integrative approaches in occupational therapy*. New York: Haworth Press.

McCarron, L. T. (1982). *McCarron Assessment of Neuromuscular Development*. Dallas: Common Market Press.

McCarron, L. T., & Dial J. G. (1979). *Haptic Visual Discrimination Test*. Dallas: Common Market Press.

Miller, L. J. (1988a, 1982) *Miller Assessment for Preschoolers: Manual*. San Antonio: The Psychological Corporation.

Miller, L. J. (1988b). *Miller Assessment for Preschoolers: Seminar administration and interpretation manual*. San Antonio: The Psychological Corporation.

Ottenbacher, K. (1982). Sensory integration therapy: Affect or effect? *American Journal of Occupational Therapy, 36*, 571–578.

Ottenbacher, K. (1988). Sensory integration—myth, method, and imperative. *American Journal on Mental Retardation, 92*(5), 425–426.

Ottenbacher, K. (1991). Research in sensory integration: Empirical perceptions and progress. In A. G. Fisher, E. A. Murray & A. C. Bundy (Eds.), *Sensory integration: Theory and practice*. Philadelphia: F. A. Davis.

Reynolds, P. D. (1971). *A primer in theory construction*. New York: Macmillan.

Schaaf, R. C. (1985). The frequency of vestibular disorders in developmentally delayed preschoolers with otitis media. *American Journal of Occupational Therapy, 39*(4), 247–252.

Seig, K. (1988). A. Jean Ayres. In B. R. J. Miller, K. W. Sieg, F. M. Ludwig, S. D. Shortridge, & J. VanDeusen (Eds.), *Six perspectives on theory for the practice of occupational therapy*. Rockville, MD: Aspen Publications.

Wells, M. E., & Smith, D. W. (1983). Reduction of self-injurious behavior in mentally retarded persons using sensory-integrative techniques. *American Journal of Mental Deficiency, 87*, 664–666.

Wilbarger P., & Wilbarger J. L. (1991). *Sensory defensiveness in children two to twelve: An intervention guide for parents and other caretakers* (p. 3). Santa Barbara, CA: Avante Educational Programs.

SECTION 5

Autism

LISA A. KURTZ

KEY TERMS

Behavior Modification or Operant Conditioning

Behavioral Deficits

Cognitive Deficits

Communication Deficits

Pervasive Developmental Disorders

Sensory Integration

Sensory Processing Disorders

Upon completion of this section the reader will be able to:

1. *Recognize the typical neurologic, developmental, and behavioral characteristics of autism.*
2. *Understand the principles behind occupational therapy assessment and intervention strategies in relation to autism.*

The treatment of autistic children poses many challenges to the occupational therapist. The term "autism" was first used by Dr. Leo Kanner (1943) to describe a group of severely mentally handicapped children who shared a characteristic pattern of behaviors that included social aloofness with withdrawal, the inability to communicate with others, an intense desire for sameness in the environment, and a tendency to engage in elaborate repetitive and often stereotypical routines to the exclusion of normal imaginative play. Typically, these deviant behaviors were present even in early infancy. Parents of autistic children described their babies as either overly passive or excessively irritable. They failed to cuddle or to mold to their mother's arms and often resisted being held even during feeding. Although Kanner commented that the parents of these children tended to appear cold and unloving, he speculated that the condition is inborn (Kanner, 1943).

Since Kanner's time, research has attempted to define the etiology and best treatment methodologies for autism. Still, many questions remain unanswered. One area of current debate concerns the diagnostic classification of autistic disorders. Although children with the full clinical picture of Kanner-type autism are fairly easy to recognize, autistic-like features are common in a variety of other syndromes such as mental retardation, vision and hearing impairment, and degenerative diseases including Rett syndrome and tuberous sclerosis (Percy et al., 1990). Both the severity of dysfunction and the nature of associated sensory and motility disturbances can be highly variable from child to child. Onset is usually, but not always, before the age of 3 years. Current classification considers autism to be one of several neurologically based conditions included under the category of **pervasive developmental disorders** (American Psychological Association, 1987). Diagnosis is based on the presence of behavioral symptoms in three areas:

Qualitative impairment in reciprocal social interactions
Qualitative impairment in verbal and nonverbal communications
Markedly restricted repertoire of activities and interests

Deviant development must be identified in all three areas for the child to fit the classification of "pervasive developmental disorder."

Incidence and etiology

Autism is a relatively rare condition. It occurs in about 4 of every 10,000 births and is three times more common in boys than in girls. A genetic component is suggested in at least some forms of the condition, since the parents of one autistic child have a 9.7% chance of producing a second affected child (Ritvo et al., 1989). Also, autism is more prevalent among identical than fraternal twins (Smalley et al., 1988). Numerous etiologic factors have been implicated in autism. In most cases, a specific cause cannot be identified. However, most researchers now agree that autism is caused by some form of brain damage or abnormality in brain development. Eighty percent of autistic children have abnormal electroencephalograms (EEGs), and 25% develop seizure disorders by adolescence (Batshaw, 1991). Evidence also exists that prenatal environmental influences, neurophysiologic abnormalities, neurotransmitter alterations, and other biochemical abnormalities may be involved (Reber & Batshaw, 1992; Gaffney et al., 1989; Goodman, 1989; Ornitz, 1985).

Developmental characteristics of autism

Cognitive deficits

Most autistic children demonstrate **cognitive deficits** such as global developmental delay; 35% test in the mildly retarded range of intelligence, 15% in the moderately retarded range, and 20% in the severely to profoundly retarded range (Batshaw, 1991). Performance may be strikingly uneven, with better skill for tasks requiring visual perception and rote memory than for those that demand symbolic or logical reasoning (Reber & Batshaw, 1992). Those children not classified as mentally retarded often exhibit language-based learning disabilities. Some autistic children demonstrate isolated areas of exceptional ability or "splinter skills," often involving memory, music, numerical calculations, or the ability to perform spatial manipulations. However, because autistic children lack judgment and imagination in their thinking, these skills are not typically applied to adaptive interactions with their environment.

Communication deficits

Severe **communication deficits** affecting both expressive and receptive language are one of the hallmark features of autism. About 50% of autistic children fail to develop useful, spoken language (Coleman, 1989). Gestural communication, including the ability to learn sign language, may also be affected. Those children who do learn to talk tend to use language in rote, stereotyped patterns rather than using functional communication. Often they repeat phrases or songs in a repetitive, sing-song fashion. Speech patterns may be entirely normal when the child is echoing something he or she has just heard, but highly deviant when the child is attempting to speak with communicative intent. Bizarre features such as pronomial substitutions ("you" instead of "I"), reversals ("pasghetti" instead of "spaghetti"), and abnormalities of pitch, rhythm, or intonation are common (Wing, 1985).

The understanding of spoken language is similarly affected. Young autistic children may react to speech no differently from the way they react to any other sound, and are typically late in responding to their name. They tend to respond better to those commands that are very brief or concrete in nature than to those that are abstract or that involve multiple steps. Often, understanding can be improved by pairing language with a concrete, visual cue.

Social and behavioral deficits

The bizarre and rigid behavior patterns of autistic children can be striking manifestations of **behavioral deficits**. Many children become obsessed with certain rituals or routines that they have developed, such as lining up small objects in a row, smelling everything that they touch, and organizing their belongings in a particular order. Rather than playing with toys, the child may form an intense attachment to an unusual object, such as a piece of string or an empty can retrieved from the trash, and may stubbornly refuse to be separated from the object (Figure 13-40). Some children wear clothes only of a certain color, or eat only two or three different foods. Many are fascinated by such visual stimuli as spinning objects and flickering lights, and can stare at these for hours on end. Any effort to interrupt the child's routine may result in extreme agitation, temper tantrums, or even self-mutilation.

Social interaction may be disordered in a variety of ways. Often the child avoids or averts eye contact, pulls away when touched or held, and appears oblivious to parents' efforts to interact on an emotional level. Some autistic children may even treat people as if they are inanimate objects and simply climb over them to obtain a desired object. Children who speak may show little desire to initiate communication except to fulfill some specific, concrete purpose. Limitations in imagination result in an absence of representational or pretend play.

Other behavioral abnormalities that may be associated with autism are stereotyped movements such as hand flapping or head banging, sleep disturbance, short attention span, hyperactivity, and aggression (Reber & Batshaw, 1992).

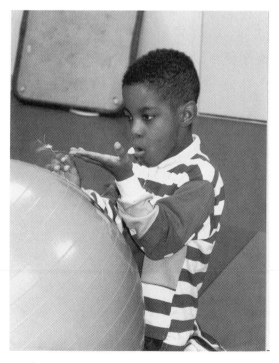

FIGURE 13-40. *Obsessive rituals are common among autistic children; this boy perseverates by blowing a piece of string to the exclusion of normal play.*

Sensory processing disorders

Sensory processing disorders are common among autistic children, who appear driven to self-induce certain forms of stimulation. Typically, there is a preference for input from the proximal senses (vestibular, somatosensory, olfactory, gustatory) over the distal senses of vision and hearing (Ramm, 1988). Both hypo- and hyperreactive levels of sensitivity may be observed, often alternating in the same child. Evidence of hyporeactivity may include such behaviors as failure to orient to novel sights or sounds, disregard of painful stimuli, absence of startle reflexes, and failure to become dizzy after prolonged spinning. Examples of exaggerated reactions to sensory stimuli are tactile defensiveness and gravitational insecurity.

Ayres (1979) described three aspects of disordered sensory processing that may be found in this population. First, there is inadequate registration of stimuli, which causes the child to ignore certain relevant aspects of the environment. Second, faulty modulation results in perceptual distortions including under- and overreactivity. Finally, because sensory input fails to trigger positive affective responses, the child avoids novel sensorimotor activities because mastery of those activities is not intrinsically pleasurable. All these factors influence the child to lack motivation, initiative, and self-direction in the type of sensorimotor play that is so crucial to adaptive learning in the normal child.

Treatment and prognosis

Autism is a chronic developmental disability that requires lifelong management. Currently, no single effective medical treatment is available, although pharmacotherapy can provide symptomatic relief for certain associated problems such as hyperactivity, aggression, and sleep disturbance (Reber & Batshaw, 1992; Gilberg, 1990). Numerous innovative approaches to therapy, including psychotherapy, sensory integration, holding therapy, play therapy, and behavior modification have been used with inconclusive results. Most authorities agree that effective management of the autistic child requires a comprehensive, multidisciplinary program provided in a highly structured, special education setting. Specific behavioral interventions, intensive speech/language therapy, training in social skills, occupational and physical therapy, and intensive family support and training are often cited as important components of such programs (Reber & Batshaw, 1992; Coleman, 1989; Wing, 1985).

Despite the variable course seen in autism, only a small percentage achieve the ability to live independently or to be self-employed as adults. As one might expect, the presence of significant mental retardation, associated neurologic handicaps, and the failure to develop meaningful language by 5 years of age are factors that have been associated with poorer outcomes.

Role of occupational therapy

Occupational therapy assessment and treatment of autistic children can be difficult, given the extreme variability in presenting symptomatology, learning style, and potential for response to intervention. Only a small percentage of high-functioning autistic persons possess the ability to comprehend and cooperate in formal standardized testing. More often, the therapist must rely on informal play observation, parent/teacher questionnaires, or performance on criterion-referenced measures of behavior to obtain information about the child's developmental maturity, sensorimotor responses, and functional capabilities. Because no singular method of therapy has been proven effective, the therapist must often use a trial-and-error approach to determine the treatment strategies that work best with an individual child. Bloomer and Rose (1990) describe seven traditional frames of reference for occupational therapy as applied to autism and advocate that therapists may appropriately use a variety of techniques drawn from these approaches. Many factors, ranging from the therapist's level of specialist knowledge to the amount of time and resources available for therapy may determine the initial decision regarding which approach to use. The two methodologies most frequently used by occupational therapists are sensory integration therapy and behavioral therapy.

Sensory integration therapy

The first major premise of the **sensory integration** theory is that learning is dependent on the ability to derive sensory information from the environment and from bodily movement, to process and integrate this information within the central nervous system, and to use it to plan and organize behavior. Second, when children have deficits in processing and integrating sensory input, problems in planning and producing behavior occur which interfere with conceptual and motor learning. Finally, it is hypothesized that providing opportunities for enhanced sensory input in the context of a meaningful activity requiring an adaptive response will result in improved central nervous system integration of sensory input and, in turn, improved conceptual and motor learning (Fisher & Murray, 1991).

Children with autism demonstrate a variety of sensory processing disorders and often show patterns of dysfunction similar to those of dyspraxic children (Ayres, 1979). The therapist choosing to use a sensory integrative approach to therapy must use creative approaches to determine the child's ability to register, modulate, and act on sensory input. Ayres and Tickle (1980) developed a useful instrument, the Response to Sensory Input, and found that autistic children who orient to certain types of

stimuli and who are hyperresponsive show greater gains in therapy than those who are hyporesponsive (Figure 13-41).

Cammisa (1991) describes other criterion-referenced methods of sensory integrative assessment for children who are difficult to test. One of the more difficult aspects of treating autistic children using sensory integration procedures is the need for clinical sensitivity in differentiating self-stimulation from self-direction. Because autistic children tend to lack the "inner drive" to master their environment, the therapist may need to be more imposing than is normally recommended for sensory integration procedures.

Behavioral therapy

Behavioral therapy, also referred to as **behavior modification or operant conditioning**, is concerned with improving specific behaviors or skills through the structured manipulation of reinforcement. Behavioral theorists believe that all behavior is learned. If desired patterns of behavior are rewarded and undesired patterns of behavior are punished or ignored, behavior can be gradually shaped into whatever pattern is desired by the person in control of the punishments and rewards (King, 1987). Critical elements of the success of behavioral approaches are the need to identify reinforcers that are meaningful to the child and the importance of immediacy and consistency in reinforcement so that the child learns that targeted behaviors are associated with predictable consequences. There is considerable evidence that behavioral therapy approaches can be effective in increasing communication and social competence in autistic persons (Werry & Wollersheim, 1989; Howlin & Rutter, 1987; Lovaas, 1987). However, some authorities are critical of the fact that this approach fails to address the underlying causes of maladaptive behavior. Also, changes are limited to those behaviors targeted for modification, without generalization to other aspects of the child's behavior.

CASE STUDY

Mark was 4 years, 7 months old when first referred to occupational therapy for improvement of functional motor, play, and self-care skills. Diagnosed with pervasive developmental

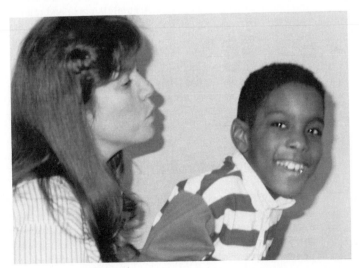

FIGURE 13-41. *Immediate orientation to certain stimuli, such as a puff of air to the back of the neck, may predict positive response to therapy using sensory integrative procedure.*

disorder at age 3 years, 3 months, he attended a special needs preschool where he received individual speech therapy.

Background medical history revealed no significant perinatal complications. He had suffered from recurrent otitis media without the need for myringotomies and had bilateral exotropia, which was surgically repaired when he was 1 year of age. Corrective lenses had been prescribed for mild astigmatism, but Mark's parents were unsuccessful in coaxing him to wear the glasses.

Developmental history included normal achievement of early motor milestones but delayed speech and language development. Psychological testing indicated low average intellectual functioning with a pattern of disordered language behaviors, poor attention span, perseveration, resistance to transitions, and inconsistent social responsiveness. No focal abnormalities were found on neurologic evaluation.

Discussion

Although Mark was high functioning compared with many autistic children, he was felt to lack the comprehension needed to respond to the Sensory Integration and Praxis Tests. Instead, assessment consisted of the following:

1. Parental history of sensorimotor development
2. Clinical observations of sensory and neurodevelopmental responses
3. Selected items from the Gesell Preschool Test
4. Developmental Test of Visual Motor Integration
5. Motor-Free Visual Perception Test
6. Southern California Postrotary Nystagmus Test

Evaluation results indicated a highly uneven developmental profile, with strengths in visual discrimination and symbol recognition and weakness in social and play interactions, self-care independence, and gross and fine motor coordination. Skills were judged to range from the 2 years, 6 month- to 5 years, 6 month- level. Evidence of sensory integrative dysfunction included highly attenuated postrotary nystagmus, poor modulation of sensory input with severe tactile defensiveness and mild gravitational insecurity, poor body awareness, poor bilateral coordination, and poor postural motor planning.

Mark's parents participated in setting short-term goals that were meaningful to them. Of primary concern was Mark's severe tactile defensiveness, which interfered with his participation in such routine tasks as taking a bath or having his hair cut and which often led to temper tantrums that were highly distressing to his parents. They also wished to see Mark become more independent in self-care skills, particularly toileting and dressing. The therapist concurred with these objectives, but also desired to see Mark develop more purposeful play patterns than his characteristic patterns of jumping, climbing, or other gross sensory stimulation.

The therapist decided to treat Mark twice per week using a combination of behavioral and sensory integration intervention strategies, with the following goals established for the initial 2-month period of therapy:

1. To increase parent's ability to create an environment at home that optimally stimulates the development of functional skills

2. To reduce the incidence of tactile defensive behaviors
3. To increase independence in toileting and dressing
4. To increase body awareness and motor planning skills
5. To encourage Mark to initiate representational play schemes

A typical therapy session might proceed as follows:

1. First, Mark is welcomed to therapy and encouraged to remove his outer clothes and to go to the toilet. Behavioral strategies include verbal and tactile cuing to increase attention to task, verbal task analysis, backward chaining of the targeted self-care skill, and social reinforcement of cooperation.
2. Mark is engaged in an activity that provides firm touch or strong proprioceptive input in an effort to inhibit tactile defensiveness. For example, he is asked to pretend that he is a sandwich by lying between two mats (bread slices); his mother adds lettuce, mayonnaise, and tomato, then squeezes the bread after each "ingredient."
3. Mark is engaged in play that encourages goal-directed responses to sensory input. Activities are selected and designed to enhance body awareness, bilateral integration, motor planning, and representation. He particularly enjoys obstacle courses.
4. Again using behavioral strategies, Mark is assisted in putting away play materials, washing his hands, and donning his clothes, thus terminating the session.

After 2 months of therapy, Mark was independent in dressing and toileting except for managing small fasteners and wiping himself after a bowel movement. He required frequent verbal prompts and had not generalized these skills to apply at home. There was some evidence of reduced tactile defensiveness. Before therapy, Mark had refused all "messy" games such as playing in sand or playing with fingerpaints. After therapy he played with fingerpaints for up to 10 minutes drawing simple representational pictures, although strong social reinforcement was necessary to engage his cooperation. Also, his mother happily reported that he had cooperated for his first haircut without the need to use physical restraint. His motor skills as measured on the Gesell Preschool Test had matured by 6 to 12 months, and he demonstrated greater self-direction in play. For example, before therapy, Mark's efforts to amuse himself consisted of random physical activity. Now, although he still lacked the ability to initiate a creative scheme, he was able to amuse himself for up to 20 minutes by repeating and elaborating on a game used in therapy, such as setting up and negotiating an obstacle course.

Summary

The pervasive developmental disorders of childhood, including autism, represent a heterogeneous group of neurologically based conditions that lead to deviations in cognitive, emotional, and sensorimotor development. Although the prognosis for autistic persons to lead independent lives as adults generally is poor, much can be done to improve the quality of their lives. Approaches to occupational therapy intervention, including sensory integration therapy and behavior modification, have been presented.

References

American Psychological Association. (1987). *Diagnostic and statistical manual of mental disorders* (3rd rev. ed.). Washington, DC: American Psychiatric Association.

Ayres, A. J. (1979). *Sensory integration and the child*. Los Angeles, CA: Western Psychological Services

Ayres, A. J., & Tickle, L. S. (1980). Hyper-responsivity to touch and vestibular stimuli as a predictor of positive responses to sensory integration procedures by autistic children. *American Journal of Occupational Therapy, 34*(6), 375–381.

Batshaw, M. L. (Ed.). (1991). *Your child has a handicap: A complete sourcebook of daily and medical care*. Boston: Little, Brown & Co.

Bloomer, M. L., & Rose, C. C. (1990). Frames of reference: Guiding treatment for children with autism. In J. A. Johnson (Ed.), *Developmental disabilities: A handbook for occupational therapists* (pp. 5–26). Binghamton, NY: Haworth Press.

Cammisa, K. (1991). Testing difficult children for sensory integrative dysfunction. American Occupational Therapy Association. *Sensory Integration Special Interest Section Newsletter, 14*(2), 1–3.

Coleman, M. (1989). Young children with autism or autistic-like behavior. *Infants and Young Children, 1*(4), 22–31.

Fisher, A. G., & Murray, E. A. (1991). Introduction to sensory integration theory. In A. G. Fisher, E. A. Murray & A. C. Bundy (Eds.), *Sensory integration theory and practice* (pp. 3–26). Philadelphia: F. A. Davis.

Gaffney, G. R., Kuperman, S., Tsai, L., & Minchin, S. (1989). Forebrain structure in infantile autism. *Journal of the American Academy of Child and Adolescent Psychiatry, 28*(4), 534–537.

Gilberg, C. (1990). Autism and pervasive developmental disorders. *Journal of Child Psychology and Psychiatry, 31*(1), 99–119.

Goodman, R. (1989). Technical note: Are perinatal complications causes or consequences of autism? *Journal of Child Psychology and Psychiatry, 31*(5), 809–812.

Howlin, P., & Rutter, M. (1987). *Treatment of autistic children*. New York: John Wiley & Sons.

Kanner, L. (1943). Autistic disturbances of affective contact. *Nervous Child, 2*, 217–250.

King, L. J. (1987). A sensory integrative approach to the education of the autistic child. In Z. Mailloux (Ed.), *Sensory integrative approaches in occupational therapy*. New York: Haworth Press.

Lovaas, O. I. (1987). Behavioral treatment and normal educational and intellectual functioning in young autistic children. *Journal of Consulting and Clinical Psychology, 55*, 3–9.

Ornitz, E. M. (1985). Neurophysiology of infantile autism. *Journal of the American Academy of Child Psychiatry, 24*(3), 251–262.

Percy, A., Gilberg, C., Hagberg, B., & Witt-Engerstrom, I. (1990). Rett syndrome and the autistic disorders. *Neurologic Clinics, 8*(3), 659–676.

Ramm, P. A. (1988). The occupational therapy process in specific pediatric conditions. In H. L. Hopkins & H. D. Smith (Eds.), *Willard and Spackman's Occupational therapy* (7th ed., pp. 628–674). Philadelphia: J. B. Lippincott.

Reber, M., & Batshaw, M. L. (1992). Autism. In M. L. Batshaw & Y. M. Perret (Eds.), *Children with disabilities: A medical primer* (3rd ed., pp. 407–420). Baltimore: Paul H. Brooks.

Ritvo, E. R., Freeman, B. J., Pingree, C., Mason-Brothers, A., Jorde, L., Jenson, W. R., McMahon, W. M., Peterson, P. B., Mo, A., & Ritvo, A. (1989). The UCLA—University of Utah epidemiologic survey of autism: Prevalence. *American Journal of Psychiatry, 146*(2), 194–199.

Smalley, S. L., Asarnow, R. F., & Spence, M. A. (1988). Autism and genetics: A decade of research. *Archives of General Psychiatry, 45*, 953–961.

Werry, J. S., & Wollersheim, J. P. (1989). Behavior therapy with children and adolescents: A twenty-year overview. *Journal of Child and Adolescent Psychiatry, 28*(1), 1–18.

Wing, L. (1985). *Autistic children: A guide for parents and professionals* (2nd ed.). New York: Bruner/Mazel.

Bibliography

Alberto, P. A., & Troutman, A. C. (1982). *Applied behavior analysis for teachers: Influencing student performance*. Columbus, OH: Merrill Publishing.

Blechman, E. (1985). *Solving child behavior problems at home and school*. Champaign, IL: Research Press.

Cohen, D. J., Donellan, A. M., & Paul, R. (Eds.). (1987). *Handbook of autism and pervasive developmental disorders*. New York: John Wiley & Sons.

Grandin, T. (1984). My experiences as an autistic child and review of selected literature. *Journal of Orthomolecular Psychiatry, 13*, 144–174.

Grandin, T., & Scariano, M. M. (1986). *Emergence: Labeled autistic*. Novato, CA: Arena Press.

Miller, L. K. (1980). *Principles of everyday behavior analysis* (2nd ed.). Monterey, CA: Brooks/Cole Publishing Co.

Nelson, D. L. (1984). *Children with autism and other pervasive disorders of development and behavior: Therapy through activities*. Thorofare, NJ: Slack.

Ornitz, E. M. (1976). The modulation of sensory input and motor output in autistic children. In E. Schopler & R. J. Reichler (Eds.), *Psychopathology and child development: Research and treatment* (pp. 115–133). New York: Plenum Press.

Petit, K. (1980). Treatment of the autistic child: A demanding challenge. American Occupational Therapy Association. *Sensory Integration Special Interest Section Newsletter, 3*, 1–3.

Rimland, B. (1987). Holding therapy: Maternal bonding or cerebellar stimulation? *Autism Research Review International, 1*, 3.

Rutter, M. (1985). Infantile autism and other pervasive developmental disorders. In M. Rutter & L. Hersov (Eds.), *Child and adolescent psychiatry: Modern approaches*. Oxford: Blackwell Scientific Publications.

Schopler, E., & Reichler, R. J. (1979). *Individualized assessment and treatment for autistic and developmentally disabled children. Vol. 2, Teaching strategies for parents and professionals*. Austin, TX PRO-ED.

Wing, L. (Ed.). (1976). *Early childhood autism* (2nd ed.). Oxford: Pergamon Press.

Wolkowicz, R., Fish, J., & Scaffer, R. (1977). Sensory integration with autistic children. *Canadian Journal of Occupational Therapy, 44*, 171–175.

SECTION 6

Neural tube defect: Spina bifida

JUDITH ATKINS

LEARNING OBJECTIVES

Upon completion of this section the reader will be able to:

1. *Define spina bifida and myelomeningocele.*
2. *Discuss the cause and incidence of spina bifida.*
3. *Define and discuss the orthopedic, neurosurgical, and urologic problems associated with myelomeningocele.*
4. *Develop an occupational therapy treatment plan for a child born with myelomeningocele.*
5. *Identify the need for a multidisciplinary or interdisciplinary approach to the care and treatment of a child with this neural tube defect.*

Spina bifida, also used interchangeably with the term myelomeningocele, is a complex congenital malformation of the central nervous system. This diagnostic group of children requires a coordinated ***interdisciplinary approach*** in management and care. Treatment of myelomeningocele begins within 4 to 6 hours after birth with the neurosurgeon's repair of the defect and continues throughout the child's life. Once thought to be a devastating condition with a poor prognosis for independent living and a productive lifestyle, the diagnosis of myelomeningocele no longer carries this burden. Early intervention, improved surgical procedures, and a well-defined interdisciplinary team approach have proved successful in most cases. Clinically, a high percentage of children with this condition have normal to nearly normal intelligence, can ambulate, attend regular school, and pursue higher education or employment.

A well-defined treatment program is carried out with contributions from the neurosurgeon, orthopedist, urologist, occupational therapist, physical therapist, social worker, pediatrician, nurse specialist, educator, and parent. Emphasis on various treatment techniques changes as the child progresses or complications occur.

Etiology and definition of terms

Lindseth (1990) states that "neural tube defects are divided into four subtypes: meningocele, myelomeningocele, lipomeningocele and rachischisis" (Lindseth, 1990, p. 508).

Meningocele is a cyst involving only the meninges. It may require neurosurgical excision and closure but causes no orthopedic or neurologic abnormalities. These children rarely need occupational therapy, and their development is generally within normal limits.

Myelomeningocele is defined as a hernial protrusion of the cord and its meninges through a defect in the vertebral canal. It involves dysplasia of the spinal cord and meninges. All affected children require a neurosurgical excision and closure and all have some degree of permanent, irreversible neurologic disability. The defect most frequently occurs in the lumbar or lumbosacral spine.

A *lipomeningocele* is a lesion in which the sac contains lipoma.

A *rachischisis* is the complete absence of the skin and sac, with exposure of the muscle and the presence of a dysplastic spinal cord without evidence of a covering.

Myelomeningocele is the most common of these subtypes and the defect most frequently seen in clinical practice. Therefore, myelomeningocele is discussed at length in this section.

Myelomeningocele

The actual cause of myelomeningocele is unknown. Several theories exist, however, including a vitamin deficiency, a hereditary component, and other exogenous factors. It is known that the defect occurs very early in pregnancy, generally between the third and fourth weeks of gestation and usually before the mother realizes she is pregnant. Literature supports that the defect occurs between 1 and 2 of 1000 live births in the United States with a higher incidence (3 to 4 of 1000 live births) in England and Ireland. Studies of spina bifida and anencephaly suggest that the risk of having a second child with a neural tube defect is about 5%. Therefore, parents facing a subsequent pregnancy are considered at risk and are offered amniocentesis between the 10th and 14th weeks of pregnancy.

Pregnancies positive for a neural tube defect have a higher than average level of α-fetoprotein in the amniotic fluid. Parents are then given the option to terminate the pregnancy. Ultrasound pictures of the fetus are usually done at the same time. Although ultrasound testing is prevalent in the practice of obstetrics, it is not conclusive in diagnosing myelomeningocele and hydrocephalus. In clinical practice, cases have also been documented in which ultrasonography did not indicate any abnormalities. Women considered at risk for a child with myelomeningocele are counseled to have both the amniocentesis and detailed ultrasonography for examination of the fetus.

One of the most important observations regarding myelomeningocele is that the disease is no longer considered static or nonprogressive. It has a tendency to undergo progressive neurologic degeneration characterized by increasing levels of paralysis and decreasing upper extremity function. The neurologic deterioration can be very slow and insidious or very rapid and dramatic. It is believed by most clinicians that there are three major reasons for or areas of deterioration and subsequent loss of function. These areas are hydrocephalus and associated hydrosyringomyelia, Arnold–Chiari deformity, and tethered cord syndrome.

Neurosurgical and neurologic concerns

Hydrocephalus is an accumulation of cerebrospinal fluid accompanied by dilatation of the cerebral ventricles and an enlarged skull. It is extremely common in children with myelomeningocele. It is reported in all the current literature that at least 90% of all children with myelomeningocele have hydrocephalus. Degree of hydrocephalus, success of shunting procedures, and complications related to the hydrocephalus also seem to correlate with intellectual function and perceptual motor abnormalities. Most children with myelomeningocele are shunted within the first 2 weeks of life. Many present with hydrocephalus at birth whereas others demonstrate an increased head size following closure of the back. Most of these children receive a ventriculoperitoneal or ventriculoatrial shunt. In very young children, parents are instructed to look for such signs as increased head size, nausea and vomiting, and marked irritability as indications of possible shunt malfunction. In older children, the symptoms become more subtle such as intermittent headaches, short attention span, increased scoliosis, increased paralysis, decreased school performance, increased irritability, and decreased upper-extremity strength.

Hydrosyringomyelia is a combination of a hydromyelia and syringomyelia. Problems often associated with hydromyelia and syringomyelia are loss of motor function in the lower extremities, spasticity, scoliosis, and increased weakness of the hands and upper extremities. Many times, shunt replacement resolves these symptoms. This is why it is extremely important to evaluate affected children periodically and to pay close attention to the above symptoms. It usually occurs in the school-age population, when clinic or physician visits are less frequent as are therapy evaluations. Parents must be made aware of the potential problem and contact their treatment center if there is a question about the symptoms just mentioned.

Arnold–Chiari deformity, or malformations of the posterior fossa, frequently occur in children with neural tube defects. Symptoms in the infant include apnea episodes, stridor, nystagmus, upper extremity spasm or weakness, swallowing difficulties, and depressed or absent cough reflex. Spastic weakness of the upper extremities may be present. Some children require surgical decompression of the posterior fossa and upper spinal region. However, most symptoms usually resolve on their own after placement of the ventriculoperitoneal shunt for treatment of hydrocephalus.

Tethered cord syndrome may also be seen in children with myelomeningocele. Associated with this condition is pain in the lower lumbar spine in the area of the myelomeningocele or pain in the buttock and posterior thigh. Also associated are increasing spasticity and loss of function in the lower extremities. This becomes more obvious with ambulators when the children and their parents observe increased difficulty with ambulation and changes in gait. Some children require a surgical release to relieve symptoms and restore function.

Urologic concerns

Most children with myelomeningocele have urinary (neurogenic bladder) and bowel incontinence. Since the nerves to the bowel and bladder emerge at the sacral level of the spinal cord, even children with a low lesion such as S1-2 may experience bowel and bladder incontinence.

Recurrent urinary tract infections and renal failure have been major causes of death in children with myelomeningocele. In addition, social stigmas are associated with incontinence and the difficulties that poor management pose at school, home, and workplace.

Many children are managed for urinary incontinence by Credé's method and intermittent catheterization. When the child is old enough, he or she is taught to do intermittent self-catheterization using a clean technique. Some children are candidates for bladder augmentation and an artificial sphincter placement. Others may have a vesicostomy or other type of urinary diversion.

Bowel management is generally done by the use of suppositories. Parents are taught very early, generally when the child is age 2 to 3 years, to initiate a bowel program that will continue throughout life.

Orthopedic concerns

Orthopedic management of children with myelomeningocele is critical and best done at a treatment center experienced in the care of children born with a myelomeningocele defect. Orthopedic treatment/management can be divided into the following anatomic areas: (1) spine, (2) hips, (3) knees, and (4) feet.

Spine

The biggest concern associated with the spine is scoliosis. Scoliosis reportedly occurs with varying degrees of severity and deformity in 80% of all children. As stated by Lindseth (1990),

> . . . in addition to idiopathic scoliosis that may occur in these children, three major abnormalities of scoliosis have been reported to date: (1) unequal skeletal growth caused by congenital malformations of the spine, (2) mechanical instability caused by absent or deficient posterior elements of the spine and by paralysis, and (3) neurologic abnormalities caused by hydromyelia and tethered cord. (pp. 515–516)

The scoliosis may be one or a combination of the above. Progression of scoliosis may be anticipated as the child grows and orthopedic treatment may include such things as polypropylene body jackets and ultimately a spinal fusion. Surgical treatment may be done when the scoliosis begins to interfere with sitting, standing, or mobility.

According to Lindseth (1990, p. 520), "uncompensated lumbosacral scoliosis that results in a fixed obliquity of the pelvis is a common and severely handicapping deformity in patients with myelomeningocele." With this deformity we see the development of ischial decubitus ulcers and difficulty in maintaining balance in the sitting position.

Lumbar kyphosis reportedly occurs in 8% to 15% of children with myelomeningocele. Lindseth (1990, p. 521) states, "children with extensive kyphosis are unable to wear braces, have trouble sitting in a wheelchair, and often have ulcerations over the prominent kyphos." Progression of kyphosis or a severe kyphosis at birth may cause breathing difficulty, eating difficulty, and failure to thrive. Surgical correction is technically difficult but necessary in some cases. Correction is followed by the child wearing a molded body jacket for a period of at least 1 year.

Although lumbar lordosis is common in children with my-eloimeningocele, it is rarely corrected surgically and does not cause a major disability in itself.

Hips

Function of the hips and the types of problems that are seen in children with myelomeningocele depend on the level of paralysis. Treatment—preventative or corrective—depends on the treatment facility and the orthopedic surgeon. Most of these children are placed prone following closure of their back with hip and knee flexion and 60 degrees of abduction. The hips are then maintained in this reduced position while the spine heals. When the back is healed and the child can tolerate it, he or she is placed in an abduction splint such as the Frejka pillow until 3 months to 1 year of age, depending on the treatment center. As the child grows, dislocation of the hip is not necessarily an indication for treatment surgically. It may be deemed necessary, however, to provide range of motion so that the child can sit satisfactorily in a wheelchair, lie comfortably in bed, or use an orthosis for standing and walking. Lindseth (1990, p. 526) states, "even in a unilateral dislocation, a dislocated hip does not prevent standing in an orthosis, sitting, or lying down unless an associated adduction contracture is present." Contractures of the hip are frequently associated with muscle imbalances around the joint and therefore are more difficult to manage.

Knees

The function of the knee in children with myelomeningocele is important for ambulation. It is important to have absence of deformity and stability at this joint. The common types of deformities seen are extension/hyperextension contractures, flexion contractures, and valgus rotational deformities. Physical therapy is indicated in treatment of these deformities and surgical treatment may also be indicated.

Feet

Foot deformities, common among those with myelomeningocele, may interfere with shoe wear, brace wear, ambulation, and wheelchair positioning. Equinovarus deformities are reportedly the most common but other deformities may be present, depending on the level of paralysis. Physical therapy is used in management of foot contractures but surgical correction may be indicated when the child is old enough for braces and shows a readiness to be in a standing position.

Fractures

Another common orthopedic concern with the child with myelomeningocele is fractures. Fractures frequently occur after cast immobilization; femoral and tibial fractures are most common.

Due to the insensitivity of the skin and the possible development of pressure sores, many of these children are effectively treated with soft casts following a fracture. Because of the lack of pain and sensation, frequently neither parents nor the child can pinpoint the time of the fracture. Parents notice swelling, local warmth, erythema, and fever, which causes them to seek treatment.

Decubitus ulcers

As with the paraplegic population, decubitus ulcers in children with myelomeningocele are common. Frequently seen are ulcers of the heels in ambulators (lumbar level paralysis). Thoracic-level-paralyzed children frequently develop ischial decubitus ulcers, necessitating the use of pressure relief cushions for those using a wheelchair as their main means of mobility.

It is extremely important in the treatment of these children to know the level of lesion. Abilities and expected levels of **_independence_** directly relate to the level of paralysis, degree of deformities, and complications associated with this diagnosis.

Occupational therapy's role in treatment

The occupational therapist has a great deal to offer the child with myelomeningocele. As stated before, occupational therapy is a key discipline in the successful rehabilitation process of these children. By nature of their disability, they are at risk for developmental delay, sensory integration problems, fine motor problems, positioning needs, activities of daily living (ADL) problems, and behavior problems. Particular attention must be given to the fact that the occupational therapy needs of children with myelomeningocele change with different age levels. Different evaluations and treatment are indicated during infancy, preschool age, school age, and adolescence/adulthood.

Occupational therapy should include evaluation and treatment in many areas. Type of treatment facility and area of the country may create some variation in the occupational therapist's role on the team. In my experience with this diagnostic group, occupational therapy has contributed in the areas outlined.

Developmental assessment and treatment

All children with myelomeningocele should be seen prior to discharge from the hospital. At that time, an informal assessment should be done and normal developmental patterns should be discussed with the family. A home program should be given for developmental stimulation with appropriate activities for the first 3 months of life. These children should then receive a formal developmental assessment at 3 months of age. **_Developmental assessments_** should be repeated every 3 months until the child reaches age 2 years. Formal evaluations should be done at least yearly thereafter until the child reaches school age (5 years). Psychometric testing by the school should be recommended at age 5.

Any type of formal developmental assessment, such as the Gesell Developmental Tests and the Bayley Scales of Infant Development, can be done. The important thing to remember is that the child should be reevaluated with the same tool so that a true comparison can be made. Home programs should be given with emphasis on the areas of deficit. It is important to remember that complications (shunt malfunction, meningitis) can occur at any age level and the child may be at risk for additional delay, loss of function, or new problems.

If ongoing treatment is indicated, the treatment plan for the child with myelomeningocele should reflect the results of the evaluation and developmental treatment the same as for any child experiencing developmental delay.

Upper extremity evaluation and treatment

Children with myelomeningocele require a thorough and comprehensive evaluation of their upper-extremity strength, coordination, and overall function. Problems with hemiparesis can be picked up in infancy by specific attention to early grasp and hand patterns. Much of the assessment during infancy and preschool center around observation of play and hand function. When the child becomes old enough for more formal assessments, evaluations used with any diagnostic group to determine hand function should be considered. Dynamometer and pinch meter readings should be taken regularly to record decreased strength. As suggested earlier, loss of grip strength can be indicative of complications such as shunt malfunction.

Hand function and upper extremity use become critical for the myelomeningocele population since upper-extremity strength and coordination directly affect successful transfer activities, independence in self-care, self-catheterizaton, wheelchair use, and school performance. Studies have shown that children with myelomeningocele have decreased fine motor coordination.

Activities of daily living

Evaluations should be done at appropriate developmental stages in ADL such as eating, dressing, grooming, and bathing. Very few children with myelomeningocele have eating problems related to swallowing except for those with severe Arnold–Chiari deformities. Most eating problems center around introduction of solids or a large weight gain. Oral motor assessments should be done when indicated, with treatment dependent on the results of such examinations.

Independence in dressing, grooming, and bathing should be assessed at the appropriate age levels. Techniques to accomplish these tasks are similar to those practiced by spinal cord injury patients, particularly if the patients have thoracic level myelomeningocele. It is important to stress good skin inspection and not to encourage independence until the child is mature enough to examine his or her own skin and assume responsibility for skin care. Parents should be instructed that their children should avoid hot bath water and hot slides in playgrounds.

Sensory integrative evaluation and treatment

Many myelomeningocele children exhibit sensory integrative problems, poor fine motor coordination, and immature sensory systems. Evaluations such as the Sensory Integration & Praxis Test (SIPT), Purdue Pegboard, and Frostig Developmental Test of Visual Perception can be used and treatment recommended according to the therapist's findings.

School performance should be discussed and families should be alerted to signs and problems.

Equipment

Children born with myelomeningocele use many different types of equipment such as braces, wheelchairs, walkers, and crutches. Occupational therapists can effectively evaluate and make recommendations for the following **equipment needs** and positioning needs. Equipment should be provided to improve function, provide support, help prevent deformity, and ease care for the family.

Wheelchairs. Fifty to sixty percent of all myelomeningocele children use a wheelchair, either as their primary means of mobility or for distance. High-strength, lightweight wheelchairs are particularly suitable for these children because they are durable and have growth potential. Removable armrests should always be considered for independent transfers as well as swing-away detachable footrests. Elevating leg rests may be needed for adolescents and young adults due to dependent edema. Wheelchairs can also be used by ambulators who are unable to do distance walking. A person prescribing a wheelchair should be knowledgeable as to product availability, features, and maintenance requirements. The family and the child should play a key role in the selection process. Power wheelchairs may be needed for college or work environment.

ADL equipment. Children with myelomeningocele benefit from transfer tub seats, hand-held shower hoses, mirrors for self-catheterization and skin inspections, and reachers. Selection of the particular type of equipment needed should be done in conjunction with the ADL evaluation.

Developmental/recreational equipment. Floor sitters and tables can enhance development of sitting, balance, and fine motor skills. Hand-propelled tricycles are an important consideration for the social leisure area. Younger children may benefit from a crawler or creeper to enhance prone mobility.

Prevocational planning

There is also a need for prevocational evaluations and vocational planning. Perceptual motor difficulties may interfere with driving and job placement.

Summary

Children with myelomeningocele have many neurologic, orthopedic, and urologic problems. Since the cause of the defect is unknown, parents may feel extremely guilty and grief-stricken. The defect is obvious at birth, with intervention started with the neurosurgical repair of the defect immediately after birth.

Although some predictions regarding independence level and function can be made based on the level of lesion, many uncertainties cause the prognosis to remain guarded. What we do know is that with a comprehensive interdisciplinary approach at the time of birth, children with myelomeningocele can be guaranteed a chance for independence and productive living. Occupational therapists, by nature of their educational background in both physical and psychosocial dysfunction, provide parents with the information, guidance, and understanding necessary to meet and deal with the challenges identified with each age group.

Reference

Lindseth, R. (1990). Myelomeningocele. In R. T. Morrissy (Ed.), *Lovell and Winters Pediatric orthopedics* (3rd ed., Vol. 1, pp. 507–538). Philadelphia: J. B. Lippincott.

Bibliography

Dunn, D., & Epstein, L. (1987). *Decision making in child neurology.* Philadelphia: B. C. Decker.

Morrissy, R. T. (Ed.). (1990). *Lovell and Winters's pediatric orthopedics* (3rd ed., Vols. 1 &2). Philadelphia: J. B. Lippincott.

Sharrard, W. J. (1979). *Pediatric orthopedics and fractures* (2nd ed., Vol. 2). London: Blackwell Scientific Publications.

S E C T I O N   7

Seizure disorders

JUDITH ATKINS

KEY TERMS

Absence Seizures	*Myoclonic Seizures*
Anticonvulsive Drugs	*Simple Partial Seizures*
Atonic Seizures	*Tonic-clonic Seizures*
Developmental Delay	*Status Epilepticus*
Partial Complex Seizures	

LEARNING OBJECTIVES

Upon completion of this section the reader will be able to:

1. *Define the different types of seizures seen in pediatrics.*
2. *Develop an occupational therapy treatment plan for a child with a seizure disorder.*
3. *Identify and discuss common behaviors and problems associated with school performance seen in a child with a seizure disorder.*

Before a pediatric occupational therapist can successfully treat children with seizure disorders, it is important to review brain anatomy and physiology and to learn how the brain controls different parts of the body. It is also important to understand some of the different types of seizures and their effects on the child. A therapist must be familiar with the **anticonvulsive drugs** used to control the seizure activity and their possible effects on the patient. It is also important to understand how such a diagnosis affects the patient, parents, teachers, and community.

The purpose of this section is to review the above-mentioned criteria, to discuss the population with seizure disorders, and to discuss treatment goals, techniques, and other pertinent facts.

Few children in a pediatric practice present with an isolated diagnosis of seizure disorder. Most frequently seen is a secondary diagnosis of seizure disorder accompanied by a primary diagnosis of cerebral palsy, tuberous sclerosis, hydrocephalus, encephalitis, or other condition. The seizure activity as well as the motor and sensory defects contribute to the child's **developmental delay** (slow physical and mental maturity), poor school performance, difficulties with independence in activities of daily living, and, later, with work performance. Parents can be overwhelmed with fears that may be associated with seizure disorders. Therefore, a pediatric occupational therapist must consider both the evaluation of the child and the environment in which the child lives.

Classification and definition of seizures

Pertinent to the diagnosis of seizure disorders are such things as family history, birth history, medical history, and developmental history. Also included is a detailed account of the seizure event. Length of time, type of activity (behavior observed), how the seizure began, and the child's behavior after the seizure all are important when describing seizure activity—whether you are a health care professional working with the child, a teacher, or a parent—and are pertinent to the diagnosis.

Other diagnostic tools are laboratory tests, electroencephography (EEG), videomonitoring, CT scan, and magnetic resonance imaging (MRI).

A seizure defined by Zierdt (1989, p. 8) "is a sudden uncontrolled episode of excessive electrical activity in the brain." This produces an alteration in behavior, consciousness, movement, perception, and sensation. Nonmedical terms for seizures frequently used by parents are fits, spells, attacks, and convulsions. It is important to remember that seizures are not a disease but a symptom or sign of a disorder.

Some seizures have definite causes; others are classified as idiopathic and have no known cause. Some common causes of seizures are fever, infection, trauma, hemorrhage, and birth asphyxia. Other causes are brain tumors, toxicity, metabolic imbalance, and prenatal problems. Hereditary diseases such as tuberous sclerosis, degenerative diseases such as Batten disease, and congenital anomalies also are contributors.

Seizures vary in type and severity. International classification is partial, generalized, and unclassified.

Partial seizures

Partial seizure means that the seizure is focal in origin and involves a specific part of the body. Partial seizures are further divided into the following:

Simple partial seizures

The child does not lose consciousness in a **simple partial seizure**. It can be focal motor (a big jerk), focal sensory (abnormal visual phenomena), or autonomic (feelings of unreality, memory disturbances). A child may have feelings of fear, anger, or excitement.

Partial complex

A **partial complex seizure** is also focal and does affect consciousness. The child may engage in abnormal but purposeful-appearing activity such as pulling on or fumbling at clothes. He or she may not recall this behavior when regaining consciousness. An aura may precede the seizure and postictal confusion or drowsiness may follow. These seizures can evolve into generalized seizures.

Generalized seizures

Generalized seizures usually occur without warning and affect the entire brain. There is nearly always a loss of consciousness. In children, these seizures are divided into four types.

Absence seizures

Very brief in nature, **absence seizures** usually last less than 10 seconds but may occur as often as 100 times per day. In school children, parents and professionals often mistake this seizure for daydreaming or staring. No aura or warning precedes onset. Seizure is sudden, affects the entire brain, and causes rapid loss and regaining of consciousness. No postictal confusion occurs. The child may drop objects, blink, or jerk.

Myoclonic seizures

Brief tonic muscle spasms without loss of consciousness characterize **myoclonic seizures**. A sudden mild or massive jerk may occur. These seizures are frequently associated with more severe and progressively worsening conditions. Infantile spasms are a specific type of myoclonic seizure that occurs in infants.

Atonic or drop seizures

Manifested by a brief involuntary, sudden loss of muscle tone, **atonic seizures** may cause a sudden slumping of the body with inability to stay in an upright position. Atonic or drop seizure is frequently associated with injury and bruising due to falls without warning. It can lead to head and facial injuries in both the ambulatory child and the child who uses a wheelchair. These children need protective headgear, padded laptrays, and other protective measures. The atonic seizure is rare and is usually associated with more severe or progressive forms of epilepsy.

Tonic-clonic seizures

The whole brain is affected in **tonic-clonic** seizures. In the past they have been termed "grand mal" seizures. Usually no warning occurs and the child may sustain injury from falling with loss of consciousness. The tonic-clonic seizure may be characterized by tongue biting, excessive drooling, and incontinence. The body may be rigid or may stiffen during the tonic phase with jerking during the clonic phase. It is usually followed by a long period of confusion, headache, and/or deep sleep. After the seizure, the child may complain of headache, sore muscles, or exhaustion.

Unspecified seizures

Febrile seizures

Seen in healthy babies, usually in children ranging in age from 6 months to 5 years, febrile seizures are characterized by a fever over 38.3°C (101°F). These seizures are usually associated with infections such as otitis media or urinary tract infection. A seizure that occurs in conjunction with such infections as meningitis, encephalitis, and trauma are *not* considered febrile seizures.

Status epilepticus

A life-threatening disorder, **status epilepticus** is a seizure that continues or reoccurs in rapid succession over a prolonged period of time. It is reported that when the seizure lasts more than 10 minutes, emergency help should be called. Seizures of this type lasting more than 1 hour can cause permanent brain damage. Status epilepticus is a frightening experience for the families and health care professionals working with these children.

Factors affecting seizures

It is known that certain factors can increase the potential for seizures. These factors include but are not limited to such things as inadequate or improper dosage of **anticonvulsive drugs**, trauma, illness, stress, and fatigue. Regulation of anticonvulsive medication requires regular checks by the physician with such tests as serum blood levels being done. The choice of drug depends on such things as type of seizure, age of patient, and risk of noncompliance. Many anticonvulsive drugs have side effects. Possible side effects are overgrowth of gums, hyperactivity, lethargy, irritability, poor sleep patterns, impaired memory, and decreased attention span. Many of these problems may also be associated with the primary diagnosis of the child.

It is important to note what to do when a seizure occurs while an occupational therapist is working with a child. It is vital that the therapist remain calm, stay with the child, protect the child from injury, and facilitate breathing, if necessary. Do not restrain the child or put anything into his or her mouth. Also, make good observations as to length of time, behavior before seizure, behavior during the seizure, and other pertinent information. If a child is having a tonic-clonic seizure, turning him or her to the side to allow saliva or vomitus to drain facilitates breathing.

Occupational therapy evaluation and treatment

As mentioned previously, few children are seen by an occupational therapist in the pediatrics department of a hospital with seizure disorder as their primary diagnosis. Usually, seizure disorder is a secondary diagnosis. Children diagnosed with a seizure disorder often have significant developmental delay that requires occupational therapy intervention. The following types of evaluation or treatment may prove beneficial to this diagnostic group.

Developmental assessment and treatment

Children with seizure disorders are at risk for developmental delay. The delays may be mild to severe. It is extremely important that from the time the diagnosis is made, these children receive a formal developmental assessment. Depending on the age of the child, the type of assessment tool may vary. The goal of the assessment is to determine the exact areas of delay and the developmental problems that the child is experiencing. After this is done, a treatment plan can be developed. The child may require regular treatment sessions, referral to a community program, or a home activity program that the parents can follow. Parents need instruction on normal development to effectively work with their child.

In addition to developmental delay, many children with seizure disorders also have abnormal muscle tone, which interferes with performance and successful completion of developmental tasks. These children may be hypotonic or hypertonic, or may experience fluctuating tone. They may also have ataxia. It is important to assess and document tone because choice of activities will reflect treatment of these areas as well as general development.

The occupational therapist should follow developmentally delayed children for a period of time to monitor progress, determine developmental levels, and intervene when indicated. As stated by Quinn (1988),

> . . . there are several standard infant scales used by professionals to assess the development levels of very young children. Intelligence cannot be accurately determined during infancy, but you can determine rate of progress (p. 113).

Delays seen in infancy have been shown to correlate with later retardation, particularly if delays are moderate or severe.

Sensory integration evaluation and treatment

Every child is different, but certain patterns that affect learning have been identified as more prevalent among children with seizure disorders or epilepsy. As stated by Quinn (1988, p. 133), "these include perceptual/motor problems, delayed verbal skills, and deficits in memory and attention." We also know that certain seizure medications affect the learning process by causing such side effects as irritability, hyperactivity, short attention span, and distractibility. Frequent seizures can interfere with a child's ability to process and receive information and stimuli, and may disrupt attention. Difficulties in concentration and memory may also be seen. In addition, personality changes and poor fine motor skills may contribute to poor school performance.

Occupational therapists can assess the child's skills in visual perception, design copying, motor planning, toleration of touch, and movement in space. Sensory motor development and sensory motor skills can be assessed using such evaluation tools as the Sensory Integration and Praxis Test, Frostig Developmental Test of Visual Perception, Motor-Free Visual Perception Test, and Developmental Test of Visual Motor Integration (Berry). These are only a few of the available sensory integrative tests.

The occupational therapist works closely with the parents and the school (depending on the age of the child) to enhance performance and improve successful completion of tasks.

Fine motor assessment and treatment

Because many children with seizure disorders experience developmental delay and muscle tone abnormalities, problems frequently are manifested in the fine motor area. Children have difficulty performing self-help skills such as buttoning, self-feeding, and grooming. This area also affects quality of handwriting, speed of writing, and general school performance. The fine motor area should be evaluated in the same manner as with any other child.

Activities of daily living

Developmental delay and coordination problems directly affect a child's independence in the activities of daily living (ADL) area. At the appropriate developmental levels, function and independence in ADL should be assessed. Children with seizure disorders may experience problems with coordinated suck and swallow and present with eating difficulties. As infants, the oral motor area should be assessed; later self-feeding should be evaluated. Independence in grooming, dressing, toileting, and bathing also should be evaluated. Treatment planning should reflect deficit areas.

Equipment needs

Children with atonic or drop seizures may need protective headgear. Many types of headgear are commercially available, but depending on the type of seizure, age of the child, and the activity level, care must be taken to match product to child's need.

Depending on degree of disability and intellectual level, children with seizure disorders may also need to be evaluated for adaptive equipment as it relates to their positioning and mobility needs. Children with severe seizure disorders and other associated diagnoses need adapted strollers and adapted wheelchairs. Type of wheelchair and seating system necessary depend on such things as activity level, type of seizures, functional abilities, deformities present, muscle tone, and the environment in which equipment will be used. Each child requires an individual assessment and matching results of assessment with product availability. Some children with severe atonic or tonic-clonic seizures may need wheelchairs for safety. Padded laptrays may be needed to guard against injury.

Behavior

Behavior problems frequently accompany seizure disorders and other developmental disabilities. Medication may complicate this problem. Early intervention assists parents to set limits, enforce rules, assign responsibilities, and reinforce positive behaviors. In severe cases, a formal behavior modification program may be indicated.

Summary

Many fears and negative attitudes are associated with seizures and seizure disorders. Seizures can be controlled in a high percentage of children with good seizure management and a healthy lifestyle. In children in whom seizure disorder is severe and associated with an equally disabling diagnosis, occupational therapists can improve quality of life by providing equipment, handling techniques, and activities to enhance maximum potential. In the less severe cases, occupational therapists can provide the assessment tools and treatment planning that will improve school performance, enhance self-esteem, and promote independent living.

References

Quinn, P. (1988). When epilepsy is not the only problem: Assessing special needs. In H. Reisner (Ed.), *Children with epilepsy: A parents' guide* (pp. 113–146). Kensington, MD: Woodbine House.

Zierdt, M. (1989). *Syllabus for seizure disorder workshop.* Unpublished manuscript.

Bibliography

Dunn, D. W., & Epstein, L. G. (1987). *Decision making in child neurology.* Philadelphia: B. C. Decker.

Reisner, H. (Ed.). (1988). *Children with epilepsy: A parents' guide.* Kensington, MD: Woodbine House.

Swaiman, K. F. (Ed.). (1989). *Pediatric neurology, principles and practice* (Vols. I & II). St. Louis: C. V. Mosby.

CHAPTER 14

Psychiatric disorders in childhood and adolescence

LINDA L. FLOREY

LEARNING OBJECTIVES

Upon completion of this chapter the reader will be able to:

1. *Identify risk factors associated with psychiatric disorders.*
2. *Describe common characteristics of attention-deficit hyperactive disorder, conduct disorder, mood disorders, anxiety disorders, and schizophrenia, and discuss the impact of these disorders on play and socialization.*
3. *Identify the primary assumptions of the occupational behavior frame of reference and explain the focus on play and socialization.*
4. *List typical evaluations used with toddlers, preschool and school-age children, and adolescents.*
5. *List the components of a measurable treatment goal.*
6. *Identify treatment principles and relate principles to treatment programs.*

Over one third of the occupational therapy work force is practicing with children and adolescents, and nearly 20% of therapists are working in the school system (American Occupational Therapy Association [AOTA], 1990). The size of the work force treating children and working in school settings reflects the impact of the 1975 passage of the Education for All Handicapped Children Act (Public Law 94–142), in which occupational therapy is listed as a related service. The number of occupational therapists working with children will likely increase in the future, after implementation of the 1986 Amendments to the original act, Public Law 99–457, in which occupational therapy is one of the primary developmental services. In contrast, the proportion of practitioners working with mental health problems continues to decline (AOTA, 1990). Although the age range of the children with whom occupational therapists work is not broken down by health problems, it would be a fallacy to assume that the numbers of therapists working with children with significant emotional problems is declining or will continue to decline.

Children and adolescents with notable psychopathology are identified in the mental health system but they are present in foster care and group homes in the child welfare system, in detention centers in the juvenile justice system, in the pediatric wards and clinics of the health care system, and in special education classes in the education system (National Mental Health Association [NMHA], 1989).

In the health care system in which a number of occupational therapists practice, children may have suffered bruises, fractures, or head trauma as a result of impulsive or aggressive behavior or as a result of self-inflicted or other abuse. Children with chronic medical conditions and brain damage are at increased risk for developing psychiatric disorders (Offord & Fleming, 1991). Since "student" is the major role in childhood, a large proportion of children with psychopathology are in the education system. Within the lexicon of special education, these youngsters are referred to as seriously emotionally disturbed (SED) and comprise the fourth largest handicapped group served under Public Law 94–142 (U.S. Department of Education, 1987).

According to the National Mental Health Association Report

(1989), the SED population is the most underserved group of students with handicaps. There are several reasons for this. There is lack of systematic identification of this population due to varied interpretations in definition and eligibility criteria. There is reluctance to label children SED because of the stigma associated with the term. Additionally, school districts may not have the services in place or may be resistant to paying for services needed for this group of children due to funding constraints (NMHA, 1989; Forness, 1988). As a result, a number of children in the school system with significant emotional problems may not be identified at all or may be misidentified as "learning disabled."

Occupational therapists working with children and adolescents in a number of different service settings are likely to encounter youngsters with significant emotional problems within their scope of practice. The intent of this chapter is to acquaint the reader with major psychiatric disorders in childhood and adolescence, to present an overview of an occupational therapy frame of reference for intervention, and to discuss assessments and treatment programs drawn from this frame of reference, which may be used with this population.

Psychopathology in childhood and adolescence

Epidemiology

Epidemiology is the study of the distribution of a disease or disorder in a population and the factors that influence that distribution. The immediate yield of epidemiologic studies is the prevalence of the disease or disorder and the identification of risk factors with which it is associated. The long-term yield of such studies is to provide a foundation for planning prevention and intervention services to eliminate or treat the disorder (Gould et al., 1981; Offord & Fleming, 1991).

The incidence of psychopathology in childhood and adolescence may vary owing to characteristics of the sample, sampling methods, case selection, and assessment procedures. Despite variations, it is conservatively estimated that at least 12% of children and adolescents have diagnosable mental disorders. In addition, many others exhibit broad indicators of dysfunction such as substance abuse, teen pregnancy, and school dropout, which are risk factors associated with mental disorders (Zigler & Finn-Stevenson, 1991). The problem is national in scope and constitutes a major public health concern. The most serious consequences of mental disorders are suicide, serious harm to others, and the need to remove children from their homes (Zigler & Finn-Stevenson, 1991).

The incidence of psychiatric disorders according to age and sex tends to vary with the specific disorder. In general, these disorders are less prevalent in the preadolescent age group, more prevalent among boys than girls in the 4- to 11-year age range, and more prevalent among girls than boys in the 12- to 16-year age range. Overall, psychiatric disorders are less common in boys than in girls (Offord & Fleming, 1991).

Risk factors associated with psychiatric disorders are chronic medical conditions that limit typical childhood activities, brain damage, poor school performance, parental psychiatric disorders or deviance, poor parenting, marital discord, and

family dysfunction (Offord & Fleming, 1991). The causes of disorders are much more difficult to determine. A number of theoretical models or perspectives have been advanced to explain cause, and many of these are mutually exclusive. They are psychodynamic, psychoanalytical, and behavioral models, among others. Etiology is being increasingly conceptualized from a biopsychosocial perspective (Garfinkel et al., 1990). This includes consideration of constitutional factors, physical disease and injury, and temperamental and environmental factors as well as family factors (Barker, 1988). One factor may play a lead role in a specific disorder but generally a multiplicity of biopsychosocial vulnerabilities or stressors are implicated.

Classification of mental disorders

The absence of focus on the etiology of mental disorders is a hallmark of the *Diagnostic and Statistical Manual of Mental Disorders,* (DSM III-R). The DSM III-R is one of the current systems by which psychiatric disorders are assessed. It uses a descriptive approach for mental disorders in which identification of a disorder is based on clinical features or identifiable behavioral signs or symptoms (see Chapter 17, Section 1).

Psychopathology in children and adolescents is primarily classified within the section "Disorders Usually First Evident in Infancy, Childhood, or Adolescence" in the DSM III-R. However, the essential features of mood disorders and schizophrenia are the same regardless of the person's age and are included in different sections within that text. Other diagnostic categories, such as adjustment and personality disorders, may be appropriate for children as well. The major disorders and their primary features are listed in Table 14-1. A basic description, overview of psychiatric treatment focus, and expected outcome are presented for attention-deficit hyperactivity disorder, conduct disorder, mood disorders, anxiety disorders, and schizophrenia.

The first four disorders are discussed in this section because of their high incidence despite variations in epidemiologic studies (Costello, 1989). Schizophrenia is not prevalent in children but is included here because symptomatology is so deviant that it can be disturbing and puzzling if one encounters a child with this disorder. Since autism, child abuse and neglect, and eating disorders are covered, respectively, in Chapter 13, Section 5; Chapter 15; and Chapter 17, Section 3 of this text, they will not be included in this chapter.

Attention-deficit hyperactivity disorder

Attention-deficit hyperactivity disorder (ADHD) is classified in DSM III-R as one of the three disruptive disorders of childhood. Children with this disorder display inappropriate degrees of inattention, impulsiveness, and hyperactivity compared with other children of the same age. They have difficulty remaining on task and focusing attention generally but may be able to attend to tasks they find enjoyable. These children have difficulty inhibiting impulses in social behavior and in cognitive tasks and have great difficulty getting any task completed. They may be inattentive in games, are often intrusive, and have difficulty getting along with their peers. Children with ADHD often are unpopular with age mates and are underachievers in school work. ADHD is more prevalent in boys than in girls, and the most common age of referral is between 6 and 11 years (Weiss, 1991).

TABLE 14-1.   *Major Psychiatric Disorders in Childhood and Adolescence*

Disorder	Primary Feature
Developmental Disorders	
Mental Retardation	Disturbance in acquisition of cognitive, language, motor, or social skills
Pervasive Developmental Disorder	
Autistic Disorder	
Specific Developmental Disorders	
Other	
Disruptive Behavior Disorders	
Attention-Deficit Hyperactivity Disorder	Behavior that is socially disruptive and often more distressing to others than to those with the disorder
Conduct Disorder	
Oppositional Defiant Disorder	
Anxiety Disorders	
Separation Anxiety Disorder	Anxiety is the prominent feature
Avoidant Disorder of Childhood or Adolescence	
Overanxious Disorder	
Post Traumatic Stress Disorder	
Mood Disorders	
Depressive Disorders	Disturbance of mood involving either elation or depression
Bipolar Disorders	
Schizophrenia	Disturbances in affect and form of thought. Failure to achieve expected level of social development
Eating Disorders	
Anorexia Nervosa	Gross disturbance in eating behavior
Bulimia Nervosa	
Pica	
Rumination Disorder of Infancy	
Tic Disorders	
Tourette's Disorder	Tic is the primary feature
Chronic Motor or Vocal Tic Disorder	
Transient Tic Disorder	
Elimination Disorders	
Functional Encopresis	Disturbance in bladder or bowel elimination
Functional Enuresis	

(*From* Diagnostic and Statistical Manual of Mental Disorders, [*3rd ed., rev.*]. [*1987*]. *Washington, DC: American Psychiatric Association.*)

The most prominent features of ADHD vary with age. In preschool children, gross motor overactivity, inattention, and impulsiveness are common. In older children, excessive fidgeting and restlessness are more common than overactivity. Adolescents with this disorder tend to present as more impulsive and display attentional difficulties and motor hyperactivity (Greenhill, 1990; Wender, 1990).

Children displaying the symptomatology of ADHD were once classified as having minimal brain damage, minimal brain dysfunction, and hyperkinetic syndrome. The changes in terminology reflect the changing concepts of etiology of this disorder (Greenhill, 1990). The etiology of ADHD is unknown. Children may have a biologic vulnerability to ADHD, but psychosocial and environmental factors may also be prominent (Weiss, 1991).

Children with ADHD are typically treated along three dimensions: (1) medication, (2) adjustment of the school program, and (3) behavioral techniques such as parent training. They may also require counseling around issues of poor self-esteem related to school failure. Many children and adolescents continue to be disabled by the core symptoms of the syndrome and are at risk for developing antisocial personality disorder, criminal behavior, and more psychopathology (Weiss, 1991).

Conduct disorder

Conduct disorder is another of the disruptive disorders of childhood. Children with this disorder display a persistent pattern of conduct in which the basic rights of others and age-appropriate societal norms or rules are violated (DSM III-R). Physical aggression is common. Children with conduct disorder initiate fights and can be physically cruel to people and animals. They may steal and the stealing may involve confrontations with other children. Often there is a history of truancy from school and episodes of running away from home. Children with conduct disorder typically have low self-esteem and to hide this may portray themselves as tough and uncaring. Conduct disorder is more prevalent in boys than in girls. Learning disabilities are common in children with this disorder, and the degree of learning disability often corresponds to their overall degree of maladaptation (Lewis, 1990; Lewis, 1991).

Children with conduct disorder were once classified as having sociopathic personality disorders. Although these children frequently get into trouble with the law, it is important to distinguish conduct disorder, a diagnostic term, from "delinquent," which is a legal term (Lewis, 1990).

There is no single cause of conduct disorder. Children with behavior problems tend to display symptoms that place them on the border of several neurologic, psychiatric, and psycho-educational categories. A multiplicity of biopsychosocial stressors and vulnerabilities are associated with antisocial behaviors. Each of these contributes to maladaptation and each may need to be addressed in a comprehensive program (Lewis, 1990; Lewis, 1991).

No one particular approach to treatment is shown to be more effective than any other. Treatment may focus on medical, psychodynamic, cognitive, behavioral, family, and environmental vulnerabilities of each child (Lewis, 1990). Some older children may require a structured residential program to contain their behavior while treatment progresses.

The course of conduct disorder is variable. Children with this disorder are at risk for alcohol and drug abuse. Early onset is associated with greater risk for antisocial personality disorder in adulthood (DSM III-R).

Mood disorders

Mood disorders in children and adolescents are classified into two major types: bipolar and unipolar depressive disorders. In bipolar disorder, a combination of manic and depressive symptoms are found (Weller & Weller, 1991).

Manic episode

An elevated, expansive, or irritable mood is characteristic of a manic episode. In addition, increased talkativeness, flight of ideas, increased activity, distractibility, and inflated self-esteem or grandiosity are common. These symptoms are more typical of older children and adolescents. Young children present with irritability and emotional lability. There may be excessive involvement in activities that are potentially dangerous (Weller & Weller, 1991).

Depressive episode (bipolar episode)

The primary features of a depressive episode are depressed mood for at least a 2-week period and diminished interest or loss of pleasure in almost all activities. Associated symptoms are somatic complaints, sleep disturbance, difficulty in concentrating or thinking, and psychomotor agitation or slowing. Most children describe themselves in negative terms such as "dumb" or "stupid" (Weller & Weller, 1991). Adolescents experience hopelessness and feelings that things will never change for the better. The most serious complication is suicidal thoughts, including recurrent thoughts of death or actual attempts at suicide (Weller & Weller, 1991).

If symptoms of mania or depression are mild, depressive disorder may be incorrectly viewed as an adjustment reaction or personality disorder. If symptoms are so severe that the child is confused or psychotic, schizophrenia or organic brain syndrome may be diagnosed (Carlson, 1990).

The etiology of bipolar disorders in children is unknown, although it is believed that family genetic factors play a significant role. The treatment of choice is pharmacologic. Specifically, lithium may be effective. Clinical issues relevant in the use of lithium are the frequency, severity, and duration of the episodes in addition to the support system available to the child or adolescent.

Major depressive episode (unipolar depressive disorder)

The symptoms of a major depressive episode are the same as those that characterize a depressive episode in a bipolar disorder (just described). Other disorders in childhood and adolescence that may include depressive features are organic conditions, child neglect and abuse, anxiety disorders, adjustment disorders, conduct disorders, and substance abuse. Numerous etiologies may lead to the expression of depressive symptoms. Genetic, biologic, psychological, and environmental factors have been implicated (Weller & Weller, 1990).

Treatment of a major depressive episode focuses on a biopsychosocial approach, which may include psychopharmacology, psychotherapy, educational assessment and planning, and social skills training. Prompt treatment is advocated to reduce complications of poor school performance, poor peer relationships, and drug abuse. Early age of onset may indicate a poorer prognosis. Children and adolescents are at high risk for recurrence of the illness. Suicidal behavior remains the most serious aspect of a depressive disorder (Weller & Weller, 1990).

Anxiety disorders

An anxious mood is the most prominent feature of this group of disorders. **Anxiety** is defined as emotional uneasiness or apprehension or dread associated with anticipation of danger (Livingston, 1991). Anxiety may manifest itself in a variety of ways. The child may report feeling nervous or afraid. Difficulty in breathing or increased heart rate may be noted. Other signs include blotching and rashes of the skin, muscle tremor, and behavioral signs such as clingy, needy, dependent, or withdrawn behavior (Livingston, 1991). Anxiety disorders are more common in girls (Bernstein, 1990). The following are classified as anxiety disorders: separation anxiety; avoidant, overanxious, and reactive attachment disorders; and phobias (Livingston, 1991; Bernstein, 1990).

Separation anxiety disorder

In separation anxiety disorder there is excessive anxiety about separation from parents or loved ones. Children with this disorder have recurrent worries of harm befalling loved ones, and they may be reluctant to go to sleep or may have nightmares involving separation themes. School refusal or phobias may be associated with separation anxiety disorder. In school refusal, children often complain of physical problems. The physical problems are more frequent when separation is anticipated. Separation anxiety disorder may be familial and it may precede the onset of panic disorder or agoraphobia in adulthood (Bernstein, 1990).

Avoidant disorder

The key feature in avoidant disorder is avoidance of contact with strangers. Because "stranger anxiety" is a normal hallmark of development, children must be at least 2½ years of age before this diagnosis can be made. Children's avoidance of strangers interferes with social adaptation and peer relationships (Bernstein, 1990).

Overanxious disorder

Children with overanxious disorder demonstrate excessive worries about past and future events and especially about competence, performance, and approval. These children are extremely self-conscious, have excessive needs for reassurance, and often have somatic complaints. They may be perfectionistic and obsessive and generally are unable to relax (Bernstein, 1990).

Reactive attachment disorder

Reactive attachment disorder develops in infants and young children who have received grossly inadequate emotional nurturing. They generally demonstrate anxiety and protest, which is followed by depression and detachment from others. The core feature here is a disturbance in social relatedness, which is expressed in withdrawal and detachment or indiscriminate and excessive relatedness (Livingston, 1991). Chronically physically ill children who must undergo invasive medical procedures and who are repeatedly separated from their parents are prime candidates for this disorder.

Phobias

Phobias occur when specific fears are associated with avoidance behavior resulting in functional or social impairment. Common phobias in children are fear of animals, blood, the dark, fire, germs, heights, insects, and closed spaces (Livingston, 1991).

Although the precise cause of anxiety disorders is difficult to determine, there is evidence that biologic factors play a role (Bernstein, 1990). Behavioral interventions, psychopharmacology, and psychotherapy have been used with children and adolescents with anxiety disorders. Overall prognosis is good but phobia states, other anxiety disorders, and depressions may present as dysfunctional outcomes of these disorders in adulthood (Bernstein, 1990).

Schizophrenia occurring in childhood

Schizophrenia is very rare in young children but may emerge in adolescence. The classic symptoms of this psychotic disorder are hallucinations, delusions, and thought disorder; in children or adolescents, a failure to achieve an expected level of social development may be present (Pomeroy, 1990). Other characteristic symptoms are marked social isolation or withdrawal, peculiar or odd behavior, blunted or inappropriate affect, peculiar content and style of communication, and magical thinking. Ritualistic and stereotyped behavior is also common. Some children with schizophrenia have marked impairments in speech, motor, and social areas before diagnosis. Another group of children may not report frank hallucinations or delusions but may demonstrate fleeting psychotic-like symptoms in addition to age-inappropriate magical thinking, mood liability, social problems, and mild delusions. These disorders more typically resemble adult schizotypal or borderline personality disorders. At this time, however, there is no appropriate diagnostic criteria for children displaying this symptomatology (Pomeroy, 1990).

Because schizophrenia in childhood is a rare disorder, little information is available on its etiology and pathology. Psychopharmacologic agents are used in treatment but they may not have a dramatic effect in some psychotic children. Treatment responses in adolescence are more marked. Behavioral intervention, individual therapy that focuses on anxiety reduction, impulse control, and family support are also viable treatments. Out-of-home placement may be necessary (Pomeroy, 1990).

Play and socialization: A focus for intervention

Frame of reference

The focus on the broad parameters of play and socialization in working with emotionally disturbed children and adolescents is drawn from the occupational behavior frame of reference. A frame of reference targets and colors the lens through which phenomena are viewed. Different frames of reference may be used simultaneously if the basic premises of each are compatible. Some theoretical orientations, however, are incompatible. For example, the neurobiologic and neurophysiologic bases of sensory integration are compatible with the biologic base of occupational behavior, which views humans as spontaneous stimulus-seeking beings. The psychoanalytic perspective in which people are conceptualized as reactive with the goal of tension reduction is not compatible with occupational behavior. When more than one frame of reference is used in occupational therapy, one assumes the lead or organizing role. The frame of reference used for assessment and treatment of emotionally disturbed children in this chapter is occupational behavior. The reader is referred to Cronin (1989), Martin and Alessi (1990), and Nelson (1984) for treatment based on other models used in child and adolescent psychiatry (see Chapter 4).

Overview of occupational behavior

Mary Reilly developed the major assumptions of the **occupational behavior frame of reference**. She wrote,

> Play in a chronological or longitudinal sense, we believe, is the antecedent preparation area for work. In a cross sectional sense we have found it clinically useful to see our adult social recreation pattern as a sublatent support to a work pattern. The entire developmental continuum of play and work we designate as occupational behavior. (Reilly, 1969, p. 302)

Florey and Michelman (1982), expanding on the work of Matsutsuyu (1971), Moorhead (1969), and others, identified major knowledge bases within this frame of reference:

> Occupational behavior is guided by at least three interdisciplinary knowledge bases. The biological base acknowledges man as a spontaneous, stimulus seeking being. The bases of social psychology and anthropology acknowledge man as a tool user, a problem solver and an achiever. The sociological base acknowledges man as occupying life roles acquired in the process of socialization. (Florey & Michelman, 1982, p. 302)

Occupational behavior focuses on the developmental continuum of play and work and how these phenomena are incorporated into occupational roles throughout the life cycle.

Occupational roles represent the major activity in which a person engages on a regular or routine basis (Matsutsuyu, 1971). Work and play phenomena are interwoven throughout occupational role, with one assuming more prominence than the other at different stages in the cycle. For example, a toddler engages in play for most of the day, whereas a first-grader takes part in both play and work activities such as school and chores during the course of a day. The distinction between play and work is not absolute because what is work and what is play depends on the perspective of the individual.

There is a developmental progression in occupational role from player to student to worker, homemaker or volunteer to retiree (Moorhead, 1969). The occupational role of preschool children is that of player, since play is the major activity during this period. Work activities are focused on learning the basics of dressing and other self-reliant behaviors and on beginning chores and responsibilities.

In childhood and adolescence, the major activity is attending and mastering academic tasks. The occupational role during this period is student. The dominant theme is work with the emphasis on productive activity in school and on displaying self-reliant behavior and completing chores at home. Paid part-time work may be done during this time period. Play activity takes up less time than in early childhood but is critical for mastering cooperation, teamwork, and competition.

In adulthood, the major activity is work. **Work** refers to any productive activity, paid or unpaid, which is done for oneself, one's family, or society. The roles of homemaker and volunteer are included as occupational roles because they represent productive activity (Moorhead, 1969). Play during this period is conceptualized as leisure and is individual or family-focused.

The occupational role in later adulthood is the retiree role and is characterized by a lack of expectations for engagement in specific activities. Work activities are at a minimum and may consist of volunteer or homemaking tasks. The majority of time is open for engagement in leisure activities. Persons may be at risk for psychiatric disorders during this period if they have not built up a pattern of satisfying leisure activity that includes social contacts with others (Florey & Michelman, 1982).

The roles of student and worker emanate from the social institutions of school and work. Many expectations for role performance are formally taught through these vehicles. The roles of player, homemaker, and retiree are taught and learned through informal systems. Socialization in role occurs in a variety of ways but primarily through sequential experiences in play, family living, school, and recreation. Sequential experiences center on the acquisition of a broad spectrum of interests, skills, and habits, which are organized throughout the life cycle into changing occupational roles (Moorhead, 1969). Thus, it is conceptualized that adult work and social recreation roles evolve from childhood play, games, crafts, and chores. Developmental literature in the psychosocial fields supports this assumption and indicates that the child's experience in roles of family member, student, peer group member, and beginning worker almost totally influences his or her ability to function adaptively in adult occupational roles (Moorhead, 1969).

Developmental focus in occupational behavior

In the occupational behavior frame of reference, a major focus is on determining the extent to which injury or illness has disrupted or impoverished occupational behavior and on identifying steps to ameliorate dysfunction and to foster progression. An understanding of human development throughout the life cycle is fundamental. The occupational therapist must know the typical expected stages of progression in behaviors, skills, or processes to sequence tasks or situations at levels that patients can understand and master.

In working with children, knowledge of growth and development in many domains is necessary. Emotionally disturbed children may display a combination of normal, immature, and pathologic behaviors, and it is important to distinguish each one as it makes an impact on the child's ability to function. These children may also use negative behavior to mask or cover immature skills. Knowledge of social and emotional stages and progression in these stages are particularly important in working with children with psychiatric disorders. It is in this domain that they experience difficulty and that problems are most evident.

Play is a major activity of childhood and a primary arena in which social relatedness is learned, rehearsed, and mastered. Preschool children move through different stages in their play relationships with others. These stages reflect increased awareness of others and increasing ability to share adult attention and to share materials. The beginning stages go from solitary play to onlooker play, in which playing by oneself or with adults is replaced by an active interest in watching other children. Children then begin to engage in **parallel play**, in which they engage in activity alongside one another with little sharing of materials. They then display associative and **cooperative play**, in which they become more adept at taking turns and sharing toys and materials (Knox, 1974).

For the school-age child, the occupational role during this period is the student. The role of student, however, comprises much more than the mastery of the three "Rs" (Havinghurst, 1973). This is a critical period in children's lives. It is a period in which the cornerstones of competence and confidence are formed and in which children leave their home and parents for most of the day and enter the expanded environment of the school and the peer group. The school is the principal socialization agent. In school, children must learn to work with teachers—adults other than their parents whom they must listen to and obey and gain favor with. Gaining favor takes on a new perspective as teachers are recognizing them not for being cute and loving but for demonstrating intellectual and physical competence (Mussen et al., 1963). Children are being judged against a standard of achievement and measured against their peer group. Grades are the concrete product of that measurement.

In the peer group, children must learn to interact with age mates, to deal with hostility and dominance, to relate to a leader and to be a leader. Children learn to work with a group and to form best friends. They learn to cooperate and also to compete. Through their peers, they learn to develop a concept of themselves based on their own assets, skills, talents, and attributes. During middle childhood, children strive to be the fastest, the bravest, the smartest, the funniest, and they develop images of themselves based on how they compare with others. Through their experiences with peers, children gain information about their own roles and status and they form attitudes and values (Mussen et al., 1963).

The knowledge of expectations and stages in the social and emotional realm of behavior is particularly important in working with children and adolescents with psychiatric problems. The developmental tasks of Havinghurst (1973) and the psychosocial stages of Erikson (1963) are presented in Chapter 5, Section 2.

The reader is also referred to Chapter 5 for a thorough presentation of human development and is encouraged to review stages in motor and cognitive development.

Play development

Play is a major activity of childhood and one of the most intriguing and puzzling phenomena confronting students of human behavior. It is so ordinary and commonplace in the lives of children that every "man on the street" has an opinion, yet scholars from such diverse fields as philosophy, psychology, sociology, anthropology, and medicine engage in dialogue and debate the form, function, causes, and definitions of play (Mitchell & Mason, 1948). Gilmore (1971) puts it in this way, "Certainly everyone knows what play is not, even if everyone can't agree on just what play is" (p. 311). Play is a process, an attitude, and a behavior. For a discussion of play from an occupational therapy perspective, the reader is referred to Chapter 8, Section 3.

The focus in this section is to describe developmental changes in aspects of play behavior. Because play serves as a processor of biopsychosocial domains, different levels of skill and maturity are reflected in play. Throughout development, there are major changes in interests, skills, relationships with peers, and ability to process rules (Florey, 1971; Knox, 1974). It is particularly important for the occupational therapist to know these changes to determine whether a particular play behavior is "typical" or "immature" compared with chronologic age.

Knowledge of different sequences in play also guides expectations for activities used in the treatment process. For example, if a 2- or 3-year-old is given a collage project consisting of paper, glue, and macaroni, the child will likely be caught up in squeezing the glue bottle and dumping and scattering the container of macaroni, regardless of the paper. Children of this age are more process- than product-oriented; this is typical behavior. If a child of 6 years reacts to the materials in this way, he or she is demonstrating immature behavior. There are no specific developmental tests of play.

Changes in play behavior and sequences of play have been developed by Takata (1974) in her listing of play epochs, Knox (1974) in her play scale, and Florey (1971) in her developmental classification of play. Studies/sources used to determine sequences are found in the work of each author. The developmental classification of play from birth through 11 years of age, developed by Florey, represents changes in play from birth through 5 years of age and changes in play from 6 through 11 years. The classification is based on the definition of play as overt observable motor responses to human and nonhuman objects. The objects formed the major categories and were subdivided into types of objects specified in the developmental studies used. Human objects included parents, peers, and the body itself. Nonhuman objects were identified with respect to the extent to which they changed shape or form when manipulated. Type I objects represented creative or unstructured media, type II represented constructional media, type III represented toys or play equipment. See Florey (1971) for the chart on changes in play from birth to 11 years.

If a response required a human object for it to occur at all, such as sharing or cooperating, it was placed in the human object category. All other responses were placed in the nonhuman object category, although it was acknowledged that it was not necessarily real nor describable to separate responses (Florey, 1971). This classification scheme, the sequences identified in Takata's epochs and Knox's play scale serve as guides for observing play and provide a gross interpretive structure for play behavior.

Impact of psychiatric disorders on play and socialization

Children may display elements of advanced and immature play simultaneously. When children are under stress, they frequently exhibit elements of immature behavior. Psychosocial stressors such as the birth of a sibling or change in schools may trigger "baby talk," dependency on adults, engagement in activities with younger children, and overall behavior characteristic of an earlier stage. This is typical and the behaviors gradually disappear as the painful event is mastered. Children with psychiatric disorders tend to display odd patterns of relating to others, however, and they may exhibit difficulties in task initiation and completion, which reflect more the pathology of the disorder than basic immaturity.

General descriptions of behavior typical of children with specific disorders are provided to acquaint the reader with the effect of psychopathology on social, play, and task behaviors. The descriptions were developed from composites of patients and are generalized for the purpose of illustration. They do not reflect the wide range of individual differences in children nor the variable nature of children's actions and responses in situations. These vignettes involve children playing a table game with a peer and making a simple craft project in the presence of a peer. The vignettes were developed with input from the occupational therapy staff at the UCLA Neuropsychiatric Institute & Hospital.

Attention-deficit hyperactivity disorder

CASE STUDY

Stevie is loud and intrusive. He can't stick with a decision about which game to play, so choices have to be narrowed down for him. He has difficulty waiting his turn in a board game and often grabs pieces of the game, such as the spinner or the dice. He does not pay attention and is constantly fidgeting. When he is sitting, he appears to be in constant motion. He is physically intrusive with his peers and does not seem aware of this. He interrupts frequently.

While doing a craft project, Stevie is unable to listen to directions. He has difficulty sequencing simple steps and becomes frustrated. He grabs at tools and materials and interferes with the work of his neighbor. He requires step-by-step instruction by a helpful adult nearby to accomplish the project. Peers often complain that Stevie "doesn't listen" and that he is intrusive.

Conduct disorder

CASE STUDY

Tom does not give his peer a chance to respond to a choice of games and makes a choice for both of them. He is used to taking over and getting his own way. He selects the color he wishes to play in the table game, then gives his peer and the occupational therapist the remaining choices. If he is not winning, he often cheats and may attempt to cover his cheating by accusing his peer. Tom is bossy and controlling with his peers and is not liked by them. Although he understands the directions on a simple project, he becomes frustrated and stops working, labeling the project "babyish" or "stupid." He needs to be coaxed to finish his project and often doesn't show pleasure or pride in successful completion of an activity.

Mood disorder, manic episode

CASE STUDY

Annie decides on a game and begins to open the box, but another game in the cabinet "catches her eye" and she quickly takes that game out. Choices need to be focused for her and she objects to the process, since narrowing choices interferes with her "independence." She chatters constantly. She asks questions, does not wait for the answers, and is apt to comment on various materials in the room or tell you what's on her mind. She is very easily distracted.

Annie is able to play a game with frequent reminders as to rules and taking her turn and often apologizes for needing reminders. She has better ideas for a project than the one presented to her and rattles off a list of materials she will need. She is very convincing in describing what she wants to produce but is unable to articulate a plan for accomplishing her production. She objects to completing the project given her but works quickly and makes mistakes because of her speed.

Although Annie is intrusive and demands a great deal of attention from those around her; she is not disliked by her peers. She is fun and uninhibited and her peers regard her excessive talking as something she can't help.

Mood disorder: Depressive episode

CASE STUDY

Mary is very compliant. She selects a game immediately but she doesn't seem interested in any of the games and is just doing what is asked of her. If her peer wants another game, she defers. She does not have difficulty with game concepts. She takes turns and is not invested in winning the game. She seems embarrassed if she wins. Mary doesn't initiate much conversation with peers or adults, but she is usually responsive when asked questions. She follows directions on craft projects and usually works slowly. At times she seems preoccupied and stares into space but can be easily directed back to the task at hand.

The most striking impression of Mary is that she seems to be going through the motions. She expresses no pleasure, seems to be having no fun, and displays little if any spontaneity. She is not disliked by her peers because she does little to provoke or annoy them. However, she is not popular with peers.

Anxiety disorder

CASE STUDY

Paul is very concerned about doing the right thing and asks for further instructions in choosing a game, for example, "Is one better than another?" He frequently asks the adult whether he is playing the game correctly and is concerned that he moves game markers and manipulates game pieces properly. He is quick to point out any mistakes or instances of cheating on the part of his peers. He is the target of nicknames by his peers such as "teacher's pet," and "prissy face." His concern with correctness and neatness carries over to craft projects. Paul asks a lot of questions although he has a grasp of the process. He needs reassurance and becomes visibly anxious when executing such "final" motions as cutting a piece of copper along the line and applying paint to paper.

Paul complains of flu-like symptoms occasionally. He doesn't seem to enjoy the process of engaging in activities and doesn't seem pleased with or proud of his final product. He is not well liked by his peers because of his anxious and somewhat rigid manner.

Schizophrenia

CASE STUDY

Ryan does not respond to the opportunity to select a game but does not object when one is brought to him. He does not initiate or direct comments to anyone, but occasionally he responds to questions asked of him. He speaks spontaneously but his speech is odd and often not related to immediate events. He obeys simple directions such as "Ryan, move your marker here," but is unable to spontaneously participate in game playing. Eye contact is poor.

Ryan is preoccupied with cars. He plays with cars and draws the same car the same way every time. When given a craft project of copper tooling with a mold, he disregards the mold and draws a car on the copper with a copper tool. He appears upset at the suggestion that the piece of copper on which he drew a car be placed on a mold and changed to duplicate the image on the mold. He will perform the operation when another piece of copper is placed on the mold and the process is initiated for him.

Ryan's looking "upset" is the closest he comes to displaying emotions. He looks neither happy nor sad but appears blank. He is neither liked nor disliked by his peers. They regard him as "weird" but they don't tease him.

Occupational therapy intervention

Occupational therapy intervention includes the process of assessment, the development of measurable treatment goals, and the designing of treatment programs. Individual and group treatment programs are based on principles that provide direction and coherence in meeting patient goals. Occupational therapy intervention usually occurs within the context of an interdisciplinary team and within a milieu or environment in which expectations for behavior or behavior management principles are identified.

Interdisciplinary team

The number and composition of the interdisciplinary team varies from setting to setting. In the school system, the team is likely to include representatives from special education, psychology, speech and language, counseling, and occupational therapy, in addition to the parents. In a mental health setting, the team is likely to include representatives from child psychiatry, psychology, nursing, special education, speech and language, social work, recreation therapy, and occupational therapy. Each member of the team contributes a unique focus with the goal of formulating a broad information base and of providing an integrated treatment approach. Members of the team meet initially to develop a treatment plan, or in the school system an Individual Educational Plan (IEP), and meet regularly thereafter to determine progress and need for revision of the plan.

It is important that the occupational therapist report his or her information in a concise, descriptive manner, free from occupational therapy or psychiatric jargon. When the team is beginning to work with a child, it is much more relevant to know how and under what circumstances a particular behavior is evident than to simply report that the child is angry, depressed, happy, anxious, or out of control. It is also important for the occupational therapist to have a frame of reference that guides practice. However, it is not helpful to communicate patient information in terms that the team doesn't understand. It is necessary to communicate how skills or behaviors, with which the frame of reference is concerned, are manifest in patients. For example, the information that a child isolates and distances himself or herself from peers can be related to specific problems the child is having in play and socialization.

Many areas of information and focus are shared among team members. For example, nearly all are interested in communication, play, and socialization patterns. However, the purpose of the communication or interaction may be different for each professional, for example, communicating feelings, negotiating chores and expectations, making a school report, and making a friend. The occupational therapist may develop programs with other professionals based on areas of shared interest and expertise, such as a vocational planning group with school personnel, a social skills group with nursing, or recreational therapy.

Behavior management

Another shared focus of the team is the development of some system of managing behavior in group settings. Identification of behaviors that are not tolerated because they have negative consequences and identification of behaviors that are encouraged because they have positive consequences are crucial in developing treatment goals. These systems range from labeling behaviors that lead to restriction of privileges to formal approaches based on principles of behavior modification such as token economy. **Token economy** is a total unit system in which tokens or points are earned for specific behaviors in situations and then traded for tangible rewards such as food, small games, and favorite TV programs (Nelson, 1984). The occupational therapist must know the overall system of milieu management and incorporate elements of the system into each person's occupa-

tional therapy program. For example, if the occupational therapist is working within a token economy system in which group members earn points for participation in their occupational therapy program, the therapist determines the criteria for successful participation, such as sharing materials, sharing attention, and working for a specified amount of time. Some criteria may be the same for all, whereas other criteria can be individualized for each patient, such as the amount of time each is expected to work independently or without interruption.

Expectations for social behavior may be situation-specific. For example, in addition to obeying rules of "good conduct" in the school, a student is expected to raise his or her hand to be called on in class. The occupational therapist will need to determine the overall rules of conduct in occupational therapy. This usually includes expectations for use of materials and tools, for sharing materials and attention, for getting along with others, and for cleaning up after an activity or event. These expectations vary according to the developmental levels and abilities of the children in the session.

Occupational therapy assessment

Occupational therapy assessment is a comprehensive process of obtaining information that is derived from specific evaluation methods. It is made up of measurable, data-based information, which is reported objectively (Cook, 1991). The purpose of assessment is identification of strengths and weaknesses from which goals and treatment strategies may be drawn. Children and adolescents with psychiatric disorders may exhibit a number of problems stemming from biopsychosocial vulnerabilities. The nature of the disorder implies that problems are focused in the behavioral, affective, or interpersonal areas and these areas should be evaluated first, with respect to individual and interpersonal aspects of play and daily living routines.

Screening for visual–motor and motor problems is routinely done because children with behavior and emotional problems frequently demonstrate deficits in these skill areas. Four types of evaluations are suggested for this population: structured observation, interviews, standardized tests, and checklists and inventories. Observation underlies all forms of evaluation. Whether administering a norm- or criterion-referenced test or conducting an interview, the occupational therapist is always observing responses to the evaluative situation. It is also a primary way to judge response to treatment.

Structured observations involve setting up a particular event or activity to be observed and recording, as objectively as possible, the specific behaviors exhibited. An observation guide or checklist is sometimes used to facilitate recording of a specific behavior such as decision making. *Interviewing* is another method of evaluation of emotionally disturbed children and adolescents. The accuracy of the information obtained may be questionable, but how the child chooses to report activities and events should be recorded. The interview is an important source of information about how children communicate information and how they view their own experiences. For example, some children report that they have "millions" of friends but are unable to name any friends or any activities or games they play with these other children. The occupational therapist may wish to verify information by looking through the medical chart or by interviewing the parents or primary guardian.

Standardized tests are the third type of evaluation, which provide information regarding performance with reference to a normal standard. *Checklists and inventories* are self-administered and provide information relevant to the area being sampled, such as play interests.

The assessment process varies with respect to age. Some evaluations are not given routinely but are administered when more information is needed or when another evaluation indicates problems in an area, for example, administering a visual–perceptual test following identification of deficits with a visual–motor screening test. The following section describes evaluations appropriate for different age groups. Some evaluations are well known to occupational therapists, and the purpose, format, and guidelines for administration are published in other texts. Information on these evaluations is not given here, but the reader is referred to *Pediatric Occupational Therapy* (Dunn, 1991), *A Therapist's Guide to Pediatric Assessment,* (King-Thomas & Hacker, 1987) and *Occupational Therapy for Children* (Pratt & Allen, 1989) for evaluation information. Evaluations that are not widely known are described in the following section.

An evaluation of the child's play is done with toddlers, preschool, and school-age children. It is important to note that an evaluation of play yields, at best, a snapshot of this area. Play is multidimensional, complex, and inner-directed, and it assumes different forms throughout the developmental continuum. The occupational therapist cannot replicate the variety of situations required to evaluate a child's repertoire of play. He or she can select areas and set up situations to evoke samples of play knowing that the information will be incomplete.

Evaluations used with toddlers and preschool children

The purpose of evaluations with the toddler and preschool-age group is to determine the level of function in play and social behaviors, in overall development, and in visual–motor skills.

Play and social behavior

With younger children two evaluative situations are used, one structured and one unstructured. In *structured play,* the child is seen alone and is given a sample of a simple project such as an animal macaroni collage and materials to construct one. A choice of animal stencils is provided as well as different kinds of macaroni and beans. Attention span, process–product orientation, attention to detail, and manipulation and construction are assessed here. In *unstructured play,* the child is provided with a range of toys and materials suitable for sensorimotor, dramatic, and constructive play. The child is seen alone in one session and with a peer in another session. What the child does with materials and how he or she engages with the therapist and a peer are evaluated with respect to the Preschool Play Scale developed by Knox or the developmental play classification developed by Florey (1971). This may be reported in a format such as that appearing in the display.

Interviewing the parents using Takata's Play History is extremely useful in providing a picture of immediate and past play experiences. In a psychiatric inpatient setting, the occupational therapist must determine the timing of this evaluation. On admission, many members of the team need to talk with the parents, so the parents may be overwhelmed with giving information and with the admission process in general. The occupational therapist should check with the team to determine the timeliness of interview sessions with the parents.

Developmental evaluations

Developmental evaluations provide an indicator of functional level, regardless of chronologic age. A number of useful tools are available for this kind of evaluation. The Miller Assessment for Preschoolers is a standardized screening tool used to identify children ages 2 years, 9 months to 5 years, 8 months who are at risk for school-related problems. The Gesell Preschool Test yields a developmental level with respect to motor, adaptive, language, and personal–social behavior for children ages 2½ through 6 years (King-Thomas & Hacker, 1987).

Visual–motor tests

The Berry-Buktenica Developmental Test of Visual-Motor Integration (VMI) is a developmental test of visual–motor integration that provides age norms and describes the developmental sequence for design copying of geometric forms. It is used with children from 2 through 15 years of age (King-Thomas & Hacker, 1987). If children score below the norm for their chronologic age in this area and if they demonstrate motor problems in the developmental testing, the Motor-Free Visual Perception Test (MVPT) is administered if the child is 4 years or older. The MVPT focuses on visual perception not requiring a motor response (King-Thomas & Hacker, 1987).

Evaluations used with school-age children

The purpose of evaluations with the school-age group is to determine their level of function in play and social behavior and visual–motor skills. Developmental assessment is done when immaturity in skills is suspected.

Play and social behavior

Children are interviewed individually with respect to their play interests, play activities, and friends before hospitalization and then are seen with a peer in game and task/craft activities. Questions target play preferences, interests, friends and playmates, types of activities in which the family may engage, and after-school activities. Children are asked to describe a "typical day." A semistructured interview focuses on a "typical weekday" and a "typical weekend day" prior to hospitalization. The yield of this information is to determine patterns in daily living, school, chores, and time management in addition to play activities. Whenever possible, this information should be validated by the parents or guardian of the child. Children are seen alone and are presented with a craft project and observed with respect to making decisions, following directions, using tools and materials correctly, and solving problems. They are given copper tooling molds, copper and tools, and a cardboard frame for the project. If there are restrictions on use of sharp objects or materials, another simple 2- to 3-step project can be selected.

Children are then seen with a peer and asked to select and play a board game. They are observed with respect to decision making, knowledge of rules and object of the game, and how they accept winning or losing, as well as how they interact socially with the peer. The outcome of the game and task assessment may be recorded in a format such as shown in the displays.

Visual–motor and motor assessments

The Visual Motor Integration Test (VMI) is used to assess visual–motor integration. This was discussed in the previous section on evaluations used with toddlers and preschool-age

FORMATS FOR DISPLAYING RESULTS OF PLAY AND GAME EVALUATIONS*

For use with children under 6.

I. PLAY SKILLS:

A. Initiation of Play with Materials/Toys when seen Individually:

    ☐ 1. Does not choose play materials independently

    ☐ 2. Independently chooses play materials

B. Play Interests when seen Individually:

The child showed the most interest in the following play materials/toys:

_____

_____

C. Pattern of Play with Materials/Toys: (check one)

    ☐ 1. Touches, mouthes, holds, throws/picks up, bangs, shakes, and carries objects.

    ☐ 2. Empties/fills, scribbles/draws, squeezes/pulls, combines/takes apart, and arranges in spatial dimensions.

    ☐ 3. End products important (not always realistic), specific goals evident.

    ☐ 4. Makes recognizable products, uses tools to make things (ie, scissors, stencils), like small construction, attends to details (ie, eyes, fingers).

    ☐ 5. Other: _____

D. Pattern of Play with Peers: (check one)

    ☐ 1. Child spends most of his time watching others play, giving suggestions or asking questions occasionally.

    ☐ 2. Child plays alone, away from other children and with different toys.

    ☐ 3. Child plays alone, but beside other children and with similar toys.

    ☐ 4. Child plays with other children and all engage in similar (if not identical) activity. No division of labor and no organized goal or outcome is planned.

    ☐ 5. Child plays with other children for the purpose of making some material product, striving to attain some competitive goal, dramatizing an adult or group life situation, or playing a formal game.

    ☐ 6. Other _____

Comment: _____

_____

_____

For use with children over 6.

II. PLAY AND GAME SKILLS:

A. Self-Reported Play Interests:

The child reported enjoying to play with the following (prior to this hospitalization): _____

_____

B. Observed Play Interests:

The child showed the most interest in the following play materials when seen individually: _____

_____

C. Past Friendships (Self-Reported):

When asked whom he/she spent the most time playing with, the child's list included: _____

(continued)

FORMATS FOR DISPLAYING RESULTS OF PLAY AND GAME EVALUATIONS* (*continued*)

D. Structured Games:

	Performs Unassisted	Performs with 1–2 Prompts	Requires Constant Adult Assistance
1. Decides which game to play			
2. Knows the rules			
3. Knows the object			
4. Takes turn in correct sequence			
5. Follows rules			
6. Accepts winning/losing			

Comments: _____

_____

* Taken from evaluations used at the UCLA Neuropsychiatric Institute and Hospital.

---

children. If problems are evident in this area, further visual–perceptual evaluations as well as the Bruininks-Oseretsky Test of Motor Proficiency (BOTMP) are given. This test is designed to assess gross and fine motor skills for children ranging in age from 4½ to 14½ years (King-Thomas & Hacker, 1987).

Developmental assessment

In working with school-age children and with adolescents, if there is a question of maturity in communication, daily living skills, socialization, or motor skills, the Vineland Adaptive Behavior Scales (Vineland) should be used. It is not routinely administered due to time constraints. The Vineland is designed to be used with children from birth to 18 years, 11 months, and employs a semistructured interview administered to the parent or caretaker of the child. This evaluation should be administered by therapists with graduate degrees and experience in assessment and test interpretation (King-Thomas & Hacker, 1987).

Evaluations used with adolescents

The purpose of evaluations with the adolescent age group is to determine level of function in socialization, task performance, daily living skills and time management, and visual–motor skills. Occupational areas may be evaluated if the adolescent wishes to gain information about himself or herself in this area. Developmental assessment is done when immaturity in skills is suspected.

Time management, daily living skills, task performance, socialization

Adolescents are interviewed with respect to their interests, activity patterns, and friends prior to hospitalization. This is done using the "typical weekday" and "typical weekend day," semistructured interview format. The adolescents are asked to describe a "typical weekday"; the occupational therapist then probes for and clarifies information regarding daily living skills, chores and responsibilities, school and after-school activities, and peer and friendship patterns.

Adolescents are asked to fill out the Neuropsychiatric Institute (NPI) interest checklist. This is a self-administered, structured checklist that yields information regarding the ability to discriminate interests and to identify clusters of interest (Asher, 1989). The adolescents are given a choice of three 2- to 3-step craft projects and are asked to complete one project. They are observed with respect to making decisions, following directions, using tools and materials correctly, and solving problems.

The frequency and content of social interactions with peers and adults in the hospital setting are assessed by observations made on the inpatient unit and in occupational therapy settings such as the kitchen and workshop areas. The observations are summed and recorded on a 3-point frequency scale as in the social interaction section of the display. Comments regarding specific behaviors and style are noted.

Visual–motor, motor, and developmental assessments

The VMI is used to assess visual–motor integration and if problems are evident, fine and gross motor skills are evaluated using the BOTMP. The Vineland is used when there is a question of maturity in communication, daily living, socialization, or motor skills. These evaluations are described in the previous sections.

Vocational surveys

Adolescents who are interested in learning more about their career interests, skills, and abilities are given career inventories. The COP System Interest Inventory (Edits, 1974) is a self-administered inventory that yields an individual interest profile with respect to 14 career clusters.

The Career Ability Placement Survey (Edits, 1976) is a self-administered timed survey that yields a score in eight primary abilities. These are mechanical reasoning, spatial relations, verbal reasoning, numerical ability, language usage, word knowledge, perceptual speed and accuracy, and manual speed and dexterity. The scores yield a career profile in which the adolescent's present abilities are compared with those required on jobs in the same 14 career clusters used in the COP System Interest Inventory. The results of these surveys are used to assist the

FORMATS FOR DISPLAYING RESULTS OF EVALUATION OF SOCIAL INTERACTION AND TASK PERFORMANCES*

For use with children and adolescents.

III. SOCIAL INTERACTION:

	Frequently	Sometimes	Rarely
A. Makes Eye Contact			
B. Initiates Contact with Peers			
C. Initiates Contact with Adults			
D. Listens to Others			
E. Accepts Praise from Others			
F. Complies with Requests Made by Adults			
G. Complies with Requests Made by Peers			
H. Isolates Self from Others			
I. Demands Adult Attention Excessively			
J. Disrupts Peers			
K. Dominates Peers			
L. Needs Limits Set			

Comments: _____

_____

_____

_____

For use with children over 6.

IV. TASK PERFORMANCE EVALUATION:

	Frequently	Sometimes	Rarely
A. Initiates Tasks			
B. Indepedently Makes Decisions			
C. Organizes Work			
D. Concentrates on Task (Indicate Time)			
E. Asks for Instructions			
F. Follows Verbal Instructions			
G. Follows Written Instructions			
H. Sequences Two or More Steps			
I. Retains Information			
J. Independently Solves Problems			
K. Accepts Feedback			
L. Delays Gratification			
M. Demonstrates Ability to Use Tools			
N. Completes Tasks			

Comments: _____

_____

_____

_____

*Taken from evaluations used at the UCLA Neuropsychiatric Institute and Hospital.

adolescent in identifying and relating current skills and interests to a sample of career clusters.

Development of treatment goals

The next step in the intervention process is to summarize and prioritize evaluation findings to guide treatment. The findings are summarized to reflect strengths as well as problem areas. The problem areas become the focus for goals; the strengths are used to facilitate goal achievement. For example, if an adolescent has problems in socialization with peers and strengths in task skills, a goal of teaching a step in a craft project to a peer incorporates both elements.

Goals should be drawn from the problem areas and stated in measurable terms. Goals stated in measurable terms are specific to the individual patient and describe an action or behavior that can be observed and measured. It is then possible to determine whether a goal has been achieved (Brands, 1977). For example, goals of "increasing peer socialization" or "increasing self-esteem" are vague and unmeasurable. The target areas of socialization and self-esteem are too broad and the expected action of "increasing" has no beginning nor end.

Measurable goals should address the who, what, when, and how of patient expected behavior in occupational therapy. The "who" identifies the key person; this is usually the patient. The "what" component describes the behavior in which the patient is expected to engage. This is indicated by an action verb such as attend, identify, seek out, or verbalize. The "when" specifies how frequently or how long the behavior is expected to occur during each treatment session. For example, an initial goal may focus on the child attending to a game for 5 minutes, whereas a goal drawn further in the treatment process would focus on the child attending for 20 minutes. The "how" of the goal indicates under what circumstances the behavior is to take place such as with or without prompting or intervention from staff. The components of the treatment goals, the behavior, the frequency or duration, and the circumstances all may be revised to reflect change in the patient's skills and abilities. Goals are modified throughout the treatment process and are paced to encourage increasing levels of difficulty, responsibility, and behavioral control.

Treatment principles and programs

In 1969, Reilly developed overall program specifications or treatment principles to guide the design and provision of services for psychiatric patients. The focal treatment principle is that occupational therapy must build a culture or milieu to examine, evoke, and reconstitute healthy skills and behaviors. She identified six specifications critical to the occupational therapy milieu:

1. That broad principles of organization such that behaviors required in personal, group, and job tasks would be associated with materials and tasks and games found in a workshop or recreation deck
2. That developmental stages present in skill acquisition would be evident in the program
3. That there would be natural decision-making areas
4. That competency would be acknowledged and curiosity aroused
5. That normal living experiences would be performed at normal times
6. That within a balanced pattern of daily living, daily events

would be tailored to individual interests, abilities, age, sex, and occupational role

Reilly urged that occupational therapy develop a milieu in which skills and behaviors could be initially taught, re-evoked, and practiced according to the level of the patient but in a context that focused on patient action rather than discussion.

Florey (1986) identifies specific elements needed in the treatment milieu for children and adolescents. She designates that play and task milieus be built in which there are opportunities for association with peers and adults. A variety of craft projects and activities that vary in complexity should be available to the patients. The play milieu provides variety and novelty, opportunities for exploration, limitation and repetition, and playful role models. The task milieu provides systematic instruction, which should be within the patient's cognitive ability, offers a moderate degree of difficulty, and provides knowledge of results or feedback. Models for craftsmanship should be provided.

The content of **treatment programs** within the milieus should reflect a range of activities and events present in normal play development to the greatest extent possible. For example, clubs are popular with children aged 8 through 12 years. Social skills training taught within the format of a club with a club T-shirt and a club handshake is appealing to children. They are receptive to information taught within this type of group structure. A Cub Scout Den chartered under the Boy Scouts of America is another example of embedding treatment goals within natural childhood activities.

The treatment principles and the characteristics of the play and task milieus establish the parameters for the development of treatment programs for children and adolescents. Patients may be seen individually and in small groups. Individualized treatment goals are designed and implemented within the context of the treatment programs. For example, having one child wait his or her turn and follow directions in a game situation and having another child initiate positive social interaction with a peer both can be accomplished within an existing play group. The content of the activities, tasks, and situations in the treatment groups are selected and paced to encourage increasing levels of skill, responsibility, interpersonal responsiveness, and emotional control. The overall programs, their descriptions, and objectives follow. They represent some of the existing occupational therapy treatment programs at the UCLA Neuropsychiatric Institute & Hospital. Descriptions of the programs have been published previously (Florey, 1986).

Treatment programs for children

Exploratory play group

A variety of play materials is provided in a semistructured play environment.

Objectives. To promote exploration of the play environment, appropriate use of objects in play, simple imitation of peers and adults, parallel play, beginning problem solving, and attention to a task.

Constructive play group

A variety of semistructured to highly structured activities is provided, which vary in complexity and in the number of steps and tools required to complete the activity.

Objectives. To promote sharing and turn taking, spontaneous interaction with others in a developmentally appropriate manner, and problem solving and skills in tool use.

Imaginary play group

Simple imaginary play focuses on learning how to role play and to engage in associative play with peers. *Complex imaginary play* focuses on using objects and events in cooperative play with peers.

Objective. To promote sequencing actions in time within the context of a role.

Game-playing group

A variety of simple to complex board games is provided in a structured setting.

Objectives. To promote cooperative play, make group decisions, follow rules, take turns solving problems, and accept winning or losing.

Skill-building group

Criteria for participation individually or in a small group are determined by delayed performance skills such as fine motor, sequencing, or visual perceptual skills.

Objective. To improve skill and competence in the identified deficit areas.

Social skills groups/clubs

Patterned after the format of a community club, structured group sessions focus on role modeling and rehearsal to learn and practice social skills.

Objectives. To listen to others, to include others in play, to initiate and maintain conversation, to express positive feelings to peers and adults, to identify feelings in others, to express negative feelings to peers and adults, to generate alternative solutions to interpersonal problems, to think of behavioral alternatives and possible consequences before acting, and to identify the consequences of one's behavior.

Cub scout program

The Cub Scout program is chartered under the Boy Scouts of America and is a combination of Cub Scout and Webelow den and pack meetings.

Objectives. To assess and develop membership, fellowship, and leadership skills, to develop basic skills in physical abilities, civic responsibilities, and craftsmanship, and to determine readiness for transition to community programs.

Girl scout program

The Girl Scout program is chartered under the Girl Scouts of America and is run as a scout troop.

Objectives. To assess and develop membership, fellowship, and leadership skills, to develop basic skills in physical abilities, civic responsibilities, and craftsmanship, and to determine readiness for transition to community programs.

Treatment programs for adolescents

Arts and crafts workshop

A variety of creative, semistructured, and structured activities and media that vary in complexity is available.

Objectives. To explore interests and a variety of media, to provide an arena for exercising choice and decision making, to increase the concentration span and the ability to organize and solve problems, and to recognize abilities and strengths in skill areas.

Cooking group

Cooking incorporates the various components involved in the gathering of ingredients, preparation of a full meal, and division of tasks in a cooperative fashion.

Objectives. To promote the development of daily living skills, socialization, and cooperation in daily tasks.

Practical skills group

Criteria for participation in practical skills are determined by basic identified deficits in daily living and community skills.

Objectives. To learn practical skills such as filling out identification forms, reading maps, using the Yellow Pages, using public transportation, writing checks, and living within a budget.

Social skills groups

A variety of situations is provided in which modeling, role playing, group discussions, and feedback are used.

Objective. To promote development of and practice in age-appropriate social skills.

Occupational exploration/development group

Interests and skills related to work-related tasks and worker roles are discussed, with assignments to volunteer worker positions within the hospital when indicated by interdisciplinary treatment plan.

Objectives. To identify personal likes, dislikes, interests, capacities, and skills and to relate to occupational goals; to learn the basic skills in applying for and securing part-time employment.

Meeting with parents

The occupational therapy treatment programs for children and adolescents also may involve meetings with individual parents. The purpose of these meetings includes identifying a child's or adolescent's strengths and problem areas from an occupational therapy perspective, providing suggestions for play activities and community resources that can be used in the home setting, and helping parents to help their children structure time and play activities.

Summary

Occupational therapists who work with children and adolescents are likely to come in contact with those who display psychopathology. The most prevalent psychiatric disorders in childhood and adolescence are ADHD, conduct disorder, mood disorder, and anxiety disorder. Certain risk factors are associated with psychiatric disorders in childhood, such as chronic medical conditions, brain damage, poor school performance, and family dysfunction. The occupational behavior frame of reference was identified as the primary conceptual base from which occupational therapy intervention was drawn. This frame of reference emphasizes an understanding of normal development and the parameters of play and socialization in working with emotionally disturbed children.

Occupational therapy intervention consists of three steps: (1) the assessment process, which is achieved through structured observations, interviews, and standardized tests or checklists; (2) the development of treatment goals, which are measurable and specific to the patient; and (3) the designing of treatment programs (individual and group), which are modified and paced throughout the treatment process.

Treatment programs for children and adolescents are drawn from occupational behavior. Examples are constructive play groups and skill-building groups for children and arts and crafts groups and cooking groups for adolescents.

The preparation of this manuscript was partially supported by the U.S. Department of Health and Human Services, Maternal and Child Health Bureau, Grant #MCJ009048.

References

American Occupational Therapy Association. (1990). *Member data survey*, Rockville, MD: Author.

American Psychiatric Association. (1987). *Diagnostic and statistical manual of mental disorders* (3rd rev. ed.), Washington, DC: American Psychiatric Association.

Asher, I. E. (1989). *An annotated index of occupational therapy evaluation tools*, Rockville, MD: American Occupational Therapy Association.

Barker, P. (1988). *Basic child psychiatry* (5th ed.). Oxford: Blackwell Scientific Publications.

Bernstein, G. (1990). Anxiety disorders. In B. Garfinkel, G. Carlson & E. Weller (Eds.), *Psychiatric disorders in children and adolescents* (pp. 64–83). Philadelphia: W. B. Saunders.

Brands, A. (Ed.). (1977). *Individualized treatment planning for psychiatric patients*. Rockville, MD: U.S. Department of Health and Human Services, 1990.

Carlson, G. (1990). Bipolar disorders in children and adolescents. In B. Garfinkel, G. Carlson, & E. Weller (Eds.), *Psychiatric disorders in children and adolescents.* (pp. 21–33). Philadelphia: W. B. Saunders.

Cook, D. (1991). The assessment process. In W. Dunn (Ed.), *Pediatric occupational therapy* (pp. 35–74). Thorofare, NJ: Slack.

Costello, E. (1989). Developments in child psychiatric epidemiology. *American Academy of Child and Adolescent Psychiatry, 28,* 836–841.

Cronin, A. (1989). Children with emotional or behavioral disorders. In P. Pratt & A. Allen (Eds.), *Occupational therapy for children* (pp. 563–579). St. Louis: C. V. Mosby.

Dunn W. (1991). *Pediatric occupational therapy*. Thorofare, NJ: Slack.

Edits (1974). *COP system interest* survey. San Diego, CA.

Edits (1976). *Career Ability Placement Survey*, San Diego, CA.

Education for all Handicapped Children Act (Public Law 94–142), 1975. 20 U.S.C. §1401.

Education of the Handicapped Act Amendments of 1986 (Public Law 99–457), 20 U.S.C. §1400.

Erikson, E. (1963). *Childhood and society*, New York: W. W. Norton & Co.

Florey, L. (1971). An approach to play and play development. *American Journal of Occupational Therapy, 25,* 275–280..

Florey, L. (1986). Child and adolescent psychiatry. In S. Robertson (Ed.), *Scope: Workbook* (pp. 113–116). Rockville, MD: American Occupational Therapy Association.

Florey, L. (1986). The depressed adolescent. In S. Ryan (Ed.), *The certified occupational therapy assistant* (pp. 177–181). Thorofare, NJ: Slack.

Florey, L., & Michelman, S. (1982). Occupational role history: A screening tool for psychiatric occupational therapy. American Journal of Occupational Therapy, *36,* 301–308.

Forness, S. (1988). Planning for the needs of children with serious emotional disturbance: The National Special Education and Mental Health Coalition. *Behavioral Disorders, 13,* 127–139.

Garfinkel, B., Carlson, G., & Weller, E. (1990). Preface. In B. Garfinkel, G. Carlson & E. Weller (Eds.), *Psychiatric disorders in children and adolescents* (pp. XV–XVI). Philadelphia: W. B. Saunders.

Gilmore, J. B. (1971). Play: A special behavior. In R. E. Herron & B. Sutton-Smith (Eds.), *Child's play* (pp. 311–325). New York: John Wiley & Sons, pp. 311–325.

Gould, M., Wunsch-Hitzig, R., & Dohrenwend, B. (1981). Estimating the prevalence of childhood psychopathology. *American Academy of Child Psychiatry, 20,* 462–476.

Greenhill, L. (1990). Attention-deficit hyperactivity disorder in children. In B. Garfinkel, G. Carlson & E. Weller (Eds.), *Psychiatric disorders in children and adolescents* (pp. 149–182). Philadelphia: W. B. Saunders.

Havinghurst, R. (1973). *Developmental tasks and education*. New York: David McKay.

King-Thomas, L., & Hacker, B. (1987). *A therapist's guide to pediatric assessment*. Boston: Little, Brown & Co.

Knox, S. (1974). A play scale. In M. Reilly (Ed.), *Play as exploratory learning* (pp. 247–266). Beverly Hills, CA: Sage Publications.

Lazare, A. (1973). Hidden conceptual models in clinical psychiatry. *New England Journal of Medicine, 7,* 345–351.

Lewis, D. (1990). Conduct disorders. In B. Garfinkel, G. Carlson & E. Weller (Eds.), *Psychiatric disorders in children and adolescents* (pp. 193–209). Philadelphia: W. B. Saunders.

Lewis, D. (1991). Conduct disorder. In M. Lewis (Ed.), *Child and adolescent psychiatry: A comprehensive textbook* (pp. 561–573). Baltimore: Williams & Wilkins.

Livingston, R. (1991). Anxiety disorders. In M. Lewis (Ed.), *Child and adolescent psychiatry; A comprehensive textbook* (pp. 673–685). Baltimore: Williams & Wilkins.

Martin, S., & Alessi, N. (1990). Formulating a role for occupational therapy in child psychiatry: A clinical application, *American Journal of Occupational Therapy, 44,* 871–882.

Matsutsuyu, J. (1971). Occupational behavior: A perspective on work and play. *American Journal of Occupational Therapy, 25,* 291–294.

Matsutsuyu, J. (1983). Occupational behavior approach. In H. L. Hopkins & H. D. Smith (Eds.), *Willard and Spackman's Occupational therapy* (6th ed., pp. 129–134.). Philadelphia: J. B. Lippincott.

Mitchell, E., & Mason, B. (1948). *The theory of play*. New York: A. S. Barnes.

Moorhead, L. (1969). The occupational history. *American Journal of Occupational Therapy, 23,* 329–334.

Mussen, P., Conger, J., & Kagan, J. (1963). *Child development and personality*, New York: Harper & Row.

National Mental Health Association Speaks. (1989). *Students with serious emotional disturbance underserved in special education*. Alexandria, Va: Author. (Available from NMHD, 1021 Prince Street, Alexandria, VA 22314)

Nelson, D. (1984). *Children with autism*, Thorofare, NJ: Slack.

Offord, D., & Fleming, J. (1991). Epidemiology. In M. Lewis (Ed.), *Child and adolescent psychiatry: A comprehensive textbook* (pp. 1156–1168). Baltimore: Williams & Wilkins.

Pomeroy, J. (1990). Infantile autism and childhood psychosis. In B. Garfinkel, G. Carlson & E. Weller (Eds.), *Psychiatric disorders in children and adolescents* (pp. 271–290). Philadelphia: W. B. Saunders.

Pratt, P., & Allen, A. (Eds.). (1989). *Occupational therapy for children*. St. Louis: C. V. Mosby.

Reilly, M. (1969). The educational process. *American Journal of Occupational Therapy, 23,* 299–307.

Takata, N. (1974). Play as a prescription. In M. Reilly (Ed.), *Play as exploratory learning* (pp. 209–246). Beverly Hills, CA: Sage Publications.

U.S. Department of Education. (1987). *Ninth annual report to Congress on implementation of Public Law 94–142: The Education of All Handicapped Children Act*. Washington, DC: U.S. Government Printing Office.

Weiss, G. (1991). Attention deficit hyperactive disorder. In M. Lewis (Ed.), *Child and adolescent psychiatry: A comprehensive textbook* (pp. 544–561). Baltimore: Williams & Wilkins.

Weller, E., & Weller, R. (1990). Depressive disorders in children and adolescents. In B. Garfinkel, G. Carlson & E. Weller (Eds.), *Psychiatric disorders in children and adolescents* (pp. 3–20). Philadelphia: W. B. Saunders.

Weller, E., & Weller, R. (1991). Mood disorders. In M. Lewis (Ed.), *Child and adolescent psychiatry: A comprehensive textbook* (pp. 646–664). Baltimore: Williams & Wilkins.

Wender, P. (1990). Attention-deficit hyperactivity disorder in adolescents and adults. In B. Garfinkel, G. Carlson, & E. Weller (Eds.), *Psychiatric disorders in children and adolescents* (pp. 183–192). Philadelphia: W. B. Saunders.

Zigler, E., & Finn-Stevenson, M. (1991). National policies for children, adolescents and families. In M. Lewis (Ed.), *Child and adolescent psychiatry: A comprehensive textbook* (pp. 1178–1189). Baltimore: Williams & Wilkins.

CHAPTER 15

Child abuse and neglect

CAROLE J. SIMON

LEARNING OBJECTIVES

Upon completion of this chapter the reader will be able to:

1. *Understand the definition of abuse and neglect of children.*
2. *Recognize the context within which abuse and neglect may flourish.*
3. *Develop an awareness of the indicators of abuse and neglect.*
4. *Understand the role of the occupational therapist in identifying, reporting, treating, and preventing abuse and neglect of children.*

KEY TERMS

Emotional Maltreatment   Physical Neglect

Mandated Reporter   Sexual Abuse

Physical Abuse   Temperament Traits

Case Studies

Case 1

A 3-year-old boy who is demonstrating rigidity and spasticity is referred to occupational therapy. He whimpers when approached, but communicates only at an infantile level. His history indicates repeated visits to emergency rooms with various explanations: "fell out of high chair," "stumbled down the stairs," "injured when car brakes were applied abruptly." The therapist discovers that the youngster is currently living with a foster family who reports he has limited self-care skills. His history includes normal birth and early development. However, repeated battering from his biologic family interrupted this progression. Much work is ahead for the occupational therapist to help this child to reach his highest potential. The therapist recognizes her own frustration that this child who once had so much potential may never attain independence.

Case 2

The occupational therapist in an early intervention center notes many skin discolorations, bruises, and scars that look like cigarette burns on the 2-year-old boy that he is beginning to treat. After disrobing the child for a quick diaper change, he notes further skin damage on the buttocks that looks as if the child has been dunked in scalding water. The child's behavior suggests to the therapist that he is reluctant to be touched, handled, or even approached. The therapist feels a flash of anger toward whomever caused these injuries.

Case 3

While working in a school system, the occupational therapist became aware of a brother and sister in first grade who were withdrawn, looked very dirty, and were offensive to be near because they smelled so bad. They seemed to be absent from school more than they were present. They did not respond to the stimuli in the classroom, nor did they participate willingly in classroom activities. Despite their frequent absences, a parent frequently came to take them home in the middle of the day. Clearly, these children were not learning in school as they should be. The therapist later learned that the youngsters had been used for childhood prostitution in their family home. They were subsequently placed in foster care in another state.

The therapist was shocked that such an episode could have happened to children in her work setting.

Discussion

Consider the feelings engendered by the above scenarios. As the occupational therapist addresses the many issues raised, there are both professional and personal needs to be met. To become useful to abused children and their families, it is important to gain an understanding about the dynamics and complexities of child abuse and neglect, as well as a knowledge of the law, the health and welfare systems involved, and a sensitivity to one's own values and attitudes.

Statistics about numbers of children abused on a yearly basis are misleading. A daily review of the newspaper often reveals at least one incident that led to harm or death of a child. Reported cases number over 1 million, but many cases are unreported. Occupational therapists may or may not know they are treating a child who has been abused. Handicapped children are at an especially high risk for abuse because of the additional stressors that act on the caretakers. Vigilance is important to detect and prevent harm to the children.

Attention to issues of child abuse is relatively recent. Since the early 1960s, articles have been published, child abuse laws have been passed, and education of medical personnel has supported recognition of the signs of a battered child who comes into the emergency room. Before 1960, many episodes of abuse were considered personal and cultural codes of disciplinary conduct. Also, before child labor laws, youth were mistreated and exploited in business and industry.

A lack of clear understanding exists about what constitutes abuse and neglect. Definitions vary from state to state, sometimes even from town to town.

Public Law 93–247, the Child Abuse Prevention and Treatment Act, defines child abuse and neglect as the physical or mental injury, sexual abuse, negligent treatment, or maltreatment of a child under the age of 18 by a person who is responsible for the child's welfare under circumstances that indicate that the child's health or welfare is being harmed or threatened. State laws stipulate further definition and can refer to a child or children in an individual family, a group of children in an institution or group home, or all children in society as a whole. *Child abuse* refers to an act of commission by a parent or caretaker that is not accidental and either harms or threatens to harm a child's physical or mental health or welfare. *Child neglect* refers to an act of omission, which may be the failure of a parent or those legally responsible for the child's welfare to provide for the child's basic needs for food, clothing, shelter, hygiene, medical attention, or supervision.

Socioeconomic conditions may mimic neglect as parents cope with their sparse resources. Cultural or religious practices may appear abusive when viewed by an outsider. In either event, society maintains a responsibility to protect its children. The laws identify mandated reporters who are immune to prosecution as they document and forward names to the proper authorities to safeguard the well-being of the children in their care. Each state has child welfare or child protective services; each facility has practices established to responsibly report abuse or neglect.

Occupational therapists must familiarize themselves with these policies.

Conditions contributing to abuse and neglect

Lack of maturity, limited knowledge about child development, poor parenting skills, low self-esteem, a history of child abuse, and dysfunctional family dynamics may be characteristics of the abuser. Maternal age was found to relate to the type and severity of child maltreatment (Zuravin, DePanfilis, & Masnyk, 1991). Children of teenagers are more likely to suffer from inadequate health care, personal hygiene, and nutrition; injuries were more likely to be severe. Sometimes parents have unreasonable expectations and requirements of a child because of lack of understanding of skills that are appropriate considering a child's maturational level.

Frustration with toilet training has been known to be instrumental in the inflicting of severe punishment such as sitting the child on a hot stove or putting him or her in scalding water. Another example is a severe reprimand of a very young child for not correctly using eating utensils. A belief in the use of force to "teach the child to mind" promotes abuse, not the desired behavior.

Parenting skills may not have been modeled anywhere in the abuser's life, so there is limited ability for love and discipline. Parents who are immature or unskilled may not be able to pick up the cues and communications offered to them by their children, and thus may not be able to respond to their needs. They may simply be emotionally unprepared for the demands of parenthood. This unpreparedness may be compounded by a history of abuse in their own background. (Although it is often true, it does not necessarily follow that an abused child will become an abuser as an adult.) Low self-esteem, a sense of isolation, lack of support or community involvement, and limited strategies to gain resources all contribute to risk for abuse or neglect. When the father is the abuser, the mother may deny or ignore the situation for fear of losing shelter and food for the family, thus perpetuating the abuse situation.

Characteristics of children may predispose them to risk of abuse or neglect. They may be unsoothable, hard to feed, averse to cuddling, hyperactive, passive, withdrawn, impulsive. If the parents are unable to recognize these as ***temperament traits***, they may feel their children are difficult or that they do not like them as parents. Thomas and Chess (1977) have identified temperament dimensions that describe an easy-going child, a slow-to-warm-up child, and a difficult child. These dimensions include rhythmicity of biologic functions, activity level, approach to or withdrawal from new stimuli, adaptability, sensory threshold, predominant quality of mood, intensity of mood, distractibility, and persistence/attention span. If any of these traits are extreme and if the parent or caregiver is also predisposed to extremes of temperament, one can see the dangers of the relationship. If, on the other hand, there is a "good fit" of temperaments, such as an "easy" parent with a "difficult" child, or a parent with a a difficult temperament with an easy child, reduced stress will be apparent and risk will be reduced.

Socioeconomic stressors may be abundant and subserve abuse and neglect; however, these maltreatments of children exist in every stratum of society. Nevertheless, the effort required of the breadwinner to support a family with diminished resources may create a volatile atmosphere with the child as the scapegoat and recipient of the frustration and anger. At the same time it is important to avoid misidentifying neglect, when families are doing the best they can with limited resources.

Drug and alcohol abuse has increased the conditions of abuse or neglect that prevail for children. When parents are seeking or are "on" substances, little or no effort or attention remains for the needs of the children. Nutritional, emotional, and shelter needs are often unmet. Supervision is often nonexistent. Moreover, children may be forced to assume the role of parent for both their siblings and the substance abuser, thus losing their childhood. In addition, the loss of control that comes with substance abuse enhances possibilities for pregnancy and can result in poor prenatal care. Male substance abusers who father children may have defective sperm that create handicapping conditions in the infants (Joffe, 1979; Wazigi, Odem, & Polakoska, 1991).

Handicapped children are at risk for child abuse and neglect. The extra demands on the parents' time, the special attention needed and travel required for treatment, the emotional upheaval, and sheer fatigue of parents contribute to the risk. The demands of rearing a handicapped child are unrelenting. Abuse and neglect can be reduced if professionals and other parents can give support, respite care can be found, and alternatives can be provided for frustration and anger.

Indicators of abuse and neglect

Physical abuse

The physical indicators of *physical abuse* may be unexplained bruises and welts anywhere on the body, which may reflect the shape of the object used to inflict harm, such as a belt buckle, an electric cord, or a hand. They may be in various stages of healing and may appear regularly after a weekend or vacation with the abuser. Unexplained burns may be in the shape of an iron, an electric burner, a cigar, a cigarette, or an immersion (socklike, glovelike markings), on buttocks or genitals. Rope burns may appear on arms, legs, neck, or torso. The burns may be infected, indicating a delay in treatment. Fractures or dislocations of unexplained origin may be evident in various stages of healing. Fractures are especially telltale if they are multiple or spiral in nature. Unexplained lacerations or abrasions on the mouth, lips, gums, eyes, and external genitalia, and bald patches on the scalp may be in various stages of healing.

The behavioral indicators of physical abuse show up as wariness of adult contacts, apprehension when other children cry, or behavioral extremes of aggressiveness or withdrawal. The child may act as if deserving of punishment, and he or she may be frightened of the parents and afraid to go home. The child may report injury by his or her parents. He or she may demonstrate a vacant or frozen stare, lie very still while surveying surroundings, and not cry when approached by the examiner. The child may respond to questions in monosyllables, show inappropriate or precocious maturity, and display manipulative behavior to get attention. This child is capable of only superficial relationships, indiscriminately seeks affection, and has a poor self-concept.

Physical neglect

Physical indicators of *physical neglect* are poor growth pattern, failure to thrive, underweight, persistent hunger, poor hygiene, and inappropriate dress. Wasting of subcutaneous tissue, unattended physical problems or medical needs, abdominal distention, and bald patches on the scalp may be found. There may be abandonment of the child or a consistent lack or supervision, especially in dangerous activities or for long periods of time.

Behavioral indicators of physical neglect may manifest as begging or stealing food, early arrival at and late departure from school, rare or poor attendance at school, and constant fatigue, listlessness, or falling asleep in class. The child may seek affection inappropriately and assume adult responsibilities and concerns. Alcohol or drug abuse may begin as well as delinquent behavior. The child may state that there is no caretaker.

Sexual abuse

Physical indicators of *sexual abuse* may be discerned by difficulty in sitting or walking; torn, stained, or bloody underclothing; pain, swelling, or itching in the genital area; and pain on urination. Bruises, bleeding, or lacerations may be present in the external genitalia, vagina, or anal area, and vaginal or penile discharge may be present. Venereal disease, poor sphincter tone, and pregnancy all may appear.

Behavioral indicators of sexual abuse may be identified as bizarre, sophisticated, or unusual sexual behavior or knowledge. The child may be unwilling to change for gym class or to participate in physical education class. He or she may exhibit withdrawal, fantasy, or infantile behavior, have poor peer relationships, become delinquent, or run away. He or she may report sexual assault by the caregiver. A change in school performance may occur.

Emotional abuse

Physical indicators of *emotional maltreatment* may become apparent as speech disorders, lags in physical development, failure to thrive, or hyperactive, disruptive behavior. Behavioral indicators include habit disorders (sucking, biting, rocking), conduct and learning disorders (antisocial, destructive), neurotic traits (sleep disorders, inhibition of play, unusual fearfulness), and psychoneurotic reactions (hysteria, obsession, compulsion, phobias, hypochondria). Behavior extremes of compliant, passive or aggressive, or demanding or overly adaptive behavior, such as in inappropriately adult or infant behavior, may exist. Mental and emotional developmental lags and suicide attempts may be seen.

Other indicators

Play behaviors can also be indicative of abuse. Deficits in developmental play and play imitation were found in a comparison of abused and nonabused children ages 1 to 5 years (Howard, 1986). The social interaction on which much play is based can be interrupted by maltreatment. The use of play in this context can have important implications for the occupational therapist.

A variety of psychiatric disorders has been suggested to have their genesis in childhood abuse. Posttraumatic stress disorder, multiple personality, and borderline personality disorder have been reported with high rates of childhood abuse (Chu & Dill, 1990; Ogata et al., 1990; Westin, Ludolph, Misle, Ruffins, & Block, 1990). The use of dissociative defenses in the presence of the psychological need to escape overwhelming experiences or trauma and abuse seems to make painful events less intense. This decreased intensity can come about through dissociative alterations in perceptions (depersonalization and derealization), can be forgotten (psychogenic amnesia), or can even be completely disowned as someone else's experience (multiple personality) (Chu & Dill, 1990). Antisocial behaviors of delinquency and criminality may also be sequelae of childhood abuse.

Role of the occupational therapist

The role of the occupational therapist in the area of child abuse and neglect is manifold. As an educator, the therapist may develop inservice groups, support groups, or individualized information to promote good parenting skills. Imparting solid knowledge about normal growth and development and realistic expectations about developmental milestones may deter an abusive reaction. Helping the parents recognize the strengths of their child and understand and respond to the child's signals and cues will improve the relationship and communication. Children with handicapping conditions may have more difficulty in demonstrating their needs and desires.

The occupational therapist may be able to interpret ambiguous gestures as meaningful to start the improved communication process. It is also important to help the caregiver develop new strategies to use at times of great emotional stress. Examples of strategies are leaving the room, taking a walk, eating a snack, calling a friend or professional, or some other diversion that may be preplanned for use when the stressful moment occurs. Establishing an atmosphere of respect for the parent and his or her dilemma helps the caregiver to validate him- or herself and live up to the therapist's expectations. The role of the occupational therapist therefore takes on the dimension of one who prevents escalation of potentially abusive situations by recognizing and diffusing stressors.

Another role to be fulfilled is that of the "hands on" therapist who remediates problems brought about through abuse or neglect. The emphasis may be in the physical or psychosocial domain, but at all times the whole child must be considered in addition to the family dynamics. A thorough evaluation of the child's developmental, functional, and adaptive behaviors will identify specific needs to be met by the treatment plan. Treatment approaches include neurodevelopmental treatment techniques, sensory integration techniques, and social–emotional support. Methods of service delivery may be direct, consultative, or monitoring. The occupational therapist may discover that more service is required than is being allowed and must become a strong advocate for the provision of appropriate services to both the child and the caretaker, parent, or foster parent.

With a good knowledge base and keen observational skills, the occupational therapist may be the professional who recognizes that abuse or neglect is occurring. In many states, occupational therapists are mandated reporters. A ***mandated reporter*** is one who in the practice of his or her profession comes in contact with children, and must make a report or see that a report is made when he or she has reason to believe that a child is an abused child.

Children in our care often have handicapping conditions that limit their resistance to assaults and make them unable to communicate verbally or nonverbally that the episode occurred. The therapist may note that abuse has occurred in the family setting or in the institutional setting. Responsible reporting to the proper authorities will bring help to the child through the child protective services of the particular locale.

A final role that an occupational therapist may fulfill is that of a children's advocate who promotes social change through laws and policies. Children do not have a vote; they must rely on adults to safeguard their welfare. Occupational therapists can contact their legislators to alert them to specific needs they have discovered in their communities. Through their work, they can develop community-based support for new laws and expanded policies.

Summary

Child abuse and neglect are prevalent. Since the 1960s laws have defined and identified maltreatment of children and the reporting procedures to be followed to protect them. Conditions that contribute to abuse and neglect include predisposing characteristics of both the abuser and the abused, as well as the stresses of society such as socioeconomic issues and substance abuse. Occupational therapists provide service to the child and the family to alleviate and remediate the abuse. The occupational therapist must become aware of his or her own skills, emotions, and values regarding child abuse and neglect.

References

Chu, J. A., & Dill, D. L. (1990). Dissociative symptoms in relation to childhood physical and sexual abuse. *American Journal of Psychiatry, 147,* 7.

Howard, A. C. (1986). Developmental play ages of physically abused and nonabused children. *American Journal of Occupational Therapy, 40,* 691–695.

Joffe, J. M. (1979). Influence of drug exposure of the father on perinatal outcome. *Clinics in Perinatology, 6*(1), 21–36.

Ogata, S. N., Silk, K. R., Goodrich, S., Lohr, N., Westen, D., & Hill, E. M. (1990). Childhood sexual and physical abuse in adult patients with borderline personality disorder. *American Journal of Psychiatry, 147,* 8.

Thomas, A., & Chess, S. (1977). *Temperament and development.* New York: Brunner/Mazel.

Wazigi, R. A., Odem, R. R., & Polakoski, K. L. (1991). Demonstration of specific binding of cocaine to human spermatozoa. *Journal of the American Medical Association, 266*(14), 1956–1959.

Westen, D., Ludolph, P., Misle, B., Ruffins, S., & Block, J. (1990). Physical and sexual abuse in adolescent girls with borderline personality disorder. *American Journal of Orthopsychiatry, 60*(1), 55–66.

Zuravin, S., DePanfilis, D., & Masnyk, K. (1991, October). The effect of maternal age on the type and severity of child maltreatment. *Interdisciplinary research symposium on child abuse and neglect: Focus on the young parent.* Symposium at Temple University, Philadelphia, PA.

Bibliography

Finkelhor, D. (1984). *Child sexual abuse: New theory and research*. New York: The Free Press.

Giovannoni, J. M., & Becerra, R. M. (1979). *Defining child abuse*. New York: The Free Press.

Haugaard, J. J., & Reppucci, N. D. (1988). *The sexual abuse of children*. San Francisco: Jossey-Bass.

Helfer, R. E., & Kempe, R. S. (1987). *The battered child*. Chicago: University of Chicago Press.

Wohl, A., & Kaufman, B. (1985). *Silent screams and hidden cries: An interpretation of artwork by children from violent homes*. New York: Brunner/Mazel

CHAPTER 16

Neurologic and orthopedic conditions: congenital deficiencies

JUDITH ATKINS

Upon completion of this chapter the reader will be able to:

1. *List the clinical signs and symptoms associated with 12 orthopedic and neurologic diagnoses commonly seen in pediatric practice.*
2. *Develop an occupational therapy treatment plan for the same 12 diagnoses.*
3. *Discuss the need for occupational therapy involvement and its impact on positive outcomes.*
4. *Identify which of these 12 diagnoses also present with potential developmental delay and other associated problems.*

Orthopedic and neurologic conditions seen in pediatrics differ from what is seen in adult physical dysfunction. Similarities exist in such diagnoses as traumatic head injury and traumatic spinal cord injury. Evaluation and treatment goals are often the same, with consideration given to the developmental level of the child and the impact of the injury on the child's function. This chapter covers neurologic and orthopedic conditions generally seen only in pediatrics due to their **congenital or hereditary** nature. Only those diagnoses more frequently seen are included. First the diagnosis is described, then its clinical signs and symptoms. An outline of occupational therapy evaluations and treatment goals are given as they relate to the diagnosis.

Obstetric brachial plexus palsy

Children with obstetric brachial plexus palsy are usually products of normal, uncomplicated pregnancies. The injury occurs at birth and the problem is isolated to the affected arm. The incidence of obstetric paralysis has decreased but is still a possibility during a difficult delivery. As stated by Bayne and Costas (1990, p. 602), "the cause of nerve injury in obstetrical palsy is traction, usually due to fetal malposition, cephalopelvic disproportion, or the use of forceps." There are three types of brachial plexus injuries:

Type I: C4, C5, C6, or Erb's palsy
Type II: The entire plexus, or Erb–Duchenne–Klumpke palsy
Type III: C8, T1, or Klumpke's palsy

Erb's palsy is reportedly the most common and is characterized by adduction, internal rotation, and contracture of the shoulder with loss of extension of the elbow. "Mild involvement includes the supraspinatus and infraspinatus muscles with extensive involvement also including the deltoid, external rotators, and elbow flexors" (Bayne & Costas, 1990, p. 602). It is stated that about 80% of children with obstetric brachial plexus injury completely recover by 12 months of age.

Occupational therapy

Occupational therapy for obstetric brachial plexus palsy consists of early splinting at birth with the arm positioned in 90 degrees external rotation and 70 to 80 degrees abduction and 5 to 10 degrees humeral flexion. The elbow is in 60-degree flexion, the forearm in neutral rotation, the wrist in neutral position, and the hand in a functional position. In addition, parents are instructed in passive range-of-motion exercises for the child. As the child regains function, bilateral activities are used to encourage active range of motion and use of the extremity.

Older children with residual deformity and lack of function are also considered for splinting and range-of-motion exercises. Surgical correction may be indicated and may involve muscle transfers, however, with the occupational therapist splinting the arm and working on reeducation of muscles following the surgery.

Radial deficiencies

The most common radial deficiency seen in occupational therapy practice is the radial **clubhand**. Clinically, the child may have partial or complete absence of the radius in the forearm. This causes the hand to be displaced radially. The thumb, when present, is usually not normal. Stiffness or lack of range of motion of the middle joints of the digits, particularly the index and long fingers, may also be present. The deficiency may be unilateral or bilateral. Radial clubhands are frequently associated with syndromes and other congenital anomalies such as radial aplasia thrombocytopenia (TAR) syndrome.

Treatment of the radial clubhand is influenced by the severity of the deficiency and the age of the patient. The intent of treatment is to improve alignment, stability, and function of the hand and upper extremity.

Occupational therapy

The occupational therapist evaluates range of motion and function of the clubhand. Stretching exercises and early splinting are usually indicated. Splints are designed to hold the hand in a central position over the wrist allowing the child to use his or her fingers and elbow. Some children with radial clubhand require surgical correction to improve function of the hand with pollicization of the index finger. Splinting and exercises are both indicated after surgery. The occupational therapist is also asked to provide an exercise program after surgery. In bilateral cases, one extremity may be surgically corrected and results documented before consideration of surgery for the other hand. Many children use lateral flexion of the hand against the forearm to grasp objects and accept their deformity; thus, independence would be compromised if the hand were surgically corrected.

Syndactyly

Syndactyly, a **webbing** of the fingers, is commonly seen in children. It is often associated with another syndrome such as Apert syndrome. Syndactyly is surgically corrected. Simple syndactyly involves only skin. In complex syndactyly, bones of adjacent fingers are fused.

Occupational therapy

The occupational therapist is asked to evaluate function before and after surgery. The therapist needs to assess range of motion, grasp patterns, and use of the hand as it relates to developmental level. Children with associated syndromes may have difficulty in function related to developmental delay rather than limitations caused by the syndactyly. Splinting after surgery may be indicated, with the splint maintaining the newly created web spaces.

Arthrogryposis

As stated by Bayne and Costas (1990, p. 580), "arthrogryposis multiplex congenita is not a specific disorder, but a symptom complex of congenital joint contractures associated with neurogenic and myopathic disorders." It is usually not considered progressive and the contractures are present at birth. There is limitation in active and passive range of motion. The problems vary in severity either with all extremities affected or with more involvement in upper extremity movement. The cause of arthrogryposis is unknown. Often the shoulders are adducted and internally rotated, the elbows fixed in extension, and the forearm pronated. The hands and wrists are generally flexed with ulnar deviation. Many children with arthrogryposis have normal and above-normal intelligence.

Occupational therapy

Treatment for arthrogryposis begins in the neonatal period with aggressive stretching, **range-of-motion exercises**, splinting, and possible serial casting. The occupational therapist must follow children with this condition closely to determine function and method of use of the upper extremities in play and purposeful activity. Surgery can in some instances improve function. Elbow releases and muscle transfers may be indicated at the elbow to provide the patient with active elbow flexion. Surgery is usually done on one side only, for the prime purpose of improving function. The occupational therapist's evaluation of passive and active range of motion combined with evaluation of function and grasp patterns is extremely helpful to the hand surgeon. Evaluation of development is important as well as family composition and compliance. All are essential to a successful postsurgery course. The therapist provides splinting and range-of-motion exercises as well as an activity program after surgery.

Children with arthrogryposis are referred to occupational therapy for activities of daily living (ADL). The goal of the hand surgeon is to provide the child with an upper extremity that can be brought to the mouth for self-feeding and that can be used for toileting. It may be necessary to provide the child with adapted equipment that provides independence in self-feeding, toileting, bathing, grooming, and dressing. The occupational therapist may also need to provide consultation in the classroom for assistance in writing and performing other fine motor tasks.

Children with severe forms of arthrogryposis and limited range of motion and function in the lower extremities may benefit from special seating systems and wheelchairs for independent mobility at home and at school. Self-propelling a manual wheelchair is impossible for these children due to upper extremity involvement; therefore, they can benefit from power-driven wheelchairs. These chairs may need to interface with environmental controls.

Osteogenesis imperfecta

Osteogenesis imperfecta is characterized by **brittle bones** that are osteoporotic and easily fractured. It varies in types and severity. Short stature, scoliosis, and a typical misshapen skull with a wide intratemporal measurement and a small triangular face are also seen with this diagnosis. Incidence of fractures decreases as the child's age increases.

Occupational therapy

Children with osteogenesis imperfecta are generally referred to occupational therapy during the neonatal period. Because of the fragile state of their bones, they may fracture with a simple change in position from prone to supine. The occupational therapist can provide the patient with a padded, specially constructed bed that allows the parent or nurse to turn the patient safely, thus preventing fractures.

It is also important to assess the development of children with osteogenesis imperfecta. Due to environmental restrictions and immobility from fractures, these children are at risk for developmental delay. Parental bonding may be adversely affected because of the parents' fear of handling and the restrictions placed on the child. It is important to outline a treatment plan that incorporates activities to enhance normal development and, later, independence.

The occupational therapist may be asked to modify and consult on car seat options for children with osteogenesis imperfecta. It is important to remember that federally approved car seats cannot have padding added behind or under the patient. Foam rolls may be used to the side of the patient.

Children with severe forms of osteogenesis imperfecta may not remain ambulatory. These children require adaptive equipment such as a wheelchair for independent mobility. Due to fractures and contractures, consideration must be given to such features as elevating legrests and removable armrests. Children with a history of upper extremity fractures are candidates for powered mobility.

Muscular dystrophy

Muscular dystrophy is a noninflammatory inherited disorder characterized by progressive degeneration and weakness of the skeletal muscle. The types of muscular dystrophy are divided by severity of muscle weakness and pattern of genetic inheritance. The most common type of muscular dystrophy in pediatric practice is **Duchenne muscular dystrophy**. Transmission is usually by a recessive gene and the disorder is primarily seen in males. It is generally diagnosed when the child is between the ages of 18 and 36 months. Because muscular dystrophy is not evident at birth, some families have had two to three children before the oldest child is diagnosed. It is not uncommon for a family to have more than one child with this disorder.

Initially, children with muscular dystrophy appear normal and are ambulatory, active children. Parents begin to notice a weakness and frequent falling, and the child may complain of muscle cramps. As the weakness progresses, walking becomes increasingly more difficult. Initially, upper extremity involvement is limited to the shoulder girdle. Eventually the child loses elbow and shoulder stability and strength; later, hand function. Respiratory failure is a common cause of death in these children.

Occupational therapy

Due to the degenerative nature of muscular dystrophy, occupational therapy intervention cannot prevent muscle weakness or loss of function. Occupational therapy can assist affected children to remain independent longer in self-care activities with the use of adaptive equipment. Therapists can also provide equipment for comfort, ease of care, and independent mobility.

Affected children require a wheelchair for independent mobility at home and at school. Due to the loss of upper extremity function, powered mobility is indicated. Even children with severe scoliosis and significant deformity can successfully use a power-driven wheelchair with a standard joystick. Removable armrests are needed for ease of transfer. Children with muscular dystrophy develop flexion contractures of the hips and knees. Equinovarus deformities occur in the feet. These contractures cannot be prevented; therefore, it is imperative to support the deformity and provide comfort while the child is sitting. A seating system and wheelchair must be matched to each child's particular need. As scoliosis progresses, the child will need lateral supports. Some children benefit from the use of chest straps.

Consideration should also be given to the use of slings and other movable arm supports so that the child can continue to self-feed, write, and turn pages of a book. Built-up utensils may prove beneficial because of loss of grip strength. Occupational therapists can offer assistance to families, helping them to cope with changes in function, in school issues, and in transportation needs.

Congenital dislocated hips

Congenital dislocation of the hip (CDH) refers to any manifestation of **hip instability** ranging from neonatal instability to established dislocation. CDH has several causative factors. According to Herring (1990, p. 816), "factors include ligamentous laxity, response of female fetuses to maternal hormones that induce ligamentous relaxation, prenatal and postnatal positioning, and certain genetic factors." Neonatal screening is done for this defect. It occurs more frequently in firstborn children. Parental complaints that might be indicative of this condition are such things as difficulty in diapering, shortening of the thigh, a limp in the ambulatory child, toe walking, or in-toeing. Various tests are done to confirm the diagnosis such as physical examination and radiographic evaluation. Children with the diagnosis of congenital hip dislocation are generally of normal intelligence with normal developmental milestones.

Occupational therapy

Treatment of congenital hip dislocation varies according to the facility and the physician. Very young children may be treated successfully with an abduction harness or splint. Occupational therapy is indicated for children who are admitted to the hospital and placed in skin traction. These children are referred to occupational therapy for evaluation and developmental treatment. Since children with congenital hip dislocation are placed in an extremely restrictive environment at a very young age, they are at risk for developmental delay. A certain amount of regression and withdrawal occurs with hospitalization and confinement to bed. The certified occupational therapy assistant can be extremely effective in carrying out treatment for the child with this type of condition.

After the hips are successfully reduced, the children are placed in a body cast for 6 to 12 weeks. The child is casted in a position of 120 degrees of hip flexion and moderate abduction.

During the casting period, the occupational therapist can assist the family in securing equipment for transporting the child, such as a wagon or adapted wheelchair for the larger child. Car seats must also be modified to accommodate the cast and the position of the lower extremities. A regular car seat can be modified, but commercially manufactured car seats are now available for these children.

The occupational therapist can assist the family with a treatment plan and a home program with activities to encourage development and enhance upper extremity function. The therapist can also assist with clothing modifications.

Legg–Calvé–Perthes disease

Legg–Calvé–Perthes disease occurs most frequently in children 4 to 8 years old and more often in boys. It is a disorder of the hip but an initial symptom of the disease is knee pain. The cause is unknown. One theory is that for unknown reasons the vascular supply to the proximal femur is interrupted, which causes necrosis and a flattening of the weight-bearing surface. Children with this disease tend to be extremely active and to prefer gross motor activities over fine motor activities. Treatment of the condition consists of non-weight bearing during the healing process. More severe cases that do not respond to treatment or those children who did not have the benefit of early diagnosis are hospitalized and placed in skin traction. Following traction, children with Legg–Calvé–Perthes disease are casted in what is called a **broomstick cast**. The legs are casted to the hips and abducted, with a bar between the casts to maintain the desired amount of abduction.

Occupational therapy

Children with Legg–Calvé–Perthes disease are generally referred to occupational therapy during their hospitalization. While in skin traction, children are seen supportively with the treatment plan focusing on their developmental level and age-appropriate activities. These children are often seen by a certified occupational therapy assistant during their hospitalization. Before discharge the child is referred to occupational therapy for a cast wheelchair. A manual wheelchair with a cast board is used to support the broomstick cast. A home activity program is given to the parents, as well as suggestions for clothing adaptations. Referral is made to the automotive safety program so the parents can be advised and supplied with the necessary child restraints for safe transport.

Torticollis

Congenital muscular torticollis is frequently seen in pediatric practice. It is due to a contracture of the sternocleidomastoid muscle. The head is tilted toward the involved side and the chin rotated toward the contralateral shoulder. Congenital torticollis may also be associated with abnormalities of the cervical spine, such as hemivertebrae. This type of deformity is seen in Klippel–Feil syndrome.

Occupational therapy

Children with torticollis are referred to occupational therapy for stretching exercises and splinting. Splinting consists of a soft or hard collar that can be removed for exercise. Parents are given a home program and can easily carry out the desired exercises. These children also benefit from bed positioning and activities to encourage active range of motion.

Juvenile rheumatoid arthritis

Juvenile rheumatoid arthritis (JRA) differs from rheumatoid arthritis seen in adults. JRA is defined as the group of diseases that has a chronic **synovial inflammation** of unknown cause. Onset occurs before the age of 16 years and there is objective evidence of arthritis in one or more joints for 6 consecutive weeks. Mosca and Sherry (1990, p. 297), define "arthritis as a swelling of the joint or limitation of motion with some combination of heat, pain, and tenderness." Other possible clinical signs are fever, difficulty with movement in the morning, and rash.

Occupational therapy

Occupational therapy is an essential part of the treatment of children with JRA. Occupational therapy can aid in preventing joint injury and future contractures through the use of **therapeutic splinting**. When splinting a child with this diagnosis, consider the following:

Range of motion of joints—active and passive
Joints involved and maximum pain-free range
Present deformities and potential tendencies to future deformities (boutonnière, swan neck)
Age of patient, activity level

Common types of splints used with children with JRA are resting pan, cock-up, knee extension, and foot dorsiflexion. Dynamic splinting may also be indicated in some cases. When working with arthritis patients, it is important to realize that after joint changes have occurred, correction and maintenance of correction become difficult.

Another area in which occupational therapy is involved is ADL. The therapist can help the family and the patient with problems of ADL to increase independence without damage or pain to affected joints. Adaptive equipment may be indicated for the child to continue to effectively use such things as eating utensils and writing devices. Children with significant lower extremity involvement and contractures may benefit from powered tricarts at school.

The field of occupational therapy can provide specific joint protection techniques that will aid in prevention of injury or contracture. The therapist instructs the child in ways to perform daily living activities with a minimal amount of stress to the involved joints to reduce pain, preserve joint structures, and conserve physical resources (energy).

Parents and patients should be provided with written and verbal information regarding rheumatoid diseases and justification for treatment with specific information on the above-stated goals.

For children who are candidates for hand surgery, dynamic splinting and active and passive range-of-motion programs are needed following surgery. Activity suggestions to enhance function must also be provided.

Spinal muscular atrophy

Spinal muscular atrophy is defined as an autosomal recessive disease with **chronic progressive degeneration**. Spinal muscular atrophies can be classified into four groups according to age of onset and distribution of weakness. The commonly seen group in pediatrics is acute infantile spinal muscular atrophy or Werdnig–Hoffmann disease. Symptoms are manifest by the age of 6 months, the disease progresses rapidly, and weakness and lack of spontaneous movement are apparent. Many affected children die by the age of 2 years. Those who survive the first year may have a life expectancy of 10 years. Affected children have weakness, hypotonia, and atrophy. Some never gain head control or independent sitting. Scoliosis and its progression are also problems.

Occupational therapy

Occupational therapy can help to prevent contractures through proper positioning and selected equipment designed to provide the necessary support. Since children with spinal muscular atrophy are alert and interact with their environment, it is important to have equipment that will enhance function. Older children attend school and need to interface with their environment. Some of these children are on prolonged ventilatory support, which also has to be transported.

Many infants with spinal muscular atrophy have eating difficulties. Difficulty relates to weakness, fatigue, and coordination of suck and swallow. It is necessary to do an oral motor assessment with appropriate treatment. A gastrostomy tube may be indicated to maintain nutrition and prevent aspiration.

Parents also need to be given home programs that relate to handling, positioning, and maximizing function.

Hydrocephalus

Hydrocephalus can be seen as a single diagnosis or associated with another condition. Children with hydrocephalus have excessive **cerebrospinal fluid** (CSF) within the ventricles or subarachnoid space. An imbalance exists between the amount of CSF absorbed and that produced. This causes increased intracranial pressure; if left untreated, this condition can result in brain damage and loss of function. Causes of hydrocephalus include midline tumors, congenital malformations, hemorrhage, and inflammation. Affected children have increased head circumference and require a ventriculoperitoneal shunt. Prognosis depends on the underlying etiology and the timeliness and success of shunt placement. Children with hydrocephalus show damage that ranges from major neurologic deficits to mild neurologic deficits to no deficits at all.

Occupational therapy

Developmental assessments and occupational evaluations should be done for all children with hydrocephalus. Treatment is based on areas of deficit. Oral motor assessments are also indicated because many of these children are at risk for feeding difficulties as well as developmental delay.

Hydrocephalic children benefit from positioning and adaptive equipment. Children with major neurologic deficits require seating systems and mobility bases for transportation or independent mobility.

Children with milder neurologic deficits may exhibit sensory integrative problems and poor school performance. The usual types of evaluations used are indicated based on age of child and clinical signs.

Independence in activities of daily living are evaluated followed by appropriate intervention and treatment. Behavior is also a consideration, as is prevocational assessment and programming.

Summary

Occupational therapy can provide evaluation results that aid in diagnosis, provide treatment to improve development, enhance function, fabricate splints, provide adapted and positioning equipment, and provide sensory integration treatment. Through working closely with the physician, family, and other members of the health care team, the occupational therapist can improve the quality of life for children with neurologic and orthopedic conditions.

References

Bayne, L., & Costas, B. (1990). Malformations of the upper limb. In R. T. Morrissy (Ed.), *Lovell and Winter's pediatric orthopaedics* (3rd ed., vol. 2, pp. 563–609). Philadelphia: J. B. Lippincott.

Herring, J. A. (1990). *Congenital dislocation of the hip.* In R. T. Morrissy (Ed.), *Lovell and Winter's pediatric orthopaedics* (3rd ed., vol. 2, pp. 815–850). Philadelphia: J. B. Lippincott.

Mosca, V. S., & Sherry, D.P. (1990). Juvenile rheumatoid arthritis and the seronegative spondyloarthopathies. In R. T. Morrissy (Ed.), *Lovell and Winter's pediatric orthopaedics* (3rd ed., vol 2, pp 297–324). Philadelphia: J. B. Lippincott.

Bibliography

Dunn, D., & Epstein, L. (1987). Decision making in child neurology. Philadelphia: B. C. Decker.

Morrissy, R. T. (Ed.). (1990). *Lovell and Winter's pediatric orthopaedics* (3rd ed., vol. 2). Philadelphia: J. B. Lippincott.

Sharrard, W. J. (1979). *Pediatric orthopedics and fractures* (2nd ed, vol. 2) London: Blackwell Scientific Publications.

Swaiman, K. F. (Ed.). (1989). *Pediatric neurology principles and practice* (vol. I). St. Louis: C. V. Mosby.

UNIT VII

*Implementation
of occupational therapy
with adults*

CHAPTER 17

Mental health

SECTION 1A
Psychiatry and mental health

DIANE GIBSON and GAIL Z. RICHERT

LEARNING OBJECTIVES

Upon completion of this section the reader will be able to:
1. *Define descriptors of mental health and mental illness.*
2. *State the purpose and two characteristics of the* DSM-III-R.
3. *List at least three typical reactions of students entering psychiatry.*

Definitions of mental health and illness

Although the terms *mental health* and *mental illness* are common in everyday speech, they are difficult to define because their definitions vary in different situations and different cultures. No single criterion defines mental health, and the terms seem abstract. Happiness, contentment, self-confidence, and self-esteem, and their opposites—unhappiness, anxiety, vulnerability, and low self-esteem—are examples of concepts that the beginning occupational therapist must put into operation in behavioral terms on a continuum from healthy to ill.

Mental health has been characterized by several enduring **behavioral descriptors** such as the following:

1. *Ability to organize thoughts, feelings, and actions* in a manner appropriate to society; this holistic criterion involves the effective integration of biologic, physiologic, psychological, and social systems necessary to allow complex functional performance.
2. *Positive attitude toward self*, in which the person experiences a sense of security, identity, belonging, and meaningfulness
3. *Growth and self-actualization*, in which the person searches for new developments; the individual is aware of feelings and can integrate them with the intellect while interacting openly with the environment.
4. *Balance of moods and feelings* in the face of life stresses; values are held consistently yet flexibly in handling conflict and frustration.
5. *Autonomy and responsibility for one's decisions and actions*; valuing self-determination implies a balance between dependence and independence as well as respect for others' choices.
6. *Accurate perception of reality*, including the ability to empirically test sensory assumptions about the physical world as well as perceive social reality via empathy and sensitivity to others
7. *Mastery of work, leisure, and self-care skills* at a level that is appropriate for the person's age and culture; emotional mastery also includes the ability to cope with loneliness, aggression, frustration, and stress without being overwhelmed (Johada, 1958; Swartzberg & Tiffany, 1988, p. 19).

The ability to meet the above criteria is not viewed against strict adherence to specific standards but from a view of what is reasonable to expect given a person's background and life experience. It is important to remember that stress and life crises are universal, and the ability to cope and to learn from disruption provides the insight and strength to weather future problems. If we think of mental health and mental illness as being at opposite ends of the continuum from the descriptors of health just described, then as we examine mental illness we may expect to see negative self-attitude, disorganization, stalemated growth, a sense of being overwhelmed by stress, dependency, poor reality testing, and lack of skills in work, leisure, and self-care. Although these global descriptors of mental illness are useful, they do not define specific disorders with the objectivity necessary for precise diagnoses.

Manual of mental disorders

The *Diagnostic and Statistical Manual of Mental Disorders* (3rd ed, revised; *DSM-III-R*) is a valuable handbook that provides objective and observable behavioral criteria for presently accepted psychiatric disorders. The *DSM-III-R* (1987) defines mental disorders as,

> . . . distress (a painful symptom) or disability (impairment in one or more important areas of functioning) or with a significantly increased risk of suffering death, pain, disability, or an important loss of freedom. (p. xxii)

According to the *DSM-III-R*, mental disorders do not involve expected responses to particular events such as death of a loved one, nor do they involve deviant behaviors of a political, religious, or sexual nature. The *DSM-III-R* represents a significant attempt to describe clinical features of disorders in an atheoretical manner. Objectively described symptoms clustered into syndromes provide clinicians with a means to observe behavior from a consistent and common viewpoint, thus allowing greater clarity in diagnosing disorders, treatment planning, and research. For example, the ***diagnostic criteria*** for 301.83, borderline personality disorder (p. 349), "must include five of the following: (1) a pattern of unstable and intense relationships; (2) impulsiveness in two areas that are potentially self-damaging; (3) affective instability; (4) inappropriate, intense anger; (5) recurrent suicidal threats; (6) persistent identity disturbance; (7) chronic feelings of emptiness or boredom; and (8) frantic efforts to avoid abandonment."

Psychiatric occupational therapy has been a formal, specialized area of practice for about 70 years. It grew from a strong belief in the human capacity to be self-healing through engagement in activity. Emphasis since the beginning of occupational therapy has been on goal-oriented performance and concepts of mastery, competence, exploration, and independence. Occupational therapists plan treatment interventions based on theoretical models appropriate to the person's diagnosis. These interventions take into account the person's goals, interests, and values. This section combines elements that the authors consider significant for the student and beginning clinician to understand in basic practice. Psychiatric practice is changing dramatically at this time; hence, current knowledge and technology can be seen as a snapshot during this evolutionary period.

Reactions of students entering psychiatry

The student experiencing the first exposure to psychiatry commonly feels anxious and overwhelmed. Understanding typical reactions of students is helpful in reducing a feeling of isolation and fear resulting from prejudices gained from novels, television, and public opinion (Stuart & Sundeen, 1986). Most students may remember the neglect and abuse associated with *One Flew Over the Cuckoo's Nest* (Kesey, 1977) or the horrifying inner world of psychosis described in *I Never Promised You a Rose Garden* (Green, 1964). They naturally worry about whether they will witness similar situations and question whether they will have the strength and ability to deal with them.

A student or therapist who is unfamiliar with psychiatry faces several uncertainties. The student may not be able to distinguish the staff from the patients and yet is expected to mingle freely with the patients. Lack of hospital gowns and uniforms prevents easy role identification. In addition, many patients do not demonstrate observable or tangible illness. In the psychiatric setting, the student has few physical accoutrements, such as the goniometer or the stethoscope, and must rely on an ability to empathize and communicate. As a result of ***role ambiguity*** and intangible experiences, students feel inadequate and painfully self-conscious.

Unsure of their communication skills, students worry about damaging a patient's treatment by saying the wrong thing. Also many students in their early 20s are still consolidating their own identity and may fear the identification of emotional illness in themselves. Simultaneously, clinical supervisors expect students to develop personal insight and awareness of the impact of their behavior on others. To accomplish this, however, the intern usually experiences painful insights about him- or herself and has to reveal personal inadequacies to supervisors. Novice clinicians also may be apprehensive about being assaulted physically or rejected on a psychological basis by patients. See the display for a list of some typical reactions of students entering psychiatry.

Because students often feel acute stress, they occasionally exhibit discomfort by hesitating to leave their supervisor or classmates, by not being able to understand or remember instructions, or by forgetting personal items. Another means of dealing with uncertainty is for the student to assume a facade of professionalism. In this case, cool and formal behavior functions as a barrier to establishing contact with a patient. Being aware that everyone has feelings of uncertainty in this new experience

---

TYPICAL REACTIONS OF STUDENTS ENTERING PSYCHIATRY

1. Uncertain about how to relate to patients with emotional illness
2. Fearful of saying wrong thing to psychiatric patients
3. Identify psychiatric symptoms or illness in self
4. Painful self-consciousness
5. Afraid of physical violence and unpredictable patient behavior
6. Anxious without physical tasks and specific techniques to use
7. Unsure of skills
8. Afraid of staff discovering fears and anxiety
9. Vulnerable to painful observations and insights about self
10. Uncertain of occupational therapy role

and being tolerant of the self for those feelings can ease the initial stress.

General stress reduction techniques may prove beneficial. Group discussion of students' first impressions, observations, and feelings provides an opportunity to share experiences and thus negates the idea, "I'm the only one feeling this way." Role playing difficult or ambiguous encounters encourages students to review their interactions and to develop optional means of relating to patients; it is also a time for others to observe problems and make suggestions. Maintaining a process-oriented record for analysis of the patient–student interaction is a useful tool, particularly if attention is given to nonverbal as well as verbal communication. Observing body language, that is, noting the symbolic meanings in actions, facial expressions, and body gestures of tension, helps students learn the importance of nonverbal messages.

References

American Psychiatric Association. (1987). *Diagnostic and statistical manual of mental disorders* (3rd ed., rev.). Washington, DC: Author.

Green, H. (1964). *I never promised you a rose garden.* New York: Rinehart & Winston.

Johada, M. (1958). *Current concepts of positive mental health.* New York: Basic Books.

Kesey, K. (1977). *One flew over the cuckoo's nest.* New York: Penguin Books.

Stuart, G. W., & Sundeen, S. S. (1986). *Principles and practice of psychiatric nursing* (3rd ed.). St. Louis: C. V. Mosby.

Swartzberg, S. L., & Tiffany, E. G. (1988). Psychiatry and mental health. In H. L. Hopkins & H. D. Smith (Eds.). *Willard and Spackman's occupational therapy* (7th ed.). Philadelphia: J. B. Lippincott.

SECTION 1B
The evolution of occupational therapy

DIANE GIBSON

KEY TERMS

Activity Analysis	*Neuroscience*
Habit Training	*Symbolic Behavior*
Moral Treatment	*Use of Self*

LEARNING OBJECTIVES

Upon completion of this section the reader will be able to:

1. *Describe the purpose of moral treatment and its impact on occupational therapy.*
2. *Describe how the emphasis on somatic treatment influenced occupational therapy during the 1940s and 1950s.*
3. *Define the importance of Eleanor Clarke Slagle on the reestablishment of professional identity during the 1970s and 1980s.*
4. *List three significant civil rights of the mentally ill.*

The process of identifying the foundational beliefs of occupational therapy leads toward a stronger identification with its values. Incorporation of values strengthens professional identity and leads to further seeking of knowledge and skills (Gillette, 1983).

The hope of moral treatment

Occupational therapy traces its inception back to the beliefs and values flowing from ***moral treatment***, a political–social–religious philosophy that emerged during the early 1800s. Bockoven (1963), a brilliant humanistic physician and writer, deduced that the origin of moral treatment rested in the 18th century assumption that the goals of science and humanitarianism were indistinguishable and that applications of science could solve the riddles of mental illness. Eighteenth-century science was dedicated to uncovering universal laws that, conceptually parallel with darwinian thinking, were presumed to influence human behavior just as they controlled evolution. Since a person could not completely control his or her behavior and held qualities and traits in common with others, he or she could be seen as equal to others; therefore, acts of irresponsibility could be forgiven (Bockoven, 1963, p. 11). These ideas fit well with those professing enlightened liberal philosophy, whose political extension began to view criminals, paupers, and psychotics with compassion rather than disdain.

Moral treatment was a collection of values and beliefs that formed seminal concepts for occupational therapy and was also significant in the development of American psychiatry. The word "moral" may arouse resistance in the contemporary reader because 20th-century clinicians ascribe to a belief in cultural and moral relativity rather than absolutism in treating patients. We are trained to look at function, that is, the impact of a person's behavior on health and disease, not to judge moral behavior. The early psychiatrist and occupational therapist used "moral" as the equivalent of "emotional" or "psychological," however, carrying with it the connotations associated with "morale," such as hope and confidence.

Nevertheless, middle class society, from which early mental health practitioners were drawn, espoused a clear sense of ethical behavior, as evidenced in 19th-century writings such as the works of Dickens, *Harper's Bazaar*, and even the *McGuffey's Readers*. The word "moral" implied a responsibility to care for those less fortunate with compassion and understanding, particularly those who were considered innocent or whose aberrations were due to willful or excessive indulgence in passion (Bockoven, 1963, p. 12).

In the late 18th and early 19th centuries, three physicians, Phillipe Pinel in France, William Tuke in England, and Benjamin Rush in America, established retreats for the "insane," which turned the old concept of "madhouse" into a new concept of an *asylum*. Within 30 years of the introduction of moral treatment, 18 hospitals had been built according to high standards set by private philanthropy in Philadelphia, Boston, New York, and Hartford. During this period, caretakers were taught that even the most insane patients were sensitive to manifestations of interest and goodwill. Another asset of moral treatment was the emphasis it placed on comfortable, homelike settings sheltered by wide lawns and trees. Monotony was considered a deterrent to health, whereas the converse, participation in a wide variety of activities, was valued as leading patients back to healthy habits.

Freedom and self-expression were encouraged in the milder, gentler society of the first half of the 19th century. Emerson encouraged self-reliance, whereas New England preachers spoke about a "loving God" as opposed to the "vengeful God" of earlier puritanism. After visiting Boston State Hospital in 1842, Charles Dickens reported that patients there participated in numerous activities including fishing, gardening, indoor and outdoor games, and carriage rides in the open air. Dickens was particularly surprised about the self-respect that was inculcated and encouraged in patients by the superintendent's attitude toward them. He made special note that the superintendent and his family dined with the patients and mixed among them as a matter of course (Bockoven, 1963).

Breakdown of moral treatment

During the latter half of the 19th century, American leaders of moral treatment died without leaving inspired leaders to carry the movement forward. After the Civil War, a rapid growth in population, which was due essentially to the immense influx of poverty-stricken immigrants, put a severe strain on the ability of hospitals to absorb patients. Hospital living quarters deteriorated along with compassion so clearly valued by earlier clinicians, "... barren dormitories adjoining even more barren dayrooms whose furniture consisted of crude benches along the walls" (Bockoven, 1963, p. 22); racial and xenophobic prejudice also produced an environment filled with callousness, leading to patient apathy and a presumption of incurability.

Exposing the horrors and suffering endured by the mentally ill warehoused in asylums at the turn of the century, Clifford Beers wrote *A Mind Which Found Itself* (1908). He eloquently described the sodden routine and insensibility as products of the stigma due to belief in incurability of the mentally ill. Assumptions regarding incurability and the absolute role of heredity in causing mental illness have been "as effective as the medieval belief in demon possession in denying (patients) their rights not only to the means of recovery but to decent standards" (Bockoven, 1963, p. 31). Failure to recognize the damaging effect of the incurability myth led to a passive acceptance of low standards in hospitals and pessimistic expectations regarding the individual patient's recovery. In 1900, pay for both physicians and attendants was very low, physicians' case loads were high, and attendants were asked to work a 70-hour work week with a few hours off each Saturday (Bockoven, 1963, p. 27).

Reemergence of moral treatment and the beginnings of occupational therapy

Moral treatment reemerged as the basis for psychiatric practice during the early 20th century owing to the vitality and seriousness of purpose characterized by leaders in both psychiatry and occupational therapy. The founders of occupational therapy were strong people whose views of treatment were greatly affected by the moral-social values prevalent in 19th-century society. They had been introduced to darwinian philosophy and as a result believed that humans, like animals, successfully interact and adapt to their environment. Adolf Meyer (1921), a great leader of American psychiatry, said that a mentally healthy individual is

> ... an organism that maintains and balances itself in the world of reality and actuality of being in active life and active use, that is, using and living and acting its time in harmony with its own nature and the nature about it. (p. 5)

The mentally ill, therefore, were those who could not adapt to their world because of defective habits that prevented them from dealing effectively with the responsibilities of adulthood. Since mental illness was assumed to be caused by a lack of holistic adaptation to the environment as exemplified by poor habits, wasn't it equally understandable that a **habit training** regimen of balanced work, rest, and nutrition could cure mentally ill patients? This assumption was incorporated into the model, enthusiastically used by early occupational therapists.

Adolf Meyer (1921) recognized the benefits of *doing* and our human need for competence and mastery when he wrote:

> It has been interesting to see how groups of a few excited patients can be seated in a small circle of two or three settees and kept wonderfully contented picking the hair of mattresses, or doing simple tasks not too readily arousing the desire for big movements and uncontrollable excitement and yet not too taxing to their patience. Groups of patients with raffia and basket work, or with various kinds of handwork and weaving and bookbinding and metal and leather work, took the place of bored wall flowers and of mischief-makers. A pleasure in achievement, a real pleasure in the use and activity of one's hands and muscles and a happy appreciation of time began to be used as incentives in the management of our patients, instead of abstract exhortations to cheer up and to behave according to abstract or repressive rules. (p. 3)

The work ethic was a powerful incentive during the time of moral treatment, and it provided an important means for feelings of competence, achievement, and self-esteem. A hospital annual report noted:

> There is no employment in which the patient so cheerfully engages as in haymaking. From twenty to thirty workmen were often in the field at one time, all busily employed. At one of my daily visits to the hayfield, I found *four homicides* mowing together, performing their work in the best manner, and all cheerful and happy (Bockoven, 1963, p. 78).

The emphasis on work meshed well with institutional life, because the hospital was a self-contained community that depended on patients and staff working together. Eleanor Clarke Slagle, a pioneer occupational therapist and colleague of Adolf Meyer at Johns Hopkins Hospital in 1913, continued to stress work and self-care (Slagle, 1922). A habit-training program required patients to get up, wash, dress, clean up the ward, use appropriate table manners, and occupy themselves in basic craft activities. Gradually, patients were expected to "graduate" to occupations requiring a greater emphasis on work beyond the ward, including gardening, field or diary work, and construction of woven rugs for the hospital. Slagle and Meyer were instrumental in developing occupational concepts, such as the use of carefully planned goals and methods for promoting health through occupation (Tiffany, 1988, p. 363).

William Rush Dunton, Jr., a psychiatrist who worked at the

Sheppard and Enoch Pratt Hospital in Baltimore added specificity to core concepts of occupational therapy by analyzing various kinds of activities and matching them with the categorized needs of patients. For example, he analyzed activities in terms of their creativity, physical effort, social potential, and intellectual demand. He presumed that the manic patient would respond best to a quieting, repetitive activity, whereas the paranoid patient would profit from concrete occupations that would deemphasize delusions and fantasies. Depressed patients were thought to respond to stimulating activity, whereas schizophrenic patients should be involved in social interaction with others who produced simple, structured projects (Dunton, 1928).

Dunton's analysis established the basis for **activity analysis** (see Chapter 9, Section 3) and observation of the individual patient in reaction to the notion that mental illness was not so much due to poor habit training as it was to neurologic and unconscious etiology. Dunton (1918) was instrumental in establishing principles for the new field. Despite the changes and growth of occupational therapy over the years, many of his principles remain valid for clinicians today. He held that patient work should be interesting, should serve a useful end, should lead to an increase in the patient's knowledge, and should never be carried to the point of fatigue. The patient's needs should be studied before initiating the activity, and the cure, not the project, should be the primary concern.

Dr. Herbert Hall, a general practitioner; George Barton, an architect whose personal experience with tuberculosis led him to set up convalescent workshops for patients; and Susan Tracy, a nurse, joined forces with Dunton and Slagle to form the beginnings of the professional organization called the National Society for Promotion of Occupational Therapy. These leaders (except Tracy) met during 1917 at Barton's Consolation House in Clifton Springs, New York, where they stated the purpose of the society to be "the advancement of occupation as a therapeutic measure, the study of the effects of occupation upon the human being and the dissemination of scientific knowledge of this subject" (Hopkins, 1988, p. 22). Continuing their pursuit of disseminating the benefits of occupational therapy, the founders instituted the *Archives of Occupational Therapy* in 1922, which was renamed *Occupational Therapy in Rehabilitation* a decade later, as well as several seminal books laying out basic principles (Dunton, 1928; Haas, 1925).

By the time of the Great Depression in the 1930s, moral treatment had steadily declined again because of its presumed ineffectiveness and lack of sophistication. It was perceived as being culturally bound to the work ethic of the 19th century in addition to its implications of paternalism and institutional oppression. Symptomatic treatment, in which the occupational therapist attempted to match the correct activity with the patient's symptoms, was the essence of treatment. During this period, the occupational therapist was identified as an aide to the psychiatrist who provided a referral on which to base treatment. Activities were broad-based and variously involved music, art, recreation, work, drama, and arts and crafts. Economic hard times of the 1930s and lack of a guiding philosophy unique to occupational therapy led to a temporary diminution of occupational therapists. During this period, clinicians began to examine individual patient needs as opposed to focusing on the undifferentiated approach to the patients, which was consistent with habit training. Activities, selected with thoughtful care, were observed to be beneficial in the alleviation of a specific individual's symptoms.

Psychological and somatic treatment

With the advent of psychoanalytic thought, occupational therapists were taught to examine the nature of activities in relation to their ability to sublimate guilt, to provide an outlet for aggression and hostility, to express fantasy, and to experience creativity. From a present-day perspective, occupational therapists had forgotten the original value of seeing the patient in a holistic manner with attention to the needs for competence and mastery in a mind–body synthesis. They were becoming sensitive to patients' feelings and **symbolic behavior** (in which behavior, for example, hand washing, symbolizes guilt rather than the face value, cleansing the hands), however, and developing awareness of their own reactions and emotions. Furthermore, the occupational therapists' knowledge and acceptance of scientific inquiry (after many years of being guided primarily by intuition and common sense) as well as the acceptance of psychodynamic concepts were conducive to becoming valued members of psychiatric teams.

Concurrent with the development of psychoanalytic techniques in hospital, psychiatry, and somatic treatments, including electroconvulsive therapy (ECT), insulin shock and psychosurgery were used extensively. The physiologic basis for improvement in patients following ECT treatment was not understood; yet its use has continued until the present for severely depressed patients. Psychosurgery, particularly lobotomies, was undertaken in the 1940s and 1950s in the treatment of combative patients before the introduction of psychoactive medications. The role of the occupational therapist was to provide safe, diversional activities that might help recovering patients regain memory loss and occupy their day. As a result of somatic therapies, especially the antipsychotic drugs known as phenothiazines, which were introduced in the mid-1950s, patients previously too disturbed to participate in craft or group activities became amenable to occupational therapy as they were moved out of back wards.

In the 1990s, the complex, interactional cause involving biochemical, genetic, and environmental determinants is becoming more clear, although knowledge is well behind much of today's physical medicine in scientific understanding. Mid-20th century psychiatrists used both somatic and psychological techniques that sometimes worked, despite lack of scientific verification. This fact explains why psychoanalytic concepts, originally explicated by Freud in relation to middle class Victorian women, were applied across the board to all mental disorders, including severely disturbed hospitalized patients. In a comparable manner, electroconvulsive therapy (ECT) was used to treat a large variety of diagnoses, many of which are no longer thought to be responsive to these modes.

Manual of mental disorders

The first edition of the American Psychiatric Association's (APA) *Diagnostic and Statistical Manual of Mental Disorders (DSM)* appeared in 1952. Rather than attempt to discuss causality of mental illnesses, an impossibly difficult task given the subjectivity and theoretical allegiances in the field, the APA authors wisely chose to describe disorders in behavioral terms, thus lending greater objectivity and clarity to the diagnostic process. Reflecting the influence of Adolf Meyer, the *DSM-I* viewed mental disorders as representation of the personality to psychological, social, and biologic factors. Since the first *DSM,* three successive manuals have been published, each representing a snapshot of psychiatric thinking of the time. The manuals have had critical influence on the standardization of psychiatric concepts, which has been important to the growth in clinical practice and research.

Psychodynamic applications

Occupational therapy entered a spirited and vital period following the publication of Gail and Jay Fidler's *Introduction to Psychiatric Occupational Therapy* in 1954 and *Occupational Therapy: A Communication Process in Psychiatry* in 1963. These publications were the first to be authored by an occupational therapist since the 1920s. The Fidlers presented professional occupational therapy as an updated, sophisticated field that used psychoanalytic beliefs and techniques in facilitating symbolic activities, group communication processes, and projective techniques. They suggested that patients could experiment with new skills and means to handle emotions in the occupational therapy laboratory.

Participating in the Boiling Springs Conference (1956), Gail Fidler and others recommended that psychiatric occupational therapists set about learning how to (1) lead groups in a manner based on a thorough knowledge of group dynamics; (2) use oneself as a treatment tool in interpersonal dynamics between patient and therapist; (3) use a broad scope of activities; (4) create a therapeutic milieu; (5) contribute to the psychodynamic formulation of patients' behavior through the use of personality, social, and skills evaluation; (6) develop treatment goals as supplementary to psychotherapy; and (7) bridge the gap between community living and the hospital (West, 1959).

The above recommendations were significant in redirecting the field away from a rigidly controlled, impersonal emphasis on symptoms and matched activities to a more demanding and creative approach. Conversely, Mosey (1986) states that the emphasis on the use of self-concept encouraged therapists to stop using crafts and activities because, presumably, the *use of self* was more easily applied in a "speaking" than a "doing" format. It was not until the 1970s and 1980s and a return to original concepts of purposeful activity that therapists became comfortable with integrating verbal orientation with activity.

Gail Fidler (1969) had helped set the stage for this integration by introducing the concept of a task-oriented group. In task-oriented groups symbolic activities could be combined with discussion, thus helping patients communicate unconscious feelings.

Occupational therapists had always shown an ability to organize and direct the therapeutic milieu, as witnessed in the days of Slagle when they established the patient's routine by dividing the patients' day into segments of work, play, and rest. With the demise of moral treatment, however, they retreated from patient wards, sometimes to the dark basements of the hospitals where they waited for patients to be brought to them. As occupational therapists became more confident in the use of activity and in the role of team member, they emerged from the cellar to play an integral part in the ward environment. By the late 1970s, occupational therapists were leading groups in activities of daily living, discharge planning, prevocational exploration, and assertiveness training.

Community movement

Maxwell Jones (1953), a British psychiatrist, published *The Therapeutic Community,* which stimulated clinicians to create a social environment in which the patient could be an active participant in treatment by becoming involved in solving the daily problems of the treatment community. Patients developed independence and mastery by planning activities, developing rules and regulations, and investigating relevant issues in their environment. The environment fostered self-direction, dignity, and trust. The occupational therapist and other team members assisted in establishing a social climate dedicated to enhancing interpersonal skills, reality orientation, and functional independence. Experience in therapeutic community settings was conducive to the evolution of group treatment and the conscious structuring of group experiences for a therapeutic effect. The size of the group, the task of the group, and its homogeneity or heterogeneity were now recognized as notable determinants in group treatment.

The massive move of institutionalized mentally ill began in the 1950s with the establishment of the Joint Commission on Mental Illness and Health in 1955, which proposed a major shift from hospital to community, reorientation of hospital psychiatrists, lay person participation, and shared federal, state, and local funding. The National Institute of Mental Health was established by the Community Mental Health Act in 1963 to fund community mental health centers. Prompted by the growing awareness that treating individuals in the community could reduce the cost and agony of hospitalization, this legislation provided a monumental impetus to deinstitutionalization and, together with the impact of neuroleptic drugs, moved thousands of chronically mentally ill persons out of state hospitals where they had resided for years.

The community mental health movement opened up new forms of treatment that could be practiced with modifications in both inpatient and outpatient settings. Occupational therapists began applying behavioral approaches, such as reinforcement regimens and operant conditioning techniques to treat the long-term mentally ill. They also became familiar with new approaches, such as gestalt therapy, transactional analysis, and token economies. This period of American psychiatry was marked by optimism, exploration, and vitality. Freudian psychoanalysis had not proved beneficial in treating chronic or severely disturbed patients who could not manage verbal interchange or emotional insight.

The 1960s ushered in a time of great social concern led by President John F. Kennedy and followed by President Lyndon B. Johnson, whose Great Society legislation funded numerous health and social programs. Medicare and Medicaid legislation sponsored insurance funding for the elderly and the poor. Social unrest and demands for change characterized society, particularly among civil rights activists, young antiwar protesters, and women who, questioning their traditional lifestyles and subservience to men, began to request equal rights in the workplace and the home. Betty Friedan's work *The Feminine Mystique* (1963) jolted middle class women into an expanded awareness of the narrow nature of their housebound mores and stimulated them to push the workplace and even their husbands into a reexamination of women's place in American society. These invigorating thoughts and powerful feelings permeated professions occupied by women, including occupational therapy. Occupational therapists felt more comfortable with experimentation, with questioning authority, and eventually with questioning their own personal and professional identities. The climate was ripe for change, and the subsequent years witnessed a proliferation of theory, research, treatment methods, and even new disciplines.

Specialized disciplines arose and gathered strength around a modality of expression such as art, dance, music, and drama. Although each discipline appeared to splinter off from the domain that previously "belonged" to occupational therapy, these disciplines, entitled *creative art therapies* or *expressive art therapies*, were directed largely toward analytically based treatment whereas skill acquisition of broad-based community living skills became the priority of occupational therapy. Therapeutic recreation and vocational counseling also emerged as new specialized professions. The growth of these fields challenged occupational therapists to define carefully its own purpose and theories in addition to sorting out how to best negotiate a practice territory that had previously been only theirs.

A. Jean Ayres (1961) and Lorna Jean King (1974) began to explore the role of neurophysiology in childhood perceptual motor dysfunction and regressed schizophrenic patients, respectively. In psychiatric occupational therapy, King fomented an interest in sensory integrative techniques for treating regressed schizophrenic patients. Outlining a series of perceptual motor deficits that she discovered by observing chronic patients, King promulgated the use of gross motor interventions that were necessary to neurodevelopment before involving social adaptive measures. King's research in the 1960s and 1970s presaged the broad-spectrum interest and research in the neurosciences of the 1990s.

Continuing the drive toward professionalization of the field, the American Occupational Therapy Association (AOTA) provided active leadership in several influential ways. The Mental Health Special Interest Group (SIG) was formed in the early 1960s to disseminate information about psychosocial occupational therapy and to provide an opportunity for peer exchange and discussion of standards. The AOTA supported this effort by publishing a regular national newsletter, holding annual meetings at the national conference, and providing consultation and encouragement for state level SIG meetings.

In 1964, the AOTA appointed a psychiatric consultant to strengthen the skills and knowledge of occupational therapists in the field. Workshops were given throughout the country on object relations, supervision, group process, and evaluation. Recently, the AOTA has again acted with responsiveness to the needs of psychosocial occupational therapists by employing a consultant to provide information and encouragement in dealing with short-term care, changing roles, and new evaluation technology.

Table 17-1 provides a timeline of the evolution of occupational therapy.

Establishing purpose and identity

Despite the support of the AOTA, many occupational therapists practicing in psychiatry spoke of inability to define their practice. As a result of inarticulation and of their feelings of being in an auxiliary and defensive position in relation to core members of the treatment team, they spoke and behaved in defensive terms. At the same time, they truly believed that activity was a wellspring in the healing process; they had heard patients themselves reveal the joyous feelings of competence or the gradual return of memory following useful productivity. Attention is paid to the awareness of their need for a more solid theoretical foundation rather than on the intellectual floundering that these occupational therapists experienced. They recognized that the collection of ideas, good intentions, and intuition was an insufficient base on which to construct a strong professional identity, especially when women were still struggling against a subservient societal role.

After trying to gain status and recognition by identifying with medicine and requesting that the American Medical Association (AMA) approve occupational therapy curricula and that physicians prescribe occupational therapy, many leaders in the field assumed admirable initiative by defining various frames of reference for guiding treatment practice.

In 1967, several of the occupational therapist leaders met in Albion, Michigan, where they scrutinized a variety of divergent theories in an attempt to build a unifying occupational theory. Following this meeting, the *American Journal of Occupational Therapy* (*AJOT*) invited clinicians to publish their concepts of psychiatric practice in the September–October 1968 issue. The authors—Diasio, Tempone and Smith, Mosey, Watanabe, and Mazer—directed readers' attention to several then-current concepts including ego psychology, learning theory, and recapitulation of ontogenesis. This publication involved critical discussions and authors' responses that greatly stimulated thinking and discussion in the field in addition to forecasting the ambitious series of writings and research in the next decade.

Occupational therapists practicing in psychosocial settings continued to question their purpose. Were they employed to treat the disease or its symptoms? Should they emphasize the sequelae (consequences or aftereffects) of the disease? Was it more significant to focus on basic living skills to enable the patient to return to the community with an effective means of coping? Or was it more important to indicate the patient's occupational role such as housewife, student, or worker, and subsequently focus on the values and performance patterns that would allow him or her to return to that role? The occupational therapist's answers to these questions determined the relevant frame of reference, evaluation methods, and treatment or rehabilitation technology. The task of defining purpose, theory, and practice was enormous—almost overwhelming; however, a number of occupational therapists were excited by the challenge. The domain of occupational therapy was seen variously as dealing with the sequelae of disease, occupational roles and behaviors, daily living skills, and central nervous system (CNS) pathology.

Mary Reilly (1974) developed the occupational behavior frame of reference, which was based on earlier principles of the work–play–rest sequence in moral treatment as developed by Meyer and Dunton. She and her colleagues redirected the focus from habit training or diagnosis as the primary concern to occupational roles played out by each person in society. The occupational behavior framework designated the work–play continuum as most important in understanding human development. Healthy functioning of the working adult was viewed as dependent on successful influences of play experiences in childhood. The roles of worker, retiree, student, and so on, became "occupational behaviors," which were fundamental to health (Matsutsuyu, 1971). This orientation was organized around the value of activities or occupations in the establishment of healthy behaviors. As such, it was not concerned with medical model

TABLE 17-1.   *Evolution of Occupational Therapy*

Date	Event	Impact on Occupational Therapy
19th Century	Philosophy of Moral Treatment	Early OTs emphasize "good habits," balance of work, play, and nutrition and adjustment to hospital life. Focus is on cultural values, not individual needs or symptoms.
1917	National Society for Promotion of Occupational Therapy, organized in Clifton Springs, NY	Founders of OT (Dunton, Slagle, Barton, Hall, Tracy) publish tenets of field and begin education classes.
1920s	First occupational therapy publications	Founders establish basic principles.
1930	Moral treatment declines; neurologic deficits are viewed as causes of mental illness.	OT declines due to lack of support and economic depression.
1930–1950	Psychoanalytic influence on psychiatry	OTs become aide to psychiatrist; focus is on symptoms and nature of activity in treatment.
1950s	Somatic treatments: electroshock, insulin shock, psychosurgery, psychoactive drugs used to treat psychotic patients	Disturbed patients become more amenable to OT. Hospital stay shortens.
1952	*DSM* published	OTs learn to describe and classify behaviors in relation to diagnosis.
1953	Publication of *The Therapeutic Community* (Maxwell Jones)	Patients are expected to plan and use social environment in therapeutic process.
1954	Fidlers publish *Introduction to Psychiatric Occupational Therapy*	Psychoanalytic theory is introduced to OTs.
1956	Boiling Springs Conference	OT enters more dynamic period. Focus changes from strict use of crafts to symbolic meanings and relationships.
1960s	Projective batteries developed	OTs begin to use evaluation techniques.
	The Women's Movement	OTs question traditional ideas and relationships and search for professional identity.
	Formation of new associations in recreation, dance, art, music therapy, drama	OTs question breadth of role and professional purpose.
1960	Behavioral treatment introduced in psychiatry	OTs use behavior modification, gestalt therapy, and transactional analysis.
	Perceptual motor research (Ayres)	OTs become aware of perceptual dysfunction in psychoses.
	Psychiatric Special Interest Group (PSIG) established	PSIG provides peer exchange and dissemination of information and standards.
	O'Connor v. Donaldson Supreme Court Decision	Patient cannot be committed unless dangerous to self or others; treatment is mandated for committed patients.
1963	Community Mental Health Act	OTs use group techniques to discuss ideas and feelings.
	Fidlers publish *Occupational Therapy: A Communication Process*	Different forms of occupational therapy—analytic, supportive, directive—are established.
1967	Albion, MI, meeting of mental health occupational therapists	New professionalism is encouraged via exploration of knowledge base.
1968	*AJOT* publishes four frames of reference.	OTs begin to use conceptual models on which to base treatment.
1970s	OTs question domain of the field	Purposes of field defined as sequelae of disease, living skills, occupational roles and behaviors, CNS pathology.
1970	Proliferation of frames of reference	Identified theories are analytical, occupational behavior, acquisitional, sensory integration, developmental, cognitive disabilities, model of human occupation.

(continued)

TABLE 17-1. *Evolution of Occupational Therapy (continued)*

Date	Event	Impact on Occupational Therapy
	Diversification of work settings	OTs expand areas of service delivery from hospitals to schools, private practice, outpatient agencies, and home visits.
	Expansion of practice technology	OTs begin using assertiveness training, stress management, gestalt and transaction techniques and meditation.
1970	Wyatt v. Stickney Supreme Court Decision	Treatment rights of hospitalized patients are defined and enumerated.
1973	Rehabilitation Act (P.L. 93–112) and Amendments (P.L. 93–516) 1974	Vocational rehabilitation of the handicapped, including mentally ill persons is provided.
1974	Souder v. Brennan Supreme Court decision	Patients can no longer work without pay.
	Education of All Handicapped Children Act (P.L. 94–142) 1975 and Amendments (P.L. 99–457), 1986.	Laws are provided for education for handicapped children; including funding for occupational therapy.
1976	Mental Health Task Force Report	OTs identify professional uncertainty and call for theory building, research, and graduate-level training.
1978	OT: 2001, Scottsdale Conference	Leaders call for philosophical base, research, and decision about technical or professional field.
1980s	Publication of many OT books and journals	OT begins renaissance of theory, research, and re-identification with lost roots of founders.
1980s	Growth of consumerism	OTs recognize self-help groups and support consumers' rights to self-determination
1986	AOTA conducts national seminars in program development (SCOPE).	OTs refine skills in innovative programming.
1988	AOTA conducts national seminars in clinical reasoning (FOCUS).	OTs link practice to therapy through clinical reasoning.
1990	Economic constraints stem rising health care costs.	OTs adapt to shorter lengths of stay and downsizing of programs by reexamining technology and moving to outpatient programs.
1991	Neuroscience research in etiology of mental illness	Role of rehabilitation is questioned in view of biochemical findings.

elements such as disease or sequelae. Furthermore, it removed occupational therapists from dependency on physicians and allied itself more with sociologic and anthropologic thinking.

In 1980, Gary Kielhofner and Janice P. Burke built on Reilly's occupational behavior model and developed a now widely known comprehensive occupational therapy theory, the *Model of Human Occupation*. During the 1980s and 1990s, this model, which is based on conceiving of the human being as an open system with three hierarchical subsystems—the volitional subsystem, the habituation subsystem, and the performance subsystem—was further refined and clarified for easier use by practicing occupational therapists.

Lorna Jean King (1974), on the other hand, stated that pathology, particularly pathology of the CNS, should be a prime consideration in the treatment of chronic schizophrenic patients. Treating this disorder with gross motor, balancing, and bilateral exercises was seen as beneficial sensory integrative treatment of the CNS, which must precede any social adaptation within the environment.

Another clear and useful theory that became exceedingly popular with clinicians during the 1970s was the *developmental theory* developed by Mosey (1970) and also by Llorens (1986).

Building on the concept of recapitulation of ontogenesis, Mosey outlined stage-specific tasks that each person must acquire in the maturational process. Health is defined as having successfully learned age-appropriate skills, whereas the converse is true of ill health or dysfunction. Treatment used the provision of simulated individual–environment interactions that are necessary for learning of skills at the indicated stage. For example, parallel play activities may be appropriate for an older child who has regressed to preschool behavior following an illness. In *Three Frames of Reference for Mental Health* (1970), Mosey described not only the developmental frame of reference but also the acquisitional model, which students will recognize as behavioral, and the object relation model, which is similar to the analytic frame of reference explicated earlier by the Fidlers.

Claudia Allen (1985), in developing the cognitive disabilities frame of reference, contributed valuable guidelines for treating patients who suffer from deficits related to brain functioning. Determining the patient's cognitive level and providing an appropriate environment and occupational treatment has been viewed as particularly beneficial for psychotic and organically impaired patients.

During the 1970s and continuing into the 1980s, occupational therapy experienced a renaissance in proliferation of theory development and frames of reference that linked theory to practice. The field was gradually emerging from an institution-based technical practice into a theory-based profession. Diversification of work settings occurred as therapists began to take more risks and perceived themselves less dependent on the security of institutional practice. Therapists gained entrance to school systems when federal law mandated that all handicapped children had a right to public education. Moving into outpatient programs, private practice, home health systems, and prison systems, they expanded their methodologies from a sole focus on crafts to a broad spectrum of educational and training modes including assertiveness training, stress management, problem solving, relaxation training, and other specialized content.

The late 1970s witnessed leaders' responses to the energy implicit within the recent theory-building years. The AOTA supported a mental health task force in 1976 (Report of the Mental Health Task Force) and held the Scottsdale Conference in 1978 in which academicians and clinicians called for a philosophical base, research, and graduate level education.

Shortly thereafter, occupational therapists in the field who saw themselves struggling to define their practice spoke of their pride and relief when a number of mental health books and journals were published. These publications dealt with theory and its application, program descriptions, research studies, and case studies. This immense dissemination of information, which allowed therapists to feel less isolated and provided opportunities for intellectual sharing, was further supported by the AOTA, which conducted nationwide seminars in program development (SCOPE, 1986) and clinical reasoning (FOCUS, 1988). These cumulative efforts resulted in a new, stronger professional image for occupational therapists who could better articulate their treatment role as they interacted with members of the multidisciplinary teams.

Civil rights of the mentally ill

Just as the Civil Rights Movement in the United States affected the rights of African-Americans and women during the 1960s, it also protected the hospitalized mentally ill. In 1960, the Supreme Court case of O'Connor v. Donaldson held that an involuntarily held person has a right to receive treatment and that if that person is not dangerous to self or others, he or she cannot be confined to a hospital (Lancaster, 1988). Treatment rights were further guaranteed in the 1970 U.S. Supreme Court case of Wyatt v. Stickney, in which treatment rights were defined to include individualized treatment plans and treatment in the least restrictive setting. Most states now provide patients with the right to uncensored communication, visitation, privacy, and standards of the Joint Commission on Accreditation of Healthcare Organizations (JCAHO) mandate a clean and safe environment and the right to wear their own clothing. Mentally ill patients have the right to be treated with respect and dignity and to be informed of their rights and of the treatment given to them. In addition, patients who used to work long hours in institutional cafeterias or laundry rooms no longer are allowed to work without pay as a result of the 1974 Souder v. Brennan Supreme Court decision.

Civil rights for the handicapped, a category in which the mentally ill were included, were further extended by several more important pieces of legislation, the Rehabilitation Act of 1973, the Education of All Handicapped Children Act of 1974, the Fair Housing Amendment Act of 1988, and the Americans with Disabilities Act of 1990. These laws not only protect the physically and mentally handicapped, they also provide treatment and rehabilitation opportunities for such persons and lead to growth potential in occupational therapy.

Consumerism

Patients and their families have played an increasingly strong part in determining the shape of care. Because less blame has been attributed to families for causing mental illness and because the public has had better access to mental health information, consumers and their families have formed local and national self-help groups, such as the National Alliance for the Mentally Ill (NAMI). The goal of this organization is to influence lawmakers and funding sources to improve treatment, to conduct research, and to provide education. In a comparable manner, Alcoholics Anonymous (AA) and Narcotics Anonymous (NA) have provided solace for its members as well as political advocacy. Occupational therapists will do well to integrate their aftercare planning with such self-help groups in the 90s.

Two important trends, economic constraints and **neuroscience** research, have had an enormous impact on the practice of occupational therapy in the early 1990s. These phenomena are reviewed in greater depth in Chapter 17, Section 1C. Briefly, rising costs in health care have led to shorter lengths of hospital stay, rigid monitoring of admission and discharge criteria, as well as third-party analysis and curtailment of perceived unnecessary treatment procedures. Diversional activity and nonspecific treatment goal setting have been rejected in a massive cost control effort by insurance carriers.

Neuroscience research has caused a major revolution in the etiologic understanding of mental illnesses, particularly psychiatric disorders. Although findings in neuroscience place new emphasis on genetic and biochemical causes of psychiatric diseases, practical information and application of the findings are yet unknown. Occupational therapy's role undoubtedly will become important in assisting patients with information processing and cognitive retraining.

References

Allen, C. (1985). *Occupational therapy for psychiatric diseases. Measurement and management of cognitive disabilities.* Boston: Little, Brown & Co.

American Journal of Occupational Therapy. (1968). Special section: Theories of psychiatric occupational therapy, *22,* 397–546.

American Occupational Therapy Association. (1986). *SCOPE.* Rockville, MD: Author.

American Occupational Therapy Association. (1988). *FOCUS.* Rockville, MD: Author.

American Psychiatric Association. (1952). *Diagnostic and statistical manual of mental disorders.* Washington, DC: Author.

Americans with Disabilities Act of 1990. (Summer, 1990). *American Rehabilitation,* 2–32.

Ayres, A. J. (1961). The development of body scheme in children. *American Journal of Occupational Therapy, 15,* 3.

Beers, C. (1908). *A mind that found itself.* New York: Doubleday, Doran & Co.

Bockoven, J. S. (1963) *Moral treatment in American psychiatry.* New York: Springer.

Diasio, K. (1968). Psychiatric occupational therapy: Search for a conceptual framework in light of psychoanalytic ego psychology and learning theory. *American Journal of Occupational Therapy, 22,* 400–414.

Dunton, W. R. (1918). The principles of occupational therapy. *Public Health Nurse, 10,* 320.

Dunton, W. R. (1928). *Prescribing occupational therapy,* Springfield, IL: Charles C Thomas.

Fidler, G. (1969). The task-oriented group as a context for treatment. *American Journal of Occupational Therapy, 23,* 1, 43–48.

Fidler, G. S., & Fidler, J. W. (1954). *Introduction to psychiatric occupational therapy.* New York: Harper & Row.

Fidler, G. S., & Fidler, J. W. (1963). *Occupational therapy: A communication process in psychiatry.* New York: MacMillan.

Friedan, B. (1963). *The feminine mystique.* New York: W. W. Norton & Co.

Gillette, N. (1983). Preface. In G. Kielhofner (author) *Health through occupation: Theory and practice in occupational therapy.* Philadelphia: F. A. Davis.

Haas, L. J. (1925). *Practical occupational therapy.* Milwaukee: Bruce.

Hopkins, H. L. (1988). An historical perspective of occupational therapy. In H. L. Hopkins & H. D. Smith (Eds.), *Willard and Spackman's Occupational therapy* (7th ed.), Philadelphia: J. B. Lippincott.

Jones, M. (1953). *The therapeutic community.* New York: Basic Books.

Kielhofner, G., & Burke, J. P. (1980). A model of human occupation. Part I. Conceptual framework and content. *American Journal of Occupational Therapy. 34,* 572–581.

King, L. J. (1974). A sensory integrative approach to schizophrenia. *American Journal of Occupational Therapy, 28,* 259–536.

Lancaster, J. (1988). *Adult psychiatric nursing.* New York: Medical Examination Publishing Company, 622–624.

Llorens, L. A. (1986). *Application of developmental theory for health and rehabilitation.* Rockville, MD: American Occupational Therapy Association.

Matsutsuyu, J. (1971). Occupational behavior: A perspective on work and play. *American Journal of Occupational Therapy, 25,* 291–294.

Mazer, J. (1968). Toward an integrated theory of occupational therapy. *American Journal of Occupational Therapy, 22,* 451–456.

Meyer, A. (1921). The philosophy of occupational therapy. *Archives of Occupational Therapy, 1,* 1–10.

Mosey, A. C. (1968). Recapitulation of ontogenesis. *American Journal of Occupational Therapy, 22,* 426–438.

Mosey, A. C. (1970). *Three frames of reference for mental health.* Thorofare, NJ: Slack.

Mosey, A. C. (1986). *Psychosocial components of occupational therapy.* New York: Raven Press.

Reilly, M. (1974). *Play as exploratory learning,* Los Angeles: Sage.

Report of the Mental Health Task Force (1976). *Occupational Therapy Newspaper, 30,* 6–7.

Slagle, E. C. (1922). Training aides for mental patients. *Archives of Occupational Therapy, 1,* 14.

Tempone, V., & Smith, A. (1968). Psychiatric occupational therapy within a learning theory context. *American Journal of Occupational Therapy, 22,* 415–425.

Tiffany, E. G. (1988). Psychiatry and mental health. In H. L. Hopkins & H. D. Smith (Eds.). *Willard and Spackman's Occupational therapy* (7th ed.). Philadelphia: J. B. Lippincott.

Watanabe, S. (1968). Four concepts basic to the occupational therapy process. *American Journal of Occupational Therapy, 22,* 439–450.

West, W. L. (Ed.). (1959). *Changing concepts and practices in psychiatric occupational therapy.* New York: American Occupational Therapy Association.

SECTION 1C
Trends affecting occupational therapy

DIANE GIBSON

KEY TERMS

Destigmatization

Employee Assistance
   Programs

Managed Care

Neuroimaging Techniques

Residential Treatment
   Centers

Utilization Review

LEARNING OBJECTIVES

Upon completion of this section the reader will be able to:

1. *Describe three results of cost containment that will affect occupational therapy during the 1990s.*

2. *Describe two neuroscience research findings and discuss their role in destigmatization.*

3. *Define an employee assistance program.*

4. *List three different outpatient programs and their advantages to patients.*

Future trends

Psychiatry and the wider domain of mental health programs will continue to be characterized by extensive change during the 1990s. Changes are evolving currently in medical economics in which the rapid increase in cost is making an impact on how long and by whom patients may be treated, on the rise of agencies external to the clinic mandating the extent and kinds of treatment to be used, and on modifications in the roles of health care providers. Biochemical research and developments in psychopharmacology have provided new understanding of the cause of many psychiatric disorders as well as new medications to control unwanted symptoms. A gradual destigmatization of the mentally ill is transforming public opinion; and concurrently employee assistance programs (EAPs) are being used widely within businesses to provide employees with nondiscriminatory, accessible mental health counseling.

Occupational therapists and their clinical colleagues will see a changing mix of patient population during the next 10 years. Moreover, they will treat increasing numbers of aged men and women, indigent persons, children, and AIDS victims. Finally, the extraordinary shortage of occupational therapists will continue during the next decade, thus forcing changes in professional roles and treatment programs. It behooves the occupational therapist to follow these trends to adapt to the rapidly changing service delivery system and the demands of newly created roles in health care.

Rising health care costs

The National Mental Health Association (NMHA) cites that one in five adults suffers from mental illness (*Special Report of the Federation of American Health Systems Review*, 1988). It estimates that 29 million Americans, or 19% of those over age 18, suffer from mental illness. These illnesses include anxiety disorders such as phobias, panic, and obsessive-compulsive disorders; alcohol and drug abuse; depression; and schizophrenia. Although the incidence of mental illness is high, only one in five mentally ill persons is treated.

Newspapers and magazines report alarm on the part of employers, the government, and the consuming public over the exorbitant rise in health care costs. Sharfstein (1990) noted that expenditures in 1990 for health care services exceeded $660 billion, or 12% of the Gross National Product (GNP), and that health care spending will continue to increase at a rate of 12% to 15% annually for the next 5 years. These costs were disproportionately accounted for by the increase in adolescent and substance abuse hospitalizations compared with adult hospitalizations.

The understandable concern of third-party payors including commercial insurance companies, government programs such as Medicare and Medicaid, and Blue Cross have led to a number of responses predicated on the need to restrict, limit, and control mental health costs (Morris & Peck, 1990). Baum (1991) has stated,

> ... increase in health care costs is affecting the gross domestic product and, thus, the net profits of U. S. corporations, which is prompting the control of health care costs we see today. This trend will continue as more companies build systems to self-insure their employees to control costs. Occupational therapy is affected in that as industry contracts directly with health maintenance organizations (HMOs) and preferred provider organizations (PPOs), the assurance of inclusion of our services is difficult unless such services have been deemed primary and cost effective. (p. 487)

Managed care companies act as intermediaries between insurance companies and hospitals by investigating the need for admissions and for continued hospital stay according to stringent criteria (Sharfstein & Beigel, 1985). The purpose of managed care, along with ***utilization review*** in which the frequency of services used is compared with set standards and procedures, is designed to shorten lengths of hospital stay and to cut costs paid to hospitals and practitioners. HMOs and PPOs originated from an attempt to control costs and monitor quality of care. In the health care field, a great debate presently rages in which managed-care proponents claim that health care professionals have ignored the costs of their services and have continued to perform the kinds of treatment they like best with the kinds of patients they like best. Clinicians, on the other hand, claim that managed care is a euphemism for breaking down both quality and quantity of care with the specific result being premature hospital discharges of seriously ill patients or inability of similar patients to gain access to the hospital in the first place.

In some cases, outcome research studies have indicated that short-term hospitalizations may be most beneficial to patients who can more easily return to family and community roles after only brief stays (Talbott & Glick, 1988). Chronic schizophrenia patients have not improved more significantly in long-term (30 to 90 days) than they did in short-term (under 30 days) treatment periods (Talbott & Glick, 1988).

The changing medical economic market has caused further turbulence in institutional life as we enter the 1990s.

> Layoffs, institutional reorganizations, and changes in staffing and productivity expectations are all occurring in response to changing reimbursement patterns and efforts to contain health care costs, and all this is happening while trying to compete in a market-driven environment. (Schell, 1990, p. 5)

Ultimately, occupational therapy survivors will acknowledge the reality and persistence of the new economic scene and adapt to shorter lengths of stay as well as to other forces with typical resiliency and creativity.

Diversification of treatment settings

The range of available treatment settings has enlarged and become increasingly diversified during the last decade (Gibson, 1990). Halfway houses, quarterway houses, ***residential treatment centers*** (RTCs), partial hospital programs, psychosocial programs, and even mobile treatment units now constitute options in outpatient care not dreamed of 30 years ago. Such programs are planned to provide extensions of inpatient care within a continuum for the seriously mentally ill or to provide viable options for clients who do not need the safety and level of supervision found within hospital settings. The advantage of such extensive options is the opportunity to match the client's need with the most appropriate program in addition to the lesser expense afforded by outpatient compared with inpatient settings.

Neuroscience research

Neuroscience research regarding mental illness etiology has expanded exponentially in the last 10 years (Farber, 1989; Gibson, 1990). The neuroscientific revolution, which has already become part of public awareness through news media, has evolved from the application of new technology and new science to some of the old problems of psychiatry, such as depression/anxiety and the degenerative neuropathologies of middle and late life (Smith, 1988). Brain scanning and other ***neuroimaging techniques***, such as positron emission tomography (PET), nuclear magnetic resonance (NMR), and computed tomography (CT), are bringing about a renaissance in the sciences of neuroanatomy and neurophysiology.

Neurochemical and genetic research has determined that many mental disorders such as schizophrenia, severe depression, manic depression, and alcoholism are caused by an interaction of biochemical and genetic determinants and of environmental stressors. Regarding schizophrenia, a core hypothesis is that acute positive symptoms such as hallucinations, delusions, and thought disorder are caused by the presence of excessive dopamine in the presynaptic neurons (Brown & Mann, 1985). Neuroleptic drugs are used to block the presynaptic dopamine receptors and thus diminish acute psychotic symptoms. MRI has revealed enlarged ventricles in the brains of schizophrenic patients (Pardes, 1991). These findings, including newly emerging etiologic data about depression, alcoholism, and Alzheimer's disease, are encouraging because they suggest possible cures or amelioration of painful symptoms. Researchers are expecting that medications prescribed to treat chemically dependent persons will stabilize their biochemistry in the same way that insulin benefits diabetics.

A positive collateral effect is the removal of blame from the families of patients who previously have been attacked vigorously as uncaring or overprotective. As researchers conclude specific roles of brain biochemistry, their findings are leading to increasingly specialized use of psychopharmacology. As a result, the future psychiatrist necessarily will focus on differential diagnoses and prescription of psychoactive medications.

Changing patient mix

Baum (1991) states that occupational therapists will have to concern themselves with treating an ever-increasing population of elderly people in the next 50 years. Community-based prevention and long-term care in the community rather than the nursing home, will focus on disability reduction and rehabilitation. Women in the work force who support aging parents will need special programs and accommodations in the business world to adapt to this phenomenon. Children will receive increased attention in the next decade due to greater awareness of at-risk populations, health promotion programs, managing children of working parents, and new treatments for infants surviving at 26 weeks' gestation. Occupational therapy's role within the school system has been consolidated and should grow, given these developments. People afflicted with AIDS will grow in number and will require the services of occupational therapists as will the number of persons abusing alcohol and cocaine.

Destigmatization

As a result of heightened public awareness and the breakdown of traditional myths surrounding mental illness, psychiatric patients are beginning to feel less stigmatized (***destigmatization***). Psychiatric problems and drug addiction can be treated rather than viewed as permanently incurable. New state laws are being enacted that prevent patient abuse and protect civil liberties. As information is disseminated through public media, help lines, community education, and self-help groups such as Alcoholics Anonymous (AA) and Narcotics Anonymous (NA), fear of and prejudice toward those with mental illness are diminishing. This allows people with psychiatric disorders to feel more like those suffering from physical problems. Patients and their families play an important role in openly accepting and discussing their experiences, thus reducing misunderstanding. Interest in wellness and a sense of responsibility for one's rights and health have prompted growth in public health workshops and subsequent growth in awareness of mental health concepts. Occupational therapists give lectures and seminars in stress management, assertiveness training, and balancing of work and play. In doing so, they are teaching public health components while simultaneously destigmatizing mental illness and building awareness of mental health.

Employee assistance programs

Employee assistance programs were developed during the past decade as a means of cutting back on employer costs resulting from alcoholism and drug abuse, which manifested in lower productivity, more absenteeism, and poor morale in the workplace. The EAP philosophy assumes that employees can and should be treated in their working and living environments if at all possible. These programs in business have grown dramatically because employees enjoy the confidentiality and ease with which they are provided quality counseling and referral to needed professionals. In some cases, EAPs act as key referral agents to inpatient and outpatient services and therefore may be a significant link in the psychiatric continuum of settings. As EAPs continue to demonstrate quality mental health services for the worker, they will help to produce a healthier work force, one in which persons with disabling mental illness will be treated as compassionately as a person with cancer.

Shortage of occupational therapists

A critical and frustrating shortage of occupational therapists in mental health services has existed since the late 1980s and will continue to be a problem during the 1990s. Although occupational therapy began in hospital psychiatry 75 years ago, clinicians are choosing to work in private practice, home health, general hospitals, and rehabilitation centers in 1990. Between 1977 and 1986, the proportion of registered occupational therapists working in mental health decreased by 11.3% (AOTA Member Data Survey). Various solutions to the shortage have been attempted including abolishing positions, filling vacant positions with other allied health personnel, and employing contract occupational therapists to treat patients and supervise paraprofessional staff. These solutions are not beneficial to the field of occupational therapy because they change the complexion of treatment and do not allow representation of occupational therapy on treatment teams. Additionally, fewer fieldwork supervisors who are critically needed for completion of occupational therapy education are available for supervision.

Lower salaries in mental health work compound the problem in an area already perceived to be less desirable than other areas because of the ambiguity and lesser status of this practice area. In the near future, mental health occupational therapists will concentrate on consultative contractual services in addition to providing functional assessments and supervision.

Directions for the future

Given the extensive changes occurring in psychiatry reviewed in the previous section, what can occupational therapists do to continue effective and efficient treatment as well as to maintain the viability of their roles? Some suggestions follow.

1. *Emphasize functional assessments* that delineate present strengths and deficits in relation to posthospital roles related to work, leisure, self-care, and family life. "Doing" in therapy is a unique characteristic of occupational therapy and as such represents an important difference from other fields. Occupational therapists can ensure their growth and survival by providing valid performance assessments using standardized tests. Repeated assessments to predict community adjustment and select appropriate housing and vocational discharge plans will play an important role. By focusing on the patient's discrete levels of functioning in

emotional, interpersonal, cognitive, and motor areas, the occupational therapist can assist the interdisciplinary team in identifying the performance areas that facilitate patients' successful postdischarge adjustment in the community (Gibson, 1990). Occupational therapists will become valuable assets to insurance carriers and managed-care use reviewers who are interested in measures that predict anticipated lengths of stay and outcome measures.

2. *Use psychoeducational modules* that are an efficient and effective method of delivering treatment, such as stress management, assertiveness training, interpersonal skills, activities of daily living, and discharge planning. These modules should be broken down into single-session segments and offered on a pretest and posttest basis with an emphasis on transferability to postdischarge living. Behavioral and learning principles can be easily used and adapted for short-term treatment.

3. *Undertake outcome studies* that will potentially validate the importance of purposeful activity in establishing or re-establishing skills essential for community living. As direction for the future, this recommendation has been made many times in the past. In fact, research throughout occupational therapy is increasing, although not at a sufficient rate nor with sufficient exposure in journals to increase the visibility and credibility of the profession. Outcome studies linking theory to practice content will establish credibility with reimbursement and funding offices which in turn will make an indirect positive impact on our professional self-esteem as well as our ability to attract new occupational therapists to mental health.

4. *Resolve staff shortages* by
   a. implementing multifaceted actions such as continuing education programs for reentry candidates;
   b. establishing career ladders and master clinician designations;
   c. enhancing psychiatric arena by reducing the ambiguity of treatment concepts and clarifying the function of occupational therapy;
   d. offering continuing education programs to fieldwork supervisors and senior clinicians that address assertiveness training and negotiation with formal and informal power bases in organizations; and
   e. providing a mental health information exhibit for use by occupational therapy schools.

The cited directions for the future do not stand separately but should be seen as interlocking and dynamic suggestions that speak to our need to develop and integrate theory, research, credibility, and professional self-confidence. See the display for a summary of future trends.

References

American Occupational Therapy Association. *Data survey* (1977, 1982, 1986, 1990). Rockville, MD: Author.

Baum, C. (1991). The environment: Providing opportunities for the future. *American Journal of Occupational Therapy, 45*(6), 487–490.

Brown, R. P., & Mann, J. J. (1985). A clinical perspective on the role of neurotransmitters in mental disorders. *Hospital and Community Psychiatry, 36,* 141–149.

Farber, S. D. (1989). Neuroscience and occupational therapy: Vital connections. *American Journal of Occupational Therapy, 43,* 637–645.

Gibson, G. (1990). The challenge of adaptation: Shaping service delivery to meet changing needs. *Hospital and Community Psychiatry, 41*(23), 267–269.

Morris, J., & Peck, J. (1990). Shifts in economic trends may underscore impact on future mental health. *Business and Health, 4*(5), 58.

Pardes, H. (1991). From the president. *Psychiatric News,* July 5.

Schell, B. A. (1990). From the chair. Administration and management. *SIS Newsletter, 6*(1), 5.

Sharfstein, S. (1990). Managed mental health care. *1992 APA annual update.* Approved for publication. Washington, DC: American Psychiatric Association.

Sharfstein, S. S., & Beigel, A. (Eds.). (1985). *The new economics and psychiatric care.* Washington, DC: American Psychiatric Press.

Smith, C. U. M. (1988). Biology and psychiatry. *Journal of the Royal Society of Medicine, 81,* 439.

Special report. (1988). New directions in mental health care. *Federation of American Health Systems Review, 21*(3), 10–11.

Talbott, J. A., & Glick, I. D. (1988). The inpatient care of the chronic mentally ill. In J. R. Lion, W. N. Adler & W. L. Webb, Jr. (Eds.), *Modern Hospital Psychiatry* (pp. 352–370). New York. W. W. Norton & Co.

SECTION 1D
Practice settings

GAIL Z. RICHERT and DIANE GIBSON

FUTURE TRENDS SUMMARY

- Extensive change throughout the 90s
- Significant neuroscience research
- Increase in employee assistance programs (EAPs)
- Increased numbers of aged, indigent, AIDS victims, children at risk, alcohol and cocaine abusers
- Shortage of occupational therapists
- Economic cutbacks
- Decrease in inpatient beds
- Increase in numbers of outpatients
- Movement of OTs from institutions to community

KEY TERMS

Case Manager	*Health Promotion*
Community Mental Health Centers	*Hospital Admission Criteria*
Community Rehabilitation Program	*Partial Hospitalization Program*
Community Residence	*Private Practice*
Consultant	*Quarterway House*
Continuum of Care	*Role Blurring*
Halfway House	*Transitional Living Continuum*

Upon completion of this section the reader will be able to:
1. *List two criteria for admission to an inpatient hospital.*
2. *Identify current trends in mental health practice.*
3. *Identify current mental health practice settings.*
4. *Describe alternative mental health practice models.*

Trends

As previously mentioned in Chapter 17, Section 1C, significant changes in mental health service delivery have occurred in recent years. These trends have made the most severe impact on the mentally ill population: practice settings, service delivery, and mental health professionals, including registered occupational therapists (OTRs). According to the National Institute of Mental Health, there has been a recent trend away from hospitalization of the mentally ill (AOTA, 1990, p. 12). Yet in the 1990 Member Data Survey of the American Occupational Therapy Association, 55.1% of mental health occupational therapists were reported to be in hospital-based practices (Table 17-2). With decreasing lengths of stay in general and psychiatric hospitals, there is a trend toward provision of services in outpatient and nontraditional settings. Therapists' reluctance to move toward practice outside the hospital often relates to unclear professional practice roles, noncompetitive salaries, and few role models (Adams, 1990, 1991).

The proportion of occupational therapists and assistants in mental health continues to decline among practitioners. Most OTRs work with adults (67.4%), whereas 24% work with children and adolescents and 8.2% work with the elderly. Mental retardation and schizophrenic and affective disorders are the most common primary patient health problems treated by occupational therapists (Table 17-3).

With the trend toward outpatient and nontraditional or alternative practice models, increasing emphasis is on the **continuum of care** for psychiatric services. This means that service may begin with short-term inpatient hospitalization and proceed to residential, then outpatient care. When these services focus on those in a particular diagnostic group such as schizophrenia, they may be designed as a product or service line and are marketed as a continuum of care for that population.

Practice settings

Hospitals

Typical hospital settings are psychiatric units of general hospitals, private psychiatric hospitals, and federal- and state-funded public hospitals. The hospital setting is reserved for critically ill patients who must be treated in a controlled milieu offering 24-hour supervision. **Hospital admission criteria** are danger to self or others and severe disorganization that has rendered the patient unable to care for himself or herself (Gibson, 1988).

Since the level of pathology is significantly greater in inpatients than outpatients, hospitalized patients typically may be disorganized, acutely paranoid, delusional, violent, or possibly

TABLE 17-2. *Profile of Occupational Therapists in Mental Health*

Primary Work Setting	Percent	
	1990	1986
College, 2-year	0.3	0.3
College/university, 4-year	1.9	1.4
Community mental health center	5.8	6.4
Day care program	2.2	2.3
HMO, PPO, IPA	0.2	0.1
Home health agency	0.4	0.2
Hospice	0	0
General hospital:		
Neonatal intensive care unit	0	—
Psychiatric unit	21.1	—
Rehabilitation unit	0.2	0.8
All other	6.7	21.3
Pediatric hospital	0.4	0.4
Psychiatric hospital	26.7	30.4
Outpatient clinic (freestanding)	0.9	1.1
Physician's office	0	0.1
Private industry	0	0.2
Private practice	2.5	2.0
Public health agency	0.4	0.4
Rehabilitation center at hospital	1.0	1.4
Research facility	0.2	0.1
Residential care facility, group home or independent living center	9.2	9.3
Retirement or senior center	0	0.2
School system (incl. private school)	11.3	10.1
Sheltered workshop/supported environment	1.7	1.3
Skilled nursing facility or intermediate care facility	3.8	5.9
Vocational or prevocational program	0.8	0.8
Voluntary agency (eg, Easter Seal/U.C.P.)	0.4	0.4
Other	1.9	3.0

Dashes indicate category not included on 1986 Member Data Survey.

self-destructive. As a result, the occupations planned, the unit environment, and the relationship with the patient need thoughtful planning tailored to his or her level of functioning at the time of treatment. Acute care emphasizes symptom reduction, medication, diagnosis, and discharge planning.

The occupational therapist works side by side with other unit personnel in providing a safe, stable, daily routine for the patient in crisis. Daily activities, balanced diet, and regular sleep periods are important for reducing the sense of subjective chaos experienced by hospitalized persons. Within the humane hospital atmosphere, care must be taken to provide for the safety of both patients and staff. Hence, policies and procedures pertaining to suicide prevention, behavioral monitoring, and aggression management are mandated to control destructive behavior when a patient is not able to manage his or her behavior from within. *Regression* in the form of evasion of responsibility, dependency, and obliviousness to others becomes a potential danger when patients remain unnecessarily long in an institution (Drake & Sederer, 1986; Wing, 1962).

Delayed return to social and vocational roles and loss of social supports are conducive to lowered self-esteem and further

TABLE 17-3. *Profile of Occupational Therapists in Mental Health*

	1990 (%)	1986 (%)
Primary Health Problem Patient		
Adjustive Disorder	5.1	5.7
Affective Disorder	22.0	17.9
Alcohol/Substance use Disorders	4.8	5.1
Anxiety Disorders	0.6	1.4
Eating Disorders	1.0	0
Mental Retardation	29.7	27.7
Organic Mental Disorders	4.5	7.3
Personality Disorders	3.4	3.6
Schizophrenic Disorders	24.7	27.4
Other Psychotic Disorders	0.6	1.1
Other Mental Health Disorders	3.6	2.8
Age Range of Patients		
Less than 3 years	1.5	*
3–5 years	3.1	
6–12 years	10.3	
13–18 years	9.5	
19–64 years	67.4	
65–74 years	5.3	
75–84 years	2.0	
84 + years	0.9	
Practitioners in Mental Health		
OTRs	16.9	22.1
COTAs	27.8	39.5

* *1986 data not comparable.*

Except for practitioners in mental health, table is based on OTRs only. Silvergleit, I. (1991). Member data survey. American Occupational Therapy Association, Research Information and Evaluation Division.

risks of institutionalization. These detriments must continually be weighed against the patient's pathology and the difficulties that may result from return to the community. Experience has demonstrated that many patients can shorten hospital stays by moving to **community residences** offering support programs. A **transitional living continuum**, illustrated in Table 17-4, demonstrates varying levels of pathology and the levels of functioning that commonly accompany the range of housing and program offerings.

Residential facilities

Quarterway houses and **halfway houses** are outpatient residences that are placed 25% and 50% in conceptual distance, respectively, from the hospital toward the community. Viewed within a continuum of care beginning with the hospital, these housing facilities and their associated programs represent decreasing supervision and increasing options for individual autonomy (see Table 17-4). Although the severity of their symptoms diminishes rapidly during successful hospital treatment, most patients need the support provided by carefully planned aftercare. The degree of residual impairment in occupational functioning determines the level of care needed. For example, a patient with chronic schizophrenia who takes medication and

follows a daily schedule with prompting might be referred to a quarterway house, whereas a depressed person who is able to volunteer part-time and participate in community meetings may be referred to a halfway house. Typically, these residences are directed by a mental health professional such as an occupational therapist who supervises a number of paraprofessional employees (Wilberding, 1991).

Community mental health centers

The National Institute of Mental Health was mandated by the community Mental Health Act of 1963 to establish **community mental health centers** (CMHCs) nationwide as part of a national movement to take more responsibility for the mentally ill. CMHCs were to be formed in homogeneous catchment areas of 75,000 to 200,000 people and to include essential services. Today they are administered and staffed by professionals and citizens and have boards of directors composed of community leaders that serve as advising or governing bodies. Frequently the centers are federally or state funded. Services of CMHCs are outpatient therapy, medication monitoring, crisis intervention, and services for children, adolescent, elderly, and chemically dependent populations. Often residential programs are affiliated with CMHCs as well as day programs such as partial hospitalization and community rehabilitation.

Along with a multidisciplinary treatment team including psychiatrists, psychologists, nurses, social workers, and other rehabilitation staff and community members, the occupational therapist provides various community-based services, including those that maximize the client's independent functioning in homes or residential programs and those that facilitate use of community resources for leisure and recreation. Through activity and psychoeducation, the clinician focuses on establishing healthy patterns, decreasing stress, and maintaining a balance among work, leisure, and self-care to avoid hospitalization (Tiffany, 1983). In addition, the occupational therapist may provide program development and prevention services to the public. As a case manager, the occupational therapist facilitates access to a whole range of services, including vocational and prevocational services, sheltered workshops, social and leisure activities, housing placement and programs designed according to client functional level, and individual programs for enhancing daily living skills (Moeller, 1991).

Partial hospitalization programs

Because of economic concerns, increased attention and growth have recently been seen in **partial hospitalization programs** (Cuyler, 1991). Third-party payors, although denying reimbursement for inpatient hospitalization, will consider the less expensive alternative of a partial hospitalization program. As a result, partial hospitalization programs have recently gained much popularity in CMHCs and in general and private psychiatric hospitals (Weiss & Dubin, 1982).

The American Partial Hospitalization Association (AAPH) defines partial hospitalization as a "time-limited, ambulatory treatment program that offers intensive, coordinated, and structured clinical services within a stable therapeutic milieu" (AAPH, 1991, p. 1). Partial hospitalization embraces day, evening, night, and weekend treatment programs that may be free-standing or part of a broader mental health or medical system but may also

TABLE 17-4. *Transitional Living Continuum**

	Client Characteristics	Housing Characteristics	Program
Outpatient	Holds job/volunteers Has leisure skills Uses support systems	Lives independently	Individual/group psychotherapy
Supervised apartment	May need help solving problems Takes meds independently Holds job/volunteer work	Staff on call Shared apartment living May look together LOS as needed	Individual/group psychotherapy Support groups
Halfway house	May hold job or volunteer Takes meds independently No substance abuse	24-hour staffing Clients expected to cook and clean for themselves 3–6 months LOS Community meetings	Individual/group psychotherapy Community trips Psychosocial programs involving ADL/pre-vocational training
Quarterway house	Follows simple directions Follows written schedule with support No substance abuse	24-hour supervision Clients assist with cooking/cleaning 1–2 years LOS	Community meetings Community trips Structured daily activities Sheltered workshop
Hospital	Harmful to self or others Psychotic Disorganized Needs medication management	24-hour supervision Locked doors Meals/housekeeping provided	Individual/group psychotherapy Rehabilitation therapies (OT, RT, art, dance, music therapies) Structured daily schedule Community meetings Medication Family therapy

* *Continuum goes from least restrictive to most restrictive.*

LOS, length of stay.

be a separate unit representing a significant link within the continuum of care of mental health services (AAPH, 1991). In addition to the treatment of the acutely and chronically ill psychiatric patient, partial hospitalization may offer programs for children and adolescent, adult and geriatric populations and for special diagnoses such as for schizophrenia, borderline personality disorder and head trauma patients (Norman & Crosby, 1990).

Within a therapeutic milieu and a multidisciplinary treatment team, occupational therapists provide assessment and evaluation, individual and group direct services, and program development. Treatment emphasizes daily structure, normalizing of behavior, and the acquiring of skills for adaptive functioning in the community. These services usually focus on activities of daily living such as meal planning, shopping, and preparation; time and stress management; and community awareness through trips into the community, sexuality education, prevocational and vocational programs, leisure and social event planning particularly for weekends, and use of community resources for sports, picnics, or hobbies (Richert & Canosa, 1985; Richert & Merryman, 1988). Other treatment services are problem solving and goal planning, task skills using various modalities such as ceramics or leatherwork, communication skills such as assertiveness training, and creative self-expression using writing, art, music, or movement modalities. In addition, other disciplines may be part of the treatment team including recreational, art, and dance/movement therapists and vocational counselors.

With such treatment team diversity, there may be considerable **role blurring** among the disciplines that causes anxiety

and ambiguity yet provides challenges and opportunities for creative practice and program development. Occupational therapists in this setting need to be flexible and adaptable and to possess a strong professional identity, because they might provide services traditionally associated with other disciplines such as group therapy, mental health psychoeducation, and psychodrama.

Efficacy studies indicate that partial hospitalization is as effective as inpatient units in the treatment of psychotics without violent or suicidal tendencies and is superior to outpatient treatment for chronic schizophrenics. In a classic outcome study, occupational therapy is demonstrated to have been an effective treatment modality (Linn et al., 1979).

Psychosocial or community rehabilitation programs

Psychosocial or **community rehabilitation programs** have been developed over the last 40 years as structured, daily, social alternatives to the more dominant medical model programs. The "clubhouse" of Fountain House in New York emphasizes belonging and security for the person who has spent time in psychiatric hospitals and, in response to younger, more motivated individuals, the "high expectancy" or "schoolhouse" approach of Horizon House in Philadelphia emphasizes learning skills to enable graduation to independent living. Principles include skills acquisition, self-determination, normalization, commitment of staff, deprofessionalization of services, unlimited participation, work-centered process, and social rather than medical supremacy (Cnaan, et al., 1988). Communuity rehabilitation programs provide daily, evening, and weekend programs for prevocational and vocational skill development through work programs or units (clerical, food preparation, maintenance, and industrial arts), supported employment, work adjustment training, and job placement, and leisure programs for building skills and social networks.

Often grant-supported through federal or state funds, community rehabilitation programs frequently have low staff ratios and mostly nonprofessional staff (Anthony, 1980). Limited opportunities exist for professional staff such as occupational therapists but these opportunities may include administrative or managerial positions, private practice components, or consultation (Harwood & Wenzel, 1990). Today, the International Association of Psychosocial Rehabilitation Services (IAPSRS) provides broad-based support for staff working in this area.

Alternative practice models

The practice of occupational therapy in nontraditional settings is no different from that in hospitals (Michael & Adams, 1991). Standards of practice are simply transferred to different practice settings. For occupational therapists to respond positively to the needs for practice in nontraditional settings, it is important to identify some viable practice models. Three professional roles for current and future community practice are consultant, generalist/case manager, and private practice therapist (Bruhn, 1991; Ethridge, 1986).

As a **consultant**, an occupational therapist gives expert advice or information on organizational, program development, supervisory, or clinical issues or any combination of these to persons seeking this service. According to the 1990 Member Data Survey, one third of occupational therapists consider consultation as their secondary employment function (Silvergleit, 1991). Often services are sought for new programs or for those undergoing significant changes or transitions. For example, psychosocial or community rehabilitation programs are often grant-supported and in need of focused, short-term consultation for program development and clinical issues by professional staff like occupational therapists. Likewise, new programs just beginning, like partial hospitalization programs, may require either brief consultation or ongoing supervision for its staff unfamiliar with such programs. In addition, consultants may provide direct services in unique ways in inpatient, hospital settings (Litterst, 1987; Watanabe & Watson, 1987; Wittman & Gibson, 1988).

The role of **case manager** is one in which the professional coordinates services; analyzes fiscal benefits; advocates for essential services; advises the client, family, or caregiver; and monitors the use of resources. Case managers require extensive clinical experience (3 to 5 years), professional autonomy, and excellent communication and organizational skills (Dufresne, 1991). Frequently, this role is filled by occupational therapists working with the chronic mentally ill (Klasson, 1989; Saltz, 1991). Case managers can also be hospital staff members who refer, monitor, and coordinate patient services to facilitate communication among treatment team members. For example, in a large psychiatric hospital, the occupational therapist coordinates the rehabilitation services department's multidisciplinary services of art, dance/movement, occupational and recreational therapy, and vocational counseling and reports to the treatment team directly.

The role of occupational therapy in mental health **private practice** may involve consultation, case management, and direct services on a contract basis with agencies, hospitals, private practices, or contractors, so that the therapist is self-employed on either a part-time or full-time basis. Direct services may be provided in a hospital, facility, or home environment. Twenty percent of mental health occupational therapists are self-employed (Silvergleit, 1991).

Some alternative practice settings have been identified for fieldwork education interns and include a homeless women's dinner program (Del Vecchio & Kearney, 1990), shelters, soup kitchens, youth programs, geriatric day care centers, and free clinics (Jackson, 1990). Prisons can also be practice settings (Michael, 1991).

Health promotion is predicted to have a major effect on practice in the next few years. Companies, institutions, and agencies have employee assistance programs (EAPs) to assist their employees in handling personal and job-related stressors and problems by identifying, confronting, diagnosing, treating, and following up employee health problems. Major contributions of occupational therapists are analysis and enhancement of daily living skills, adaptation of work and home environments, task analysis and instruction in work simplification, energy conservation, identification and elimination of architectural barriers, instruction in adaptive devices, modification of the work unit, and promotion of a milieu supportive of occupational role performance (Maynard, 1986).

References

Adams, R. (1990). The role of occupational therapists in community mental health. *Mental Health Special Interest Section Newsletter, 13*(1), 1–2.

Adams, R. (1991). The pros and cons of nontraditional practice. *Mental Health Special Interest Section Newsletter, 14*(2), 5–6.

American Association for Partial Hospitalization. (1991). Standards and guidelines for partial hospitalization. (Available from American Association for Partial Hospitalization, 411 K Street NW, Suite 1000, Washington, DC 20005).

American Occupational Therapy Association (22 November, 1990). *OT Week.*

Anthony, W. A. (1980). *The principles of psychiatric rehabilitation* (pp. 213–231). Baltimore: University Press.

Bruhn, J. G. (1991). Occupational therapy in the 21st century: An outsider's view. *American Journal of Occupational Therapy, 45*(9), 775–780.

Cnaan, R. A., Blankertz, L., Messinger, K. W., & Gardner, J. R. (1988). Psychosocial rehabilitation: Toward a definition. *Psychosocial Rehabilitation Journal, 11*(4), 61–77.

Cuyler, R. N. (1991). The challenge of partial hospitalization in the 1990's. *The Psychiatric Hospital, 22*(2), 47–50.

Del Vecchio, A. L., & Kearney, P. C. (1990). Homeless women's dinner program: Adapting traditional interventions to a nontraditional environment. *Mental Health Special Interest Section Newsletter, 13*(1), 4–6.

Drake, R. E., & Sederer, L. I. (1986). Inpatient psychosocial treatment of chronic schizophrenia: Negative effects and current guidelines. *Hospital and Community Psychiatry, 37,* 897–900.

DuFresne, G. M. (7 March, 1991). A position statement: The occupational therapist as case manager. *OT Week,* 11–13.

Ethridge, D. A. (1986). Issues and trends in mental health practice: An update. *Mental Health Special Interest Section Newsletter, 9*(3), 1–2.

Gibson, D. (1988). Activity therapy in hospital psychiatry. In J. Lion,

W. Webb & W. Adler (Eds.), *Hospital psychiatry* (pp. 181–207). Baltimore: Williams & Wilkins.

Harwood, K. J., & Wenzel, D. (1990). Admissions to discharge: A psychogeriatric transitional program. *Occupational Therapy in Mental Health, 10*(3), 79–100.

International Association of Psychosocial Rehabilitation Services. (1990). (Available from International Association of Psychosocial Rehabilitation Services, 5550 Stenett Place, Suite 214, Columbia, MD 21044.)

Jackson, S. H. (1990). Education for community practice. *Mental Health Special Interest Section Newsletter, 13*(1), 4–6.

Klasson, E. M. (1989). A model of the occupational therapist as case manager: Two case studies of chronic schizophrenic patients in the community. *Occupational Therapy in Mental Health, 9*(1), 63–90.

Linn, M. W., Caffey, E. M., Klett, C. J., Hogarty, G. S., & Lamb, H. R. (1979). Day treatment and psychotropic drugs in the aftercare of schizophrenic patients. *Archives of General Psychiatry, 36,* 1055–1066.

Litterst, T. A. (1987). Work: A central element in acute short-term psychiatric programming. *Mental Health Special Interest Section Newsletter, 10*(2), 45.

Maynard, M. (1986). Health promotion through employee assistance programs: A role for occupational therapists. *American Journal of Occupational Therapy, 40*(11), 771–780.

Michael, P. S. (1991). Occupational therapy in a prison? You must be kidding! *Mental Health Special Interest Section Newsletter, 14*(2), 3–4.

Michael, P. S., & Adams, R. (1991). From the guest editors. *Mental Health Special Interest Section Newsletter, 14*(2), 1.

Moeller, P. (1991). The occupational therapist as case manager in community mental health. *Mental Health Special Interest Section Newsletter, 14*(2), 4–5.

Norman, A. N., & Crosby, P. M. (1990). Meeting the challenge: Role of occupational therapy in a geriatric day hospital. *Occupational Therapy in Mental Health, 10*(3), 65–78.

Richert, G. Z., & Canosa, R. A. (1985). Sexuality education in a partial hospitalization program. *International Journal of Partial Hospitalization, 4*(1), 49–61.

Richert, G. Z., & Merryman, M. B. (1988). A model for vocational services. *International Journal of Partial Hospitalization, 4*(1), 49–61.

Saltz, D. L. (28 March, 1991). Bringing it all together. *OT Week.*

Silvergleit, I. (1991). *Member data survey.* Rockville, MD: American Occupational Therapy Association.

Tiffany, E. (1983). Psychiatry and mental health. In H. L. Hopkins & H. D. Smith (Eds.). *Willard and Spackman's Occupational therapy* (6th ed., pp. 267–333). Philadelphia: J. B. Lippincott.

Watanabe, D. Y., & Watson, L. T. (1987). Psychiatric consultation-liaison: Role of the occupational therapist. *Mental Health Special Interest Section Newsletter, 10*(2), 1,6,7.

Weiss, K. J., & Dubin, W. R. (1982). Partial hospitalization: State of the art. *Hospital and Community Psychiatry, 33*(11), 923–928.

Wilberding, D. (1991). The quarterway house: More than an alternative to care. *Occupational Therapy in Mental Health, 11*(1), 65–91.

Wing, J. (1962). Institutionalization in mental hospitals. *British Journal of Social and Clinical Psychology, 1,* 38–51.

Wittman, P. P., & Gibson, R. W. (1988). The case of the broken copy machine: What can we do? *Mental Health Special Interest Section Newsletter, 13*(4), 4–5.

Bibliography

Asher, K., & Weisman, E. (1988). *Case management: Guiding patients through the healthcare maze.* Chicago: Joint Commission on Accreditation of Healthcare Organizations.

Torrey, E. F. (1986). Continuous treatment teams in the care of chronically mentally ill. *Hospital and Community Psychiatry, 37*(12), 1243–1247.

SECTION 1E
Program planning, development, and implementation

GAIL Z. RICHERT

KEY TERMS

Assertiveness Training	Program Evaluation
Cognitive Rehabilitation	Program Implementation
Competency-Based Curriculum	Program Planning
	Protocol
Directive Group Therapy	Psychoeducation Modular Group
Discharge Planning	
Environment and Systems Analyses	Stress Management
	Treatment Group Continuum
Program Development	

LEARNING OBJECTIVES

Upon completion of this section the reader will be able to:

1. *Define the following: program planning, program development, program implementation, and program evaluation.*

2. *Describe the program development process in a facility and in a clinical setting.*

3. *Identify the components and one example of a treatment group protocol.*

4. *Describe three ways to organize and structure treatment groups.*

5. *Identify three priorities for services in acute care psychiatry.*

6. *Identify patient education books and resources.*

7. *Delineate patient functional levels in two examples of treatment group continua.*

8. *Describe components of a cognitive rehabilitation program.*

Definitions and process

Program planning and development are essential components of mental health occupational therapy in public, private, and forensic psychiatric hospitals, psychiatric units in general hospitals, residential facilities, community mental health, and outpatient programs. All these practice settings have unique needs and demand unique programs. General principles govern the design of rehabilitation and occupational therapy services, however, and it is essential for occupational therapists to be familiar with these because employers frequently seek these skills and use occupational therapists for their experience in and knowledge of program design, planning, and development (Fidler, 1984; Gibson, 1988; Mosey, 1986, pp. 481–485).

Recognizing the need to develop programs to meet the needs of the mentally ill along a continuum of care, the American Occupational Therapy Association, under the leadership of Susan C. Robertson, developed a ***competency-based curriculum*** called *Mental Health SCOPE: Strategies, Concepts, and Opportunities for Program Development and Evaluation* in 1986, which was delivered in numerous locations throughout the country. Its purpose was to assist occupational therapy personnel in diverse settings to effect change in service delivery. Using a curriculum rich in resource material, leaders in mental health occupational therapy facilitated a process for clinicians to develop an integrated plan designed for their particular setting.

Program development has many meanings. In a sequence of levels, it refers to a particular treatment program like community living skills to a full complement of programs under an occupational therapy program, and to a full range of services within a comprehensive program in a particular facility. Finally, it can refer to the total scope of services in a city, state, or country, such as a state mental health program (Kirkland, 1986).

On a broader scale, the program development process begins with an ***environmental and systems analysis*** of a particular facility. This is a data gathering or needs assessment process. Although the facility's documents such as mission and philosophy statements and strategic plans are important, face-to-face input with key leadership such as disciplinary leaders, administrators, peers, and colleagues is also important. This initiates the collaborative process that enables staff to get to know each other better through engaging in purposeful activity (Gibson, 1989a). Occupational therapy's mission statement, statement of philosophy, classification of personnel, and standards of practice are then developed after gathering the more global information (AOTA, 1983, 1989; Evans, 1985; Schell, 1985; Shriver & Foto, 1983). Identification of patient demographics, length of stay, diagnoses, and functional levels allows selection of an appropriate frame of reference and begins the program planning process. The type of service delivery, such as inpatient or outpatient services and individual or group services, is then identified.

Program implementation includes documentation, communication, and coordination. Usually one person is identified as the coordinator or manager of this process, although others may have input into it. ***Program evaluation*** measures the goals of the program and may include outcome studies, quality assurance, and utilization review. Based on analysis of results, further changes may be needed and the process begins again (Fig. 17-1.)

Content and practice areas

The focus of program development is on the process of organizing and implementing occupational therapy services to meet the evaluation and treatment needs of specialized patient populations. Although entry-level occupational therapists generally do not have primary program planning and development responsibilities, their participation in the process is essential for their own sense of involvement and power; managers in turn gain new ideas from a committed and involved staff (McGourty, 1990). Content areas for programs are the same or similar to those for practice and include performance areas (activities of daily living,

---

Environment and Systems Analysis

1. Description of the community
2. Overview of mental health services
3. Your program and your facility

Program Planning

1. Goals and objectives
2. Strategies for change
3. Program development

Program Implementation

1. Principles of marketing
2. Implementation and collaboration

Program Evaluation

1. Goals of evaluation
2. Methods of evaluation
3. Designing your evaluation plan

FIGURE 17-1. *Program planning, development, and implementation. (Adapted from Robertson, S. C. [1986].* Mental Health SCOPE: Strategies, Concepts, and Opportunities for Program Development and Evaluation. *Rockville, MD: American Occupational Therapy Association.)*

---

work, and leisure or play activities) and performance components (sensorimotor, cognitive integration and cognitive components, and psychosocial skills and psychological components; AOTA, 1989).

When the goal of program development includes the implementation of group treatment, the reasoning process begins with the development of a group protocol, which is a format for treatment that includes structure and content components (Howe & Schwartzberg, 1986). The process of developing a ***protocol*** is a challenging one that includes clinical decision making (planning) and clinical reasoning (implementation) along with group process and critical elements of a group plan (Haiman, 1989). The protocol sets the parameters for the treatment process and contains the following:

I. Structure or format
   A. Name—title that should include the primary group goal rather than the modality, as in task skills versus ceramics or leather
   B. Time—length of group
   C. Space—requirements of room size
   D. Size—maximum and minimum number of patients

II. Definition (Purpose or general goals, philosophy, frame of reference [Medicare requirement])

III. Goals (Behavioral and special [Medicare requirement]). Goals are related to practice and include performance areas and performance components.

IV. Criteria for patient selection

V. Leadership and approach
   A. Staff qualifications to provide leadership
      1. Qualifications specific to a person in a discipline such as an occupational therapist, nurse, physician, or social worker if the group is to be co-led
      2. Other related or general qualifications, such as a knowledge of group dynamics that other disciplines would be expected to have
   B. Modalities used such as ceramics, basketry, or woodworking
   C. Methodology—group structure

VI. Evaluation
   A. Forms used such as patient surveys, questionnaires, or pretests and posttests.
   B. Frequency of documentation and oral reports to treatment team

VII. Content (Optional for some groups like a task group but necessary in a psychoeducational group)

See the display on page 254 for a sample protocol. For other examples, see Gibson (1989b) and Brown, Harwood, Heckman, & Short (1989).

In multidisciplinary departments, it is important to maintain the autonomy of various disciplines in all aspects of program development (Fidler, 1984). Disciplinary boundary issues can be resolved at the onset by attending specifically to V, Leadership and Approach, in the previous protocol. For example, in a stress management group with occupational and recreational therapist coleaders, the skills, knowledge, similarities, and differences of each are recognized. Both leaders have a knowledge of stress management, relaxation techniques, and anatomy and physiology, and an understanding of group dynamics; their differences are identified here:

I. Specific qualifications for an occupational therapist
   A. Extensive knowledge and ability to analyze patient's cognitive task skills
   B. Extensive knowledge of and ability to analyze/adapt and structure activities for the functional level of the group members

II. Specific qualifications for a recreational therapist
   A. Extensive knowledge of how leisure choices and leisure lifestyle can play a vital role in improving a person's stress management
   B. Extensive knowledge and skill in adapting physical activities so that participation in the activity can serve as a stress management technique

In ***directive group therapy***, a nurse and an occupational therapist are coleaders and both are expected to have a knowledge of group dynamics. The occupational therapist adapts and structures treatment modalities consistent with the patient's functional level and the treatment plan. In turn, the nurse adapts knowledge of the therapeutic milieu and psychotropic medications consistent with the nursing care plan (see the sample protocol display).

Program organization

There are several ways to organize and structure treatment groups that relate to special patient populations, including patient length of stay, patient functional level in a given performance area or performance component, and patient diagnosis.

Length of hospital stay in acute care psychiatry

Although the number of beds in acute care psychiatry remains constant, the incidence of hospital admissions has increased, and lengths of stay have decreased, creating high rates of turnover. Acuity has increased in both psychiatric and physical symptomatology, including multiple system diseases like AIDS, chemical dependency, and head trauma, which results in an increase in dually diagnosed patients. Social problems such as homelessness and poverty complicate discharge efforts, whereas cost-containment initiatives of third-party payors and managed care programs result in increased recidivism when patients are discharged too quickly. These external pressures have produced demands for faster and more effective treatment and cost containment, and competition for limited resources.

Fine (1987) notes other clinical trends in mental health service. One trend is the remedicalization of psychiatry with advances in psychopharmacology and the neurosciences. Another is the increased interest in functional capabilities and renewed commitment to functional performance and skills in daily living. The *DSM-III-R* has expanded Axis V to incorporate patient's current and past level of functioning supporting occupational therapy's historic focus (American Psychiatric Association, 1987; Bonder, 1990).

Novak (1988) has identified three priorities for occupational therapy services in moving the patient toward independent functioning in acute care psychiatry. These are evaluation, patient education, and discharge planning, and they can be used as the basis for treatment planning as well as for program development. Although evaluation can be conducted in a group setting, it is usually done on an individual basis. Evaluation is addressed in Chapter 17, Section 1G.

Patient education is the second priority of inpatient acute care service. Historically, the primary unit of occupational therapy treatment in mental health has been the group. Fidler (1969) identified the task-oriented group, and Mosey (1970a, 1970b) identified groups that were designed consistent with the patient's interactional skill level. Kaplan (1988) identifies a highly structured approach called *directive group therapy* for minimally functioning patients who are defined as disorganized, disturbed, psychotic, and dependent due to neurologic disorders, mental retardation, or organic causes. Today, in the fast-paced settings of acute care psychiatry, groups may serve the dual purposes of assessment and treatment (Munoz & Schweikert, 1988; Sheffer & Harlock, 1980).

The ***psychoeducation modular group*** meets the educational therapeutic needs of short-term patients. It is an educationally oriented, time-limited group in which each session is self-contained with specific content, an identified task, and final processing. Patients who meet established criteria are individually referred and may enter and leave the groups at any point. The complete sequence of groups ends in 4 to 5 weeks after twice-weekly meetings and then may begin again. For example, ***stress***

THE SHEPPARD AND ENOCH PRATT HOSPITAL
REHABILITATION SERVICES DEPARTMENT
DIRECTIVE GROUP THERAPY

I. *Format*
 A. Time: 45 minutes, 3 times a week
 B. Space: small group room
 C. Size: 3–6 patients

II. *Definition*
 Directive group therapy is a form of group treatment designed to meet the needs of acutely ill, minimally functioning patients who represent a wide range of diagnoses, ages, and problems and who have extreme difficulty taking care of themselves, even with supervision. They are unable to function and have serious impairment in judgment and communication skills.

III. *Purpose*
 This group assists the psychotic or organically impaired individual to reorganize his behavior to a basic level of competence in a supportive environment.

IV. *Goals*
 A. Engage in positive, goal-directed activity in a structured, unit-based group setting.
 B. Increase attention and concentration through successful completion of a task.
 C. Increase frequency of appropriate verbal responses.
 D. Decrease impulsive behavior.
 E. Follow one–two step verbal instructions on task projects.
 F. Increase initiation.

V. *Criteria for Patient Selection*
 A. Cognitive functioning
  1. Can imitate familiar schemes or follow one direction at a time (cognitive levels 3–5 according to the Allen Cognitive Level Test)
  2. Can attend to a task for 15–45 minutes most of the time; may need redirection
  3. Demonstrates concrete or confused thinking
  4. Has difficulty making decisions and problem solving
 B. Interpersonal/psychological functioning
  1. Functions at the project level of group interaction
  2. Often has difficulty initiating, responding to, or sustaining verbal interaction
  3. Often unaware of the needs of others

VI. *Leadership and Approach*
 A. Staff qualifications to provide leadership
  1. Qualifications specific to an occupational therapist (OTR)
   a. Knowledge of and ability to analyze cognitive task skills
   b. Knowledge of and ability to analyze/adapt and structure activities for the functional levels of group members
   c. Knowledge of the therapeutic use of various treatment modalities
  2. Qualifications specific to a nurse (RN)
   a. Knowledge and development of patient's nursing care plan (NCP) and how it relates to patient's current functioning
   b. Knowledge of the therapeutic milieu and how patients function in it
   c. Knowledge of medications and how they affect patients' functioning
  3. Knowledge of group dynamics
 B. Modalities—simple, familiar tools and materials, such as paper, pencil, glue and scissors.
 C. Methodology—short-term, structured group tasks and exercises

VII. *Evaluation*: Effectiveness to be evaluated through leader's regular processing of group's activities and periodic reports to the treatment team.

(*This group is based on Kaplan, K. [1988]. Directive group therapy: Innovative mental health treatment. Thorofare, NJ: Slack.*)

management takes place over a 5-week period in 10 contained, educational modules. These modules incorporate the psychological, environmental, and physical components of stress and include structured discussion, written and physical group exercises, self-assessments, audiotapes, role play, and role modeling. The topics include the following:

Week 1—stress components and stress signals
Week 2—self-awareness and communication skills
Week 3—time management and nutrition
Week 4—relaxation and exercise
Week 5—stress management, goal development, and implementation

A stress management program can also be developed to help patients improve situational coping skills while making a transition from inpatient to outpatient status (Courtney & Escobedo, 1990). This provides a continuum of care during a transitional phase when patients are particularly vulnerable to relapse.

Another example of a psychoeducation modular group is **assertiveness training**, in which the content is covered in 4 weeks with twice-weekly meetings:

Week 1—personal rights and distinctions among passive, aggressive, and assertive behavior
Week 2—verbal components including initiating and maintaining conversation, giving compliments, expressing anger, and refusing demands as well as nonverbal components
Week 3—active listening skills
Week 4—impact of assertiveness on others and transfer of new skills

This group uses structured role play, goal setting, log keeping and review, and pretest and posttest evaluations.

Another aspect of patient education is a readily accessible library of educational, readable books, which have been written for the mass media. These books can be made available to patients who are interested in education about their illness (see Patient Bibliography).

Discharge planning, the third priority for occupational therapy services, facilitates the transition from inpatient to outpatient treatment. Given the decreasing length of stay, this service is offered frequently in individual or group sessions. An outline facilitates the problem-solving process that each patient uses to consider, note, and discuss nine major life areas:

- daily structure
- education
- finance
- legal situation
- leisure
- living arrangement
- outpatient treatment
- relationships
- transportation

These areas provide the structure for involvement in the discharge planning process. For those not yet ready to problem solve, the important question, "How will you know when you are ready for discharge?" can be posed. Patients scheduled for discharge during the week are expected to discuss their plans, whereas other patients discuss aspects of their plans that are in

place at that time. Mutual problem solving is encouraged. The clinician uses knowledge of patient treatment needs and of community resources such as the Alliance for the Mentally Ill, Alcoholics Anonymous (AA), Narcotics Anonymous (NA), Depression and Related Affective Disorders Association (DRADA), and other relevant local support groups including those for homosexuals or people with physical or social problems (Schwartzberg & Abeles, 1986). Frequently, the discharge planning group is co-led with other disciplines, which gives added richness to a patient's discharge plan.

After programs are developed, continual evaluation and modification are essential since patient populations and staffing change. When modifying program content, it is important to be flexible, to maintain realistic expectations in goal setting and time constraints, to set a congruent philosophy, to incorporate group values, and to collaborate with peers and evaluate group dynamics in relation to unit dynamics (Bradlee, 1984).

Functional level: Treatment group continuum

Program development dilemmas may center around uniting or segregating acute/chronic or high/low functioning patient populations within the same program. These concerns can be resolved by developing a track or continuum of service (Agacinski & Stein, 1984). A **treatment group continuum** is a sequence of treatment groups designed according to a patient's functional level. These groups are sequenced according to patient performance areas and performance components. An example of this is a task skills continuum, based on the Allen Cognitive Level Test (ACL) score (Allen, 1985). Using the cognitive disabilities frame of reference, the environment in each group is structured and adapted to ensure the successful functioning of patients, whatever their cognitive deficits may be. Whereas Task Skills I focuses on patients with the severest deficits who need the most environmental adaptation (levels 3 and 4), Task Skills II focuses on patients on mixed levels (levels 3, 4, 5), some of whom are not as dysfunctional but need rehearsal in serial imitation and overt trial-and-error problem solving. In addition, some patients (level 5) may work on interpersonal skills and increasing self-esteem or mastery through assisting others. Patients with minimal cognitive deficits (levels 5 and 6) use modalities in Task Skills III primarily for interpersonal/social and emotional behavioral goals such as learning sharing, assertiveness, mastery over the environment, and appropriate expression of feelings (Table 17-5).

In a similar manner, the developmental and cognitive disabilities frames of reference are used to develop a model for vocational services called the *vocational continuum*. This continuum provides both prevocational and vocational services, which are sequential and stage-specific. These services support

TABLE 17-5. *Task Skills Continuum*

Group	ACL Score
Task skills I	3.5–4.9
Task skills II	3.5–5.9
Task skills III	5.0–5.9

ACL, Allen Cognitive Level Test.

TABLE 17-6.   *The Vocational Continuum**

	Level of Cognitive Functioning
Prevocational Continuum	
Cognitive Task Skills I	Level 4
Problem Solving	Levels 4 to 5
Vocational Adjustment	
Work Therapy	
Cognitive Task Skills II	Levels 5 to 6
Vocational Continuum	
Cooperative Skills	Levels 5 to 6
Vocational Preparation	
Vocational Experience—patients in:	
1. Paid employment	
2. Volunteer employment	

* *Data from the Sheppard and Enoch Pratt Hospital, Adult Day Hospital*

(From Richert, G. Z., & Merryman, M. B.: The vocational continuum: A model for providing vocational services in a partial hospitalization program. Occupational Therapy in Mental Health, 7[3], 1–20.)

progression and skill acquisition while allowing for patient regression when necessary. The prevocational continuum includes group services in problem solving and cognitive task skills according to the patient's level of cognitive functioning, which is determined by the ACL score. The vocational continuum includes group services for cooperative social skills and vocational preparation as well as support for patients already engaged in paid or volunteer employment (Richert, 1990; Richert & Merryman, 1987; Table 17-6).

Diagnosis: Cognitive rehabilitation

Since 1989, when a joint United States Congressional proclamation declared the 1990s the "decade of the brain," public attention has focused on the neurosciences, and the National Institutes of Health (NIH) targeted certain areas for special attention and research funding. The American Occupational Therapy Association, acknowledging the need for a neuroscience knowledge base for its expanding membership, initiated "Neuroscience Foundations of Human Performance" as part of its self-study series (Royeen, 1990). The response was dramatic and by April 1991, 3000 association members were already participating (AOTA, 1991).

Cognitive rehabilitation illustrates the biopsychosocial practice model as it evaluates and defines the relationships between physical rehabilitation and mental health specialties in occupational therapy. As such, it is perfectly suited for application to treatment of schizophrenia, a severe emotional disorder characterized by the failure to function and multiple structural abnormalities of the brain (Fine, 1990). Positive symptoms of schizophrenia are characterized by prominent delusions, hallucinations, formal thought disorder, and bizarre behavior; the patient may respond to antipsychotic medications. Negative symptoms, by contrast, are characterized by a flattening of affect, a lack of pleasure, attentional and cognitive impairments, lower levels of function, and cerebral atrophy (Fine, in press). The principles of the cognitive rehabilitation model, originally proposed for the treatment of the brain-injured adult (Abreu & Toglia, 1987), are now applied to the treatment of the schizophrenic.

Andreason's Scale for the Assessment of Negative Symptoms (SANS) (1983) is used to evaluate important areas of attentional and information processing deficits known to impede occupational performance in schizophrenics (Fine, in press). This is followed by the dynamic investigative method of assessment, which involves evaluation of learning potential or the individual's maximum level of function. It includes investigating response to cues (prompting) and modification of the task and of the environment (Toglia, 1989).

Treatment strategies are taught, rehearsed, and applied in several contexts, ultimately requiring the individual to self-monitor and self-regulate. Characterized as Task-Oriented Learning Treatment (TOLT), the program begins with individual treatment that uses tasks, games, or computer software to focus on skill acquisition. Treatment then progresses to psychoeducation in a structured and graded Life Skills Curriculum (LSC), which addresses personal goal setting, social skills, self-care, time and stress management, leisure planning, and community resources (Fine & Schwimmer, 1986). Patients proceed to a sequenced combination of both, and, finally, to a rehabilitation program that emphasizes social skills training, minimizes talk, and emphasizes tasks.

References

Abreu, B. O., & Toglia, J. P. (1987). Cognitive rehabilitation: A model for occupational therapy. *American Journal of Occupational Therapy, 41*(7), 439–448.

Agacinski, K., & Stein, D. (1984). A two track system enhances therapeutic gains for the chronically mentally ill in a day hospital population. *Occupational Therapy in Mental Health, 4*(2), 15–22.

Allen, C. A. (1985). *Occupational therapy for psychiatric diseases: Measurement and management of cognitive disabilities.* Boston: Little Brown & Co.

American Occupational Therapy Association. (1983). Purposeful activities. *American Journal of Occupational Therapy, 37*(12), 805–806.

American Occupational Therapy Association. (1989). Uniform terminology for occupational therapy (2nd ed.) *American Journal of Occupational Therapy, 43*(12), 808–815.

American Occupational Therapy Association. (April 4, 1991). Decade-of-the-brain activities under way at NIH. *OT Week*, p. 5.

American Psychiatric Association. (1987). *Diagnostic and statistical manual of mental disorders* (3rd ed., rev.). Washington, DC: Author.

Andreason, N. O. (1983). *The scale for the assessment of negative symptoms* (SANS). Iowa City: University of Iowa.

Bonder, B. R. (1990). Disease and dysfunction: The value of Axis V. *Hospital and Community Psychiatry, 4*(9), 959–964.

Bradlee, L. (1984). The use of groups in a short-term psychiatric settings. *Occupational Therapy in Mental Health, 4*(3), 47–57.

Brown, C., Harwood, K., Heckman, J., & Short, J. (1989). *Mental health protocols for occupational therapy.* Bethesda, MD: Chess Publications.

Courtney, O., & Escobedo, B. (1990). A stress management program: Inpatient to outpatient continuity. *American Journal of Occupational Therapy, 44*(4), 306–310.

Evans, A. (1985). Roles and functions of occupational therapy in mental health. *American Journal of Occupational Therapy, 39*(12), 799–802.

Fidler, G. S. (1969). Task-oriented group as a context for treatment. *American Journal of Occupational Therapy, 23*, 43–48.

Fidler, G. S. (1984). *Design of rehabilitation services in psychiatric hospital settings.* Laurel, MD: RAMSCO Publishing Company.

Fine, S. B. (1987). Looking ahead: opportunities for occupational therapy in the next decade. *Occupational Therapy in Mental Health, 7*(4), 3–50.

Fine, S. B. (1990). Clinical casebook II: Psychosocial issues and adaptive capacities. In C. B. Royeen (Ed.), *AOTA Self-study series: Assessing function.* Rockville, MD: American Occupational Therapy Association.

Fine S. B. (in press). Neurobehavioral perspectives in schizophrenia. In J. Van Deusen (Ed.), *Body image and perceptual dysfunction in adults.* Philadelphia: W. B. Saunders.

Fine, S. B., & Schwimmer, P. (1986). The effects of occupational therapy on independent living skills. *Mental Health Special Interest Newsletter, 9*(4) 2–37.

Gibson, D. (1988). Activity therapy in hospital psychiatry. In J. Lion, W. Adler & W. Webb (Eds.), *Modern Hospital Psychiatry* (pp. 179–207). New York: W. W. Norton & Co.

Gibson, D. (1989a). Requisites for excellence. Structure and process in delivering psychiatric care. *Occupational Therapy in Mental Health, 9*(2), 27–52.

Gibson, D. (Ed.) (1989b). Group protocols: A psychosocial compendium. *Occupational Therapy in Mental Health, 9*(4).

Haiman, S. (1989). Preface: Selecting group protocols: Recipe or reasoning? *Occupational Therapy in Mental Health, 9*(4), 1–14.

Howe, M. C., & Schwartzberg, S. L. (1986). *A functional approach to group work in occupational therapy.* Philadelphia: J. B. Lippincott.

Kaplan, K. L. (1988). *Directive group therapy: Innovative mental health treatment.* Thorofare, NJ: Slack.

Kirkland, M. (1986). Introduction. In S. Robertson (Ed.), *Mental health SCOPE: Strategies, concepts and opportunities for program development and evaluation* (pp. 9–13). Rockville, MD: American Occupational Therapy Association.

McGourty, L. K. (1990). Program development with entry-level staff. *Administration and Management Special Interest Section Newsletter, 6*(2), 3–4. American Occupational Therapy Association, Rockville, MD.

Mosey, A. C. (1986) *Psychosocial components of occupational therapy.* New York: Raven Press.

Mosey, A. C. (1970a). The concept and use of developmental groups. *American Journal of Occupational Therapy, 24,* 272–275.

Mosey, A. C. (1970b). *Three frames of reference for mental health.* Thorofare, NJ: Slack.

Munoz, J. P., & Schweikert A. P. (1988). A program for inpatient psychiatry. *Mental Health Special Interest Section Newsletter, 11* (3), 3–4, Rockville, MD: American Occupational Therapy Association.

Novak, E. S. (1988). Improving payment for occupational therapists in mental health through effective documentation strategies. *Acute care psychiatry: Practical strategies and collaborative approaches: Proceedings* (pp. 17–22.). Rockville, MD: American Occupational Therapy Association.

Richert, G. Z. (1990). Vocational transition in acute care psychiatry. *Occupational Therapy in Mental Health, 10*(4), 43–61.

Richert, G. Z., & Merryman, M. B. (1987). The vocational continuum: A model for providing vocational services in a partial hospitalization program. *Occupational Therapy in Mental Health, 7*(3), 1–20.

Robertson, S. C. (Ed.). (1986). *Mental health SCOPE: Strategies, concepts and opportunities for program development and evaluation.* Rockville, MD: American Occupational Therapy Association.

Royeen, C. B. (Ed.). (1990). *AOTA Self-Study Series: Neuroscience foundations of human performance.* Rockville, MD: American Occupational Therapy Association.

Schell, B. A. (1985). Guide to classification of occupational therapy personnel. *American Journal of Occupational Therapy, 39*(12), 803–810.

Schwartzberg, S. L., & Abeles, J. (1986). Occupational therapy. In L. J. Sederer (Ed.), *Inpatient psychiatry: Diagnosis and treatment,* 2nd ed. (pp. 308–323). Baltimore: Williams & Wilkins.

Sheffer, M., & Harlock, S. (1980). Use of drawings in occupational therapy patient evaluations. *Journal of Rehabilitation, 46,* 44–49.

Shriver, O. T., & Foto, M. (Compilers for AOTA Commission Practice). (1983). Standards of practice for occupational therapy. *American Journal of Occupational Therapy, 37*(12), 802–804.

Toglia, J. P. (1989). Approaches to cognitive assessment of the brain-injured adult: Traditional methods and dynamic investigation. *Occupational Therapy Practice, 1*(1), 36–55.

Bibliography

Cotton, D. H. G. (1990). *Stress management: An integrated approach to therapy.* New York: Brunner/Mazel.

Griffin, R. M. (1990). *Protocols for adapting activities to the changing needs of people with dementia.* Bethesda, MD: Chess Publications.

Robinson, A. M., & Avallone, J. (1990). Occupational therapy in acute inpatient psychiatry: An activities health approach. *American Journal of Occupational Therapy, 44*(9), 809–814.

Patient bibliography

Beatty, M. (1987). *Codependent no more: How to stop controlling others and start caring for yourself.* Center City, MN: Hazeldon.

Burns, D. D. (1980). *Feeling good: The new mood therapy.* New York: William Morrow & Co.

Colgrove, M., Bloomfield H., & McWilliams, P. (1981). *How to survive the loss of a love.* Allen Park, MI: Leo Press.

Fieve, R. R. (1989). *Moodswing.* New York: William Morrow & Co.

Finney, L. D. (1990). *Reach for the rainbow: Advanced healing for survivors of sexual abuse.* Park City, UT: Changes Publishing.

Forward, S., & Buck, C. (1988). *Betrayal of innocence: Incest and its devastation* (rev.). New York: Penguin Books.

Kline, N. S. (1987). *From sad to glad.* New York: Ballantine Books.

Norwood, R. (1989). *Women who love too much.* New York: Simon & Schuster.

Stearns, A. K. (1985). *Living through a personal crisis.* New York: Ballantine Books.

Woititz, J. G. (1983). *Adult children of alcoholics.* Deerfield Beach, FL: Health Communications.

SECTION 1F
The therapeutic process

DIANE GIBSON and GAIL Z. RICHERT

KEY TERMS

Adverse Reactions	*Milieu Therapy*
Ambiguity	*Multiaxial System*
Coping Mechanisms	*Overinvolvement*
Cultural Relevance	*Psychopharmacology*
Diagnostic and Statistical Manual of Mental Disorders (DSM-III-R)	*Role Blurring*
	Self-Disclosure
Flexibility	*Treatment Team*

The patient

When persons are no longer able to adapt constructively to stresses, they develop painful symptoms and an inability to function in significant areas of life. Healthy persons use anxiety as a warning signal that something is wrong and proceed to resolve the underlying problem through the use of positive **coping mechanisms**. They think about the problem in a clarifying way, thus altering their perception of the stressor as dangerous and threatening. Or they may seek social support and reassurance from a friend, thereby reducing a sense of isolation.

In contrast, a person who becomes mentally ill uses destructive coping mechanisms to ward off the unwanted anxiety; however, this action evades the underlying problem rather than solves it. The destructive coping mechanisms, such as paranoia, denial, regression, and hostility, are examples of symptoms that, when classified in syndromes (a pattern of symptoms), can be evaluated for medical diagnosis.

At the present time, most clinicians and scientists believe that the etiology of mental illness is multidetermined by an interaction of genetic and biochemical factors, environmental stressors, and the level of coping skills available.

A common misconception about mental illness is that people can avoid mental illness if they "try harder" or "have stronger willpower." Unfortunately, persons suffering from depression, schizophrenia, or other diseases are dealing with their illness as well as they can. Another misconception is that mental illness classifies people rather than disorders. We occasionally hear, "she's a schizophrenic," as opposed to "she's a person with schizophrenia." A third misconception is that persons sharing the same mental disorder are all alike. Although they may have similar defining characteristics of the disorder, they may differ significantly in other aspects affecting treatment. Awareness of these misconceptions can assist the student in maintaining respect for the person's uniqueness, an important aspect of psychiatric care.

Diagnostic and Statistical Manual of Mental Disorders

The **Diagnostic and Statistical Manual of Mental Disorders** (*DSM*), first published in 1952, has been continuously updated according to changing definitions and criteria used to describe mental illnesses. Published by the American Psychiatric Association, it has been used nationally and internationally. The great value of the *DSM* has been the standardization of terminology that has enabled clinicians to speak a common language. Furthermore, its emphasis on behavioral descriptions has facilitated a sound basis for research and administration.

The diagnosis for each patient is based on several axes that determine varying kinds of information. The **multiaxial system** is based on a biopsychosocial approach and is atheoretical regarding etiology. Typically, the psychiatrist makes the diagnosis using input from team members.

Axis I: Clinical syndromes—(all psychiatric disorders) and Axis V codes (conditions not attributable to mental disorders)

Axis II: Developmental disorders and personality disorders—disorders beginning in childhood or adolescence and persisting in a stable form into adulthood

Axis III: Physical disorders and conditions—disorders that may affect medical treatment and outcomes

Axis IV: Severity of psychosocial stressors—documents the severity of psychosocial stressors, such as death of spouse, loss of job, on a scale of 1 to 7 in which numbers are associated with descriptors (eg, mild, moderate, extreme)

Axis V: Global assessment of functioning—assesses psychological, social, and vocational functioning on the Global Assessment Functioning (GAF) scale at the time of evaluation and during the past year

All of the presently known mental disorders are classified on Axis I and Axis II listed in the display below.

Descriptive criteria for each diagnosis involve identifiable behaviors (such as disorientation or agitation), thus diminishing the possibility of subjectivity and inference on the part of the clinician. The text describes each disorder in terms of essential criteria, associated features, age of onset, course, impairment, complications, prevalence, sex ratio, familial pattern, and differential diagnosis.

The following case study illustrates how definition and diagnostic criteria of *DSM-III-R* are applied to a person suffering from a borderline personality disorder.

DSM-III-R CLASSIFICATIONS

Axis I Syndromes and Disorders

- Organic and mental
- Psychoactive substance abuse disorders
- Schizophrenic disorders
- Delusional (paranoid) disorders
- Psychotic disorders not classified elsewhere
- Mood (affective) disorders
- Anxiety disorders
- Somatoform disorders
- Dissociative disorders
- Gender and sexual disorders
- Impulse control disorders not classified elsewhere
- Adjustment disorders

Axis II Syndromes and Disorders

- Developmental disorders
- Personality disorders

CASE STUDY

Ms. A is a 45-year-old, white, divorced female who has been hospitalized for emotional illness three times before the present hospitalization. Although she had been doing some part-time secretarial work, she had recently regressed and exhibited signs of impulsive and self-destructive behavior. She repeatedly cut herself, took over-the-counter drugs, and threatened to kill herself.

At home, she would isolate herself and spend long hours lying in bed while she ruminated negative thoughts and thoughts about suicide. Several times she drove her car in an erratic and dangerous manner, and she inquired how to procure a gun. Friends from her church brought her to the hospital when they recognized the extent of her depression and suicide ideation. Other symptoms were insomnia, overeating, and severe anxiety, which interfered with concentration and an inability to organize her life and daily routine.

She reported that she had been sharing an apartment with a woman with whom the relationship had been good at the beginning, but had shifted to anger and resentment.

Abandoned by her mother, Ms. A lived with her grandmother until she attended college. She married an abusive and rejecting man who ultimately left her after 17 years of marriage. Hospitalization for depression and a suicide attempt occurred following her mother's death. Before her admission, Ms. A had successfully held a job as a secretary for years and regularly participated in church activities.

Using the *DSM-III-R*, Ms. A's psychiatrist diagnosed her as having 301.83, borderline personality disorder (BPD), on Axis II. She met the criteria for this diagnosis by exhibiting unstable relationships, impulsiveness leading to self-damaging acts, affective instability, intense anger, suicidal acts and self-mutilating cutting, and chronic feelings of emptiness. On Axis IV, separation from her husband and death of her mother yielded a rating of 4 or "severe" for psychosocial stress, whereas suicidal behavior and lack of friends yielded a rating of 5 or "serious" on Axis V, the global assessment functioning scale.

Bonder (1990b) has carefully delineated how occupational therapists might collaborate with psychiatrists in using *DSM-III-R* as a common tool. Psychiatrists' roles involve diagnosing patients from a medical vantage point in addition to providing medications for symptom relief and verbal therapy. By contrast, the occupational therapist teaches performance skills, facilitates patients' awareness of personal goals, interests, and feelings, and modifies the environment to promote individual success. These two roles, as well as the roles of other team members, can be cooperatively integrated in treatment, despite the fact that they use different models through the employment of the various *DSM-III-R* axes. Axis IV and Axis V represent a great potential for the occupational therapist to demonstrate skill in performance assessment and adaptive training.

Patient–therapist relationship

People who are ill enough to require hospitalization or participate in outpatient programs using occupational therapists have severe problems. Earlier life experiences and relationships may have been abusive, filled with neglect or hostility. Genetic and biologic causes of psychotic disorders may have resulted in confusion, delusions or hallucinations, and poor reality testing. Understandably, the patient may view human relationships as destructive and resulting in unpredictability and distrust. Being admitted to a psychiatric unit heightens the person's fears and anxieties and makes the person ask, "What will happen to me here?" "Will they help me get better?" "Do they understand how I feel?"

During the admission stage, the occupational therapist uses many interpersonal attitudes and abilities, learned during academic training and life experiences to establish rapport and develop trust with the patient. One important facet of the emerging and ongoing relationship is the creation of a genuinely caring environment in which the therapist demonstrates concern and respect for the patient despite hostile or threatening language or behavior. This does not mean that the therapist is intrusive, paternalistic, or authoritarian in manner.

Throughout the relationship, the therapist builds trust by listening sensitively to the patient's comments and ideas even if they seem strange or inappropriate. Listening to the hidden meaning rather than only to the words is essential to learning the patient's perspective about himself or herself and others. Similarly, observing the nonverbal behavior may reveal incongruent feelings with the spoken word. For example, a teenager may say, "I really don't want to hang out with those sicko kids," while wistfully watching them play a card game.

Acknowledging pain, disappointment, anger, and rejection rather than attempting to deny or talk the patient out of these feelings is a way of letting the patient know he or she is understood and accepted, thus reducing the sense of isolation and uniqueness. Students may think they are supporting the patient by saying, "no need to feel depressed," when in fact they may be trying to prevent intolerable feelings within themselves. The therapist's attempts at reassurance denies the importance of the feelings and problems raised by the patient and thereby trivializes them (Mosey, 1986, p. 20). Offering hope, however, is valuable to patients when depression and confusion begin to lift during treatment. Statements of hope for a brighter, healthier life are more easily accepted when related to small increments in performance and when spoken in a simple manner. For example, "Donna, you moved a step ahead today when you spoke assertively in the role play," is a specific notation regarding having reached a goal and thus represents hope. Other patients' positive feedback as well as their hopeful statements about their own changes are also immensely useful in establishing hope.

The ability to tolerate ***ambiguity*** when working with psychiatric patients is essential. Nuances in meaning and intangible, not yet understood exchanges with patients underlie therapeutic questions such as, "What is he saying?" "Why does he behave like that?" The uncertainty creates mystery and a challenge to learn more regarding the dynamics of the patients' pathology. Holding off on the formation of opinions and remaining flexibly open allows the therapist to consider openly new observations over time when developing the treatment picture. Furthermore, a rigid, cookbook approach may elicit an impersonal and inflexible position in determining acceptable patient behavior, which alienates patients when it is applied to scheduling.

Tolerating ambiguity is not to say that the therapist does not follow institution rules or set limits on unacceptable behavior. In fact, clear understanding of and adherence to rules regarding safety, respectful treatment for self and others, and designated norms within the therapeutic milieu are necessary to provide order and safety. Students may say, "Supervisors instruct from varying and conflicting viewpoints—how am I to learn such awesome skills?" Acquiring subtle clinical skills, which are so important to excellent care, are neither quickly accomplished nor completely attained. See the display below for a summary of patient–therapist relationship guidelines.

Throughout the treatment stage, the therapist serves as a role model for the psychiatric patient. Since many patients were deprived of a healthy interpersonal environment in which their self-perception, social skills, and coping mechanisms were strengthened, the patient–therapist relationship provides an ideal opportunity for the patient to experiment and practice healthy responses in a safe, nonjudgmental arena. The teacher/mentor bond with the patient facilitates interchanges that help to correct aberrant perceptions about the world and to modulate behavior to bring about desired responses from others. Even in short-term settings, patients profit from role playing new behaviors, such as assertiveness or social skills, then receiving peer feedback regarding expressed ideas, feelings, and nonverbal behavior.

In one assertiveness training group, a patient revealed an altered perception of his parents' objection to his coming home late at night when he said, "You helped me see my folks' point of view when you said they were worried about my safety rather than just being nasty." Within a dyad or group format, the therapist can also support the development of problem-solving skills when approaching difficult problems. Such exploratory questions as, "What do you think the critical issue is?" "What steps are necessary?" "What might be the best time and place for you to deal with this problem?" are useful in leading the patient to think in a cause-and-effect manner. Patient group interaction can be supportive and assistive in developing new options that the individual patient can think about. In addition, the resulting altruism and caring are beneficial and a healthy spinoff in small groups in which patients share their problems and suggestions with each other.

Self-disclosure on the part of the therapist serves to humanize the relationship and allow the patient to observe how much alike all people are regardless of status and role. Self-disclosure can incorporate humor and humility, thus reducing

the despair experienced by many patients. Self-disclosure should incorporate a point to be made for learning rather than serve the self-aggrandizing needs of the therapist. Leader vignettes about "how frustrated I became with the motor vehicle administration" or "how I dealt with the school principal" in addition to metaphors and jokes stimulate spontaneity while enriching and warming the relationship.

Self-disclosure and a sense of closeness to a patient do not indicate overinvolvement as some new therapists might think. ***Overinvolvement*** means preoccupation and loss of objectivity regarding patient care, which eventually results in loss of effectiveness (Mosey, 1986, p. 207). Good supervision, watching out for the danger signs, and healthy interest outside the clinical setting diminish the potential of overinvolvement. Overinvolvement may lead to *burnout,* a condition in which the once idealistic neophyte therapist becomes exhausted and disillusioned due to inability to recognize needed personal and energy limits.

Treatment intervention

Treatment strategies, once primarily encompassing crafts or work activities, have become more elaborate and sophisticated as occupational therapy theorists and researchers have successfully conceptualized the purpose, the content, and the process of the field. For many years, practicing mental health occupational therapists suffered defensively when other practitioners asked, "What does an occupational therapist do?" or "Why is what you do of value to the patient?" Lack of articulation regarding the core principles often leads to poor professional self-image and unassertive stances within psychiatric hospitals and community settings.

Nelson (1988) suggested that occupation is the doing of or engagement in activities, tasks, and roles that embody purpose and meaning from the performer's point of view. Christiansen (1991) elaborated on Nelson's ideas by defining occupation in a hierarchical format, which includes activities, tasks, and roles.

Activity is a specific goal-oriented behavior and basic unit of performance. Examples of activity are the voluntary movements, speech, and gestures. *Tasks* are a set of activities that can be broken down and analyzed in terms of their complexity, structure, and purpose. Driving a car is an example of a task involving a number of activities, such as turning the key and stepping on the accelerator. *Roles,* such as homemaker, student, worker, and retiree, define the behaviors and social expectations.

Treatment strategies in the 1990s fall into five major categories:

1. Use of occupation as a therapeutic medium;
2. Education and training;
3. Sensory and neuromotor remediation;
4. Modification of physical environment; and
5. Application of technologic aids (Christiansen, 1991, p. 37).

A particular patient's treatment involves one or more of these treatment categories, depending on the nature and severity of the illness as well as the frame of reference and the setting. For example, a depressed patient whose activities of daily living and work skills are intact may profit from "education and training" in assertiveness and values clarification in contrast to a patient with chronic schizophrenia who may benefit from "sensory and neuromotor" treatment coupled with activities of daily living (ADL) practice.

PATIENT–THERAPIST RELATIONSHIP GUIDELINES

Demonstrate respect and caring by listening more than talking.

Acknowledge patients' unpleasant feelings, complaints, and problems rather than denying or judging them.

Offer hope through noting incremental improvement related to goals.

Learn to live with ambiguity—it represents opportunities for growth and challenge.

Role model interpersonal and problem-solving skills to allow patients to emulate, experiment, and practice healthy behaviors.

Use self-disclosure to illustrate points and yield spontaneity and clarity in relationships.

Occupational therapists historically have defined health as having achieved mastery in work, leisure, and self-care as well as self-acceptance and interpersonal satisfaction. It follows that remediation of dysfunction in these areas will lead to improvement in skills and attitudes that contribute to satisfying life performance. The most effective interventions use the following guidelines, which are essential to contemporary occupational therapy and which differentiate it from modalities used by other mental health professionals.

Guidelines for Treatment

1. The use of occupations (used synonymously with activities) focuses on "doing" rather than "receiving" in the sense that emphasis is on participation, involvement, and productivity.
2. Occupations reflect and relate to real-life roles and situations as much as possible to prepare the patient for return to his or her anticipated role and environment. The total schedule represents a balance in work, rest, leisure, self-care, and sleep.
3. Occupations provide "here and now" social and task situations in which patients give and receive regular feedback and positive reinforcement from peers and therapist.
4. Occupations include a broad range of purposeful human involvement. They may be goal-oriented or nondirected, work- or leisure-oriented, or symptom-reducing and skill-developing in nature. Examples are creative, expressive, and symbolic activities; sports, games, and crafts; discussions; exercises; work; and organizational tasks.
5. Occupations incorporate the patient's or patient groups' responsibility to make their own decisions. Growth toward independence and self-determination is fundamental to rehabilitation.
6. The use of occupations is designed to foster growth in competence and mastery, in curiosity and self-awareness, and in creativity.
7. Occupations are selected and graded to meet the patient's interests, needs, sex, age, cultural background, and level of skill. The patient as an agent of change must participate in determining the treatment goals as well as in making the choice regarding occupations and other interventions.
8. Occupations are selected based on high probability of success, thus ensuring a sense of achievement. Consideration is given to capability of task completion, provision of correct materials, equipment, and instructions (Gibson, 1988).

Occupations enable patients to practice their capacity for experiencing, responding, controlling, and creating a reservoir from which to draw in coping with problems of everyday life (Gibson, 1988). Barris, Kielhofner, and Watts (1983) focus on occupation when they maintain that competence and confidence result from "doing." Through doing people develop their potential while both giving and receiving from their culture.

Competence and its byproduct, self-esteem, evolve from direct and repeated real encounters with task experiences. Task groups are designed to provide the doing that results in validation of efficacy of action via verbal and nonverbal feedback from patient peers and staff (Fidler & Fidler, 1978). In a similar vein, Gibson (1988) has stated:

> The intrinsic gratification of accomplishment and even the sheer pleasure of moving to music or creating a painting are subtle aspects of the human experience which contribute to self-esteem.

Patients say, "It feels good to dance," or "I'm pleased I could draw the flower the way I see it." The inherent drive toward mastery is powerful. It explains the joy and gratification of being a cause, of having an effect, and of accomplishing something within one's own resources. Motivation of this kind lies behind the desire of the occupational therapist to learn group techniques or the patient's desire to speak assertively in the training group. (p. 189)

Occasionally the occupational therapist meets lively resistance from psychiatric patients who do not want to involve themselves in "doing" experiences. This is a difficult situation for the well-meaning young therapist, who may interpret the patient's behavior as a personal attack. It is important to remember that early negative feedback from others and lack of success in manipulating nonhuman objects have left these patients with a sense that "to do is to verify one's incompetence." Hence, rationalizations such as "activities are dumb and boring" are used to defend against failure. This point demonstrates the importance of grading the activity to meet the patient's functional level, interests, and goals to ensure motivation and success.

Additionally, the patient must be allowed choices in activity selections that have social and **cultural relevance**.

> Cultural relevance was exemplified by the case of a depressed woman who refused to discuss her feelings and problems with her psychiatrist as she improved, yet regularly attended a cooking group in which she demonstrated pleasure in cooking and serving others. Her psychiatrist hesitated in discharging her until she understood her open feelings and problems. Her husband, a blue-collar worker, explained that he and his wife were happy that she was now well and could return home to cook for the family. The definition of health included functional work skills, not verbal skills or insight into problems, which are middle class values. (Gibson, 1988, p. 190)

Group leadership

Treatment in psychiatry most frequently occurs within the context of groups due to the nature of the problems and goals in this area. Hence, it is imperative for the student to gain insight and skills in group leadership. The most important member of any group is its leader, who bears responsibility for communicating goals and purpose, creating the normative culture, setting the physical and social structure, and enhancing interaction. How the group responds is determined by the way the therapist plans, structures, and communicates with the members. Leading groups, particularly verbal groups rather than task groups alone, may intimidate beginning therapists who are unsure of the subtleties of interpreting or limiting patients' responses. Although some therapists have a flair for communicating spontaneously with little inhibition and are able to rapidly establish rapport with a patient group, personality is not the key factor in leading groups; technical knowledge and skills acquired through experience and supervision are important. An experienced group leader can make this process look easy.

The leader has immeasurable power and influence in the group and consequently must not underestimate this influence (Glass, 1971). The leader's statements determine the norms, such as empathy, support, and genuineness, which play a vital role in providing a therapeutic environment. Implicitly, the leader uses this influence by commenting, "Yes, I can see what you mean," or "I can imagine how confused you must have been." Patients in the group pick up on the content as well as the manner in which the leader makes such statements and seek to emulate the occupational therapist in interactions with other people. When a patient attempts to make a scapegoat of another patient, the leader sets limits and establishes nondestructive norms by saying, rapidly and directly, "In this group, we are careful not to say things which unnecessarily hurt others."

In a comparable manner, the leader structures the group experience by stating the expectations of meeting times, purpose, time frames, and new member orientation. These expectations are stated clearly during the initiation of the group as well as throughout the life of the group. Experienced leaders inform the group about the nature of their role and even explain simply the rationale behind their actions, thus reducing apprehension and uncertainty. When the group is resistant, the leader may say, "I don't know what's happening; if I were silent as you are now, I might be feeling unsure or disappointed. Can you tell me what you're feeling?" Letting the group in on your experience allows members to identify with your discomfort and invites them to share in responsibility for the group.

Self-disclosure is as valuable a tool in group work as in the patient–therapist relationship if the content is relevant to the point being made and contributes to spontaneity and openness (Yalom, 1975). In group work, self-disclosure tends to build cohesiveness within the group because it helps establish a sense of universality, and a feeling of not being alone. "I handled that kind of situation by . . . " is an example of leader openness that permits a sense of identification as well as relevance. Humor in self-disclosure, even if it is slightly self-deprecating, provides an awareness that the leader is human and can accept mistakes. Humor in self-disclosure adds levity to group experience, a balancing ingredient during the bad times of a psychiatric hospitalization.

At times, the therapist may not understand the unreasonable hostility or irrelevant reaction of a particular patient. The reaction may be due to *transference*, a phenomenon in which the patient projects feelings, thoughts, and wishes toward a person from the past onto the therapist. It is best not to interpret the transference, but to be aware of it to understand the reactions rather than accept it in a personal way. The power of listening is a great therapeutic tool; listening shows more respect than talking. When a therapist listens to the patient's complaints, frustrations, and hopelessness, he or she shows concern for the patient and, in doing so, shares a bit of strength with the patient. Thoughtful, active listening to the meaning of what the patient says permits the therapist to understand the nuances of patient dynamics. In addition, it grants greater significance to comments when the leader does speak.

Flexibility is a hallmark of an experienced group leader (Kaplan, 1988). Most therapists treat seriously ill patients in short-term settings where the turnover of patients is constant and patient crises are the rule. Flexibility in changing the group exercise or the manner in which the therapist leads the group depends on many things—group and individual pathology, the ability of the group to complete the assigned task, and even the way the leader is feeling. When a selected activity does not work, the leader might say, "Perhaps this wasn't the best choice; let's try something different," or "I don't get the impression you want to do this; could you tell me about what's going on?" Flexibility means offering choices to patients, which is an important antidote to perceiving oneself as helpless and childish. Offering choices rather than maintaining a rigid schedule of exercise and

---

GROUP LEADERSHIP GUIDELINES

The group leader
  Recognizes the great influences of the leader in a group
  Communicates the group's purpose, schedule norms, limits, and termination procedures initially and in ongoing manner
  Sets limits on inappropriate speech or behavior directly and clearly as it occurs in the patient group
  Uses self-disclosure when relevant to the therapeutic point
  Uses humor to add spontaneity and levity to group discussion
  Admits own mistakes openly, thus reassuring patients that they can make mistakes and be accepted
  Understands the transference phenomenon in interpreting patients' reactions
  Listens carefully and nonjudgmentally to patient statements
  Turns questions back to group members in order to build participation and cohesiveness
  Responds flexibly and offers choices when group session is not working

---

activities implies that patients' opinions are valued and "that they are necessary in shaping the form the group takes" (Kaplan, 1988, p. 72). Flexibility in choice may run from choosing to conduct the group outside the building to choosing between two games yielding similar objectives. Whatever the choice, the primary issue is empowerment and respect of the patient. See the display above for some group leadership guidelines.

Environment

Milieu therapy

Milieu therapy on inpatient psychiatric units refers to the social processes in a hospital environment that affect patients therapeutically. The term is used interchangeably with therapeutic milieu and therapeutic community (Oldham & Russakof, 1987). The five processes in milieu therapy are containment, support, structure, involvement, and validation or affirmation of a member's individuality (Gunderson, 1978).

Containment refers to several physical components such as seclusion, wet packs, locked doors, and provision of food, shelter, and medical care to prevent patients from harming themselves or others and to reinforce their own internal controls. *Support*, ensuing from the belief that patients benefit from warmth and respect within a relatively stress-free environment, includes physical provisions for escort or cigarettes as well as verbal provisions for direction, advice, reality testing, and education. Both containment and support were advocated by late 18th century pioneers in moral treatment (Gunderson, 1983).

Structure refers to the organization of time, space, and activity and may include the use of privilege/responsibility levels, behavioral contracts, isolation, and the regulation of sleeping, eating, and hygiene times. *Involvement* refers to the insistence that patients attend to and interact with the social environment to strengthen their sense of self and to modify maladaptive interpersonal patterns. This concept arose in the 1950s with the concept of the therapeutic community introduced by Maxwell Jones (1953, 1956). *Validation* refers to processes that affirm individuality; it includes acceptance of regression, incompetence, and symptomatology as meaningful expressions of the inner self. The inclusion of these three processes brought the milieu from a treatment background to a definable treatment in its own right (Gunderson, 1983).

Milieu therapy is found in addiction programs, in chronic schizophrenic units where behavior modification or token economies might be used, and in short-term psychiatric units (Levenson, 1977; Oldham & Russakof, 1987). A controlled milieu is the chief difference between inpatient and outpatient treatment, but outpatient programs such as partial hospitalization programs may also have a therapeutic milieu. This is generally more difficult to sustain since patients voluntarily arrive and depart daily. Communication components of the therapeutic milieu include unit reports or team meetings, community meetings, and therapeutic activities for patients and staff. In addition, treatment planning and discharge planning conferences as well as staff, administrative, and policy and educational meetings are for staff only (Leeman, 1986).

The role of occupational therapy in the therapeutic milieu, especially in inpatient psychiatry, is to build cohesiveness and to structure patient needs through provision of the patient's daily or weekly schedule, therapeutic groups, and various treatment modalities including movement and tasks to balance verbal psycho-

therapy groups. This reinforces the value of a balanced routine and lifestyle (Schwartzberg & Abeles, 1986). The five processes of milieu therapy can also be used to organize occupational therapy unit-based groups and to integrate them with others in patient treatment (Maves & Schulz, 1985).

Multidisciplinary treatment team

The concept of the multidisciplinary **treatment team** has long been one in which various mental health disciplines working together assess and treat the patient more effectively than each one could working individually. Although this concept is a common and often articulated one, much is required to attain effective team functioning. Mental health has a long and distinguished history of contributions to interdisciplinary collaboration and, in fact, has led other health fields in this area (Hertzman, 1984).

In today's fast-paced health care market, demand for some disciplines is declining; for others it is expanding. This may create competition among team members as well as **role blurring** in which the boundaries among disciplines become unclear as staff try to fill traditional roles of other disciplines. The first and most important aspect of effective team functioning is to identify interdisciplinary role functions. Table 17-7 identifies potential treatment team members according to education (lowest level), national certification, state regulation, and accountability. Second, it is important to support one another by acknowledging each person's particular skills and talents, independent of discipline, and commenting on a job well done. This can be a

TABLE 17-7. *Mental Health Disciplines*

Discipline	Education	National Certification	State Regulation	Accountability
Occupational therapy	Baccalaureate degree or Masters degree and field-work education	American Occupational Therapy Certified Board (OTR)	Licensure—38 states; certification—4 states; registration—3 states; trademark—2 states	Functional assessment and activities to promote function and adaptation.
Art therapy	Master's degree and internship	American Art Therapy Association registration (ATR)	None	Preverbal psychotherapy through art
Dance/movement therapy	Master's degree and internship	American Dance Therapy Association registration (DTR and ADTR)	None	Preverbal psychotherapy through movement
Nursing	Staff nurse—associate diploma or baccalaureate degree Clinical specialist—master's degree	American Nursing Association (RN)	Licensure—50 states	Nursing care and therapeutic milieu
Psychology	Doctorate in clinical psychology and internship	American Board of Professional Psychology (ABPP)	Licensure—50 states	Psychological testing, assessment, and psychotherapy
Psychiatry	Doctorate in medicine and psychiatric residency	American Board of Psychiatry and Neurology	Licensure—50 states	Medical care
Recreational therapy	Baccalaureate degree and internship	National Council for Therapeutic Recreation (CTRS)	Licensure—3 states; registration—1 state	Restoration, mediation, or rehabilitation of independent functioning in leisure
Social work	Master's degree includes fieldwork	Academy of Certified Social Workers (ACSW)	Licensure and vendorship—37 states	Family assessment, intervention, and discharge planning
Vocational counseling	Baccalaureate degree; master's degree with internship preferred	Commission Rehabilitation Certification (CRC)	Licensure—10 states	Work readiness evaluation and training and career counseling

stimulating and challenging process as treatment team members continue to understand and improve their clinical skills and be the teachers of one another (Hertzman, 1984).

The third aspect of successful team functioning is education. Co-leadership of groups among disciplines and didactic education or orientation of new staff and interns and residents lead to a better understanding of occupational therapy. The fourth aspect of team functioning is management of conflict resolution, which involves a systematic approach to problem solving such as recognizing the problem, determining optimal time and persons for resolutions, defining and prioritizing the problem, identifying solutions and supporting, implementing, and evaluating the plan (Hertzman, 1984).

Regarding treatment team accountability, the psychiatrist and the psychologist focus on psychopathology and psychodynamics, the social worker on social systems, and the occupational therapist focuses on performance. With the advent of *DSM-III* and *DSM-III-R*, performance has been separated from symptomatology (Axis I, II, III) and appears separately in its own right on Axis V. This gives added importance for functioning as an

TABLE 17-8. *Pharmacotherapies Commonly Used in Psychiatry**

	Antidepressants	Antipsychotic Agents	Antimanic Agents (Lithium Salts)	Antianxiety Agents	Anticonvulsants
Indication	Mental depression, attention deficit disorder, bulimia, obsessive-compulsive disorder (Anafranil)	Psychotic disorders	Bipolar disorder, mental depression	Anxiety; anxiety associated with depression; alcohol withdrawal; panic disorders	Anticonvulsant, anti-neurologic, antimanic, antipsychotic
Common trade name	Tricyclics: Elavil, Anafranil, Norpramin, Sinequan, Tofranil, Pamelor, Vivactil Tetracyclic: Ludiomil	Thorazine, Prolixin, Loxitane, Serentil, Moban, Trilafon, Mellaril, Navane, Stelazine	Lithium carbonate	Xanax, Klonopin, Tranxene, Librium, Valium, Ativan, Serax	Tegretol
Adverse reactions	Skin rash, anticholinergic effects, fast, slow, or irregular heartbeat, nervousness, extrapyramidal syndrome	Akathisia, hypotension, photosensitivity, tardive dyskinesia, extrapyramidal syndrome	Cardiovascular-fainting, fast or slow heartbeat, irregular pulse; leukocytosis—usually tired or weak; weight gain.	Confusion, mental depression, aphasia, blurred vision, dizziness, habitual/addiction potential	CNS toxicity—blurred/double vision, nystagmus, behavioral changes, especially in children, severe diarrhea, aplastic anemia (rare)
Indication	Mental depression	Psychotic disorders, severe behavioral disorders		Anxiety	Epilepsy, bipolar disorder
Common trade name	Wellbutrin	Haldol		BuSpar	Depakene
Adverse reactions	CNS stimulation, fast or irregular heartbeat, seizures (higher doses) contraindicated in patients with seizure or eating disorders	Extrapyramidal syndrome		Chest pain, confusion, depression, fast or pounding heartbeat, sore throat, or fever (all rare)	Behavioral, mood, or mental changes, hepatotoxicity, opthamalogic effects, pancreatitis
Indication	Mental depression, obsessive-compulsive disorder	Schizophrenia			
Common trade name	Prozac	Clorazil			
Adverse reactions	Skin rash or hives, dizziness, lightheadedness, chills or fever, joint or muscle pain, dry mouth	Tachycardia, hypotension, fever, hypersalivation, weight gain, blood dyscrasia (rare but significant)			
Indication	Mental depression				
Common trade name	MAO inhibitors: Nardil, Parnate				
Adverse reactions	Orthostatic hypotension—severe sympathetic stimulation, peripheral edema, diarrhea				

* *Ingrid Baramki, RPh, MS, Sheppard and Enoch Pratt Hospital, Baltimore, MD; adapted from USP-DI 1991 (11th ed.) Drug Information for the Health Care Professional by authority of the United States Pharmacopeial Convention, Inc.*

indicator or disorder and supports occupational therapy's traditional focus on function (Bonder, 1990a).

Psychopharmacology

Psychopharmacology has been an important part of medicine since the mid 1950s and continues to play an important role in symptom reduction and management of psychiatric patients. Although the physician prescribes psychoactive agents and the nurse administers them, the treatment team as a unit shares responsibility for feedback to the physician about their efficacy. Therefore, the occupational therapist needs basic knowledge of the indications and **adverse reactions** of various medications to evaluate and treat the patient more effectively, reassure the patient who may be upset and provide some education, and provide feedback to the treatment team and physician about their efficacy (Mosey, 1986). Table 17-8 identifies some of the most commonly used psychopharmacologic agents. A useful reference for the clinician is the *Physicians' Desk Reference* (*PDR*), which gives a comprehensive account of all medications. The following are some common adverse reactions and appropriate interventions for clinicians (Mosey, 1986, pp. 479–481).

Akathisia (involuntary motor restlessness). Provide simple, short-term, nonsedentary activities.

Convulsions. Learn facility procedures for management. Some patients have an aura and can predict when a convulsion is coming; encourage the patient to share this with you and get him or her into a safe, prone position immediately.

Dizziness, faintness, and weakness. Find a safe place for the patient to sit or lie down. Encourage resumption of activities when episode is over.

Drowsiness. Engage patient in meaningful, interesting activity.

Dry mouth and throat. Provide water and low-calorie, caffeine-free drinks. Chewing gum or hard candy may help.

Increased appetite or weight gain. Provide low-calorie snacks and encourage a restricted diet and regular exercise.

Orthostatic hypotension (a sudden drop in blood pressure due to rapid postural changes causing dizziness and faintness). Assist patient to avoid rapid postural changes from sitting, bending, and standing.

Photosensitivity (sensitivity to the sun). Limit time outdoors if necessary. Patient's face should be covered with a sunscreen lotion and hat and limbs covered with a sunscreen lotion or clothing.

Tardive dyskinesia (repetitive involuntary movements primarily affecting the face and mouth, including tongue protrusion, smacking and sucking lip movements, and facial grimaces). The limbs and trunk may be involved. Tardive dyskinesia is the most serious side effect of antipsychotic medications, and the treatment of choice is to discontinue the medication.

Extrapyramidal syndrome (EPS). The side effects are classified into three categories and include parkinsonian syndrome, dystonias, and akathisia. Parkinsonian syndrome consists of masklike face, tremor at rest, rigidity, shuffling gait, and motor retardation and its symptoms are identical with those of Parkinson's disease. The dystonias consist of a broad range of bizarre movements or tongue, face, and neck (Fisher, 1991). Medication can be prescribed.

References

American Psychiatric Association. (1980). *Diagnostic and statistical manual of mental disorders* (3rd. ed.). Washington, DC: Author.

American Psychiatric Association. (1987). *Diagnostic and statistical manual of mental disorders* (3rd ed., rev.). Washington, DC: Author.

Barris, R., Kielhofner, G., & Watts, J. (1983). *Psychosocial occupational therapy* (2nd ed.). Baltimore: Waverly Press.

Bonder, B. R. (1990a). Disease and dysfunction: The value of Axis V. *Hospital and Community Psychiatry, 41*(9), 959, 964.

Bonder, B. R. (1990b). *Psychopathology and function.* Thorofare, NJ: Slack.

Christiansen, C. (1991). Occupational therapy: Intervention for life performance. In C. Christiansen & C. Baum (Eds.), *Occupational therapy: Overcoming performance deficits.* Thorofare, NJ: Slack.

Fidler, G., & Fidler J. (1978). Doing & becoming: Purposeful action and self-actualization. *American Journal of Occupational Therapy, 32,* 305–310.

Fisher, P. J. (1991). Psychotropic medications. In B. R. Bonder (Ed.), *Psychopathology and function* (pp. 155–183). Thorofare, NJ: Slack.

Gibson, D. (1988). Activity therapy in hospital psychiatry. In J. Lion, W. Adler & W. Webb (Eds.), *Modern Hospital Psychiatry* (pp. 179–207). New York: W. W. Norton & Co.

Glass, S. (1971). *The practical handbook of group counseling.* Baltimore: BCS Publishing Co.

Gunderson, J. G. (1978). Defining the therapeutic process in psychiatric milieus. *Psychiatry, 41,* 327–335.

Gunderson, J. G. (1983). An overview of modern milieu therapy. In J. G. Gunderson, O. A. Willis & L. R. Mosher (Eds.), *Principles and practice of modern milieu therapy* (pp. 1–13). New York: Jason Aronson.

Hertzman, M. (1984). A psychiatrist's experience with occupational therapy in a short-term general hospital unit. *Occupational Therapy in Mental Health, 4*(3), 101–114.

Jones, M. (1953). *The therapeutic community.* New York: Basic Books.

Jones, M. (1956). The concept of a therapeutic community. *American Journal of Psychiatry, 112,* 647–650.

Kaplan, K. (1988). *Directive group therapy: Innovative mental health treatment.* Thorofare, NJ: Slack.

Leeman, C. P. (1986). The therapeutic milieu and its role in clinical management. In L. C. Sederer (Ed.), *Inpatient psychiatry: Diagnosis and treatment* (2nd ed., pp. 219–239). Baltimore: Williams & Wilkins.

Levenson, A. I. (1977). Theoretical issues in short-term treatment. *National Association of Private Psychiatric Hospitals, 9*(1), 12–66.

Maves, P. A., & Schultz, J. W. (1985). Inpatient group treatment on short-term acute care units. *Hospital and Community Psychiatry, 36*(1), 69–73.

Medical Economics Company. (1991). *Physicians' desk reference.* Oradell, NJ: Author.

Mosey, A. C. (1986). *Psychosocial components of occupational therapy.* Thorofare, NJ: Slack.

Nelson, D. L. (1988). Occupation: Form and performance. *American Journal of Occupational Therapy, 42*(10), 633–641.

Oldham, J. M., & Russakof, L. M. (1987). *Dynamic therapy in brief hospitalization.* Northvale, NJ: Jason Aronson.

Schwartzberg, S. L., & Abeles, J. (1986). Occupational therapy. In L. I. Sederer (Ed.), *Inpatient psychiatry: Diagnosis and treatment* (pp. 308–323). Baltimore: Williams & Wilkins.

Yalom, I. (1975). *The theory and practice of group psychotherapy,* New York: Basic Books.

Bibliography

Faulk-Kessler, J., Mamich, C., & Pearl, S. (1991). Therapeutic factors in occupational therapy groups. *American Journal of Occupational Therapy, 45*(1), 59–66.

Peloquin, S. M. (1988). Linking purpose to procedure during interactions with patients. *American Journal of Occupational Therapy, 42*(12), 775–781.

Peloquin, S. M. (1989). Sustaining the art of practice in occupational therapy. *American Journal of Occupational Therapy, 43*(4), 219–226.

Peloquin, S. M. (1990). The patient-therapist relationship in occupational therapy: Understanding visions and images. *American Journal of Occupational Therapy, 44*(1), 13–21.

SECTION 1G
Service delivery

GAIL Z. RICHERT

KEY TERMS

Assessment	Functional Assessment
Clinical Reasoning	Quality Assurance
Discharge Planning	Reevaluation
Documentation	Synthesis Approach
Evaluation	Treatment Plan
Frame of Reference	

LEARNING OBJECTIVES

Upon completion of this section the reader will be able to:

1. *Identify three stages of clinical reasoning.*

2. *Define the synthesis approach.*

3. *Identify six frames of references in mental health, appropriate patient populations for which they are used, and suggested instruments.*

4. *Identify and describe the seven standards of practice of occupational therapy in mental health.*

5. *Define assessment and evaluation.*

6. *Name and give examples of seven types of instruments.*

7. *Develop a method to screen and select instruments.*

8. *Give examples of functional assessments used in mental health.*

9. *Describe the treatment planning process according to the case method of problem solving.*

10. *Identify four purposes of documentation.*

11. *Identify three methods of evaluating program effectiveness.*

In 1988, under the leadership of Susan C. Robertson, the American Occupational Therapy Association's Division of Continuing Education developed the second part of a competency-based curriculum for occupational therapists providing direct services in assessment and treatment. This curriculum was used as the basis for workshops given nationally and was called *Mental Health FOCUS: Skills for Assessment and Treatment* (Robertson, 1988a). Today, the foundations of this curriculum continue to be relevant for clinicians in mental health.

Fine (1991) reminds occupational therapists to start with the patient's experience of his or her condition rather than with the tools of practice. In striving for patient functional adaptation and positive treatment outcome, the clinician must draw out the patient's experience of his or her tragedy and integrate this with preexisting patterns for self-regulating activity.

Clinical reasoning

The concept of **clinical reasoning**, which links practice with theory, is widely used in occupational therapy. In the application of theory to practice, clinicians have two models at their disposal. In the *medical model*, based on the scientific approach, symptoms are viewed as related to disease entities. Disease is observed to be separate from the ill person. The *meaning-centered model*, which comes from physical anthropology and considers the patient to be part of his or her difficulty or disease. The essential perspective for the occupational therapist is to engage the patient in the treatment process, because he or she is part of both the problem and the solution in the meaning-centered model (Mattingly, 1988). The clinical decision-making process has three key stages: (1) defining the problem, (2) determining what could be done to improve patient function, and (3) deciding what treatment should be provided. The **frame of reference** or practice model defines the parameters of reasoning and is integral to defining the problem and determining what can be done to improve function (Robertson, 1988b).

Frames of reference

Establishing the link between theory and practice is part of the clinical reasoning process and begins with the selection of a frame of reference. The clinician determines his or her own professional beliefs about mental disorder and whether it is biologically or environmentally based or a combination of both. The next step—evaluating the patient—usually begins with a screening and chart review to assess the patient's level of functioning. The clinician then selects a frame of reference that is appropriate, given the clinician's perspective and the patient's preliminary screening data including demographics, diagnosis, and history.

A method for determining a frame of reference is the **synthesis approach** in which the Allen Cognitive Level Test (ACL) is administered. The ACL is a performance-based, standardized leather-lacing task in which the patient's task performance is scored on levels 1 through 6 (Allen, 1985). If the patient is on the lower level of the test (low 4 or below), it is determined that the patient has significant learning problems and the cognitive disabilities frame of reference could be considered. If, however, the patient is in the middle or high 4 level, he or she could benefit from other frames of reference (Denton & Skinner, 1988).

Currently, many frames of reference are being used in occupational therapy; these are discussed at length in Chapter 4, Section 3. Many frames of reference are also being used in mental health (Bruce & Borg, 1987; Levy, 1986). It is important to remember that certain commonalities exist among all frames of reference, regardless of which one is selected (Borg & Bruce, 1991):

1. Emphasis on a partnership between the patient and the therapist; assessment is viewed as an opportunity for shared learning and integration
2. Support for a combination of interview and task or structured and unstructured components
3. Identified need for an initial and ongoing assessment process.

Six frames of reference are selected and presented in Table 17-9 (Mosey, 1986, pp. 375–384). These frames of reference are acquisitional (Mosey, 1986, pp. 443–449; Stein, 1982), cognitive disabilities (Allen 1985, 1988a), developmental (Mosey, 1986, pp. 407–415), model of human occupation (Kielhofner, 1985), psychoanalytic (Mosey, 1986, pp. 385–393), and sensory integration (King, 1974, 1982, 1990). Other frames of reference commonly used are lifestyle performance profile (Fidler 1982a, 1988) and role acquisition, an acquisitional frame of reference

TABLE 17-9. *Frames of Reference in Mental Health*

Acquisitional	Cognitive Disabilities	Developmental	Model of Human Occupational	Psychodynamic (Psychoanalytic)	Sensory Integration/ Neurodevelopmental
Theoretical base					
Watson, Skinner, Azrin, others, and learning theory	Piaget, neurology, neurophysiology, cognitive and normal development	Ayres, Arieti, Piaget, Freud, Erikson, Maslow, White, others	White Reilly, von Bertalanffy, McClellan, others	Freud, Jung, Sullivan, others	Ayres, Rood, Farber, and neurosciences
Theorist					
Mosey (Role Acquisition)	Allen	Mosey (recapitalization of ontogenesis), Llorens, Reed	Kielhofner, Burke, Igi, Barris, Florey, others	Fidler, Mosey (Reconciliation of Universal Issues)	King—adapted for a psychiatric population Wilbarger
Function/dysfunction continuum					
Seven categories with continua Based on frequency of maladaptive/adaptive behaviors	Continua of 6 cognitive levels in routine task behavior	Seven adaptive skills continua with sequential skill components	Maladaptive vs. adaptive cycles	Vaguely defined symptoms produced by unconscious conflicts Function restored when needs are brought to consciousness and met	Vaguely defined Related to ability to integrate sensory input
Patient population					
Chronic schizophrenia, obsessive compulsive disorders, others Patients experiencing difficulties in role transitions	Affective and schizophrenic disorders, dementia, CVA, TBI, organic brain syndrome, AIDS, substance abuse, others	All patients who have not mastered the developmental stages	All ages and diagnoses	Personality disorders Patients with maladaptive intrapsychic content and markedly altered life situations	Chronic schizophrenia, geropsychiatric patients Sensory affective disorders
Assessment format and process					
Behavioral observation scales Interview, behavioral Functional assessment Questionnaires Self-report measures	Interview, task history Performance-based tests of voluntary motor actions	Interview for mastered life tasks Performance observation Standardized and non-standardized tools	History taking Interview Observation Standarized and nonstandarized test	Interview, open-ended Projective tasks Focus on inference	Interview Performance of a structured task
Suggested instruments					
Bay Area Functional Performance Evaluation (BAFPE) Comprehensive Evaluation of Basic Living Skills (CEBLS) Comprehensive Occupational Therapy Evaluation (COTE) Functional assessment Milwaukee Evaluation of Daily Living Skills (MEDLS)	Allen Cognitive Level Test (ACL) Chart review Lower Level Test (LCL) Routine Task Inventory (RTI)	Bay Area Functional Performance Evaluation (BAFPE) Group Interaction Skill Survey (Mosey, 1986, p. 325) Interpersonal Skill Survey (Mosey, 1986, p. 324) Survey of Task Skill (Mosey, 1986, p. 322)	Bay Area Functional Performance Evaluation (BAFPE) Occupational Case Analysis and Interview Rating Scale (OCAIRS) (Kaplan and Kielhofner, 1989) Occupational Performance History Interview (OPHI) (Kielhofner, Henry, and Walens, 1989) Role Checklist	Azima Battery Activity Configuration Bay Area Functional Performance Evaluation (BAFPE) House-Tree-Person (HTP) Magazine Picture Collage	Clinical observation SBC Adult Psychiatric Sensory Integrative Evaluation Draw-a-Person Nurses' Observation Scale for Inpatient Evaluation (NOSIE)

(Adapted from L. Levy [1986], A. C. Mosey [1986], C. Neilson [Outline for FOCUS, 1988], S. Robertson [1988a].)

that is a combination of action-consequence, activities therapy, and occupational behavior (Mosey, 1986, pp. 450–476, 1988).

Standards of practice

The standards of practice for occupational therapy services were established by AOTA in 1978 and revised in 1992 (see Appendix B). This document provides guidelines for clinicians providing service delivery.

Referral

Between the 1950s and the 1960s, occupational therapists and physicians advocated changing from a prescription to a referral system, which mandated the clinician to translate diagnostic information into specific goals and processes or to evaluate functioning (Hemphill, 1982, p. 5). Today, many referral systems exist, and referrals may originate from other treatment team members as well as from the physician. It is important to note, however, that in some cases, a physician referral may be required as in services provided for Medicare (Department of Health and Human Services, 1988).

Assessment and evaluation

Assessment and evaluation are both used in fact-finding procedures that precede setting treatment objectives. **Assessment** is the sum of evaluation procedures and yields a composite picture of patient functioning. **Evaluation** refers to data gathered from specific procedures (Smith & Tiffany, 1988).

Using the *Uniform Terminology for Occupational Therapy* (2nd ed.) found in Appendix C, occupational performance areas and occupational performance components are assessed and evaluated as follows:

I. Performance areas
   A. Activities of daily living
   B. Work activities—home management, care of others, educational and vocational activities
   C. Play or leisure activities
II. Performance components
   A. Sensory motor—sensory integration, neuromuscular, and motor
   B. Cognitive integration and cognitive components
   C. Psychosocial skills and psychological components—psychological, social, and self-management

When examining assessment and evaluation tools, it is important to identify the points of view. These include the following (Borg & Bruce, 1991):

1. Insider or subjective point of view, which is the patient's perspective and includes interviews, projective tests, activity configurations, self-rating scales, journals, and media experiences
2. Outsider or objective point of view, which is the perspective of the assessor or the objective third person and includes structured interviews, behavioral rating scales, and structured tasks
3. Combination of the subjective and objective points of view, which includes both personal history and a specific task. The patient and the assessor independently rate the pa-

tient's skills. An example is Schroeder-Block-Campbell Adult Psychiatric Evaluation (Schroeder, Block, Campbell, Trottier, & Stowell, 1978).

After identifying assessment points of view, the clinician reviews the different types of instruments used in mental health including (Borg & Bruce, 1991):

1. *Self-report formats*—people describe or rate their own thoughts, feelings, or behaviors. These include checklists, true–false questionnaires, and performance scales. Some examples are Interest Checklist (Matsutsuyu, 1969), Role Checklist (Oakley, Kielhofner, Barris, & Reichler, 1986; Oakley, Kielhofner, & Barris, 1988), an activity configuration (Mosey, 1986), and Activity Laboratory Questionnaire (Fidler, 1982c), which follows Activity Laboratory (Fidler, 1982b). These formats have an insider or subjective point of view.

2. *Self-monitoring*—people self-monitor changes in thoughts, feelings, or behavior. These may include paper-and-pencil formats and unstructured activities, structured self-reports, checklists, and graphs. Examples are the use of daily journals or activity configurations. These have an insider or subjective point of view.

3. *Behavior observation scales*—the assessor observes and rates a sample of individual behavior viewed as necessary for daily functioning. Examples of these scales are Bay Area Functional Performance Evaluation (BaFPE; Williams & Bloomer, 1987), Comprehensive Occupational Therapy Evaluation (COTE; Brayman & Kirby, 1982), Comprehensive Evaluation of Basic Living Skills (CEBLS; Casanova & Ferber, 1976), Nurses' Observation Scale for Inpatient Evaluation (NOSIE; Honigfield, Gillis, & Kleitt, 1966) and Parachek Geriatric Rating Scale (Parachek & King, 1986). These have an outsider or objective point of view.

4. *Projective tests*—the person responds verbally or nonverbally to a stimulus, and the assessor makes inferences about the responses. These tests include drawing, sentence completion, word association, and play techniques. Examples are Magazine Picture Collage (Lerner & Ross, 1977; Lerner, 1979), Azima Battery (Azima, 1982) and variations of Draw-A-Person including House-Tree-Person (Buck & Jolles, 1972). These assessments were commonly used in the 1950s and 1960s. They have a subjective/objective or individual/assessor point of view.

5. *Psychometric techniques*—the person's responses are treated as correlates of human traits. These techniques include personality inventories like Minnesota Multiphasic Personality Inventory (MMPI) and Myers-Briggs Type Indicator, interest inventories like Strong-Campbell Interest Inventory, and attitude, value, and opinion scales. These tests are primarily used by psychologists rather than occupational therapists and may be part of a patient's history or current evaluation. They have a subjective/objective or individual/assessor point of view.

6. *Biopsychological assessment*—the person's thoughts and emotions are related to bodily states. This type of assessment includes self-report behavior scales, interviews, and others. Some examples are Allen Cognitive Level Test (Allen, 1985, 1988a), Schroeder-Block-Campbell Adult Psychiatric Sensory Integration Evaluation, and Draw-a-Person, which serves not only as a projective, but also as an indicator of

body image and maturational and neurologic change (King, 1982). These assessments have a subjective/objective and individual/assessor point of view.

7. *Interview*—the assessor asks questions and the person responds. Interviews may be structured or loosely structured, but some form of interview is common to all frames of reference. Interviewing is an important component of any assessment, and the numerous methods used to conduct them are influenced by the practice setting, immediate environment, the person's characteristics, the interviewer's beliefs and frame of reference, and the dynamics of the therapeutic relationship (Chapter 17, Section 1F). An example of an occupational therapy interview is Occupational Role History (Florey & Michelman, 1982). Interviews have a subjective/objective and individual or assessor point of view.

Given the current availability of so many assessments and evaluations, how does the clinician begin the selection process? Having identified previously a frame of reference according to professional beliefs and the patient's preliminary screening data (demographics, diagnosis, history) and level of functioning, the clinician selects an instrument compatible with the frame of reference. Table 17-9 suggests some possibilities. In addition, case studies in Chapter 17, Section 1H illustrate the clinical reasoning process in selecting a frame of reference with specific patients in various practice settings with a range of ages and diagnoses.

Even within a given frame of reference, screening and reviewing the range of evaluation tools can still present dilemmas to the clinician. To screen assessments, Michael and Kaplan (1988) suggest using *Uniform Terminology for Occupational Therapy* (2nd ed.), which provides a framework for organizing and retrieving instruments suitable for particular clients (see Appendix C). Once screened, instruments may be examined according to patient population, reliability, validity, standardization, and time and equipment needed (Maurer, 1988). Several comprehensive resources exist for mental health instruments including Asher (1989), Hemphill, (1982, 1988), and Kielhofner (1985).

An important and recent trend has been mental health leadership's focus on function (Bonder 1990, 1991; Dickie & Robertson, 1991) and functional assessment (Allen, 1988b; Denton, 1988; Gibson, 1990; Hemphill, Peter & Weiner, 1991; Levy, 1990). This direction evolved in response to economic pressures in the field, particularly in acute care psychiatry, which presses clinicians to return patients to the community after shorter periods of institutionalization. To prepare patients for discharge as soon as possible, **functional assessments** are used to predict community adjustment and to select appropriate housing and vocational placement (Gibson, 1990). Some functional assessments identified by mental health leaders are the Allen Cognitive Level Test, the Bay Area Functional Performance Evaluation, Comprehensive Evaluation of Basic Living Skills, Comprehensive Occupational Therapy Evaluation, Independent Living Skills (Johnson, Vinnecombe & Merrill, 1980), Milwaukee Evaluation of Daily Living Skills (Leonardelli, 1988a, 1988b), Parachek Geriatric Rating Scale, Routine Task Inventory (RTI; Allen, 1985), Kohlman Evaluation of Living Skills (KELS; McGourty, 1979, 1988) and Scorable Self-care Evaluation (SSCE; Clarke & Peters, 1984).

Treatment plan development and implementation

After the frame of reference is identified and data are gathered through assessment and evaluation, Pelland (1987) suggests that the **treatment plan** proceed according to the case method of problem solving:

1. *Analyze the data*. This may result in an identified need for data or in referral to another discipline or service.
2. *Identify strengths and weaknesses*. During this process, functional capabilities and limitations are identified as well as the biopsychosocial factors that enable or inhibit function. These factors may lead to the need for more data, referral to another discipline, or referral to occupational therapy.
3. *Develop the treatment plan*. The findings are summarized and short- and long-term goals, intervention plans, and plans for further data collection are identified. Treatment planning may vary according to the practice setting. It may be done collaboratively with the treatment team, or the coordinating role may be assigned to one of the team members.
4. *Implement the treatment plan*. Plans are prioritized in accordance with patient goals, prognosis, and length of stay (Fig. 17-2).

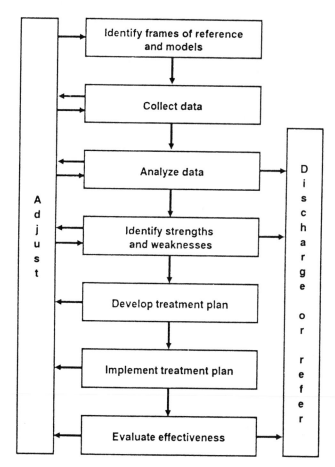

FIGURE 17-2. *A conceptual model of treatment planning.* (*From Pelland, M. J. [1987]. A conceptual model for instruction and supervision of treatment planning.* American Journal of Occupational Therapy, 46 *[6], 351–359.*)

It is essential to involve the patient in the occupational therapy treatment planning process, a generic belief that is supported by the Code of Ethics (see Appendix A) as well as health care standards set by the Joint Commission on Accreditation of Healthcare Organizations (JCAHO), the Commission on Accreditation of Rehabilitation Facilities (CARF), and the American Physical Therapy Association (APTA) (Nelson & Payton, 1991).

Another essential component of this process is family or caregiver involvement, especially with the safety issues and environmental adaptation needed by the cognitively disabled psychiatric patient (Allen, 1989). Sometimes this is accomplished best through a home evaluation in the patient's own environment followed by subsequent education of both the patient and the family or caregiver. A home evaluation results in a smoother transition for the patient to appropriate residential placement.

Discharge plan

Discharge planning represents the culmination of the treatment planning process and, in acute care psychiatry, begins with data gathering. Discharge planning is an integral part of the treatment planning process as well as a team effort. In some settings, one member of the team may be designated as accountable. The occupational therapist has a key role in providing patient and family or caregiver education to facilitate transition to the community. Guidelines for effective discharge planning include a summary of assessment and treatment results, a home program, if applicable, and aftercare recommendations and referrals to appropriate support groups, community resources, and programs to promote effective community transition (see Appendix E). Aftercare programs may include occupational therapy services such as stress management, assertiveness training, activities of daily living, and vocational transition groups.

Reevaluation

The effectiveness of the patient's treatment is evaluated at appropriate and regular intervals according to goal achievement (**reevaluation**). If necessary, the treatment planning process is repeated and appropriate referrals are made. After discharge, the clinician may continue to treat the patient as part of aftercare services.

Documentation

The Guidelines for Occupational Therapy Documentation identify four purposes: a legal record, an information source, facilitating communication, and data for treatment, research, education, and reimbursement (see Appendix E). As a legal document, it must meet state and federal guidelines including those for Medicare and Medicaid. The Medicare law is usually the most stringent, and adherence to its requirements usually suffices to meet standards often set in other guidelines (Acquaviva & Steich, 1988; Department of Health and Human Services, 1988). Other Medicare guidelines are physician prescription, general supervision of a certified occupational therapy assistant, and practical improvement in the person's level of functioning within a reasonable period of time. **Documentation** also resolves professional malpractice issues and is used to assign disability status based on functional capacity gleaned from the medical record by Social Security Administration representatives. Therefore, occupa-

tional therapy, which frequently documents functional status, can make a significant contribution to the functional capacity assessment.

As long as the primary criteria for coverage are met and the recording documents patient function, the form of documentation is of secondary importance. In acute care psychiatry, where rapid patient turnover necessitates recording that meets Medicare criteria and is short in length, there is considerable debate about documentation form among clinicians. One form is the problem-oriented medical record (POMR), which uses SOAP notes. Here, recording is organized around subjective data (S), objective data (O), assessment (A), and plan (P) (Kettenbach, 1990). An adaptation of the POMR that has specific, measurable, and attainable functional goals has been developed for use in a multidisciplinary department (Lang & Mattson, 1985).

Quality review

Each clinician is responsible for reviewing systematically the quality of outcomes and services according to professional consensus and recent developments in research and theory. One way to evaluate programs is to use a **quality assurance** format involving a problem-solving process. This is used by JCAHO to monitor and evaluate the quality and appropriateness of patient care. Other aspects of quality assurance include peer review, which monitors professional standards, and program evaluation, which is conducted by accrediting agencies like CARF and JCAHO (Joe, 1988).

For the clinician who desires to start a departmental quality assurance plan, JCAHO has developed a generic plan, easily adaptable to any practice setting (Brinson, 1988). Another system, Continuous Quality Improvement (CQI), measures, directs, and improves the quality of services on a continuous basis (Stoffel & Cunningham, 1991). Three methods for demonstrating treatment effectiveness in mental health occupational therapy are progress toward goals, patient satisfaction questionnaires, and behavioral rating scales that measure patient level of skill performance at the beginning and end of treatment (Thien, 1987).

References

Acquaviva, J. D., & Steich, T. J. (1988). Occupational therapy documentation in mental health. In S. Robertson (Ed.), *Mental health FOCUS: Skills for assessment and treatment* (pp. 1-169–1-177). Rockville, MD: American Occupational Therapy Association.

Allen, C. K. (1985). *Occupational therapy for psychiatric diseases: Measurement and management of cognitive disabilities.* Boston: Little, Brown, & Co.

Allen, C. K. (1988a). Cognitive disabilities. In S. C. Robertson (Ed.), *Mental health FOCUS: Skills for assessment and treatment* (pp. 3-18–3-33). Rockville, MD: American Occupational Therapy Association.

Allen, C. K. (1988b). Occupational therapy: Functional assessment of the severity of mental disorders. *Hospital and Community Psychiatry, 39*(2), 140–142.

Allen, C. K. (1989). Treatment plans in cognitive rehabilitation. *Occupational Therapy Practice, 1*(1), 1–8.

Asher, I. E. (1989). *An annotated index of occupational therapy evaluation tools.* Rockville, MD: American Occupational Therapy Association.

Azima, F. J. C. (1982). The Azima Battery: An overview. In B. Hemphill

(Ed.), *The evaluative process in psychiatric occupational therapy* (pp. 57–61, 339–341). Thorofare, NJ: Slack.

Bonder, B. R. (1990). Disease and dysfunction: The value of Axis V. *Hospital and Community Psychiatry, 41*(9), 959, 964.

Bonder, B. R. (1991). *Psychopathology and function.* Thorofare, NJ: Slack.

Borg, B., & Bruce, M. A. (1991). Assessing psychological performance factors. In C. Christensen & C. Baum (Eds.), *Occupational therapy: Overcoming human performance deficits* (pp. 539–586). Thorofare, NJ: Slack.

Brayman, S. J. & Kirby, T. (1982). The comprehensive occupational therapy evaluation. In B. Hemphill (Ed.), *The evaluative process in psychiatric occupational therapy* (pp. 211–226, 383–388). Thorofare, NJ: Slack.

Brinson, M. H. (1988). Getting started: Perspectives on initiating a quality assurance program. In S. C. Robertson (Ed.), *Mental health FOCUS: Skills for assessment and treatment* (pp. 3-128–3-130). Rockville, MD: American Occupational Therapy Association.

Bruce, M. A., & Borg, B. (1987). *Frames of reference in psychosocial occupational therapy.* Thorofare, NJ: Slack.

Buck, J., & Jolles, I. (1972). *House-tree-person projective technique.* Los Angeles: Western Psychological Services.

Casanova, J. S., & Ferber, J. (1976). Comprehensive evaluation of basic living skills. *American Journal of Occupational Therapy, 30*(2), 101–105.

Clarke, E. N., & Peters, M. (1984). *Scorable self-care evaluation.* Tucson, AZ: Therapy Skill Builders.

Denton, P. (1988). Assessing the patient's functional performance. *Hospital and Community Psychiatry, 39*(9), 935–936.

Denton, P. L., & Skinner, S. T. (1988). Selecting a frame of reference/ practice model. In S. C. Robertson (Ed.), *Mental health FOCUS: Skills for assessment and treatment* (pp. 100–108). Rockville, MD: American Occupational Therapy Association.

Department of Health and Human Services, Health Care Financing Administration. (1988). Medicare guidelines for occupational therapy services. In S. C. Robertson (Ed.), *Mental health FOCUS: Skills for assessment and treatment* (pp. 3-113–3-115). Rockville, MD: American Occupational Therapy Association.

Dickie, V. A., & Robertson, S. C. (1991). Perspectives on human functioning. *Hospital and Community Psychiatry, 42*(6), 575–576.

Fidler, G. S. (1982a). The life-style performance profile: An organizing frame. In B. Hemphill (Ed.), *The evaluative process in psychiatric occupational therapy* (pp. 43–47). Thorofare, NJ: Slack.

Fidler, G. S. (1982b). The activity laboratory: A structure for observing and assessing perceptual, integrative, and behavioral strategies. In B. Hemphill (Ed.), *The evaluative process in psychiatric occupational therapy* (pp. 195–207). Thorofare, NJ: Slack.

Fidler, G. S. (1982c). Appendix V: Activity laboratory questionnaire. In B. Hemphill (Ed.), *The evaluative process in psychiatric occupational therapy* (pp. 379–380). Thorofare, NJ: Slack.

Fidler, G. S. (1988). The life-style performance profile. In S. C. Robertson (Ed.), *Mental health FOCUS: Skills for assessment and treatment* (pp. 3-35–3-40). Rockville, MD: American Occupational Therapy Association.

Fine, S. B. (1991). Resilience and human adaptability: Who rises above adversity? 1990 Eleanor Clarke Slagle Lecture. *American Journal of Occupational Therapy, 46*(6), 493–503.

Florey, L. L., & Michelman, S. M. (1982). Occupational role history: A screening tool for psychiatric occupational therapy. *American Journal of Occupational Therapy, 36*(5), 301–308.

Gibson, D. (1990). The challenge of adaptation. Shaping services delivery to meet changing needs. *Hospital and Community Psychiatry, 41*(23), 267–269.

Hemphill, B. J. (Ed.). (1982). *The evaluative process in psychiatric occupational therapy.* Thorofare, NJ: Slack.

Hemphill, B. J. (Ed.). (1988). *Mental health assessment in occupational therapy: An integrative approach to the evaluative process.* Thorofare, NJ: Slack.

Hemphill, B. J., Peter, C. Q., & Weiner, P. C. (1991). *Rehabilitation in mental health: Goals and objectives for independent living.* Thorofare, NJ: Slack.

Honigfield, G., Gillis, R. D., & Kleitt, G. J. (1966). NOSIE-3, a treatment-sensitive ward behavior scale. *Psychological Reports, 19,* 180–182.

Joe, B. E. (1988). Quality assurance. In S. C. Robertson (Ed.), *Mental health FOCUS: Skills for assessment and treatment* (pp. 1-178–1-185). Rockville, MD: American Occupational Therapy Association.

Johnson, T. P., Vinnecombe, B. T., & Merrill, G. W. (1980). The independent living skills evaluation. *Occupational Therapy in Mental Health, 1*(2), 5–18.

Kaplan, K., & Kielhofner, G. (1989). *Occupational analysis interview and rating scale.* Thorofare, NJ: Slack.

Kettenbach, G. (1990). *Writing S.O.A.P. notes.* Philadelphia: F. A. Davis.

Kielhofner, G. (Ed.). (1985). *A model of human occupation: Theory and application.* Baltimore: Williams & Wilkins.

Kielhofner, G., Henry A. D. & Wallens, D. (1989). *A users' guide to the occupational performance history interview.* Rockville, MD: American Occupational Therapy Association.

King, L. J. (1974). A sensory integrative approach to schizophrenia. *American Journal of Occupational Therapy, 28*(9), 529–536.

King, L. J. (1982). The person symbol as an assessment tool. In B. J. Hemphill (Ed.), *The evaluative process in psychiatric occupational therapy* (pp. 169–194). Thorofare, NJ: Slack.

King, L. J. (1983). Occupational therapy and neuropsychiatry. *Occupational Therapy in Mental Health, 3*(1), 1–12.

King, L. J. (1990). Moving the body to change the mind: Sensory integrative therapy in psychiatry. *Occupational Therapy Practice, 1*(4), 12–22.

Lang, E., & Mattson, M. (1985). The multidisciplinary treatment plan: A format for enhancing activity therapy department involvement. *Hospital and Community Psychiatry, 36*(1), 62–68.

Leonardelli, C. A. (1988a). The Milwaukee evaluation of daily living skills (MEDLS). In B. Hemphill (Ed.), *Mental health assessment in occupational therapy* (pp. 151–162). Thorofare, NJ: Slack.

Leonardelli, C. A. (1988b). *The Milwaukee evaluation of daily living skills: Evaluation in long-term psychiatric care.* Thorofare, NJ: Slack.

Lerner, C. (1979). The magazine picture collage: Its clinical use and validity as an assessment device. *American Journal of Occupational Therapy, 33*(8), 500–504.

Lerner, C., & Ross, G. (1977). The magazine picture collage: Development of an objective scoring system. *American Journal of Occupational Therapy, 31*(3), 156–161.

Levy, L. L. (1986). Frames of references for occupational therapy in mental health. In S. Robertson (Ed.), *Mental Health FOCUS: Skills for assessment and treatment in mental health:* Application Supplement (pp. 17–24). Rockville, MD: American Occupational Therapy Association.

Levy, L. L. (1990). Activity, social role retention, and multiply disabled aged: Strategies for intervention. In D. Gibson (Ed.), *Evaluation and treatment of the psychogeriatric patient.* Binghamton, NY: Haworth Press.

Matsutsuyu, J. S. (1969). The interest checklist. *American Journal of Occupational Therapy, 23*(4), 323–328.

Mattingly, C. (1988). Perspectives on clinical reasoning for occupational therapy. In S. C. Robertson (Ed.), *Mental health FOCUS: Skills for assessment and treatment* (pp. 1-81–1-88). Rockville, MD: American Occupational Therapy Association.

Maurer, P. A. (1988). How to review mental health assessments. In S. C. Robertson (Ed.), *Mental health FOCUS: Skills for assessment and treatment* (pp. 1-115–1-123). Rockville, MD: American Occupational Therapy Association.

McGourty, L. K. (1979). Kohlman evaluation of living skills. KELS Research, Box 33503, Seattle, WA 98133.

McGourty, L. K. (1988). Kohlman evaluation of living skills (KELS). In B. Hemphill (Ed.), *Mental health assessment in occupational therapy* (pp. 133–146). Thorofare, NJ: Slack.

Michael, P. S., & Kaplan, K. (1988). Screening and evaluation instrument. In S. C. Robertson (Ed.), *Mental health FOCUS: Skills for assessment and treatment in mental health* (pp. 1-109–1-114). Rockville, MD: American Occupational Therapy Association.

Mosey, A. C. (1986). *Psychosocial components of occupational therapy.* New York: Raven Press.

Mosey, A. C. (1988). Role acquisition: An acquisitional frame of reference. In S. C. Robertson (Ed.), *Mental health FOCUS: Skills for assessment and treatment* (pp. 3-60–3-77). Rockville, MD: American Occupational Therapy Association.

Nelson, C. E., & Payton, D. D. (1991). The issue is—a system for involving patients in program planning. *American Journal of Occupational Therapy, 45*(8), 753–755.

Oakley, F., Kielhofner, G. B., & Barris, R. (1988). The role checklist. In B. Hemphill (Ed.), *Mental health assessment in occupational therapy* (pp. 75–91, 250–253). Thorofare, NJ: Slack.

Oakley, F., Kielhofner, G., Barris, R., & Reichler, R. (1986). The role checklist: Development and empirical assessment of reliability. *Occupational Therapy of Research, 6*(3), 157–170.

Parachek, J. F., & King, L. J. (1986). *Parachek geriatric rating scale* (3rd ed.). Center for Neurodevelopmental Studies, 8434 North 39th Avenue, Phoenix, AZ 85051.

Pelland, M. J. (1987). A conceptual model for instruction and supervision of treatment planning. *American Journal of Occupational Therapy, 46*(6), 351–359.

Robertson, S. C. (Ed.). (1988a). *Mental health FOCUS: Skills for assessment and treatment.* Rockville, MD: American Occupational Therapy Association.

Robertson, S. C. (1988b). Reasoning in practice. In S. C. Robertson (Ed.), *Mental health FOCUS: Skills for assessment and treatment* (pp. 1-48–1-50). Rockville, MD: American Occupational Therapy Association.

Schroeder, C. V., Block, M. P., Campbell, I., Trottier, E., & Stowell, M. S. (1978).

Schroeder, Block, Campbell adult psychiatric sensory integrative evaluation (2nd experimental edition). La Jolla, CA: "SBC" Research Associates, Psychiatric Occupational Therapy.

Smith, H. D., & Tiffany, E. G. (1988). Assessment and evaluation: An overview. In H. L. Hopkins & H. D. Smith (Eds.), *Willard and Spackman's Occupational therapy* (7th ed.). Philadelphia: J. B. Lippincott.

Stein, F. (1982). A current review of the behavioral frame of reference and its application to occupational therapy. *Occupational Therapy in Mental Health, 2*(4), 35–62.

Stoffel, V. C., & Cunningham, S. M. (1991). Continuous quality improvement: An innovative approach applied to mental health programs. *Occupational Therapy Practice, 2*(2), 52–60.

Thien, M. H. (December, 1987). Demonstrating treatment outcomes in mental health. *Mental Health Special Interest Section Newsletter,* American Occupational Therapy Association.

Williams, S. L., & Bloomer, J. (1987). *Bay Area functional performance evaluation* (2nd ed.). Palo Alto, CA: Consulting Psychologists Press.

Bibliography

Kuntavanish, A. A. (1987). *Occupational therapy documentation.* Rockville, MD: American Occupational Therapy Association.

Lynch, J. J., & Stein, F. (1986). Evaluating occupational therapy psychiatric care through medical documentation. *Occupational Therapy in Mental Health, 6*(3), 53–66.

Payton, O. D., Nelson, C., & Ozer, M. (1990). *Patient participation in program planning: A manual for therapists.* Philadelphia: F. A. Davis.

SECTION 1H
Case studies in psychiatry

GAIL Z. RICHERT

LEARNING OBJECTIVES

Upon completion of this section the reader will be able to:

1. *Identify six frames of reference used in mental health occupational therapy practice.*

2. *Describe six mental health patients in various practice settings treated using appropriate frames of reference.*

3. *Identify assessment, treatment, and discharge planning strategies according to patient diagnosis, functional level, and frame of reference.*

4. *Analyze case studies as practice models.*

Case studies

The six mental health case studies that follow are organized in the same way with the six different frames of references presented.

CASE STUDY 1*

Practice Setting: Private psychiatric health system, quarterway house

Diagnosis: 295.70 Schizoaffective disorder, 305.90 mixed substance abuse, in remission

Frame of Reference: Acquisitional or learning/behavioral

Initial Assessment and Evaluation: Chart review, interview, behavioral observation, functional assessment, Bay Area Functional Performance Evaluation (BAFPE), cooking evaluation

Demographics and History

Ms. Price is 42 years old with a 24-year history of psychiatric problems. She avoided hospitalization for most of those years and received extensive training as an artist. At 38, however, she entered the hospital with delusions about being poisoned, losing her soul, not sleeping, and with pronounced negative symptoms of social withdrawal, amotivation, and poverty of speech.

Setting, Program, and Service Delivery

Ms. Price was admitted to the quarterway house for long-term rehabilitation after a 2-year, intensive inpatient hospitalization. The program provides a structured milieu and 24-hour staff supervision under the direction of an occupational therapist. Service delivery is on an individual and group basis, with an emphasis on learning through repetition

* Deborah Wilberding, MOTR/L The Sheppard and Enoch Pratt Hospital, Baltimore, MD 21285

of practice, functional behavioral reinforcement, and illness management.

Assessment Findings

Ms. Price had an average to low-average IQ. Her BAFPE results indicated her overall performance was below normal limits but fell within the average patient range in all areas except for motivation, which was below the patient range. Organization was within normal limits. She showed much frustration and made self-deprecating comments during the test. She was socially isolated and negativistic, had difficulties initiating conversations, but showed a sense of humor and had a supportive family. Ms. Price had significant ADL deficits in self-care, budgeting, household maintenance, meal planning and preparation, and time management. Her leisure interests and work history were limited. She was cooperative, could follow written instructions, responded to behavioral reinforcement, and had begun to express interest in her artwork. Her cooking evaluation showed serious deficits in safety awareness, concentration, attention to detail, knowledge of nutrition, and hygiene. Ms. Price was able to work at an average pace, follow a simple recipe, and problem solve. She enjoyed eating and was overweight.

Treatment Plan, Goals, and Objectives

Problem 1. Passivity

Goal: To follow daily schedule
Objective: Resident will attend planning meeting and follow written schedule with no more than two prompts from staff daily.
Goal: To get up in the morning on time and take morning medications
Objective: Resident will get up with alarm clock and take morning medications independently.
Goal: To pursue vocational/leisure activities
Objective: Resident will participate in scheduled leisure activities.
Objective: Resident will begin a volunteer job in addition to her day program.

Problem 2. Lack of independent living skills

Goal: To develop consistent independent living skills
Objective: Resident will do her laundry as scheduled, using written instructions.
Objective: Resident will develop safe cooking practices. Restricted to supervised use of kitchen only. 1:1 Training. Assigned cooking times.
Objective: Resident will complete all assigned house chores using written checklists.
Objective: Resident will maintain appearance, change clothes daily, sleep in nightwear, and dress for work appropriately.

Problem 3. Negativity

Goal: To express positive aspects of both self and program
Objective: To orient new residents to the program. Resident will attend communication group twice per week.

Problem 4. Alcohol abuse—two occurrences

Goal: To have no reoccurrences of alcohol abuse

Objective: Resident will attend Alcohol Education and weekly support group per signed contract. Level promotion is contingent on keeping her contract.

Problem 5. Lack of initiation in discharge planning

Goal: To develop discharge plan
Objective: Resident will follow discharge plan and complete all visits.

Course of Treatment

Ms. Price progressed to the point of self-budgeting and self-medicating, and had graduated off the credit reinforcement system, performing at the least restrictive privilege level. She had obtained a volunteer job in the community and was taking tennis lessons weekly. She had developed friendships outside the house from this involvement. Ms. Price had acquired safer cooking skills and maintained 14 months of sobriety. She was able to travel independently using a cab, bus, train, or plane. She remained stable, with her delusional ideas subsiding, after months of regular medication administration and illness education.

Discharge Plan

After 30 months of rehabilitation, Ms. Price was discharged to a supervised apartment program off-campus.

CASE STUDY 2[†]

Practice Setting: Private psychiatric health system, inpatient adult unit
Diagnosis: 295.70 Schizoaffective disorder
Frame of Reference: Cognitive disabilities
Initial Assessment and Evaluations: Chart review, interview, behavioral observation, Allen Cognitive Level Test (ACL), and home evaluation

Demographics and History

Mr. Peter is a 71-year-old, single, retired technician who currently lives in a subsidized efficiency apartment. He has a long history of schizoaffective/psychotic disorder with delusions of impending doom and suicidal ideation.

Setting, Program, and Service Delivery

Mr. Peter is admitted for the second time to a short/intermediate-term adult unit. The program has a therapeutic milieu with a multidisciplinary treatment team. Occupational therapy service delivery is on an individual and group basis with both unit-based and centralized treatment programs.

Assessment Findings

Mr. Peter's eye/hand and gross motor coordination, reflexes, and flexibility are impaired. He has contractures of the fourth and fifth digits of his dominant right hand secondary to surgery for a pinched nerve 2 years ago. His score on the ACL is 4.1/6.6, demonstrating significant cognitive impairments including decreased attention span, poor problem-

† Gail Z. Richert, MS, OTR/L, The Sheppard and Enoch Pratt Hospital, Baltimore, MD 21285

solving skills, and poor short-term memory. He has difficulty modulating his affect, which is blunted and at times labile. His judgment is impaired. Although he is friendly and has a sense of humor, speech content is often delusional.

Mr. Peter is dependent on his married sister who lives nearby and on a previous employer with whom he has daily telephone contact. Leisure interests are very limited. He reports significant ADL deficits in self-care, meal planning, and preparation, money, time, and stress management. He lives independently; however, he is dependent on his sister for transportation and daily meal preparation. Although he is able to use some compensatory techniques with his nondominant hand, there are safety issues with oven use. This discovery necessitated a home evaluation while Mr. Peter was in the hospital.

Treatment Plan and Short-Term Objectives

Problem 1. Symptoms of psychosis—persecutory delusions

Goal: To develop coping strategies to manage symptoms
Objective: Patient will express delusions and irrational fears to a staff member. Individual staff only.
Objective: Patient will label a calendar for regular medication administration at home.

Problem 2. Impaired cognitive task/problem-solving skills

Goal: To develop compensatory skills for poor short-term memory
Objective: Patient will follow his daily written schedule of activities with assistance.

Problem 3. Impaired daily living skills

Goal: To improve performance in safe oven use
Objective: Patient will protect both hands with heavy oven mitts during oven use.
Objective: Patient will use nondominant hand and dominant hand as an assist in placing/removing TV dinners from the oven.
Objective: Patient will use dominant hand as an assist in fine motor activities.
Goal: To improve personal hygiene
Objective: With one prompt, patient will attend each group with a clean shirt.

Problem 4. Social isolation and withdrawal

Goal: To increase peer contact
Objective: With one prompt, patient will modulate his affect when interacting with peers each session.
Objective: Patient will attend geriatric day hospital after discharge.

Course of Treatment

Initial assessment determined the need for a home evaluation, which was conducted 12 days after admission. Recommendations were made to Mr. Peter's sister to purchase oven mitts and provide some supervision rather than cooking for the patient, since he was adamant about returning to his apartment after discharge. Mr. Peter was referred to task and ADL groups in which the environment was structured and adapted commensurate with his level of cognitive functioning. He was generally cooperative, motivated, and likable and

felt safe in the hospital environment. His mood stabilized with regular medication administration. Mr. Peter had difficulty modulating the intensity of his affect when interacting with peers. In response to prompting in communication skills, he decreased verbal frequency and egocentric speech. He related to others through telling jokes.

Mr. Peter learned to follow his hospital schedule with assistance and needed prompting and numerous one-step directions for task completion. He expressed a desire to be independent in all ADLs and was appreciative of the staff's interest. He practiced safe oven use and used his dominant hand as an assist in meal preparation and in dressing.

Discharge Plan

After 18 days, Mr. Peter was discharged to return to his apartment with daily support from his sister and to attend the geriatric day hospital for daily structure, medication monitoring, and social interaction. He planned to continue the Meal Planning and Preparation group on an outpatient basis to gain increased competence in safe oven use.

CASE STUDY 3[‡]

Practice Setting: State psychiatric hospital
Diagnosis: 296.340 Major depression, recurrent with mood congruent psychotic features
Frame of Reference: Mosey's recapitulation of ontogenesis (developmental)
Initial Assessment and Evaluations: Kohlman Evaluation of Living Skills, Street Survival Skills Questionnaire, perceptual motor screening, chart review, interview, Phieffer's Short Portable Mental Status Questionnaire, Draw-A-Person, and a 4-step task

Demographics and History

Ms. Jones is a 28-year-old divorced, female with 12th-grade education. Patient has a history of short-term psychiatric hospitalizations for suicidal attempts and substance abuse. She lives with her mother and was last employed for 3 years as a switchboard operator.

Setting, Program, and Service Delivery

Ms. Jones is admitted voluntarily to an admission ward and transferred to an adult continued care ward after stabilization of behavior. The program has a therapeutic milieu with a multidisciplinary treatment team. Occupational therapy services are provided on an individual and group basis on the ward, in a centralized rehabilitation building, and in hospital-wide programs.

Assessment Findings

Ms. Jones has no deficits in sensory integration skills. She displays minimal abilities in the cognitive skills areas of problem solving and coping skills. Patient is able to enter into an intimate relationship but was unable to sustain this dyadic interaction skill as evidenced by her divorce and dependency on mother for cooking and laundry. Most of her

[‡] Beth Kist, OTR/L, Springfield Hospital Center, Sykesville, MD 21784

leisure time is spent alone and patient was unable to identify leisure resources. Group interaction skills are limited to project group involvement. Patient has deficits in the self-identity areas of self-confidence, accepting self-responsibility, and viewing self as influencing events. She is able to identify weaknesses but not strengths. Sexual identity skills are not assessed, although her divorce status indicates problems in sustaining heterosexual relationships. When asked to draw a whole person, Ms. Jones draws a small, misshapen, faceless figure of no specific gender.

Living skills are adequate with some impairment noted in cooking. Ms. Jones is able to follow written directions for a pencil, paper, and ruler task; however, attention to detail is poor.

Treatment Plan and Short-term Objectives

Problem 1. Poor self-concept

Goal: To develop coping skills
Objective: Patient will be able to identify solutions to problems.
Objective: Patient will make one positive statement about self each week. Interaction group referral.

Problem 2. Limited interaction skills

Goal: To increase interaction skills
Objective: Patient will actively participate in group activities.
Objective: Patient will interact assertively with peers.
Objective: Patient will find others for group. Interaction group referral.

Problem 3. Impaired living skills

Goal: To improve meal preparation skills
Objective: Patient will prepare a different part of meal each week.
Objective: Patient will actively participate in meal planning. Cooking group referral.
Objective: Patient will attend day program for prevocational training. Community referral.

Course of Treatment

Occupational therapy services were provided over a 7-month period. The role of the therapist was to select appropriate learning experiences and to provide support, encouragement, and reinforcement of behaviors that were needed to learn subskills. Goals and objectives were mutually agreed upon by patient and therapist. Initially, Ms. Jones was referred to an interaction group. She regularly attended group and occasionally assisted staff with finding others for group. Although her participation in social games was good, she had difficulty expressing positive feelings. She was able to identify shortcomings but needed encouragement to identify problem-solving strategies. She eventually started to identify solutions to problems but was slow to follow through.

Ms. Jones was also referred to a task group (parallel group) that focused on practicing prevocational skills through craft activities. Her attendance was regular and her attention to detail improved. She developed some insight into her work capabilities and need for a structured work setting. She began attending a community day program twice a week where she was involved in the clerical unit and at-

tended a cooking group (project group). Attendance was sporadic, and she had some difficulty working with peers to complete tasks. Involvement in meal planning improved, and she was able to reach 80% of her objectives while she made much progress toward her goals. Prior to discharge, Ms. Jones was ward president and led weekly meetings, indicating an improvement in her self-confidence and interaction skills.

Discharge Plan

She was discharged to supervised housing. Aftercare plans included attending a day program 5 days a week, referral to Department of Vocational Rehabilitation, and bimonthly mental health clinic appointments.

CASE STUDY 4[§]

Practice Setting: A federal biomedical research hospital
Diagnosis: 290.00 Primary degenerative dementia of the Alzheimer type, senile onset, uncomplicated
Frame of Reference: Model of Human Occupation
Assessment: Assessment of Motor and Process Skills, Medical Record Review, Daily Activities Questionnaire, Interest Checklist, Internal/External Locus of Control Scale, Interview Role Checklist, Self-Assessment of Occupational Function

Demographics and History

Mrs. Ball is a 70-year-old who has been widowed for 18 years. She has one 54-year-old married son who lives locally. Her primary occupational roles are home maintainer and caregiver. Her occupational functioning was intact until 1 year ago when she began experiencing problems with her memory.

Setting, Program, and Service Delivery

Mrs. Ball is admitted to an 8-bed inpatient unit where patients voluntarily participate in drug research studies of about 4 months' duration. An occupational therapist is part of a multidisciplinary team of research experts. The occupational therapist assesses and treats patients within the confines of the research protocols and shares results with the patients, their families, and the primary investigator.

Assessment Findings

Performance. Mrs. Ball's motor skills are intact except for a mild intention tremor in her right upper extremity. She displays deficits in process skills such as problem solving and initiating activities. She expresses herself well; however, her speech is sometimes circumstantial.
Environment. Six months ago, Mrs. Ball sold her home of 35 years and moved into a private apartment in a supported residential facility that provides routine recreational activities both on and off the premises, maid service, and all meals in a communal dining room. She has had emotional difficulty adjusting to her new resi-

§ Frances Oakley, MS, OTR/L and Bonnie Koch, MA, OTS, National Institutes of Health, Bethesda, MD 20892

dence. She has a supportive family and supportive staff at the residential center, and is financially secure.

Volition. Mrs. Ball shows signs of decreased self-confidence, which is a contrast to her premorbid personality. She searches for compliments and seeks constant reassurance in what she does. She feels she can be successful at making things happen in her life and highly values independence. In general, she reports decreased involvement in interests and feels self-conscious about her intention tremor, which has forced her to abandon specific interests.

Habituation. Mrs. Ball has no normal routine or present occupational roles. The disrupted roles of home maintainer and family member are very valuable to her. Her priorities include effectively organizing her time and resuming these valued occupational roles.

Occupational Performance/Output. Mrs. Ball is independent in all Personal ADL but requires assistance with the Instrumental ADL of shopping, money management, and cooking. She does not initiate interaction with others or pursue interests or recreational activities unless prompted. She lacks meaningful occupational roles to organize her daily life and to provide a source of identity, self-confidence, meaning, and purpose.

Status of Occupational Functioning. Mrs. Ball's life history pattern appears to be one of competent occupational performance until the onset of Alzheimer's disease. Her motor and process skills deficits have adversely affected her ability to independently enact occupational roles, interests, and Instrumental ADL. Her ability to remain independent has been significantly compromised.

Treatment Plan and Objectives

Overall Objectives. Modify and structure the hospital and home environment to maximize Mrs. Ball's occupational performance. Since Alzheimer's disease is a progressive illness, reassess her occupational performance about every 6 months and provide feedback and recommendations to continue to maximize her functioning.

Specific Objective/Plan

Environment. To facilitate transition from the hospital to the home, share findings with Mrs. Ball, her family, and (with her permission) the residential center staff and involve them in intervention strategies.

Volition. Increase positive feedback and provide opportunities for success and independent decision making. Encourage and support Mrs. Ball's involvement in interests by providing adaptations to permit her to engage in the interests affected by tremor.

Habituation. Assist Mrs. Ball in developing and following a daily schedule. Encourage involvement in valued roles via environmental modification. Support involvement in the occupational therapy work program during hospitalization. Decrease maid service at home to allow her to reestablish the home maintainer role.

Skills. Provide opportunities to use skills. Redirect circumstantial speech. Cue as needed to support Mrs. Ball's impaired processing skills.

Output. Encourage continued independence in Personal ADL. Provide needed Instrumental ADL support.

CASE STUDY 5[‖]

Practice Setting: Veterans Administration Hospital (VA), acute care psychiatric unit
Diagnosis: 300.14 Multiple personality disorder
Frame of Reference: Psychodynamic
Initial Assessment and Evaluations: Staffing, chart review, group behavioral observation, the Goodman Battery, and Magazine Picture Collage

Demographics and History

Mr. Ray is a 22-year-old veteran who currently attends a local university. He was in the military 3 years ago, where his enlistment lasted for only 4 months, after which he was discharged because of mental illness with the diagnosis of manic depression. The patient claims to remember only the last 2 weeks of his military experience. At that time, he said he awoke in a military hospital in a distant location. The patient does not recall enlisting in the military and was surprised to find that he had done such a thing. This is Mr. Ray's first admission to the VA hospital. He has had numerous admissions, however, to a local community mental health center since his medical military discharge. He has had several diagnoses since that time, including psychotic depression, schizophrenia, and borderline personality disorder.

Setting, Program, and Service Delivery

Mr. Ray is admitted to an acute care psychiatric unit of the VA hospital that contains 20 beds and is staffed by a multidisciplinary treatment team. Occupational therapy services are provided via primary therapist referral and include individual and group interventions. Services are offered both on the unit and in the occupational therapy clinic.

Assessment Findings

Mr. Ray is appropriately dressed and appears to be a typical university student. He is physically intact, socially appropriate, and articulate. He mentions during his staffing, that he has had some recent experiences with what he calls "missing time." He complains of headaches, admits to hearing voices arguing inside his head, and states that he cannot seem to meet academic goals or organize his time in productive ways. He says that people whom he doesn't know seem to know him but call him by a different name.

Mr. Ray generally stays isolated on the unit. He attends occupational therapy group sessions willingly and is often helpful to other patients; however, the content of the patient's conversation and contributions in group are guarded and superficial. During Magazine Picture Collage evaluation, he talks to himself frequently and demonstrates a variety of conflicting facial expressions and behaviors, such as smiling and tearing out a picture, then immediately frowning and crumpling up the picture. It is apparent through group discussions that he does not recall memories from his youth and early teenage years. When asked to complete a figure drawing as part of the Goodman Battery, Mr. Ray draws a crude form (self) with bare feet and no hands. Later in the week, he brings the therapist a well-executed pencil portrait

‖ Peggy L. Dawson, M. Ed, OTR, University of Missouri–Columbia, Columbia, MO 65211

that he finds in his journal. Patient disavows any knowledge of this portrait.

Treatment Plan and Short-term Objectives

Problem 1. Lack of insight and understanding of current diagnosis

Goal: To become aware of other parts of his personality
Objective: To acknowledge the behaviors and products of independent parts of himself
Objective: To remember his early years through his personalities

Problem 2. Lack of success in good attainment

Goal: To learn to use rather than repress the talents and resources of his alternate personalities
Objective: To coordinate personal priorities with those of his alternate personalities
Objective: To ask for and accept help from alternate personalities while completing tasks

Course of Treatment

Initially skeptical of his diagnosis, Mr. Ray accepted it because he was presented repeatedly with evidence that there were acting parts of his personality unknown to him. Through poetry, painting, and myth writing, he acknowledged his forgotten early memories and history of child abuse. His alternate personalities helped him in certain daily tasks such as cooking and writing papers. They also caused much disruption by outwardly insisting on their preferences and expressing strong views that contradicted each others' views and those of Mr. Ray.

Mr. Ray was determined to succeed in treatment. He performed several projective tasks such as nonobjective art and journaling with his left hand to discover important symbols in his life.

Discharge Plan

After 4 weeks of intensive occupational therapy and psychotherapy, Mr. Ray was discharged to continue his schooling. He moved out of the dorm and into a private apartment. He participated in outpatient treatment with both psychiatry and occupational therapy to increase goal-directed behaviors and to encourage cooperation with alternate personalities.

CASE STUDY 6[¶]

Practice Setting: University hospital, inpatient unit and outpatient satellite clinic
Diagnosis: 296.2 Major depression, 300.01 panic disorder
Frames of Reference: Sensory integration, cognitive disabilities
Initial Assessment and Evaluations: Allen Cognitive Level Test (ACL), Routine Task Inventory (RTI), Sensorimotor History, and Ayres Clinical Observations

[¶] Sandra K. David, OTR/L The Medical College of Georgia Hospital and Clinics, Augusta, GA 30912

Demographics and History

Mrs. Amy is 27 years old with a developmental history including a 34-week gestation followed by 4 weeks of tube feeding with restraints (deprivation of experiences that facilitates normal development), colic, a 6-month delay in walking, ocular abnormalities corrected by glasses, and sexual abuse by nonrelatives during childhood. She attended 2 years of college. Her supportive family lived an 8-hour drive away. There is no history of substance abuse. Her psychosocial problems included marital discord and learned avoidance of affective issues. She works in a technical position.

Service Delivery

Mrs. Amy is treated as an inpatient for 7 weeks and for 3 years as an outpatient.

Program

During treatment, activity requirements are matched to the current capabilities of the patient. A significant score difference between the level of function and the ACL test requires further evaluation. Sensory processing abnormalities are detected as defensive behaviors that significantly affect the emotional perception and function in everyday life. The protocol for treatment of sensory defensiveness includes the following:

1. Severe defensiveness in three sensory systems
2. A supportive discharge environment
3. Education and training in a sensory diet
4. Voluntary participation in the treatment program
5. A contract clarifying responsibilities for treatment goals
6. Active patient participation in treatment
7. Training in sensory normalization techniques to improve the patient's ability to regulate arousal
8. Treatment of underlying problems

Assessment Findings

Mrs. Amy has decreased kinesthesia; gravitational insecurity; severe tactile, visual, and auditory defensiveness; poor self-esteem; impulsivity; passivity; and ineffective coping skills. There is a difference between her functioning (RTI score = 5) and her cognitive abilities (ACL score = 6).

Course of Treatment

Mrs. Amy's unrelieved distress during hospitalization led to evaluation and entry to the sensory defensiveness protocol. She learned the self-initiated normalization techniques and the sensory attributes of the environment (eg, bright light). At discharge, she was having fewer panic attacks.

Initially, outpatient treatment was once weekly, then gradually reduced to once monthly. During periods of simultaneous unexpected change, Mrs. Amy was seen for 2 to 3 weekly treatments. Her outpatient treatment continued the inpatient work and consisted of sensory integrative and cranial sacral therapy. As treatment progressed, her panic attacks decreased. Her "sensory diet" became refined and integrated into her daily routine. As her underlying sensory processing inefficiencies improved, her adaptive responses became smoother.

A continued improvement in Mrs. Amy's sensory processing was evident by her ability to adjust her level of arousal to meet environmental demands. Her functioning was at ACL 6. After 3 years of outpatient treatment, Mrs. Amy developed effective coping strategies and was panic-free. She identified changes in her interaction style and improved her observation of herself and others. She accurately recognized that her thinking was no longer "black and white," or "all or nothing" and identified various factors leading to panic symptoms. Table 17-10 summarizes Mrs. Amy's case history.

TABLE 17-10. *Case History Summary (Mrs. Amy)*

Behavior Prior to Treatment	Behavior After Treatment
Decreased Kinesthesia	
Frequent bruising (bumping into furniture/doorways)	Seldom bumped into objects
	No bruising on arms or legs
	Improved body scheme
Tactile Defensiveness	
Wore soft clothes, 3–4 layers (100% cotton)	Wore clothes of varying materials and textures
Avoided light touch	Engaged comfortably in light touch activities (eg, shopping, church, standing in lines)
Maintained large personal space	Maintained normal body space
Intolerance of textures (newspapers, embossed materials)	Routinely read newspaper
Auditory Defensiveness	
Distracted by high and low frequencies	Filtered high and low frequency noise appropriately
Low tolerance to sudden noises	Tolerated sudden noises
Low tolerance to simultaneous conversations	Filtered simultaneous conversations
Overwhelmed by multiple sounds in the environment	Rarely became overwhelmed by multiple sounds in the environment
Visual Defensiveness	
Overwhelmed by multiple visual stimuli (shutdown)	Rarely became overwhelmed by multiple visual stimuli
Fell asleep when reading	Improved reading endurance
Other	
History of multiple nightly awakenings since childhood	Seldom awoke during the night
Described self as clumsy	Described self as "not accident prone anymore"
Poor sense of self-competence	Sense of self-competence (active participation in community groups)

Special thanks to Sandra David, Peggy Dawson, Beth Kist, Fran Oakley, and Deb Wilberding for their clinical wisdom and insight and their eagerness to share these with others. Also, special thanks to Ingrid Baramki, Gary Jackson, Kathy Kannenberg, Susan Robertson, and the clinical medical library and word processing staff at The Sheppard and Enoch Pratt Hospital.

Bibliography

Duncombe, L. W., Howe, M. C., & Swartzberg, S. L. (1988). *Case simulations in psychosocial occupational therapy* (2nd ed). Philadelphia: F. A. Davis.

Perry, S., Frances, A., & Clarkin, J. (1990). *Innovated approach for treatment of psychiatric patients. A DSM III-R; casebook of treatment selections.* New York: Brunner/Mazel.

SECTION 2

Substance abuse: Drug addiction and alcoholism

NANCY L. BECK

KEY TERMS

Alcoholics Anonymous
Detoxification
Group Process
Maladaptive Behavior

Multidisciplinary Medical Team Model
Partial Programs
12-Step Model

LEARNING OBJECTIVES

Upon completion of this section the reader will be able to:

1. *Sensitize readers to the magnitude and ramifications of addictions in society.*
2. *Explore the design of an occupational therapy program for substance abusers.*
3. *Identify and explore the occupational therapy treatment process.*

Working with patients who are compulsively and pathologically addicted to substances—drugs or alcohol—is exciting, rewarding, and at times frustrating for occupational therapists (OTR). It is important to understand the nature of these addictions, to remain goal-directed and focused in treatment, and to develop the skills necessary to effectively facilitate recovery from the addiction.

Overview of addiction

Addiction can affect persons of any age, sex, race, religion, or socioeconomic background. The all-encompassing quality of an addiction affects the user's behavior and thought processes. Supporting the addiction and obtaining the addictive substance (drugs or alcohol) becomes the primary motivating factor for the user, often to the exclusion of everything else. Obtaining the substance and experiencing the euphoria of use drive the user into activities that can leave a trail of damaged or broken relationships with family, friends, employers, and society.

As a result, the road to recovery is a continuing process of rebuilding and using healthy strengths, restructuring positive behaviors and actions, and facing the emotional and physical consequences of the addiction. This arduous process of self-evaluation and behavioral change can be difficult and frightening for the recovering addict. Resistance to making these changes is common and recidivism is high. The addict may need multiple attempts at sobriety to learn and use the tools needed to maintain sobriety.

Current trends in governmental subsidies and funding for addiction programs are strongly affecting the kind and length of programming available. Prevention, education, research, and lower cost programs are being emphasized. Declining funding for long-term care and inpatient treatments has given rise to short-term partial and outpatient programs. Funds are also being allocated for addiction-related issues that are causing tremendous strains on society, such as AIDS, codependencies, and the effect of addiction on families. Research supported in part by the National Institute for Drug Addiction and Alcoholism and other nationally based addiction organizations is being focused on efficacy studies of treatment, methods of prevention, and a search for the physiologic basis of addiction.

Growing public anger and fear directed toward addiction and addiction-related crimes have given rise to governmental and private prevention campaigns to reduce addiction. Three studies conducted in the 1980s—the New Zealand study, the Vermont study, and the Midwestern Prevention Project—showed that community-based prevention programs are effective in reducing alcohol-related problems (Friedl, 1991). Despite the changes from these programs, addiction remains one of the major killers and causes of trauma in the United States. Prisons are overcrowded with addiction-related offenders and punishment for these offenses has become increasingly severe, such as imprisonment for "driving under the influence" (of alcohol).

Although there is a strong movement for carrying out more punitive measures for addiction-related crimes, the number of addiction programs is growing. Many new programs are focused on special populations such as children, teenagers, the elderly, and children of alcoholics and drug addicts (Moyers, 1991). This is indicative of the expansiveness of addiction. These addiction programs are not limited to drug and alcohol addictions, but include addictions such as compulsive gambling, sexual abuse, eating disorders, nicotine addiction, and others that are rapidly becoming major issues in mental health care (Custer, 1985; Kieffer, 1982).

The contribution that occupational therapy can make addresses the core issues of addiction, which can facilitate the learning and growth needed to transform the habits of addiction into habits of health. The systematic and practical methods used in occupational therapy add strength and quality to the process of recovery.

Service settings

Although the model for delivery of service varies in some ways according to the setting, basic ingredients are recognized as essential: a strongly collaborative treatment team that works specifically with the substance abuse patients, a well-structured program that allows only small amounts of unplanned time, and good follow-up plans that include continued support and treatment or both when the patient leaves the setting.

Hospital for substance abusers

Many hospitals or clinics are completely devoted to the treatment of substance abusers with some specialization in the treatment of those with either drug addiction or alcoholism. The mission of these free-standing addiction hospitals frequently is multi-leveled, including inpatient treatment, some continued aftercare treatment program, outpatient treatment, 12-step support groups like Alcoholics Anonymous (AA) and Narcotics Anonymous (NA), public education, and research.

The biggest and most lucrative service offered by hospitals is usually the inpatient programming, which is built on variations of two treatment team models: a 12-step model and a multidisciplinary medical team model. ***The 12-step model*** uses the structure of the 12 Steps and 12 Traditions of Alcoholics Anonymous groups as the foundation of the program. The treatment team may be composed of addiction counselors (recovering substance abusers certified to work in treatment centers), psychiatrists, nurses, activities therapists, social workers, and perhaps psychologists and occupational therapists. ***The multidisciplinary medical team model*** emphasizes comprehensive patient assessments, individualized treatment planning with clearly defined treatment outcomes, 12-step support group involvement, and a wide range of clinical options to assist patients with the social, psychological, and medical problems that often accompany addiction (Cristoforo, 1991; AA World Series, 1952).

In addition to occupational therapists, the multidisciplinary team may include physicians, psychiatrists, psychologists, addictions counselors, family therapists, activities, or adjunctive therapists (eg, recreation, art, movement, horticulture, music, expressive therapists), AIDS counselors, social workers, and nurses. The strength of the team is in the members' ability to work collaboratively to help the patients work through the denial of the suffering that the addiction has caused them and to understand the rapidly fluctuating feelings and behaviors they are experiencing. Good collaboration is essential not only for helping the staff and patients stay focused on the goals and objectives of treatment, but also for helping the patients trust the staff to help them make the behavior and habit changes needed for recovery from the addiction.

When the entire hospital is devoted to the treatment of addiction, it enjoys certain advantages over hospitals with a more multifaceted mission. The single focus helps in the definition of training and education, treatment approaches, and research development, and often serves as a strongly unifying factor among staff. All staff members at every level have some understanding and contribution to make to the common mission (Jones, 1953)

Addictions unit in a psychiatric hospital

Psychiatric hospital units share some of the properties of a single-focused hospital, but with notable differences. Although the program is frequently a multidisciplinary medical team model, there is a greater emphasis on medical and psychiatric services. Patients with addictions who are admitted to psychiatric hospitals frequently have become suicidal or suffer from dysthymia, depression, or personality disorders that require the more intense course of medical and psychiatric services (Allen, 1985; Korpell, 1984; Spitzer & Williams, 1987).

Detoxification

The first phase of most treatment for addiction is ***detoxification***. Reactions to detoxification vary from a mild period of discomfort to severe physical and emotional distress. The primary emphasis in treatment in this phase is to make the patients comfortable, to focus attention away from their discomfort, and to prepare them for the more intense treatment of the addictions programs.

Detoxification can take place in a variety of settings including a short-term unit in a general medical-surgical hospital, an addictions unit in a psychiatric hospital, a free-standing addictions hospital, or an outpatient addiction program. The role of the occupational therapist in the detoxification phase of treatment is minimal. Excluding the medical treatments, most of the treatment and treatment preparation can be performed effectively by addictions counselors and activity therapy personnel.

Partial programs

Partial or day hospital programs have been an established mode of treatment in mental health for many years. Patients attend the program during the day and go home at night or work during the day and attend the program at night or on the weekend. **Partial programs** cost less to run than inpatient programs and have long been considered both an alternative to inpatient care and a good postdischarge plan for supportively easing patients back into the community. Although partial programs have not been used extensively as a vehicle for treatment among addiction providers, the trends in funding allocations are generating a growing interest in these less costly programs.

As the inpatient lengths of stay decrease because of cuts in governmental and insurance funds, patients are being discharged in more fragile states of recovery from their addictions. Entering a partial program can give them the extra time needed to learn and practice the skills for maintaining abstinence from chemicals.

Although the treatment team in a partial program is usually small and may or may not include an occupational therapist, a strong collaborative team is needed.

Outpatient programs

Outpatient programs treat patients by individual appointments and in family units. Substance abusers meet with the outpatient therapist for continued support after discharge or as a preadmission consultation. Therapists are addiction counselors, psychologists, social workers, nurses, AIDS counselors, and others, including OTRs trained in counseling.

Alcoholics Anonymous

Alcoholics Anonymous (AA) is a self-help support group founded in 1934. It is used both as an alternative to hospitalization and as a follow-up support system after hospitalization. AA, with its 12 Steps and 12 Traditions, marks the beginning of a system for the treatment of alcoholism and other addictions that gives dignity, respect, and hope to those who are recovering. The principles of AA have been used to give birth to many other addiction-related, self-help support groups such as Narcotics Anonymous for drug abusers, Al-Anon for spouses of alcoholics, Alateen for teen children of substance abusers, Cocaine Anonymous, Gamblers Anonymous, and Overeaters Anonymous. In recognition of the positive strength of the self-help support groups, treatment programs in hospitals and communities frequently include them as an essential component of inpatient

programming and as a part of the aftercare plans for patients. Although OTRs do not work professionally with AA, it is important to understand how AA works to help patients accept the support of AA (Thomson, 1975; AA World Series, 1952).

Other treatment settings

There are a myriad of other types of settings such as halfway houses, prisons, and community centers for treatment of substance addiction. Occupational therapists are needed and at times are present in these settings.

Program design

Frame of reference

The first step in defining the role of the occupational therapist in a treatment center for addiction is to determine a frame of reference that is effective in guiding OTRs as they work with patients (Rogers, 1986). This system for treating patients needs to be consistent with the basic concepts or model of occupational therapy and to be able to encompass the problems and issues specific to addiction (Mosey, 1986). In addiction, the best frames of reference assume that patients have the ability to learn adapted behaviors and change their life habits as a result. Other factors to consider in choosing a frame of reference are the mission and philosophy of the treatment center, the type of setting, and the expected role of occupational therapy within the structure of the setting. Hence, the frame of reference needs to be compatible with the profession, the patient's needs, and the overall mission of the center (Levy, 1986).

The frame of reference determines the design of the program. Maintaining the integrity of the frame of reference throughout will guide the therapist in choosing treatment procedures including evaluative tools, treatment plan procedures, treatment methods, and the means by which he or she communicates with other professions.

Using the behavioral frame of reference, which draws from the theoretical base of Skinner, Watson, and others, the treatment of an alcoholic might appear as follows.

Example

The focus of treatment is on unlearning maladaptive behaviors and learning predetermined functional behaviors through experiencing an adapted environment (Levy, 1986). The data for evaluation are collected through observation of the patient's behavior; for example, a male alcoholic might be observed in a social setting. The results are measured against behaviors considered appropriate and those considered inappropriate by the treatment team. For instance, when the alcoholic was observed socializing, he talked only about the exciting things that happened while he was drinking. This action was determined by the treatment team to be an action leading to drinking—hence, a **maladaptive behavior**. As a result of this analysis, a problem area is defined and a treatment plan including long- and short-term goals and treatment methods is developed to address the problem.

The identified problem was that the patient continues to revel in the excitement of his addiction. The long-term goal is for the patient to find enjoyment in appropriate social interaction. The short-term goal is to stop the glorified alcohol use stories.

Possible treatment methods are for the occupational therapist to redirect the alcoholic's interests into appropriate structured group activities, to confront and inhibit the "glory stories," and to model appropriate social interactions. After reevaluation, another short-term goal is determined by the occupational therapist and the treatment team with proper adjustments made to the environment to facilitate further movement toward the long-term goal. For example, reevaluation shows that the patient has stopped talking about alcohol use and has become agitated and short-tempered. The new goal is to have the patient practice appropriate outlets for anger through high-energy use and relaxation activities. If the patient exhibits maladaptive behaviors, his privileges at the hospital may be dropped. The constant reevaluation continues until the patient demonstrates appropriate behavior for a predetermined length of time and the long-term goal is met.

Collaboration

While the whole treatment team may be working on the same overall goal, each team member is working on goals that are specific to their knowledge base and perhaps working from varying frames of reference. The collaboration between them provides the continuity of treatment needed to facilitate the patient's goal attainment. In addiction treatment centers, collaboration is essential due to the fluctuating emotions and mood swings of the patients. Because of the nature of the frame of reference in the previous example, it would be necessary for the entire treatment team to share the same frame of reference for goal attainment to be possible. The behavioral frame of reference would be very appropriate in a setting using AA as the structure on which the program is built, because AA is founded on the premise that substance abusers can change their drinking behaviors with the continual reinforcement of support of their peers.

Compatibility

Frames of reference should not vary among different professions in the same setting. Compatibility facilitates good communication. Other frames of reference—developmental, model of human occupation, and self-actualization—are used by occupational therapy and could be compatible for use in hospital and partial program settings. When choosing a frame of reference, consideration must be given to the treatment center and patient needs.

Program design summary

The design of an occupational therapy program for substance abusers is structured by the frame of reference chosen as the guide for treatment. It is crucial that the frame of reference be consistent with the philosophical base of occupational therapy and can address the special needs of substance abusers. Strong collaboration among the treatment team members is essential for working effectively with substance abusers. Communication with others is based on the frame of reference used in occupational therapy programming; thus, it is necessary that it be compatible with the rest of the treatment team.

Role of occupational therapy in addiction treatment

The occupational therapist has an important role in the treatment of addiction. In addiction treatment centers, therapy from other disciplines has a highly verbal content, which needs to be balanced with concrete practical experiences. Involvement in activity in occupational therapy gives patients the opportunity to can practice the skills they are learning.

Treatment methods

Although individual sessions are used for reviewing significant issues with patients, groups are the primary mode of treatment used in working with addicts. Addicts tend to view their environment from a skewed perspective and usually have the skills to express their views with logically sequential thought patterns. They also tend to have poor social integration skills that can take the form of egocentric social habits or they may swing toward self-denial as they interact with others. In all these circumstances, the group itself becomes a therapeutic tool for the addict when the therapist uses the group to provide feedback and reality test the thoughts, feelings, and actions presented during the group meeting.

Goals of treatment

In general, most occupational therapy treatment for addicts is focused around issues relating to their communication skills, leisure skills, emotional outlets, and understanding of what motivates them to action. The specific goals for each patient are individualized according to the patient's specific needs.

Types of groups

All the groups used in occupational therapy are task-oriented, ranging from parallel play to cooperative groups. "The emphasis in the task group is the achievement of an identified end product: either specific decisions, recommendations or tangible results" (Borg & Bruce, 1991, p. 6). Whether the end product is a poem written by the addict, a craft, or a list of community resources, substance abusers benefit greatly from the tangible quality of the task groups. For example, a completed craft project may serve as a symbol of achievement to a patient who otherwise feels like a failure; the poem may be the only way the patient has of expressing real feeling; the list of resources may be the link to healthy leisure pursuits. The task and the process by which the task is achieved differentiate occupational therapy from the more verbal psychological group therapy methods used by other treatment teams.

Modalities

Occupational therapy modalities are limited only by the knowledge and imagination of the therapist. Using skills in activity analysis and activity adaptation, the modality possibilities are endless. The therapist can structure the use of popular games like Pictionary and Outburst to be an avenue for controlled emotional outlet, a method for promoting family interaction, or an avenue for understanding competitive social interaction patterns. If the therapist's creative planning needs assistance, numerous activity resources are available. Some are written by occupational therapists and some by psychologists, social workers, and recreation therapists (Borg & Bruce, 1991; Hughes & Mullins, 1981; Kaplan, 1988; Korb, Azok, & Leutenberg, 1989).

As Kaplan (1988) suggests, the activities should never be attempted without a clear plan and goal for how they will be used. Substance abusers with higher cognitive function tend to ask questions about the relevance of the activity to their recovery process. Having a clear plan and a realistic goal for the activity is necessary to help the patients understand the rationale for doing the activity and to successfully engage them in the activity. For example, if the activity is a blindfolded trust walk, the patients should know that the goal is to work on issues related to trust. It involves them in the therapeutic process of the group and helps them focus on their feelings and reactions to trust in relationships with others. Their investment in the group makes a difference in how much they gain from doing the activity.

Processing the group

The activity alone is frequently not enough. Short-term hospitalizations prohibit the use of learning by repetition over a long period of time. Patients need to understand what is happening to them in treatment to enable them to use the skills when they leave the program. The therapist must help them make the link between doing the activity and recovering from the addiction. If the link is not made, occupational therapy becomes simply a nice thing that happened to them when they were in the hospital. A link that seems obvious to the therapist is not always clear to the concrete thinking of the substance abuser. The patient needs to be able to understand the link as his or her own. Hence, the therapist must facilitate the patient's learning by using activities and ***group process*** to tap into his or her internal belief systems. Evidence that the learning is taking place will come as the patient begins to verbalize the changes in his or her own words.

The skills the therapist needs to effectively facilitate this linkage are derived from a synthesis of three areas of knowledge: knowledge of the dynamics of the patient, knowledge of the dynamics of the illness, and knowledge of dynamics of the activity. The patient dynamics come from assessment and evaluation. The dynamics of the illness comes from texts and from experience working with substance abusers, and the dynamics of activity comes from the knowledge base of occupational therapy.

For example, a cocaine addict, who is a 25-year-old medical student, puts high personal demands on himself, is suicidal and lonely, and has been referred to an occupational therapy craft group. The dynamics of the illness indicate that expected behaviors may be irritability, attempts to work on several projects at once without completion of any of them, short attention span, grandiosity, high rate of recidivism, and denial of problems. The patient needs to be involved in the treatment plan and needs a short-term project with an adult theme that will be of interest to him. The challenge of the therapist is to take this information, discuss it with the patient, help the patient define a meaningful goal that is related to his addiction, and choose a project. Throughout the group meeting the therapist's brief interactions are related to the goal and the progress that the patient is making on the project. The interactions are at times supportively confrontational when needed for redirection and encouragingly supportive concerning the task. At the end of the group meeting the therapist facilitates the patients through a group discussion of the progress they are making in the goals they have chosen for themselves (Scaffa, 1991).

Use of self

The therapist's role is that of a catalyst by which the patients are able to recognize their maladaptive behavior exhibited in the performance of the activity and develop new patterns of thoughts and behaviors that are conducive to recovery from an addiction. As a catalyst, the therapist needs to have integrity with the group to elicit trust from the patients. Integrity comes when the therapist is honest, consistent, and direct with the patients and believes in the benefits of the therapeutic use of activity. Substance abusers generally have a history of lying during their addictions and thus frequently recognize insincerity. If the therapist has only a vague understanding or confidence in the purpose of activity, the substance abuser recognizes it very quickly and the effectiveness of treatment is lost. The mood swings of substance abusers require a certain amount of emotional consistency from the therapist to help them learn how to modulate the extremes of their emotional reactions.

The following case study reflects a standard procedure for treatment including the setting identification, patient demographics, frame of reference, assessment findings, treatment plan, course of treatment, and discharge (Denton, 1987).

CASE STUDY

Bob is a 28-year-old black male with a cocaine addiction who is in a partial program setting. The frame of reference is the model of human occupation.

Bob works as a secretary and technician with critically ill infants in a hospital from 3 PM to 11 PM. He was recently fired from a second job due to excessive absenteeism. He said it gave him more time to spend with his children. He is a father of two (a 9-year-old daughter and a 2-month-old son) by his fiancé of 13 years. She is not addicted and has threatened to leave him. He has been abusing cocaine for 1½ years, using cocaine from 2 AM to 8 AM every day. His past interests were weightlifting, swimming, basketball, and reading the Bible, but he has not participated in any of them in the last year. He spends a lot of time by himself because he is "often used by others." He says he has thought about suicide, "no one that uses coke hasn't thought about it." He says, "the only therapy I need is my Bible."

Assessment findings

Using the occupational history and interest checklist procedures, the assessment reveals an analysis showing that overall internal organization of the patient has been seriously disrupted by the addiction and that Bob is functioning at the exploratory behavior level. In the area of volition, he feels the addiction and other people have control over his life and he is looking for a cure from an outside source, in the Bible, and to some degree in treatment. In the area of habituation he is experiencing a role performance imbalance evidenced by the use of his time in that the addiction and work conflict with his desire to spend time with his family and the pursuing of his interests. A review of his skills shows that impulsive responses have created loss of a job and threatened his home. His environment review shows little interaction with others.

Treatment plan

1. Bob will not use cocaine from day 1 of treatment monitored through daily urinanalysis.
2. Bob will plan and pursue leisure activities in the community with his family after 2 weeks.
3. Bob will work consistently every day while in treatment.
4. Bob will identify and use five constructive outlets for his feelings.

Course of treatment

Treatment began with Bob's involvement in structured activities involving education work roles and exploration of leisure pursuits. He completed an inventory of how he uses his time and participated in activities of his interests such as sports. The therapist helped Bob to process his experiences in the activity groups and gave him homework assignments to do between sessions at home, at work, and with his family. Treatment was gradually expanded as his functioning became healthier; he was discharged when he demonstrated goal attainment.

Outcome evaluation

Bob was reevaluated at periodic intervals during his treatment and through a self-report 6 months after discharge.

Summary

Substance abuse is an illness that has devastating ramifications not only for the abuser, but also for generations of families of abusers and for the incredible number of victims of addiction-related accidents and crimes. Funding for addressing the issues of addiction is now being funneled in many directions including prevention, research, inpatient, partial, and outpatient treatment programs. Recent trends show the emergence of treatment programs for compulsive gambling, nicotine addiction, and other addictions.

The activities used in occupational therapy provide the means by which the substance abuser is able to tangibly assess his or her thoughts and behaviors and practice behaviors that lead to recovery from the addiction. Using a wide range of activities, the therapist structures and plans treatment to be specifically relevant to each patient. With a synthesis of three areas of knowledge—patient dynamics, dynamics of the illness, and dynamics of activity—therapists are armed with tools needed to become a catalyst for effectively facilitating the patient's treatment in occupational therapy. Occupational therapy has proved to be effective in decreasing the need for hospitalization for many other kinds of patients.

In addiction treatment settings, occupational therapy can be a strong, stable, goal-directed process that promotes healthy living habits and quality life experiences. Knowledge skills and understanding of addiction are key ingredients in working with substance abusers.

References

Alcoholics Anonymous World Series, Inc. (1952, 1953). *Twelve steps and twelve traditions.* New York: The AA Grapevine.

Allen, C. K. (1985). *Measurement and management of cognitive disabilities.* Boston: Little, Brown & Co.

Borg, B., & Bruce, M. A. G. (1991). *The group system.* Thorofare, NJ: Slack.

Bruce, M. A., & Borg, B. (1987). *Frames of reference in psychosocial occupational therapy.* Thorofare, NJ: Slack.

Cristoforo, C. (Ed.). (1991). *25 years in review. Eagleville Quarterly, 4*(3), 2.

Custer, R., & Milt, H. (1985). *When luck runs out.* New York: Fax on File Publications.

Denton, P. L. (1987). *Psychiatric occupational therapy: A workbook of practical skills.* Boston: Little, Brown & Co.

Friedl, S. (1991). Community-based research on preventing alcohol-related problems. ADAMHA News, 17(3), Rockville, MD: U.S. Department of Health and Human Resources.

Hughes, P., & Mullins, L. (1981). *Acute psychiatric care.* Thorofare, NJ: Slack.

Jones, M. (1953). *The therapeutic community.* New York: Basic Books.

Kaplan, K. L. (1988). *Directive group therapy.* Thorofare, NJ: Slack.

Kieffer, S. N., (Eds.). (1982). *Addictive disorders update: Alcoholism, drug abuse, gambling.* New York: Human Sciences Press.

Korb, K., Azok, S., & Leutenberg, E. (1989). *Life management skills.* Beachwood, OH: Wellness Reproductions, Inc.

Korpell, S. (1984). *How you can help: A guide for families of psychiatric hospital patients.* Washington, DC: American Psychiatric Press.

Levy, L. (1986). Frames of reference for occupational therapy in mental health. In S. C. Robertson (Ed.), *SCOPE* (pp. 17–24). Rockville, MD: American Occupational Therapy Association.

Mosey, A. C. (1986). *Psychosocial components of occupational therapy.* New York: Raven Press.

Moyers, A. (1991). Occupational therapy and treatment of the alcoholic's family. *Occupational Therapy in Mental Health, 11*(1), 45–64.

Rogers, J. (1986). Articulating a frame of reference in occupational therapy. In S. C. Robertson (Ed.), *SCOPE* (pp. 25–32). Rockville, MD: American Occupational Therapy Association.

Scaffa, E. (1991). Alcoholism: An occupational behavior perspective. *Occupational Therapy in Mental Health, 11*(2/3), 99–111.

Spitzer, L., & Williams, J. B. W. (Eds.). (1987). *Diagnostic and statistical manual of mental disorders III-R.* Washington, DC: American Psychiatric Association.

Thomsen, R. (1975). *Bill W.* New York: Harper & Row.

SECTION 3

Eating disorders: Anorexia nervosa and bulimia nervosa

NANCY L. BECK

KEY TERMS

Aftercare Programs

Angry Counterdependent
    Phase

Approaching Relating
    Phase

Binge Eating

Body Image

Depressed Needy Phase

Food Management

Maintenance Phase

Perfectionism

Vocational Rehabilitation

LEARNING OBJECTIVES

Upon completion of this section the reader will be able to:
1. *Describe the emerging illness of eating disorders.*
2. *Discuss the dynamics of treatment for eating disorders.*
3. *Explain the role of occupational therapy in treatment.*

Although eating disorders were recognized as a problem as early as the late 1800s, treatment specific to the eating disorders, anorexia nervosa and bulimia nervosa, has been in existence only since the 1970s. The 1970s saw a rising public interest in becoming thin. Marks (1984, p. 45) suggests that teenagers in general and people with eating disorders specifically have been influenced by the "gaunt high-fashion models and the pervasive notion that thin is in" ever since the 70s. Most anorexics and bulimics identify dieting and external pressure to remain thin as major contributors to the onset of their illness. Further progression of these illnesses reveals their serious and often life-threatening qualities as well as the contributing psychological components that surface during treatment (Anderson, 1979; Hornyak & Baker, 1989; Johnson & Connors, 1987; Marks, 1984).

Profile of patients with eating disorders

Until the 1980s bulimia was considered a facet of anorexia nervosa because many anorexics exhibit bulimic behaviors such as binging and purging, excessive exercise, and so on. Research and treatment of eating disorder patients have served to distin-

guish bulimia as a disease with its own properties (Johnson & Connors, 1987).

Anorexia nervosa

The essential features of patients with anorexia nervosa are a refusal to maintain body weight over a minimum normal weight for age and height, a weight loss of 15% or more of the original body weight, an intense fear of gaining weight or becoming fat (even though underweight), a fear that weight gain is out of the patient's control, a distorted body image, amenorrhea (in females), and no physical illness to cause the weight loss. The weight loss has most frequently resulted in difficulty in concentration, coldness, lowered vital signs, weakness, and low potassium levels. Starvation and suicide are primary causes of death among anorexics (American Psychiatric Association, 1987; Garner & Garfinkle, 1985).

Anorexia nervosa is more prevalent among females (about 95%) and begins in early or late adolescence. Occasionally onset of the illness is as late as age 30, but this is rare. Usually some kind of stressful life situation precipitates the onset. *DSM-III-R* (American Psychiatric Association, 1987), Johnson and Connors (1987), and Sullivan and Everstine (1989) refer to the preponderance of earlier sexual trauma as a precursor to the development of anorexia.

The pre-illness personality in anorexics is characterized by a tendency toward **perfectionism** and perseverance and not very much insight into or understanding of her eating habits as being abnormal. Anorexic bulimics who engage in self-induced vomiting have some recognition of the abnormality of that behavior, but deny recognition of abnormality in the practice of starvation. Frequently, anorexics are considered model children who are well behaved and are high achievers in school (Anderson, 1979).

Bulimia nervosa

The essential features of patients with bulimia nervosa are recurrent episodes of **binge eating** (rapid consumption of a large amount of food in a short period of time) usually lasting less than 2 hours; a feeling of lack of control over eating behavior during the eating binges even with the awareness that their eating habits are abnormal; self-induced vomiting; use of laxatives or diuretics; strict dieting or fasting or vigorous exercise to prevent weight gain; and persistent overconcern with body shape and weight. Physical symptoms that result from purging—especially vomiting—are electrolyte imbalances and cardiac and kidney dysfunction. Other signs of bulimia nervosa are consumption of high-caloric, easily ingested foods during a binge; secretive eating during a binge; ending the binge because of abdominal pain, onset of sleep, or interruption by another person; repeated crash dieting; and frequent fluctuations in weight of more than 10 pounds due to alternating binges and fasts (*DSM-III-R*, 1987; Marks, 1984).

Bulimia most often begins in late adolescence or young adulthood. White females are most vulnerable, with a rather high incidence among college women (30% or more of all college women). Boys and men affected by bulimia usually become involved because of sports activities like wrestling in which they need to maintain a certain weight for a position on the team (Levenkron, 1982). The illness usually lasts about 2 to 5 years before treatment is sought. Only 35% of bulimics are below the normal weight range. Most are within the normal weight limits or above. It is common for the mothers and sisters of bulimics to be overweight. Although bulimics tend to have higher premorbid body weight than anorexics, both are relentlessly preoccupied with food and weight (Johnson & Connors, 1987).

Bulimics tend to have a crippling degree of self-sacrifice that impairs their ability to function effectively in interpersonal relationships. They are more apt to care for plants and pets and "mother" other people than to become involved in the give and take of an interpersonal relationship (Hall & Cohn, 1982). They are prone to depression with suicidal thoughts or self-mutilation. Although bulimics are generally more socially outgoing than anorexics, they too abuse food to ignore their own fears and emotions. They often binge in response to feelings such as anger, boredom, loneliness, competition, or fear of success or failure. Regardless of the feeling, the expression of it is turned inward and becomes self-defeating.

Perfectionism among bulimics is also self-defeating. For example, an absolute promise like "I will not binge" is very difficult to fulfill and often broken; this leads to feelings of guilt, anger, and dissatisfaction with self. Unlike most anorexics, however, bulimics usually have some degree of insight into the abnormality of their eating habits. Although they feel powerless over controlling the habits, they are more apt to seek treatment (Hall & Cohn, 1982; Johnson & Connors, 1987).

Common factors among anorexics and bulimics

The eating patterns of anorexics and bulimics are symbolic of their attempts to maintain control over an aspect of their lives when their environment has become unmanageable. They generally view those who want to help them or who have a relationship with them as trying to take away their control. This fosters feelings of distrust toward others like family members, friends, and therapists.

The ritualistic and secretive behavior of bulimics and anorexics is an example of their attempt to maintain control over their bodies and their environment. For example, Hall and Cohn (1982) describe the ritualistic behavior as follows:

> Covering my tracks was second nature to me. . . . During one period, I went to the same grocery daily to buy large quantities of binge food. I told the checkers that I was a nursery school teacher buying snacks for the children. My rituals included a preoccupation with scales, mirrors, and trying on clothes. I used to weigh myself before and after binges to be sure that I gained no weight. I used to empty my closet and try on all my clothes, checking myself in a full-length mirror to be sure that the clothes still fit and I was not getting any fatter. . . . I could not pass any mirror without fully checking myself out first. (p. 11)

Other rituals are measuring all food eaten to control calorie intake, arranging food on the plate so it looks like more than it is, eating systematically to maintain control over food consumption, and trying fad diets.

Both bulimics and anorexics have a great deal of difficulty with self-identity. They often look to others for validation and feelings of self-worth as evidenced by the common practice of assuming the perfect little girl role. Hsu (1986) attributes the pursuit of thinness to a misguided striving for specialness, acceptance, and individuality. The result has been an absorption with appearance and self-criticism. As they turn their feelings inward,

it is common for bulimics and anorexics to harbor feelings of neediness, deprivation, rejection, anxiety, and anger. Their lack of self-assertion and individuation inhibits their expression of these feelings. Normal growth and maturation for developing social and vocational interests and for trusting in themselves enough to be able to manipulate their world outside the structured family and school settings are thwarted.

Treatment settings

Anderson (1979) and Garner and Garfinkle (1985) suggest that a strong team-oriented intensive program using a variety of methods is necessary to stop the cycle of aberrant eating habits and to promote a healthier and happier lifestyle. Although the literature does not define the treatment team specifically, many professions have emerged as having an important contribution to make to the treatment of eating disorders. Besides occupational therapy, nursing, medicine, nutrition counseling, psychology, psychiatry, social work, creative arts therapy, and family therapy are recognized as important components of treatment. Collaboration among the treatment team members is essential to provide the atmosphere, environment, and support needed to treat patients effectively.

Outpatient, inpatient, and intensive day hospital programs are the primary treatment settings for those with eating disorders. The latter two programs are needed for the more severely involved patients who need close observation and support to work on their treatment issues.

Inpatient programs are needed for those who are in significant medical difficulty, who have a significant risk of suicide or self-mutilation, who are too weak to provide their self-care, whose family cannot provide an adequate psychological environment for improvement to occur, and who need to interrupt the binge/purge cycle (Johnson & Connors, 1987).

Day hospital is a newer treatment program process that involves intensive treatment much like the inpatient programming, but the patients go home at night. Day hospital processes support the theory that the patients need to practice learned behaviors in both simulated and natural settings. It decreases the degree of distancing from the dysfunctional living situations. Consequently, patients are addressing their environmental obstacles from the early stages of treatment. Inpatient programs can address these issues directly only through family therapy and day passes that allow the patients to test their new skills before they leave the inpatient phase of treatment. Day hospital programs are cost-efficient and can accommodate more patients, thus increasing availability to patients. The flexibility in programming allows for a natural aftercare process by decreasing days of attendance as the patient's condition improves (Piran & Kaplan, 1990).

Follow-up or *aftercare programs* are very important to the success of treatment. As in an addiction, the process of a patient changing her habits and lifestyle (in this case, eating habits and patterns rather than alcohol or drug intake) is very difficult. Recidivism is high and continued support is needed. Partial or day hospital and outpatient programs are important aftercare programs for inpatients because they allow the patient to gradually and supportively take steps toward becoming independent. Support systems like Overeaters Anonymous (OA), patterned after the 12-step program of Alcoholics Anonymous, are frequently begun and encouraged while the patient is in the intensive phase of treatment (in both inpatient and day hospital programs). Many inpatient programs have OA groups on the grounds of the hospital and also give passes to patients to attend OA meetings near their homes. The purpose is to help the patients establish healthy support systems before they leave the hospital.

Vocational rehabilitation is another important follow-up process identified by Kerr (1990). Most patients have not yet entered the work arena or have made poor work choices. As a result of the illness those who have held jobs have experienced strained work relationships, underproductivity, long periods of absenteeism, and termination. Although these issues begin to be addressed in the treatment setting, getting and maintaining a job that is appropriate for the patient require the continued support of professionals and organizations designed to assist patients in vocational choices and work stability.

Treatment

Treatment is a process of stabilizing the patients medically, breaking the dysfunctional behavioral patterns, and transferring the management and control of eating and functioning to the patient. Generally this is done in a supportive and nurturing atmosphere that progresses toward a more challenging and insight-oriented treatment process. Because eating disorder patients have such fragile self-identities and because they look to others for validation of themselves, it is important to provide a supportive environment in which they feel safe to begin to explore the feelings that they have kept protected and hidden through eating and starving. As they begin to communicate their feelings with the members of the treatment team and their peers, the learning and maturing begin.

The course of treatment is characterized by a period of close monitoring to prevent starvation, binging, and purging, after which there is gradual expansion of privileges and choices in treatment. The early stages are frequently determined by weight gain for the anorexics (they gain privileges as they gain and maintain weight) and controlled eating for the bulimics. During the initial stage of treatment, patients may be confined to bed rest and may be unable to attend treatment groups. The intent is to ensure that food intake is used to build strength and not to abuse or purge. The progression of privileges is based on the gradual introduction of activity. Resistance and denial of the problems are high.

Although patients with eating disorders are anxious to be in less restricted stages of treatment, they also resist treatment groups that are geared toward addressing their problems. Hence, gaining privileges in the middle stages of treatment is dependent on group attendance and participation. As patients begin to address their treatment issues, they are frequently given the responsibility of monitoring themselves by keeping a diary or receiving credits for participation in treatment groups. The diaries are used as therapeutic tools and serve as a record of the progress the patients have made. Anderson, Morse, and Santmeyer (1985) identify the last phase of treatment as the "***maintenance phase***," at which time the controls are returned to the patient. It is a time when patients have begun to internalize the structure and controls of the program and are encouraged to make food, exercise, and activity choices. The staff monitoring is

less intense and patients have more freedom (Anderson, 1979; Meyers, 1989; Naitove, 1986; Piran & Kaplan, 1990).

Although treatment is described here as a steady progression of improvement, it rarely appears that way. Patients who are asked to make dramatic changes in their behavior patterns rarely follow a smooth course of treatment. Each time a patient gains privileges, makes progress, or faces a major challenge like going to a family meeting or grocery store, there is the possibility of a regression in treatment. The fear of success or failure is frightening and often creates a psychological atmosphere conducive to returning to the old coping mechanisms of abnormal eating habits. These occasional episodes of starving, hoarding food, binging, and purging can be used in treatment as a means to explore acceptance of self as a whole person with both positive and negative qualities.

Since control issues are a primary focus for bulimic and anorexic patients, it is important that the patient is treated with dignity and is involved in the treatment process. The patients need to understand and be a part of what is happening to them. A patient, as retold by Meyers (1989), recalls her treatment and her relationship with her occupational therapist:

> She saw me, not as an eating disorder, but as a fellow human being. I appreciated that, because if she had bought into the label, I wouldn't have had to accept any responsibility. We both knew I had that problem, but it wasn't the focus, I was a whole person who needed to make some changes in my behavior. As my treatment progressed, my therapist was there to coach as needed and she was also there to be my cheerleader as I experienced success. I did the work, but my therapist provided the opportunities and was there to challenge and encourage me. (p. 38)

The key to the success of the treatment process for eating disorders is gaining the patient's trust and engaging her in treatment decisions.

Establishing a relationship with the patient

The good patient–therapist relationship is all-important for the treatment to be successful. It is not an easy task, however. Meyers (1989), Piran and Kaplan (1990), and Deering (1987) describe the stages in developing a therapeutic relationship as follows. The first phase is the ***angry counterdependent phase***. It usually occurs in the early stages of treatment as the patients are becoming stabilized medically, monitored closely, and gently guided toward becoming honest about their feelings toward themselves and others. Patients often indiscriminately direct their anger about themselves toward everything and everyone.

The ***depressed needy phase*** appears next. This is a time when the patient begins to seek help and demand attention and validation from the therapist. The patient realizes that the illness has control over her and feels a sense of hopelessness and helplessness. The last phase, the ***approaching relating phase***, is the beginning of the patient's acceptance and trust in herself and the therapist. It is the product of the steady, supportive, and consistent work that the therapist has done with the patient up to this point.

It is important for the therapist to be honest and supportively confrontive throughout the course of treatment. Confrontation challenges the patient to accept and work through her issues. It is always tempered by the patient's ability to hear and understand the content of the issues being presented. For example, a patient in the first stage of treatment, who is dealing with the issues of denial of illness, needs supportive nurturance and gentle probing to begin to accept her illness. In later stages when the patient–therapist relationship is well established, the patient may be able to understand the greater challenges of facing the more intimate and painful aspects of her life.

During the course of treatment the extreme feelings of self-deprecation, anger, and guilt that the patient feels and expresses can be misdirected toward the therapist. The patient's propensity for denying the illness and testing the sincerity of the therapist can be frustrating for the therapist. The treatment team can be an important source of encouragement and support for each other as well as for the patient.

Frames of reference and assessment

The selection of assessment tools is determined by the theoretical frame of reference on which the occupational therapy program is designed. Rockwell (1990) concludes that no one frame of reference or methodology is preferable to another for treating patients with eating disorders; however, her limited study of the frames of reference indicates that there is a strong tendency for occupational therapists to emphasize psychoanalytic, cognitive, and familial issues in the treatment of eating disorders. Kerr (1990) describes the use of the model of human occupation and suggests the use of assessments related to the frame of reference such as the Role Checklist and the Activity Laboratory Questionnaire. She also uses several other assessments designed and tested by the day hospital program to assess the issues specifically related to eating disorders. As the treatment of patients with eating disorders continues, further research will expand and define the use of frames of reference in occupational therapy.

Treatment concerns in occupational therapy

The literature indicates that the primary areas of treatment in occupational therapy revolve around body image issues, nutrition and food management, social and sexual relationships, communication skills, leisure issues, work skills, and discharge planning (Garner & Garfinkle, 1985; Hsu, 1986; Kerr, 1990; Meyers, 1989).

Body image is a fundamental aspect of the treatment of patients with eating disorders. It is at the base of the delusional thought processes. No matter how thin these patients become, they always view themselves as fat. This concept drives them toward starvation and kindles their obsession with food and losing weight. Treatment is often a painful process of reality orientation and adjustment using a variety of activities to help patients make the adjustment.

For example, Meyers (1989) describes an activity of having the patients trace their bodies on a sheet of paper and compare the pictures with their perceptions of themselves. Body image is also related to personal appearance and dress. As described earlier, clothes are very important to the patient. The occupational therapist helps the patients to choose age-appropriate clothes and to feel comfortable in a variety of clothes. As the patient gains weight, she needs new clothes. A shopping trip for clothes can be very difficult; however, with support and guidance from the therapist, it can be an important turning point in the adjustment to a new body image.

Healthy exercise is another important adjustment that patients may need to make with their physician's approval. A controlled and guided exercise program can be very helpful in improving muscle tone and body weight as their bodies grow. Included in this process is education on how to exercise properly instead of the punitive exercise regimens the patients used during their illness.

Food management is another very painful yet important experience for patients with eating disorders. They need practice and education in almost every aspect of meal preparation: nutritional education, money management, meal planning, food shopping, meal preparation, eating, socializing while eating, and cleaning up after the meal. There are many creative ways to help patients work on issues related to food management.

Communication skills development of patients with eating disorders is facilitated through the use of assertiveness training, relaxation techniques, and alternative creative expressive activities. Learning to assert themselves and provide self-nurturance are key components in promoting positive relationships with their spouses and families and in developing other social relationships.

Learning how to enjoy and use leisure time is a major task. It takes time and practice. Idle, unproductive time may have led to binging and other destructive behaviors in the past. It is important to help patients explore and develop interests in nonfood-related activities to help reduce the anxiety associated with food.

The therapist can create many ways to simulate a work situation so that patients can address the work problems they are having. Prevocational assessments and exploration are helpful while the patient is in the intensive phase of treatment. Work for some, however, may come later after discharge in an aftercare setting, allowing the intensive treatment phase to be focused on the immediate medical and psychological aspects of recovery.

The occupational therapist has a strong role in the discharge of the patient. A thorough assessment of education, leisure, and vocational strengths and weaknesses can be used to facilitate follow-up recommendations for management and continued care.

Occupational therapy treatments generally need to be directly related to the patient's illness and processed with the patient so that she understands their purpose, usefulness, and relevance to recovery. For example, the therapist needs to facilitate the patient's understanding of how an activity such as learning and working on a craft can symbolically represent real life situations. It gives the patient an opportunity to work side by side with other people, use problem solving and work skills, and prove that completion and follow-through are possible. Although the patient often rejects or is highly critical of the finished product, with the therapist's encouragement the patient will recognize this behavior and work toward accepting the end product as it relates to acceptance of herself. The processing of the activity is critical to facilitating this understanding. As with an addiction, the patient needs guidance from the therapist and feedback from her peers to benefit from the use of activities. (Processing activities are also discussed in Chapter 17, Section 2.)

Summary

Eating disorders are relatively new phenomena in health care, and occupational therapy has been in the forefront of programming and research from the early stages.

Anorexics are characterized among other things by their restrictive eating habits and low body weight. Bulimics are characterized by a near-normal body weight and some degree of insight into their illness and the habitual patterns of binging and purging the body of food. Both are relentlessly obsessed with food and weight issues. Both illnesses can be life-threatening and require professional help to break the dysfunctional behavioral and psychological patterns of existence.

The most common settings for treatment are the outpatient and inpatient treatment settings. Day hospitals are emerging as a more cost-efficient and more available setting for treatment. An intensive phase of treatment with a strongly collaborative treatment team is needed to stabilize patients medically, break the cycle of the obsessional activities, and lay the groundwork for patients to gain happier and healthier patterns of living and relating to others. Since anorexics and bulimics tend to have a high rate of recidivism, continued care through follow-up or aftercare programs is an essential component of treatment. The latter involves organizations such as OA, outpatient care, day hospital, and vocational rehabilitation.

Treatment occurs best in a supportive and nurturing atmosphere that progresses toward a more challenging insight-oriented process as the patient improves. Occupational therapists have an important role in all phases of treatment. The occupational therapist begins contact with the patient during the first phase of treatment, when the patient is on bed rest and closely monitored on the unit. These individual contact sessions are supportive and gently confrontive. The patient gains privileges in the second phase of treatment and begins group treatments with peers in occupational therapy in which she struggles to face the challenges of self-acceptance and discovering healthier patterns of living. During the maintenance phase of treatment, the patient is given the opportunity to take control and responsibility for her food intake and activity participation in preparation for discharge.

The therapist's relationship with the patient is a key ingredient to the success or failure of treatment. Eating disorder patients have a long history of impaired relationships with difficulties in trusting others and communicating their feelings. When the therapist is honest, consistent, empathetic, and supportive, the patient will feel safe enough to trust the therapist to help her.

References

American Psychiatric Association. (1987). *Diagnostic and statistical manual of mental disorders* (3rd rev. ed.). Washington, DC: Author.

Anderson, A. (1979). Anorexia nervosa: Diagnosis and treatment. *Weekly Psychiatric Update Series. 3,* 1–8. Princeton, NJ: Biomedia Inc.

Anderson, A. E., Morse, C., & Santmyer, K. (1985). Inpatient treatment for anorexia nervosa. In D. M. Gardner & P. Garfinkle (Eds.), *The handbook of psychotherapy for anorexia nervosa and bulimia.* New York: Guilford Press

Deering, C. (1987). Developing a therapeutic alliance with the anorexia nervosa client. *Journal of Psychosocial Nursing, 25*(3), 11–17.

Garner, D., & Garfinkel, P. (1985). *Handbook of psychotherapy for anorexia nervosa and bulimia.* New York: Guilford Press.

Hall, L., & Cohn, L. (1982). *Understanding and overcoming bulimia. A Self-help Guide.* Santa Barbara, CA: Gurze Books.

Hornyak, L., & Baker, E. (Eds.). (1989). *Experimental therapies for eating disorders.* New York: Guilford Press.

Hsu, L. K. (1986). The treatment of anorexia nervosa. *American Journal of Psychiatry, 143*(5), 573–581.

Johnson, C., & Connors, M. (1987). *The etiology and treatment of bulimia nervosa: A biopsychosocial perspective.* New York: Basic Books.

Kerr, A. (1990). Occupational Therapy. In N. Piran et al. (Eds.), *A day hospital group treatment program for anorexia nervosa and bulimia nervosa.* New York: Brunner/Mazel.

Levenkron, S. (1982). *Treat over and overcoming anorexia nervosa.* New York: Warner Bros.

Marks, R. (1984, January). Anorexia and bulimia: Eating habits that can kill. *RN, 47*(1), 44–47.

Meyers, S. (1989). Occupational therapy treatment of an adult with an eating disorder: One woman's experience. *Occupational Therapy in Mental Health, 9*(1), 33–48.

Naitove, C. (1986). *"Life's but a walking shadow": Treating anorexia nervosa and bulimia.* New York: Guilford Press.

Piran, N., & Kaplan, A. (1990). *A day hospital group treatment program for anorexia nervosa and bulimia nervosa.* New York: Brunner/Mazel.

Rockwell, L. (1990). Frames of reference and modalities used by occupational therapists in the treatment of patients with eating disorders. *Occupational Therapy in Mental Health, 10*(2), 47–63.

Sullivan, D., & Everstine, L. (1989). *Sexual trauma in children and adolescents: Dynamics and treatment.* New York: Brunner/Mazel.

SECTION 4

Stress management

MAUREEN E. NEISTADT

KEY TERMS

β-Endorphins

External Physical Stressors

General Adaptation Response

Internal Physical Stressors

Mental Imagery

Progressive Relaxation

Social Environmental Stressors

Stress

Stressor

LEARNING OBJECTIVES

Upon completion of this section the reader will be able to:

1. *Define the terms stress and stressor.*

2. *List categories of common stressors.*

3. *Describe the general adaptation response.*

4. *List 12 stress management techniques.*

5. *Outline a stress management program for a clinical population.*

Stress is the collection of physical and emotional changes that are felt in response to a perceived challenge or threat. These changes produce a certain amount of wear and tear on the body over time. Stress affects health. Too little stress in our lives can lead to boredom, malaise, and, in extreme cases, confusion and disorientation. Too much stress can lead to or exacerbate illness and disability, causing a decrease in functional abilities. Stress management programs, by relieving anxiety, can promote wellness and help people to function optimally. Consequently, occupational therapists offer structured stress management programs for many clients, including those with cardiac, mental health, neurologic, and pain problems (Courtney & Escobedo, 1990; Lysaght & Bodenhamer, 1990; McCormack, 1988; Neistadt, 1987; Stein & Nikolic, 1989; Strong, Cramond, & Maas, 1989; Trombly, 1989a).

Many occupational therapists also practice stress management techniques themselves to help them cope with work-related pressures and demands. This section looks at the elements of an effective stress management program: an examination of common stressors; the neurophysiologic effects of the stress response; a conceptual model for stress management techniques; and guidelines for choice among these techniques.

Common stressors

Any agent or circumstance capable of triggering stress reactions is called a **stressor** (Selye, 1974, 1978). It is important to be aware of the many and varied stressors so that when we or our clients feel too stressed or tense, we can accurately identify the causes of those feelings. Knowing the sources of stress can help to predict and control the amount of stress we feel in our lives (Aronson & Maschia, 1981; McQuade & Aikman, 1975; Miller, Ross, & Cohen, 1982; Pelletier, 1977; Selye, 1974, 1978).

The potential stressors encountered in everyday lives fall into three major categories: external physical, internal physical, and social environmental. Some of these stressors can cause direct biologic trauma and illness in addition to triggering stress reactions.

External physical stressors

External physical stressors include noise, crowding, poor lighting, inadequate ventilation, and environmental pollutants. Research has shown that excessive or continuous noise (90 decibels or higher) at home or work can cause high blood pressure and hearing loss (Raloff, 1982a, 1982b). Crowding can make people irritable and aggressive. Poor lighting and ventilation have been reported to cause eye irritation, headaches, nausea, and drowsiness in workers (Raloff, 1981a, 1981b). Environmental pollutants have been correlated with a wide range of health problems. Short-term exposure to many of the chemicals in crafts, ceramics, and woodworking supplies used in some occupational therapy clinics can cause health problems ranging from headaches to respiratory distress. Longer-term exposure

can cause more serious health problems (McCann, 1979; *Science News*, 1981). Daily exposure to external physical stressors makes a baseline coping demand on our nervous systems, and additional stressors make demands on a nervous system already engaged in responding to larger environmental stressors.

Internal physical stressors

The internal neurobiologic environments, known as **internal physical stressors**, also affect stress responses. Patterns of neurologic organization—expressed in individual biorhythms, relative brain hemispheric lateralizations, and different personalities—partially determine our susceptibility to stress. Also, chemicals that we ingest can affect our nervous system's reaction to potential stressors.

Blood levels of enzymes, hormones, and other body chemicals fluctuate daily in conjunction with circadian rhythms or biorhythms. These are normal cycles of change in metabolism that occur daily and are indicated by fluctuations in body temperature, pulse, and breathing rates, blood chemistry assays, and sleep patterns (Dale, 1976). Changes in work schedules or normal sleep patterns can disrupt circadian cycles and deplete a person's ability to cope with stressors. For example, nurses work a variety of shifts that change frequently or abruptly and thus may experience the greatest disruptions of biorhythms (Czeisler, Moore-Ede, & Coleman, 1982). Such schedule irregularities have been correlated to a high number of stress-related errors on the job (Hilts, 1980).

Geschwind and coauthors (1982, 1985) have found that left-handedness, or motor dominance of the right hemisphere, is associated with a statistically higher incidence of dyslexia, headaches, allergies, and autoimmune diseases. Speculation exists that this pattern of cerebral organization may result in a compromised immune system and thus more susceptibility to environmental stressors.

Herbert (1982, 1983) and Kagan (1984) have claimed that overvigilance of the right hemisphere may be linked to excessive timidity and fearfulness or depression in some people. Their research has suggested that inability to screen out extraneous nonverbal stimuli can result in a neurologically overwhelmed person who is extremely susceptible to stressors.

Individual patterns of brain organization express themselves in behavioral styles or personalities. Kabosa, Hilker, and Maddi (1979) have identified three personality factors that distinguish stress-prone and stress-resistant people. Stress-resistant people see change as a challenge, feel they have control over their environment, and have a sense of commitment and purpose about their lives. Stress-prone people see change as a threat, feel helpless in controlling their environment, and have a sense of alienation about their lives.

Friedman and Rosenman (1974) have identified a stress-prone, type A personality as hard-driving, achievement-oriented, hostile, and highly sensitive to time pressures. Type A personality might be seen as a reaction formation to the stress-prone feelings identified by Kabosa et al. (1979). This behavior pattern has been correlated with an increased risk of heart disease.

Certain chemicals that most people ingest regularly can interfere with the nervous system's ability to cope with other stressors. For example, caffeine and nicotine, as sympathomimetics, produce many of the same physiologic reactions seen during a stress response and thus sap the nervous system of the energy needed to cope with other stressors. As little as 250 mg caffeine can cause headache, tremors, nervousness, insomnia, and irritability (Pelletier, 1977). One 5-oz. cup of coffee contains from 110 to 150 mg of caffeine; one 5-oz. cup of tea contains from 9 to 50 mg of caffeine, depending on the preparation method and length of brewing time (Union Hospital, 1982). Caffeine can be found not only in coffee and tea, but also in cola, cocoa, baked goods, frozen dairy products, soft candy, gelatins, puddings, and some nonprescription drugs.

Central nervous system depressants like alcohol and diazepam (Valium) inhibit the ability of the nervous systems to react constructively to stressors. Abuse of these and other drugs can cause somatic symptoms, disrupt social relationships, and increase levels of stress.

Social environmental stressors

Social environments can also be a source of stressors. Major life changes that alter social roles and relationships—marriage, divorce, job change, serious illness, death of a loved one—can increase susceptibility to stress, especially when several of these changes occur within a brief period of time. Studies have shown that for some people, multiple major life changes within 1 year's time correlate with a higher risk of injury or illness (Holmes & Rahe, 1967; Rahe, 1979). Other studies have shown that widowed middle-aged men have a significantly higher mortality rate than married men of the same age, and that separated and divorced women have an increased mortality rate for some diseases (Bower, 1986; Helsing, Szklo, & Comstock, 1981). The link between major stressors and illness appears to be the immune system. For instance, Kiecolt-Glaser and colleagues (as reported in Miller, 1968) have found bioassay evidence of depressed immune function in medical students during examination periods. This has been correlated with an increased incidence of infectious diseases like colds during that same time period (Miller, 1986).

Minor changes or day-to-day aggravations also can act as stressors. Lazarus (1981) has identified three minor "hassles" rated as most annoying by adults aged 18 to 64 years: (a) misplacing or losing things, (b) being concerned about physical appearance, and (c) having too many things to do. Other common annoyances listed by survey subjects were economic pressures, household chores, and crime. These vexations can have a cumulative effect and are magnified during periods of major life changes. Major life changes, in addition to their immediate impact, can create a "ripple effect" of continuing minor hassles.

Changes in social roles caused by major life changes necessitate changes in daily activities. A divorce, for example, may force both partners to assume chores and financial obligations that had previously been shared. The duration, frequency, intensity, and context of these relatively minor hassles influence how potent they are as stressors. Clusters of stressful events have been correlated with an increased incidence of accidents and job-related errors (Sheehan, O'Donnell, Fitzgerald, Hervig, & Ward, 1981–1982).

The lack of an active social network of family and friends contributes to stress responses and decreases life expectancies by denying people emotional support and nurturing. Without a network, a person lacks an important source of practical information and assistance. A social network can provide information about employment opportunities and medical care, and assis-

tance like grocery shopping and small loans (Berkman, 1982; *Science News,* 1980).

A person's sense of involvement with his or her network may be as important as the existence of that network. One study found that feelings of isolation, even in the presence of a social network, contributed to a higher incidence of cancer and higher mortality rates in women (Miller, 1986).

Some people in our social environments may be stress carriers. Those who fail to clearly communicate their expectations or a plan of action and then get angry at others for not doing things the "right" way can provoke stress reactions. Stress carriers often question in a manner that puts people on the defensive and they give nonconstructive criticism that undermines the recipient's self-confidence.

Stress response

Occupational therapy clients are particularly prone to some of the stressors just mentioned. Illness and disability themselves are major life changes and can cause social roles changes and generate a host of minor aggravating changes in daily activities. Hospital routines can be extremely disruptive to some clients' biorhythms. Changes in appearance or behavior can leave a client constantly fearful of rejection. The larger society that our clients hope to join is not always socially and physically accessible to them.

On the other side of the therapeutic relationship, therapists have to deal with some trying job-related stressors that can easily lead to burnout, chronic fatigue, and irritability caused by too much stress. Time pressures are intense in many settings, with demands for direct treatment, documentation, inter- and intra-department communication, and continuing education being made constantly and simultaneously. Since the establishment of the Medicare prospective payment system and similar cost-containment procedures from other insurers, many clinics are experiencing drastic changes in types of caseload and client/staff ratios. Inadequate space is an issue in most occupational therapy clinics and the client's constant need for empathy can be emotionally draining.

Stressors do not automatically trigger stress responses in everyone. How a person responds to any potential stressor is a matter of interpretation. A minor change in routine may be upsetting to one person, but insignificant to another. Our bodies respond to potential stressors only when we interpret them as significant. When we do respond, our physiologic reactions are the same, regardless of whether the stressor is viewed as positive or negative. For instance, whether a move to a new house or apartment is viewed as devastating or exciting, our bodies would need to organize a stress response to deal with the demands of relocation. The emotional labels we attach to stressors influence our ability to work through the stages of our stress response.

General adaptation response

Selye (1974, 1978) describes the body's stress reaction as the **general adaptation response**. This response occurs in three stages: the alarm reaction, the adaptive or resistive stage, and the exhaustion phase. Not everyone experiences all three stages; the exhaustion phase is reached only when the person either gets stuck in the alarm stage or goes through the alarm and adaptive stages too often.

Alarm reaction

The alarm reaction is the fight-or-flight response that prepares a person to meet a challenge or threat. During this stage, the cerebral cortex activates the reticular activating system to generally alert the organism. The cortex also activates the sympathetic nervous and endocrine systems by way of the hypothalamus. The sympathetic system releases adrenalin from its nerve endings to effect increases in heart rate, blood pressure, perspiration, muscle tone, and cell metabolism. Blood vessels just under the skin constrict and digestion is slowed. The endocrine system releases hormones from the adrenal and thyroid glands, which increase the body's supply of glucose and help cells to accelerate their metabolism. In addition, the hypothalamus triggers the release of β-endorphins from the pituitary. **β-*Endorphins*** are endogenous opiate proteins that elevate mood and decrease pain perception. They have also been linked to suppression of the immune system (Shavit et al., 1985). Figure 17-3 provides more details about this stage.

Adaptive or resistive stage

In the adaptive or resistive stage, the body returns to its preexcited state and recovers from the physiologic strains of the alarm stage. Stress-prone or overstressed persons who may interpret even normal events as negative stressors often are unable to reach this particular stage. They get stuck in the alarm reaction until their bodies enter the exhaustion phase. People who are able to successfully move to the adaptive stage may also reach the exhaustion phase if there are too many stressors in their lives.

Exhaustion phase

The exhaustion phase is a reaction to the constant high metabolic demands of the alarm stage. During this phase, the neurophysiologic ability to respond to stressors effectively is no longer present.

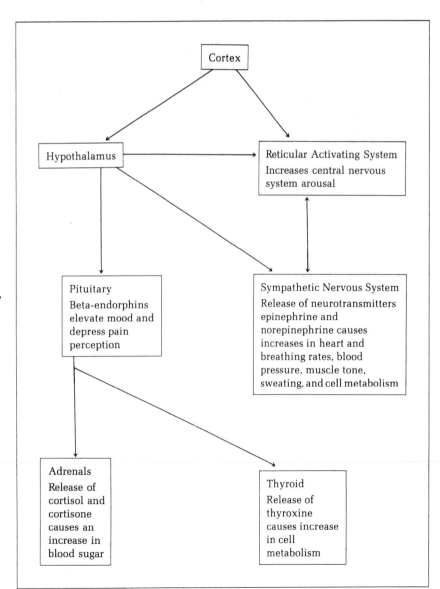

FIGURE 17-3. *Stimulation pathways of the alarm stage.*

Chronic stress

The constant physiologic demands of chronic stress have been linked to many diseases and disorders. A continual state of stress-linked alertness can deplete the neurotransmitters used to record and store new information, thus making it difficult to learn. Constantly elevated blood pressure can lead to hypertension, which is a risk factor for stroke. Increased muscle tension can result in headaches and low back pain. Changes in circulation can aggravate heart disease, Raynaud's disease, and diabetes; changes in the digestive process can affect ulcers (Miller et al., 1982). Some people experience ventricular fibrillation in response to stressful situations of interpersonal conflict, marital separation or threat of it, bereavement, business failure, and public humiliation (Reich, DeSilva, Lowin, & Murawski, 1981). Uncorrected ventricular fibrillation can lead to heart failure and death within minutes. Chronic stress can also depress the functioning of the immune system, increasing vulnerability to disease and compromising recovery (Farber, 1989).

Stress management techniques

Stress management techniques have been developed to help relieve chronic stress and its detrimental effects. These techniques are learned behaviors that interrupt the nervous system's stress reactions. Different techniques influence nervous system processing at different levels. Table 17-11 lists some common stress management techniques according to the level of nervous system on which they have their greatest impact.

A brief description of the various techniques and hints about teaching them follow. Many excellent resources that describe these techniques in more detail are available (Aronson & Maschia, 1981; Benson, 1975; Harris, 1969; Jacobsen, 1938; McQuade & Aikman, 1975; Miller et al., 1982; Pelletier, 1977; Trombly, 1989b; Wall & Neistadt, 1982).

Aerobic exercise

Aerobic exercise involves slow, repetitive, rhythmic contractions of the large muscles of the legs and arms. Examples are walking, running, bicycling, and swimming. This type of exercise is called "aerobic" (in the presence of oxygen) because muscles use aerobic metabolism to get energy for this type of movement. In aerobic metabolism, muscles use oxygen to break down carbohydrates into carbon dioxide, water, and adenosine triphosphate (ATP), an energy-releasing compound. The muscle demand for oxygen inherent in this cycle forces the body to increase the efficiency of its systems for oxygen supply (pulmonary system), oxygen delivery (cardiovascular system), and oxygen use (musculoskeletal system). Consequently, if aerobic exercise is done regularly, breathing capacity improves and heart muscle becomes stronger, resulting in increased stroke volume and a decreased heart rate. In addition, circulation improves, blood pressure decreases, and overall muscle strength increases (Cooper, 1977). These physiologic changes also stimulate alterations in brain biochemistry that can increase deep sleep and improve mood (Carr et al., 1981; McCann & Holmes, 1984).

Aerobic exercise, therefore, can have an immediate stress management effect by allowing a person to actively work off built-up tensions. If done regularly, aerobic exercise can make a person more stress-resistant by improving their overall health and mood. Anyone planning to start an aerobic exercise program first should be seen by a physician for a complete checkup; all exercise programs should begin gradually and work slowly toward increased difficulty to avoid injuries. Specific guidelines for setting up individualized aerobic exercise programs are available from other sources (Cooper, 1977).

Autogenic training

Autogenic training is a meditative process that uses autosuggestion or self-hypnosis and mental imagery to achieve relaxation. Autosuggestions typically involve imagining sensations of physi-

TABLE 17-11. *Stress Management Techniques*

Nervous System Level/ Stress Function	Stress Management Techniques	Client Skills Needed	Environmental Resources Needed
Cortex (interpretation of events, control of emotional reactions, planning of behavior)	Autogenic training, biofeedback, communication skills, mental imagery, time management, verbalization	Abstract thinking, concentration, delay gratification, sequencing	Cost of equipment (biofeedback), time and quiet*
Hypothalamus (autonomic nervous system and endocrine system control)	Deep breathing / Laughter, meditation	Concentration, concrete thinking / Concentration, delay gratification	Time and quiet*
Reticular activating system (alertness levels)	Aerobic exercise, dark and quiet room, vestibular stimulation	Concentration, sensorimotor skill	Rocking chair (vestibular stimulation), equipment (exercise), time, quiet, and space*
Peripheral nervous system (sensory input and motor output)	Aerobic exercise / Progressive relaxation exercises	Concentration, sensorimotor skill	Equipment (exercise) / Time*

*Relevant to all techniques in category

cal heaviness and warmth to achieve muscle relaxation and vaso-dilation, respectively. Imagining oneself in settings where one would feel warm, comfortable, and heavy can facilitate these autosuggestions.

Autogenic training involves six steps: (1) assuming a mental stance of open passivity, (2) physical relaxation of muscles, (3) inducing overall feelings of warmth, (3) cardiac regulation and respiratory control, (5) inducing a sense of warmth in the abdominal region, and (6) a cool-down. Learning this process requires daily practice over many months. Autogenic training is not recommended for clients who are agitated or hallucinating (Courtney & Escobedo, 1990). Only those who have been specifically trained in this technique should consider teaching it (Miller et al., 1982; Pelletier, 1977).

Biofeedback

Biofeedback refers to a collection of devices and techniques that increase a person's awareness of subtle changes in body functions like heart rate and muscle tension. Biofeedback training is a process of learning to use information from those devices and techniques to control body functions. For instance, a person might learn to consciously slow his or her heart rate by monitoring the pulse while attempting to relax (changes in pulse rate reveal which thoughts or behaviors are most effective in reducing heart rate).

Biofeedback training helps to change the characteristic bodily responses to stressors. Through biofeedback training a person can learn to modify the autonomic nervous system's response to stressors and decrease the detrimental health effects of prolonged stress. Features of biofeedback are discussed in Chapter 9, Section 6.

Communication skills

Many stressful situations are caused by misunderstandings from unclear communication. Practicing effective communication skills like clarifying expectations, defining needs honestly, and providing tactful and constructive feedback can decrease the number of stressful misunderstandings. It is also helpful to examine the most troublesome interpersonal exchanges from the perspective of transactional analysis, a psychological theory and method of diagramming social interactions that helps identify a person's hidden agendas. Information from such an analysis can be used to change a person's behavior or modify reactions to the behavior of others. Further details are provided in other sources (Berne, 1964; Harris, 1969).

Deep breathing

Deep (diaphragmatic) breathing involves slowly inhaling and exhaling to slow down the general pace and work off tension in the shoulders, trunk, and abdomen. Because this technique involves quiet concentration on a rhythmic body function, it is also a form of meditation.

The process begins with focusing on normal breathing in a quiet and comfortable place. This is followed by a period of deep inhalation and slow exhalation. During inhalation, the abdominal muscles should be relaxed. During exhalation, the abdominal muscles should be contracted. It is often helpful to rest a hand lightly on the abdomen during this process. During inhalation,

the abdomen should puff up; during exhalation, the abdomen should flatten. Just a few minutes of deep breathing can be very relaxing.

Deep breathing technique is relatively easy to learn, requires no equipment, and can be done anywhere as long as the person is able to ignore outside distractions. It is a quick and easy way to relax at any time of the day. This technique is not recommended for clients with chronic obstructive pulmonary disease (Courtney & Escobedo, 1990).

Laughter

The healing power of humor has received much attention from health care professionals over the past few years. Some writers have suggested that laughter may stimulate the release of *endorphins*, the brain's endogenous opiates, thereby helping to alleviate pain and stress (Cousins, 1979). It is important for therapists to remember that therapy does not have to be solemnly serious to be effective.

Meditation

Meditation involves focusing attention on a rhythmic, repetitive word, phrase, or sensation (eg, breathing, heart rate) to achieve relaxation. Benson (1975) has suggested that this mental process blocks the stress response of the sympathetic nervous system by activating the anterior hypothalamus, which controls the parasympathetic nervous system. This technique requires considerable mental discipline and can take many months to learn.

Mental imagery

Mental imagery techniques use both passive and active daydreaming to interrupt habitual stress patterns. Passive techniques can offer temporary escape from a stressful situation, giving the nervous system a reprieve. Imagining oneself in a calm and pleasant setting like a deserted beach or forest are examples of passive techniques.

More active methods of imagery can change stress patterns by expanding the perspective from which stressful situations are viewed or by exploring alternative ways of responding. The blowup technique, for instance, involves imagining all the worst possible, most exaggerated consequences of a problem. After that exercise, the original problem looks harmless and mild in comparison to the overblown speculations. Mental role playing of difficult interpersonal interactions allow the practice of different behavior patterns in response to stressful situations (Wall & Neistadt, 1982). These techniques are not recommended for clients who are hallucinating (Courtney & Escobedo, 1990).

Progressive relaxation exercises

Jacobsen's **progressive relaxation** exercises involve systematically tensing and relaxing all muscle groups in the body, one group at a time, from head to foot. This technique teaches the difference between muscle tension and muscle relaxation by exaggerating the contrast between the two tone states. The learning sequence for this technique is (1) systematic tensing and relaxing of muscle groups to verbal cues, (2) systematic relaxing of muscle groups to verbal cues, and (3) relaxation of muscle groups by autosuggestion. Progressive relaxation exercises re-

Purpose: To give you a graphic representation of your patterns of time use.

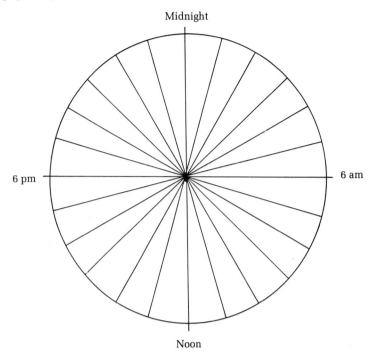

Directions: Use two charts—one for a typical weekday and one for a typical weekend day. On each chart, fill in each hour with what you do during that time.

Analysis:

Rest and Relaxation	Responsibilities
How many hours do you spend sleeping? _____ How many hours do you spend resting? _____ How many hours do you spend relaxing, doing something just because you enjoy it? _____	How many hours do you spend fulfilling responsibilities to others? (Job, childcare, homemaking, meetings, etc.) _____ How many hours do you spend on self-maintainance tasks? (Dressing, grooming, meals, chores, etc.) _____
Total: _____	Total: _____

Do the totals from these two columns match? What changes might you make in your life to achieve a more satisfactory work/play balance?

FIGURE 17-4. *Pie of life.*

quire mental discipline and daily practice, and can take months to learn completely (Jacobsen, 1938). The first step in the learning sequence can be used to provide temporary relief from excess muscle tension but is not recommended for clients with upper motor neuron lesions and spasticity. Because these exercises involve isometric muscle contractions, they are not recommended for clients with hypertension or cardiac disease (Courtney & Escobedo, 1990; Smith & Lukens, 1983).

Time management

Time management techniques include realistically scheduling and organizing time, setting priorities about task accomplishment, making lists, setting limits, and accepting the fact that everything cannot be done at once. Changing schedules or daily routines to avoid stressful situations is also a form of time management (Lakein, 1973).

Verbalization

Talking to friends and acquaintances about stressors can help to ventilate pent-up feelings and to find new solutions to old problems. Friends can offer different perspectives, new suggestions, and support, all of which are helpful in extricating a person from feeling stuck with a problem situation.

Vestibular stimulation

Slow, rhythmic, rocking or rotary motions of the head produce mild vestibular stimulation and can have a calming influence on the nervous system. These motions are part of rocking in a rocking chair and of aerobic exercise. The physiologic mechanism for the relaxing effect of these motions may be reticular activating system's activation of the parasympathetic nervous system (Farber, 1982).

General guidelines for choice of technique

Self-assessment

Guided self-assessment of individual stressors and stress reactions is the first step in designing an appropriate stress management program. The guiding can be done by someone else or by structured forms that the person can fill out independently. The Holmes-Rahe Life Change Index (Holmes & Rahe, 1967) or the Stress Management Questionnaire (Stein & Nikolic, 1989) can help to identify stressors. Other forms are available to help people assess their physical, emotional, and behavioral stress responses (Aronson & Maschia, 1981; Miller et al., 1982; Vitaliano, Russo, Carr, Maiuro, & Becker, 1985; Wall & Neistadt, 1982). Care should be taken to interpret scores on formal stress scales as gross, relative indications of stress levels and behavior patterns only. If scores on these instruments are taken too literally, they can become self-fulfilling prophecies. On the Holmes-Rahe scale, for instance, the statistical correlation between higher scores and the risk of illness or injury, although positive, is relatively weak. A list of the categories of stressors mentioned earlier might be a more useful, less restrictive, and less suggestive way to structure a person's self-assessment. The "pie of life" is a very useful way for a person to look at both time management strategies and the work/play balance in his or her daily activities (Fig. 17-4).

General factors

Some stressors can be avoided; others cannot. Some general factors to consider in suggesting stress management techniques for clients or deciding on such techniques for oneself are the following:

Learning style (concrete versus abstract)
Level of financial and interpersonal resources
Lifestyle and daily routine
Amount of time available to learn a new technique

For example, if a cardiac client cannot afford to purchase a biofeedback unit for home use, it would not be useful for an occupational therapist to spend the client's hospitalization time teaching him or her to use such a unit for stress control. Meditation takes many months to learn properly and could not be taught within a short hospital stay. Deep breathing techniques, on the other hand, are relatively easy to learn, require no outside equipment, and can generally be taught fairly quickly.

Conclusion

Effective stress management programs can be part of individual or group therapy sessions and are particularly helpful for clients with stress-related illnesses or with high stress levels that seriously impede their functional progress. Although not all clients need formal stress management training, it is important to remember that all clients are in stressful situations by virtue of their illness or disability. All clients are therefore tense and anxious to a certain degree. Occupational therapists need to keep this in mind and to do their best to help their clients relax during any treatment session. Explaining procedures and making clients partners in the treatment process will go a long way toward relieving their stress and helping them to achieve their maximal functional potential.

References

Aronson, S., & Maschia, M. (1981). *Stress management workbook*. New York: Appleton-Century-Crofts.

Benson, H. (1975). *The relaxation response*. New York: Avon Books.

Berkman, L. F. (1982). Social network analysis and coronary heart disease. *Advances in Cardiology, 29,* 37–49.

Berne, E. (1964). *Games people play*. New York: Grove Press.

Bower, B. (1986). Social isolation: Female cancer risk? *Science News, 129,* 166.

Carr, D. B., Bullen, B. A., Skrinar, G. S., Arnold, M. A., Rosenblatt, M., Beitins, I. Z., Martin, J. B., & McArthur, J. W. (1981). Physical conditioning facilitates the exercise-induced secretion of beta-endorphin and beta-lipoprotein in women. *New England Journal of Medicine, 305,* 560–563.

Cooper, K. (1977). *The aerobics way*. New York: Bantam Books.

Courtney, C., & Escobedo, B. (1990). A stress management program: Inpatient-to-outpatient continuity. *American Journal of Occupational Therapy, 44,* 306–311.

Cousins, N. (1979). *Anatomy of an illness as perceived by the patient*. New York: Bantam Books.

Czeisler, C. A., Moore-Ede, M. C., & Coleman, R. H. (1982). Rotating shift work schedules that disrupt sleep are improved by applying circadian principles. *Science, 217,* 460–3.

Dale, A. (1976). *Biorhythm*. New York: Pocket Books.

Farber, S. (1982). *Neurorehabilitation: A multisensory approach*. Philadelphia: W. B. Saunders.

Farber, S. (1989). Neuroscience and occupational therapy: Vital connections—1989 Eleanor Clarke Slagle lecture. *American Journal of Occupational Therapy, 43,* 637–648.

Friedman, M., & Rosenman, R. H. (1974). *Type A behavior and your heart*. New York: Alfred Knopf.

Geschwind, N., & Behan, P. (1982). Left-handedness: Association with immune disease, migraine, and developmental learning disorder. *Proceedings of the National Academy of Science USA, 79,* 5097–5100.

Geschwind, N., & Galaburda, A. (1985). Cerebral lateralization: Biological mechanisms, associations, and pathology: I. A hypothesis and program for research. *Archives of Neurology, 42,* 428–459.

Harris, T. A. (1969). *I'm ok, you're ok.* New York: Avon Books.

Helsing, K. J., & Szklo, M., & Comstock, G. W. (1981). Factors associated with mortality after widowhood. *Public Health, 71,* 802–809.

Herbert, W. (1982). Sources of temperament: Baseful ar birth? *Science News, 121,* 36.

Herbert, W. (1983). Depression: Too much vigilance? *Science News, 124,* 84.

Hilts, P. (1980). The clock within. *Science, 80,* 61–67.

Holmes, T. H., & Rahe, R. H. (1967). The social readjustment rating scale. *Journal of Psychosomatic Research, 11,* 213–218.

Jacobsen, E. (1938). *Progressive relaxation.* Chicago: University of Chicago Press.

Kabosa, S. C., Hilker, R. R., & Maddi, S. R. (1979). Who stays healthy under stress? *Journal of Occupational Medicine, 21,* 595–598.

Kagan, J. (1984). *The nature of the child.* New York: Basic Books.

Lakein, A. (1973). *How to get control of your time and life.* New York: Signet Books.

Lazarus, R. (1981). Little hassles can be hazardous to your health. *Psychology Today, 15,* 58–62.

Lysaght, R., & Bodenhamer, E. (1990). The use of relaxation training to enhance functional outcomes in adults with traumatic head injuries. *American Journal of Occupational Therapy, 44,* 797–802.

McCann, I. L., & Holmes, D. S. (1984). Influence of aerobic exercise on depression. *Journal of Personality and Social Psychology, 46,* 1142–1147.

McCann, M. (1979). *Artist beware.* New York: Watson-Guptill Publications.

McCormack, G. L. (1988). Pain management in occupational therapy. *American Journal of Occupational Therapy, 42,* 582–590.

McQuade, W., & Aikman, A. (1975). *Stress.* New York: Bantam Books.

Miller, J. A. (1986). Immunity and crises, large and small. *Science News, 129,* 340.

Miller, L. H., Ross, R., & Cohen, S. I. (1982). Stress: What can be done? *Bostonia Magazine, 56,* 3–80.

Neistadt, M. E. (1987). An occupational therapy program for adults with developmental disabilities. *American Journal of Occupational Therapy, 41,* 433–438.

Pelletier, K. (1977). *Mind as healer, mind as slayer.* New York: Delta Press.

Rahe, R. H. (1979). Life change events and mental illness: An overview. *Journal of Human Stress, 5,* 2–9.

Raloff, J. (1981a). Basement parking and high rise CO_2. *Science News, 120,* 316.

Raloff, J. (1981b). Building illness. *Science News, 120,* 316.

Raloff, J. (1982a). Occupational noise—the subtle pollutant. *Science News, 121,* 347–350.

Raloff, J. (1982b). Noise can be hazardous to your health. *Science News, 121,* 377–380.

Reich, P., DeSilva, R. A., Lowin, B., & Murawski, B. J. (1981). Acute psychological disturbances preceding life threatening ventricular arrhythmias. *Journal of the American Medical Association, 246,* 233–235.

Science News (Staff). (1980) Social ties and length of life. *Science News, 118,* 392.

Science News (Staff). (1981). Beware the supplies of arts and crafts. *Science News, 119,* 325.

Selye, H. (1974). *Stress without distress.* New York: Signet Books.

Selye, H. (1978). *The stress of life.* New York: McGraw-Hill.

Shavit, Y., Terman, G. W., Martin, F. C., Lewis, J. W., Liebeskind, J. C., & Gale, R. P. (1985). Stress, opioid peptides, the immune system, and cancer. *Journal of Immunology, 135,* 834s–837s.

Sheehan, D. V., O'Donnell, J., Fitzgerald, A., Hervig, L., & Ward, H. (1981–1982). Psychosocial predictors of accident/error rates in nursing studies: A prospective study. *International Journal of Psychiatry and Medicine, 11,* 125–36.

Smith, D. A., & Lukens, S. A. (1983). Stress effects of isometric contraction in occupational therapy. *Occupational Therapy Journal of Research, 3,* 222–242.

Stein, F., & Nikolic, S. (1989). Teaching stress management techniques to a schizophrenic patient. *American Journal of Occupational Therapy, 43,* 162–169.

Strong, J., Cramond, T., & Maas, F. (1989). The effectiveness of relaxation techniques with patients who have chronic low back pain. *Occupational Therapy Journal of Research, 9,* 184–192.

Trombly, C. A. (1989a). Cardiopulmonary rehabilitation. In C. A. Trombly (Ed.), *Occupational therapy for physical dysfunction* (3rd ed., pp. 581–603). Baltimore: Williams & Wilkins.

Trombly, C. A. (1989b). Biofeedback as an adjunct to therapy. In C. A. Trombly (Ed.), *Occupational Therapy for Physical Dysfunction* (3rd ed., pp. 316–328). Baltimore: Williams & Wilkins.

Union Hospital. (1982). Caffeine and your health. *What's News,* March 4, 2.

Vitaliano, R., Russo, J., Carr, J., Maiuro, R., & Becker, J. (1985). The ways of coping checklist: Revision and psychometric properties. *Multivariate Behavioral Research, 20,* 3–26.

Wall, N., & Neistadt, M. E. (1982). *Stress: A study guide to accompany the slide-tape program "stress."* Boston: AIM for Health.

SECTION 5

Pain management

JOYCE M. ENGEL

KEY TERMS

Acute Pain	*Pain Assessment*
Chronic Pain	*Relaxation Training*
Discrimination Training	*Respondent Behavior*
Gate Control Theory	*Sensory Decision Theory*
Operant Conditioning	*Social Modeling*

LEARNING OBJECTIVES

Upon completion of this section the reader will be able to:

1. *Give two basic definitions of pain.*
2. *Identify two theories of pain.*
3. *Assess the effects of pain.*
4. *Explain a minimum of three approaches for pain intervention.*

Pain and disability are staggering problems in terms of both human suffering and economic loss. At least 15% to 20% of Americans have acute pain and between 25% and 30% have chronic pain. Of the persons with chronic pain, one half to two thirds are either partially or totally disabled for periods of days (eg, from headache), weeks, and months (eg, from reflex sympathetic dystrophy), and some are permanently disabled (eg, from low back pain, cancer pain). Pain costs the American people over $65 billion per year including costs for surgery, loss of income, medication, hospitalization, disability payments, and litigation settlements (Bonica, 1990a). The costs of human suffering are inestimable. The presence of pain may affect a person's performance of physical and emotional daily living skills and may disrupt occupational roles.

Defining pain

The word pain refers to an endless variety of qualities that are categorized under a single linguistic label (Melzack, 1975). Pain has typically been conceptualized as a neurophysiologic event that involves a complex pattern of emotional and psychological arousal, including sensations of noxious stimulation, psychological trauma, and resultant tissue damage, behavioral avoidance, and complaints of subjective distress (Parker & Cinciripini, 1984). The Task Force on Taxonomy of the International Association for the Study of Pain recommended that pain be defined as "an unpleasant sensory and emotional experience associated with actual or potential tissue damage, or described in terms of such damage" (Mersky, 1986, p. S217). This definition conveys the multidimensional and subjective nature of pain (Turk, Meichenbaum, & Genest, 1983, p. 82).

Although definitions of pain are varied, most authors agree that acute and chronic should be differentiated (Fordyce, 1976; McCaffery, 1979). This differentiation is essential for the occupational therapist's use of appropriate assessment and intervention strategies (Katz, Varni & Jay, 1984). *Acute pain* and its associated physiologic, psychological, and behavioral responses are almost invariably caused by tissue damage or irritating stimulation in relation to bodily insult or disease (Katz et al., 1984). The duration of acute pain is usually limited in time to 6 months or less (Sternbach, 1974). Acute pain serves a biologic or adaptive purpose by directing attention to injury, irritation, or disease and signaling the necessity for immobilization and protection of an injured area such as a laceration (Katz et al., 1984).

Chronic pain may begin as acute pain or may be more insidious and exist without a known time limit (beyond the time for normal healing). It may vary in its duration (continuous or intermittent) and intensity (mild to severe). Chronic nonmalignant pain does not appear to serve a biologic purpose and is often experienced in the presence of minimal or no apparent tissue damage as in low back pain (Johnson, 1977).

Psychopathology or environmental factors may have a profound influence on chronic pain (Bonica, 1990a). Chronic recurrent pain is characterized by intense episodes of pain interspersed with pain-free periods as in migraine headaches (Turk et al., 1983).

The literature may provide characterizations of pain, but certainly not a clear definition of what pain is. Classifications of a variety of pain syndromes have been outlined by the International Association for the Study of Pain (Mersky, 1986).

Pain syndromes

The most frequently treated types of recurrent painful conditions seen by occupational therapists based on 1986 estimates are described in the following text.

Headache pain

Bonica (1990b) estimated that 29 million Americans experience severe disabling headache and spend $4 billion annually to relieve it. Headaches account for an additional $12 billion a year in indirect costs such as missed workdays, compensation, litigation, and quackery.

Migraine headaches are characterized by recurrent attacks varying in frequency, intensity, and duration. These attacks are typically unilateral and may be accompanied by anorexia, nausea, and vomiting and preceded by neurologic symptoms (photosensitivity) and mood disturbances (irritability). A strong genetic predisposition has been suggested in the origin of migraine, and females are more frequently affected than males (Speer, 1977).

Tension headaches are described as a steady, nonthrobbing ache, and may be characterized as tightness of the forehead, temples, or the back of the head, a "bandlike" sensation about the head that may progress to a caplike distribution, and muscular cramping of the neck and upper back areas. Tension headaches may be fleeting and are often characterized by frequent changes in site and intensity (Diamond & Dalessio, 1982).

Low back pain

About 21 million Americans experience low back pain (Bonica, 1990b). About 3.7 million of these are partially or totally disabled. The total annual cost (health care plus indirect costs) attributable to low back pain is about $20 billion.

The most common causes of low back pain are injury or stress, resulting in musculoskeletal and neurologic disorders (eg, muscle spasm, sciatica). Pain may also result from infections, degenerative diseases, and malignancies (Bonica, 1990b).

Arthritis pain

Bonica (1990b) estimated that 24 million Americans have painful arthritis and 11.5 million are at least partially disabled. The total annual cost attributable to arthritis is about $17 billion.

Rheumatoid arthritis is characterized by inflammation, a dull ache, and structural changes in the affected joints (Spencer, 1988). These symptoms may occur in young to older persons.

Osteoarthritis is characterized by a progressive dull ache and swelling typically affecting the fingers, elbows, ankles, knees, and hips, and may be exacerbated by movement (Spencer, 1988). It occurs when there has been strain on the joint or accompanies the aging process.

Cancer pain

Cancer pain, especially bone and cervix, affects about 1.1 million Americans annually (Bonica, 1990b). The pain may result from the tumor, the debilitating effects of the disease, or the medical procedures (eg, bone marrow aspirations).

Myofascial pain

Myofascial pain syndrome refers to a large group of muscle disorders characterized by highly sensitive trigger points within muscles or connective tissue (Sola & Bonica, 1990). This common complaint is perceived as a continual dull ache often located in the head, neck, shoulder, and lower back regions. Myofascial pain may result from sustained muscle contraction, trauma, or weakness.

In most people with the above-described complaints, usually the pain not the underlying pathology prevents them from achieving a productive and satisfying life (Bonica, 1990b).

Theories of pain

Gate control theory

Ideally theories of pain transmission should explain the range of pain phenomena (Weisenberg, 1977). To date, no single pain theory adequately accounts for the realm of pain experiences. Melzack and Wall (1965) offered a variation of the specificity (pain resulting from direct stimulation of specific pain receptors in the periphery) and pattern (nerve impulse patterns coded at the periphery) theories to explain pain transmission, which is called the *gate control theory*. They suggested that skin receptors have specific physiologic properties by which they may transmit particular types and ranges of stimuli in the form of impulse patterns. According to this theory, pain is modulated by a "gating" mechanism located in the spinal cord that can increase or decrease the flow of nerve impulses to the brain (Bockrath, 1985; Engel, 1988a).

Specifically, afferent (sensory) impulses can travel to the dorsal horn along large (A fiber) and small diameter (A-delta or C fiber) nerves associated with pain impulses. At the dorsal horn, these impulses encounter a gate thought to be substantia gelatinosa cells. This gate, which may be presynaptic or postsynaptic, may be closed, partially open, or open. When the gate is closed, pain impulses cannot proceed. If the gate is at least partially open, pain impulses stimulate T (transmission or trigger) cells in the dorsal horn, which then ascend the spinal cord to the brain resulting in pain perception. After the pain impulses are perceived, higher central nervous system structures (brain stem, thalamus, cerebral cortex) can modify pain by influencing T-cell activity. These structures can alter such factors as attention span, memory, and affect, thereby contributing to the determination of a person's unique pain perception (Bockrath, 1985; Schechter, 1985).

Although certain aspects of the gate control theory remain controversial (eg, physiologic and anatomic bases of the gate), this theory has been critical in furthering multidimensional pain assessment and research. The gate control theory of pain suggests that psychology has much to offer in both understanding and treating pain. Motivational and cognitive processes are examined in terms of their contribution to the pain experience (Turk & Genest, 1979).

Sensory decision theory

Sensory decision theory also places pain within the realm of psychology (Chapman, 1978). Pain is viewed as a perceptual process with an imperfect relationship to sensory input. Chapman hypothesized that before a stimulus gives rise to a response, the observer must process the input through the attentional filter and central organization mechanisms before making a decision about what response will be given. Sensory input, beliefs, expectations, memory of previous events, and potential costs and rewards all have impact on a person's pain experience.

Respondent and operant theory

To further differentiate types of pain, Fordyce (1976) proposed that pain be examined as respondent or operant behavior. Pain behavior can be classified as *respondent behavior* if its onset and incidence were due to antecedent tissue damage. This acute trauma leads to an unconditioned stimulus such as tissue irritation or damage, which automatically produces an unconditioned response such as overactivation of the sympathetic nervous system (Bonica, 1977). Through repeated pairing of the unconditioned stimulus and external stimuli (place or thing), the external stimuli alone may come to elicit the response. This conditioned stimulus can evoke a *conditioned pain response* (Linton, Melin & Götestam, 1984).

Since pain is a private experience, there is no way to know when someone else perceives an aversive stimulus. Conditioning arguments must therefore be stated as hypothetical contingencies that could operate if the person were experiencing pain. When pain exists, analgesics, avoidances of specific activities, and attainment of specific body postures may result in a reduction of pain perception. As such contingencies operate, the occasion is set for negative reinforcement since the pain has become discriminative. A particular person, place, or comment can function as a discriminative stimulus. The consequence may be positive reinforcement by attention or solicitation (eg, administering medication, taking over chores). Stimulus generalization may occur when the person talks about pain at inappropriate times. In addition, sedentary activities may be positively reinforced by the enjoyment received. An inherent reinforcer in sedentary activities is the lowering of pain intensity and avoidance of pain-provoking activities (Fordyce, 1976; Linton et al., 1984).

Social modeling theory

Social modeling, or learning through observation of the behavior of others, is another proposed theory of pain transmission. *Modeling* refers to the concept that a person can anticipate and learn from the consequences of behavior without having to personally experience them (Bandura, 1977). Bandura hypothesized that most learning occurs through modeling. In persons with chronic pain the probability is relatively high that other members of the family have also suffered from chronic pain (Stone & Barbera, 1970; Violon & Giurgea, 1984). The relationship between pain behaviors and possible modeling influences or a genetic predisposition toward painful conditions (migraine headaches) is not clear and needs to be further researched.

These theories about pain transmission illustrate the complexity of the phenomenon of pain and its multiple dimensions. Such theories are important to the occupational therapist because they speculate about the causes of pain and direct the clinician toward effective means of relief. As more is learned about pain and pain transmission, it appears that multidimensional assessment and treatment are necessary to achieve adequate pain control.

Pain assessment

Whatever intervention methods (pharmacologic or psychological) are used, effective management of pain depends on accurate and multifaceted *pain assessment*. Proper assessment requires the use of valid and reliable instruments for determining pain effects before and after treatment. Several methods for pain assessment have been used to measure clinical pain. Each of these general types of assessment are discussed separately in the text that follows.

Behavioral

Behavioral assessment may be used to identify behaviors in need of change and to identify environmental or organismic variables that control the occurrence of specific pain behaviors (Fordyce, 1976; Keefe, 1982). Behavioral psychologists have broadened their view of behavior to include not only overt but covert and physiologic responses (Sanders, 1979). Assessment techniques therefore typically focus on these three major categories of pain behavior, which may be incorporated into occupational therapy evaluation.

Overt

Overt motor behavior or observable pain responses (pain medication use, limpness) are commonly targeted for assessment as are well behaviors. Persons experiencing pain may rub the pain site, grimace, and demonstrate atypical body posturing. A behavioral interview of the client and a person who is close to the client (partner, family member, employer) is often used to assess these

behavior patterns (Fordyce, 1976; Keefe, 1982; Turk et al., 1983). This interview, as well as daily activity diaries, can aid in the analysis of both situational specificity and temporal consistency of behavior (Keefe, 1982; Potts & Baptiste, 1989). Clients may be poor or biased self-observers, however. Indirect assessment of pain may then be pursued; this includes physical parameters (range of motion), job absenteeism, a decreased activity level including rest, and number of physician visits/hospitalizations. These measures combined with behavioral observations of the client's performance of physical daily living skills, work activities, and play may provide a more accurate and complete appraisal of the person's functional status (Caruso & Chan, 1986; Flower, Naxon, Jones & Mooney, 1981; McCormack & Johnson, 1990).

Covert

Self-reports of pain responses, as illustrated in the display, have also been investigated since pain is considered by many to be a primarily subjective phenomenon (Keefe, 1982). Graphic rating or visual analogue scales (VAS) have been used to measure the client's perceived pain intensity. This pain scale is a line that represents a continuum with the ends marked for the two extremes of a pain experience such as "no pain" and "worst pain imaginable." The person is asked to rate pain intensity on the line. On a similar rating scale, the client is asked to indicate pain intensity on a scale of 1 to 10 or 1 to 100 with the highest number

---

SAMPLE DAILY PAIN DIARY TO BE COMPLETED BY CLIENT BEFORE AND AFTER TREATMENT

A. Date and day of week: _____

B. Location of pain: _____

C. Time pain began and ended: _____

D. How severe did the pain get? (Circle one number):
   1 = mild pain
   2 = discomforting
   3 = moderate pain
   4 = horrible pain
   5 = excruciating pain

E. Where were you? _____

F. What were you doing? _____

G. Who was with you? _____

H. What were you feeling and thinking prior to and during the severe pain?
   _____
   _____
   _____
   _____

I. What was your *usual* pain intensity? (5, highest; 1, lowest)
   (Circle here: 1, 2, 3, 4, 5)

J. How did you try to reduce pain?
   (Example: Took 2 aspirin, rested 1 hour, used icepack)
   _____
   _____

K. How effective was this? (Circle one number):
   0 = did not help at all
   1 = helped very little
   2 = helped somewhat
   3 = helped a lot
   4 = stopped the pain

equal to "the most excruciating pain possible" and 1 equal to "the least amount of pain detectable." The person then assigns a numerical value to the perceived pain.

Rating scales are easy to use but have major problems. These scales typically attempt to measure only one component (pain intensity) of a multidimensional phenomenon (including pain frequency and duration). In addition, rating scales are prone to response biases. Finally, the distances between responses on VAS are unknown, but are typically treated statistically as if they were equal (Lodge & Tursky, 1981).

Pain questionnaires were developed to address dimensions other than intensity of the pain experience. For example, the McGill Pain Questionnaire (MPQ) provides a subjective report of the sensory (eg, pressure), affective (eg, fear), and evaluative (eg, overall intensity) components of the pain experience (Melzack, 1975). Vocabulary or language limitations of the client, however, may limit the usefulness of this instrument.

Finally, pain assessment is further complicated in that the private nature of pain has demanded the use of self-report measures. Verbal report of a private stimulus, however, may be influenced by earlier conditioning (Skinner, 1974), distortion according to the client's motives, attitudes, and self-interests such as escape from demands (Kazdin, 1980; Strong et al., 1990), and is dependent on the client's cooperation and effective language skills.

Physiologic

Physiologic pain responses are the third major category used in the behavioral assessment of pain. Hyperactivity of the sympathetic nervous system is considered one of the major psychophysiologic mechanisms of chronic pain (Bonica, 1977). Changes in these physiologic indicators may also be seen with other subjective phenomenona (anxiety), making it difficult to detect a pattern of responses unique to pain (Stewart, 1977).

In addition, Sternbach (1974) and McCaffery (1979) have suggested that a process of adaptation of physiologic pain responses exists, which results in the physiologic parameters returning to near normal. Another major problem in using physiologic responses as measures of pain is that overt, covert, and physiologic responses typically do not correlate highly and research has not yet determined which is the most valid measure (Katz et al., 1984).

Cultural and familial

Cultural and familial influences are other important factors to be considered by the occupational therapist in pain assessment and treatment, especially when the pain etiology is not clear (MacRae & Riley, 1990; Parker & Cinciripini, 1984). Each culture has a unique system of transmitting values and attitudes to its members. As a person becomes acculturated, he or she learns what the culture expects and accepts as appropriate behavior (Baptiste, 1988; Niemeyer, 1990). With the process of acculturation the child may be rewarded, ignored, or punished for emitting pain behaviors. By adulthood, these responses and consequences may be well ingrained (Weisenberg, 1977).

Recommendations

The assessment of pain remains a complex problem. The clinician is cautioned against oversimplification during evaluation. Physical, psychological, cognitive, social, and motivational aspects of pain require repeated assessment in varied settings and with regard to the client's age (Engel, 1988b). Continued assessment of the interacting cluster of overt, covert, and physiologic responses appears warranted. Independent and unannounced periodic observations of overt pain behaviors by a trained person could function as a reliability check for indirect measures of pain occurrence (pill counts, bed rest) compared with the client's pain diary and activity diary recordings. In addition, the use of automated devices (eg, mercury switch-activated timers measuring time spent standing) and archival data (eg, job absenteeism) may also be compared with the client's reports to assess the reliability of record keeping, to indicate other possible treatment benefits, and to check compliance with treatment recommendations.

Management of pain

The choice of treatment for pain control depends on objective findings (eg, abnormal myelogram), pain occurrence (incidence, duration, intensity), the client's overt, covert, and physiologic pain responses, and the clinician's training. A variety of pain control options are available. Each of the general methods are discussed separately.

Pharmacologic

Medication management is typically the initial treatment of choice. Antipyretic analgesics (aspirin and acetaminophen) are frequently used in the treatment of mild intensity pain due to their high level of effectiveness, low level of toxicity, and limited abuse potential (Schechter, 1985).

Nonsteroidal antiinflammatory agents (ibuprofen) have been primarily used in the treatment of osteoarthritis, rheumatoid arthritis, and inflammation of musculoskeletal origin. Stomach upset and ulcers may result from their use (Schechter, 1985).

Codeine is the drug of choice for pain of moderate intensity that cannot be relieved by antipyretic analgesics. Side effects of codeine include drowsiness, lethargy, constipation, respiratory depression, and some risk of addiction (Schechter, 1985).

Morphine is the standard with which the analgesic properties of all opioid drugs are compared and remains unsurpassed in the relief of severe pain. An additional benefit of morphine appears to be its mood-altering effect (euphoria), which allows the person to perceive a sensation that it is no longer identified as pain. Side effects of morphine are drowsiness, nausea and vomiting, and respiratory depression (Schechter, 1985).

Schechter (1985) recommended that medication for acute pain be prescribed in anticipation of pain and for prevention of its recurrence. When pain medication is administered regularly and prophylactically in a time-contingent manner, the client need never experience pain, thereby preventing chronic pain and the need for higher doses of narcotics than necessary to relieve existing pain. Mood-altering drugs have also been found to be helpful in the treatment of adult chronic pain. These drugs may help to reduce pain by alleviating anxiety, potentiating narcotic analgesia, and affording their own analgesic effect. Antidepressants have proved effective in alleviating reactive depression and pain complaints, including their associated sleep disturbances and fatigue. The major and minor tranquilizers have been used to control anxiety, a precipitating pain factor (Tollison, 1982; Ward, 1990).

Surgical

Chronic, intractable pain has been viewed not as a symptom, but as a functional disease of the central nervous system. Surgical procedures for pain relief have developed over the past 80 years. For years, traditional neurosurgical procedures focused on transecting a peripheral nerve, nerve root, or central tract. Time and experience have proved that this approach rarely achieves long-term pain relief, however, and may result in increased pain or new pain complaints (Howell, Luna & Miakowski, 1985). Present neurosurgical pain-relieving procedures focus on interrupting pain pathways at three major levels: the peripheral level (first-order neurons), the spinal level (second-order neurons), and the brain level (third-order neurons; Howell et al., 1985).

First-order neurons transmit pain impulses from the receptor, along the peripheral nerve, and into the dorsal horn. Procedures such as a nerve block (injection of a local anesthetic into or around a peripheral nerve), neurectomy (excision of a peripheral nerve), sympathectomy (surgical interruption of the sympathetic nerve pathways), and rhizotomy (surgical division of the nerve root as it enters the spinal cord) interrupt pain pathways at the level of the first-order neurons. First-order neurons synapse with second-order neurons within the dorsal horn.

Second-order neurons send axons to the opposite side of the spinal cord. Pain impulses therefore ascend to the thalamus along the lateral spinothalamic tract on the other side. A cordotomy interrupts the lateral spinothalamic tract at the level of the second-order neurons. Second-order neurons synapse with *third-order neurons* in the thalamus. These sensory neurons transmit pain impulses to the cerebral cortex where pain perception occurs.

Stimulating electrodes in the thalamus may interrupt pain pathways at the level of the third-order neurons for adults with intractable pain (Howell et al., 1985). About 60% to 80% of adult clients experience some relief following these procedures, but pain returns in 30% to 50% of clients within 3 months (Schechter, 1985).

Behavioral strategies

Behavioral methods for chronic pain management have appealed to the health care community for numerous reasons. Behavioral methods can help identify the problems of clients with chronic pain in a precise and objective manner, especially with regard to the socioenvironmental factors that may control pain behaviors. In addition, increasing dissatisfaction with the results of medically based treatments and the recognition of complex interactions of pharmacologic, physiologic, and psychological factors in the perception and elaboration of pain have prompted the growing interest in behavioral strategies for pain control (Keefe, 1982).

Operant conditioning (acquisition or elimination of a response as a function of environmental contingencies of reward and punishment) is indicated as a treatment for persons with chronic nonmalignant pain who are (1) receiving excessive pain-related medications; (2) not participating in routine physical activities of daily living (deactivation); (3) engaging in too much postural guarding; (4) demonstrating inappropriate pacing for task completion; (5) displaying excessive concern about the pain complaint; and (6) engaging in excessive health care use (Fordyce, 1990). A coordinated, goal-directed, interdisciplinary team (physician, clinical psychologist or psychiatrist, occupational therapist, physical therapist, vocational specialist) services may be offered on an inpatient or outpatient basis with the scope and intensity of medical, psychosocial, and vocational services matched to the client's needs (Commission on Accreditation of Rehabilitation Facilities, 1992). Examples of operant techniques for the elimination or reduction of pain behaviors are provided in the following text.

Medication intake

To encourage discontinuation of analgesics, muscle relaxants, and tranquilizers, their use is shifted from a pain-contingent to a time-contingent basis. Fordyce (1976) recommended that following baseline, the medications be delivered in a color- and taste-masking liquid medium ("pain cocktail") at fixed time intervals, with the systematic reduction of the proportion of active ingredients over time. By providing adequate medicinal coverage on a time-contingent basis, the learned behavioral chain between overt pain expressions and medication intake is abolished (Grzesiak, 1982). Linking detoxification to a reactivation program (physical retraining, social support) facilitates this process (Fordyce, 1990).

Physical activity

Increasing the client's activity level is the cornerstone of most chronic pain management treatment programs and is a major area of occupational therapy intervention. Intervention involves positively reinforcing (praising) the client's attempts at physical activity or exercise. Activity increases are done on a gradual basis with the client working to "tolerance" (gradual increase in task completion) as opposed to "pain" before a scheduled rest period. Resting at the time of the pain onset/elevation is avoided because it may reinforce pain behaviors (Fordyce, 1976; Grzesiak, 1982). Group or individual progressive mobility, strengthening, and endurance exercises/activities are routinely scheduled daily to assist the client in achieving maximal functional status. Modalities (heat or cold) may be applied to prepare the client for exercise. Specific guidelines for reactivation have been outlined by Fordyce (1990). Proper use of posture, body mechanics, energy conservation, and joint protection techniques are emphasized as means of pain reduction (Caruso & Chan, 1986; Giles & Allen, 1986). Adaptive equipment and splinting may be prescribed to enhance independent performance of activities of daily living (Tyson & Strong, 1990).

Communication of pain

Discrimination training is directed at enhancing stimulus control so that the client discusses pain with appropriate people (such as health care professionals) at appropriate times and places. People interacting with the person experiencing chronic pain are instructed to avoid giving attention and sympathy for both verbal and nonverbal expressions of pain and to praise the client's achievements and efforts to cope with pain. Social skills training may also be used by the occupational therapist, during which the client is taught and reinforced for using behaviors in social contacts not revolving around the pain experience. Involvement of the partner or a significant other in stress or anger management, resolution of sexual dysfunction, and goal-setting skills may make up part of the total treatment package (Fordyce, 1990).

Relaxation and self-instruction about feelings and images

Relaxation training

Self-regulation of pain perception teaches the person with pain to respond to possible antecedents (eg, muscle tension) and the pain occurrence. This approach emphasizes the occupational therapist instructing the client in specific methods for altering pain perception. **Relaxation training** may involve teaching the client to systematically contract and relax the major skeletal muscle groups (progressive muscle relaxation), the silent repetition of phrases about the ideal physiologic state of the body (autogenic training), or the purposeful use of images to achieve a desired goal (guided imagery). The potential benefits of these approaches are reduction of acute anxiety, distraction from pain, alleviation of skeletal muscle tension, reduction of fatigue, improved sleep, enhancement of other pain-relief measures, and a sense of control over pain (McCaffery, 1979; Turner & Romano, 1990). Evidence suggests that *relaxation rehearsal* may be helpful in the reduction of the person's perceived pain frequency, intensity, or duration (Engel & Rapoff, 1990a; Strong et al., 1989).

Biofeedback

Relaxation training may include the use of biofeedback to facilitate the client's learning voluntary control of musculoskeletal and vascular responses that may precipitate a pain episode. Biofeedback has been used effectively for a wide variety of pain complaints, most notably headache, low back, neck, and shoulder pain, and temporomandibular joint syndrome (Blanchard & Ahles, 1990; Engel & Rapoff, 1990b).

Cognitive restructuring

Cognitive restructuring includes educational and training components. Clients are educated about the role of cognitions and emotions in pain and the interrelationships among pain, stress, and tension. Clients are taught that emotional reactions to and behaviors after an event depend to a large extent on a person's thoughts. Together, the clinician and the client examine whether negative thoughts are realistic. Distorted negative thoughts are then replaced with more realistic positive ones. Studies are needed to support the efficacy of this approach (Turner & Romano, 1990).

Distraction

Increased pain awareness may result from a lack of distracting activities. It is therefore advantageous for persons experiencing pain to learn how to distract themselves more effectively when exposed to noxious stimuli (painful medical procedures such as injections) and low environmental stimulation, and during periods of minimal activity. Clients cannot attend as much to pain when they are concentrating on something else. Cognitive distraction techniques therefore involve the person actively redirecting attention to something other than pain (doing a puzzle, counting the number of ceiling tiles) or focusing inward (eg, imagining a pleasant scene or reminiscing), but not directly on the pain. Involvement in purposeful activity has been demonstrated to improve pain tolerance (maximal level of noxious stimulation that a person is willing to tolerate; Heck, 1988; McCormack, 1988). A balance of work, recreation, and social activities is of value in distracting attention away from pain (Hanson & Gerber, 1990; Heck, 1988).

Social support

The importance of social support in facilitating behavior change cannot be underestimated. Support groups may assist the person suffering from pain by helping them realize that others have endured similar circumstances, may provide a neutral place to express feelings, and may provide opportunities for learning coping strategies. Support groups can ease the transition from terminating treatment to self-management.

Cutaneous stimulation

Transcutaneous electrical nerve stimulation

Transcutaneous electrical nerve stimulation (TENS) is a noninvasive pain relief measure consisting of cutaneous (skin) stimulation. A TENS unit consists of a battery-powered generator that sends a mild electrical current through electrodes placed on the skin at or near the pain site, stimulating A fibers. TENS use has had some success in relieving acute and chronic painful conditions caused by pathology in nerve structures, the skeleton, muscles, pain of ischemic origin in the extremities, and angina pectoris. Typically, paresthesia is evoked in the painful area by electrical stimulation via surface electrodes of large cutaneous afferent nerve fibers at 30 to 100 Hz. TENS use is contraindicated in clients with pacemakers. In addition, the unit should not be placed on the anterior aspect of the neck to avoid stimulation of the carotid nerves and possible hypotension. Skin irritation is another possible side effect and, in rare instances, an aggravation of the pain complaint. Individual adjustment of the technique and client demonstration of appropriate TENS use are critical. Reevaluation of client status after 3 months is recommended (Sjölund, Eriksson & Loeser, 1990).

Massage

Massage regulates muscle through reflex and mechanical actions. Stimulation of peripheral receptors in the skin is produced by repetitive rhythmic movements of the therapist's hands (stroking, kneading, rubbing) or devices in a centripetal direction. This stimulation induces muscle relaxation and arteriole dilation or constriction, increases local blood circulation, improves muscle flexibility, loosens scar tissue, and increases emotional well-being. Massage may be used in preparation for exercise and to improve performance. Conditions that may respond to massage are arthritis, sprain, strain, muscle spasm, bursitis, and contusion. It is contraindicated in the presence of an acute inflammatory process, thrombophlebitis, lymphangitis, acute burn, dermatitis, malignancy, advanced arteriosclerosis, nephritis, and severe debilitation (Lee, Itoh, Yang & Eason, 1990).

Thermotherapy

Heat from hydrocollator packs penetrates the skin superficially. The 71°C to 79°C pack is applied to the pain site over layers of terry cloth for 20 to 30 minutes. Heat may also be applied with a hot water bottle, an electric heating pad, or a chemical pack. These devices may be useful in reducing muscle spasm, spasticity, bursitis, and tendinitis. Edema, swelling, and tissue damage may be aggravated by heat. Because packs may be heavy and bulky, they may not be suitable for tender regions. Heating pads should not be used by persons with impaired sensation.

Paraffin therapy produces increased skin tissue temperature while decreasing the temperature of subcutaneous tissue. Paraffin may be helpful in relieving arthritis of the small joints of the hands and feet. It is contraindicated where there is a skin opening, rash, infection, or dermatitis (Lee et al., 1990).

Cryotherapy

In addition to heat, cold can also improve pain control by elevating the pain threshold (the minimal level of noxious stimulation at which the person first reports pain). Like heat, cold can reduce muscle spasm secondary to joint or skeletal pathology and spasticity. Edema, swelling, and tissue damage may be decreased by cold. Joint stiffness, however, may be aggravated. Cold can be applied via packs, sprays, or a stick for massage. Contraindications to cryotherapy include vascular insufficiency, an anesthetic area, Raynaud's phenomenon, and intolerance to cold (Lee et al., 1990).

A variety of other physical agents (ultrasound, diathermy, whirlpool therapy) that have the benefits of heat or cold are available. Evaluation by a physical therapist would help to determine whether the client is an appropriate candidate for such approaches. The occupational therapy practitioner is cautioned to comply with federal and state laws and American Occupational Therapy Association statements when using physical agent modalities.

Vibration

Vibration may mask the discomfort of low-intensity shock and reduce the perceived pain intensity. Electric and battery-operated vibrators of varying shapes and sizes may be used with or without heat, cold, or medication (McCormack, 1988). Good relief from this approach has been reported for chronic postherpetic neuralgia (Crue, Todd, & Maline, 1975) and phantom limb pain (Russell cited in McCaffery, 1979). Anecdotal reports of low back pain relief have also been noted (McCaffery, 1979).

Conclusion

Occupational therapists have a core role in providing therapeutic activities that enable the client with pain to develop the skills and tolerances necessary for the attainment of self-care, vocational, and leisure goals. Due to the complex nature of pain, a "cure" is not readily available. Treatment efforts therefore cannot simply emphasize the reduction of the pain experience.

Ideally, interventions need to focus on improving functional levels and coping strategies, while being sensitive to the client's belief and value systems. Additional data to support the effectiveness of the above-described treatment approaches and their durability are needed. Finally, future research must also address the social significance of treatment goals and the social appropriateness of treatment procedures.

References

Bandura, A. (1977). *Social learning theory.* Englewood Cliffs, NJ: Prentice-Hall.

Baptiste, S. (1988). Chronic pain, activity and culture. *Canadian Journal of Occupational Therapy, 55* (4), 179–184.

Blanchard, E. B., & Ahles, T. A. (1990). Biofeedback therapy. In J. J. Bonica (Ed.), *The management of pain* (2nd ed., pp. 1722–1732). Philadelphia: Lea & Febiger.

Bockrath, M. (1985). Fundamentals. In K. W. Carey et al. (Eds.), *Pain* (pp. 6–24). Springhouse, PA: Springhouse Corporation.

Bonica, J. J. (1977). Neurophysiological and pathologic aspects of acute and chronic pain. *Archives of Surgery, 112,* 750–761.

Bonica, J. J. (1990a). History of pain concepts and therapies. In J. J. Bonica (Ed.), *The management of pain* (2nd ed., pp. 2–17). Philadelphia: Lea & Febiger.

Bonica, J. J. (1990b). General considerations of chronic pain. In J. J. Bonica (Ed.), *The management of pain* (2nd ed., pp. 180–196). Philadelphia: Lea & Febiger.

Caruso, L. A., & Chan, D. E. (1986). Evaluation and management of the patient with acute back pain. *American Journal of Occupational Therapy, 46*(5), 347–351.

Chapman, C. R. (1978). Pain: The perception of noxious events. In R. A. Sternbach (Ed.), *The psychology of pain* (pp. 189–190). New York: Raven Press.

Commission on Accreditation of Rehabilitation Facilities. (1992). *Standards manual for organizations serving people with disabilities.* Tucson, AZ: Author.

Crue, B. L., Jr., Todd, E. M., & Maline, D. B. (1975). Postherpetic neuralgia—conservative treatment regimen. In B. L. Crue, Jr. (Ed.), *Pain: Research and treatment* (pp. 289–292). New York: Academic Press.

Diamond, S., & Dalessio, D. (1982). *The practicing physician's approach to headache* (3rd ed.). Baltimore: Williams & Wilkins.

Engel, J. M. (1988a). Pain treatment. In J. Havranek (Ed.), *Physical capacity assessment and work hardening therapy: procedures amd applications* (pp. 9–19). Athens, GA: Elliot & Fitzpatrick.

Engel, J. M. (1988b). Pediatric pain [Monograph]. *Vanguard Series in Rehabilitation, 1*(1), 1–44.

Engel, J. M., & Rapoff, M. A. (1990a). A component analysis of relaxation training for children with vascular, muscle contraction, and mixed-headache disorders. In D. C. Tyler & E. J. Krane (Eds.), *Advances in pain research therapy* (Vol. 15, pp. 273–290). New York: Raven Press.

Engel, J. M., & Rapoff, M. A. (1990b). Biofeedback-assisted relaxation training for adult and pediatric headache disorders. *Occupational Therapy Journal of Research, 10*(5), 283–299.

Flower, A., Naxon, E., Jones, R. E., & Mooney, V. (1981). An occupational therapy program for chronic back pain. *American Journal of Occupational Therapy, 35*(4), 243–248.

Fordyce, W. E. (1976). *Behavioral methods for chronic pain and illness.* St. Louis: C. V. Mosby.

Fordyce, W. E. (1990). Contingency management. In J. J. Bonica (Ed.), *The management of pain* (2nd ed., pp. 1702–1710). Philadelphia: Lea & Febiger.

Giles, G. M., & Allen, M. E. (1986). Occupational therapy in the treatment of the patient with chronic pain. *British Journal of Occupational Therapy, 49,* 4–9.

Grzesiak, R. C. (1982). Cognitive and behavioral approaches to management of chronic pain. *New York State Journal of Medicine, 82*(1), 30–38.

Hanson, R. W., & Gerber, K. E. (1990). *Coping with chronic pain: A guide to patient self-management.* New York: Guilford Press.

Heck, S. A. (1988). The effect of purposeful activity on pain tolerance. *American Journal of Occupational Therapy, 42*(9), 577–581.

Howell, J. S., Luna, M. L., & Miakowski, C. A. (1985). Nonpharmacological therapies. In K. W. Carey et al. (Eds.), *Pain* (pp. 38–72). Springhouse, PA: Springhouse Corporation.

Johnson, M. (1977). Assessment of clinical pain. In A. K. Jacox (Ed.), *Pain: A source book for nurses and other health professionals* (pp. 139–166). Boston: Little, Brown & Company.

Katz, E. R., Varni, J. W., & Jay, S. M. (1984). Behavioral assessment and management of pediatric pain. In M. Hersen, R. M. Eisler & P. M. Miller (Eds.), *Progress in behavior modification* (Vol. 18, pp. 163–193). New York: Academic Press.

Kazdin, A. E. (1980). *Research design in clinical psychology.* New York: Harper & Row.

Keefe, F. J. (1982). Behavioral assessment and treatment of chronic pain: Current status and future directions. *Journal of Consulting and Clinical Psychology, 50*(6), 896–911.

Lee, M. H. M., Itoh, M., Yang, G. W., & Eason, A. L. (1990). Physical therapy and rehabilitation medicine. In J. J. Bonica (Ed.), *The management of pain* (2nd ed., pp. 1769–1788). Philadelphia: Lea & Febiger.

Linton, S. J., Melin, L., & Götestam, K. G. (1984). Behavioral analysis of chronic pain and its management. *Progress in behavior modification, 18,* 1–42.

Lodge, M., & Tursky, B. (1981). The workshop on the magnitude scaling of political opinion in survey research. *American Journal of Political Science, 25,* 376–419.

MacRae, A., & Riley, E. (1990). Home health occupational therapy for the management of pain: An environmental model. *Occupational Therapy Practice, 1*(3), 69–76.

McCaffery, M. (1979). *Nursing management of the patient with pain.* Philadelphia: J. B. Lippincott.

McCormack, G. L. (1988). Pain management by occupational therapists. *American Journal of Occupational Therapy, 42*(9), 582–590.

McCormack, G. L., & Johnson, C. (1990). Systems for objectifying clinical pain. *Occupational Therapy Practice, 1*(3), 21–29.

Melzack, R. (1975). The McGill Questionnaire: Major properties and scoring methods. *Pain, 1,* 277–299.

Melzack, R., & Wall, P. (1965). Pain mechanisms: A new theory. *Science, 50,* 971–979.

Mersky, H. (1986). Classification of chronic pain: Description of chronic pain syndromes and definitions of pain terms. *Pain* (Suppl. 3), S217.

Niemeyer, L. O. (1990). Psychologic and sociocultural aspects of responses to pain. *Occupational Therapy Practice, 1*(3), 11–20.

Parker, L. H., & Cinciripini, P. M. (1984). Behavioral medicine with children: Applications in chronic disease. *Progress in Behavior Modification, 17,* 136–165.

Potts, H., & Baptiste, S. (1989). An occupational therapy medico-legal programme for chronic pain patients. *Canadian Journal of Occupational Therapy, 56*(4), 193–197.

Sanders, S. H. (1979). Behavioral assessment and treatment of clinical pain: Appraisal of current status. In M. Hersen, R. M. Eisler & P. M. Miller (Eds.), *Progress in behavior modification* (pp. 249–291). New York: Academic Press.

Schechter, N. L. (1985). Pain and pain control in children. *Current Problems in Pediatrics, 15*(5), 3–67.

Sjölund, B. H., Eriksson, M., & Loeser, J. D. (1990). Transcutaneous and implanted electrical stimulation of peripheral nerves. In J. J. Bonica (Ed.), *The management of pain* (2nd ed., pp. 1852–1861). Philadelphia: Lea & Febiger.

Skinner, B. F. (1974). *About behaviorism.* New York: Alfred Knopf.

Sola, A. E., & Bonica, J. J. (1990). Myofascial pain syndromes. In J. J. Bonica (Ed.), *The management of pain* (2nd ed., pp. 352–357). Philadelphia: Lea & Febiger.

Speer, F. A. (1977). *Migraine.* Chicago: Nelson-Hall.

Spencer, E. A. (1988). Functional restoration: Neurologic, orthopedic, and arthritic conditions. In H. L. Hopkins & H. D. Smith (Eds.), *Willard and Spackman's Occupational therapy* (7th ed., pp. 461–515). Philadelphia: J. B. Lippincott.

Sternbach, R. A. (1974). *Pain patients: Traits and treatment.* New York: Academic Press.

Stewart, M. (1977). Measurement of clinical pain. In A. K. Jacox (Ed.), *Pain: A source book for nurses and other health professionals* (pp. 107–137). Boston: Little, Brown, & Company.

Stone, R., & Barbera, G. (1970). Recurrent abdominal pain in childhood. *Pediatrics, 45,* 732–738.

Strong, J., Ashton, R., Cramond, & Chant, D. (1990). Pain intensity, attitude and function in back pain patients. *Australian Occupational Therapy Journal, 34*(4), 179–183.

Strong, J., Cramond, T., & Maas, F. (1989). The effectiveness of relaxation techniques with patients who have chronic low back pain. *Occupational Therapy Journal of Research, 9*(3), 184–192.

Tollison, C. D. (1982). *Managing chronic pain: A patient's guide.* New York: Sterling Publishing.

Turk, D. C., & Genest, M. (1979). Regulation of pain: The application of cognitive and behavioral techniques for prevention and remediation. In P. C. Kendall & S. D. Hollon (Eds.), *Cognitive-behavioral intervention: Theory, research, and procedures* (pp. 287–318). New York: Academic Press.

Turk, D. C., Meichenbaum, D., & Genest, M. (1983). *Pain and behavioral medicine.* New York: Guilford Press.

Turner, J. A., & Romano, J. M. (1990). Cognitive-behavioral therapy. In J. J. Bonica (Ed.), *The management of pain* (2nd ed., pp. 1711–1721). Philadelphia: Lea & Febiger.

Tyson, R., & Strong, J. (1990). Adaptive equipment: Its effectiveness for people with chronic lower back pain. *Occupational Therapy Journal of Research, 10*(2), 111–112.

Violon, A., & Giurgea, D. (1984). Familial models for chronic pain. *Pain, 18,* 199–203.

Ward, N. G. (1990). Pain and depression. In J. J. Bonica (Ed.), *The management of pain* (2nd ed., pp. 310–319). Philadelphia: Lea & Febiger.

Weisenberg, M. (1977). Pain and pain control. *Psychological Bulletin, 84,* 1008–1044.

CHAPTER 18

Functional restoration

SECTION 1

Preliminary concepts and planning

ELINOR ANNE SPENCER

> so much
> depends upon
> a red wheel
> barrow
> glazed with rain
> water
> beside the white
> chickens
>
> William Carlos Williams (1964)

The outward simplicity and inherent complexity of Williams's poem is analogous to the impact of debilitating disease or injury on a person's life. Although the poem conveys an initially simple and colorful image, through it surges an underlying current of symbolism that adds meaning and dimension to the words. So, too, the process of functional restoration after a disabling condition embodies the totality of human potential.

Functional restoration is the primary objective of rehabilitation. Assisting a person to build or restore his or her life to its fullest use and satisfaction is a philosophical mandate of occupational therapy. Thus, the occupational therapist is an essential member of the rehabilitation team.

Traditionally, occupational therapists have directed their efforts toward enabling patients and clients to achieve maximal performance in daily functions regardless of the disease, injury, and resulting dysfunction. Evaluation and treatment methods have developed from a disease orientation based on a medical model. During its growth as a profession, occupational therapy progressed from an allied medical profession to an allied health profession. ***Therapeutic intervention*** is used to prevent further disability, to reverse current disability, or to improve ability. An outgrowth of the disease orientation is a disability orientation; an outgrowth of the health orientation is an ability orientation.

Health care professionals, including occupational therapists, are in the midst of a positive, health-oriented movement directed toward assisting people with taking responsibility for their own health. Occupational therapists have long contributed to the promotion of health through a commitment to habilitation, rehabilitation, and prevention.

The effects of disability are reflected in psychosocial and physical responses reaching into all areas of a person's life, often requiring adjustments in life patterns. The extent and quality of adjustment depend on the premorbid context of the person's life, the prognosis of the functional outcome, and the goals set by the patient, family, and rehabilitation team.

Impact of trauma and disease

Trauma and disease that result in physical and mental disabilities can be devastating to a person's life. The onset can be *sudden* or *gradual*. The course can be *nonprogressive* or *progressive*. The manifestations of disability may be *temporary* or *permanent*.

Sudden onset of external trauma is characteristic of spinal cord injury, brain injury, fractures, peripheral nerve injury, and amputation. These injuries are often caused by accidents involving cars, sports, industrial machinery, falls, or weapons, and they usually affect the young adult or middle-aged population. Although the manifestations may result in permanent limitations, the injuries are generally nonprogressive. Sudden onset also is characteristic of internal trauma from such neurologic causes as a cerebrovascular accident (CVA, stroke). The symptom complex may take several hours to develop until the stroke is "completed." After the attack, clinical signs generally do not increase; however, there can be a subsequent CVA.

A gradual or insidious progressive onset is seen in diseases such as multiple sclerosis (MS), Parkinson disease, arthritis, myasthenia gravis (MG), and amyotrophic lateral sclerosis (ALS). These diseases tend to have an inconsistent but progressive pattern of remissions and exacerbations. When in remission, the disease process is quiescent or at rest; when in exacerbation, the disease process is active, and the person experiences increased symptoms. The severity of the exacerbation is unpredictable, as is the duration of remission. During these periods, the person may show marked differences in functional ability. The progressive aspects of a condition may be primary causes of disability. Secondary effects (contractures, decubitus, or weakness) may result from initial deficits caused by the disease or trauma. For example, spasticity may be a primary disability resulting from CVA, and contracture may be a secondary disability resulting from the spasticity. Whereas impaired sensation may be a primary deficit resulting from a spinal cord lesion, a decubitus ulcer or serious skin breakdown may result from prolonged pressure on the desensitized area, causing a secondary deficit.

With an effective rehabilitation program suited to the person's needs, a person suffering from temporary disability from orthopedic or neurologic conditions can be assisted in returning to independent living. A more complex and challenging situation is the person suffering permanent or progressive disability. In this case, the long-term functional and psychological implications may not be recognized or accepted by the person or family in the early stages of recovery. Unanswered questions, unmet needs, and unresolved problems contribute to the development of long-term denial that leads to anger, depression, and rejection of both individual potentials and therapeutic programs.

The immediate or eventual difference between what was and what is may result in confusion, fear, questions, insecurity, feelings of inadequacy, or disequilibrium. A previous level of life adjustment and understanding may be replaced by unknown and unfamiliar or unacceptable conditions or situations. To establish a relationship that will help the patient regain self-acceptance, the occupational therapist must determine the psychosocial significance of the patient's medical condition and what its impact will be on his or her lifestyle.

Disability can have a variety of effects on the educational development of a person. For example, a student with congenital anomalies or with disabilities resulting from injury or disease may be compelled to use a wheelchair. This student depends on such environmental adaptations as ramps, curb cuts, and wide doorways for access to school, classrooms, and other functional areas. The occupational therapist can greatly assist the school in enhancing the environment by advising the school on how to meet the needs of the disabled student.

The person suffering a brain injury may have damage to perceptual or intellectual centers in the brain that hinder visualization, communication, and retention of information necessary for learning, thus preventing continuation of academic studies without appropriate adaptation. A student who becomes disabled suddenly may not have developed the ability or interest in pursuing academic goals, although such goals may offer outlets to compensate for the loss of normal physical function and mobility. The student or adult experiencing remissions and exacerbations resulting in fluctuating functional abilities is challenged to maintain a positive attitude toward using and improving those capacities.

The economic implications of disability can be devastating for both the patient and the family. Financial assistance is available according to age, extent of financial assets, type of illness or disability, duration, vocational or educational prognosis, governmental benefits, private insurance coverage, and liability coverage. Without financial aid, rehabilitation costs can drain individual or family resources. Possible expenses include outlays for surgery, special treatment, assistive devices, wheelchairs, special home equipment, home modifications, adapted transportation aids, home health care, personal care attendant, outpatient treatment, follow-up, and adaptation of the employment site.

Functional implications

The effects of trauma and disease influence the total life experience of the person. The extent to which adjustments are essential to ensure continued success in personal relationships and the achievement of life goals varies with the extent and course of the disease or injury and the resulting dysfunctional manifestations. As the daily patterns of a familiar lifestyle change, the patient and family are forced to adjust to an unfamiliar and imposed combination of independent and dependent levels of function dictated by the course of the disease or injury. The familiar patterns of personal behaviors and social interactions influence how these challenges are met. An accurate analysis of the biopsychosocial context by the therapist is essential to determine the *functional implications* of the patient's condition.

Temporary or permanent disability takes on a unique meaning for each patient. Age, developmental stage, previous ability, achievements, lifestyle, family status, self-concept, interests, and general responsibilities affect attitudes such as understanding, acceptance, motivation, and emotional response. The process of rebuilding or rehabilitating begins with guidelines set by the person before the trauma or disease. Preceding experiences, abilities, and problems affect the rehabilitation process by enhancing or hindering the accomplishment of goals. Thus, the therapist learns as much as possible about these factors for the patient.

As an example, a child born with a congenital disability experiences early life development with the disability, which becomes part of the body image as the child grows. The congenitally disabled adult thus shows a high level of developmental integration because of a lack of experiential guidelines to normal functioning. In contrast, the adolescent or adult who has experienced life as an able-bodied person knows the implications of loss of function. It appears that the higher the physical, mental, or social achievement the person has reached before disability, the greater the challenge in accepting the loss and developing positive alternative goals compatible with the balance of permanent functional deficits and assets. The stage of development and the age of the person can be both advantageous and disadvantageous to necessary adjustments.

Another concept relating to the functional implications of trauma or disease is that of the transitions from *ability* to *disability* and then back to *ability* during rehabilitation. Although the first contact the occupational therapist has with a patient may be after the trauma or disease, the therapist must first consider the previous functional life of the patient. The patient with a sudden imposed disability maintains the self-concept, self-awareness, and responses of an able-bodied person. Thus, the actual functional limitations and implications may be unrecognized or denied. For the patient suffering remissions and exacerbations of a progressive disease, the self-concept may be more flexible, even tentative or bordering on dependent. The positive trend of rehabilitation is to focus on ability rather than disability and to assist the person who has limitations to become aware of his or her functional potential and to explore these resources in therapeutic programs. It is essential for the therapist to assist the patient in making the transitions. When the patient has suddenly, and possibly unknowingly, made the transition from the ability context to the disability context, therapeutic intervention directs the patient into an integration of both aspects of function into adaptive, ability-oriented performance.

Figure 18-1 illustrates the ability–disability–ability pattern. Areas in which changes from premorbid patterns may have occurred are listed, as are those affected by trauma and disease and those requiring adaptation for optimal function after formal rehabilitation.

The life experiences listed in Figure 18-1 are global. The functional restoration needed by the patient experiencing limitations from disease or trauma, although specifically related to such special programs as therapeutic activity, activities of daily living (ADL), homemaking, avocational pursuits, or vocational pursuits, must be geared toward the context of the individual patient to be acceptable and appropriate to the patient's particular interests, abilities, and goals. Program planning that does not directly involve the patient's input and commitment will not serve the person well upon discharge and thus will not encourage continued rehabilitation. It is crucial to work directly with the patient to remain aware of the patient's abilities, activities, and priorities with regard to functional limitations, implications, and potential gains.

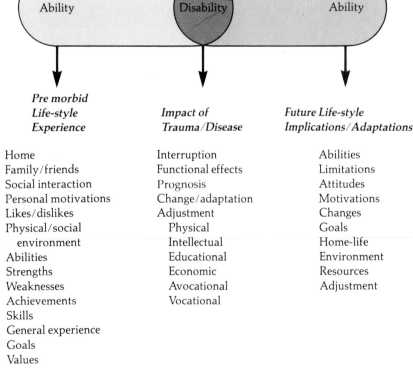

Changing Disability to Ability

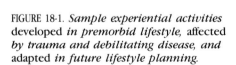

FIGURE 18-1. *Sample experiential activities developed in premorbid lifestyle,* affected *by trauma and debilitating disease, and* adapted *in future lifestyle planning.*

Pre morbid Life-style Experience	*Impact of Trauma/Disease*	*Future Life-style Implications/Adaptations*
Home	Interruption	Abilities
Family/friends	Functional effects	Limitations
Social interaction	Prognosis	Attitudes
Personal motivations	Change/adaptation	Motivations
Likes/dislikes	Adjustment	Changes
Physical/social	Physical	Goals
environment	Intellectual	Home-life
Abilities	Educational	Environment
Strengths	Economic	Resources
Weaknesses	Avocational	Adjustment
Achievements	Vocational	
Skills		
General experience		
Goals		
Values		

Factors affecting rehabilitation process and outcome

Personal development

The premorbid level of development in all areas of function provides the person suffering from dysfunction with ways to deal with the effects on his or her present life, which has suddenly come to be made up of unfamiliar events, people, patterns, and procedures. The prognosis is determined in part by the premorbid characteristics the person has to invest in the process of rehabilitation. A person fortunate enough to have had the resources to develop a strong sense of values and self-esteem, personal independence and achievement, healthy physical activity, social interaction, optimal work habits, and motivation for productive activity brings a healthy background to the challenge of rehabilitation. On the other hand, a person with poorly conceived or developed skills, poor work habits, and unhealthy attitudes toward personal performance or responsibility brings poorly developed resources to the rehabilitation challenge and process. Negative personal attitudes can combine with negative social attitudes toward illness or disability to thwart the effect of rehabilitation resources. Thus, longstanding personal attitudes and biases can deter the positive gains from a therapeutic program. For example, the fear of the unknown path ahead may be reinforced by a growing dislike of self due to the disability. This can result in denial or rejection of the reality of long-term infirmity or physical limitation. The patient or the family that harbors the belief that disabled people are "not normal" (ie, are less intelligent, less socially acceptable, less physically attractive, less functionally capable, and less significant than nondisabled people) is forced to adjust perspectives to accept the reality of long-term disability. Nonacceptance leads to rejection of therapy as a means of adapting to disability and achieving ability, rejection of association with disabled people in a therapeutic milieu or within the community, and development of dependency patterns due to decreased self-value and lesser independent function.

Recognizing, accepting, and working through negative personal attitudes with the patient are crucial parts of rehabilitation. Generally, biases necessitate supportive understanding by professionals working with the patient. During the initial interview covering the previous experience of the patient, respect must be given to the patient's personal development. The value of the therapist will be in the flexibility of attitude available to meet the variety of cultural variables that may be presented by the patient and the family.

Social interaction

Social interaction is essential for healthy human development, whether a person is gregarious or shy. At some point, a person has need of others. When tragedy occurs, friends and family rally, but the duration of their commitment to the needs of the traumatized person will depend on the nature of the disability, the demands it makes on people, the ability to give and the personality of the individual, and the duration of need. The sequelae of disability (disfigurement; assistive devices; pathologic motor patterns; the presence of tremors, drooling, or peculiar voice patterns; or deviations in normal behavioral or intellectual patterns) present a challenge to continuing social contact.

The difficult adjustments experienced by a person in a rehabilitation program may be influenced by personal or social attitudes, concepts, associations, taboos, experiences, or dreams. Words take on a new meaning; personal associations may positively or negatively affect the rehabilitation process.

In the social milieu, the disabled person is faced with a new arena of behavior, one in which gains in self-awareness are challenged by a complex environment. Strong self-concepts and self-acceptance are essential for expanding perceptions and reactions to include others and for being able to function effectively within a group. Here, as well as in the nonhuman environment, gains in the ability to function will depend on the type and level of opportunities available. To interact with a group, the patient must be able to perform at the level expected by the group; otherwise, the patient will not be included as a significant member.

Role of occupational therapy

Occupational therapy practice has been influenced by changing medical concepts and practice with regard to life-support systems; diagnostic accuracy; awareness of and referral to allied medical, health, and therapeutic services; the effect of drugs on human behavior and function; and the technical development of diagnostic, therapeutic, and adaptive equipment.

Occupational therapists and occupational therapy assistants have participated in the growth within therapeutic services by joining team efforts with physicians and other professionals and by developing specific techniques. A rich variety of specific treatment approaches is available to the clinical occupational therapist and assistant. Because the therapeutic approaches and modalities used must be appropriate to a person's needs, specific approaches and techniques are often combined into an eclectic grouping. Methods developed and researched for use with children are being modified for use with adults with similar needs; approaches in psychiatry and physical dysfunction are combined when the clinical signs call for a melding of treatment objectives and techniques. Examples of global approaches that have been adapted for use in a variety of situations are the sensory-integration approaches and the neurophysiologic techniques.

Therapeutic perspectives have progressed from localized specific treatment of an injured part to a comprehensive consideration of psychosocial, environmental, educational, and vocational implications. This is particularly emphasized in the rehabilitation programs, where a patient may be involved in sensory integration, group treatment, adapted recreation, ADL, work-simulated tasks, and homemaking programs leading to independent living. The traditional concern of the occupational therapist with assisting the patient in functional development within the context of the "whole person" maintains its strong focus in the rehabilitation programs, whether in the hospital, in the ambulatory clinic, or in the community.

Principles of functional restoration

The rebuilding of a lifestyle demands a creative, realistic, and practical day-to-day adaptive approach to daily living skills, activities, and tolerance. The patient knows the meaning of *ability* in functioning but must learn the meaning of *disability*. The therapist can challenge the patient to become an independently functioning person, both mentally and physically, and aid the patient in maintaining a balance in all abilities, no matter how well or how poorly developed.

The following principles are basic to functional restoration through occupational therapy:

Correlation of the program with the medical condition of the patient, general assessment information, motivation level, and stated goals of the patient, the family and home situation, other treatment programs and services the patient is receiving, the medical and functional prognoses, and joint planning for admission, treatment, and discharge

Use of therapeutic relationships during evaluation and treatment sessions between patient and therapist or assistant, patient and patient, patient and group, patient and family, and treatment team, patient, and family

Use of the environment to aid in adjustment and adaptation by the patient for functional living, including (1) adjusting the setting for effective evaluation of functional level, (2) adapting the level of external stimuli for tolerance and interaction, (3) adjusting for successful and satisfying daily living activity, and (4) ensuring self-worth through productive and social activity

Use of therapeutic positioning of the body for evaluation, treatment, and rest using equipment appropriate for the patient's need and level of function and using the principles of body mechanics

Use of a variety of evaluation techniques, including observation, interviews, standardized tests, and performance tests

Use of purposeful activity during evaluation and treatment

Use of activity analysis in the choice of activity for evaluation and treatment and in the choice of treatment method as related to the therapeutic value of the selected activity

Correlation of physical treatment procedures with the patient's level of receptivity, behavior, and potential

Use of ADL in evaluation and treatment to provide body awareness and acceptance, daily exercise, and indication of independent skill level and assistance needed

Use of adaptive devices and equipment to obtain maximal involvement in functional physical activity, provide independence in daily self-care, and provide self-esteem and self-worth in task completion

Use of work simplification and energy conservation techniques for motivation, accomplishment, and productivity; maximal achievable independent living functions; and task accomplishment

Use of community resources for successful community reentry, continued level of independence after discharge, social stimulation and benefit, and independence in continuing rehabilitation goals

Components of therapeutic intervention

Environment

Occupational therapy is based on the belief that people are capable of relating to the human and nonhuman environments in a manner that is self-directed, purposeful, meaningful, and satisfying. Throughout the developmental continuum from birth to death, humans grow by adapting to the challenges and stresses confronted in daily living. Adaptation is enhanced, thwarted, encouraged, or delayed by the person's unique abilities to progress through the myriad learning experiences toward integra-

tion of sensorimotor and cognitive awareness and function necessary to accomplish meaningful tasks.

The occupational therapist's greatest challenge is to motivate a person toward self-direction and achievement for personal satisfaction. To this end, the occupational therapist organizes the patient's immediate environment to provide opportunities for achievement of independent and productive functions.

To reach independence at any level, the disabled person must achieve enough control over the natural and the human-made environments to achieve his or her goals with self-respect and satisfaction. Although there may be limitations that render the patient "handicapped" in specific situations, the extent to which the person with temporary or permanent disability can accomplish his or her goals depends on this control. The following are helpful in gaining self-confidence and strength to cope with the challenges of the environment:

- Determining what one can do independently
- Determining what one can do with assistance
- Determining what one cannot do without assistance
- Ability to ask for assistance and get it
- Knowing whom to ask for assistance
- Ability to instruct the person giving assistance
- Ability to adjust to changes imposed by disability (appearance, special equipment, changes in abilities)
- Development of knowledge of available resources (people, services, equipment, construction)
- Development of knowledge of rights
- Development of knowledge and acceptance of physical and mental tolerance

The environment consists of all people (human environment) and things (nonhuman environment) surrounding a person. Human performance is greatly affected by environmental influences and the way a person interprets them. The person encumbered by disability and its accompanying emotions may find on reentry that a previously known environment is now unfamiliar and unknown. Instead of having a safe, familiar, and comforting feeling for the person, it may have an unfriendly, unsafe, unwelcoming, or even hostile aspect. The environment is continually changing during the recuperation of the disabled person; this phenomenon may represent an overwhelming and continuing challenge and may pose an obstacle to adaptation.

In adapting to the familiar environment with a different body and mind, the person may be in the situation of having to adjust to the old with decreased adaptive ability and to adjust to the new with even less ability to adapt. The recovering patient, however, may actually be more aware of the adaptive challenges of the environment through a sudden slowing down of all physical and mental adjustment mechanisms.

Dunning (1972) suggests that occupational therapists are managers of space (to promote stimulation), people (to encourage social interaction), and tasks (to develop skills). In this role, the therapist analyzes the effects of the surroundings on a person in terms of the person's response. Deficits found during the initial interview and evaluation cue the therapist to changes needed in the environment, either to stimulate or to inhibit the person's behavior or adaptation. The therapist must assist the patient in adjusting to the challenges of the environment by increasing appropriate performance within it.

The occupational therapy program provides the patient with activities to create awareness of self in time and space, develop awareness of the environment, and reveal behavior changes and development of abilities. To enhance these awareness areas, the occupational therapist should use the following objectives in planning the treatment program: (1) encourage movement and performance, and (2) involve the patient with those nearby and with the environment to provide opportunities, channel abilities, facilitate action, and eliminate barriers to function. Through a program of normal activities in an appropriate environment, the therapist helps the patient establish a new self-image and accept changes in physiology, feelings, and appearance. The therapist also aids the adjustment in preparation to reenter the home and community and to assume healthy attitudes toward self and family.

Environmental influences can have positive or negative effects on the evaluation and treatment of the person with physical or neurologic dysfunction. The following elements can structure the environment for success:

- *Atmosphere.* The area used for evaluation and treatment should have adequate comfortable space, lighting, and temperature. The therapist initially orients the patient to the meaning of the room, its contents, its location, and its functions and introduces the patient to the other people there. The therapist controls the visual and auditory stimuli to relieve any anxiety or confusion.
- *Sensory bombardment.* Excessive, unexpected sensory impulses (visual, auditory, tactile, proprioceptive, or kinesthetic) can confuse, fatigue, or frighten the patient. Therefore, the therapist controls *all* the stimuli.
- By using voice and body in a supportive, nonthreatening way, the therapist becomes a *therapeutic tool.*
- An acceptable *level of achievement,* commensurate with the patient's interests, is necessary as positive feedback.
- In some situations, familiar objects may be threatening early in the treatment. Therefore, *unfamiliar activities and exercises* may be better for initial evaluation and treatment.

The occupational therapist assists in providing an optimal living environment. Arrangement of furniture in the room, bed location in relation to the door and to other patients, accessibility of personal items, proximity to the emergency call button, and accessibility and ease of use of the bathroom all contribute to or detract from mental, physical, and emotional well-being. Wherever the patient eats and socializes (own room, cafeteria, or dining room), the facilities should be accessible and should encourage independent functioning; the patient should be placed with compatible persons during meals and for social functions.

In the occupational therapy room, depending on the goals of the treatment program at a given time, the patient should be allowed to work in a secluded area if he or she desires or to work in proximity to others who could have a therapeutic effect.

Family members and friends can have various effects on the patient; some may be encouraging and may stimulate functional recovery, whereas others may be patronizing or pitying and thus may retard progress. The objective of stressing environmental interaction is to assist the patient in adjusting to the return home and in using skills to adapt to the environment for maximal function and minimal stress.

Able-bodied people tend to limit their perception of the environment to what they know or where they are rather than noticing the conditions to which the disabled person must adapt.

Aspects of the environment to be evaluated are the responsibilities of the patient and others sharing the immediate surroundings; the expectations of the patient for performance and role; others' expectations and roles; housing design; location of living quarters; type of neighborhood; use of private or public transportation; and location of community resources.

Relationships

The relationship between the therapist and the patient is crucial to the patient's reception of the resources available. Because the patient is confronted by the need to make myriad adjustments in the initial phases of trauma or disease, the therapist must recognize the impact of evaluation and treatment methods on the patient's level of awareness and acceptance of the debilitating condition and its implications. Essential to the establishment of an effective and functional relationship is awareness by the therapist of his or her personal limitations and biases. The therapist must maintain objectivity toward the patient and not feel personally rejected if the patient balks at program procedures. Working closely with the patient and listening to the patient's views of the situation allows the patient adequate self-expression and self-awareness. In the progression of health care from the acute care facility to outpatient services to postdischarge follow-up visits, the objective of therapeutic involvement is to assist the patient in gaining maximal independence and personal control of all aspects of daily living. This includes being able to maintain and establish effective relationships with family, friends, service providers, and others.

In her distinction between the *sick role* and the *disabled role,* Daniels (1981) states that choice of role affects the type and value of health care given to and received by the patient. Daniels describes the patient in the sick role as receiving care focused on noncontinuing or acute illness, with the medical treatment directed by a physician. In this role, the person "acts sick" and responds to the authority of the physician, lacking the knowledge and experience to care for himself or herself.

During the initial acute care phase of disability, a person may respond to this sick role due to the overwhelming nature of the symptoms and hospitalization. The patient avoids anxiety and uncomfortable feelings of confusion and helplessness by reaching out for protective denial of the implications to use as a crutch or as a retreat from reality. The unwanted reality may be severe damage to body parts and bodily functions implying undesirable long-term personal and social changes. Vargo (1978) states that, in this denial stage, "the individual is not emotionally prepared to accept the reality and the implications of the disability and consequently will deny that such a disability exists" (p. 32).

Daniels (1981) states that the sick role should not be applied to a disabled person because this can result in undertreatment (not enough information being provided to the patient regarding the medical condition and treatment), overtreatment (too much or inappropriate care being given), or mistreatment (decisions regarding the medical condition and treatment being made without consulting the patient). To avoid these errors, the health care providers should use the disabled role. Daniels describes this as a continuous process in which the treatment is centered on the patient and the patient's goals, coordinating the care with lifestyle and working through cooperation. In this role, the patient seeks rehabilitation, accepts disability as a personal characteristic, and, through growing knowledge of the disability, takes an authoritative role in his or her own care.

The disabled role is often difficult to follow in a general hospital setting, where care is directed toward acute medical intervention. A disabled person hospitalized for acute distress, however, should be allowed to carry out as much self-care as possible because being treated for the long-term disability rather than for the acute illness constitutes overtreatment; and "interrupted established routines can injure the self-sufficiency of the disabled person" (Daniels, 1981). This advice, of course, refers to the patient who has already been through the process of rehabilitation and has been living in the community as a disabled person.

The hospitalization of the newly disabled patient may terminate during the denial stage, with the patient unreconciled to the implications of disability and unprepared to leave the sterile protection of the medically oriented environment. In acknowledging the patient's difficulty in accepting alternatives to prior decisions and actions, Heijn and Granger (1974) state that the occupational therapist "introduces unfamiliar devices and techniques that substitute for actions that have become difficult or impossible due to functional loss" which may be "direct nonverbal confrontation with existing deficits" necessitating "recognition of the permanence of the impairment" (p. 28).

After the period of autocratic denial of disability and unsuccessful attempts to regain the past, the affected person begins to recognize the facts regarding the condition and passes into a period of bitter mourning when the fantasy of denial can no longer be maintained. Medical changes begin to plateau, and the patient sees that his or her new life does not fit into old patterns. During this depression, the patient may consider suicide or wish for death, become uncooperative toward care, and hurt both family members and those most able to aid the patient in improving the condition.

Heijn and Granger (1974) state that "a patient must be able to mourn his losses to see the options in a restricted life" (p. 29). A patient puts limited effort into learning new methods when insisting on holding onto past and out-of-reach methods. In adjusting to a new body image, the patient must accept a new or adapted lifestyle and indeed may wish to change it. The strength for these life changes is won by developing a new sense of self-worth through participation in experiences that allow abilities to grow and to be accepted.

Self-worth is developed through trial and result, whether successful or unsuccessful. One's concept of ability is proved through accomplishment of tasks and recognition by oneself and others. When the opportunity to repeat the same successful performance is removed by inability to perform a part or all of the task, one may doubt one's future ability, and the gradual destruction of self-confidence and motivation may begin. Then, self-worth must be regained by the acceptance of one's actual ability.

When the patient is no longer in the hospital, the relationship with the therapist becomes a formal resource to the patient. For example, in the outpatient situation, the patient has returned home and comes to the hospital for specific evaluation or treatment. The patient may be referred to as a "client" rather than as a "patient" due to this change in the relationship. Responsibility falls on the patient and family for continued connection with the hospital as a resource rather than as a temporary home. On returning home, the patient is likely to become more cognizant of the importance of rehabilitation objectives previously presented in the confines of the hospital. The patient has the oppor-

tunity to integrate hospital gains with the challenges of increased control of use of time in the home environment. The occupational therapist may visit the patient in the home to ensure that the social and physical aspects of the environment are conducive to further gains in the person's independent functioning. Here, the therapist becomes an important link in the continuity of care as well as a resource if there are further needs.

Performance

One of the basic practices of occupational therapy is the use of performance as feedback to assist the patient in becoming involved in self-initiated, purposeful activity (Figure 18-2). Adaptive techniques to assist in the achievement of independent functions (self-care, social interactions, planning and initiating tasks) are often employed.

As a treatment facilitator, performance provides the experience of *doing*, from which the patient can gain an indication of whether and how well he or she is able to accomplish the task. Thus, the patient gains feedback for self-awareness. Performance of a specific movement, such as repetitive reaching or supination, may increase function for use in task completion. To effect a feeling of self-worth, what a person does must be meaningful to the person. Since people value the opinions of others, the patient will also derive self-worth when significant people recognize accomplishments.

Humans progress through life experiences and growth in a delicate balance of physical and psychological impressions, reactions, effects, and behaviors. These impressions are interdependent and interchanging and stand in a cause-and-effect relationship to function. The mind and the body work together in providing feedback from function to effect change, adaptation, and improvement in the ability to relate to people, things, and tasks. As the person is motivated to act, the mind designs the task for the body to perform. The nature of performance determines the sensory feedback, which motivates for continuation or for change in the performance. The performer gains an awareness of social and personal acceptance that is dependent on the quality and appropriateness of the performance.

The Activity Factor. The theory expressed by Reilly (1962) that "man, through the use of his hands as they are energized by mind and will can influence the state of his own health" (p. 1) has long guided the occupational therapist in the use of manual activity for therapeutic purposes. The therapeutic value of the activity, or the **activity factor**, depends on its meaning to the person performing it. Activity provides the patient with information about what he or she is capable of doing.

Ayres (1979) suggests that doing the activity is a more meaningful way to improve human functioning than is thinking or talking about the activity. She further suggests that the brain needs information from gravity, movement receptors, muscles, joints, and the skin of the entire body for effective integration: "The interaction of the sensory and motor systems through all their countless interconnections is what gives meaning to sensation and purposefulness to movement" (p. 46). Ayres describes purposeful activities as things that begin, continue, and end. In the process of purposeful activity, one follows through to the purpose one wants by doing something *with* something, *to* something, or *for* something (Ayres, 1979).

First gained in the initial contact, information is reviewed periodically with the patient throughout rehabilitation. Insight

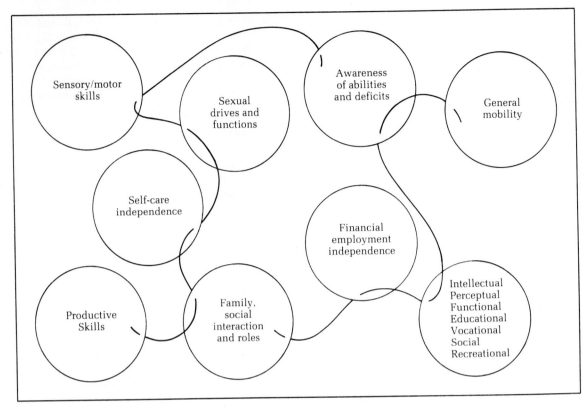

FIGURE 18-2. *For the patient, the experience of and feedback from performance in one area of function can facilitate motivation and accomplishment in another. The timely interrelation of tasks is connected by the thread of achievement.*

into the patient's interests with regard to educational and vocational pursuits, home life, lifestyle, responsibilities, and leisure activities must be gained. Areas to explore include feelings and plans related to family, social contracts, physical and mental potential, life goals for achievement, competitiveness, interest in creative activity, skills, and plans.

The types of activity in which the patient has shown interest may become important in the adjustment to disability. It is important to find out what sort of association and objective the patient had or expects to have with an activity. For example, if one patient is interested in sports, is it to compete with skill or ability, to participate socially, to dream of being outstanding, to describe or review, or to enjoy watching a game either in person or on television? If another patient's interest is in music, does this person wish to perform well, to perform adequately, to listen, to be knowledgeable in discussions, or to attend performances? Are the patient's favorite leisure activities socializing with friends at home or at community events, camping with family or friends, traveling, or engaging in such solitary outdoor activities as fishing?

Diagnostic Aspects. Performance in an activity appropriate to the patient's rehabilitation level and goals can show the patient and the therapist what functional level the patient is able or willing to achieve. Regardless of negative feelings about the medical condition, the patient is able to experience specific feelings about the level of achievement. Activity allows myriad opportunities for self-expression. Depending on how it is designed and presented by the therapist, activity provides informa-

tion regarding quality of performance, level of task completion, skill, talent, insight, strength, tolerance, and ability.

Restorative Aspects. In the process of achieving adaptive behavior through the use of activity, the patient assists in realistic planning through self-staging and gradual accomplishment and begins to adjust to people and to the environment. The patient begins to see himself or herself as a functioning member of society, regains independent functioning, and begins to reach out to family and peers.

In providing adjustment to disability through the use of therapeutic activities, the occupational therapist assists the patient in learning:

- Physical, mental, and emotional abilities and limitations
- How to compensate for physical dysfunction
- The limits of physical and mental tolerance
- How to compensate for disability by using substitutes for familiar functions
- How to cope with emotional frustrations caused by lost or decreased function
- The social, economic, interpersonal, and familial implications of dysfunction
- How to cope with economic problems caused by long-term disability (cost of hospitalization, expense of continuing treatment and assistive devices and equipment, decrease in job opportunities, and the necessity to be dependent on others in previously independent areas of function)
- How to adapt to a new functional level of achievement

- How to use leisure time functionally
- How to organize, adjust to, and accept a new lifestyle

Personal and Environmental Adaptation. Seeing oneself as having less self-worth as a result of disability is a normal reaction to loss. This is confirmed by the social signs of difficulty in acceptance and "forgiveness" of disability, such as in attention to making the environment accessible to the physically disabled. Feelings of anger and helplessness against these attitudes can be channeled positively into assisting the community to recognize disabled people as citizens with equal human rights. Community, state, and national organizations of disabled people provide peer support and channels for action for those interested in becoming involved in changing attitudes.

In considering the impact of disability from a social point of view, it is interesting to note Vargo's (1978) comment that, although *disability* is regarded as an observable impairment in the functioning of a body part, a *handicap* is a function of the interaction between people and their total environments. A society's political and fiscal priorities will determine whether people will be able to manage in spite of their disabilities. In a totally accessible society, a disabled person is not handicapped; in a society filled with stairs, curbs, visual identifications of locations, and auditory warning signals, handicapping situations confront every disabled person (Vargo, 1978).

Housing accessibility for the physically disabled person is complex. The home itself may be difficult to get into and out of, regardless of its inhabitants' limitations. It may also have architectural idiosyncrasies that make it difficult for the disabled person to perform daily activities previously done independently. Checklists to aid in complete evaluation and recommended measurements for access areas (entrance hallways, rooms, and garages) are provided through many resources (see Chapter 8, Section 2A).

Wheelchair users should be instructed in how to determine if a building and its functions are accessible or adaptable. Considerations of the accessibility or challenges presented by any building will become a natural part of planning. Nationally accepted standards of accessibility are available on request from the American National Standards Institute. Federal and state laws stipulate accessibility regulations and provide enforcement mechanisms for demanding proper construction of public buildings. These are used both in constructing new buildings and in renovating existing ones to ensure equal access by all people, regardless of disability.

Community Reentry and Functional Recovery. The fact that a person was a part of a neighborhood, school class, or working team before disability entails many adjustments in returning to these familiar friends and formerly comfortable places; residual disabilities may render this person limited in relation to former abilities. How the newly disabled person feels with old friends and in making new friends while using a wheelchair, for example, will depend on the acceptance of the wheelchair as an important part of functioning. As another example, the middle-aged man returning to work as a hemiplegic, recovered enough from his stroke to perform somewhat modified tasks with his fellow workers, may have to accept a slower pace of physical performance and intellectual functioning.

Referral to occupational therapy services

The *referral* is the basic request for services to be provided to a patient by an occupational therapist. This request also may be called a *consultation* or an *order*. The form and concept of the request for services varies among facilities and programs and may range from recommendations regarding a specific problem to a request for a complete assessment and treatment program for functional restoration. The frequent lack of specific instructions in the referral allows the occupational therapist to choose from a variety of individualized approaches and techniques in determining the methods of data gathering, treatment provision, and coordination with other involved professionals.

Referrals to occupational therapy are likely to come from physicians, therapists, nurses, psychologists, social workers, counselors, employers, teachers, or administrators.

Assessment planning and process

The occupational therapy assessment and treatment components are thoroughly identified in the *Uniform Terminology for Reporting Occupational Therapy Services* adopted by the American Occupational Therapy Association (AOTA) (see Appendix C). Briefly, **assessment** includes screening, consultation, and evaluation. Evaluation areas include (1) independent living and daily living skills and performance, (2) sensorimotor skills and performance, (3) cognitive skills and performance, (4) psychosocial skills and performance, (5) therapeutic adaptations, and (6) specialized evaluations (special training required for administration). Occupational therapists use a variety of evaluation procedures to gain an accurate historical and clinical picture of the functional capacities in these areas. Specific approaches vary from setting to setting.

In preparation for the formal functional assessment of a person, the therapist or assistant develops pertinent identifying information regarding the subject. Information gathered includes the reason for the referral, relevant background of the individual, medical and nonmedical information, the specific information or program requested by the referring party, and the type and location of the referral source. A referral signature is an essential part of the patient's permanent record (see Chapter 11, Section 2). The therapist first reviews the documentation received on the patient and then determines the time available for the assessment, which may be determined by the referring party or reimbursement source. If time is limited, it may determine the extent and type of evaluation tools used. If it is unlimited, the therapist must ensure that the assessment is relevant to the needs of the patient. In no case should the patient go through hours of evaluation, which, although providing interesting information, is not appropriate or necessary for determining treatment needs or delineating the manifestations of the condition or the prognosis.

Usually, a comprehensive assessment includes enough methods of evaluation to provide the patient with alternatives in performance, thus making the process tolerable and even enjoyable. Throughout the evaluation, it is essential to derive accurate, factual information. The more the patient understands and becomes involved in the procedure, the more progress will be made.

A coordinated team effort can minimize the time required for the assessment process and maximize the information gained from it. Working out roles among occupational therapy staff and interdisciplinary staff is essential to avoid unnecessary overlap and to provide the most accurate, economical, and effective procedures. The occupational therapy assistant participates under the supervision of the occupational therapist, particularly in the use of standardized tests and evaluations. Specific role delineations with regard to both assessment and treatment provided by the occupational therapist and the occupational therapy assistant are identified in detail in the *Entry-Level OTR and COTA Role Delineation* by the AOTA (see Appendix F). The therapist and the assistant collaborate in the assessment conclusions.

The occupational therapy assessment includes all results derived from specific evaluation procedures and provides a composite picture of a person's functional capacity and behavior. The methods used may be structured, standardized, or nonstandardized. In addition, the therapist uses observation as well as interviews to derive the composite meaning from the assessment process. The four methods—observation, interview, structured or standardized evaluation and testing, and nonstandardized assessment of performance—are described further below.

Observation

The preliminary approach to the patient is observation, which begins with the first contact. The therapist must continually be aware of how the therapist, the environment, and the tests are affecting the patient. Signs of the mental and physical condition should be observed closely. Observation requires no previous contact with either the chart or with other people and can be used effectively in the absence of other information.

By observing the patient's facial expression, the therapist can detect paralysis, drooling, spasticity, or confusion as well as alertness, fatigue, happiness, sadness, or pain. The position of the arms and legs can indicate spasticity, flaccidity, deformity, or pain. The sitting position can give indications of muscle imbalance, discomfort, or lack of voluntary control. Splints or slings also indicate some deficit in normal function. When walking into the room, the patient may display a gait produced by the use of braces, crutches, a prosthetic limb, a cane, or a walker or reveal a degree of paralysis not necessitating these aids. The skin may exhibit the effects of exertion or anxiety by appearing sweaty or red or becoming pale and clammy. Undue pressure from a splint or brace produces red or ulcerated marks or sores on the skin. If the therapist asks the patient to perform a task, the response can reveal hearing loss, muscle weakness, or incoordination.

Interview

The interview is a chance to get to know how the patient feels about what has happened, the effects on life and family, and the crucial priorities of the situation. Little may be known about the patient or the patient's condition. The interview (combined with observation) is the opportunity to find out information helpful to the therapist in planning the therapeutic program. Informal discussion leads to ease with the therapist and with the environment.

The attitude of the therapist must be accepting if trust and confidence are to be inspired. The interview need not be rigidly formal or completed in a single session. The initial contact marks only the beginning of the relationship. This beginning is crucial

to the establishment of a good therapeutic environment, incorporating atmosphere, privacy, duration, acceptance, freedom of expression, and comfort (see Chapter 7).

Structured and standardized evaluation and testing

Structured and standardized evaluation and testing procedures are objective methods with which to judge performance levels. Frequently, these methods are broken down into specific tests to be completed with specific equipment and in conformity with specific procedures. Examples include using a goniometer to measure passive and active range of motion (ROM), using a dynamometer to gauge grip strength, using a pinch gauge to register prehension pressure, or using an aesthesiometer to determine two-point discrimination.

Standardized tests for coordination include dexterity tests, such as the Crawford Small Parts Dexterity Test (Figure 18-3), the Pennsylvania Bimanual Work Sample, the Minnesota Rate of Manipulation Test (Figure 18-4), and the Bennett Hand Tool Test. These tests and many others have norms or standardized measurements for comparing results. At times, however, the norms relate to normal performance and thus have selected use for the physically disabled person. Each test has a specific purpose and method of administration. If the norms are to be used in reference to the test score, administration of the test must be according to the instructions. For example, a quadriplegic, lacking a normal level of physical movements and sensory functions of the hands, may perform much lower on a coordination test if speed is an important factor, whereas if the speed factor is removed, this person may perform with a high level of accuracy and tolerance. From the many tests available, it is essential to select those that

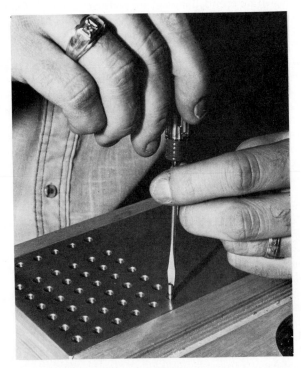

FIGURE 18-3. *Crawford Small Parts Dexterity Test. A timed, standardized, bimanual coordination test using small screws and a small screwdriver to complete transfer pattern to a metal plate.*

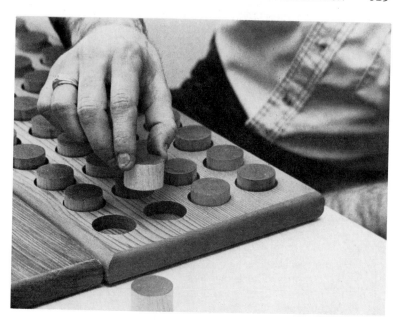

FIGURE 18-4. *Minnesota Rate of Manipulation Test. A five-part, timed, standardized test using unilateral and bilateral object manipulation patterns for transfer of wooden disks.*

will reveal the needed information so that explicit information can be given to team members as needed.

Treatment centers use a variety of specific tests to measure performance according to norms. Further information on specific tests can be found in Chapter 7.

Nonstandardized assessment

In assessing general performance, the therapist evaluates how well the patient accomplishes a specific task. What are limitations of strength, coordination, or ROM as indicated by ability in reaching for, grasping, or placing objects? How well is the patient adjusting to limitations? This can be evaluated by observing the character of social interactions with other patients, mental tolerance of the social context and activity of the occupational therapy room, and ability to work with a family member or the therapist in reviewing self-care abilities in light of eventually going home, where the assistance of a family member may be needed.

Performance testing also involves the assessment of problem-solving ability in accomplishing a task comprising several steps. For example, a woodworking project may be used to test the perceptual–motor abilities of the patient with brain damage. The therapist observes the method of planning the project, signs regarding visual perception, eye–hand coordination, concept of verticality, and proper use of tools.

In performance testing, it is essential to set up the task so that, although difficult, it is within the patient's ability. The use of a familiar task in evaluation may be threatening because it causes the patient to become acutely aware of the loss of ability. Performance testing must include a balance of success along with evaluation of functional deficits. Otherwise, the client may become overly discouraged or negative toward the occupational therapist, and such an attitude can hinder progress.

Documentation

Accurate documentation is essential in the accumulation of specific testing results, impressions, and interpretations. Forms vary from setting to setting and are often under revision. A sample worksheet for general information gained from the interview or performance testing is shown in the display. As stated, this is simply a structured format to assist the therapist in gathering and noting specific information for the overall assessment report. In many program settings, there are restrictions as to forms that are included in the formal chart documentation; therefore, the therapist devises forms to assist the informal gathering of information. The form presented in the display on pages 616 and 617 is helpful in noting information for subsequent inclusion in the formal report, for communication to other occupational therapists or assistants working with the patient, and for general reference regarding the progress of the patient. Additional specific evaluation forms may be used, such as those for perceptual testing, ROM testing, strength testing, and testing of self-care independence. The use of forms depends on the individual needs of the patient.

Treatment planning and process

Specific functional areas designated in occupational therapy treatment are described in the *Uniform Terminology for Occupational Therapy*, 2nd edition (see Appendix C). They include the *occupational performance areas* of ADL, work activities, and play or leisure activities as well as the *performance components* of sensory motor, neuromuscular motor, cognitive integration, and psychosocial skills.

The *Standards of Practice* (see Appendix B), also developed by the AOTA, provides a guideline for the implementation of the treatment programs. Recommendations for documentation, standards of assessment and treatment, program design, discharge planning, reevaluation, and quality assurance are included in this resource.

The person referred to occupational therapy for functional services may actually fear the achievement of functional independence. In this case, there may be an underlying resistance to all positive approaches from others and to potential gains. The challenge for the occupational therapist and the occupational therapist assistant is to establish effective therapeutic intervention by developing an environment and relationships that will assist the patient to develop therapeutic performance.

SAMPLE OCCUPATIONAL THERAPY WORKSHEET

Admission Date: _____

Discharge Date: _____

Occupational Therapy Worksheet

Name: _____

Address: _____

Age: _____ Education: _____

Occupation: _____

_____

Marital Status: _____

Children: _____

Other: _____

House: Surroundings: _____

    #Floors: _____

    Kitchen: _____

    Architectural Barriers: _____

Admission Date: _____ Room # _____

Diagnosis: _____ Duration: _____

Pertinent History: _____

O.T. Referral/Order: _____

_____

Dr.: _____ Date: _____

Precautions: _____

Entrance: _____

Bedroom: _____

Bathroom: _____

Physical Evaluation:

    Upper Extremities: (ROM, strength, coordination, sensation, muscle tone, movement patterns, endurance)

_____

    RUE: _____

_____

    LUE: _____

    Bilateral: _____

_____

    Functional Deficits: _____

    Trunk and Lower Extremities: (Mobility, sensation, muscle tone, sitting/standing tolerance, balance, gait)

_____

Mental Functioning Evaluation: (attention, awareness, judgment, behavior, retention, reception, abstract reasoning, cognition, problem solving)

_____

Perceptual Functioning Evaluation: (visual, auditory, motor planning, stereognosis, proprioception, perceptual motor correlation)

_____

_____

Functional Activity Evaluation:

    ADL: (position, balance, transfers, mobility, assistive devices used, motivation, perceptual deficits)

    Hygiene/Bathing/Grooming: _____

_____

    Dressing: _____

_____

    Self-feeding: _____

    Writing/Reading: (signature, tracing, copying, spontaneous writing and reading, dominance, field cut, neglect, eyesight)

_____

    Homemaking: (food preparation, clean-up, safety, home modifications, assistive devices, positioning, responsibilities, financial management, work simplification, energy conservation)

_____

_____

_____

(continued)

616

SAMPLE OCCUPATIONAL THERAPY WORKSHEET (*continued*)

Attitudes: (emotional status, self-concepts, behavior)

_____

Interests: (vocational, avocational, and social skills and abilities)

_____

_____

Orthotic and Assistive Equipment: (type, date given, recommendations)

_____

_____

Summary of Findings: (deficits, functional limitations, potentials, attitudes)

_____

_____

_____

_____

_____

Treatment Plan:
   Objectives: _____

   _____

   _____

   Methods: _____

   _____

   _____

   Duration/Frequency: _____

   Expected Outcome: _____

   _____

Date: _____   _____ OTR
                                                    Signature

---

When the occupational therapist develops the treatment plan, the patient is the prime component and must be included when choosing methods to achieve functional gains. This includes initial planning, changes based on progress, and feedback regarding performance. This consideration encourages the patient to take an increasing role in planning therapeutic activities and adaptations. If the therapist sees the patient first in the outpatient or home environment, prime consideration for the patient's views and maximal involvement with program planning is even more essential. In taking gradual steps toward responsibility in planning and self-evaluation, the patient develops self-awareness, confidence, creativity, problem solving ability, and responsibility for his or her own health. The following are some ways in which the patient can be included in the treatment planning and implementation:

- Encouraging the patient to participate in the initial evaluation procedures and results and to assist with the treatment plan design
- Providing the patient with factual information from the assessment results to use in planning the course of treatment
- Involving the patient's interests, major current concerns, abilities, and long-term goals in the plan
- Planning short-term goals with the patient; obtaining commitment from the patient if feasible
- Planning treatment modalities to include positive feedback to the patient to increase self-awareness and satisfaction from gains

- Planning long-term goals with the patient with regard to implications of disability, financial boundaries, and medical and functional prognosis
- Encouraging the patient to develop the ability to design treatment goals, to set priorities among treatment objectives, and to take responsibility for the program

Beginning the treatment program with a short-term goal that is significant to the patient helps establish an effective relationship between the therapist or assistant and the patient. Use of passive ROM or demonstrations aids in the teaching of active movements and encourages functional patterns. New or adaptive techniques and equipment should be demonstrated by the therapist in the same manner that the patient is expected to perform so that the patient can imitate the expected motion. Involvement in therapeutic exercise and activity provides increased productivity and a sense of purpose to the therapeutic regimen. The engagement of the patient in problem solving, planning, and evaluation to meet treatment objectives aids in the accomplishment of the objectives. With appropriate and therapeutic feedback with regard to performance, the patient increases self-awareness and can relate the daily progress to the goals. The treatment plan itself should relate to the eventual goal of going home and being responsible for the continuity of care. Patient and family involvement in treatment facilitates continuity in the home after discharge from formal institutional programs. Long-term accomplishments are effected by day-to-day efforts in a succession of intermittent but progressive gains.

Independence of the patient in self-care activities is an area of concern and adaptation shared by the nurse and the occupational therapist. Self-care represents the most significant aspect of self-awareness and self-acceptance. During the initial stage of denial, the patient is effectively able to deny responsibilities, the body, and its functions. Concern is focused on physical sensations, such as pain, positioning, and movement. The patient relinquishes responsibility for care of the body and may even be afraid of it since the frightening effects of disease or trauma have made it an unknown.

During therapy sessions, movement is incorporated into self-care programs. The responsibility for assistance in independent self-care falls generally to the occupational therapist in collaboration with the nurse. The occupational therapist assesses the self-care problems. For example, inability to distinguish objects of different shapes or colors or to relate to vertical or horizontal positions may make the patient unable to determine the front, back, or sleeve of a shirt. A person with a flaccid arm cannot handle eating utensils in the usual manner and thus may have to learn how to cut meat using one hand, switch the fork to the nondominant hand, or use a plate guard. The occupational therapist analyzes these problems, determines the approach for handling them, and teaches techniques to be used in performing each activity. These techniques are then used in the patient's daily program.

With the physically disabled person, ADL generally comprise those necessary for basic self-care independence: bathing, hygiene, elimination, grooming, dressing, and eating. Consideration is given to such items as eyeglasses, hearing aids, dentures, prostheses, splints, slings, braces, and adapted clothing. The patient's abilities should be evaluated both with and without the adapted equipment to accurately assess levels of independence. For example, a patient who is unable to button without the use of a hand splint is considered independent with the hand splint but dependent without it. This is also true when special utensils or other equipment are required for eating without the assistance of another person.

The disabled person learns how to choose and retrieve clothing from drawers and cabinets, how to apply and secure assistive devices, how to use catheters, tampons, or suppositories as necessary, how to manage such items as soap, washcloths, nail clippers, combs, toothpaste, and make-up. In the process of eating, the patient learns the use of napkins, utensils, glasses, and cups as well as how to take food from a serving dish and use salt and pepper.

Included in self-care is the use of the telephone, including how to dial the telephone, answer it, take a message, and call for help. Those who need special equipment learn how to use it and how to obtain special operator assistance.

In some instances, the patient can accomplish self-care and eating tasks by performing them in a different manner rather than by learning how to use special devices or equipment. When devices are necessary (elastic shoelaces, Velcro closures, or elastic thread), or when a new skill must be mastered (one-handed shoe-tying or meat-cutting), all possibilities should be explored to ensure minimal reliance on, but maximal effectiveness of, the special equipment or the acquired skill. Effectiveness in self-care provides the patient with independence, which not only aids the patient but also helps in family relationships. The accomplishment of self-care tasks leads to further successes, enhances motivation, and provides daily physical exercise.

The general mobility of the patient is a concern and adaptation shared by the nurse, the physical therapist, and the occupational therapist. Since the patient must assume optimal position for function, an adapted transfer technique from bed to wheelchair or to walker or crutches may be necessary. Although the physical therapist may decide which technique the patient should use, a coordinated team effort is needed to assist the patient in the same technique to aid in learning; therefore, the occupational therapist needs to know transfer techniques.

Specific restoration of functional ability may precede or follow the development of self-care activity. Body exercise and sensory awareness developed during the accomplishment of daily tasks are correlated with specific activities also directed toward the restoration of functional ability. These activities include specific exercises to improve strength, ROM, coordination, and function.

The terms *exercise* and *activity* are used here interchangeably since it is believed that activity provides exercise and exercise can be provided through activity. An exercise modality may consist of a measured movement or a combination of movements.

Occupational therapy emphasizes active rather than passive exercises and uses the abilities of the patient to the maximum. Although assistive equipment (suspension slings, wheelchairs, lapboards, and splints) may help the patient passively, the *purpose* of their use is to achieve the maximal level of independent and active functioning. For example, the suspension sling may facilitate arm movement for a quadriplegic, enabling the patient to bring both hands together, to eat independently, to use a button board for practice, to write a letter, or to type schoolwork. A variety of assistive equipment may be needed to encourage arm and hand function and to prevent fatigue during exercise activities.

The treatment room provides an atmosphere of activity, with emphasis on productive achievement and encouragement to try. Activity is geared toward what is interesting, purposeful, and acceptable to the patient so that the patient can see its relation to the overall rehabilitation goals. The patient may reject a treatment situation because of inability to do things done competently in the past. The patient may resent doing familiar tasks in an inferior way, performing the games of a child painfully and laboriously, or being unable to function to an expected or desired standard. For some of these reasons, the patient may become belligerent and refuse to participate in the therapy program. The occupational therapist must make every effort to involve the patient in planning appropriate treatment programs and activities.

The occupational therapist discusses vocational plans with the patient and focuses training objectives on areas related to vocational interests, aptitudes, and goals. For example, a patient who is attending school may wish to improve handwriting and note-taking skills. Job tasks may be simulated for the patient who can return to work. If new vocational goals are set, such as bookkeeping or mechanical drawing, proficiency in performing these tasks may be gained by using hand splints, special techniques, or adaptations.

In a hospital program, the occupational therapist may work with a vocational rehabilitation counselor in the formulation of vocationally oriented treatment. In a rehabilitation center, the vocational program may be separate from occupational therapy but may follow the prevocational exploration program provided by the occupational therapist. A vocational readiness program may be provided by the therapist or assistant on an outpatient basis, or the patient may be referred to a facility specially equipped to provide vocational testing and work-simulated tasks to determine realistic vocational areas for consideration by the patient. Many training programs in occupations are adapted to the needs of people with physical limitations.

Avocational interests are explored to give the patient an interest in daily activity. Hobbies such as reading, writing, painting, and drawing can be pursued even though physical limitations may require use of adapted equipment. Avocational pursuits can also develop into economic benefits for the patient.

The occupational therapist can assist the patient in making satisfactory adjustments to a disability and in restoring self-confidence by concentrating on accomplishments and capabilities and also by providing opportunities for social interaction. The patient should be encouraged to participate in recreational programs and in the patient governing bodies active in many rehabilitation facilities.

To ease the fear of taking part in outside social activities because of looking different, the patient should be encouraged to go on outings, such as bowling, baseball games, and movies, while still in the hospital. These activities make the patient begin to function as a member of a community in preparation for discharge. Upon discharge, each person should be encouraged to participate in social and community affairs and to attend functions that were attended before the injury or onset of disease.

The team approach

The ideal treatment approach to the patient with multiple problem areas, who is cared for by several people or programs, is the **team approach**, in which formal and informal interaction are encouraged among all people working toward developing and implementing a unified treatment program. This team includes the patient and family as well as specialists in the health field.

Team members are important sources of information and support for one another. For example, a patient may develop signs of extreme fatigue, such as sweating and difficulty in breathing, while in the occupational therapy area. The occupational therapist contacts the physician or the nurse for assistance in determining the cause and seriousness of the symptoms. The occupational therapist contacts the physical therapist to determine, for example, techniques for safe and successful transfer from one chair to another, whether the patient will be safe standing to perform a woodworking project, or whether the patient can safely stand and walk in the kitchen for assessment of homemaking skills.

Occupational and physical therapists should coordinate muscle testing, ROM, sensory testing, and assessment of physical tolerance and balance. The speech therapist and occupational therapist work together in designing treatment for the aphasic patient. Realistic vocational planning by the counselor is aided by the occupational therapist, who assesses the functional abilities of the upper extremities, the intellectual level of functioning in applied tasks, and the general physical tolerance. The physician aids in developing realistic planning in terms of the prognosis and the patient's mental approach to rehabilitation.

In the rehabilitation approach, there generally are overlaps in evaluation and treatment among physicians, nurses, occupa-

tional therapists, physical therapists, speech therapists, social workers, and vocational rehabilitation counselors. Overlaps can be useful in providing carry-over of activities and exercises and continual monitoring of the patient's progress. Good communication among team members is necessary to encourage coordination rather than antagonism over who does what. For example, the occupational therapist works with the physician, heeding the medical precautions on correct body positioning, optimal mental and physical tolerance of activity, and progression of pathologic symptoms. A coordinated self-care program involves the cooperation of nurses and occupational therapists in planning daily hygiene, grooming, dressing, and eating programs. The occupational therapist coordinates the morning dressing program and general exercise activities with the physical therapy program so that physical gains are maintained throughout the day and fatigue is avoided. The speech therapist aids team members in effective communication skills for patients who have speech deficits. When dealing with the patient and family, the social worker needs to know the treatment programs and progress to interpret and convey this information to the family and to assist the patient in understanding the daily program. The vocational rehabilitation counselor relies on the occupational therapist's evaluation of functional ability to determine the need for further education, job return, training, placement, or relocation.

A functional delineation of roles among team members is essential for optimal communication and effective rehabilitation. The specific roles of each member of the team may vary in different treatment settings.

Discharge planning

With the development of the team approach and the growth of rehabilitation, **discharge planning** has grown from the concept of placement or referral of a person after discharge to actual preparation for discharge by the patient and the rehabilitation team. The result of a well-coordinated team effort is effective referral for community reentry, with all team members contributing to the plan. The most important member of the team is the patient.

Preparation includes medical considerations (continuation of medication, follow-up visits, plans for future treatment), provision of assistive equipment for home exercise functions and independence in daily living, counseling the family on the patient's self-care and general activity, and a home visit to determine the presence of architectural barriers and to evaluate the patient's potential for functioning there.

Discharge planning begins with the referral of the person to the treatment setting where the anticipated treatment program is to take place. Thus, the first information regarding discharge questions or expectations will appear in referral materials. The program that follows referral may diverge from the initial expectations and may result in further discharge planning. Thus, discharge planning becomes a continual process based on the condition of the patient at any given time rather than simply a plan of where to go when a given program is completed.

After the referral information is gathered, evaluation occurs. This includes all team members and the gathering of pertinent information for appropriate and optimal treatment of the patient, including information about the patient's home environment, lifestyle, educational level, and occupation. The patient and the team can create a treatment plan that will assist the patient in preparing to go home. Since the total treatment plan is geared toward meeting the needs of the patient on discharge, therapy can be seen as important for realistic discharge planning rather than as a program that bears no relation to the most crucial problems of returning home.

Publications are available to aid the family and the recovering patient in postdischarge home programs that continue the rehabilitation process. Since recovery may continue over a period of years, professional programs are transferred to the patient and family to incorporate into daily routines.

In planning long-range needs and placement, the therapist and the patient must consider the following possible limitations: no home to return to after discharge; no financial coverage for outpatient services; no transportation available for outpatient services; or no family member to provide attendant care or homemaking services in the home after discharge.

Consumer groups provide many types of support and many opportunities for disabled people. National organizations established to benefit victims of a particular disease and to engage in specific relevant research projects publish information for professionals and consumers, hold educational meetings, and provide a forum for discussions.

Consumer groups, which may include able-bodied friends and professionals, provide initial socialization opportunities at meetings. A person can meet others with the same disability or with similar problems. Discussions focus on common concerns, such as the legal rights of the disabled, architectural and accessibility laws, building codes, transportation needs, housing, employment, and educational opportunities. Attending such meetings can be encouraging and informative for both the patient and the therapist. Such meetings may be held in rehabilitation centers or hospitals, thus making preliminary information and experience available early in the adjustment process.

Summary

The process of functional restoration after a disabling condition embodies the totality of human potential. Assisting a person to build or restore his or her life to its fullest use and satisfaction is a philosophical mandate of occupational therapy practice. The occupational therapist works with the patient, family, and other professionals in a coordinated interdisciplinary team from admission of the patient to a therapeutic program to achieving the optimal level of independent living at discharge. Through this process, health professionals collaborate in a health-oriented approach to daily living.

Individual effects of disability are reflected in psychosocial and physical responses by a person, reaching into all areas of life and often requiring adjustment of familiar life patterns. Trauma and disease may result in dysfunctional manifestations through a sudden or gradual pathologic process. Disability may be nonprogressive or progressive, temporary or permanent. The functional implications of the problem may be denied by the patient initially and require long-term intervention for acceptance of self and redirection of physical energies. Attitudes of people experiencing disability are affected by age, previous ability, achievements, lifestyle, family, status, self-concept, interests, and general responsibilities. The patient goes through a process from ability to disability to a regaining or refinding of ability during rehabilitation. Attitudes have a significant effect on the rehabilitation

process and its outcome. The disabled person draws on all personal resources.

The occupational therapist has a large variety of approaches, methods, and tools to use in assessing the deficits and potentials of a functionally limited person and designing appropriate treatment programs for functional restoration. The occupational therapist uses the concept and components of a therapeutic environment, therapeutic relationships, and therapeutic performance to improve function. The activity factor is crucial to the constructive aspects of performance and the regaining of function through purposeful activity. Activity can aid in diagnostic, therapeutic, and restorative program objectives.

Personal and environmental adaptations are crucial to reentry into the world of purpose and accomplishment. Architectural access to one's own home as well as to the buildings in the environment is essential. Functional recovery progresses through the final stages of community reentry.

The initial contact between the patient and the occupational therapist is facilitated by a referral to services. Although this may come from virtually any professional on behalf of the patient, specific program and reimbursement restrictions may be incurred. The assessment process is related to the treatment process. Assessment requires the appropriate involvement of the occupational therapist and the certified occupational therapy assistant, as designated by the AOTA role delineation. Treatment content is identified by both the AOTA *Uniform Terminology* and the AOTA *Standards of Practice*. The assessment is performed using nonstructured, nonstandardized, and standardized methods as well as by observation and interview. How the patient responds to the assessment and treatment procedures depends on the therapeutic relationship between the therapist and the patient and the degree of participation of the patient in the planning and implementation of the program. This aspect is essential to encourage the development of individual responsibility for continued rehabilitation on the part of the patient through the practice of problem-solving abilities.

There are many types of programs in which the occupational therapist provides services. Whatever the specific program, correlation of occupational therapy objectives and techniques with other programs in which the patient is involved is necessary for effective progress. Discharge planning is a team effort that involves the patient and assists the patient in developing healthy attitudes toward community involvement as a consumer and in maintaining healthy attitudes and activities in the independent environment.

This section is dedicated to the memory of my dear friend and colleague Patricia A. Curran, who provided constant editorial assistance and encouragement in professional and technical writing.

Appreciation is extended to Lois Rosage, Linda Strathdee, and Jean Blanchard for critical review and to Laura Tasheiko and Blue Hill Memorial Hospital in Blue Hill, Maine for technical assistance.

References

Ayres, A. J. (1979). *Sensory integration and the child* (p. 46). Los Angeles: Western Psychological Services.

Daniels, S. (1981). In disability and sickness: A theory. *Project Health, 1,* 1.

Dunning, H. (1972). Environmental occupation therapy. *American Journal of Occupational Therapy, 26,* 292.

Heijn, C., & Granger, C. V. (1974). Understanding motivational patterns:

Early identification aids rehabilitation. *Journal of Rehabilitation,* *40*(6), 26–29.

Reilly, M. (1962). Occupational therapy can be one of the great ideas of 20th century medicine. *American Journal of Occupational Therapy,* *16,* 1.

Vargo, J. W. (1978). Some psychological effects of physical disability. *American Journal of Occupational Therapy, 32*(1), 32.

Williams, W. C. (1964). In M. C. Richards (Ed.), *Centering* (pp. 79–80). Middletown, CT: Wesleyan Press.

SECTION 2

Neurologic, arthritic, orthopedic, cardiac, and pulmonary conditions

ELINOR ANNE SPENCER

KEY TERMS

Adaptive Techniques	Joint Protection
Daily Living Performance	Lifestyle
Dysfunction	Pathology
Functional Deficits	Potential
Functional Restoration	Therapeutic Approaches
Impact	

LEARNING OBJECTIVES

Upon completion of this section the reader will be able to:

1. *Identify the characteristics of neurologic, arthritic, orthopedic, cardiac, and pulmonary diagnoses and conditions commonly seen by the occupational therapist.*

2. *Identify clinical manifestations of dysfunction as presented by patients in the designated diagnostic groups.*

3. *Describe specific areas of evaluation and treatment appropriate for specific diagnoses.*

4. *Explain the functional impact and implications of certain disease categories.*

5. *Describe specific therapeutic techniques and adaptations for use with manifestations of dysfunction.*

The focus of this section is on major diagnostic and symptom complexes in neurologic, arthritic, orthopedic, cardiac, and pulmonary conditions commonly seen by the occupational therapist

in clinical and community settings. Specific conditions call for modifications in the application of general concepts presented. Assessment and treatment techniques may be associated with specific symptomatology in the text but may not be limited to those specified.

The occupational therapy program consists of three major areas: (1) *identification* of functional capacities and deficits through evaluation procedures in the assessment process, (2) *development* of functional capacities through the use of specific activities, and (3) *integration* of functional abilities into daily tasks. The occupational therapist and the certified occupational therapy assistant work together with the patient to plan and implement an appropriate program of *functional restoration*. The specific value of this program for the patient is enhanced by effective communication with all people involved with the rehabilitation. Nonprofessional as well as professional people, family, and friends are often included in the comprehensive approach to optimal functional restoration, regaining of a satisfying lifestyle, and setting and implementing of a positive future perspective. Components of the occupational therapy program include setting a therapeutic environment for function, facilitating therapeutic relationships, and establishing programs directed toward therapeutic performance.

Neurologic conditions

Perhaps the most complex manifestation of *functional deficits* and the most difficult rehabilitation challenges arise from neurologic conditions. Neurologic dysfunction is caused by damage to the nervous system but may affect other body systems as well. Major sites of lesions in the nervous system are the brain, the spinal cord and nerve roots, the myoneural junction (between the spinal cord and the muscles), and the extremities. The specific clinical manifestations are determined by the location, type, and extent of the lesion. Symptom complexes are identified as the outcome of trauma or disease. Table 18-1 lists various neurologic conditions according to the location of the lesion, the resulting pathologic or diagnostic condition, the course of the lesion, and the gross areas of clinical manifestation.

The course of a neurologic condition may be *nonprogressive* or *progressive*. Sudden onset of cerebrovascular accident (CVA) (stroke) or head injury, spinal cord injury, Guillain-Barré syndrome, polio, or peripheral nerve injury leaves immediate clinical signs. The symptoms of these trauma and disease effects are *stationary*—they do not increase. The maximal severity of the symptoms occurs at the time of onset. *Progressive* neurologic diseases include MS, Parkinson disease, MG, and ALS, among others. In the course of these diseases, which are discussed in this section, symptoms worsen over time, progressively diminishing functional capacity. Although there may be a similarity in the clinical assessment and treatment of specific deficits associated with these progressive diseases, the long-term pattern of treatment and personal psychological adjustment may differ.

Cerebrovascular accident

A CVA is a lesion in the brain commonly referred to as a stroke, an insult, or a shock because of its sudden onset. It results in paralysis of one side of the body (hemiplegia) or of both sides (bilateral hemiplegia). The lesion is characterized by an inter-

TABLE 18-1.   *Correlation of Location of Lesion with Resultant Pathological Condition, Course, and Organic Manifestations*

Location	Pathologic Condition	Course of Pathology	Manifestations
Brain	Cerebrovascular accident	Nonprogressive	Intellectual
	Head injury	Nonprogressive	Personality
	Multiple sclerosis	Progressive	Sensorimotor
	Parkinson disease	Progressive	Emotional
			Communication
			Physiologic
			Functional
Spinal cord	Amyotrophic lateral sclerosis	Progressive	Physical, physiologic, motor communication
	Poliomyelitis	Nonprogressive	Sensorimotor
	Guillain-Barré syndrome	Nonprogressive	Physiologic
	Spinal cord injury	Nonprogressive	Functional
Myoneural junction	Myasthenia gravis	Progressive	Motor communication
Extremity	Peripheral nerve injury	Nonprogressive	Physical, functional

Note: bracketed manifestations apply to all pathological conditions listed in the group.

ruption of the blood supply to the brain tissues in a particular location, caused by thrombus, embolus, anoxia, hemorrhage, or aneurysm. Precipitating factors may include hypertension, arteriosclerosis, or congenital artery wall weakness. Hypertension and arteriosclerosis contribute to the vessel breakdown or occlusion in the older adult, whereas congenital vascular weakness can result in an aneurysm, a common cause of hemiplegia in the young adult.

Vascular disease can cause a complete CVA with a full picture of hemiplegia or temporary symptoms from a transient ischemic attack (TIA) caused by vascular insufficiency. The TIA may result in brief and spotty impairment of neurologic functions; it is frequently a warning of the likelihood of a more serious CVA in the future. The treatment of the patient with either a complete CVA or a TIA should be geared not only toward rehabilitation of the present problem but also toward prophylactic techniques to prevent further TIA or CVA.

Other causes of hemiplegia include external trauma (a blow on the head or striking the head during a fall), heart attack, and brain and spinal tumors. In these cases, the character of the condition may differ slightly from the cerebrovascular lesion, but because many of the symptoms are similar, evaluation techniques and treatment procedures used in cases of CVA can be applied.

The lesion in the brain that causes hemiplegia usually occurs in one hemisphere and affects the contralateral limbs and face. The result is designated right or left hemiplegia, according to the side of the body involved. It is essential to distinguish between the location of the CVA and the location of the hemiplegia: should the CVA occur in the left hemisphere, the hemiplegia will be on the right side of the body, and vice versa.

Depending on which side of the brain is involved, there can be, in addition to motor and sensory deficits, impairment of perceptual and cognitive functions, of premorbid personality, of motor planning and problem-solving abilities, and of judgment. Urinary continence, motivation, and a sense of social awareness and responsibility may be lost. A lesion can affect both hemispheres of the brain, causing bilateral clinical signs.

Impact

Whether the person is affected by the sudden onset of an internal CVA or by the shock of external head trauma causing hemiplegia, the results of the condition can have a devastating impact on the person's life. The adult patient may be going to school, in preparation for employment, secure in employment, nearing retirement, or retired. In all these situations, the patient may suffer the threat of not returning to the previous lifestyle or occupation. The severity of the brain damage, the premorbid health conditions, the patient's attitude toward the condition and rehabilitation, the support of the family, and the restoration of various functions are all factors in rehabilitation.

Functional restoration

Psychosocial

Whereas the patient's developmental level before the CVA was that of an adult, the effect of the CVA may reduce the physical and mental levels to those of a child. The patient may be unable to accept the arduous recuperation of lost functions through specific "childlike" activities, such as strengthening of limbs and development of coordination; learning again to read, write, and speak; or developing independence in self-care and toilet functions. The patient may be unable to cope with the multitude of problems facing the patient and family, or the patient may suffer damage to those brain tissues that control motivation and adjustment. The adult hemiplegic person tends to look back to normal functioning and impose premorbid standards on present abilities.

Sensorimotor losses are accompanied by changes in body image and personality, which affect both the patient and the family and can strain their relationship. Confusion resulting from brain trauma can leave the patient unable to establish self-direction and purposeful motivation or to understand simple conversations. The effects on the patient's personality may result in a change in values, affecting the level of performance. Because the older adult suffering a CVA has all that has been gained to lose, one of the most difficult problems for both the patient and the therapist is overcoming the belief that the patient has lived his or her life and that there is nothing left.

The following factors contribute to disorientation, confusion, malfunction, and lack of progress:

- Auditory deficit
- Receptive or expressive aphasia
- Impairment of spoken or written expression
- Deficits in learning ability
- Impairment of previously independent function
- Denial and neglect of affected extremities and other functional deficits of the condition
- Distortion of time and place affecting the patient's ability to perceive the future and to plan realistically
- Loss of tactile sensation and motor function
- Loss of proprioceptive and kinesthetic awareness, which hinders integration
- Impaired bilateral extremity function
- Apraxia (loss of voluntary motor activity), which hinders functional ability and motor improvement
- Visual–perceptual deficits, such as field cut (hemianopsia), visual neglect, or deficits in functional scanning, discrimination of color and form, and figure-ground perception

These deficits are not always present, at least not to the same extent.

Mention has been made of the devastating effect of hemiplegia on the person. Not all people, of course, react in the same way to catastrophic illnesses or disabilities. Often, the reactions reflect premorbid taboos and fears. The patient's gains from rehabilitation are, to some degree, dependent on attitudes developed before the CVA.

The patient who is lacking in motivation and is depressed is difficult to rehabilitate and may become a burden to both himself or herself and the family. Often, the patient is the breadwinner or the homemaker, and the loss of ability to carry out these responsibilities affects both the patient and the family. The family may suffer financial hardships because of the hospitalization, and this may be a further worry for the patient. At times, the family needs counseling to understand the course of rehabilitation and to solve the seemingly insurmountable problems of daily living.

The supportive benefits of group activity can be shared through the patient's learning about individual abilities and limitations in physical, communication, and social skills. In structured group activities, patients have the opportunity of working together in performing body movement exercises, projects, recreational activities, or perceptual games, thus stimulating motivation and encouragement. Group work diminishes fear of personal interaction with family and friends and aids in development of self-awareness and acceptance. Helping team members and receiving help restore self-confidence. The therapist teaches the patient to use bilateral movements to stimulate sensorimotor sensitivity and function, right and left orientation, and trunk balance. During physical activity, patients talk with each other and the therapist about what they are doing and how and what they see in the outside environment. Visual–perceptual tasks increase interest in the environment, and the change in atmosphere stimulates new interest and motivation. Group activity aids in integrating sensory, motor, and perceptual skills for improved performance in daily tasks. The peer support gained from group activity relates to social skills the patient needs to return home and to the community.

Communication

Both left and right hemiplegic patients show communication disorders in the early stages after CVA; however, the right hemiplegic person tends to retain more severe deficits in speech, verbal reception, and language because a lesion in the dominant hemisphere (usually the left) affects all language areas to some degree. Specific problems that occur are impairment in interpretation of the meaning of spoken and written words (receptive aphasia), impairment of the ability to use speech and to write communicatively (expressive aphasia), and impairment of motor function of speech (dysarthria). Distorted auditory reception, loss of hearing, and inability to locate auditory stimuli or to make meaning of them can affect the speech response. Apraxia is the impairment of the voluntary ability to use the speech mechanisms; the patient may possess these functions but be unable to use them. Despite apraxia, the patient may be able to use the tongue, lips, or speech mechanisms for automatic and reflexive actions, such as chewing or blowing.

The occupational therapist correlates the use of speech and written language in both instruction-giving and writing exercises with the objectives and functional levels recommended by the speech pathologist. Consistency in language development is important for the patient's improvement and self-confidence as well as for preventing confusion from overstimulation or overexpectation of functional ability.

Cognitive

With the disturbance in sensorimotor reception and expression, the hemiplegic patient frequently demonstrates impairment in abstract reasoning. The severity of this condition depends on the auditory, visual, and tactile abilities that remain intact. Sensory deficits may impede learning through auditory instructions, reading, imitation, and demonstration. The prognosis for restoration of independent function depends on the ability to receive and to organize information for learning and implementation. Careful evaluation of perceptual areas is essential to planning the patient's approaches to learning.

Visual

Double vision (diplopia), loss of half of the visual field (hemianopia), and neglect are three common manifestations of visual impairment. Loss of part of the visual field prevents the patient from seeing objects on the right or left side. Patients are unaware of this "cut" in the visual field until they realize that a paragraph makes little sense because they can read only half of it, until they drive their wheelchairs into the side of a doorway, or until they half dress, thinking the task has been completed.

Visual field neglect occurs when the patient ignores visual stimuli on the side of the hemiplegia when confronted with simultaneous stimuli from both visual fields. This occurs when visual fields are intact (Mossman, 1976). Distortions in the perception of spatial relations (vertical, horizontal, oblique) result in difficulty in deriving meaning from visual stimuli and in using this information in intellectual functions.

Although diplopia can be controlled by an eye patch, it is often difficult for the patient to recognize and compensate for a field cut (hemianopia). Visual cues, practice, and remembering to turn the head to the side of the limited field may be helpful.

Sensorimotor

A lesion in the brain, usually localized in one hemisphere, impairs motor function on the opposite side of the body. Complete (-plegia) or partial (-paresis) flaccid paralysis of the upper and lower musculature and facial muscles is manifested in the loss of active mobility of the involved extremities. Although passive ROM is complete initially, gradual onset of spasticity presents the threat of increased muscle tone, impeding active ROM and causing contractures and deformity. The severity of involvement depends on the location and extent of the lesion. Some patients begin to regain voluntary muscle power a few days after a CVA; others experience no return for months or years; and for some, the ability is never regained. Impairment of the dominant extremity necessitates a change of dominance and causes loss of bilateral coordination with a possibility of partial loss of strength and coordination in the sound extremity.

Sensory impairment is manifested in reduced peripheral reception of stimuli, tactile functions in the affected hand, and general sensory awareness. Manifestations of peripheral impairment include lack of sensation of cutaneous stimuli (temperature, touch, pain); inability to locate the area of stimulus; inability to identify the position of the extremity (proprioception); inability to identify a familiar object through tactile sensation (stereognosis); inability to effect the motor act (apraxia); inability to correlate purpose and accomplishment of tasks (ideational apraxia); and inability to carry out new, purposeful activities while retaining the ability to perform routine activities (ideomotor apraxia). Lack of sensory functions and impairment of sensory receptors in the extremities affect motor functions by causing lack of feedback. Bilateral integrative functions are also affected by sensory deficits.

In all sensorimotor activities, it is important to evaluate the status of sensation and sensory function in the extremities before initiating exercises, activities, self-care, or splinting. Because the objectives of treatment include sensory integration and total body awareness and adaptation, the patient must be informed of the results of the sensorimotor evaluation.

A variety of treatment modalities and approaches are used to aid in the development of isolated and voluntary function of flaccid or spastic extremities. Because synergy patterns may develop after a stroke, the patient may have asymmetric reflexes and sensorimotor behavior. Treatment techniques stemming from neurophysiologic approaches to development of volitional extremity function are effective in occupational therapy programs or in combination with physical therapy. Facilitation and inhibition techniques used appropriately can stimulate independent function.

In the early stage of hemiplegia, the extremity tends to be flaccid, and a major concern is the positioning of the extremity to prevent deformity, contractures resulting from spasticity, and edema. If visual neglect and decreased sensation are present, the patient may be unaware of the arm's position or location. Splinting the extremity helps with visual and sensory awareness of the flaccid extremity and contributes to preventing the above problems. A simple, cock-up splint can aid in wrist positioning for functional use of the extremity. A static, forearm–hand splint can be used at night and during the day when the patient is not working with the extremity in therapy, functional activities, or self-regulated ROM exercises. Snook (1979) suggests the use of a spasticity reduction splint, which incorporates the Bobath technique of using a reflex-inhibiting posture for positioning, using wrist and thumb extension, finger abduction, and extension of the interphalangeal joints. This splint is designed to provide full-pan volar support at fingers and thumb, with dorsal coverage on the forearm and carpal area of the hand. Finger separators are used to maintain finger abduction, with metacarpal flexion at 45

degrees and wrist extension at 30 degrees. A variation of the static forearm–hand pan splint is to set the wrist and fingers at maximal-extension abduction stretch beyond the point of spasticity.

The splint is removed periodically for relaxation, inhibition, and facilitation techniques as appropriate to work toward isolated volitional movements. As the patient begins to regain function, the need for a splint is reassessed to determine wearing time and design alteration, allowing the hand freedom during the day for functional activities while maintaining or allowing for regained function.

In some cases, treatment techniques do not include splinting. Attention to consistent and collaborative therapy techniques is essential for optimal success.

Function

Activities such as rolling over in bed, eating, dressing, bathing, grooming, and two-handed activities are limited by the paralysis of an arm and a leg. Not only are the specific peripheral functions impaired, but the sense of integration of the body is also affected. The patient may find it difficult to adjust to a necessary change in hand dominance. Activities requiring total sensorimotor awareness are affected. The patient may deny or neglect the functional implications of this condition and may grow to depend on others for assistance in daily functions and responsibilities. The rehabilitation program is geared toward maximizing both independence and family awareness and acceptance of the patient's level of function.

Functional activities for developing abilities are geared to the ability level of the patient in all areas previously mentioned. Treatment is directed toward the following goals:

- Maximal active ROM, strength, and coordination of the extremities
- Maximal volitional, unilateral and bilateral function of the upper extremities
- Maximal independence in self-care activities
- Use of assistive devices for increased function as needed
- Awareness and acceptance of functional ability
- Ability to achieve social interaction and basic communication (verbal or nonverbal)
- Prevocational and avocational exploration and planning as appropriate

With the left hemiplegic patient, daily exercises and activities are directed toward increasing sensory awareness and carrying over this awareness into self-care functions. Exercises and activities should develop visual and proprioceptive awareness of the involved extremity, encourage turning of the head to the affected side to include the part missing from sight because of field cut or neglect, and increase the patient's proprioceptive awareness of the involved extremity through developing bilateral functions. Although distortion in body image concepts may hinder self-care independence, the practice of self-care techniques and activities can aid awareness and integration of bilateral functions.

The patient whose limitations in function are primarily in the motor areas (flaccid or moderately spastic extremities, for instance) can learn techniques of self-care fairly easily by using the sound extremities to assist the affected ones.

The occupational therapist assists both right and left hemiplegic patients in self-care eating, dressing, bathing, and grooming tasks as soon as medically possible and incorporates these skills into the patient's daily program. The patient is also encouraged to use one-handed techniques and assistive devices, such as a rocker knife for cutting meat, Velcro attachments on clothes for ease of fastening, and elastic shoe laces. Bathing and grooming are assisted by long-handled sponges, bath mitts, and adapted nail clippers for one-handed use. Use of neurophysiologically based movement and balance techniques is correlated with self-care activities to encourage developmental patterns of reeducation of function, bilateral awareness, and adaptive behavior.

Family education regarding the patient's ability level and areas of need for assistance is essential. Sessions with the patient and the family help to show the family what the patient has achieved, can do, and needs help in accomplishing. This helps to ensure continuation of the patient's ability level upon returning home.

The level of accomplishment in all ADL by the hemiplegic patient is largely dependent on *motivational, perceptual, judgmental,* and *sensory-integrative* factors. Although both right and left hemiplegic patients suffer motor paralysis or limitations, there are distinctions in the effects of the locations of the lesions. Functional areas largely affected by a lesion in the right hemisphere of the brain are those involving motivation, perception, judgment, and sensory integration. Therefore, the left hemiplegic patient may deny the affected extremities, have visual or sensory neglect or denial, have distortions in concepts of movement and spatial relations, have lost the concept of the motor act, or lack motivation for self-improvement. These deficits may be more of a hindrance to function than are motor paralysis and physical limitation. The left hemiplegic patient also is more likely to suffer difficulties in tasks, such as seeing all the food on the plate or finding eating utensils, grooming the left side of the body, dressing the whole body, or walking, than is the right hemiplegic patient. The right hemiplegic person, while also suffering motor paralysis or impairment, usually does not incur the problems with judgment encountered by the left hemiplegic person. The right hemiplegic person, however, shows various degrees of communication disability.

The social implications for reentry into the home and community include adjustment to permanent functional deficits, dependence on assistive equipment (braces, slings, wheelchair), and financial insecurity. The person may no longer be able to drive or to work because of visual and intellectual deficits. Developing a new lifestyle may be necessary.

For the young or middle-aged adult suffering hemiplegia, the effect on vocational potential can be serious. Return to a previous vocation depends in large measure on the type of job the patient was doing, the patient's status in the company, the understanding of the employer, and the patient's ability to regain salable skills. If return to employment is feasible, the occupational therapist includes prevocational assessment and planning in the treatment program and carefully and realistically assists the patient in reviewing alternatives.

The worker who is no longer able to pursue a vocation suffers a loss in self-esteem, self-image, and status in the family and society. Prevocational evaluation for alternative job opportunities and training programs to learn new skills then become part of the rehabilitation program.

Head injury

Head injuries are caused by direct trauma to the skull, with 70% occurring in traffic accidents and falls. Other common causes are industrial accidents, wounds, or direct blows. The resulting trauma includes concussion, contusion, laceration, or compression. Although both skull fractures and brain damage may occur, one can occur without the other. The resultant *state of the brain*, rather than the state of the skull, is the most significant effect of a head injury.

A variety of neurologic symptoms and manifestations can result from head injury. Depending on the location and extent of the lesion, the symptoms may be of short duration, latent, or extended over a period of years. The outcome of rehabilitation is also related to the length of time the person was in a coma: the longer the coma, the poorer the prognosis.

Posttrauma manifestations include occasional loss of consciousness, dizziness, headache, or vertigo provoked by sudden changes in position; confusion and disorientation about time and place; convulsions; and emotional reactions, such as combativeness. Behavioral disturbances may be blatant, particularly during the initial recovery period. Personality disorders, amnesia, and delirium may also occur. These manifestations may be accompanied by intellectual deficits, blindness, diplopia, hemianopsia, olfactory dysfunction, and auditory deficits. Physical symptoms include quadriparesis, unilateral or bilateral hemiparesis, initial decerebrate rigidity, and speech deficits. Restoration of functional, intellectual, social, psychological, and physical manifestations may require years if the injury was severe.

The patient may demonstrate physical and mental deficits similar to those of a person who has suffered CVA: cognitive–perceptual–motor dysfunction, spasticity, disorientation, speech deficits, and disturbance of sensorimotor integration. Mental manifestation and personality changes are often more pronounced than those seen in CVA, even though these patients are generally much younger than stroke victims. These deficits prevent the head-injured person from effectively interacting with the environment and may hinder rehabilitation. The patient may seem to have lost contact with the surroundings and to be able to focus only on the narrow, yet overwhelming, feelings, concerns, and behaviors imposed by the sudden disability.

The functional problems of the patient with brain injury fall into four general categories: (1) cognitive, (2) behavioral and emotional, (3) communicative, and (4) physical. The clinical picture represents a pattern of fluctuating symptoms in these areas, subject to frequent change influenced by internal and external stimuli. This fluctuation is evident throughout the recovery as the patient tries to adjust to the deficits imposed by the injury, to learn to decrease and eliminate handicapping effects, and to renew self-confidence through awareness and acceptance of the immediate and future levels of function. In the early stages, therapeutic support during unknown or confusing occurrences is needed to allay anxiety until the patient gradually regains conscious control of feelings, behaviors, motivation, abilities, relationships, and daily activities.

Impact

The trauma of head injury causes significant personal impact. The patient must deal with the residual manifestations with whatever assets can be retrieved from the premorbid life experience. The following areas are common rehabilitation challenges of the brain-injured patient and are described briefly to give a general clinical picture of this patient; however, not all patients show the symptoms, nor do they show them to the same extent. Premorbid characteristics of lifestyle, body health and type, achievement, attitudes, and goals may positively or negatively affect the functional outcome. Also, since many head injuries are caused by traffic accidents and falls, there may be accompanying physical disabilities, such as amputations, peripheral nerve injuries, paralysis, or fractures, that add to the complexity of adequate treatment.

The long-term impact of brain injury may interfere with learning ability, cognitive integration, social interaction and status, self-esteem, and motivation for personal goal setting and achievement.

Functional restoration

Recovery scales have been developed in an attempt to determine prognosis and to outline programs appropriate to the patient's abilities. Information from these scales aids in the coordination of goals and methods used by team members. There is some tendency to model scales on the developmental patterns of cognitive or intellectual function, behavior, and social, motivational, and motor levels.

The Developmental Assessment of Recovery from Serious Head Injury method uses four chronologic segments of development to determine areas and levels of function:

0 to 4 years, using functions from infant scales
4 to 8 years, using items from the Stanford-Binet Intelligence Scale
8 to 12 years, using tests for basic information processing, including sequencing, left and right differentiation, and visual perception
Mature adaptive function, including concepts, skills, and information processing related to daily activity performance (Eson, Yen, & Bourke, 1978)

The Disability Rating Scale uses the following eight categories from the Glasgow Coma Scale to rate the head injury according to specific functional area: (1) eye opening, (2) verbalization, (3) motor response, (4) feeding, (5) toileting, (6) grooming, (7) level of functioning, and (8) employability (Rappaport, 1980). The Glasgow Coma Scale indicates eye, motor, and verbal response levels, whereas the Glasgow Outcome Scale consists of five stages related to the ability to work: (1) death, (2) persistent vegetative state, (3) severe physical and mental disability (cannot work), (4) moderate disability, and (5) good recovery with continuing emotional problems but can work. (Jennett & Bond, 1975; Jennett & Teasdale, 1977).

Eson and colleagues state that the quality of neuropsychologic recovery is highly variable in rate, pattern, and level of recovery of adaptive function. Levels of adaptive function are defined as follows: *early*—ADL, self-care, and rudimentary social interaction; *middle*—conceptual and information-processing skills needed for social interaction and ability to initiate and carry out sustained, planned activities directed toward a goal; and *complete or near complete*—ability to seek and maintain employment and to participate in normal adult social and recreational activities without supervision (Eson et al., 1978).

In the effort to plan and implement effective and appropriate rehabilitation for the brain-injured person, a variety of approaches have been developed by professional teams and researchers. Whatever the structure or organization of methods of treatment used by the occupational therapist, it is essential that they relate meaningfully to programs and techniques used by others in the daily care of the patient.

The program at Loewenstein Hospital Rehabilitation Center identifies three stages relative to the medical picture based on behavioral characteristics. The first phase is *postcoma*, characterized by dreamlike disorientation in time and space, causing disturbances in establishing order and relationships within environmental stimuli. The second stage is *behavioral*, characterized by increasing consciousness of the outside world but continuing disturbance in interpreting and handling stimuli, resulting in anxiety and stress fatigue. In the third phase, the patient begins to enter a period of *realism* and experiences a series of conflicting but realistic changes in self-awareness, which result in a variety of emotional responses. During this stage, the struggle to identify with the external environment satisfactorily and functionally and to integrate external and internal experiences and meanings occurs (Stern, 1978).

In its approach to rehabilitative management, the Rancho Los Amigos Hospital program describes eight progressive levels of cognitive functioning and behavioral responses based on developmental order: (1) no response (coma), (2) generalized response (inconsistent and nonpurposeful), (3) localized response (specific but inconsistent response to stimuli), (4) confused and agitated (heightened state of activity with decreased ability to process information), (5) confused, inappropriate, and nonagitated, (6) confused and appropriate, (7) automatic and appropriate, and (8) purposeful and appropriate. Beginning with the initial assessment, the treatment team determines at which level the patient is functioning and then administers treatment in accordance with this developmental pattern. (Hagan, Malkmus, & Durham, 1972). The occupational therapy approach depends on the rehabilitation program in the individual setting and the use of such scales as mentioned above.

In preparing for the functional assessment of the brain-injured patient, the therapist must think of the long-term effects of short-term care. This begins with the patient's first contact with the therapist. The initial interview should take place in an area physically comfortable, with few auditory and visual distractions. Input received during early periods may be stored for future use when the patient is more capable of volitional behavior; attention to therapeutic and functional positioning informs the patient of the therapist's concern for comfort as well as conveying the expectation of active, functional use of his or her body. Repeated abnormal functioning can contribute to later weakness and deformities of both the trunk and the extremities.

Having evaluated the effect of the physical environment, the therapist observes the patient's social reactions to the therapist and to other people in the area. Through discussion with the patient and family, the therapist obtains a picture of what the patient was like before the injury. This information helps in planning therapeutic programs related to the patient's interests. It is also important to know what accomplishments, failures, dreams, plans, and specific areas of activity played a significant role in the personal and social life before the head injury. Since the patient may suffer amnesia with regard to information about premorbid life or the injury, or experience language deficits resulting in reception or expression inadequacies, questions regarding these areas may cause anxiety, irritability, or confusion. Gentle encouragement to discuss the accident assists the patient in clarifying and accepting the medical situation and in understanding why he or she is receiving treatment. It also provides a check on the patient's accuracy of information. This helps prevent the build-up of anxieties regarding the unknowns of the past, present, and future by providing an outlet for self-expression and discussion of changing feelings and concerns.

The patient may experience the following symptoms during initial evaluation and treatment:

Postural dizziness: sensation of dizziness or disorientation caused by change of position or quick movements of the head; dizziness may also result from exertion or fatigue

Headache: intermittent or persistent headache, pain, feeling of pressure in the head

Fatigue: related to extent and length of time of physical or mental effort during activity

Eye strain: due to intensive light, contrasting colors, or movement of visual stimuli, weakness in focus or interpretation

Hypersensitivity: to sudden, loud, or multiple noises or movements in the immediate physical area

The point at which the patient is seen by the therapist—in the acute stage of trauma, the early rehabilitation phase, the outpatient stage, or during home treatment—determines the nature and extent of evaluation and the treatment programs appropriate. At all levels, continual communication between the therapist and the patient is essential with regard to changes in the treatment goals, progress, and the patient's motivation and goals.

Treatment begins with assessment of a communication method, sensorimotor deficits, orientation, and functional ability. The patient is then treated *symptomatically*, with the program directed toward self-awareness, awareness of objects, and initiation and accomplishment of purposeful activity. Development of motor strength and coordination is combined with activities to encourage social awareness and interaction with others. Graded intellectual and problem-solving tasks (reading, arithmetic, and writing) aid the patient in regaining function.

Treatment may begin with basic visual and tactile discrimination and sensorimotor activities, such as self-care skills, exercise, activities, and games. Initially, the occupational therapist works with the patient in quiet surroundings, gradually increasing the auditory and visual stimuli. The patient is provided with activity simple enough to hold his or her interest. As physical and mental tolerance increase, the therapist can expand the complexity of the environment.

Psychosocial aspects

The clinical response may be characterized by bewilderment, confusion, denial, anger, complacency, or hostility, with fluctuating changes in behavior related to the individual stage of self-awareness and the level of adaptation to self and environment. Short-term or chronic personality changes may occur, beginning with denial and vagueness in response or with hyperactivity, depending on the level of consciousness and the severity of injury to brain tissue. Disturbance in the ability to relate to the outside environment and to time outside of the present may be apparent. Expressed desires and needs may relate to self-concerns and comforts.

The patient may represent a totally new person to the family. The therapist learns about the patient *as the person the patient has become* and is challenged to help the family understand and accept that person. The family helps the therapist learn what type of person the patient was before the injury so the therapist will understand the amount and type of change that both the family and the patient are experiencing.

The patient may demonstrate loss of inhibitions, distortions in judgment, personality changes, and denial of reality. The patient may lack awareness of the meaning of the present situation. Since the patient may be unable to differentiate appropriate and nonappropriate social behavior, he or she may benefit from techniques such as behavior modification, group process, reality orientation, and other psychodynamic methods of social adjustment and self-awareness.

In working with the patient suffering manifestations of brain injury, it is important to provide an atmosphere free from overwhelming and confusing input and challenges to the sensory systems. Reassurance regarding the program's content, duration, and expectations helps the patient relax enough to respond to specific treatment techniques. The therapist can limit anxiety by talking about the physical surroundings, what is going on, and feelings about where the patient is, what the patient is doing, and how the patient is doing. This helps with reality orientation, resocialization, and environmental adaptation.

Working through the stages of denial, anger, and depression to self-awareness and acceptance requires physical and emotional endurance and often results in fatigue or decreased motivation for continuing the struggle. When the patient is able and ready to begin to deal with the realities of the situation, discussions with the therapist about the injury help reassure the patient, may clarify what has happened, put present and future goals and concerns into perspective, promote self-understanding, and help the patient adjust to changes. As adjustment occurs, the patient is able to take on more responsibility in decision making by planning and implementing daily schedules and evaluating progress.

The patient may have difficulty in adapting to people and things and may deny reality, forcing others to relate to him or her. Disturbance in self-awareness may allow fantasizing regarding both condition and behavior, and feelings of unfairness regarding the condition may be expressed. Striving for stability and control, the patient may react poorly to change and time, showing a tendency toward minimal social initiative and occasionally showing suspicion of other people who are attempting to help. Disorder in judgment may contribute to an emphasis on physical problems rather than on psychological difficulties relating to cognition and behavior.

Self-awareness develops through active involvement of the mind and body. Task-oriented individual and group projects can provide opportunities to develop and practice abilities and to reintegrate the positive and negative aspects of functioning. Group projects can extend participation in and responsibility for social activities by demonstrating productivity and skill. Group discussions provide social feedback as to acceptable and nonacceptable behaviors and provide opportunities to change behaviors as necessary or desired.

The use of videotaping during activity gives the patient a visual picture of his or her physical and social behavior, which can be viewed privately, critically, and objectively. In viewing the group, the patient is able to distinguish between himself or herself and others and to engage in cognitive development. Working within the group helps the patient practice social skills useful in developing and maintaining successful contacts with family members, friends, and strangers.

Social awareness, visual tolerance, concentration, and cognitive functioning and adaptation are stimulated by participating in group discussions and activities, listening to the radio, watching television, playing electronic games, reading books, and reading the newspaper. Gradual increase in responsibility in social and productive activities helps to increase familiarity and function in the environment. In the rehabilitation process, it is important for the patient to be able to adapt to the distractions of unfamiliar environments in the community to be socially adjusted and independent.

Communication

In using language to communicate with the patient and to stimulate functional response, it is essential that the occupational therapist follow the guidance of the speech pathologist to maintain consistency in the aspects and levels of the patient's language development.

Finding a means of response is the initial task of the occupational therapist. Use of physical demonstration followed by imitation by the patient may provide a means of communication for the patient with severe language deficits. Although unable to respond orally, the patient may be able to read and write words or symbols.

The patient who is unable to engage in normal verbal communication is often denied satisfying social interaction and opportunities for personal, educational, and social development. Selection of appropriate equipment for functional communication is preceded by an evaluation of other equipment being used, the cognitive level of function, and optimal body positioning.

Electronic and battery-operated communication aids can assist in the evaluation of deficits as well as in retraining programs to develop skills to apply to educational, vocational, and avocational pursuits. These aids are equipped with computer mechanisms that provide feedback through a visual or auditory signal, indicating physical and cognitive functional abilities and levels. Devices can be activated by a variety of sources (head turning, mouthstick, light touch, breath control, muscle contractions, and pointing). Use of communication aids by the occupational therapist reinforces the efforts of the speech pathologist in developing physical and cognitive skills and in providing consistency of newly learned techniques. Head sets are useful in minimizing auditory distractions during retraining.

The occupational therapist provides input to the rehabilitation team regarding physical ROM, strength, coordination, and endurance needed to activate the equipment as well as with regard to the patient's ability to scan visual input effectively for use of the device. Strip printers or a typewriter may be included to provide additional feedback.

With the development of computer systems, electronic aids are increasingly available and adaptable to the disabled person in treatment, at home, or at work. The use of electronic games assists both the child and the adult in adaptation of these systems for practical purposes. A variety of communication aids can be mounted on a wheelchair or on a desk table and can be powered by rechargeable batteries for practical use (see Chapter 9, Section 6).

Cognition

Memory deficits may prevent the patient from remembering or recognizing people or events from day to day; therefore, continual repetition of tasks and symbols might be necessary until memory is extended. Establishing routines of activity and expecting the patient to perform in consistent patterns may be useful, as may behavior modification techniques.

Memory is needed for visualization and learning. In working with a patient with a memory deficit, attention is given to determining the number of steps in a task the patient is able to store and retrieve. Exercises can be devised to test and practice memory for past events, types of things remembered, retention time, and carry-over to future planning. Planning and scheduling practice are increased by individual and group exercises in visualization of current events and future events and with carry-over from the day with application to planning. Organization of time is improved by the patient's taking responsibility for scheduling daily activities, accepting responsibilities with time limits, achieving carry-over of activities, and reinforcing time and space concepts.

The level of mental tolerance is related to motivation, functional deficits, and amount of adaptation required to carry out instructions. The patient may display a short attention span, distractibility, and fear of insanity, particularly when blindness, disorientation, amnesia, or a combination of physical, psychological, and intellectual manifestations are present. Techniques to increase mental tolerance include relating a task to an interest area (sports, reading, cooking, or puzzles), using repetition to provide practice of specific skills to reinforce methods of performance, and providing feedback regarding ability. The program should be graded to gradually increase skill and challenge and should use time blocks to increase physical and mental tolerance. Through the therapeutic group experience, the patient gains a broader social reality focus, learns coping skills for working with others, and practices assertiveness training for self-confidence.

Performance may be hindered by general limitations in adjusting to environmental stimuli. Controlling such strong stimuli as the bright light of the sun, loud or sudden noises, or the distracting sounds of people talking is useful. For maximal selective response to the therapist, the patient may initially require an area void of visual and auditory stimuli. As tolerance for stimuli increases, the therapist gives meaning and relevance to gradually increased stimuli and assists the patient in focusing attention while in the presence of distracting sights and sounds.

Sensorimotor aspects

The patient initially may be defensive tactually, hypersensitive, or apraxic or may demonstrate lack of coordination caused by tremor or ataxia. Spasticity may develop later in the recuperation period. Evaluation of reflex patterns revealing abnormal tone in the brain-injured patient shows three major patterns: (1) decerebrate rigidity or extensor pattern of all extremities, (2) decortication rigidity flexor pattern in the arms, or (3) a mixed pattern of upper-extremity (UE) flexion and lower-extremity (LE) extension. Increased muscle tone produces trunk rigidity, which may result in poor sitting balance. Lack of control of the trunk muscles may also result in poor sitting patterns. The patient may be sensitive to touch and may lack volitional movement.

Before functional activity programs focusing on the upper extremities can be carried out effectively, the patient must be able to maintain a functional sitting position and balance without using the arms for support. Special equipment may be necessary to achieve this, including aids for position and control. Neurophysiologic therapy techniques assist the patient in regaining head control, trunk rotation, equilibrium, trunk extension, trunk balance, and arm relaxation for independent isolated control and function.

Function

Since a patient commonly uses denial to avoid seeing the reality of an imposed traumatic situation, involvement in activity programs not only helps to increase strength, joint ROM, coordination, and cognitive function but also provides feedback to the patient regarding his or her actual abilities. The focus is on the *increase in ability*. Activities are chosen to provide the patient with the means to express anger and hostility as well as to assist in the development of speed, accuracy, and competence in productive accomplishment of specific tasks.

Participation in individual and group physical activities assists the patient in adapting to and overcoming the effects of dizziness. Activities that necessitate changing body position in space (woodworking, gardening, shuffleboard, and table tennis) help in vestibular adaptation.

Specific physical activities provide increased self-awareness and self-worth through increases in joint ROM, strength, and coordination. The programs must be correlated with other functional areas, such as perception, social interaction, behavior, and tolerance of environmental stimuli. In preparing for discharge, the patient needs to know what he or she can and cannot do safely and competently. The patient develops and practices physical functions in a compatible, supportive environment and is encouraged to learn adaptation when necessary. Decreasing symptoms such as spasticity, contracture, apraxia, tremor, and pain is part of the physical restoration program used to increase functional abilities.

While in a treatment setting, the patient learns how to live in a controlled and structured environment. In preparation for discharge, the patient must learn how to adapt to other environments as well as how to exercise control over his or her goals and behaviors and plan daily activities and responsibilities. Independent attitudes and functions, beginning with self-care skills, are developed, and the patient progresses to being responsible for scheduling time and organizing activities. The patient chooses clothes and retrieves them from drawers and closets and takes care of grooming and other needs in preparation for daily activities. Independence in the structured treatment setting prepares the patient for discharge planning.

Other commonly needed skills, including using a pay telephone and telephone book, reading a map, listening to and following directions, organizing appointments, applying for a job, and using a newspaper, can be practiced during individual and group outings.

The patient may maintain the delusion that going home will improve the condition or, conversely, that he or she is unwanted or unneeded at home. Family awareness of residual impairments and needs at discharge from the formal rehabilitation program is encouraged in predischarge orientation and guidance sessions. By attending predischarge therapy and group sessions with the patient and the therapists, the family members can see how they can assist with the program and how to welcome the patient back into family life. Sharing in group sessions with other families is helpful to both the family and the patient.

Family orientation to specific problems (memory deficits, reduced tolerance of external stimuli, physical or communications problems) is important before the patient begins resocialization with weekend visits at home. These visits often show the family and the patient what has been accomplished and how much work remains to be done.

Outings from the treatment center or from home help the patient communicate and assume socially appropriate behavior regarding activities and interaction with others. Such activities may include those available through adult programs or church groups. Community activities include such familiar tasks as crossing streets, using money, finding restrooms, reading menus, ordering food, buying things in a store, and paying bills.

The patient's educational and employment goals depend on overcoming intellectual and judgmental deficits as well as developing integrative abilities. Learning, retraining, work adjustment, and development of social skills and work habits may be necessary for vocational readiness.

The level of pretrauma intellectual functioning and the achieved educational level affect the regaining of vocational potential. In regaining the ability to return to work, the brain-injured person is more likely to be hindered by cognitive, behavioral, and social difficulties in performance than by physical deficits. Regaining a positive self-image, independence in self-care, physical and mental tolerance, successful social contact and interaction, capability in cognitive and intellectual functioning, and acceptable work habits contributes to vocational potential for the well-motivated person.

During functional retraining, the patient with vocational potential is provided with opportunities to work on familiar skills and those needed for his or her job. Levels of cognitive, social, behavioral, and physical function are determined through prevocational assessment techniques to evaluate the need for retraining or vocational redirection.

Return to work may begin on a part-time basis. Retraining and relocating may be necessary to ensure employment of the patient who is able to work in some capacity but unable to return to a previous occupation at the earlier level of performance. Although premature return to work requiring strenuous physical or mental effort is strongly discouraged, too long a rest from the routine of work may be detrimental to the person capable of employment.

Outpatient follow-up provides physical and psychological support during the transition from hospital or rehabilitation center to family and community reentry. Through this type of program, the patient can continue therapy outside the structured setting. This may help the patient adjust to less structured surroundings and develop confidence to plan daily activities and responsibilities.

Multiple sclerosis

Multiple or disseminated sclerosis is a progressive disease of the nervous system. It begins with the destruction of the myelin sheath covering the nerve fibers, which interferes with the transmission of impulses and results in fatigue. The degenerated sheath is replaced eventually by sclerotic plaques or patches that affect the white matter of the brain and spinal cord. These plaques may also be found in the gray matter of the cerebral cortex and in the cranial and spinal cord roots (Brain & Walton, 1969).

Impact

Characterized by intermittent exacerbations and remissions, MS may pursue its unpredictable course for many years. It usually affects young adults (ages 20 to 40) during their period of greatest potential and productivity. Although the cause of the disease is unknown, viral infections, pregnancy, surgery, and trauma may be precipitating factors. Change in climate, fatigue from overwork, and poor dietary habits have also been implicated. Nervous tension and irritability may precede the onset of physical symptoms, which may vary in intensity, character, duration, and location.

The clinical picture may be hemiplegia, paraplegia, or quadriplegia, and the patient's prognosis and life span are variable. Although the average life span of a person with MS may be 20 years, it can range from 3 months to 40 years; remissions can last as long as 25 years (Bannister, 1973). There may be long and almost complete remissions in the early stages of the disease. After middle age, however, the disease often progresses.

Symptoms appear in two general modes. The first is characterized by a single lesion or several isolated lesions that result in neuritis, double vision, weakness in a limb, or numbness in a part of the body. The second is insidious and is manifested as a slowly progressive weakness of one or all limbs. Accompanying spinal symptoms include spastic paraplegia, superficial sensory loss in the lower limbs and trunk, impairment of postural sensibility and sense of vibration, and spastic or atactic gait (Bannister, 1973). Decreased sexuality, loss of self-esteem, and anxiety may be evident.

Common early signs of MS include nystagmus (lateral oscillation of an eye to one or both sides), slight intention tremor in one or both upper limbs, and exaggeration of tendon reflexes. These initial symptoms may disappear over a period of weeks or months, leaving only slight residual physical signs; however, the cumulative effects of multiple lesions later cause permanent changes in personality (Bannister, 1973).

The symptoms of advanced MS include scanning or staccato speech and slurring of syllables, nystagmus, dissociation of conjugate lateral movement of the eyes, weak and grossly atactic upper limbs, paraplegia, contractures, sensory loss, incontinence, episodes of euphoria and depression, irritability, impairment of postural sensibility, and astereognosis.

Although muscular wasting or atrophy are rare, motor weakness may appear in the extremities, trunk, and face. The patient may experience a feeling of heaviness in the spastic extremities and may lose postural sensibility in limbs and trunk.

Incoordination is a frequent problem for the patient with MS. Intention tremor on involuntary movement is accompanied by muscle imbalance in hands and arms, and the tremor may develop in head movements during the later stages of the disease. When the patient must perform tasks requiring accurate movement, the tremor may increase, resulting in incoordination. Ataxia is evident in the gross movements of both the upper and the lower extremities.

The patient suffers sensory deficits manifested by numbness, impairment of positional and joint sense, fine tactile discrimination, hypersensitivity to contact, impaired postural sensibility and vibration sense, and astereognosis.

The ability to communicate orally may be hindered by dysarthria caused by spastic weakness or ataxia of the muscles of articulation. In some instances, the speech impairment may become so severe as to render the patient unintelligible.

In some cases, the patient with MS displays only ocular symptoms for many years. Although the patient's vision usually improves within a few weeks of the initial onset of symptoms, residual damage to the optic nerve is manifested in atrophy. Sporadic unilateral blindness or diplopia may occur.

The patient may exhibit some reduction in intellectual efficiency and some emotional changes; the patient may suffer wildly contrasting moods, going from euphoria to depression quickly. Conceptual thinking, memory, attention span, and judgment may be affected. These fluctuations in mental and physical ability are characteristic and must be considered during evaluation and treatment. The patient has gradual and intermittent loss of physical and mental control, resulting in emotional reactions and irritability.

Functional restoration

During evaluation and treatment, the therapist provides encouragement and support regarding the patient's fluctuating capabilities. Because the patient is prone to anxiety and tension, the occupational therapist emphasizes maintenance of functional abilities and stresses avoidance of chill or fatigue and of situations in which injury may occur. The patient may feel good at the start of the day. Energy diminishes in the afternoon, resulting in taking chances that may result in an accident. Decreased sensation, incoordination, transient blindness, and impaired judgment can create life-threatening conditions for the patient with MS. Evaluation areas include the following:

- Physical abilities of the extremities: strength, joint ROM, coordination, and balance
- Intention tremor: ataxia, paresthesia, sensory function
- Visual acuity and perception
- Level of self-care independence
- Level of functional independence and tolerance
- Psychological and intellectual functions
- Behavior, emotional stability, and adjustment to disabilities

General treatment goals include the following:

- Maintenance of passive and active joint ROM
- Prevention of spasticity, contractures, deformities, and decubitus
- Optimal functional independence
- Maximal coordination, strength, and function of extremities
- Understanding and acceptance of the nature and course of the disease
- Ability to reach maximal functional level of activity
- Awareness of and use of assistive devices as needed generally and for self-care

Treatment consists of providing the patient with exercises and activities that present graded resistance to weak muscles, prevent substitution patterns from developing, and employ repetition to encourage physical endurance. The occupational therapist must pay close attention to the fatigue factor because the patient may not recognize or admit fatigue.

The patient should be encouraged to engage in exercises and activities that employ all the extremities, but the patient may become discouraged with hand activities if sensation and coordination are poor and if intention tremor is prevalent. If the patient has the muscle power and endurance, activities should be performed from both a seated and a standing position.

The patient may need assistive devices and reeducation in ADL; the patient should be encouraged to participate in social functions to maintain the ability to relate to family and friends.

In all activities, the patient must be assisted in adjusting to the *progression* of the disability. The patient may deny the gradually worsening condition and become euphoric in an attempt to hide the lack of acceptance and to ward off depression. Euphoria may prevent acceptance of assistive devices and may cause establishment of unrealistic goals. The occupational therapist can aid in the establishment of realistic long-term and short-term goals, maintenance of self-care, and avoidance of anxiety.

Setting a daily schedule of activity that provides rest and productivity within the capability and endurance of the person with MS is essential to maintaining the optimal functional level. Activities, including self-care, homemaking, family responsibilities, education, prevocational exploration, and avocational involvement, can be explored in the treatment program. Education of the patient and family can assist all family members in adjusting to the fluctuating abilities as well as in accepting adaptation for productive and satisfying living. Community agencies, such as the Multiple Sclerosis Society, provide helpful resources and general support.

Parkinson disease

Parkinson disease is a slowly progressive condition caused by the degeneration of neurons in the substantia nigra and globus pallidus, resulting in damage to the basal ganglia of the brain. This chronic condition may be precipitated by carbon monoxide and manganese poisoning, encephalitis, senile brain changes, or arteriosclerosis.

Impact

Occurring between the ages of 40 and 80 years, Parkinson disease causes the gradual loss of physical abilities, resulting in interference with lifestyle, changes in appearance and behavior, loss of employment, and depression.

The disturbance in motor function is characterized by slowing of emotional responses and voluntary movement, muscular rigidity and weakness, slowly spreading tremor, and a shuffling gait. Symptoms may appear over a period ranging from months to years, with stationary periods of nonprogressive symptoms. The symptom complex may be variable in specific types of Parkinson disease. Gradually, the person assumes a physical attitude of immobility, with masklike facial expressions, staring eyes, and loss of free movements of the limbs and rotary movements of the spine. The arms and trunk tend toward flexion, with adduction at the shoulders. Loss of tenodesis action in the distal joints produces a tendency toward stiff wrist extension, finger flexion at the metacarpophalangeal joints, and extension at the phalangeal joints. Development of fibrous tissue in the joints causes contractures, with resultant atrophy of muscles due to decreased voluntary movement.

Movements are characteristically slow, with the patient demonstrating difficulty in initiating movement, weakness in voluntary movements, and loss of associated movements. Intrinsic movements are awkward and uncoordinated, resulting in loss of manual dexterity. General reduction of joint ROM affects oral articulation, causing slurring of speech, decreased volume, and monotone sound. There is a tendency to drool. Chest excursion may be limited due to muscular rigidity, thus decreasing the vital capacity.

Involuntary movements of the extremities are generally described as a jerky, "cogwheel" tremor or a smooth, "lead-pipe" rigidity. These common manifestations may be unequal on the two sides of the body. Tremor is characterized by rhythmic, alternating movement of the opposing muscle groups simulating a "pill-rolling" motion of the thumb and fingers at the metacarpophalangeal joints. The tremor may shift from one muscle group to another. It is usually present when the patient is at rest and diminishes when the patient voluntarily moves the limb; the tremor increases with emotional excitement, although it can be inhibited temporarily by conscious effort. As the disease progresses, rigidity becomes more pronounced, with resultant limitations in joint ROM due to contractures and muscle atrophy. The rigidity can cause muscular pain but does not result in sensory loss.

The typical gait is easily recognized: slow, with shuffling, small steps and a tendency toward lurching. The person shows a flexed or bent position, and the rigid, decreased mobility gives the appearance of the body's moving all at once, propelled by momentum and unable to stop quickly. Balance is poor. The patient is described as having a festinating gait, hurrying with small steps in a bent attitude as if trying to catch up with the center of gravity (Brain & Walton, 1969).

Functional restoration

The evaluation begins with complete assessment of the manifestations of the symptoms. The degree of involvement is noted, as is the impact on functional activities. The following areas are included:

- Passive joint ROM: presence of contractures
- Active joint ROM: characteristics of movement
- Presence and characteristics of tremor and rigidity
- Sitting and standing balance, tolerance, and characteristics
- Presence of pain or other discomfort
- Functional abilities: self-care, ADL, communication, coordination, strength, reach, grasp
- Employment status and potential
- Emotional status
- Avocational interests and abilities
- Home situation, lifestyle, social interests, and responsibilities

The goals of treatment are directed toward assisting the patient to achieve a positive attitude toward his or her abilities and to accept the gradual decrease in ability. To maintain the maximal functional level and to prevent rigidity, it is essential to involve the patient in a daily pattern of continual activity to maintain complete active joint ROM, strength, and productivity. The course of formalized treatment should be related to a home program so that the patient can continue to do activities that are meaningful. This helps prevent the patient from becoming immobile owing to depression caused by loss of abilities and skills. The treatment program is developed by both the patient and the therapist to achieve maximal use of movement and to maintain activity tolerance. Treatment goals include the following:

1. Maintain maximal independence in functional activities to prevent limitations from rigidity or tremor.
2. Maintain complete reciprocal joint ROM; prevent contractures.
3. Encourage therapeutic breathing patterns and chest expansion; integrate the breathing patterns with daily activities.
4. Encourage increase of speed and coordination in movement.

5. Encourage independence in self-care; provide **adaptive techniques** or assistive devices.
6. Develop activity tolerance and increase endurance.
7. Increase activity interests to maintain social, physical, and functional mobility.
8. Provide therapeutic group program for social participation and adaptation.
9. Educate the patient and family regarding the necessity for a home program of good physical habits, exercise, and activity to maintain mobility and motivation.
10. Provide a home program of self-care, homemaking, productive activity, recreation, and community involvement for continued mobility.

Treatment includes graded resistive exercises to increase strength and coordination, gross motor activities to encourage general mobility and to increase chest excursion, fine patterns of movement for maintenance of productive abilities, maximal independence in self-care and ADL, and encouragement of motivation, self-esteem, and socialization.

Because the gradual development of rigidity and immobility are characteristic of Parkinson disease, auditory stimulation, such as music, can be used to encourage body mobility through rhythmic marching, dancing, clapping, and singing, either individually or in groups. Participation in groups also provides needed support and encouragement to maintain mobility in spite of continuing symptoms.

Sports can be used for motivation, socialization, and movement; ball-throwing, table tennis, darts, and shuffleboard also increase strength and speed of movement in all extremities. In gross motor activities, balance, coordination, and breathing patterns are emphasized.

Manual activities can be used to maintain gross and fine motor coordination, strength, and concentration since these are required for general self-care functions. Activities should be designed to encourage good posture, increase mobility, and stimulate successful accomplishment. Manual activities can also be related to assessing and developing vocational skills to enable the patients to keep their jobs. Although patients may experience a change in job activities or responsibilities, it is essential to maintain their daily work status as long as possible.

Broadening of social contact and activity interests helps encourage continuing mobility and productivity programs at home. Patient and family education aids in ensuring the continuation of these activities. To assist the family and the patient in planning daily activity programs, the therapist can guide them to the resources of the National Parkinson Foundation, which is a valuable organization for the consumer, providing helpful information on the disease, on exercise, and on activities to maintain mobility.

Amyotrophic lateral sclerosis

Amyotrophic lateral sclerosis is a chronic, systemic disease of unknown cause that affects the corticospinal system from the cortex to the periphery. It is characterized by degenerative changes that are most evident in the anterior horn cells of the spinal cord, motor nuclei of the medulla, and corticospinal tracts. The loss of nerve cells causes progressive wasting of the muscles, particularly those in the upper extremities and those innervated by the medulla (Brain & Walton, 1969). The onset of ALS is gradual, and the disease is steadily progressive, with death generally occurring within 1 to 6 years (Alpers & Mancall, 1971). ALS is nonhereditary.

Impact

The symptoms of ALS may first occur either in muscles most used by the patient in his or her occupation or at the site of an injury (Brain & Walton, 1969). Muscular atrophy usually begins in the intrinsic muscles of the hands and the arm musculature; the patient complains of weakness, stiffness, and clumsiness of the fingers. Although the onset usually is centered symmetrically in the upper extremities, it can vary in location and severity. Thenar and finger flexor atrophy generally precede atrophy of the extensors.

Weakness extends proximally from the hands to the shoulders. From the shoulders, the weakness moves to the tongue, where atrophy and paresis of the lips, tongue, and palate cause slurred speech, which eventually becomes unintelligible. The ability to swallow is also affected. As the extensors become involved, weakness in the trunk, loss of head control, and LE paralysis occur; eventually, all reflexes are lost.

Functional restoration

ALS is treated symptomatically to maintain nutrition, to prevent fatigue, to prevent respiratory infections, and to avoid exposure to cold. Drugs can be used to control problems in swallowing, spasticity, and respiratory and urinary infections.

The rehabilitation program includes moderate activity to maintain strength through muscle reeducation and passive exercises to prevent contractures. The exercise program provides relaxation and alleviation of spasticity. Self-care techniques require the use of assistive devices to substitute for the gradual loss of motor function, including respiratory failure. Gait training with braces is used when the patient can tolerate standing.

The occupational therapist provides both physical and psychological assistance in the development of coping skills. Therapeutic techniques and activities should be used with care to maximize functional benefit and minimize fatigue. Passive ROM by the occupational therapist can provide relaxation in addition to maintaining maximal ROM in the joints. The passive ROM exercises should be followed by a short, active exercise period determined by the patient's muscle power.

Assistive equipment can help the patient to retain as much function as possible and to remain active as long as possible. A wheelchair, suspension slings, arm supports, and positioning aids can stimulate the patient to socialize, to provide self-care, and to engage in activities that provide a day-to-day enjoyment of life. Environmental control systems or attendant care may be necessary in the later stages of ALS as the patient loses mobility in the extremities.

Poliomyelitis

Because of the extensive use of effective vaccines, poliomyelitis is no longer prevalent in children's hospitals or in adult rehabilitation centers. The occupational therapist occasionally encounters a patient who has had polio, however, which complicates the current admission for treatment. Also, in a prevocational or vocational program, the therapist may need to evaluate the functional ability of a client who has had polio.

Polio, a lower motor neuron (LMN) lesion, is an acute infectious disease caused by a virus that can affect the anterior horn cells of the gray matter of the spinal cord and the motor nuclei of the brain stem (Bannister, 1973). The result is immediate, widespread or localized muscular paralysis with subsequent atrophy. The paralysis may be asymmetric and patchy, resulting in long-term paralysis in some muscles of one limb but not in others, causing an imbalance. Although the lower limbs are more often affected than the upper limbs, there may be complete or partial monoplegia, hemiplegia, paraplegia, or quadriplegia. Sensation is intact.

The symptoms include loss of cutaneous and tendon reflexes in the affected muscles, flaccid paralysis of the muscles affected, atrophy, subluxation of adjacent joints, general body weakness, respiratory and circulatory effects, and imbalance of muscle power. Contractures can occur in stronger muscles because of weakness of the antagonist muscles. Asymmetric paralysis of spinal muscles can result in scoliosis. Bone growth can be retarded in the affected limbs.

Impact

Polio results in immediate and long-term paralysis of muscles, necessitating the eventual use of substitutes for function. In extreme cases, the patient requires extensive functional devices and mechanisms for breathing; more commonly, the patient needs splints, arm supports, braces, or assistive devices for self-care and other UE functions.

Functional restoration

Medical treatment begins with immediate and complete bed rest; physical activity increases the risk of further paralysis. Hot packs are provided to relieve muscle pain, and the patient is positioned to protect the limbs from contracture and deformity. A tracheotomy may be necessary to provide an airway, and there may be a need for assistance in ventilation. Various types of respirators and ventilators are used and may be required throughout the patient's life.

During the phase in which the patient is receiving assistance in breathing, a *gentle* program of maintenance of passive and active functions is used. Massage, passive and active joint ROM with graded resistance, splinting for prevention of contractures, and functional training follow as the patient regains physical tolerance. Surgical considerations include tendon transfers and arthrodesis to improve function and correct deformities.

The prime precaution in treating the patient with polio is to avoid muscle and body fatigue. Fatigue can result in further weakness, and, if the muscles are overworked, function can be lost. Aside from this serious problem, fatigue can cause the patient to miss hours of necessary treatment because of the debilitating effects. Respiratory and cardiac stress must also be avoided. Signs of labored breathing should be looked for, and, if necessary, the treatment should be terminated. The muscle function should be continually evaluated for signs of imbalance.

To maintain and increase the ROM, endurance, and coordination, exercises and activities should be progressive and resistive and should be done symmetrically. Prevention of substitution patterns is important in the initial treatment program to encourage strengthening of weak muscles; however, when opti-

mal muscle power has been reached, the patient may have to learn to use substitution patterns to assist in independent functions.

Arm supports and splints can be used both to minimize fatigue and to aid the patient in positioning weak extremities, particularly if there is shoulder girdle involvement. The balanced forearm orthosis (ball-bearing feeder) can be used for self-feeding, hygiene, UE dexterity tasks, and other activities. Gravity can assist weak musculature. For the severely involved patient, provision of special equipment becomes essential for continuation of UE functions. Devices such as an electric wheelchair, electric page-turner, tape recorder, prism glasses, talking books, and special splinting can be helpful. With the proper equipment, the severely involved but well-motivated patient can adjust to adaptive functioning for daily activities and employment.

One of the most significant contributions the occupational therapist can make is in providing assistance through adaptive and supportive activities for maximal productivity and social involvement. Because the effect of the disease is permanent, the patient with severe UE involvement must adjust to being assisted by complicated mechanical and electronic systems that substitute for or assist with arm positioning and hand activities.

Guillain-Barré syndrome

Guillain-Barré syndrome is an acute distress of the nervous system that involves the spinal nerve roots, peripheral nerves, and, occasionally, the cranial nerves. It is characterized by a hypersensitivity response of the peripheral nervous system, resulting in polyneuritis or inflammation of the nerves after a viral infection. The disease can affect either gender at any age. The acute phase of this LMN lesion involves the rapid onset of paralysis of the limbs with accompanying sensory loss and muscle atrophy.

The initial illness, followed by flaccid paralysis, may affect all four limbs at once or may begin in the legs and spread upward to the arms. It may involve muscles of respiration. The proximal and distal muscles of the limbs are usually affected symmetrically. Reflexes are diminished or lost, sensation is impaired in the extremities, and the muscles are tender, but not all sensory modalities are impaired.

Impact

The patient with Guillain-Barré syndrome, unlike the patient with polio, has a good prognosis for recovery. The factors affecting recovery are the premorbid physical condition, motivation, extent of return of muscle function, and the character of the rehabilitation program.

The prognosis varies, and improvement may be sporadic. Almost complete recovery may be gained within 3 to 6 months or more; or the recovery may be incomplete with slight remissions, serious relapses, or a plateau. The patient may regain independent ambulation but retain some residual weakness and incoordination in all extremities, with some atrophy in the intrinsic muscles of the hands. The patient who makes slow progress may develop atrophy, which, if unattended, can hinder the effective use of the hands in manipulative tasks. The patient with weakness and incoordination of the legs may require braces to substitute for the lack of strong muscles.

Functional restoration

The patient generally benefits from an intensive rehabilitation program. With the initiation of rehabilitation techniques as soon as medical stability has been reached, activities are introduced to encourage active muscle use to prevent atrophy or wasting.

A common precaution in the rehabilitation program is the avoidance of fatigue to protect future function. Psychological support, practical use of returning musculature in productive activity, and social stimulation are essential if the patients are to become involved in the rehabilitation objectives. General rehabilitation goals include maintenance of nutrition, prevention of contractures, gradual diminution of the initial rest program, passive and active joint ROM exercises for the affected extremities, activity for muscle strengthening and coordination, restoration of sensation, increase in activity according to the patient's tolerance, splinting to prevent deformity from atrophy and disuse, a self-care program to encourage independent functions, assistive devices to encourage functional use of extremities, and development of work tolerance for prevocational preparation.

The occupational therapist designs a program geared to the *gradual* improvement of active functions. Because the patient may be totally paralyzed when referred to occupational therapy, the first consideration may be to provide splints to maintain the functional position of fingers, thumbs, and wrists to prevent contractures from poor positioning. While on bed rest, the patient can benefit from the stimulation and encouragement of light social activities, such as visits from family and friends, watching television, and supportive visits from the therapist, who engages the patient in positive conversation regarding his or her interests while performing passive ROM exercises. It is important to maintain free joint motions of the wrist and fingers for grasping activities that use tenodesis function.

Early treatment is similar to that of the spinal cord-injured quadriplegic patient. The therapist must consider maintaining full passive joint range and encouraging active range against gravity. In addition, the therapist provides psychological support and social stimulation and encourages the patient to use special devices, such as an electric page-turner, which can provide the satisfaction of reading independently yet requires a minimum of movement to operate.

As the patient improves medically and begins to regain motor power, the occupational therapist provides activities that require increasing ranges of motion, coordination, and strength. The development of strength in specific muscles encourages the strengthening of other muscles. As has been stressed, however, *care must be taken not to fatigue the patient.* Fatigue can be prevented by providing suspension slings or arm supports for positioning and for facilitation of movement for hand functions. As the power begins to return and coordination improves, care should be taken to vary activities between gross and fine, resistive and nonresistive, so that maximal gain can be derived without undue fatigue.

Specific activities of the upper extremities should encourage coordinated movements while maintaining good body alignment to minimize the development of substitution patterns. The patient who is steadily improving needs assistive devices *only* to prevent fatigue and substitution; usually, these are not needed permanently. The patient whose progress is slower, however, should be encouraged to use assistive equipment to gain strength and function.

From the beginning of treatment, self-care activities can encourage sensory and motor stimulation. Self-feeding and grooming can be started when necessary arm functions begin to return, even if a palmar cuff is needed to substitute for grasp. Dressing can be started when physical tolerance increases and the patient has sufficient active joint ROM.

As the patient regains functions, the program should be upgraded to challenge strength and coordination. The patient should be encouraged to function independently whenever possible and to ask for assistance only when needed. Along with the physical therapist, the occupational therapist monitors the regaining of individual muscle control and checks for muscle atrophy.

Because the prognosis for the return of ambulation and functional UE ability is generally good, the recovering patient is encouraged to participate in an activity program in which abilities for maximal independence can be developed. Recreational activities improve physical endurance and coordination. (For specific adaptation of activities, assistive devices, and self-care techniques, see the following section on spinal cord lesions.)

Spinal cord injury

Injury to the spinal cord results in temporary or permanent paralysis of the muscles of the limbs and the autonomic nervous system, usually manifested *below* the level of the lesion. Symptoms of a temporary nature are caused by compression of the cord without transection or puncture. Permanent paralysis is caused by fractures and dislocations that puncture or transect the spinal cord.

Spinal cord injury is caused by gunshot wounds, stab wounds, falls, automobile accidents, and sports accidents. The most common of these is the automobile accident, when forced flexion and hyperextension of the trunk results in fracture and dislocation of the vertebrae. The initial symptoms are (1) spinal shock, (2) loss of sensation, (3) flaccid paralysis of the affected extremities, (4) incontinence of bowel and bladder, and (5) decreased reflex activity below the level of the lesion followed by an increase in reflex activity. In many cases, secondary injury results from improper handling of the injured person at the scene of the accident and during transportation to the treatment facility.

Impact

The temporary or permanent implications to the injured person include the sudden interruption of the chosen lifestyle; severe loss of familiar bodily sensation, awareness, and volitional functions; and loss of bowel, bladder, and sexual controls, physical independence, psychological stability, social effectiveness, sexuality, financial security, educational goals, vocational skills and plans, avocational interests, personal expectations, and hopes for future content and planning.

Common problems that may occur periodically during rehabilitation are denial, anger, hostility, boredom, depression, lack of motivation, dependency, urinary tract infection, decubitus, weakness, atrophy, spasticity, and contractures.

Survival, disability, treatment, and function of the spinal cord-injured patient depend on the level and extent of the lesion. Quadriplegia results from injury to the cervical and, possibly, the high thoracic areas of the cord and produces sensory deficits and muscular deficiencies of the upper extremities, trunk, and lower extremities. Paraplegia occurs from injury to the thoracic and lumbar cord areas and produces sensory deficits and muscular paralysis of the trunk and lower extremities. The terms *quadriplegia* and *paraplegia* refer to paralysis of the limbs, whereas *quadriparesis* and *paraparesis* refer to weakness of the limbs.

The level of segmental innervation determines the effect of the trauma. The extent of the injury determines the functional outcome. Muscles innervated by segments at and below the level of injury are affected. The sensory and autonomic systems may be involved; functional loss may be asymmetric, depending on the location of the lesion. Although a functional estimate and expectation can be made on the basis of the level of the injury, other factors may retard or change the rehabilitation prognosis. Among these factors are respiratory complications, head trauma, other accompanying injuries, sensory loss, decubitus, damage to the vertebral column, urinary tract infections, spasm, and lack of motivation for recovery.

Functional implications

The initial program for the person with a spinal cord injury is crucial to his or her total well-being and the beginning of the rehabilitation process, which may require adjustment to lifelong disability. It is a gradual, arduous, and sometimes painful progression from total dependence to the maximal level of independence—from the shock of functional loss to the acceptance of achievable abilities. Communication, planning, and coordination among team members are essential to ensure optimal rehabilitation outcomes medically and functionally.

Both the acute care setting and the rehabilitation center provide medical care, carry out rehabilitation measures to prepare the injured person for future life involvement, provide therapy directed toward achievement of maximal levels of bodily movement and function, and implement psychological preparation for self-motivation for daily activity and goal setting. Rehabilitation is the preparation for setting and reaching achievable satisfactory goals. The initial rehabilitation period is a mere beginning to the new life the person will lead as a quadriplegic or paraplegic person upon entry into community living.

In the early care, it is essential to prevent the patient from becoming either overly discouraged or overly hopeful. In discussing the medical condition with the patient, physicians may advocate informing the patient, immediately and clearly, of the chances of walking and of the degree of permanent paralysis to expect to avoid false hope by the patient and family and to facilitate the rehabilitative process. In other cases, the physician may initially inform the patient that he or she will recover full functions or provide ambiguous answers to questions regarding functional loss to avoid psychological trauma. In the early stages of hospitalization, the patient tends to deny the extent of the injury. At this stage, denial serves as a valuable protective mechanism to avoid seeing the realities that must be faced eventually. In most cases, denial actually helps the patient through the devastating effects of the initial trauma and the long-term implications of disability.

Functional restoration

Planning begins in the acute care facility with protection of the flaccid extremities for future functioning, establishment of short-term and long-term goals, and gradual conditioning to enable the patient to tolerate an upright position. Establishment of maximal use of the upper extremities for self-care and productive activities aids the patient in acceptance of permanent paralysis and in preparation for functional wheelchair living. The therapist helps the patient develop physical and intellectual resources with which to combat the challenges of functional living and social interaction.

The goals of rehabilitation for the patient with spinal cord injury, regardless of the level of the lesion, include the following:

- Recognizing and developing physical and intellectual capacities
- Attaining the maximal level of self-care
- Resuming satisfying relationships with family and friends and redeveloping social activities
- Making realistic plans
- Understanding the condition and accepting responsibility for continuing the rehabilitation process
- Learning and following a therapeutic home program
- Learning of and using available community resources
- Resuming education and employment activities and plans

Involvement with the treatment plan helps the patient learn to take responsibility and enables the patient to develop an independent attitude toward his or her abilities. This involvement begins during acute care hospitalization, continues during early rehabilitation, and progresses further if treatment continues at a specialized rehabilitation facility.

Positioning

Exercises and activities can be done in almost any position if both the patient and the equipment are properly situated. In preparation for productive activity, the patient should be positioned for optimal biomechanical advantage in function.

Bed. Upper-extremity activities can be assisted by the use of an inclined lapboard in the supine and sitting positions with suspension slings attached to traction frames for early arm support.

To avoid the natural tendency of the flaccid extremities to yield to the pull of gravity, they are properly positioned in normal alignment using sandbags, pillows, or footboards to prevent the stretching of unused or weak muscles and the development of contractures of spastic muscles, which would limit future function of the limbs. Undue pressure on flaccid limbs from bed clothes is avoided, and the limbs should be visible to monitor positioning. Prism glasses enable the patient to see his or her extremities and to request repositioning if necessary.

Prone Position on a CircOlectric Bed. When the quadriplegic patient is prone (face down) on the CircOlectric bed, he or she can use gravity for shoulder flexion and elbow extension. A table is necessary to provide support in elbow flexion if the patient lacks lower-arm functions. For the quadriplegic person in a prone position, independent eating should be encouraged, using slings, a palmar cuff, and a nonskid mat and positioning the tray under the bed. Plate guards allow the patient to pick up the food independently.

Wheelchair. The patient is generally seated on a cut-out seatboard with a gel, water, or air cushion for hip positioning and prevention of decubitus. The chair should initially have an extended back, adjustable arm, and foot support. A lapboard, suspension slings, or a balanced forearm orthosis can be attached to the wheelchair for the quadriplegic person.

Standing Table. This device is used by the patient wearing braces to aid in trunk strengthening and balance, standing tolerance, and upright positioning. Activities done at the standing table may also be accomplished by some patients with sufficient balance by using a belt support to stand at a work table.

Skin Protection. Protection of the skin and prevention of contractures are essential for the patient with a spinal cord injury. Because sensation is lost below the level of the lesion, the patient is unable to detect pressure from external objects. In addition, because of muscle paralysis, the patient is unable to change position easily. Thus, position changes must be made initially by nurses or attendants. The skin is susceptible to injury from the shearing force of sheets, pressure from footboards used for positioning, and the gravitational effect of the immobile limbs on the mattress. Decubitus ulcers (pressure sores) develop from local anemia caused by this pressure and appear over bony prominences. Even though air mattresses and water mattresses are used and routine position changes are followed, decubitus ulcers can still occur. To avoid pressure sores, the therapist instructs the patient in the importance of turning in bed or shifting weight when seated in the wheelchair. As a patient becomes more mobile, instruction is given on how to check all vulnerable areas of the body, using a long-handled mirror to check the back, buttocks, arms, and lower extremities.

Self-care

The daily accomplishment of self-care and other independent or assisted activities helps the patient maintain joint ROM, strength, and physical and psychological endurance. The abilities and progress in these areas should be discussed with the family throughout the hospitalization and rehabilitation process so that they will encourage as much independence as possible.

The person with paraplegia is generally able to regain independent self-care activities and virtually all aspects of daily living. Depending on the level of the lesion and the manifestations, complications, and motivation for independent function, the person with quadriplegia is challenged with use of electronic assistive equipment, hand splints, and motorized or a specially equipped wheelchair to deal with disability in all four extremities.

Assistive equipment

Adaptive equipment may be required for substitution of motion, compensation for decreased trunk balance, and assistance for reduced reach and grasp and for limitation in locomotion. Assistive devices may be needed to perform the self-care activities of personal hygiene, grooming, eating, and dressing. Although assistive equipment may increase functional independence, it may decrease desired sensory and motor function. Some patients refuse all assistive equipment; others want everything, even some that is not needed.

In most cases, the wheelchair becomes a way of life for the spinal cord-injured person. Therefore, it must be prescribed for individual comfort, safety, maneuverability, and independence. A poorly fitted wheelchair can contribute to deformity, muscle disuse, decubitus, and decreased motivation for function and

socialization. The wheelchair needs of the paraplegic and quadriplegic patients are different.

The wheelchair should be ordered as soon as possible in the rehabilitation program to encourage the patient's early association with wheelchair living.

Avocational activities

Activities provided for restoration of specific UE function can become outlets for avocational needs and interests. As the spinal cord-injured person works through adjustment to wheelchair living, avocational outlets are needed for venting feelings as well as for providing a sense of accomplishment. As new patterns of movement and skill develop, the patient can apply these to pursuing leisure activities at school or in the community. Many spinal cord-injured people have benefited greatly from participation in organized sports, such as basketball, swimming, table tennis, and weightlifting. Competition contributes to resocialization, achievement, and increased sense of self-worth and confidence.

School environment

Vocational goals and discharge plans may include returning to school for the adolescent or young adult with a spinal cord injury. Therapists evaluate the campus for architectural accessibility by wheelchair to buildings, classrooms, bathrooms, cafeterias, and other areas. A system for carrying books, obtaining optimal work surfaces and heights, and note taking may be needed by the quadriplegic student. Full involvement of the wheelchair-mobile person in all aspects of the educational environment is essential to acceptance by peers.

Driving

One of the most common social problems facing the wheelchair user is the lack of adequate public transportation. Therefore, it is essential that the paraplegic person become independent in using hand controls for driving, car transfers, and placing the wheelchair in the car.

Many quadriplegic people can drive with hand controls and a steering knob, although they may need assistance getting in and out of the car, and most need help getting the wheelchair into the car. For these people, a van with a wheelchair lift is recommended. The person may need to transfer from the wheelchair to the driver's seat or passenger's seat once in the van, or the van may be equipped with clamps to secure the wheelchair in a position to allow the person to drive. Predriving evaluation and training programs are available to guide the person in using safe techniques in purchasing an appropriate vehicle and in driving.

Prevocational

The employment potential of the spinal cord-injured person is not necessarily correlated with the injury and its residual manifestations. A person with a debilitating injury is able to return to work if he or she is motivated, possesses salable knowledge and skills, is offered reassurance from family and friends, and is able to find a job, although the person may have to change former vocational goals. The occupational therapy program provides the patient with the opportunity to learn potential functional levels and to explore feasible vocational areas of interest. Prevocational evaluation determines the salable skills that the person has, can develop, or requires for vocational planning and preparation for appropriate vocational training.

Discharge planning

The patient and family are included in the rehabilitation program as soon after hospital admission as possible and are fully informed of all the stages of the rehabilitation process the patient will go through. The process begun in the hospital continues at home, in the rehabilitation facility, and in the community for as long as is necessary. The person maintains a relationship with the rehabilitation team to achieve planned goals upon discharge through outpatient programs and follow-up.

During hospitalization, the rehabilitation team may encourage the patient to go home on weekends to begin to face the adjustments that will have to be made after discharge and to use skills acquired in the treatment facility in the home environment. These visits alert the family to the patient's capabilities, progress, and general program. It is from these visits that the patient, family, and therapist can work together on home planning and architectural renovations.

Specific considerations: Quadriplegia

The initial treatment of the person with quadriplegia (paralysis in upper and lower extremities) is immobilization of the vertebral column by skeletal traction using head tongs or neck bracing. Traction is generally applied for 6 weeks, after which immobilization is continued with a neck support for 2 to 4 months (Rusk, 1971).

The patient's position while in traction is interchangeable (supine and prone) in a completely extended position for optimal protection of the spinal cord and musculature. The injured person may be placed on a Stryker frame bed, which rotates horizontally for position change to prone or supine, or on a CircOlectric bed, which can be turned from the horizontal to the vertical position on a 180-degree axis and can be stabilized at any angle, allowing placement in the supine or prone position. These special beds are used to aid in the frequent change in body position essential to protect skin and limbs from decubitus. Change of position is made every 2 hours. The tilt table is also used to assist in moving the patient passively from the horizontal to the vertical position. If not gradually acclimated to changes in space during the initial immobilization, the patient tends to become dizzy when assuming the sitting position after spending weeks in traction.

Early treatment of the quadriplegic patient in the acute stage of trauma consists of turning, massage for circulation and sensory stimulation, and passive ROM exercises to maintain freedom of joint movement and to prevent muscular contractures and decubitus. After the traction period, general conditioning exercises are provided, including proper breathing and training in rolling from side to side. Self-care is begun as soon as possible to relieve anxieties regarding nonsensitive and nonmoving body parts and to prevent dependency on others for any functions the patient is able to accomplish.

Evaluation

As previously mentioned, the level of segmental innervation determines the effect of trauma and the anticipated functional outcome. In the acute care setting, the quadriplegic patient is usually seen for initial evaluation while confined to bed. The following steps are recommended for the initial assessment of capabilities and functional deficits:

1. Review the chart for medical status, treatment prescribed, and bed position restrictions owing to the injury to the spinal cord and other areas.
2. Establish nonthreatening rapport with the patient on the initial visit, showing empathy and respect. Interview the patient about what happened, the medical situation, treatment plans, and schedule, asking for a description of concerns and priorities.
3. Evaluate active and passive joint ROM, strength, sensation, coordination, general mobility, and function of the extremities and trunk.
4. Evaluate bed position for alignment of extremities and trunk for prevention of muscle stretching, shortening, and deformity and for the patient's awareness of position requirements.
5. Examine the extremities for reddened areas, which indicate pressure.
6. Determine the functional aspects of UE sensation by requesting the patient to identify the location of and describe sensory stimuli and to identify the location of the extremity during passive positioning.
7. Determine passive and active joint ROM, identifying restrictions caused by trauma, pain, weakness, spasticity, contractures, or hypersensitivity.
8. Determine the need for hand splints to maintain body alignment for future function to prevent deformity and for sensory awareness and stimulation.
9. Assess the need for arm support to extend the functional positioning of the hands for use; assess the need for arm exercises in a supine position.
10. Talk with the patient about interests, abilities, past achievements, and primary concerns regarding the condition and its implications for the patient's life.
11. Inform the patient of the results of the evaluation and discuss the patient's personal goals; make treatment plans with the patient for short-term and long-term goals.

Treatment

Bed Phase. During all treatment in this phase, the patient should be encouraged to use *all* possible active movement to increase physical endurance, strength, and functional ability. By doing this, the patient becomes involved in the program and assumes some responsibility for rehabilitation. The therapist provides activities in which the patient is interested and psychological support throughout the treatment regime. The therapist coordinates occupational therapy with nursing and physical therapy personnel and other members of the rehabilitation team to aid the patient in gaining maximal function while suffering minimal fatigue and frustration.

Treatment considerations during the bed stage are as follows:

1. Monitor *bed positioning* daily for prevention of decubitus and contractures.
2. Gently *massage* and stimulate sensory receptors of the upper extremities for sensory awareness and tactual localization.
3. Move the upper extremities in gentle, full *passive ROM* daily to monitor changes in range, informing the patient when the extremity is moved, in which direction, and how many times. Encourage the patient to watch the extremity during massage and passive joint ROM.

4. Precede active ROM exercises by gentle *manual resistance* to joints and muscle groups in the hands and arms for sensory stimulation and motor facilitation.

5. Attach *suspension slings* to the traction bar above the bed to support the arms as well as to stimulate available active movements of the shoulders and elbows. Slings can be modified with springs to facilitate movement and to provide sensory feedback. The use of weights encourages increased muscle power. Use elbow and wrist straps to support the arms for maximal active movement and hand functions; use a palmar cuff with a pocket for insertion of a spoon or a pencil, enabling the patient to use the arms and hands in productive activity; facilitate motion of all joints of the upper extremities by using gravitational assistive devices, such as suspension slings, the balanced forearm orthosis adaptations, weights, or a bed table.

6. Use *assistive devices* to facilitate and support movement; among these devices are a common bath mitt, a universal palmar cuff device to hold a fork for eating, a plate guard to aid in arm control while eating, and arm slings or positioners. These devices encourage exercise through active arm movement, increase body awareness, encourage self-esteem by providing independent function, and decrease dependency.

7. Provide *splinting* to prevent tightening of muscles and deformity. Restriction may be necessary to prevent flexion of the elbows, wrists, fingers, and ankles. It is essential to correlate the use of splints with manual therapeutic techniques. Provide initial static hand splinting progressing to dynamic splinting to stimulate tenodesis function as appropriate. Splinting stimulates sensory awareness and assists in channeling the muscles for function.

8. Set up an *electric page-turner* on the bed table so that the patient can operate it with palm contact or with movement of the chin or shoulder if the patient lacks lower-arm function.

9. Provide *prism glasses* to prevent the patient from developing eyestrain while viewing television; reading, seeing, and talking with visitors; or watching his or her limbs as the therapist moves them when the patient is supine.

In the bed position, the following adaptations are possible:

1. Use the bed table to position objects for activities (books or visual puzzles) that can be performed by using prism glasses.

2. A table lapboard with a bottom edge can be placed over the patient's chest; this can be inclined and stabilized using projecting legs to hold reading materials and other items.

3. Commercial book holders are useful.

4. Suspension slings can be attached to the traction frames on the bed.

5. Slings, mirrors, and activities can be attached to the CircOlectric bed frame.

6. Objects for activities can be placed on a chair or low table for the patient who is prone on the CircOlectric bed. Food trays can also be placed on a chair.

During the bed stage, the patient is encouraged to adjust to the vertical position for sitting by using the tilt table. This adjustment should be accomplished gradually. When cerebral spatial adjustment and physical tolerance increase to a sufficient functional level, the patient progresses to the semireclining wheelchair and then to the fully upright position for continued adaptation to wheelchair mobility, sitting balance, and the use of the upper extremities.

The move to the wheelchair for daily treatment sessions is significant for the quadriplegic patient. This change in position requires vestibular adjustment as well as total body adaptation. The occupational therapy program changes to focus on evaluation of functional ability in this position and to direct therapeutic methods toward optimal sensorimotor performance achievements.

Wheelchair selection for the quadriplegic patient is crucial to daily health and function. A variety of chairs, controls, and accessories are available to meet the varied demands of individual capabilities, interests, and lifestyles. For the quadriplegic patient with a high cervical lesion and severely limited or nonfunctional reach and hand placement, electronic arm or head controls may be necessary. Electronic wheelchair and environmental control systems enable the severely disabled person to have independent wheelchair mobility and an element of independent function. With such systems, the disabled person can control appliances such as an electric bed, a call signal, a telephone or intercom, television, thermostat, or doors.

Quadriplegic patients with lower cervical lesions benefit from operating electric controls on wheelchairs or from using special accessories on standard nonelectric wheelchairs. For ease of maneuvering, the quadriplegic person may require knobs or plastic friction sheaths on the wheel rims for easier propulsion or a motorized chair with touch controls. The back should be higher than that of the paraplegic person's chair, since the quadriplegic person has lost trunk control and needs extra support. A brake extension may be necessary for independence in locking brakes. Heel loops and leg rests are needed for foot and leg positioning, and a safety belt may be needed for balance. Although a wheelchair with a reclining back may be used at first to compensate for the quadriplegic patient's tendency to become dizzy, it is not recommended during later periods because it can increase dependency on the reclined position, which limits UE function.

Wheelchair Phase. When the patient has progressed to sitting in a wheelchair, guidelines are determined for treatment planning. During all evaluation procedures, the therapist assists the patient in movements when necessary. Fatigue or discouragement should not be allowed. The therapist should emphasize what *can* be done and encourage the patient to accomplish it; be explicit in instructions and demonstrate when necessary; and terminate the evaluation before the patient becomes fatigued and try to end with accomplishment. In addition, it is important to talk with the patient regarding his or her interests so that the treatment program can include activities that are related to these interests and aid the patient in setting realistic long-term and short-term goals. The following evaluation areas should be examined:

1. Joint ROM: Move the joints through complete passive ROM, one at a time, being careful not to cause pain in sensitive joints, particularly in the shoulders and elbows. Give support to the flaccid or weak limbs by holding them carefully, always informing the patient of what is to be done. Measure the joint range with the goniometer. Check for spasticity and deformity in the upper extremities.

2. Muscle strength: Provide gravitational assistance if necessary to determine how much gravity the patient can resist. Give gentle resistance to joint movement to determine gross muscle strength and the presence of spasticity. Use a scale gauge to measure gross joint strength against resistance and a pinch gauge and dynamometer for grip.

3. Sensation: Note the presence of pain during passive movement. Occlude the patient's vision; touch the skin lightly with your finger and determine if the patient responds to the stimulus. Progress from distal to proximal areas. To evaluate two-point discrimination, sharp touch, and localization of stimuli, touch the skin with a sharp object, such as a sharpened dowel stick or a two-point pressure gauge. Determine first whether the patient responds to the stimulus, can localize the stimulus, and can distinguish one from two stimuli. Place an object between the patient's thumb and fingers, move it around in the palmar area, and then ask for recognition of the object by its size, shape, and texture to determine stereognostic function.

4. Position sense (proprioception): Move the body part to be tested gently in reciprocal movements and then ask the patient to identify the position of the limb when stopped. The patient may feel the movement but may be unable to identify the position without seeing it.

5. Patterns of movement: Provide the patient with a reaching or grasping task to perform, for instance, picking up a 2 × 2-inch foam block, reaching to the shoulder, or reaching for an object held in the air. Observe the pattern of movement to determine functioning muscles and the presence of spasticity. Observe any substitution patterns the patient may use to the detriment of other muscles that should be strengthened.

6. Functional activities: Determine the actual gross grasp, prehension, coordination, strength, and tenodesis function. Determine the ability to perform functional activities, such as picking up an object and placing it, reaching for an object, using two hands, writing, pushing and pulling objects, and turning the pages of a book. Use objects of various weights, sizes, and textures. Present tasks within the patient's functional ability as determined by joint ROM, muscle power, sensation, position sense, and patterns of movement already observed and evaluated. Do not ask a patient to do impossible tasks.

7. Determine the trunk control for free movement of the upper extremities in isolated asymmetric use and use in ADL.

8. Evaluate the need for assistance devices or splints for restorative exercises and activities in addition to those needed for positioning and self-care activities.

9. Evaluate self-care and all ADL, including self-feeding, grooming, toileting, bathing, dressing, writing, clerical skills, and homemaking skills. The physical plan of the home must also be evaluated.

10. Prevocational evaluation: Evaluate functions for job skills and employment potential when the patient has mastered UE functional activities and the ADL within his or her limits.

Self-Care. Although the quadriplegic patient may have little ROM and muscle strength with which to accomplish self-care tasks, it is essential that the patient use the available power to accomplish parts of tasks. Limitations in reach, grasp, strength, joint ROM, respiration, and physical endurance are common. Assistive and substitutive techniques of adaptive body positioning, use of reflexes, and assistance from an attendant help in developing skills. Long handles to extend reach, palmar cuffs to substitute for hand grip, spring clips to provide sustained grip, loops on clothing, special devices for grooming, soap on a rope, bath mitts, and adapted equipment for grooming and make-up are readily available and often make the difference between ability and handicap. Often, the most limiting factor can be the patient's refusal to participate.

Functional Restoration. All activities should increase UE joint ROM, strength, physical tolerance, grasp, and psychological adaptation. These activities should include the use of assistive equipment to increase the patient's capacity to function independently, and they should result in the realization of maximal capacities.

Specially designed tables adjust to the height of the wheelchair, angled for easy access to work surfaces or on a rotating base assist the patient in optimal mechanical advantage for task accomplishment.

Manipulation of pegs and of other objects of various sizes, weights, and textures improves the grasp, reach, and ability to place objects. These can be presented in the form of peg games (HiQ, checkers, or chess) to elicit the patient's interest. The activity teaches isolated arm and hand functions and provides the patient with experience in using assistive equipment.

Constructive activities, such as woodworking, can be adapted to provide joint ROM and strengthening of the upper arms and trunk muscles. If the patient has poor grasp, a palmar cuff, bilateral handles, or holding mitts can be used with tools for such tasks as sanding, sawing, planning, or drilling.

Activities are also provided for the pure fun of engaging in a game with another person (socialization) while at the same time assisting the patient in gaining functional use of the upper extremities. These activities, such as checkers, chess, or Scrabble, can be done in bed or in a wheelchair. Arm support may be needed, as may hand splints, but the patient is able to engage in competitive activity and receive the rewards from it.

Suggestions for adapted activities for the spinal cord-injured person, with modifications according to lesion level, include the following:

- Use of table-based power tools, such as a small jigsaw, drill press, or printing press, which can have extended handles for easy reach and control
- Use of hand-power equipment, secured if necessary to substitute for the patient's lack of control
- Vertical- and adjustable-angled chalkboards for gross arm and writing exercises
- Ropes attached to loom harnesses to enable the patient to change the shed by using the arms, if the lower extremities are paralyzed
- Special handles on the loom beater to provide supination or pronation exercises
- Use of a pulley and weight system attached to the loom beater for strengthening upper extremities by providing resistance
- Use of recreational activities, such as ball throwing, shuffleboard, and shooting pool, for gross arm exercises
- Use of manual activities, such as painting, knitting, or hooking, for sustained upper-arm strengthening and light resistive hand use

- Use of activities for sensory stimulus and light resistive hand use, such as gardening using adapted planters at wheelchair level and forming and painting ceramics
- Use of homemaking activities, such as cooking, cleaning, and ironing

All activities offer possibilities for adaptation. Some of the activities mentioned are helpful to the paraplegic patient as well as to the quadriplegic patient because they provide a means to increase strength, endurance, and balance for the trunk and upper extremities. The quadriplegic patient needs these functions for wheelchair manipulation and for performance of all activities. The paraplegic patient needs upper arm strengthening for wheelchair maneuvering over long distances, transferring, standing in braces, and walking with crutches. The build-up of maximal UE strength is essential to the paraplegic patient. Engagement in an UE activity program is crucial to the beginning of productivity from a wheelchair and leads to independence in daily living tasks, increased responsibility, and, eventually, employment. The paraplegic patient should experience all aspects of functioning from a wheelchair before leaving the rehabilitation setting.

Functional Splints. Early use of appropriate splints benefits the quadriplegic patient by providing muscle exercise, mechanical function for purposeful activity, and assurance that the patient is capable of accomplishing tasks.

The quadriplegic patient is provided with a tenodesis or flexor-hinge hand splint when he or she has achieved active hyperextension of the wrist. With active motion against resistance, the patient is able to channel movement through the splint into a strong and functional prehension grip. The tenodesis splint uses the natural function of the finger flexor tendons to tighten in wrist hyperextension and to relax in wrist flexion. Although the patient may be able to effect this function voluntarily with sufficient active wrist extension without the splint, grip sufficient for strong grasp and fine prehension may be lacking in thumb–finger prehension. The splint is applied to give power for the functional needs of prehension.

Various forms of splints are available; some are for trial and training, whereas others are for permanent use. Trial tenodesis splints may be made by the occupational therapist from thermoplastic materials. The patient is taught how to use the splint in active grasping and releasing and in coordination activities. The flexor-hinge hand splint is made by the occupational therapist or the orthotist for permanent use and is usually made of metal or high-temperature plastic. The patient may continue to use the splints if they aid in daily activities or may eventually discard them as muscle power and substitute functions are gained.

If the patient does not have active wrist extension against gravity and resistance, other types of hand–wrist tenodesis splints may be needed to provide the function of grasp. These may be controlled electronically or by carbon dioxide. The use of these devices depends on the motivation of the patient since they require tolerance to noise and the pressure of harnesses and special rigging as well as acceptance of complicated assistive equipment to substitute for natural functions.

Environmental Control Systems. The high-level quadriplegic patient who is unable to move his or her upper extremities for functional activity depends on teaching others how to perform needed physical tasks. In spite of this dependence, the severely disabled patient can find independence in environmental control and self-expression in written communication through the aid of environmental control systems. Such systems enable training and practice in functional written communication skills for use in recreational activities, educational needs, or employment functions. Electronically controlled computer systems with typewriter mechanisms, auditory systems, visual feedback, and custom adaptations can be made for positioning and operation.

Specific considerations: Paraplegia

Evaluation

Evaluation of the paraplegic patient in the initial posttrauma stage may be at the bedside if the patient is immobilized in traction and special equipment or has significant accompanying injuries. In evaluating the paraplegic patient, the therapist looks for variations in functional ability, which depend on the level of the lesion. Although the paraplegic person initially may be immobilized, he or she demonstrates full functional use of the upper extremities in active ROM, sensation, and hand use. While in bed and during the wheelchair phase, the patient becomes accustomed to depending on the arms and trunk for mobility and function to provide leg positioning.

Specific areas of evaluation during the bed phase include the following:

1. Determine status, rehabilitation goals, and treatment being provided.
2. Determine medical restrictions on movement as noted in the chart with regard to the status of the spinal cord injury and other injuries.
3. Note the body position for proper alignment of the paralyzed trunk and lower extremities.
4. Evaluate the passive and active ROM and strength of the upper extremities (which should be normal but may be weak).
5. If not medically restricted, evaluate trunk and LE movement, noting areas of spasticity, weakness, paralysis, sensory loss, substitution, and compensation.
6. Assess need for an ability to use self-care devices to perform daily activities.
7. Interview the patient with regard to accident, medical condition and its impact, lifestyle, goals, and expectations.
8. Encourage the patient to discuss premorbid achievement, avocational and vocational interests, and plans.

Treatment

Bed Phase. While confined to bed, the paraplegic patient benefits from an UE activity program to strengthen the arms and hands, to provide initial self-care assistance, to learn body image and self-awareness, to learn the extent of current functions, and to provide a sense of self-worth through accomplishment of achievable tasks on a daily basis. The longer the patient remains away from productive activity, the more difficult is his or her adjustment to the benefits of rehabilitation. The following activities and adaptations are suggested to encourage a positive attitude toward maintenance of restoration of productive abilities:

- Inclined bed table, lapboard, and prism glasses for ease in performing UE activity in bed

- Devices with extended handles for reaching and self-care; a long-handled sponge for bathing; a reacher for picking up items
- Increasing involvement in daily self-care program
- Low-exertion UE activities for active exercise of the arms while supine, such as reading, book games, and manual activities
- Activities that offer resistance in hand and arm functions to increase strength and to decrease mental frustration from inactivity, such as Theraplast, leatherwork, making models, copper tooling, macrame, loom weaving, and woodcarving

Barring the complications of decubitus and excessive spasticity, the paraplegic person is able to learn to be essentially independent in self-care. The high-level paraplegic patient may have some problems with LE dressing because of trunk instability and loss of muscle strength for balance; however, various assistive devices can help in overcoming these problems.

Self-care activity increases self-awareness, responsibility, and self-esteem. When the restrictions on mobility are removed, the patient can begin self-care activities, such as bathing in bed or in the wheelchair using a long-handled sponge to reach the feet.

At this time, if the patient is able to turn in bed and to reach a sitting position, UE dressing can be done in bed as tolerance for the sitting position increases. When the patient can sit for longer periods, LE dressing in bed may be begun. For this, a long-handled reacher may be needed.

Wheelchair Phase. Some adjustment time may be required for the patient to regain a sense of balance and body use when first moving from the bed into a wheelchair. When this is accomplished, all bathing and grooming can be done before a mirror, and UE dressing can be done in a wheelchair. It is crucial to the rehabilitation of the paraplegic person that he or she be encouraged to assume these responsibilities as functional ability is regained. Self-care activities not only provide independent functions but also provide important daily exercise in balance, strength, and coordination. Since fatigue may be experienced in the early accomplishment of these tasks, the treatment program must be coordinated with all other therapies. All rehabilitation team members are informed of the patient's level of accomplishment so that efforts are coordinated toward the achievement of maximal independence.

Since functioning from a wheelchair will, in most cases, become a way of life for the paraplegic person, it is essential that the wheelchair be equipped to meet all physical, personal, and functional needs. The wheelchair should be heavy-duty but lightweight for ease of lifting in and out of a car; it should be as narrow as possible for easy passage through doorways and maneuvering in bathrooms; it should have swing-away, removable footrests for transfer and proximity to cabinets and work areas; and it should have removable desk arms at a comfortable height for arm positioning, transfer, and proximity to tables and counters. A seatboard with a special cushion to prevent decubitus is sometimes used to maintain good positioning of trunk and hips. The foot pedals should clear 2 inches from the ground for safe travel over bumps and rough ground, the depth of the seat should extend to 2 inches proximal to the knee bend, and the back height should extend no farther than 3 inches below the axilla to allow free movement of the arms but provide needed trunk support. Pneu-

matic tires are often recommended for ease and safety over rough ground and for a comfortable ride. Because these tires need to be checked for sufficient air pressure and do go flat occasionally, however, they are contraindicated when the patient is unable to attend to these functions or does not have access to someone who can help. Hard rubber tires may be more practical in this case. In most cases, the paraplegic person will be able to propel a wheelchair both inside and outside on smooth ground with ease and less easily on rough ground.

Assistive Devices. The paraplegic person needs fewer assistive devices than does the quadriplegic person for independent living. The paraplegic patient generally uses a seatboard and special cushion for the wheelchair, a transfer board, a long-handled reacher for dressing or retrieving objects from high places or the floor, and wheelchair accessories (drink holder, ashtray, and carrying bag). The patient who is able to transfer with or without a sliding board can practice this skill in occupational therapy by transferring to a regular chair. The chair should have both a firm back and a firm seat. Working from a regular chair increases trunk and UE strength and mobility.

Activities and Skills. In the social and activity-oriented climate of occupational therapy, the paraplegic person is able to use his or her arms fully in bilateral strengthening activities, increasing UE coordination, balance, and physical tolerance for performing all productive activity from a wheelchair. The challenges of using cabinets, shelves, electrical outlets, standing electric machinery, and heavy hand tools help in developing skill and self-value in accomplishment. Group activities with peers and other patients (games, projects, discussions, planning) aid in self-awareness, social skills, and responsibility. Construction of assistive equipment, such as seatboards, tubboards for transfer, and sliding boards aid in acceptance of their use by the patient and may provide opportunities to gain skills to benefit others as well (Figure 18-5).

In many cases, the paraplegic patient will want to learn to use braces and crutches to walk; however, the braces are heavy, and walking requires much strength. Because of the cost in energy, the patient often resorts to the wheelchair for ease of travel; this occurs after a trial time that may last for months or years.

Life in a wheelchair, however, requires that all activities be done sitting. The patient will be dependent on the arms for mobility, vocation, and avocations. The resourceful paraplegic patient can do virtually anything from a wheelchair except climb steps, pass through narrow doorways, or reach appliances and counters that are too high.

The occupational therapy program consists of developing UE productivity, which will lead to prevocational and vocational planning. Skills begun in occupational therapy during hospitalization can greatly assist the paraplegic person in accepting limitations and using abilities for developing salable skills and healthy attitudes.

With training, the paraplegic person can function independently in self-care from bed and wheelchair, perform household activities from a wheelchair, transfer to and from the wheelchair, drive with hand controls, and perform vocational skills. The major problems will be those caused by architectural barriers outside of and within buildings—problems that impair mobility and make job-seeking extremely difficult.

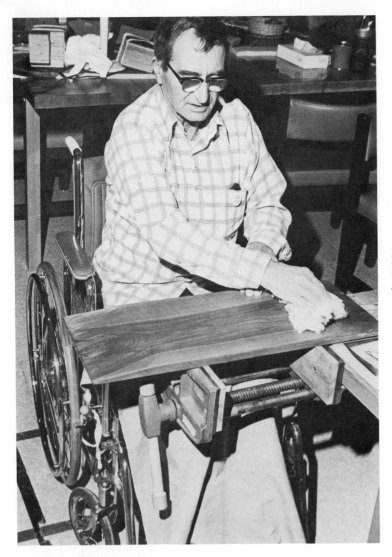

FIGURE 18-5. *Assistive equipment. Paraplegic patient works on his transfer board for upper-extremity strengthening and adjustment to wheelchair living.*

Community reentry

In the occupational therapy program, opportunities for total independence in self-care, ADL, homemaking skills, manual skills, program planning, and evaluation of functional levels and progress assist the patient in developing abilities for successful community reentry.

The spinal cord-injured person benefits from patient and family education sessions, weekend trials of self-care and social skills, group trips into the community during the formal treatment program, and education regarding the community resources available after discharge. The patient is able to participate in sports competition, social activities, conferences, workshops, and other functions designed and sponsored by and for disabled people. Due to increased efforts to eliminate architectural barriers to disabled persons, wheelchair users are finding that, where individual motivations and efforts are demonstrated, they can reenter communities in fully functioning capacities despite their physical disabilities. In an accepting society, they are disabled, but they are not handicapped.

In suffering a spinal cord injury, the person immediately becomes involved in an interruption of lifestyle content and plans. The loss may be devastating or adjustment impossible. In accepting assistive equipment, the patient must accept loss of physical function and the use of mechanical substitutes. Energy level and motivation determine the patient's priorities in the functional use of the remaining physical and mental abilities. Whether the patient can accept doing part of a task rather than the whole, accept assistance, and ask for help when needed are important elements in rehabilitation.

The person who must adjust to permanent spinal cord injury must accept continuing daily personal and social life in a wheelchair. From the onset, the person begins to make choices, which often require compromise. These are some of the choices faced by patients in planning for community reentry:

- Whether to remain immobile and dependent or to become mobile and perhaps partially independent
- Whether to use a shiny, metal, electronically operated hand splint to permit handling objects with strength and coordination or to be dependent on others to pick up objects because of a lack of hand strength, coordination, and joint ROM
- Whether to use limited energy to push the wheelchair independently or to save the energy for other functions and use an electric wheelchair

- Whether to stay home because many buildings are inaccessible to people using wheelchairs or to use community resources to determine those that are accessible and to fight to make more of the community barrier-free
- Whether to make the disability obvious to others by using helpful assistive devices for function or to remain dependent without independent functions to ensure self-worth through attention-seeking
- Whether to do part of a task or to ask someone else to do all of it

The therapist begins working with patients on adjustment, planning, and practicing new skills beginning with the evaluation. Early involvement aids patients in learning their capabilities and needs, enabling them to request help and to monitor that help effectively to strengthen them for the challenges of daily living in the community, where they may find rejection, lack of interest, and lack of help and where they must be able to use all their remaining abilities and skills to deal with the challenges facing them.

Myasthenia gravis

Myasthenia gravis (MG) is a progressive, degenerative disease that affects the myoneural junction and is characterized by severe muscle weakness. Impairment of conduction of nerve impulses to muscles occurs because of a presynaptic or postsynaptic block at the receptors on the motor endplates caused by a lack of release of the neurotransmitter acetylcholine (Bannister, 1973). Abnormalities in the thymus gland and the body's immune system are suspected of being responsible for MG.

Impact

Beginning with a gradual onset, this chronic disease is characterized by intermittent, abnormal fatigue of isolated muscle groups. In later stages, MG results in permanent weakness of some muscles and atrophy of others. Although it can occur at any age, the disease usually affects young adults, with females being more commonly affected than males.

The most common symptom of MG is abnormal muscular fatigue, most frequently in the eye muscles, where it leads to ptosis (drooping of both upper lids) and diplopia (double vision). In addition, the patient may present weakness of the facial muscles; total eye closure; retraction of the angles of the mouth; weakness of the bulbar musculature necessary for chewing, swallowing, and articulation; dyspnea (shortness of breath); weakness in the trunk and limbs, causing difficulty in balance and walking; and general fatigue. Initially, these symptoms are exacerbated when the patient is fatigued but may disappear after rest. The patient may also have a tendency toward respiratory failure and may demonstrate a high, nasal voice.

In the later stages of the disease, the patient experiences difficulty in swallowing and speaking. Eventually, the patient becomes bedridden and immobile, with severe permanent paralysis.

Remissions (decrease in symptoms) and improvement in general muscle strength and function may be marked and can last for years; however, exacerbation or attacks of weakness caused by physical exertion, infection, or childbirth can occur. These fluctuations can be sudden and of unpredictable severity.

Functional restoration

The therapist's primary concern in working with the patient with MG is to aid the patient in regaining muscle power and endurance; the therapist must take care not to cause debilitating fatigue. Because this disease is characterized by remissions, the recuperating patient may be able to regain functional abilities in the upper extremities, independence in self-care, and in some instances, the ability to walk. If physical tolerance can be maintained during rehabilitation, the patient might be able to return to a nonexerting form of work. Overexertion must be avoided, and respiratory problems must be prevented. The patient should be encouraged to employ work simplification techniques, therapeutic breathing, and energy conservation during activities.

The therapist should provide gentle, nonresistive activities that are interesting to the patient. These activities should be creative and productive and should provide psychological and intellectual stimulation to maintain a concept of self-worth. During therapy, the patient may use a respirator to maintain breathing.

In the later stages of the disease, the bedridden patient may lack ability to use his or her arms. Should this occur, the patient can benefit from assistive equipment, such as arm supports and splints, to aid in positioning for function. Electronically controlled devices that substitute for nonfunctioning arms and hands can be activated by microswitches, minute body movements, chin controls, or breath controls. These devices can enable the patient to operate a tape recorder, record player, television set, radio, or telephone. They have been produced in the United States (Prenke Romich) and in England (POSUM). Although they are expensive to buy and to repair, they enable the severely disabled person with intact intellectual abilities to communicate with the outside world and to have control over his or her immediate environment. For example, systems can be devised for activation of heating systems, windows, doors, lights, and typewriters in addition to those pieces of machinery mentioned above. A discussion of the social and intellectual stimulation that this equipment can provide to the patient severely disabled with MG appears in Dorothy Clark Wilson's book *Hilary* (1973).

Lesions of the peripheral nerves

Peripheral nerve injuries result from direct trauma to the extremity and affect all muscles innervated below the point of injury. Common causes include fractures, dislocations, crush injuries, compression, and lacerations. Primary impairments include sensory and motor dysfunction, contractures, deformity, and swelling. Continuing malfunction of the nerves can cause long-term or permanent muscle dysfunction, deformities of the hand, sensory loss, and trophic changes.

The occupational therapist encourages the patient to develop maximal functional use of the impaired extremity. Total body use is important in reintegrating the disabled extremity with the rest of the body; activities that are gradually upgraded in resistance encourage coordination, increase function, and augment general physical and mental tolerance of the condition. The occupational therapist must be careful not to overwork the patient, however; excessive exercise can cause edema in the affected extremity, creating stiffness in the joints and thus hindering ROM. For additional information, see Chapter 18, Section 4.

Arthritic conditions

Arthritis can affect a person of any age, has a variety of causes and effects, and can be of short duration or lifelong. It can result from local trauma or the aging process (osteoarthritis) or from systemic conditions (rheumatoid arthritis). Although it is commonly thought that arthritis is an affliction of the elderly, it may also be a disability of the young.

Degenerative joint disease (DJD), or osteoarthritis, is the least-feared type of the disease. DJD most commonly affects the fingers at the interphalangeal joints, causing little or no pain. Other frequently traumatized joints are the ankles, knees, hips, and elbows. DJD often occurs in people who have been active in sports or in those whose jobs have caused strain on their joints. It also accompanies the aging process, affecting the weight-bearing joints. The swelling associated with DJD is in the bony structure.

The treatment of DJD is generally local, consisting of rest of the affected joints to relieve pain and stress. Heat and therapeutic exercises may be prescribed in a gradually intensified program. The focus for the patient is on maintaining joint mobility and muscle power by carrying through a home exercise program, using assistive devices as needed to relieve joint stress, and developing individual work simplification methods to conserve joint functions in daily activities.

Other arthritic diseases involve the soft tissues surrounding the joints. Among these are lupus erythematosus, scleroderma, and rheumatoid arthritis. These diseases share the characteristics of joint inflammation, edema, decreased extremity function, and potential deformity. The occupational therapist may see all three in the clinical setting; however, the patient with rheumatoid arthritis is by far the most frequently referred. The therapist may see the patient with rheumatoid arthritis in both clinical and home care situations. Many of the methods for evaluation and treatment of arthritis are applicable to people with other conditions resulting in joint limitation and pain. Therefore, the focus of this section is on assessment and treatment methods used for rheumatoid arthritis.

Impact

Rheumatoid arthritis is a progressive, systemic disease resulting in inflammation, pain, and structural changes in the affected joints. Characterized by remissions and exacerbations, rheumatoid arthritis results in progressive limitation and deformity. Many patients are between the ages of 20 and 40 years. They exhibit swollen, reddened, and painful joints during and after excessive use. Because of the limitations imposed by the disease, the patient's functional ability, physical appearance, and mental and psychological tolerance are affected. Treatment must be geared toward assisting the patient in combating the debilitating effects of the disease and in maintaining maximal independent functions. The occupational therapist aids the patient in learning a self-directed program of joint protection and function to continue at home. Due to the intermittent nature of the disease, it may be necessary to change functional lifestyle patterns that may exacerbate the symptoms and result in joint destruction. Therefore, working with the patient to develop therapeutic, daily functional patterns is an essential part of the program. Because the disease is progressive, the patient experiences a gradual decrease in functional ease and capacity due to decreasing strength, mobility, coordination, and pain-free movement.

Functional implications

The major clinical focus in rheumatoid arthritis is the joints, where there may be subluxation, dislocation, pain, swelling, stiffness, and deformity. Functional problems caused by arthritis arise from limitations in active and passive joint movement affecting reach, grasp, and coordination. Among the causes are internal joint damage, fear of pain, actual pain, decreased strength and sensation, and deformity.

During the period of inflammation, the joints are vulnerable to deformity produced by repetitive stress causing malalignment. Muscles are strained and weakened during this time, giving less resistance to the development of deforming positions. If muscles become overstretched and shift position, they can actually maintain and strengthen the deformity. This is frequently seen in the ulnar deviation of the metacarpophalangeal joints due to lateral slippage of the long finger tendons. When this realignment occurs, continuous finger flexion encourages rather than counteracts the deformity.

The following precautions should be taken when performing physical evaluations and during treatment of the patient with arthritis:

1. In the presence of dislocation and subluxation:
   a. Avoid overactivity of the affected joints.
   b. Avoid resistive exercises.
2. In the presence of pain and swelling:
   a. Limit passive ROM of the extremity during the acute stage of the disease.
   b. Encourage active ROM with resistance (as tolerated).
   c. Do not allow fear to develop.
   d. Minimize strenuous activity and alternate activity with rest periods.
3. Avoid overexercise; work within the limits of joint pain, exertion, swelling, and general tolerance.
4. Prevent muscle atrophy.
   a. Limit exercise to the maximal ROM with regard to specific joint range.
   b. Provide an activity in which the patient can work on strengthening muscles when he or she can work against resistance.

One of the preventive surgical procedures performed to combat the symptoms of rheumatoid arthritis is synovectomy. This procedure is performed early in the course of the disease to relieve pain and swelling of the joint, release contractures, and prevent arthrodesis of joints. Other surgical procedures include arthroplasty and joint replacement and are directed toward relieving pain, aligning joints, establishing function, and increasing ROM. When a surgical procedure is considered, the occupational therapist should inform the surgeon of the patient's functional ability so that function is retained postoperatively. The patient's attitude and expectations regarding surgery are crucial to rehabilitation. Through careful evaluation of functional activities, the occupational therapist is able to determine an accurate picture of what the patient is incapable of doing because of deformity, pain, or muscle imbalance. It is important to communicate this information to the surgeon before the operation.

Functional restoration

Assessment

The occupational therapist assesses the mental and physical tolerance by chart review, observation, and discussion of the patient's progress with members of the rehabilitation team. Evaluation sessions should not be prolonged beyond the effectiveness of both the patient and the therapist. During the session, the therapist provides encouragement and support; particular areas for consideration are the patient's stated concerns and apprehensions, medical condition, and resultant functional challenges. The occupational therapist varies the tests and activities so the patient can complete them without unnecessary pain, frustration, or joint stress. It is important that the therapist emphasize the patient's abilities realistically.

The following steps should be taken:

1. Examine the extremities for signs of redness, swelling, atrophy, discoloration, surgical scars, malalignment, joint deformities, hyperflexion, hyperextension, abduction, adduction, and ulnar deviation.
2. Examine the relaxed limbs for signs of atrophy, joint limitation, and discomfort.
3. Examine splints, braces, or other special equipment. Determine the patient's ability to use and care for the devices and evaluate their effectiveness.
4. Gently move the extremities through the passive joint ROM, noting any subluxation, limitation, muscle tightness, or pain.
5. Ask the patient to move his or her extremities through all ROM actively and to indicate if there is pain.
6. Check the muscle strength by providing resistance to active ROM.
7. Provide activities that demonstrate the functional use of hands and arms:
   a. *Grasping* small objects, such as coins, paper clips, a pencil, or a key
   b. *Lifting* heavy objects, such as a hammer, using one hand, and a large can of sugar, using two hands
   c. *Reaching*, by placing a book on a shelf, turning on a faucet, or opening a drawer
8. Observe the use of the hands in task activities, such as writing, removing a letter from an envelope, counting money (either change or bills), and finding a page in a book.
9. Evaluate self-care, including: bathing, grooming, eating, transferring from one position to another, walking, and carrying needed items.

The therapist should remain alert for signs of mental, psychological, or physical fatigue. The patient's confidence can be increased by asking him or her to describe present needs, interests, and concerns and to discuss plans.

Treatment

General principles

Several basic principles of therapeutic intervention can be used when working with the patient with rheumatoid arthritis, whether in an acute care program, an outpatient program, or a home care program. It is toward these objectives that the therapist instructs the patient so that the patient can maintain the long-term attention to self-care that the disease requires.

Control of the rheumatoid process

Antiinflammatory and analgesic drugs are used to control the disease. Bed rest is essential during the acute phase and after operation in instances of severe destruction of the joints. Although procedures may succeed in retarding the rheumatoid process for a time, the patient may continue to have exacerbations of the disease. When the joints show a reduction of swelling and inflammation, the rehabilitation program can begin.

Joint mobility through range of motion

Passive and active joint ROM of all extremities are essential for functional restoration. Passive and active joint ROM techniques should be employed to determine the presence of pain and limitation. Active ROM with resistance should be encouraged only after pain, swelling, and inflammation have been sufficiently reduced to avoid any risk of deformity.

Functional training

The occupational therapist uses a functional training program to make the patient aware of both limitations and abilities. Analyzing the patient's daily activities can help the therapist provide specific self-care techniques and appropriate productive avocational activities in conjunction with joint protection.

Maintenance of muscle power

The patient with rheumatoid arthritis may exhibit weakness. Deformities may prevent functional use of muscles, and joint alignment may be continually challenged. Without adequate joint function, muscle power is reduced, but the use of a functional hand splint can properly align muscles, joints, and tendons. Activities requiring strength must be used carefully in the therapeutic program. Too much resistance can cause joint pain. The occupational therapist must avoid activity that will cause fatigue and must make the patient aware of limitations in strength.

Independence in self-care

Because of the existence of pain and joint limitations characteristic of arthritis, the patient may suffer deficiencies in self-care, may avoid dressing, or may request assistance in basic ADL. The therapist should encourage the use of self-care techniques as therapeutic exercises, employing assistive devices and special equipment to conserve energy and to avoid further joint destruction.

Increasing physical and mental endurance

The person with rheumatoid arthritis is subjected to frequent hospitalizations. Exacerbations and remissions are common, and the patient displays the frustration caused by the inability to cope with family or job responsibilities. The therapist should encourage the patient to develop a regimen of alternate rest and work that will protect joints and conserve energy. The patient should also be instructed in the principles and use of joint protection techniques. Awareness of the nature of the disease can help both the patient and the family cope with the physical limitations that result from tension, overwork, or pain.

Assistive devices

Assistive devices should be used only to increase function or to protect impaired joints. They should be lightweight, simple to operate, and acceptable to the patient. They should encourage independent function. If the patient cannot use the device easily, he or she will discard it.

Home program

The occupational therapist must stress the need for the patient to continue the therapeutic program at home. Among the elements of discharge planning are a home visit to determine architectural barriers, necessary rearrangement of furniture and toilet facilities, assistance with work space and appliances, and development of specific devices.

Specific measures

The approaches to treatment must be individualized. The outpatient may be seen for the first time at the request of a physician for the construction of resting splints or splints to protect joints and to improve function, education about energy-conservation, and provision of assistive devices. The outpatient often has a family to care for, a job to perform, or school to attend. With the implementation of various aids and programs, the patient can perform tasks with greater ease and comfort and can gain the satisfaction of accomplishing chosen activities with less pain and stress. After the remission of painful symptoms requiring medical treatment, the patient may need only a few treatment sessions. The homemaker can be assisted in organizing time and tasks to minimize tension. The employed arthritic person can be assisted in self-evaluation of job activities and can learn how to adapt equipment or arrange the work schedule. The student can learn ways to ease the strain of note-taking and of carrying books and equipment. The student should also be encouraged to participate in social activities and to engage in recreation.

The inpatient is likely to be on bed rest during the acute stage of arthritis. Evaluation and initial treatment may be accomplished during this time. During the period of inflammation, there should be little stress on the joints, and daily activities of bathing and feeding should be assisted. Bathing can be simplified with the use of a bath mitt or a long-handled sponge. For meals, the patient can be provided with a fork with a built-up handle, a serrated knife, a large-handled plastic mug, easily managed food containers, and a rubber mat upon which to place plates.

Bed positioning is extremely important to prevent deformities and to encourage the most beneficial, comfortable, and successful means of functioning. The patient should use a firm mattress and should lie flat in the supine position with the arms and hands straight at the sides. A small pillow may be used if necessary. Lightweight covers should be used to minimize weight on sensitive limbs.

Prism glasses for television viewing or seeing visitors can minimize fatigue and eyestrain during this period. A book holder can be angled for bed use, and a lapboard placed in a comfortable position can be used for reading and writing. All items should be placed within easy reach.

During the period of bed rest, the patient often suffers pain from inflammation of the joints and requires encouragement and diversion more than active exercise. Exercise, when used, should *not* include resistance.

Poor positioning of the extremities may cause pain, poor alignment, stiff joints, deformity, and general discomfort. Thus, splints may be indicated during the acute inflammatory stage of rheumatoid arthritis. Note, however, that the provision of splinting for the patient with rheumatoid arthritis is both crucial and controversial. As Hollander (1972, p. 603) wrote, "It is usually much easier to prevent a deformity in arthritis than to correct one." Some experts believe that no splint at all is preferable to a splint that causes decreased function or deformity. The purposes of splinting the arthritic joints are provision of support to diseased joints, alleviation of pain, prevention of deformity, maintenance and promotion of function, and establishment of functional alignment.

Splints are used at night to maintain the extremity in a static position, providing proper alignment of the joints without undue stress on them and establishing a functional position for daily activities. Because the wrist is the key joint for hand function, stabilization and alignment of the wrist must be done before splinting of the fingers. The splint used at night can be a volar splint that extends from the distal third of the forearm to the fingertips, with abduction and extension of the thumb. In some cases, the thumb may be left free, and the splint may terminate at the distal portion of the metacarpophalangeal joints. This construction may be necessary to prevent stiffening of the phalangeal joints in extension since they should be slightly flexed.

Daytime splints also maintain functional alignment of the wrist and fingers; however, the splints must be different types from those used at night. If the pain is at the wrist, static positioning can stiffen the joints, and thus the splint must be removed and the joints allowed full ROM several times during the day. Dynamic splinting must be controlled to prevent both pain from movement and deformity from poor positioning. The palmar aspect of the splint can terminate at the palm. Finger cuffs and rubber bands can be used to provide finger mobility, with an outrigger for positioning and resistive activity. With this type of positioning, it is essential that the wrist be stabilized to minimize trauma to the finger joints.

After the occupational therapist has constructed the splints, they should be inspected to ensure that they provide proper support and comfort. Splints should be lightweight, cover a minimum of skin, and be easily applied or removed (Figure 18-6). The patient must be advised to inform the therapist of areas of irritation and to use both passive and active ROM exercises in conjunction with use of the splint.

The importance of positioning continues when the patient is sitting in a chair, using a wheelchair, or walking. When the patient is able to sit in a chair for activity, attention should be given to proper alignment of the body. A high-backed chair should be used for trunk and head support. Feet should be placed firmly on the floor, and firm cushions should be used to raise the patient to a comfortable position. Good positioning minimizes strain, encourages mechanical advantages in function, and prevents deformities.

When the patient is in a wheelchair or is ambulatory, the occupational therapy program becomes more intensive. As soon as it is medically feasible, the patient can engage in light activities that employ maximal active ROM. Needlework, Turkish knotting, light weaving, and painting can be used to strengthen the upper extremities and to increase joint ROM and coordination. In occupational therapy, water can be used as a therapeutic medium to relax and soothe the painful extremity in preparation for passive and active joint ROM exercise and activity. Careful massage of joint and tendon areas by the therapist helps to loosen stiff areas for active movement. This limbering may be provided in the physical therapy session and is particularly beneficial if scheduled just before the occupational therapy session. In preparation

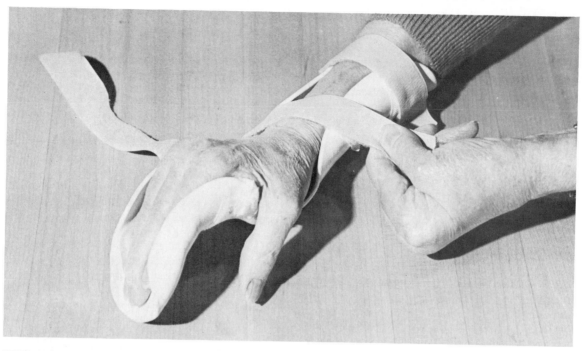

FIGURE 18-6. *Patient with rheumatoid arthritis puts on her volar splint, which provides rest and functional positioning of the hand and wrist at night on during the day.*

for functional activity, the patient benefits from warmth and from the desensitizing flotation effect of this exercise. Doing grasping exercises of increasing resistance and coordination uses the warmth and flotation to advantage.

Joint protection

Education in joint protection is an essential part of the occupational therapist's work. Because of pain and instability, some arthritic patients fear further damage to the joints and therefore avoid using them. On the other hand, an arthritic patient may deny the disability, avoid preventive precautions, and actually cause destruction and deformity.

Adopting the joint protection attitude and techniques can benefit the school-aged child with arthritis; he or she can endure writing exercises by using custom-made hand, wrist, or finger splints and large, square or rough-textured pencils for traction. Work surfaces and chair contour and height should fit the child comfortably and therapeutically to maintain stable, pain-free positioning for maximal performance.

The patient must become involved in the rehabilitation process, carrying over program principles learned during hospitalization. Among these principles of joint protection are the following:

1. Avoid positions that cause deformity. The therapist should encourage the patient to look carefully at the affected extremities to determine whether natural positions are resulting in redness, swelling, or pain. Tests for both passive and active joint ROM should be discussed with the patient so that the patient recognizes how to avoid excessive strain during daily activities.
2. Avoid sustained positions. The occupational therapist should teach the patient that maintaining a fixed position places stress on specific joints. For example, the longer a person grasps an object, the greater the likelihood of pain and stiffness on release of the object. The arthritic patient must be encouraged to change position or activities frequently, encouraging the reciprocal muscle movement to stretch tightened muscles and to relieve pressure on the joints.
3. Use the strongest joints for heavy work. Patients with arthritis must be taught to compensate for weakened joints and to try to develop bilateral capacity.
4. Do not start what you cannot stop. Arthritic patients are often characterized by ambition and a strong work ethic. These traits impair the ability to create a pace compatible with the disease. The occupational therapist must instruct the patient in energy conservation, organization of tasks, and awareness of fatigue.
5. Use joints to the greatest mechanical advantage. Certain activities can be done more easily in a standing position; among them are mopping a floor, mixing a cake, or washing one's hair. Among activities that are more easily done while seated are reading a book, working on a puzzle, doing needlework, or sewing. The crucial element here is not only putting the body in the most advantageous position but also preventing stress on other joints. If the mechanical aspects of different positioning for different activities are analyzed thoroughly by the therapist, the findings can be valuable in assisting the therapist in adapting positions and activities to increase function. Not using the body in a position that uses strong muscles and joints effectively may cause strain and even present a safety hazard.
6. The patient must be taught to respect pain. Although one can sometimes detect the signs of pain on someone's face or can learn of pain through the patient's complaint, pain itself

is highly subjective. Tolerance for pain varies, and, when there is a sensory deficit, the perception of pain may be entirely lacking. In periods when the arthritis is active, the patient may complain of severe pain, and there may be visible inflammation of joints. In the stages after acute attacks, the pain must be considered when planning activity programs. It must be conveyed to the patient that joint protection is for the purpose of improving and maintaining function rather than restricting function. This is often misinterpreted, and the patient ignores the suggestions for optimal bodily functions in the presence of arthritis. Improper use of joints can increase pain. Lack of attention to position changes and activity changes can cause pain. Denial, frustration, or tension can cause improper use of joints and put undue strain on them. The patient must plan activities to maximize function and ROM.

The occupational therapist teaches the patient the use of assistive devices and techniques that can aid in self-care and homemaking activities. For example, built-up handles, mitts, and rubber mats for cooking utensils aid the homemaker. Dressing can be assisted by the use of long-handled implements, and reachers can be used to grasp objects from the floor or from high places.

The arthritic patient's home can be made safe by the addition of railings at stairways, removal of heavy doors and scatter rugs, provision of easily managed latches on doors and cabinets, and arrangement of furniture and work areas for ease of movement and function. The occupational therapist can advise the patient in these labor-saving and safety factors.

To maintain muscle power and prevent deformity, the patient learns methods of using the muscles that maintain joint ROM, strength, coordination, and body alignment. Therapeutic use of joints keeps the patient functioning with maximal use of muscles and prevention of deformity. The most effective way of performing protective exercises for preservation of joints and prevention of deformity is to incorporate these therapeutic positions and movements into daily living activities.

A daily plan of activities schedules them according to the degree of physical stress, enabling the patient to alternate work and rest activities, gross and fine motor functions, and sitting and standing to provide therapeutic change to maintain activity tolerance and realistic productivity according to the individual patient's needs, desires, and abilities.

Orthopedic conditions

In the acute care setting, patients may be referred for occupational therapy with a variety of orthopedic problems, such as fractures, muscle tears or lacerations, bone repair or replacement, and amputations. Referral depends on such factors as the length of hospital stay, the short-term or long-term functional implications, additional problems, the extent of functional disruption of independent lifestyle patterns and expectations, and recognition of the value of occupational therapy by the orthopedic surgeon. Treatment of patients with UE conditions may be provided in an outpatient program.

Impact

The impact of a sudden fracture and the resultant temporary or permanent disability varies with the extent and complexity of the clinical manifestations. The range extends from the simple bone lesion requiring immobilization for a period of weeks to the more complex injuries involving bone, nerve, and muscle trauma. In such cases, therapeutic programs are directed toward regaining maximal functional ability through an adaptive program of daily exercise and activity. To accept the restrictions imposed on activity by casting, bracing, confinement to bed or wheelchair, and the new need for assistive devices to accomplish previously independent functions requires understanding of the condition, the course of recuperation, and the expected functional outcome on the part of the patient. When there is immediate and sudden disruption of the continuity of lifestyle patterns, the patient's acceptance is enhanced by recognizing the functional value of his or her remaining abilities.

The patient with brain or spinal cord injury may also have sustained one or more fractures of the extremities. In this case, the more severe injury may complicate the healing and general care of the fractured limbs. If the patient exhibits communication deficits, behavior disturbances, or decreased sensation, it is important that he or she understand what the therapist is doing and why. Sensitivity may be increased or decreased. If splinting or assistive devices are used in the presence of a sensory deficit, the affected extremity should be closely monitored for fit, function, and pressure areas. Alternate therapeutic approaches may be necessary to facilitate passive and active joint ROM in the presence of traction or additional therapeutic equipment.

Functional restoration

Among patients referred to occupational therapy are those with hand injuries and those with hip, back, and UE or LE fractures that confine them to bed or cause them to be placed in traction. The evaluation differs depending on the type of injury and the extent of the immobilization.

In preparing to evaluate the patient, the occupational therapist should review the medical factors pertinent to the injury and the present medical condition. These factors include the type of fracture; length and type of immobilization; alignment and progress of bony union; presence and extent of nerve involvement; presence of infection; precautions for mobility, safe joint movement, and muscle stretching; and appropriateness of removal of supporting casts, braces, or splints during activity or exercise.

Evaluation includes passive and active ROM of the joints proximal and distal to the immobilized joint; general mobility of all extremities; positioning alternatives; feasibility of the use of a wheelchair or of walking; and the existence of factors such as paralysis, trophic changes, edema, pain, fatigue, contractures, scar tissue, and psychological problems. The occupational therapist evaluates the level of functional ability and independence in ADL.

The general principles of treatment for the affected limb include the following:

- Support of the injured part to relieve trauma, to prevent further destruction of tissue, to ensure proper alignment of the extremity, and to prevent pain from joint limitation

- Prevention of disuse atrophy in the musculature surrounding the traumatized area by encouraging the patient to maintain strength, ROM, and function
- Provision of a therapeutic exercise program for reeducation of muscles and joints
- Encouragement of normal functional return after immobilization through gradual use of the extremity in unilateral and bilateral activities
- Assistance for the patient's adjustment to any cosmetic and functional changes

A patient may have pain in the extremity caused by the trauma itself or by immobilization; such a patient may not be motivated to participate in a full program of exercise and activity. The therapist encourages the patient to become involved in rehabilitation to prevent deformities, pain, and substitution of motor patterns in the weakened limb.

The patient with UE trauma may remain in the acute care setting for a relatively short time but long enough for adequate setting of the fracture, healing of surgical sites, and stabilization of medical complications. Initial casting is usually done by the physician, but the occupational therapist may be requested to assist in preparing for future adjustment by splinting in coordination with a functional exercise and activity program.

Specific considerations—upper extremity

For patients with UE injuries, the surgeon may request functional training for increasing joint ROM, strength, and coordination; provision of assistive devices for self-care; static and dynamic splinting; and supportive activities for those in traction. The general rehabilitation goal is to return the patient to a maximal level of function and independence. The injury may have caused serious damage to the sensorimotor system, resulting in the loss of extremity function by blocking the conduction of nerve impulses. Depending on the location and severity of the injury, the patient may suffer a long-term disability. The rehabilitation program focuses on return of the capacity to use the extremity and development of sensory and motor function. Physical and cosmetic changes in the extremity may cause difficulties in the patient's psychological adjustment to disability.

Shoulder disabilities can occur postoperatively in cases involving tumor, traction, immobilization, fracture, or periarthritis. Clinical signs include pain, muscle atrophy, shoulder weakness, contracture of the adductors with inability to rotate externally, fear of movement, and stiffness. After heat, massage, and whirlpool activity in physical therapy, the occupational therapy program includes graded activities to increase strength, joint ROM, and function. Examples of such activities are the floor loom, woodworking, macrame, and basketry. The patient should be encouraged to participate in recreational activities such as shuffleboard, darts, bowling, and ball games to develop full use and integration of the injured extremity. The physical tolerance and fatigue level should be the gauges for gradation of the program. Prevocational evaluation becomes part of the treatment program for the patient who will be able to return to work. The occupational therapist works closely with the vocational rehabilitation counselor in identifying specific job-related abilities. The industrially oriented program is basically one of regaining work tolerance in a graded conditioning program.

For UE injuries, activities such as using hand tools and power machinery, painting, and shoveling are used. The conditioning program should use productive work tasks, and activity time should be increased as endurance develops; however, the patient should be monitored for signs of pain, swelling, or fatigue. Home activity programs should be developed to encourage the patient to maintain a general conditioning program.

Patients who have a fractured forearm or hand may require a splint as a supportive device for strenuous activity. Unless there is peripheral nerve involvement from the injury, the orthopedic surgeon usually provides the initial splint. The occupational therapist may be asked later to provide a dynamic splint to encourage finger function. The most useful treatment is functional training in the use of the injured extremity. Productive activity is essential to the achievement of this goal. Graded manual activity and specific dexterity training in the affected hand are essential for the regaining of functional abilities. If the patient cannot regain adequate use of the hand through functional activity, counseling for alternative job training and placement may be required.

Patients who suffer residual effects from surgery (scarring or amputation) may need cosmetic adjustments. The occupational therapist counsels the patient, pointing out assets and helping the patient accept the additional trauma of cosmetic disfigurement.

Specific considerations—lower extremity

When a patient has suffered a fracture of an LE, the occupational therapy program begins with activities to provide support while the patient is confined to bed. When able to stand and put weight on the injured extremity, the patient can begin a program of standing tolerance and general reconditioning. LE active exercises include graded, resistive exercises of the extremity, coordination exercises, and use of the extremity together with the entire body.

Adaptations to the floor loom, bicycle saw, and woodworking equipment can aid in the gradual increase in strength and coordination. Work-simulated tasks designed for the injured worker offer preparation for the demands of the job.

For the patient who has had a back or leg injury, work activities include weight bearing, lifting, carrying, climbing, and bending. Activities such as lifting, carrying weights, climbing ladders, shoveling, chopping wood, pushing a wheelbarrow, and pulling heavy objects are upgraded according to the patient's tolerance. Specific activities for strengthening a limb and increasing tolerance that are used for the patient with a LE injury include balancing and exercising using adapted equipment such as a bicycle saw.

The patient with a fractured hip or hip replacement is commonly referred to the occupational therapist by the orthopedic surgeon, rheumatologist, or physiatrist. The patient benefits from supportive activities, self-care training, assistive devices, home evaluation, and home adaptation.

During the bed rest stage after surgery, the patient may benefit from supportive activities that assist in psychological adjustment and divert attention from pain. When there is medical clearance for the patient to move around in bed, the patient should be encouraged to participate in morning hygiene and self-care. Because the patient may be restricted in the use of the hip joint in flexion and resistive movements, long-handled reachers and special hooks can provide assistance in dressing. When the physician concurs, joint ROM of the hip should be encouraged during activity, but the rehabilitation process must be gradual.

The patient may be discharged from the hospital before he or she has fully recovered from the injury or surgery; therefore, a home program should be established to protect the hip from further injury and to encourage participation in exercise and self-care activities. The occupational therapist instructs the patient in both protective precautions and the use of various devices that can assist in self-care. The patient should avoid bending the hip more than 90 degrees and crossing the legs at the knees or ankles. A firm, knee-height, straight-backed chair with arm rests should be used. Reclining chairs are difficult for the patient to get into or out of, can cause the patient to fall, and thus should be avoided. Toilet seat extensions and firm pillows in low chairs can ensure proper height for adequate transfer and comfort.

The patient should be advised to sleep in a supine position to promote good alignment of the hip joints. If the patient is accustomed to turning in bed, a pillow should be placed between the legs to inhibit movement.

Other aspects of the home program include instruction and advice regarding the use of assistive devices for bathing (long-handled sponges, soap on a rope, and nonskid safety strips in the shower), for dressing (long-handled shoehorn, stocking aids, elastic shoe laces, and reachers), and for other ADL. A walker bag attached to the crutch may be used to carry small objects. Cars with low reclining seats should be avoided, although a cushion may be used to raise the seat to a comfortable height.

Cardiac conditions

The heart provides the essential thrust to the cardiovascular system by its pumping mechanism, which sends oxygen and nutrients to the body tissues and helps remove waste products. The pressure-regulated flow of blood through the circulatory system is dependent on open arteries and efficient heart valves to provide for the changing metabolic energy demands of daily activity. The action of the heart is correlated with that of the respiratory system and of the musculoskeletal system. The combined function of these three systems affects the capacity of a person to engage in exercise or activity and dictates the limits and benefits of specific activity. With cardiac disease, there is a disruption in the balance of the oxygen supply to the tissues and in the demand for sufficient amounts of oxygen to meet the metabolic requirements of functional performance. Risk factors related to coronary disease include (1) high intake of saturated fats, sodium, and cholesterol, (2) hypertension, (3) tobacco and alcohol use, (4) obesity, (5) sedentary living and lack of exercise, (6) competitive personality and stress, and (7) lack of coping mechanisms for general lifestyle control for healthy living.

Impact

The character of lifestyle components is a crucial factor in the initial prevention of heart disease, in the rehabilitation toward a productive and satisfying life after hospitalization, and in secondary prevention of further manifestations of disease. Mortality from coronary heart disease is declining due to public interest in improved diet, exercise programs, stress reduction, and self-monitoring.

The impact of cardiovascular disease on a person can result in serious physical and psychological health implications. Sudden hospitalization results in social and sensory deprivation with reduced mobility, independent function, and control. Such change results in reality loss, confusion, decreased attention span, boredom, and lethargy leading to depression regarding unresolved deprivations (Cornett & Watson, 1984). A primary psychological aspect is the fear of death and persistent anxiety with regard to participation in self-care and exercise activity after an acute episode or in the presence of pain. With the achievement of stability in the medical condition, the rehabilitation program is individually directed toward regaining mobility and productivity within the limits and dictates of the condition and prognosis. Patient and family education is essential to assist in adjustment to the illness, to encourage full understanding of the disease process and the rehabilitation program, for adequate discharge planning and resumption of a maximal level of activity within a scheduled period of time, and for secondary prevention of further manifestations of the disease process.

The role of the occupational therapist is essential to the regaining of self-esteem, functional activity, and self-regulation by the patient through performance routines and tasks. Primary functions of the therapist are orienting the patient to the varying levels of cardiac and metabolic demand of daily activity and encouraging and monitoring participation in a program of gradual augmentation of increased cardiac output for effective use of oxygen by the body through the three body systems as stimulated by the musculoskeletal system. Early mobilization to meet psychological and physical needs is essential. Patient education regarding the condition, the potential for recovery, and the treatment process serves to offset anxiety regarding threat of death, to provide a sense of control through program planning and participation, and to assist in the development and implementation of a health-oriented lifestyle. Since activity is an essential component of daily living and cardiac function, the expertise provided by the occupational therapist is a major component.

Functional implications

The purpose of rehabilitation is to enhance the capacity of the patient and family for coping with lifestyle changes that may be necessary to meet a functional level they believe will enhance quality of life. Research studies suggest mortality is decreased with increased physical activity and that exercise can effect improvement in physical and mental well-being (Fardy, 1988). Physical activity thus increases myocardial function and coronary vasodilation, decreases heart rate, increases tolerance to stress, and decreases strain associated with stress. Too sudden or too much exercise can negatively affect the cardiac patient, so it is imperative to correlate the occupational therapy program with other services provided to the patient. Initial direction from the physician and nurse reveal the patient's condition and the safe and optimal level and extent of activity recommended.

Assessment

Assessment of the cardiac patient begins with reading the patient's medical chart and discussion with appropriate team members regarding the present condition; precautions; and activity level recommendations and restrictions with regard to location and position for assessment and treatment procedures. General assessment areas include (1) evaluation of the patient's general attitude and orientation to the condition, awareness and knowledge of the disease process, and manifestations, (2) identification of the patient's premorbid lifestyle components and characteristics, (3) description of home social and physical environment, (4) identification of the patient's functional objectives, work history, present physical capacity, and endurance, and (5) observation of clinical signs, such as pallor, swelling, weakness, and shortness of breath. Initial evaluation includes determination of heart and pulse rates, which are taken before and after all activity as well as during activity if clinical signs indicate. Noting the demeanor of the patient during the interview is essential to determine the level or character of fear present and to encourage the patient by providing appropriate information regarding his or her condition and the occupational therapy role. A discussion with family members, with or separate from the patient, is beneficial to develop a comprehensive treatment plan considering the total situation and to prepare for discharge planning.

Treatment

The objective of the occupational therapy program for the cardiac patient is to stimulate and enhance cardiac output through a progressive program of purposeful activity within the level of tolerance of the patient. From the initial assessment of the medical status, the functional condition, and the premorbid characteristics of work, rest, play, and leisure, the occupational therapist develops, in conjunction with the patient, a plan for regaining control of lifestyle components. The therapist provides a therapeutic environment to promote healing and to prevent further insult to the heart.

General considerations and procedures involved in initiating an activity program with a patient include the following:

1. Determine the present status of the cardiac condition and levels of recommended activity.
2. Determine the pulse and blood pressure levels, and prepare to monitor them during the assessment and treatment processes.
3. Determine the optimal position of comfort, endurance, and maximal cardiac output before activity.
4. Begin the program and gradually build up activity within the tolerance of the patient.
5. Watch for clinical signs of excessive cardiac output, such as pallor, shortness of breath, dizziness, confusion, and patient complaint of fatigue, chest pain, and nausea.
6. Base activity on moderate and gradual upgrade in energy expenditure.
7. Plan positioning of activity and patient according to individual needs for work and rest.
8. Discuss activity, comfort, and progress with the patient.
9. Document information on a graph with patient assistance to monitor progress.

Work physiologists have established guidelines, metabolic equivalent tables, called METS, for determining levels of work based on oxygen consumption and caloric equivalents, which indicate the ratio between basal metabolism and metabolism related to specific activity performance. Activities are graded in six levels from minimal, or less than 1.5 METS, to excessively

severe, or 7 or more METS. Many excellent resources indicate a breakdown of a large variety of self-care, work, recreational, and homemaking activities according to MET level and specify position of function, such as standing, sitting, or lying (Krusen, Kottke, & Ellwood, 1971; Cornett & Watson, 1984). The following are some examples of MET levels and activities:

Minimal (less than 1.5): rest, sitting on bedside, standing at bedside (1–1.2), listening to the radio (1.45)
Light (1.5–2.5): eating (1.5), sewing (1.6), getting in or out of bed (1.65), writing (1.8), driving or propelling a wheelchair (2.5)
Moderate (2.5–3.5): playing piano (2.5–2.7), dressing (2.5–3.5), preparing meals (3), walking (3.2), taking a warm shower (3.5)
Heavy (3.5–5): having a bowel movement (3.6–4.7), making the bed (3.9), golfing (4), walking down stairs (4.5), gardening (4.5)
Severe (5–7): walking with brace or crutches (6.5), playing tennis (6), scrubbing a floor (5.3), riding a bicycle 8 to 10 mph (7)
Excessively severe (more than 7): skiing (8), mowing lawn (7.7), climbing stairs rapidly (9), having sexual intercourse (6–9)

Performance speed, air temperature, emotional tension, use of assistive devices, and locomotor problems during activity can upgrade the MET level and thus further challenge cardiac output and energy requirement.

Activity is essential to the cardiac patient to prevent respiratory complications, venous stasis or pooling, joint stiffness, and muscle weakness. It is beneficial to the patient's psychological and physical rehabilitation and well-being to regain control of his or her functional capabilities, and it is the challenge of the occupational therapist to present graded functional tasks within the realm of independent participation and psychological satisfaction. It may be frequently necessary to remind the patient that although the task may seem familiar and easy, it now may be stressful and fatiguing. Since lack of activity leads to problems of physical immobilization and depression, as well as poor cardiac output, a gradual progression of activity is recommended to improve output, reserve, and regaining of motivation for independent activity. The breakdown of activities by MET greatly helps the appropriate choosing of activity and the daily design of productive tasks at the patient's level of energy expenditure.

A cardiac rehabilitation program generally consists of some variation of four phases. Phase I is the acute care phase, when rest is imperative and activity is minimal until the patient is through the danger period and the condition is stable. During this period, there may be extensive monitoring of systems, passive ROM, breathing exercises, and gradual patient participation in self-feeding, hygiene, and limited face and hand bathing. If able, the patient may transfer with assistance from bed to chair and engage in activities from 1.5 to 2 METs toward development of sitting tolerance, UE activity, and awareness of daily scheduling of an activity and rest regimen. During this phase, the occupational therapist can be helpful in providing assistive equipment for therapeutic positioning for low-level activity. The rehabilitation program begins with phase II, when the focus extends to the build-up of strength and familiar functions through self-care, with energy conservation and work simplification methods. General exercise and mobility are increased with the resumption of walking, stair climbing, and showering, with METs limited to 3.5. Pulse rate monitoring is important here as well as in the initial stage, with patient education being an important aspect. This initial convalescent period extends into phase III, when the patient continues self-care and begins homemaking duties, including diet planning, while keeping activities within 4 to 5 METs for a period of 6 to 8 weeks. The occupational therapist may have begun a homemaking program in phase II that can be carried into either an outpatient program in phase III or a home program. In this period, a home evaluation can be done to assist the patient in modifying the environment for ease in access and in function. A build-up of energy requirement in activity is continued for endurance and for phase IV, which is the recovery or return-to-work phase. Return to work depends on the type of job and condition of the patient. Many jobs require 4 METs, and others can require 9 METs or more for short periods. METs should not exceed 7 for 6 months.

Therapists working with cardiac patients need to be informed on the MET breakdown of activity, methods of monitoring cardiac response to activity in the clinical situation, the continuing medical status and recommendations for the level of patient activity, along with precautions and clinical signs of malfunction. Resources from the American Heart Association are beneficial. For neurologic complications from cardiac disease and episodes, the reader is referred to the material in this section on neurologic conditions. Adaptive techniques and assistive devices may be required.

The cardiac patient may be seen in the general hospital, the rehabilitation center, the outpatient clinic, the nursing home, or the home environment. In each location, the opportunities for regaining of self-care, homemaking, and work capacities vary. It is essential for the occupational therapist to design an individualized program with the patient. Self-care activities performed in the hospital will be done with the nursing staff and with the family at home. Homemaking activities can be performed in the hospital unit, in the occupational therapy room, or in the patient's home. Work tasks can be simulated as well. It is essential that the occupational therapist provide the patient with an activity program that not only assists in upgrading cardiac output and productive activity but also provides diagnostic information with regard to level of progress.

Pulmonary conditions

Respiratory diseases may result from (1) obstruction of gas exchange in the lung, (2) reduction in lung volume, (3) diseases occupying the lung space, (4) vascular disease, and (5) disorders of ventilatory regulation. Manifestations of chronic obstructive pulmonary disease include narrowing of airways and plugging with secretions, as in asthma; the productive cough resulting from hypertrophy of mucous glands, as in chronic bronchitis; and the distention and destruction of alveolar walls causing reduction of tissue elasticity and collapse of airways, as experienced in emphysema. Reduction of lung volume may occur from pressure on the airways due to obesity and dysfunction of respiratory muscles due to cervical cord injury and neurologic diseases. Pneumonia, tumor, and interstitial diseases pathologically fill lung spaces. Pulmonary vascular diseases, such as pulmonary heart disease, pulmonary thromboembolism, and left heart failure affect arterial functions and weaken the cardiac system. Disordered ventilatory regulation may result in hyperventilation from injuries to the brain stem, from acute and chronic anxiety,

and from hypoxemia. Hypoventilation may result from neurologic damage to the brain stem, vascular insufficiency, or drug intake (Luce, Tyler, & Pierson, 1984). Obstructive and restrictive lung diseases can lead to severe disability, heart failure, and death. The progression of the disease is often slow.

Risk factors related to pulmonary disease include (1) irritants such as tobacco, dust, air pollution, (2) respiratory tract infections, (3) anxiety, (4) breathlessness leading to fear of activity involvement, (5) development of sedentary lifestyle, (6) loss of independent activity, and (7) depression. Warning signs of onset include (1) increased mucous, (2) change in mucous color, (3) increased wheezing, (4) increased cough or productivity, (5) dyspnea or shortness of breath, (6) fever, (7) chest pain, (8) swelling of the ankles, and (9) excessive drowsiness.

Impact

Chronic obstructive pulmonary disease is the fifth leading cause of death in the United States. Chronic respiratory diseases are the fourth largest cause of major activity limitation and the sixth leading cause of premature retirement due to disability (DeLisa, 1988). Cooper (1991) has characterized the patient with chronic pulmonary disease as entering a vicious cycle of immobility due to severe breathlessness, which leads to physical deconditioning, isolation, depression, and further impairment of exercise tolerance. This seemingly irreversible downward spiral is the challenge of the pulmonary rehabilitation program. Primary objectives of treatment are to correct the abnormal breathing pattern that increases the work of breathing, increase the energy to breathe, decrease fatigue from activity, facilitate the patient's regaining of control over his or her life and activities, and prevent further manifestations of pulmonary disease. Through the coordination of an interdisciplinary approach that includes respiratory medicine, physical therapy, occupational therapy, nursing, dietary, social service, and vocational rehabilitation, the comprehensive needs of the patient are identified. Patient education is the main aspect of orientation to the disease process and its implications. The patient works through the challenges of neuromuscular reeducation, self-care, self-awareness, homemaking, and avocational, vocational, and social activity for efficient and realistic future planning for community reentry. A program of gradual progressive exercise and activity concurrent with relaxation, smoking cessation, dietary modification, breathing patterns, and resumption of activity is shared by all disciplines with the patient as tolerated and appropriate.

The pulmonary rehabilitation program is a carefully monitored system of patient services and teaching. Fluid intake must be adequate to keep airways clear of secretions. Smoking cessation reduces the depth of inhalation needed to reverse the focus onto exhalation through a breathing program. Avoiding irritants assists in the benefit of breathing exercises through pursed-lip and diaphragmatic breathing to minimize breathing effort and maximize oxygen intake and use. Muscle endurance training is necessary to increase the capacity to exercise without undue fatigue to build endurance. The patient is taught diet control through use of a high-protein diet to meet metabolic needs of activity. Medications include oxygen, bronchodilators, corticosteroids, antibiotics, diuretics, cardiac drugs, and psychotrophic drugs. Prevention of infection by avoiding disease carriers is essential. Patients may have coexistent heart disease or other medical conditions, and frequently, a pattern of exercise or activity avoidance results in a sedentary lifestyle to minimize anxiety. Reconditioning is necessary to upgrade psychological, physical, and social abilities and performance. With the regaining of a higher level of performance, the patient regains self-esteem and self-worth. The individualized reconditioning program is modeled after the MET system for cardiac patients, providing a systematic, numeric grading and progression of all types of activity according to energy requirement and expenditure. Activity analysis and familiarity with the METs of activities are beneficial to the program. Vocational rehabilitation may follow the work begun by the occupational therapist in self-care and daily activity, leading to the development of hobbies, employment, or volunteer work. These contribute to self-sufficiency and social participation. Effective vocational reentry is enhanced by avoiding respiratory irritants at work, reducing energy output to a safe level, informing employers of limitations, and counseling for job placement as indicated.

Functional implications

Working with the pulmonary patient requires an understanding of the psychological and physical aspects of activity and inactivity. With the downward activity spiral suggested by Cooper (1991), the pulmonary patient may appear not only disinterested in but also fearful of changing the daily pattern to a more active one due to the increase of shortness of breath with activity. Increased nervousness and breathing may result in the feeling of getting stuck in a position of inspiration where too much air gets trapped in the lungs, and there results an inability to get oxygen because the lungs are too full. Pursed-lip breathing is taught to avoid this. The patient becomes a candidate for significant lifestyle changes in (1) breathing patterns, (2) relaxation patterns, (3) analysis and pacing of activities, (4) self-monitoring, and (5) healthy patterns of fluid intake. Learning the lifestyle and premorbid behaviors and values of the patient is essential to providing significant help to the patient in making these changes. Important considerations include helping the patient to minimize dependency on family and community through teaching optimal capability for carryover into ADL, self-reliance, and the development of useful activities.

Assessment

Initial pulmonary evaluation by respiratory therapists or physical therapists includes determining blood gas levels, adequacy of ventilation, ability to clear secretions, pulmonary function, physical endurance and capacity, and psychological effect (Goodgold, 1988).

The occupational therapy assessment begins with a thorough chart review to determine medical status and interdisciplinary findings. Interview and performance testing provide information on general physical performance, level of self-care and homemaking skills, and present avocational and vocational activity. Discussion with the patient regarding performance characteristics, response to stressful situations, presence of anxiety in lifestyle components, and presence of shortness of breath assist in giving indications of problem areas. Discussion of major concerns and objectives of the patient with regard to current problems and priorities can indicate areas for future planning and therapeutic intervention. An evaluation of the home and work physical and social environments may be done in preparation for

discharge or as part of outpatient or home patient assessment. Functional status assessment is essential for determining the treatment objectives and program with regard to the gradual build-up of functional capacity and endurance.

Treatment

The lack of control over breathing and fear of increased shortness of breath leads to a general avoidance of physical activity with resultant deconditioning. All activity must be coordinated with correct breathing to increase overall endurance. Breathing retraining includes pursed-lip breathing and diaphragmatic breathing, both of which can be learned from respiratory therapists and incorporated into the occupational therapy program. Pursed-lip breathing creates a resistance to the flow of air out of the lungs and slows down the breathing rate. This technique is used with stressful activities to avoid shortness of breath. Diaphragmatic breathing decreases the cost of breathing and enables the patient to engage in purposeful activities. Bronchial hygiene through smoking cessation, coughing and fluid intake, postural drainage to prevent mucous pooling in lungs, controlled coughing, and humidification in rooms are all part of the rehabilitation program. Correct breathing and relaxation are stressed with the exercise and activity programs. Bronchodilators, antibiotics, and oxygen medications may be used.

The patient learns conscious breathing and conscious relaxation along with the graded progressive activity program in bed, in a chair, and standing and walking. Reconditioning activities must be programmed individually. Psychological counseling may be needed to assist the patient in adjusting to dependency and changing social roles and in developing coping mechanisms.

In the acute care phase, the occupational therapist begins with a bed exercise and activity program, which progresses as the patient gains strength and endurance. The program includes self-care, avocational activity, ROM and strengthening activities, cognitive activity, training in relaxation and proper body mechanics, pacing for energy levels, energy conservation, and work simplification training, with particular regard for self-care and homemaking. A job analysis is done when appropriate.

It is essential that the patient learn to distinguish between relaxation and tension as well as learn the process of activity analysis for future self-monitoring and activity planning. Energy conservation involves planning ahead, rest between activities, organization of work items and location before task initiative, optimal accessibility of items and procedures, consistency of task, use of pursed-lip breathing with prolonged expiration, and use of adaptive devices and techniques for task accomplishment.

The occupational therapist focuses on a task and activity approach with the patient. Sufficient explanation to the patient regarding the essence of the correlation of breathing and pacing of rest and activity must be made for the patient to accept the possibility of a more active life within his or her limitations. With the progression of successful involvement in activity, the patient develops improved self-esteem and motivation to work toward healthier lifestyle components and behaviors. The use of the MET system of activity levels can provide an effective way to engage the patient in designing a progressive activity schedule consistent with energy levels and interests. Additional benefits of self-direction of the rehabilitation program are an improvement of self-image and self-acceptance as well as an individual effort toward increasing the level of independence in daily activity, which may include returning to gainful employment or choosing a more healthy alternative to a previous occupation.

Summary

Lesions in the brain can result from trauma, such as head injury or CVA, and from disease, such as MS and Parkinson disease. Lesions can produce temporary or permanent functional deficits. The onset can be sudden or progressive. The particular clinical manifestations, in the form of dysfunction, depend on the part of the brain affected by the trauma or lesion. Symptoms that are commonly manifested, either temporarily or permanently, are personality and behavior changes resulting in psychosocial challenges, cognitive distortions, and intellectual deficits; sensorimotor dysfunction; and disruption of functional performance. Deficits in these areas can have a significant impact on the future functioning of the patient and may require lifestyle changes with regard to family and community life.

Treatment programs are directed toward functional restoration and adaptive living. Effective functional restoration depends equally on psychosocial and physical rehabilitation. The occupational therapist makes an essential contribution in providing the patient with opportunities to develop the maximal level of functional ability, self-awareness, and acceptance through individual and social interaction and daily activity in the therapeutic environment. Programs are individually designed with the patient for maximal effectiveness.

Disease and trauma affecting the spinal cord and its pathways can result in progressive or nonprogressive dysfunctional conditions. The progressive disease ALS presents a clinical pattern of diminishing sensorimotor stability and function in the extremities, which may include the motor functions of speech. In poliomyelitis, the immediate paralyzing effects are permanent. In Guillain-Barré syndrome, although there is an immediate paralysis, there is a good prognosis for substantial return of function during an intensive rehabilitation program. The functional manifestations and permanence of the initial paralysis due to injury to the spinal cord are dependent on the segmental level of the cord lesion and the type and extent of the injury.

The occupational therapy program provides the patient with the opportunity to focus on ability through specific muscle reeducation, functional adaptation and performance, and planning based on awareness of his or her condition and capabilities. Mutual planning by therapist and patient, communication with rehabilitation team members and family, and adaptation of treatment modalities to the patient's lifestyle and preferences contribute to the potential effectiveness of the program and effective community reentry.

Diseases of the joints affect the overall mobility and function of the patient. DJD, or osteoarthritis, affects individual joints and is manifested as swelling in the bony structure. Treatment focuses on the relief of joint pain and stress. Rheumatoid arthritis, lupus erythematosus, and scleroderma are systemic diseases characterized by inflammation in the soft tissues of the joint, edema, pain, decreased function, and potential deformity. Because the patient with rheumatoid arthritis is frequently referred for occupational therapy services, assessment and treatment aspects of functional restoration with regard to this disease have been emphasized. The principles of joint protection not only aid the patient with rheumatoid arthritis but also provide an optimal therapeutic approach to all patients with joint sensitivity resulting in decreased motivation and confidence in maximal daily functional activity.

The occupational therapist provides an essential service to the patient with arthritic manifestations by providing functional adaptation opportunities through assistive splinting, assistive devices, or adaptive methods that promote effective daily exercise and activity as well as the psychosocial benefit of continued optimal performance.

Patients referred to occupational therapy with orthopedic conditions involving the trunk, the upper extremities, or the lower extremities may be seen on a short-term basis while in the acute-care setting, or the treatment may continue into or begin in the outpatient setting. Patients with orthopedic injuries may have accompanying neuromuscular deficits as well as damage to additional systems. The occupational therapist and the certified occupational therapy assistant contribute to the general functional program of the patient with particular regard to assistance in the regaining of sensorimotor, self-care, avocational, and vocational abilities. A significant aspect of the program is the assessment of the need for assistive devices and equipment for optimal function in the home as well as in the treatment setting, with specific recommendations for the provision of appropriate equipment.

A person's ability to engage fully in exercise or activity depends on the combined functions of the cardiovascular, respiratory, and musculoskeletal systems. Lifestyle characteristics may adversely impact cardiac output and put a person at risk for coronary disease. While primary prevention is the ultimate social goal, rehabilitation is geared toward lifestyle change for healthy living, gradual build-up of cardiac output tolerance, and resumption of daily activities within limits of tissue and mechanical capacity of the heart and circulatory systems. The occupational therapist participates in the daily design and upgrading of the patient's activity program leading to independence in self-care, homemaking, and vocational and avocational pursuits.

Diseases of the respiratory system affect the flow of oxygen and carbon dioxide to and from body tissue for functional use. A downward spiral of ability to engage in daily activity begins with fear of breathlessness and gradual loss of functional independence due to the energy requirement of breathing. Focus of the rehabilitation program is on breathing retraining; relaxation training; general physical conditioning; regaining of functional independence through an activity program using the MET system; development of positive self-image, self-esteem, and a healthy lifestyle; pacing of activity; energy conservation; and work simplification. Patient and family education are essential. Since there may be combined cardiac and pulmonary components, similarities may be found in the monitoring and progressive development of independent activity, with energy conservation and work simplification elements combined with patient and family education for effective community reentry.

The occupational therapist is in a unique position to provide essential services to patients in regaining a healthy perspective and involvement in life experiences after disease or trauma. Within the context of the philosophical base of occupational therapy and the availability of dynamic frames of reference, therapeutic theory, specific skills in clinical and community application of practice techniques, and adaptations are the mandates for responsible and essential therapeutic services.

This section is dedicated to the memory of my dear friend and colleague Patricia A. Curran, who provided constant editorial assistance and encouragement in professional and technical writing.

Appreciation is extended to Harmarville Rehabilitation Center in Pittsburgh and to Eastern Maine Medical Center in Bangor for photographs and library resources, to Lois Rosage, Linda Strathdee, and Jean Blanchard for critical review, to Richard Mason for consultation and resources, and to Laura Tasheiko and Blue Hill Memorial Hospital in Blue Hill, Maine for technical assistance.

References

Allen, A. (1991). Casa Colina's pulmonary rehabilitation program. *RT The Journal for Respiratory Care Practitioners, 4*(5), 25–30.

Bannister, R. (1973). *Brain's clinical neurology* (4th ed., pp. 323, 329, 347, 392–394). London: Oxford University Press.

Brain, B., & Walton, J. N. (1969). *Brain's diseases of the nervous system* (pp. 494, 525, 595, 598, 814). London: Oxford University Press.

Cooper, C. B. (1991). The use of oxygen in pulmonary rehabilitation. *RT The Journal for Respiratory Care Practitioners, 4*(5), 13–22.

Cornett, S. J., & Watson, J. E. (1984). *Cardiac rehabilitation: An interdisciplinary team approach.* New York: John Wiley & Sons.

DeLisa, J. A. (Ed.). (1988). *Rehabilitation medicine: Principles and practice.* Philadelphia: J. B. Lippincott.

Eson, M. E., Yen, J. K., & Bourke, R. S. (1978). Assessment of recovery from serious head injury. *Journal of Neurology, Neurosurgery and Psychiatry, 41,* 1036.

Fardy, P. S., Yanowitz, T. G., & Wilson, P. K. (1988). *Cardiac rehabilitation: Adult fitness and exercise testing* (2nd ed.). Philadelphia: Lea & Febriger.

Goodgold, J. (1988). *Rehabilitation medicine.* St. Louis: C. V. Mosby.

Hagan, C., Malkmus, D., & Durham, P. (1972). *Communication disorders service* (revised 11/15/74 by D. Malkmus, & K. Stenderup). Downey, CA: Rancho Los Amigos Hospital.

Hollander, J. L., & McCarthy, D. J. Jr. (1972). *Arthritis and allied conditions* (p. 603). Philadelphia: Lea & Febiger.

Jennett, B., & Bond, M. (1975). Assessment of outcome after severe brain damage: A practical scale. *Lancet, 1,* 482.

Jennett, B., & Teasdale, G. (1977). Aspects of coma after severe head injury. *Lancet, 1,* 878.

Krusen, F. H., Kottke, F., & Ellwood, P. M. (1971). *Handbook of physical medicine and rehabilitation* (2nd ed.). Philadelphia: W. B. Saunders.

Luce, J. M., Tyler, M. L., & Pierson, D. J. (1984). *Intensive respiratory care.* Philadelphia: W. B. Saunders.

Mossman, P. L. (1976). *A problem-oriented approach to stroke.* Springfield, IL: Charles C. Thomas.

Rappaport, M. (1980). *Disability rating scale for severe head trauma patients.* Presented at the Third Annual Conference on Head Trauma Rehabilitation: Coma to Community.

Rusk, H. (1971). *Rehabilitative Medicine* (4th ed., p. 321). St. Louis: C. V. Mosby.

Snook, J. H. (1979). Spasticity reduction splint. *American Journal of Occupational Therapy, 33,* 648.

Stern, J. M. (1978). Cranio-cerebral injured patients: Psychiatric clinical description.

Wilson, D. C. (1973). *Hilary.* New York: McGraw-Hill.

Bibliography

Abreu, B. C. (Ed.). (1981). *Physical manual.* New York: Raven Press.

Alpers, B. J., Mancall, E. L. (1971). *Clinical neurology* (6th ed., p. 598). Philadelphia: F. A. Davis.

American Occupational Therapy Association (1980). *Mart catalog.* Rockville, MD: AOTA.

Ayres, A. J. (1979). *Sensory integration and the child.* Los Angeles: Western Psychological Services.

Banerjee, S. N. (Ed.). (1982). *Rehabilitation management of amputees.* Baltimore: Williams & Wilkins.

Basmajian, J. V., & Wolf, S. (Eds.). (1990). *Therapeutic exercise* (5th ed.). Baltimore: Williams & Wilkins.

Boyes, J. H. (1970). *Bunnell's surgery of the hand* (5th ed., p. 240). Philadelphia: J. B. Lippincott.

Brooks, N. A. (1982). From rehabilitation to independent living. In F. J. Kottke, G. K. Stillwell, J. F. Lehmann (Eds.), *Krusen's handbook of physical medicine and rehabilitation* (3rd ed.). Philadelphia: W. B. Saunders.

Carle, T. V. (1984). The long term picture in spinal cord injury. In P. E. Kaplan (Ed.). *The practice of physical medicine.* Springfield, IL: Charles C. Thomas.

Cromwell, F. S. (Ed.). (1984). *Occupational therapy strategies and adaptations for independent daily living.* New York: Haworth Press.

Cynkin, S. (1979). *Therapy toward health through activities.* Boston: Little, Brown.

DeLisa, J. A. (Ed.). (1988). *Rehabilitation medicine: Principles and practice.* Philadelphia: J. B. Lippincott.

Demopoulos, J. T. (1984). Rehabilitation in fractures of limbs. In A. P. Ruskin (Ed.), *Current therapy in physiatry.* Philadelphia: W. B. Saunders.

Dorros, S. (1981). *A patient's view.* Cabin John, MD: Seven Locks Press.

Ehrlich, G. E. (Ed.) (1985). *Rehabilitation management of rheumatic conditions* (2nd ed.). Baltimore: Williams & Wilkins.

Erhlich, G. E. (Ed.). (1986). *Total management of the arthritis patient* (2nd ed.). Philadelphia: J. B. Lippincott.

Fardy, P. S., Yanowitz, F. G., & Wilson, P. K. (1988). *Cardiac rehabilitation: Adult fitness and exercise testing* (2nd ed.). Philadelphia: Lea & Febiger.

Field, E. V. (Ed.). (1977). *Multiple sclerosis.* Baltimore: University Park Press.

Flatt, A. E. (1983). *Care of the arthritic hand* (4th ed.). St. Louis: C. V. Mosby.

Flower, A., Naxon, E., Jones, R. E., & Mooney, V. (1981). An occupational therapy program for chronic back pain. *American Journal of Occupational Therapy, 35,* 243.

Ford, J. R., & Duckworth, B. (1987). *Physical management for the quadriplegic patient* (2nd ed.). Philadelphia: F. A. Davis.

Fraser, C. (1984). Does an artificial limb become part of the user? *British Journal of Occupational Therapy, 47,* 43.

Friedman, L. W. (1978). *The psychological rehabilitation of the amputee.* Springfield, IL: Charles C. Thomas.

Gilfoyle, E. M., Grady, A. P., & Moore, J. C. (1981). *Children adapt.* Thorofare, NJ: Charles B. Slack.

Golden, C. J. (1981). *Diagnosis and rehabilitation in clinical neuropsychology.* Springfield, IL: Charles C. Thomas.

Goodgold, J. (1988). *Rehabilitation medicine.* St. Louis: C. V. Mosby.

Gruen, H., Medsger, T. A., & White, J. F. (1980). *Joint protection training for the patient with early rheumatoid arthritis.* Basle: CIBAGEIGY.

Gurgosd, G. D., & Harden, D. M. (1978). Assessing the driving potential of the handicapped. *American Journal of Occupational Therapy, 32,* 41.

Heilman, K. M., & Valenstein, E. (1979). *Clinical neuropsychology.* New York: Oxford University Press.

Heiniger, M. C., & Randolph, S. L. (1981). *Neurophysiological concepts in human behavior: The tree of learning.* St. Louis: C. V. Mosby.

Held, J. P. (1984). Rehabilitation of head injury patients. In A. P. Ruskin (Ed.), *Current-therapy in physiatry.* Philadelphia: F. A. Davis.

Jennett, B., & Teasdale, G. (1981). Aspects of coma after severe head injury. *Lancet, 1,* 878.

Jennett, B., & Teasdale, G. (1981). *Management of head injuries.* Philadelphia: F. A. Davis.

Kaplan, P. E. (Ed.). *The practice of physical medicine.* Springfield, IL: Charles C. Thomas.

Kottke, F. J. (1982). Therapeutic exercise to develop neuromuscular coordination. In F. J. Kottke, & J. F. Lehmann (Eds.), *Krusen's handbook of physical medicine and rehabilitation* (3rd ed.). Philadelphia: W. B. Saunders.

Krusen, F. H., Kottke, F., & Ellwood, P. M. (1990). *Handbook of physical medicine and rehabilitation* (4th ed.). Philadelphia: W. B. Saunders.

Malick, M. H., & Meyer, C. M. H. (1978). *Manual of management of the quadriplegic upper extremity.* Pittsburgh: Harmarville Rehabilitation Center.

Marquit, S. (1981). *Factors in the management of Parkinson's disease.* Miami: National Parkinson Foundation.

Meyer, N. H. (1984). Concepts in head injury rehabilitation. In P. E. Kaplan (Ed.), *The practice of physical medicine.* Springfield, IL: Charles C. Thomas.

Morris, A. F., & Brown, M. (1976). Electronic training devices for hand rehabilitation. *American Journal of Occupational Therapy, 30,* 379.

Najenson, T., Groswasser, Z., Mendelson, L., & Hackett, R. (1980). Rehabilitation outcome of brain damaged patients after severe head injury. *International Rehabilitation Medicine, 2,* 133.

National Handicap Housing Institute. (1981). *Product inventory of hardware, equipment and appliances for barrier-free design* (2nd ed.). Minneapolis: Author.

Nichols, P. J. R. (1980). *Rehabilitation medicine: The management of physical disabilities* (2nd ed.). Woburn, MA: Butterworths.

O'Brien, M. T., & Pallett, P. J. (1978). *Total care of the stroke patient.* Boston: Little, Brown.

O'Sullivan, S. B., & Schmitz, T. J. (1988). *Physical rehabilitation: Evaluation and treatment procedures* (2nd ed.). Philadelphia: F. A. Davis.

Occupational therapy in the care of spinal pain patients. (1979). Downey, CA: Professional Staff Association, Rancho Los Amigos Hospital.

Olszowy, D. R. (1978). *Horticulture for the disabled and disadvantaged.* Springfield, IL: Charles C. Thomas.

Palmer, M. L. (1985). *Manual for functional training.* Philadelphia: F. A. Davis.

Payton, O. D., Hirt, S., & Newton, R. A. (1977). *Scientific bases for neurophysiological approaches to therapeutic exercise.* Philadelphia: F. A. Davis.

Pedretti, L. W. (1985). *Occupation therapy: Practice skills for physical dysfunction* (2nd ed.). St. Louis: C. V. Mosby.

Prentke Romich Company. *Electronic aids for the severely handicapped: Wheelchair control systems.* Wooster, OH: Author.

Redford, J. B. (Ed.). (1985). *Orthotics etcetera* (3rd ed.). Baltimore: Williams & Wilkins.

Reed, K., & Sanderson, S. R. (1983). *OTR concepts of occupational therapy* (2nd ed.). Baltimore: Williams & Wilkins.

Reichel, W. (Ed.). (1988). *Clinical aspects of aging* (3rd ed.). Baltimore: Williams & Wilkins.

Rowland, L. P. (Ed.). (1989). *Merrit's textbook of neurology* (8th ed.). Philadelphia: Lea & Febiger.

Roy, R., & Tunks, E. (Eds.). (1989). *Chronic pain: Psychosocial factors in rehabilitation* (rev. ed.). Baltimore: Williams & Wilkins.

Ruskin, A. P. (Ed.). (1984). *Current therapy in physiatry.* Philadelphia: W. B. Saunders.

Sacks, O. (1987). *A leg to stand on.* New York: Harper and Row.

Scheinberg, L. C., & Holland, N. J. (Eds.). (1987). *A guide for patients and their families* (2nd ed.). New York: Raven Press.

Sharpless, J. W. (1982). *Mossman's a problem oriented approach to stroke rehabilitation* (2nd ed.). Springfield, IL: Charles C. Thomas.

Silverstone, B., & Hyman, H. K. (1982). *You and your aging parent.* New York: Pantheon.

Stern, G., & Lees, A. (1982). *Parkinson's disease: The facts.* New York: Oxford University Press.

Trombly, C. A. (Ed.). (1989). *Occupational therapy for physical dysfunction* (3rd ed.). Baltimore: Williams & Wilkins.

Umphred, D. A. (1989). *Neurological rehabilitation* (2nd ed., Vol. 3). St. Louis: C. V. Mosby.

Vallbona, C. (1990). Bodily responses to immobilization. In F. J. Kottke, G. K. Stillman, & J. F. Lehmann (Eds.), *Krusen's handbook of physical medicine and rehabilitation* (4th ed.). Philadelphia: W. B. Saunders.

Wenger, N. K. (Ed.). (1985). *Exercise and the heart* (2nd ed.). Philadelphia: F. A. Davis.

Wilson, D. J., McKenzie, M. W., & Barber, L. M. (1984). *Spinal cord injury: A treatment guide for occupational therapists* (rev. ed.). Thorofare, NJ: Charles B. Slack.

Wittmeyer, M., & Barrett, J. E. (1980). *Housing accessibility checklist.* Seattle: University of Washington Press.

Wittmeyer, M. B. & Stolov, W. C. (1978). Educating wheelchair patients on home architectural barriers. *American Journal of Occupational Therapy, 32,* 557.

Wolf, J. K. (Ed.). (1987). *Mastering multiple sclerosis: A guide to management* (2nd ed.). Rutland, VT: Academy Books.

Wright, G. N. (1980). *Total rehabilitation.* Boston: Little, Brown.

SECTION 3

Amputation and prosthetic replacement

ELINOR ANNE SPENCER

KEY TERMS

Conventional Prostheses

Limb Replantation

Myoelectric Prostheses

Phantom Sensation

Postoperative Program

Preprosthetic Program

Prosthetic Replacement

Prosthetic Training Program

LEARNING OBJECTIVES

Upon completion of this section the reader will be able to:

1. *Explain the functional implications of amputation.*

2. *Identify the levels of amputation and some options for surgical intervention and prosthetic replacement.*

3. *Describe elements of postoperative early fitting, preprosthetic training, and prosthetic training programs.*

4. *Explain the prescription and the operation of the upper-extremity prosthesis.*

5. *Describe the components of an upper-extremity prosthetic training program.*

6. *Work effectively with the upper- and lower-extremity amputee in a therapeutic adaptation program.*

It's not what you've lost that counts,
it's what you do with what's left.

McGonegal, C. (Russell & Ferullo, 1981, p. 17)

To be an amputee is to be without a limb or limbs as a result of congenital deformity, injury, or disease. Age, developmental level, sex, functional ability, vocational and avocational preferences, social status, psychological status, and financial factors affect surgical decisions, preprosthetic programs, and prosthetic replacement. A child born with a congenital anomaly generally develops bodily functions and body image while adapting to the anomaly during the growth process. Therefore, a prosthesis is an addition to the natural developmental process and must be incorporated into a meaningful relationship with the body to become a functional part of it. The older child, adolescent, or adult, having passed this developmental period, suffers an amputation as a loss that disrupts both the body image and the sensorimotor integration of previously developed bodily functions and skills. The traumatic amputee and the congenital amputee must adapt to the mechanical replacement of natural function and then incorporate its use into total body function. The circumstances of the loss, its meaning to the person, and the functional consequences are thus different for the congenital and the traumatic amputee.

Regardless of the developmental level or cause of the amputation, effective **prosthetic replacement** depends on a coordinated team effort by the physician, nurse, physical therapist, occupational therapist, psychologist, social worker, prosthetist, educator or vocational counselor, patient, and family. To ensure maximal team effort in the appropriate prosthetic replacement for the amputee, the following factors are essential:

1. The amputee must be able to accept the use and appearance of the prosthetic replacement in relation to personal lifestyle and daily needs.
2. The prescribed prosthetic components and design must be appropriate to the needs and expectations of the amputee.
3. The prosthesis must fit properly before functional training and use can begin.
4. The amputee must be able to tolerate the prosthesis physically for functional wear and use.
5. Fundamental elements of the prosthetic replacement program include: assessment, prescription, preprosthetic training, prosthetic checkout and care, prosthetic training, and follow-up.

The major focus of the first part of this section is on traumatic amputation and prosthetic replacement in the upper extremity (UE). Although the discussion relates to the adolescent or adult amputee, the materials and approaches can be applied to the child amputee as appropriate. Some discussion of pediatric considerations is given at the end of the section. Because the role of the occupational therapist includes preprosthetic and prosthetic assessment and training, major attention is given to these areas. The section includes surgical considerations, postoperative program, and prosthetic replacement.

The second part of the section discusses the lower-extremity (LE) amputee. Generally, the specific preprosthetic and prosthetic assessment and training programs for the LE amputee are carried out by the physical therapist. During these periods, an LE amputee may be referred to the occupational therapist for functional standing tolerance and balance activities and for adaptation and training in self-care, homemaking, vocational, and avocational skills. To train the amputee in these skills adequately, it is necessary for the occupational therapist to have some awareness of the precautions and objectives of the **prosthetic training program**.

Upper-extremity amputation and replacement

The amputee rehabilitation program begins with the decision to amputate and ends with the successful functional and cosmetic integration of the prosthesis into the body schema. Whether the cause of the amputation is trauma or disease, the first step in the program is selection of the type and level of surgery and the psychological and physical preparation of the patient.

There are many causes of amputations. In the UE, the most common is external trauma caused by industrial machinery, burns, or firearms. Other causes are prolonged infection such as osteomyelitis, severe neuromuscular impairment such as injury to the brachial plexus, or tumors.

Before the operation, the necessity of the amputation, the expected result, the postoperative conditioning program, the possibility of difficulties in adjustment, and the prosthetic training program are explained to the patient. When feasible, presurgery exercise and activity to strengthen specific muscles that will be needed postoperatively for prosthesis operation assist both physical and psychological adjustment to the total process. Such programs include humeral and scapular range of motion (ROM) and forearm rotation.

Surgical considerations

During surgical amputations, all possible bone length, soft tissue, and skin is saved (Cummings, Alexander, & Gans 1984). This practice stems from the belief that the lower the amputation, the better the function will be both with and without the prosthesis. The importance of structural length and support of the bone, the length and strength of cut or damaged muscles, and the sensory properties of adequate skin coverage bear out the practicality and necessity of preserving tissue. Regardless of the level of the amputation, the muscles involved directly or indirectly in the function of the amputated part are affected by the loss. In addition to providing adequate tissue to withstand the pressure of the socket during prosthesis use, maximal sensation is preserved to provide sensory feedback during prosthesis function. The loss or distortion of sensation is the greatest limiting factor to prosthesis use and is discussed further in this section.

Both during and after surgery, an effort is made to form the stump in such a way as to maintain maximal function of the remaining tissue and to provide maximal use of the prosthesis. Blood vessels and nerves are pulled down, cut, and allowed to retract so that they do not interfere with the amputee's use of the prosthesis by causing pain in the stump when the device is used.

Either a *closed* or an *open amputation* may be done by the surgeon. The open amputation allows free drainage of material, minimizing the possibility of infection before closure. The immediate closed amputation may reduce the period of hospitalization, but it also reduces free drainage and increases the danger of bacterial growth. When a closed amputation is performed, either immediately or after sufficient drainage, the maximal amount of tissue is saved. Regardless of the surgical method used, however, the stump must be strong and resilient and must have a snug, comfortable contact with the socket of the prosthesis because the amputee will exert much pressure on the stump while using the device.

Levels of upper-extremity amputations

Amputations are generally defined in relation to the fingers, wrist, elbow, and shoulder. The levels indicate both the surgical level and the type of prosthetic replacement expected.

Amputations at the joints are referred to as *disarticulations* (ie, finger, wrist, elbow, or shoulder disarticulation). Amputations below the wrist across the metacarpal bones are referred to as *transmetacarpal amputations*. At this level and below, amputations are referred to as *partial hand amputations*. Should the amputation occur between the wrist and the elbow, the level is referred to as *below-elbow* (BE), and amputation between the elbow and the shoulder is referred to as *above-elbow* (AE) *amputations*. Amputations at the surgical neck of the humerus (distal to the humeral head) to the shoulder articulation are referred to as *shoulder disarticulations* (SD). Amputations above the shoulder joint involving the clavicle and scapula are referred to as *forequarter amputations* (Figure 18-7).

Although there are general types of prostheses for each level of amputation, each prosthesis is medically prescribed for the person's individual needs, and the artificial limb is custom-made and individually fitted.

The higher the amputation, the more the amputee must depend on the prosthesis for replacement of bodily function. The shorter the stump, the greater the coverage of the stump socket, thus adding weight, limiting proximal joint functions, and limiting sensory contact of the extremity. With the progressive prosthetic replacement of joint functions, the prosthesis gains weight and challenges the amputee to increasingly complex motions of the amputated and sound extremity to accomplish functional replacement.

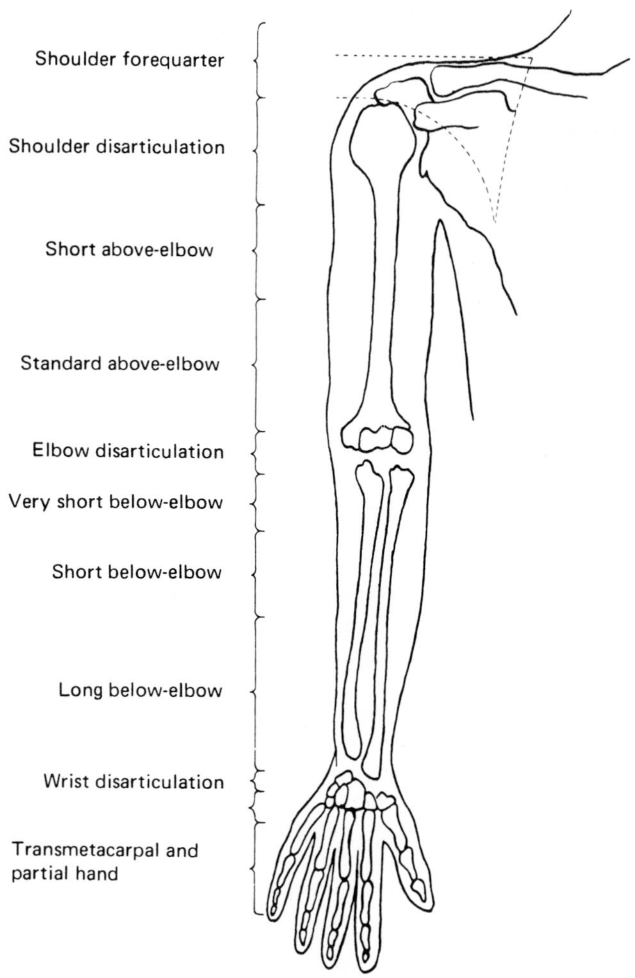

Sensation and pain

After traumatic injury and surgery to an extremity, the amputee may experience a variety of sensory changes. Initially, the patient experiences the pain of sudden trauma and then of surgery. Because the sensory representation of the amputated limb remains in the brain after the limb has been removed, a sensation of the missing part, or **phantom sensation**, can be triggered or reinforced by sensory input from elsewhere in the body (Cummings et al., 1984). The sensation may be described by the amputee as a tingling sensation, an actual sensation of the hand or foot, or a sense of gripping or clenching. Although in most cases phantom awareness is painless, it can become intolerable if sensed as actual pain. Traumatic crush injuries are prevalent causes of painful phantom sensations such as burning or cramping. Phantom pain can lead to postsurgical problems for the amputee; if serious, it may warrant surgical revision of the stump. Continuation of phantom pain can lead to difficulties in accepting, tolerating, and using a prosthesis. In addition to supportive counseling, the most effective compensations for phantom sensations are (1) early preprosthetic use of the amputated extremity in daily activity, (2) stump desensitization to build tolerance

FIGURE 18-7. *Amputation levels of the upper extremity.*

to sensory contact and to ensure prosthetic readiness, and (3) early prosthesis fitting.

Pain can also result from edema, infection, or neuroma in or around the amputation. The nerve tissue neuroma or tumor forms a painful mass in the stump. The pain increases on contact of the stump with the prosthetic socket and is unrelieved by the prosthetist's revisions of the socket. Surgical revision may be recommended.

The sensation in the stump is important in the amputee's rehabilitation. For optimal prosthesis use, adequate skin coverage is essential. The presence of scar tissue, fragile skin areas, and bony prominences can hinder the development of sensory tolerance of the pressure needed to operate the control system.

If a hand has been amputated and the patient has been fitted with a prosthetic prehension device, the patient no longer experiences functional sensation in the area that has been amputated. Although the amputee has sensation in the stump, it is functionally lost when the prosthesis is put on. Therefore, he or she will have to depend on visual cues to use the terminal device (TD) to handle objects. Sensation can also be a problem if the socket is ill fitting or if the stump is not well formed at the distal end. Therefore, the amputee must adjust to the pressure of the socket on the stump. The amputee also must become used to the pressure of the harness on the shoulders and to the weight of the prosthesis.

The amputee may also have to accept a new body image; this is difficult for some amputees because major changes in their body images will occur with the loss. Some amputees may be disturbed by this change in body concept and may have subsequent difficulties in prosthetic training. To be functionally useful, the prosthesis must be integrated into the body schema and must become a part of the person.

Partial hand options

A major consideration in the traumatic partial hand amputation is whether to leave remaining healthy hand tissue or to amputate. Decisions involve careful evaluation of the integrity of the remaining tissue as well as of sensory, motor, functional, and cosmetic aspects. Further amputation may be postponed. This area of consideration demands individual and creative design in the skillful provision of functional and cosmetic components relative to the amputee's needs.

The partial hand amputee may or may not need or want a prosthesis.

In the effort to save as much tissue as possible, the surgeon can often save parts of the hand for motor function and sensation. As shown in Figure 18-8, full function can be maintained for the grasping of tools and general coordination and sensation with partial amputation of the fingers. In this case, there is complete function of the metacarpophalangeal joints for adequate positioning of the fingers, and strength is preserved in the muscle tendons, as is fingertip sensation.

Levels of amputation are generally classified as transphalan-

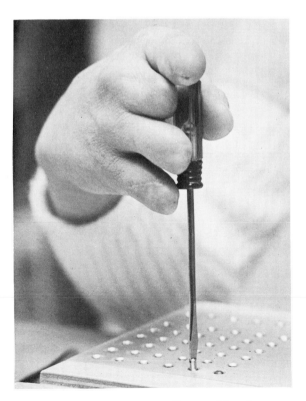

FIGURE 18-8. *Amputee grasps a small screwdriver between the partially amputated fingers and the remaining thumb.*

geal, thenar, transthenar, or transmetacarpal, with or without the thumb. Surgical reconstruction of the hand or part of it may be feasible to maintain functional structure and sensation and to avoid prosthetic or orthotic replacement.

Complete amputation of the fingers necessitates prosthetic replacement to provide grasp and prehension. Figure 18-9 shows the use of a functional replacement to enable the amputee to use tools. The amputee shown here has normal function and sensation in the thumb. Cosmetic replacement can also be provided by a glove with soft or firm fingers that can be manually positioned for function and appearance. A custom glove may fit over a passive partial hand replacement molded from the sound hand and fabricated as desired. It may be supplied with or without a zipper for ease in wearing. It can also be designed with freckles, veins, and hair to provide a natural appearance.

Limb replantation

Limb replantation, or the immediate surgical rejoining of the traumatically amputated part, has been done with varying success. Replantation has not yet proved effective in providing a functional body part. The best results have been found with simple digit replantations (Cummings et al., 1984).

Replantation has been done when immediate medical attention is available and when the amputated part of the limb can be salvaged and replaced safely. Success depends on vascular continuity and nerve and tendon repair. Fibrosis and atrophy can occur, however, and the replanted part may be limited in function and sensation.

Figure 18-10 shows an amputee who has functional amputated digits of her right hand and a hand replantation of her left arm at the wrist. In this case, a 1-inch prehension range was achieved; however, digital sensation is minimal. The amputee uses her hand as a functional assist, and she enjoys the relatively normal cosmetic look. Since amputees are likely to have different opinions regarding cosmetic value and function, it is important to find out how the amputee feels in regard to the replacement alternatives.

Postoperative program

Psychological adjustment

In assisting the amputee in adjusting to his or her condition and in becoming motivated to learn the function and care of the prosthesis, the occupational therapist must recognize the amputee's psychological reactions to the situation. If the patient feels guilt or shame regarding the amputation, his or her relationships with family and friends may be affected, presenting difficulties. The patient may be depressed and may refuse to cooperate with the training program. On the other hand, the amputee may be interested in compensating for the loss by learning as much as possible about the prosthesis, by accepting change, and by demonstrating eagerness to learn.

During the **postoperative program** and the preprosthetic period, the patient usually automatically uses the sound extremity. If the dominant extremity has been amputated and the patient is forced to use the nondominant extremity for grasp and placement of objects, the patient may have some incoordination. In this case, the patient can benefit from activities to improve the fine coordination of the previously nondominant arm.

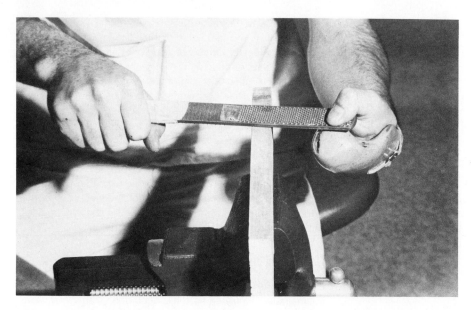

FIGURE 18-9. *This patient wears a partial hand prosthesis to hold tool for bimanual wood filing.*

The amputee who has suffered loss of the nondominant extremity may be less motivated to use the prosthesis because he or she will depend on the dominant extremity.

Becoming familiar with the prime concerns of the amputee with regard to vocational and social needs as well as self-esteem begins with the initial contact between the patient and the therapist. Careful attention is given to combining the components needed and desired by the patient. Careful initial evaluation, preprosthetic preparation, and prosthetic training in all areas of function are necessary for acceptance and use of the prosthesis by the amputee. The therapist's positive attitude toward the amputee and the stump, the patient's fears, achievement of lost function, and cosmesis through prosthetic replacement reinforce the patient's attitude. Most important is the provision of opportunities for the patient to use the prosthesis in all appropriate activities and to socialize with others in the process. Involvement of family members in the training program is essential.

Immediate and early prosthetic fitting

It is generally recognized that early fitting of the prosthetic socket and components aids in effective prosthetic adjustment, wear, and use. When the amputee is provided with a working prosthesis before the sutures are removed, it is referred to as *immediate fitting*. This postsurgical fitting is a temporary prosthesis made with a rigid cast socket to which controls and components are attached for early use training. Immediate fitting, in addition to shortening the time between the amputation and the wearing of the prosthesis, hastens the control of edema, lessens postsurgical pain, encourages conditioning of the stump, and provides more rapid use of the controls and the prosthesis. The plaster dressing and conventional harness and controls are applied at the time of surgery or during the immediate postoperative period. The plaster casts are changed as the stump shrinks. Provision of this type of immediate prosthesis encourages a

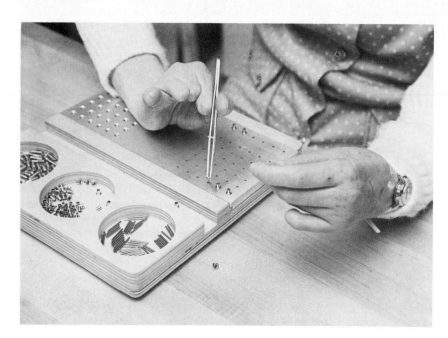

FIGURE 18-10. *Bilateral amputee uses right, partially amputated fingers to grasp tweezers. The left hand is a replantation and has limited pinch function and acceptable cosmetic value but lacks functional sensation.*

positive approach from the patient and early learning of appropriate muscle use and control movement.

Early fitting of the prosthesis is similar to that applied in the immediate fitting, consisting of a plaster cuff with components and a control system similar to those of the permanent prosthesis. Early fitting is done after healing and removal of sutures and relief of swelling. Bender (1974) states that application of the prosthesis soon after the amputation reduces pain and edema in the stump, facilitates healing, and ensures a minimal waiting time until a permanent prosthesis can be fitted. Some physicians and therapists think it is more desirable to fit several temporary prostheses rather than to wait for several months for the arrival of the permanent one.

Prosthetic replacement

The occupational therapist is a principal team member in the prosthetic training program; with sufficient expertise, the occupational therapist can recommend the type of prosthesis appropriate for the amputee. The occupational therapist monitors the amputee's adaptation through the preprosthetic and prosthetic period, checking the prosthesis for fit, comfort, and optimal function.

The most important factor in prosthetic replacement is the choice of components and control system to suit the functional and emotional needs of the amputee. Patient and family education are as essential as a therapeutic prosthetic training program directed toward return to school or employment, family, home, and community.

The prescription of the prosthetic replacement and the acute and rehabilitation program routines vary according to the treatment team, patient needs, and facility. The material included in this section gives a general view of approaches to the needs of the amputee with regard to the type of prosthetic replacement provided.

Partial hand replacement

As mentioned in the discussion of surgical considerations, the partial hand replacement often requires individual adaptive considerations according to the type and extent of the injury and the extent of the remaining functional parts. The amputee may have a prosthesis to provide the function of the thumb or the fingers to achieve a functional grip. The occupational therapist may be requested to devise a temporary adaptive device and to recommend a permanent design for an orthotist or a prosthetist to fabricate. Because the partial hand amputee may prefer to use the remaining sensation in the digits, the training program may be one of muscle reeducation, sensory discrimination, coordination, and adaptive hand use. Unilateral and bilateral activities are provided for skills training. Prevocational and avocational areas are explored with the patient through occupational therapy.

Conventional prosthesis

The **conventional prosthesis** is the traditional means of prosthetic replacement. Using a basic figure-eight or figure-nine harness across the shoulders for suspension of the plastic laminate socket, hook, or hand, the prosthesis is operated by a cable control system attached at the TD (artificial hook, hand), the socket, and the harness. The sources for the operation of the

prosthesis are within the gross movements of the affected extremity and the shoulder of the sound extremity. Control from the sound extremity can be assistive in cases of high amputations and decreased efficiency for prosthetic controls in the amputated extremity. The BE amputee uses unilateral or bilateral scapular excursion or abduction and adduction and shoulder flexion for operation of the TD; the AE amputee uses biscapular abduction and shoulder flexion for TD operation and shoulder extension for operation of the elbow lock; the SD amputee uses chest excursion for all functions.

The preprosthetic period is the time between the amputation and the fitting of the prosthesis. This is the period of getting ready for the prosthesis. In the following discussion, the program described is that in which an immediate or early fitting has not been prescribed and there is a delay between the surgery and the provision of the permanent prosthesis, during which time the stump heals and the amputee learns and applies stump wrapping for shrinkage and densitization and engages in exercises and activities to prepare for prosthetic use.

Preprosthetic training program

A successful **preprosthetic program** hastens physical and psychological adjustment to the prosthesis and minimizes problems in wearing and using the permanent prosthesis. In this period, it is important to counsel and guide the amputee regarding both the acceptance of his or her condition and the acceptance of the mechanical device that must substitute for natural motor power, sensation, and physical appearance. Counseling sessions with the amputee should also include family and friends to involve them in the training program.

Generally speaking, the longer the stump, the more the amputee can do both in the preprosthetic program and in the prosthetic training program. With a well-healed, healthy stump, the amputee has a good purchase power on the socket and security in its fit. In the case of a BE amputation, the longer the stump, the more active supination and pronation the patient is likely to have to assist in positioning the hook for grasp and placement of objects. Also, if the stump is long, either AE or BE, it is more useful to the amputee; he or she has a tendency to use it more frequently, thus maintaining normal ROM and strength.

When medically approved, passive ROM and active strengthening activities are started by physical and occupational therapists to encourage maximal use of the stump, maximal ROM, and maximal use of muscles, especially those of the arm and shoulder. A well-planned preprosthetic exercise program contributes to successful adaptation and provides strong muscles for the training in isolated motions needed for control and use of the prosthesis.

After the amputation, the loss of the weight of the missing part causes a shift in the amputee's center of gravity. Atrophy of the musculature on the side of the amputation, scoliosis, and compensatory curves may occur if the patient does not have proper exercise. Therefore, the beginning exercise program is geared toward correcting faulty body mechanics and developing substitution patterns that provide the amputee with sufficient ROM and strength to operate the prosthesis.

The first step is to establish good rapport with the patient so that it will be possible to help the patient work through the necessary adjustments and learn independence in daily living with the aid of an artificial limb. The relationship between the therapist and the patient is a very important one because the therapist must understand the patient's attitudes toward the prosthesis to help the patient accept and use it. The amputee may have fears of being different, may question the attitudes of others, and may even question himself or herself about possible inadequacies.

Before the amputee receives the prosthesis, he or she must develop strength and tolerance in the stump. Therefore, as soon as possible after the amputation, exercises are begun to maintain and, if necessary, to regain normal passive and active ROM in the joints proximal to the amputation (Figure 18-11). Since the hospital stay may be short, these exercises are designed so that they can be done in outpatient situations in the clinic. Although exercise may be painful to the patient, it is important to maintain and encourage maximal movement and use of the extremity during healing to prepare the amputee for the prosthesis, to prevent weakening of muscles through disuse, and to encourage shrinkage of the stump.

After complete healing, the stump is massaged to encourage circulation, to prevent adhesions from scar tissue, to reduce swelling, to encourage desensitization, and to prevent the patient from fear of handling the stump (Figure 18-12). Bandaging with an elastic Ace or shrinker bandage is done several times per

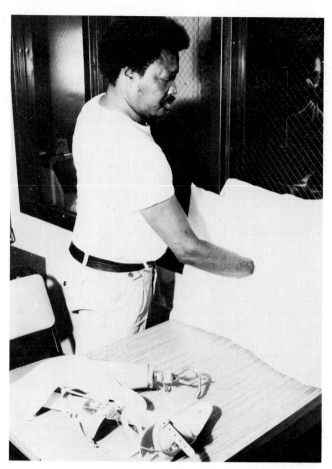

FIGURE 18-12. *To desensitize and improve pressure tolerance of the distal stump in preparation for socket contact, the amputee punches a soft pillow with increasing arm force.*

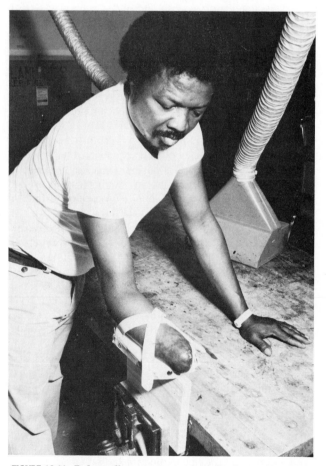

FIGURE 18-11. *Below-elbow amputee benefits by early active use of the amputated extremity in sanding with an adapted sanding block. The patient gains early awareness of the use of his arm, and pressure on the sanding block helps desensitize the stump.*

day to encourage shrinkage and shaping. Wrapping should be done carefully with attention to tightness, avoidance of unnecessary folds, and complete, even coverage of the stump to ensure comfort. Bandaging should be done from the distal to the proximal end. Care must be taken not to bandage so tightly as to produce muscle atrophy.

To encourage the use of the stump, the occupational therapist may strap utensils to it that are used in ADL. Such utensils may include a knife, fork, or toothbrush. The amputee should be encouraged to use the individual implements in ADL.

The shrinking and shaping of the stump are also hastened by provision of a temporary prosthesis in the form of a leather or plaster cuff to which utensils can be attached for functional use of the extremity.

Although the preprosthetic program can be enhanced by the use of a temporary prosthesis, the amputee's tolerance determines when it may be applied. The temporary prosthesis aids the amputee in overcoming the initial psychological shock of amputation in the following ways: it provides a temporary replacement for the length of the missing arm; it provides the patient with a degree of independence because a fork or a tool or other utensils may be attached to it to provide functional use of the amputated extremity; it aids in cosmetic lengthening of the stump; and, most significantly, it is a device with which the amputee can perform bimanual and bilateral activities. One of the most important parts of the training program lies in the amputee's early involvement in activities that show results.

At this time, the amputee should be encouraged to use the sound arm in one-handed activities, even though he or she may not be naturally motivated to do so. If the amputated arm was the dominant one, the amputee may have temporary difficulties in accepting the loss and in using the nondominant arm. In this case, the amputee may need exercises to develop coordination patterns in the remaining limb. Activities such as eating, dressing, writing, and bathing may be difficult with the nondominant hand. It is important at this time to provide a program to encourage successful one-handedness in daily activities.

In preparing the patient for prosthesis wear and in providing the prosthesis appropriate to the patient's needs and expectations, the occupational therapist must consider several important questions. First, does the patient need it? This will depend on the patient's limitations as a result of the amputation, vocational and avocational needs and interests, and attitude toward the value of the prosthesis. Second, will the patient wear it? This depends largely on the patient's attitude toward the loss of the limb and of function and the relationships of the amputee with other people. Third, does the amputee need and want function or cosmetic acceptance, or both? Finally, what is most important to the amputee in home life, at work, in hobbies, and in social life? After the preprosthetic program, or near its end, these questions are seriously considered to prescribe the appropriate prosthetic components for the maximal benefit to the amputee. At this point, the rehabilitation team comes together for consultation.

Before the prescription, the physiatrist measures the stump and examines the patient. The parts and controls of the prosthesis are determined by many factors: ROM, strength, length, skin coverage and appearance, incision site, and job requirements. At this time, if not before, the occupational therapist can acquaint the new amputee with the various components and harnessing that the amputee is likely to have and perhaps can introduce the amputee to another amputee who has completed the training program and is using a similar prosthesis successfully.

The bilateral amputee usually chooses the side with the longer stump to become the dominant side. Sometimes the amputee is trained in the use of one prosthesis at a time. Because the two prostheses have a common harness and the body must adjust to the weight and balance of both mechanical devices, however, the bilateral amputee may start the training program with both limbs, concentrating on one at a time.

Prosthetic components

The basic components of the conventional prosthesis are a plastic laminate socket, the TD, a wrist unit, the harness, and a control system. All UE prostheses have these components, with variations for individual amputation and functional levels and needs.

Plastic laminate socket

The intimate fit between the socket and the stump must be snug and comfortable to ensure tolerance and optimal prosthesis use by the amputee. The socket may be either single- or double-walled. A BE amputee has a double-walled socket consisting of an inner wall that conforms to the stump and an outer wall that provides length and contour to the forearm replacement. The wrist unit is laminated onto the distal end of the forearm socket.

Since the forearm socket can be used by both the AE and the BE amputee to carry objects (ie, a coat, a handbag, or packages), as well as to push or to pull large or heavy objects, it is made of strong plastic resins that are light and durable.

Because overall weight and bulk must be minimized for the AE or SD amputee, a single-walled forearm socket, or shell, is used for these prostheses. The socket provides length and contour to the forearm replacement. A double-walled socket is provided for the upper-arm stump.

The Munster-type socket was devised mainly for the short stump of the BE amputee to eliminate problems of fit, security, and poor leverage that were prevalent with the conventional split sockets, which are difficult to fit on this type of amputee. It consists of a single, double-walled forearm socket that extends just proximal to the olecranon process posteriorly and fits around the biceps tendon anteriorly. The socket is preflexed at about 35 degrees, thus limiting complete flexion and extension of the elbow. Even with this disadvantage in ROM, however, the fit is adequate for lifting and holding.

The more distal the socket coverage on the forearm, the more active supination and pronation the amputee will have with the prosthesis on. Extending the socket length proximally increases stability of the prosthesis for functional use.

The upper-arm unit of the AE prosthesis is a double-walled socket with the locking elbow unit laminated onto the socket. Since the AE amputee lacks independent elbow flexion and extension, these are provided mechanically by an elbow unit, which is activated, locked, and unlocked by the cable control system. A turntable at the joining of the locking elbow unit and the upper-arm socket can be manually moved for internal and external rotation of the forearm, enabling the amputee to work with the hook directly in front of the body or out toward the side. The forearm shell is attached to the locking elbow unit and the upper-arm socket (Figure 18-13).

The SD prosthesis has a supporting socket portion that sometimes extends to the anterior and posterior aspects of the shoulder, depending on the level of the amputation. Frequently, a passive abduction hinge joint is added at the shoulder for ease in manually positioning the arm and donning clothing.

Hinges provide functional alignment and positioning between the forearm and the upper-arm socket or the harness. In addition, the flexible Dacron or leather hinges used in the BE prosthesis allow active rotation of the forearm with a minimum of restriction. In the AE prosthesis, the steel hinges provide rigidity for the mechanical elbow joint to ensure strength, durability, and dependability.

A stump sock is worn by the amputee to absorb perspiration, to provide warmth, and as padding for comfort and fit of the socket. An AE amputee frequently uses the short sleeve of a T shirt in place of the stump sock. Use of an underblouse or T shirt can alleviate discomfort from the harness straps in beginning training sessions.

Terminal device

The most significant component of the prosthesis is the TD, which provides function, cosmesis, or both.

A cosmetic TD, used principally for appearance, may be as simple as a flesh-colored glove used to cover a partial hand. Aside from being used to hold light objects or to position objects by pushing or pulling, this device may have little functional value. Its psychological value, however, is unquestionable.

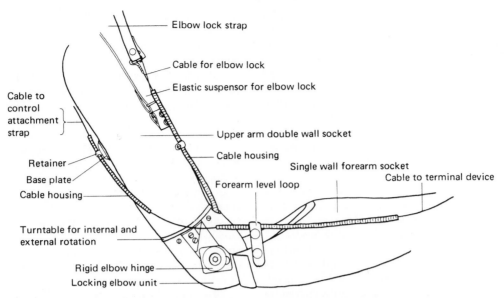

FIGURE 18-13. *Conventional right, above-elbow prosthesis with locking elbow unit.*

A second type of cosmetic TD is the functional hand that can be attached to the wrist unit of most UE prostheses (Figure 18-14) and is operated by cable control. The functional hand consists of a plastic, spring-controlled device with fingers that are controlled in flexion and extension at the metacarpophalangeal joints by the control cable of the prosthesis. The thumb can be placed manually in either of two positions: to grasp small objects or to grasp large ones. A plastic glove fits over the hand, presenting a natural appearance. The gloves are available in a variety of skin tones. Functional hands have either voluntary opening or voluntary closing mechanisms activated by cable control, and they may either lock in position or be free-wheeling or nonlocking.

The hook is the most functional of the TDs. It is made of either steel or aluminum, and it is canted, or lyre-shaped. It is either locking or nonlocking, with either voluntary opening or voluntary closing capacity (Figure 18-15). The hook may be lined with neoprene, to protect objects while the amputee is grasping them, or serrated, to improve grasp. The needs of the amputee determine the weight, length, design, and function of the hook chosen by the rehabilitation team.

Many kinds of hooks are available to provide for diverse needs. Among them are aluminum hooks required for AE and SD amputees who need minimal weight of the prosthesis, steel hooks for BE amputees requiring durability, farmers' or carpenters' hooks for ease and safety in tool handling, and narrow-opening hooks for use in laboratory or office work. Special hooks also are available for bowling and for holding a baseball mitt. Special adaptations are available for ease in grasping tools or in driving.

A series of children's hooks are available that have rubber or plastic parts to increase cosmesis and to prevent harm to objects while the child is using the prosthesis to play.

Hooks and functional or cosmetic hands are generally interchangeable through the common wrist unit attachment laminated onto the forearm socket.

Wrist unit

The TD (hand or hook) is connected to the forearm socket (or shell, as in the AE or SD prosthesis) by the wrist unit. This unit allows interchange of cosmetic and functional TDs and rotation

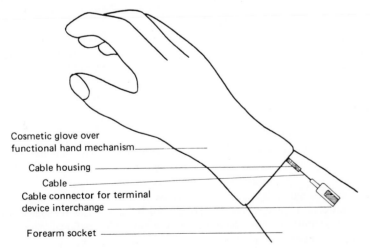

FIGURE 18-14. *Functional hand with cosmetic glove and cable attachment.*

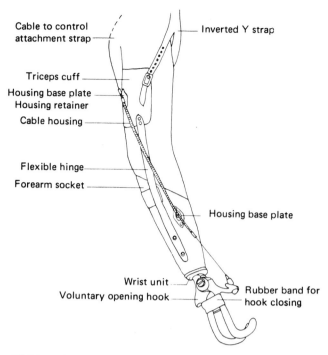

Cable to control attachment strap

Inverted Y strap

Triceps cuff

Housing base plate
Housing retainer

Cable housing

Flexible hinge

Forearm socket

Housing base plate

Wrist unit
Voluntary opening hook

Rubber band for hook closing

FIGURE 18-15. *Conventional right, below-elbow prosthesis.*

for TD position change for functional variations. There are three basic wrist units: locking, friction, and oval.

The advantage of the *locking* unit is that it prevents the hook from rotating during heavy industrial work. By pushing a button, the amputee manually operates the unit, which allows the position of the hook to be changed by rotation. The hook can easily be ejected for interchange of hook and hand.

The *friction* unit has threads, and the hook must be screwed into the unit. Although this procedure is more time-consuming than that of the locking unit, the hook can be positioned more easily for specific tasks. Either the locking or the friction unit can be used with both BE and AE prostheses.

The *oval* unit is a special thin unit for a wrist disarticulation prosthesis. It is used when the length of the components must be minimal to make the length of the amputated arm conform to that of the sound extremity.

A *flexion* unit is available for placement of the hook in three wrist flexion positions for increased function. It is a manually operated device, and it is usually prescribed for the bilateral amputee for added versatility in TD positioning. One activity that is aided by this device is shaving; it also helps in other activities close to the body.

Terminal devices and wrist units have standard connections. When the desired type of TD has been chosen, one needs simply to determine the type and size of the wrist unit to accompany it. Usually, the wrist unit is chosen according to the way in which the amputee will use the prosthesis in ADL and at work.

Harness

The harness attaches directly to the socket. Its function is to provide stable support of the prosthesis to facilitate the amputee's wearing and using of it, to provide attachment for the control cables, and to assist the cables in the operation of the prosthesis. Basically, the Dacron straps are formed in a figure-eight pattern, with extra straps added as needed for better sup-

port or additional control function. For ease in use, the figure-nine harness is used with the BE Munster prosthesis. For the wrist disarticulation amputee, a simple cuff socket and a figure-nine harness may suffice.

The shoulder saddle harness may be used for the BE amputee to minimize stress from the axillary loop used in the figure-eight harness; this stress occurs on the sound arm during heavy work. The shoulder saddle is fabricated of leather, Dacron, or polyethylene. Shaped like a saddle, it rests over the shoulder of the amputated side, and it is attached to the prosthesis anteriorly and posteriorly, bearing the weight of the axial load rather than transmitting the pull to the sound axilla (Bender, 1974). A chest strap is used to secure the saddle in position and to attach control cables.

Use of the saddle harness enables the amputee to lift heavier loads with the prosthesis and to gain complete ROM. There is less discomfort for the amputee because the saddle covers larger and stronger weight-bearing areas over the shoulder. The chest strap also distributes pressure over a larger body surface, thus preventing problems from tight pull of the axillary loop in the sensitive axillary area of the sound arm.

Control system

The control system determines the functional value of the prosthesis for the amputee. The control cable of the TD is attached to the device and to the harness. This cable is guided along the socket and cuff or the upper-arm socket by retainers that hold it in the most advantageous position for ease of function. TD operation is generally accomplished by forward flexion of the shoulder. During the training period, the amputee practices this isolated motion and eventually is able to operate the hook or hand with minimal physical strain.

For the AE amputee, this basic TD control cable also serves in flexion and extension of the mechanical elbow when the elbow unit is unlocked. It is activated by forward shoulder flexion. At times, additional joint motions are used in this cable operation because of limitation of shoulder control or strength, to provide smooth operation of the prosthesis, and to enable the wearer to achieve maximal function of the mechanical arm and hand in reaching, grasping, releasing, and holding. These motions may be shoulder abduction and adduction, scapular abduction and adduction, or shoulder flexion of the nonamputated arm.

The second basic cable operates the elbow lock. It is attached internally or externally to the elbow unit, and it extends to the anterior deltoid–pectoral strap of the harness. A combination of shoulder elevation, depression, external rotation, and extension is used both to lock and unlock the elbow unit.

Control cables for the SD and forequarter prostheses are attached to the humeral or scapular part of the upper-arm socket, and their exact design and function are determined by the needs of the individual amputee. The range of mechanical function of the prosthesis includes grasp, release, hold, push, pull, and reach, which, depending on the control by the wearer and the types of prescription components, can be extensive.

Prosthetic checkout and care

Before the amputee begins a training program, members of the rehabilitation team examine the prosthesis to make sure that it conforms to the prescription and that it is mechanically sound. In performing the checkout of the prosthesis, the occupational therapist evaluates its fit and comfort for the wearer and checks the motion and function of the components. Should adjustments be needed in any part of the prosthesis, the rehabilitation team makes recommendations to the prosthetist. The amputee should not begin the training program with an uncomfortable or mechanically mediocre device. The physician gives the final approval of the prosthesis.

At the time of the checkout, which occurs during the first training session, the occupational therapist begins to acquaint the amputee with prosthetic terminology. The amputee learns the names of the parts and their functions and learns the proper attachment of the harness and the components so that he or she can keep the prosthesis clean and can interchange the TDs efficiently.

In instructing the patient in the care of the prosthesis, the occupational therapist teaches the proper use of the hook, wrist unit, and cable system. The amputee is instructed to use just enough motion to open or close the hook, to watch for worn rubber bands, to avoid putting unnecessary strain on the cable, and to watch for spreading of the housing and excessive friction between the cable and the housing. The socket should be kept clean with soap and water; the stump socks should be washed daily; and the harness should be washed at least once a week. Leather parts can be cleaned with saddle soap. If the tips of the Dacron harness straps begin to fray, they can be sealed at the edge by singeing with a match.

The amputee should be instructed to use only cable control to operate the functional hooks and hands. Manual operation may damage the mechanism. The amputee should also be warned never to use the TD for such activities as hammering nails or removing screws because this can tear threads and damage hook neoprene.

The cosmetic gloves on the functional hand are perishable. It is important to guard the glove against tearing because it protects the hand mechanism from dirt and wetness. Also, these gloves soil easily, can be stained or marked if laid on dirty surfaces, and darken with age. Substances such as certain foods, ink, newsprint, and chemicals can damage the glove and lessen its cosmetic effect. The occupational therapist should recommend that the amputee keep the hand in a plastic bag when it is not in use. The amputee should be warned against oiling parts of the prosthesis or removing the glove from the hand and should be counseled to return to the prosthetist for any assistance needed.

Prosthetic training program

A successful training program for an amputee requires the coordinated efforts of a rehabilitation team that includes the surgeon, nurse, physiatrist, physical therapist, occupational therapist, social worker, prosthetist, rehabilitation counselor, and psychiatrist or psychologist. A coordinated effort of these people is necessary for appropriate prosthetic replacement and training in the use of the prosthesis.

At the beginning of the training program, the prosthesis should be put on over a lightweight shirt so that the occupational therapist and the amputee can see the prosthesis function and so that it is not hindered by tight clothing. The amputee should become accustomed to using the mirror as a guide to learning the correct positioning of the harness straps in back and in learning control motions.

Loose clothing is recommended for the amputee to facilitate putting on, wearing, and using the prosthesis. Clothing with front fastenings, Velcro closures, and wide shirt cuffs are helpful. The use of a button hook designed especially for the amputee can assist in fastening the sleeve button on the sound side. Sewing the buttons on with elastic thread enables the amputee to leave the button fastened when removing the shirt, even if the cuffs are narrow because the cuff will then stretch enough to allow the hand and arm to be removed from the sleeve. When putting on the shirt, the amputee should put it on the amputated side first. One-handed shoe tying and special closures can simplify dressing.

Two approaches are commonly used in training amputees. In one, the training program is directed toward developing the maximal potential level of performance. With this approach, a unilateral amputee learns fine coordination with the prosthesis so that he or she can have maximal use of it even in case of an injury to the remaining extremity. The other approach differs in that the amputee is trained to use the prosthesis only as an aid in bimanual activities. Regardless of the approach, activities should be suitable to the amputee's needs. The occupational therapist should encourage the amputee to indicate any additional and special training that he or she desires.

The training period serves as a trial of the efficiency of the prosthesis and the practicality of the components for the amputee's individual needs and permits adjustment to correct any malfunctions of the device. The length of the sessions should be increased as the amputee's tolerance and adaptation increase. The amputee must master prosthesis use before combining it with the remaining extremity in bimanual activities and before wearing it outside the clinic. Wearing it outside the clinic overnight is advised for the first out-of-clinic experience. This is preferable to having the amputee wear it at home for an entire weekend. Training with the hand should be delayed until use of the hook has been mastered unless only a hand has been provided.

The general goals of training include (1) independence in self-care and ADL, (2) return to former work or to a better job, (3) improved appearance, (4) return to hobbies and recreations, and (5) mastery of new skills.

Certain factors affecting the amputee's capacity to learn may, unfortunately, be detrimental. They include poor habits uncorrected in preprosthetic training, lack of motivation, lack of sensory feedback from the nonsensory prosthesis, time needed for training, age, inability to learn, and lack of a sense of accomplishment. The occupational therapist must attempt to minimize these factors.

The positive attitude of the amputee is important; he or she must want to learn. The amputee should be cautioned against using the opposite shoulder to control the device and should be taught to operate the prosthesis with the amputated extremity as much as possible. Control motions should be minimal to save strength and, thus, to extend the time during which the amputee can wear and use the prosthesis.

Sensation is a natural guide to motor control; we recognize objects by shape, texture, size, and movement. The amputee must often substitute vision for sensation, however (eg, using visual cues to determine the amount of hook opening). The amputee combines this with the sensation of cable tension to provide visual–sensory training, using the perception of both position and force. The proprioceptive sensation in the stump and the arm can aid here. The amputee also uses auditory cues, such as the clicks in the elbow lock, hand, and hook, for efficient operation of the prosthesis.

During the first session, it is important to acquaint the amputee with the actual function of the hook by teaching exercises for opening and closing it.

After the cable pull by shoulder flexion, the cable tension is released by shoulder extension, and the hook is pulled closed by its rubber bands, which yield 1 lb of pressure each. The standard number of rubber bands is usually three or four, although eight or more may be used for the BE amputee for added grip strength. The amputee begins training by learning to isolate the control motions needed to activate the hook. Then, using visual cues and sensing in the shoulder the resistance of the rubber bands, the amputee learns how to control the opening of the hook. To minimize the energy expenditure needed to use the hook, the amputee should be encouraged to open the hook only slightly beyond the size of the object he or she wishes to pick up—just enough to grasp it. The amputee should practice with objects of different sizes and weights. Additionally, drills requiring the grasp of objects of different forms, textures, and materials are necessary for the amputee to learn the basic motions used in operating the hook (Figure 18-16). Since some materials are light, breakable, or easily crushed (eg, a paper or plastic cup), it is important to teach the amputee to employ a minimum of pressure by maintaining tension on the cable during grasp. The amputee should also learn to operate the hook in different planes of arm movement so that he or she will achieve maximal functional use.

These drills for grip control should be extended to other components of the prosthesis. The amputee must learn how to position the TD at the wrist unit, how to operate the elbow unit, how to use the turntable, how to coordinate the elbow lock and elbow flexion and extension, and how to position the shoulder. In these drills, the use of the TD is combined with a number of gross arm functions. The amputee learns the grasp, placement, and release of objects on shelves, tables, and the floor and learns to depend on the grip of the hook or functional hand (Figure 18-17).

During this early drill period, use of the sound extremity should be encouraged. During the rest periods, the amputee should be encouraged to practice unilateral activities as well as bilateral activities. It is through these more complicated coordination activities that the prosthesis begins to be functionally integrated into the bilateral UE activities of the amputee. Although the unilateral amputee may already have become independent in ADL during the preprosthetic period, there are many things that we are accustomed to doing with two hands. For example, the amputee may find it difficult to cut meat, button a sleeve, tie shoes, or wrap a package with one hand. The prosthesis may help the amputee accomplish these things, or the occupational therapist may discover that additional adaptive devices are needed.

Whatever the problem, the occupational therapist should encourage the amputee to become skillful in the use of the hook and to devise ways to increase independence in function. Participation in woodworking, sewing, weaving, or other avocational

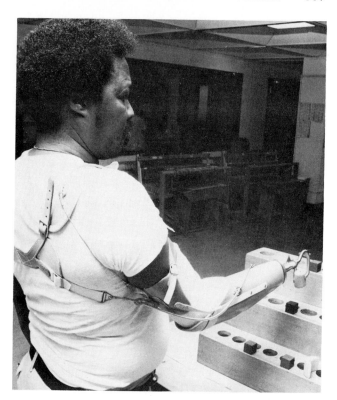

FIGURE 18-16. *Amputee practices control of hook opening and closing in grasp, release, and placement of blocks of various shapes.*

activities can be motivating for the amputee, can provide coordination and strength, can show how the prosthesis can help in doing things, and can aid in integrating the prosthesis into bodily function.

Using a worksheet checklist of activities accomplished can be helpful in recording the amputee's progress in training both in the clinic and at home. Since there are many activities the patient will do at home that cannot be simulated in the clinic, the therapist should continue to encourage the amputee to do new things at home after each training session and to report successes or difficulties with the new tasks. In this way, the therapist is able to assist the patient not only in controls, training drills, and activities but also in tasks and responsibilities in the routine of daily living. Thus, the program becomes relevant to each amputee's needs. The categories on the worksheet should include basic prehension activities, dressing and grooming (including putting on and taking off the prosthesis), eating and social skills (eg, using keys and opening an umbrella), homemaking, clerical activities, and activities related to vocational and avocational interests.

Another aid is a prosthetic training board with common objects (locks, light switches, pencil sharpener) attached to it.

Recreational activities during the preprosthetic and prosthetic training periods provide general body conditioning and assist the development of a new image for the amputee.

Because industrial accidents are a frequent cause of UE amputations, a prevocational assessment should be included in the training program to assist the amputee in recognizing capa-

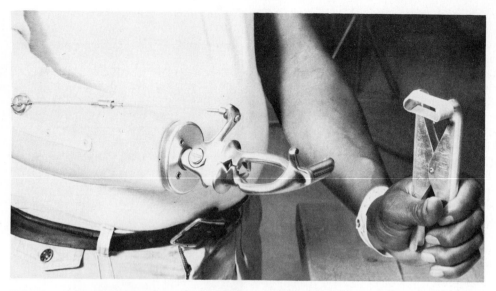

FIGURE 18-17. *During initial prosthetic training, the amputee learns to apply bands to the voluntary opening hook to increase grip pressure of the hook.*

bilities in prosthetic function and in deciding whether he or she can safely return to the former occupation or needs to consider a change of occupation and additional vocational training. Specific tasks related to the amputee's type of work should be included in the prosthetic training program; for example, assessment of safe and efficient handling of tools, power equipment, and heavy and light materials. Work tolerance can be assessed with timed, job-simulation tasks (Figures 18-18 and 18-19).

Prevocational considerations include training in general household activities. Training in the accomplishment of home-making tasks, such as meal preparation, cleaning, and household repairs, is included. Child care is also included as appropriate.

In assisting the amputee to return to the former job or to redirect his or her vocational goals, the occupational therapist works closely with the vocational counselor and the employer. Use of standardized tests and work-stimulated activities are an important part of the program for assessment of attitudes, aptitudes, work habits, and skills.

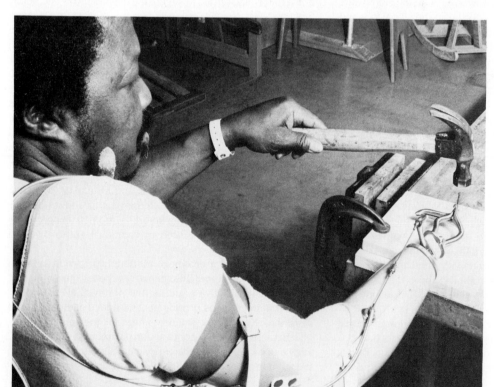

FIGURE 18-18. *The below-elbow amputee is able to position the carpenter's hook to hold a nail for hammering.*

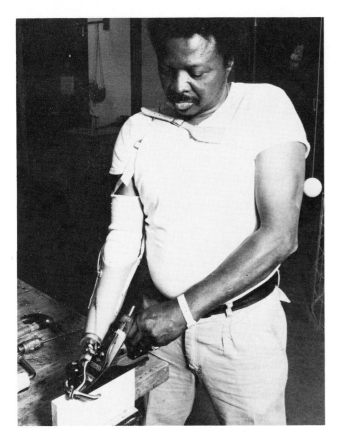

FIGURE 18-19. *Practice with bilateral grasping and use of common construction tools improves coordination and bilateral integration. Here, the amputee uses a steel carpenter's hook with serrated edges for firm grasp.*

Pediatric considerations

"Movement puts the child in relationship with his surroundings so that through this relationship the child can have an effect upon his environment as well as be affected by his environment" (Gilfoyle, Grady, & Moore, 1981, p. 1).

Depending on the nature of the condition, a child with a congenital skeletal deficiency may develop adaptively without prosthetic replacement of the missing parts and often without the need of symmetry. Although the lack of a prosthesis during this period may not be a concern for the child or the parents, a prosthesis may become necessary or desirable later so the person can participate as fully as possible in individual and group activities with peers. If the provision of a prosthesis is postponed beyond early development, there may be tremendous psychological, physical, and social problems in adjusting to wear and use.

For the congenital amputee, the prosthesis is ideally prescribed at 6 months to 1 year of age. It is prescribed as soon as possible after a traumatic amputation. This is essential for the young child to prevent the natural development of habits that might be detrimental to early adaptation and integration of a prosthetic replacement for optimal present and future function.

The training program of the child amputee must involve activities natural to the child's level of development. Early fitting during the prewalking period aids the child in developing gross bilateral coordination and balance in integrated trunk and extremity activity.

During the first year of development, from the horizontal to the vertical position in bodily reflexes, the child learns body parts, their extent, and their use through imitation, trial, adaptation, and accomplishment.

Education and training are vital for the family to encourage psychological adjustment to the prosthesis and to teach the importance of putting on and removing the prosthesis, checking the skin for irritation, and encouraging positive play activities using the prosthesis. Children are often hindered by parental distractions during training sessions, so times should be scheduled for the child alone as well as for the child and parent together. This results in effective training for prosthetic function and for family education. The most successful method of teaching a child prosthetic function is through play; consideration of the age and attitude of the child is essential.

The child with a congenital limb deficiency may first be fitted with a semirigid, passive Robin-Aids mitt, with a Munster-type socket that has preflexed elbow and figure-eight harness control. This prosthesis can be used for gross bilateral use and initial balance activities. This cosmetic device is preparatory to the functional one. At 6 months, a mechanical element is added to the prosthesis. Natural development of movement in time and space, supplemented by guidance in the use of appropriate components, can be incorporated into the child's body image and can assist functional use in further development. Between 12 and 18 months of age, the child becomes ready for a functional TD with cable control.

A Child Amputee Prosthetics Project device may be provided. This is a voluntarily opening TD made of nylon and Kraton that provides function and cosmesis and can be used until the child is 8 years old. An alternative is the voluntary opening, covered child's split hook with a protective plastisol covering. The AE amputee may use a preflexed socket until 2 years of age for ease in using the TD and for bilateral proximity in holding objects and body balance while using the prosthesis.

As the child plays wearing the cable-operated prosthesis and notices the hook opening and closing, he or she learns to control this action. With early fitting, the child generally has a hook by 2 years of age. The smallest hand is for a 5-year-old. "Children become aware of the purpose for changing the position of the forearm during the third year of life. They learn to operate the prosthetic controls and apply them to functional activities during the fourth year of life" (Shaperman, 1979, p. 304).

In her discussion of AE prosthetic training of the young child, Shaperman notes the following five developmental factors related to learning control use:

1. Ability to see some purpose for positioning the forearm and willingness to explore new uses for this positioning
2. Ability to follow oral instructions and perform drills
3. Ability to meet the physical requirements for consistent operation of the dual-control system
4. Possession of a well-fitting, well-functioning prosthesis and availability for therapy
5. Experience of some previous success in using the prosthesis (Shaperman, 1979).

Whether the child benefits from prosthetic replacement depends on functional capacity, ingenuity, integration, and family support. It is important that the child with a congenital deficiency be provided with a prosthesis before starting school. Generally, a new prosthesis is provided every 4 years to accommodate growth and functional development (Bender, 1974).

Considerations in bilateral amputees

The bilateral amputee faces not only the functional and cosmetic adjustments of the unilateral amputee but also the complete loss of sensory contact with objects while using the prostheses. Prosthetic replacement is prescribed according to the level of amputation. Particular attention is given to minimizing weight and to providing ease of bilateral operation of the elbows and TDs through the control system. For ease in putting on and removing the prosthesis by the amputee, as well as for its security and adjustment, the two prostheses are secured to a common harness system. A wrist flexion unit is helpful on one side for added mechanical positioning.

Because sensation is essential to the blind bilateral amputee, the Krukenberg surgical procedure may be done if the patient has a long BE amputation of either or both arms. This procedure involves separating the radius, ulna, and accompanying musculature to enable the amputee to achieve grasp and release through supination and pronation of the forearm. Sensation is maintained as grasp is achieved without an external prosthesis. Some amputees can achieve independence with this procedure.

Myoelectric prosthesis

Developments in the use of myoelectric controls for prosthetic and orthotic replacements of lost limb functions have been steadily increasing in clinical application. A major significance of **myoelectric prostheses** is the use of signals from the neuromuscular system to activate specific component functions.

By approaching the amputee and prosthetic replacements as a complete unit or system, research and clinical teams are integrating natural and artificial elements (Stein et al., 1980). In the effort to assist the amputee in achieving both efficient and natural function and appearance, combinations of conventional and myoelectric components may be considered within the same prosthesis, particularly for amputation or skeletal deficiencies above the elbow. Myoelectric components and controls are available for operation of the cosmetic or functional hand, wrist rotation, and elbow flexion and extension. These are available for unilateral, bilateral, BE, and AE amputees.

Preprosthetic program

Ability to isolate and control the muscle sites and to develop strength and speed of muscle contraction determines effective prosthetic use. Assessment of surface EMG muscle sites for control of a prosthesis is made using the myotester. Further training with the myotester helps the amputee develop signal levels and reliable isolation of potential myoelectric control sites. This may be done using bench-mounted units such as the TD and the wrist unit (Stein et al., 1980). A temporary plaster prosthesis may be used to determine the preliminary ability of the amputee to use myoelectric controls implanted in the socket. Efficiency of mus-

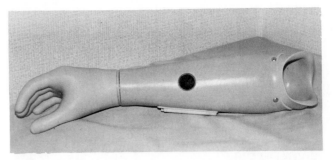

FIGURE 18-20. *Complete below-elbow myoelectric prosthesis with cosmetic/functional terminal device, external battery pack, and double-walled forearm socket.*

cle control is established through use of the temporary prosthesis until the permanent one is ready for fitting and training.

Identification of muscle sites and the number of sites required for prosthetic operation depend on the level of the amputation and the ability of the amputee to isolate and use the muscle contractions. For example, a BE amputee may use either a single site or two sites for TD operation. In the dual control, extensor muscle contraction may be used to open the TD, and flexor muscle contraction may be used to close it, thus simulating normal body associations. The AE amputee may use biceps contraction for prosthetic elbow flexion and triceps contraction for prosthetic elbow extension, with cocontraction of these muscles to open and close the hand.

Passive, manually operated shoulder, elbow, and wrist components may be used. Cosmetic and functional electric hooks, hands, and elbows are commercially available. Electronic controls and batteries are stored within the sockets or the hand of the prosthesis or externally (Figure 18-20).

Prosthetic components

A myoelectrically controlled prosthesis or component operates by using the electric potential produced by a contracting muscle to activate a battery-driven motor that operates a prosthetic component. Proportional control of the motor by regulation of the extent or speed of muscle contraction can affect the force or speed of the movement of the component (Robertson, 1979).

Myoelectric prostheses are provided to children and adults both experimentally and clinically. In both cases, the candidates are chosen for optimal success in myoelectric wear and use. Since the myoelectric prosthesis is expensive, both in initial provision and in maintenance, proximity of the amputee to the prosthetist, adequate funding, vocational appropriateness, and available prosthetic checkout and training are essential considerations. During the initial prosthetic prescription, factors such as the level of the amputation, the condition of the limb, the number of limbs involved, the extent of power, and the control in the remaining limb and body are assessed.

The following are the positive aspects of the myoelectric approach:

- Use of natural muscle stimuli for component operation
- More accurate control with less energy output from the amputee
- Elimination of the shoulder harness
- Ease in full range of isolated extremity movements

- Improved natural control and cosmesis
- Decreased body movement to control prosthesis

The negative aspects of the myoelectric approach are the following:

- High expense of controls, components, and repairs
- Requirement for skilled repair in the event of breakdown
- Limited number of suitable candidates
- Noise of component operation
- Daily battery charge required
- Lack of proprioceptive feedback from harness
- Added weight
- Efficient control sites necessary
- Muscle fatigue

Good candidates for myoelectric replacement have the following attributes:

- A healthy attitude toward the disability
- A desire for myoelectric control
- Commitment to following the procedures and fulfilling the responsibilities for myoelectric wear and care
- Healthy skin and stump for effective socket and electrode contact
- Fair muscle function in the arm to produce electrode signals for component operation

Sockets are single- or double-walled, depending on the level of amputation. Generally, the harness is eliminated and the prosthesis is self-suspended on the extremity. In the BE prosthesis, a supracondylar suspension, using bony prominences, or a Munster-type socket high on the forearm, is used for secure fit and comfort. In the Munster-type socket, there is no supination and pronation available in active movement, and elbow flexion and extension are limited. The AE socket uses atmospheric pressure suspension.

Preliminary temporary fittings assist the amputee in adjusting to prosthetic replacement and use. Early and permanent fitting of the myoelectric controls involves locating suitable sites for the electrodes; casting for electrode placement locations; providing the permanent socket with electrode emplacements; providing the component system, controls, battery pack, and on–off switch; and pigmenting. Since provision and maintenance of myoelectric controls and components are expensive, the amputee may first be provided with a conventional prosthesis with harness control to determine individual feasibility for myoelectric wear and function. To best meet the individual needs of the amputee, combinations of cable-driven and myoelectric components can be used as feasible and appropriate for optimal function and cosmesis.

Prosthetic training program

Prosthetic training is done on either an inpatient or an outpatient basis and begins with a preprosthetic program of isolating muscle contractions to produce signals for training in specific component operation. The prosthetic training program includes the following:

- Checkout of the fabrication, fit, and efficiency of the prosthesis
- Evaluation of the amputee's ability to control the prosthesis

- Specific training in general component use and coordination
- Instruction in the care and operation of the prosthesis
- Training in self-care activities
- Use of prosthetic and natural UE motions in bimanual and bilateral functional activities

The extent of daily use of myoelectric controls is dependent on conservation of the battery's energy during nonuse. This is accomplished by a manual switch that is turned on to use the controls and turned off when the amputee removes the prosthesis or during long periods when control use is not necessary. To avoid blockage between the electrode contact and the muscles, a stump sock is not worn. The amputee is taught to examine skin areas on removal of the prosthesis to monitor irritation from the socket and to keep the socket and parts clean.

Wear and successful use of the prosthesis depend on an appropriate prescription and effective training with adequate periodic follow-up and monitoring of the function of the prosthesis.

During the training program, patients share experiences and meet individual needs through group discussions. Since prosthetic replacement of function is a personal and individual adjustment, patients are encouraged to take part in planning the program by talking about individual expectations, goals, problems, and ideas regarding their prosthetic replacement.

Pediatric considerations

In providing prosthetic components to the child with a congenital or a traumatic amputation, it is essential to consider the child's developmental level. The sooner the prosthesis can be fitted, the better. Sorbye (1980) reports that children between the ages of 2½ and 4 years are the most suitable for the BE myoelectric prosthesis and that all children should be able to learn to use one. Sorbye advises that a change from the standard or split-hook prosthesis be made before the child is 4 years old to avoid problems of adjusting to a change in the prosthesis and the control system.

Candidacy for myoelectric replacement in children depends on personality, maturity, and the interest of the child and family since all will be involved in learning the system and in monitoring prosthetic wear and use with regard to training. Sorbye states: "The children teach themselves how to open and close the prosthetic hand within a few minutes from the initial application, over 2½ years of age" (Sorbye, 1980, p. 36). Training programs emphasize two-handed activities and involvement in developmental activities appropriate to the age and maturation of the child. Whether the child amputee benefits from the prosthesis depends on the child's functional capacity and ingenuity.

Endoskeletal modular system

The endoskeletal modular prosthetic system is designed primarily for cosmesis, which is provided by a central inner tubular (pylon) support covered with a soft, pigmented polyurethane foam to give natural contour and soft appearance. A nylon stocking covering is stretched over the foam. A variety of interchangeable components are available to meet the needs of the amputee. The modular arm includes a nonfunctional cosmetic hand, passively activated elbow, and shoulder units. Harness and control cables can be eliminated because the components are operated manually with the sound hand.

Lower-extremity amputation and replacement

Amputations of the lower extremities are generally more common than those of the upper extremities because of the high incidence of peripheral vascular disease and traumatic injuries to the lower limbs. The psychological reactions of the UE amputee, mentioned earlier, pertain also to the LE amputee. Since age, body build, physical and medical condition, vascular supply, and motivation are factors in the rehabilitation of the LE amputee, there are some patients for whom a prosthesis is contraindicated. These patients are encouraged to maintain maximal independence and mobility with the aid of a wheelchair, crutches, and other necessary assistive devices. The amputee for whom a prosthesis is appropriate can usually look forward to partial restoration of basic functions, independence in self-care, and the opportunity to return to work of some kind.

Role of occupational therapy

Basically, the detailed study of LE function, preprosthetic preparation, prosthetic prescription, checkout, training and the management of problems encountered by the amputee are handled by the physician and the physical therapist. There are many ways in which the occupational therapist can contribute to the functional rehabilitation of the LE amputee, however. In a general hospital or a rehabilitation center, the occupational therapist may actually work with as many or more LE than UE amputees. The occupational therapist assists with both the preprosthetic and prosthetic programs for general physical conditioning, psychological and functional adaptation to the loss of a body part, and the regaining of maximal functional independence in self-care and general mobility. To provide effective therapeutic programs for the LE amputee, the occupational therapist needs to participate with the physical therapist, the physician, the prosthetist, and other professionals in a coordinated team approach.

Preprosthetic program

Passive and active exercises of the lower extremities are performed or supervised by the physical therapist during the early postoperative period. The nurse or physical therapist teaches the amputee to bandage the stump to encourage shrinkage and forming for prosthetic fitting. Proper positioning of the body in the wheelchair is important to prevent contractures in the joints proximal to the amputation, scoliosis, and edema, all of which could hinder successful prosthetic function. In the case of a below-knee amputation, a seatboard adapted for the individual amputee can be used in a regular chair or a wheelchair to maintain the knee in passive extension, with knee flexors stretched, while the amputee is performing activities in a sitting position.

The LE amputee may be referred to occupational therapy in the preprosthetic or the prosthetic phase of training. In either case, the occupational therapist should become familiar with the medical aspects of the patient's care and the goals of the rehabilitation program. Pertinent information obtained from the chart or staff members should include the following:

- Location, type, level, and cause of amputation
- Condition of the stump and amputated extremity
- General body condition
- Any precautions and complicating conditions
- Previous prosthetic replacement, if any
- Recommendations for passive and active positioning of the joints of the amputated extremity
- Appropriate amount of standing and walking and the degree of safe support needed by the amputee

Throughout the preprosthetic and prosthetic training, the amputee may go through changes in attitude and behavior as he or she gradually realizes the extent of the loss and its effect on his or her life. Continual counseling is often necessary to help the amputee adjust to the amputation, the change in body image, and the wear and use of the mechanical device to substitute for natural function. The amputee must also adjust to working with his or her arms, gearing to abilities rather than disability, finding new interests, and socializing in the new situation.

The seatboard mentioned previously can be made by the amputee as part of an UE exercise program. It can be made of 1/2- or 3/4-inch plywood that conforms to the measurement of the inside of the chair seat; one side extends to the end of the amputee's stump. The extended side should be narrow enough to prevent interference with the comfort of the sound leg in a sitting position and at the same time should provide passive extension of the knee of the amputated leg. The seatboard should be padded sufficiently for comfort, and particular attention should be paid to such sensitive areas as the end of the stump.

In this preprosthetic phase, the amputee may come to occupational therapy either in a wheelchair or walking with crutches. A variety of treatment techniques can be used. Since balance and UE and trunk strength will be important in prosthetic use, maximal function of these areas is encouraged. Insofar as the amputee can tolerate the exercise, sitting tolerance and balance is challenged by the use of UE activities. Although at first the patient with a high above-knee amputation or bilateral leg amputations may need to hold onto the chair with one hand for support in the sitting position while using the other hand, the patient should be encouraged to depend on the trunk for balance to leave both arms free for UE activities. As UE strength and confidence in balance increase, ROM and resistance required for manual activities should be increased to further challenge trunk balance. Activities such as woodworking and weaving may be adapted to the amputee's individual needs. An activity in which the patient has a vocational or avocational interest may provide motivation so that the patient can increase tolerance of the given position and redirect energies from anxieties regarding his or her condition toward purposeful activity.

Another aspect of independence is the ability to perform self-care tasks, including bathing and care of the stump, transfers, and dressing. A unilateral amputee should have little or no difficulty in this area; however, aids such as grab bars for bath and toilet, a transfer board or tub seat for bathing, and a raised toilet seat can be helpful as the amputee adjusts to a new body image and copes with the problems of balance. Phantom limb sensations can be a complicating factor if the amputee suddenly moves to get up and forgets that he or she cannot stand on the amputated limb, even though feeling is there. Dressing is usually easier from a sitting position on the bed. Front fastenings and loose clothing help minimize frustrations.

Maximal independent function should be encouraged both with and without the prosthesis. For example, the amputee should be encouraged to stand on the sound leg in front of a table for short periods of time. This will encourage hip extension of the amputated side, and it will help the amputee develop balance; however, attention must be paid to the amount of standing time so as not to encourage scoliosis.

Therapists have found that immediate postoperative fitting of a prosthesis or the use of a temporary pylon and the working prosthesis after the amputee's scar tissue has healed is beneficial to the training program. The temporary pylon provides early replacement of the amputated limb to encourage functional activity while the stump is being conditioned and the permanent prosthesis is being made.* The pylon consists of a plaster stump socket to which a pylon is attached to provide length and base support to the amputated leg. With the pylon, the patient can stand and ambulate soon after the amputation.

At first the amputee fatigues more rapidly, even in maintaining sitting and standing positions, and until tolerance increases, energy is directed toward these basic functions.

Prosthetic training program

The LE amputee depends on the prosthesis for support in standing and walking. It is important that the prosthesis be appropriately prescribed, that it fit comfortably, and that it provide adequate functional assistance. The prescription and mechanical function of the prosthesis are checked thoroughly by the physical therapist. Function of the parts, how the amputee should put on the prosthesis, and how he or she should use it are taught by the physical therapist.

Independent locomotion depends on the fit and comfort of the prosthesis as well as on the general condition and tolerance of the amputee. Some may be able to discard their wheelchairs fairly soon. The amputee with poor tolerance of the prosthesis or a poorly fitting one, however, may need the security of the wheelchair for a long time. In either case, the occupational therapy program can benefit the amputee by encouraging work in the treatment room doing activities in a standing position when the patient can tolerate it. Even if still dependent on the wheelchair early in prosthetic training, the amputee must eventually adjust to the mechanical, insensitive prosthesis by learning to judge where it is relative to the rest of the body and must learn how to function with it.

When the amputee receives the prosthesis, most of his or her attention will be on the fit and use of it. Since the amputee needs rest from ambulation training, the amputee continues in an occupational therapy program for UE strengthening and prosthetic tolerance. The activities outlined in the preprosthetic period are continued. At this point, they are done with the prosthesis on unless the amputee is resting the stump or it has been irritated by the prosthesis. The program is geared toward encouraging acceptance of the prosthesis (to function in activities challenging UE and LE coordination and function), prosthesis tolerance, development of ADL independence, UE and LE exer-

cise, realization of capacities, and vocational and avocational guidance.

The prosthesis wearing time is gradually increased according to the comfort and tolerance of the socket in sitting and standing positions. The amputee must adjust to the sensation of bilateral weight-bearing and the sensitivity of the stump to the hard edges and base of the socket. According to individual tolerance and balance, the amputee can decrease the support used while standing. Engagement in UE activities in a standing position, which provides a wide ROM and resistance, helps to challenge and increase standing balance. Walking to cabinets to get and replace materials or tools and walking around tables and machines should be encouraged to increase functional independence. Carrying articles from place to place also challenges balance and independent function. Aids such as a cart with wheels or a tray can minimize the stress of carrying items.

In ADL, the patient learns to incorporate the prosthesis into bodily activities. The amputee learns at what point in dressing to put on the prosthesis so that it will aid, rather than interfere with, ease and speed in dressing.

An important part of the prosthetic training program is helping the amputee realize individual capabilities. In the occupational therapy environment, tasks may be set up both to improve the amputee's tolerance and function with the prosthesis and to relate to the requirements of his or her job.

Prevocational exploration

Amputation may prevent a person from returning to a former line of work, and this may be a great source of anxiety. In such cases, the occupational therapist can provide valuable information to the vocational rehabilitation counselor regarding the functional capabilities of the amputee. Information regarding interests, intelligence, physical abilities and skills, work tolerance, work habits, and general motivation for achieving new skills assists the counselor in investigating possibilities for the employable amputee in vocational planning.

Through formal prevocational performance evaluation using standardized dexterity tests, interest tests, and work-simulated tasks, the occupational therapist is able to provide an indication of motivation and readiness for vocational exploration. Through simulated work activities, the therapist is able to assess general work habits, comprehension, problem-solving ability, social compatibility, quality of work, and work tolerance.

Summary

Amputations of the upper and lower extremities may be due to congenital deformity, injury, or disease. A variety of options are available for prosthetic replacement in the attempt to meet the developmental, psychological, physical, social, and functional needs of the amputee.

In UE amputations, surgical procedures are directed toward saving as much bone and soft tissue as possible so that the amputee can gain optimal benefit from the prosthetic device. Prosthetic components are custom-prescribed by the rehabilitation team to form the most functional type of prosthesis according to the level and type of amputation. Residual sensation and pain affect adjustment to the prosthesis and eventual wear and use.

---

* For specific designs of the pylon, see Jones, M. S. (1964). *An approach to occupational therapy* (Chap. 6). London: Butterworths.

The postoperative program begins with psychological adjustment to amputation and orientation to the preprosthetic and prosthetic training program. Immediate or early fitting of a temporary prosthesis enhances general conditioning of the stump as well as psychological and functional adjustment.

The occupational therapist contributes to the preprosthetic and prosthetic training program and general adaptation of the LE amputee.

This section is dedicated to the memory of my dear friend and colleague Patricia A. Curran who provided constant editorial assistance and encouragement in professional and technical writing.

Appreciation is extended to Eastern Maine Medical Center in Bangor and to the Harmarville Rehabilitation Center in Pittsburgh for library and technical resources, to Ed Collins, Ron Gregory, and Patricia Marvin for photographs, to Barry Kaufman for line drawings, to Lois Rosage, Linda Strathdee, and Jean Blanchard for critical review, and to Laura Tasheiko and to Blue Hill Memorial Hospital in Blue Hill, Maine for technical assistance.

References

Bender, L. F. (1974). *Prostheses and rehabilitation after arm amputation* (pp. 34, 57, 157). Springfield, IL: Charles C. Thomas.

Cummings, V., Alexander J., & Gans, S. O. (1984). Management of the amputee. In A. P. Ruskin (Ed.), *Current therapy in physiatry* (pp. 212, 213, 219). Philadelphia: W. B. Saunders.

Gilfoyle, E. M., Grady, A. P., & Moore, J. C. (1981). *Children adapt* (p. 1). Thorofare, NJ: Slack.

Robertson, E. (1979). *Rehabilitation of arm amputees and limb-deficient children* (pp. 42, 44). London: Bailliere Tindall.

Russell, H., & Ferullo, D. (1981). *The best years of my life* (p. 17). Middlebury, VT: Paul S. Eriksson.

Shaperman, J. (1979). Learning patterns of young children with above-elbow prostheses. *American Journal of Occupational Therapy, 33,* 304.

Sorbye, R. (1980). Myoelectric prosthetic fitting in young children. *Journal of Clinical Orthopedic Related Research, 148,* 36.

Stein, R. B., Charles, P. D., Hoffer, J. A., Arsenault, J., Davis, L. A., Moorman, S., & Moss, B. (1980). New approaches for the control of powered prostheses particularly by high-level amputees. *Bulletin of Prosthetics Research, 10–33,* 51–62.

Bibliography

Agnew, P. J., & Shannon, G. F. (1981). Training program for a myoelectrically controlled prostheses with sensory feedback system. *American Journal of Occupational Therapy, 35,* 722.

American Occupational Therapy Association Division of Professional Development. (1979). *Orthotics/prosthetics* (Information Packet). Rockville, MD: AOTA.

Banerjee, S. N. (Ed.). (1982). *Rehabilitation management of amputees.* Baltimore: Williams & Wilkins.

Cummings, V., Alexander, J., & Gans, S. O. (1980). Management of the amputee. In A. P. Ruskin (Ed.), *Current therapy in physiatry.* Philadelphia: W. B. Saunders.

D'astous, J. (Ed.). (1981). *Orthotics and prosthetics digest reference manual.* Ottawa: Edahl Productions.

Dickey, R. E., & Stieritz, L. (1981). Amputation and impaired independence. In B. C. Abreu (Ed.), *Physical disabilities manual.* New York: Raven Press.

Ey, M. C. (1978). Experiences with myoelectric prostheses: A preliminary report. *Inter-Clinic Information Bulletin, 17,* 15.

Ey, M. C., & Helfgott, S. (1978). A temporary thumb prostheses. *Inter-Clinic Information Bulletin, 17,* 9.

Fraser, C. (1984). Does an artificial limb become part of the user? *British Journal of Occupational Therapy, 47,* 43.

Friedman, L. W. (1978). *The psychological rehabilitation of the amputee.* Springfield, IL: Charles C. Thomas.

Herberts, P., Korner, L., Caine, K., & Wensby, L. (1980). Rehabilitation of unilateral below-elbow amputees with myoelectric prostheses. *Scandinavian Journal of Rehabilitative Medicine, 12,* 123.

Madruga, L. (1979). *One step at a time: A young woman's inspiring struggle to walk again.* New York: McGraw-Hill.

Mastro, B. A., & Mastro, R. T. (Eds.). (1980). *A review of orthotics and prosthetics.* Washington, DC: American Orthotic and Prosthetic Association.

Murphy, E. F., & Horn, L. W. (1981). Myoelectric control systems—a selected bibliography. *Orthotics Prosthetics, 35,* 1.

National Amputation Foundation. (1977). *Prosthetics yes ... bionics maybe* (review of Third World Congress, International Society of Prosthetics Orthotics). Whitestone, NY: Author.

National Research Council, Division of Medical Sciences, National Academy of Sciences, Committee on Prosthetic-Orthotic Education. *Review of visual aids for prosthetics and orthotics.* Washington, DC: Author.

Pedretti, L.W. (1985). *Occupational therapy practice skills for physical dysfunction* (2nd ed.). St. Louis: Mosby.

Rosenfelder, R. (1980). Infant amputee: Early growth and care. *Journal of Clinical Orthopedic Related Research, 148,* 41.

Shaperman, J., & Sumida, C. T. (1980). Recent advances in prosthetics for children. *Journal of Clinical Orthopedic Related Research, 148,* 26.

Talbot, D. (1979). *The child with a limb deficiency: A guide for parents.* Los Angeles: UCLA Child Amputee Prosthetics Project.

Taylor, C. L. (1981). The biomechanics of control in upper-extremity prostheses. *Orthotics Prosthetics, 35,* 7.

Thompson, R. G. (1984). Evaluation of the amputee. In P. E. Kaplan (Ed.), *The practice of physical medicine.* Springfield, IL: Charles C. Thomas.

Whipple, L. (1980). *Whole again.* Ottawa: Green Hill.

SECTION 4

Hand rehabilitation

ELAINE EWING FESS

KEY TERMS

Circumferential Measurement	*Remodeling*
Edema	*Scar Maturation*
Fibroplasia	*Sensibility*
Goniometric Measurements	*Skin Temperature*
Inflammation	*Sudomotor Response*
Instrument Reliability	*Tensile Strength*
Instrument Validity	*Torque-Angle ROM*
Pain Analog Scale	*Total Active Motion*
Position of Antideformity	*Total Passive Motion*
Position of Deformity	*Volumeter*
	Wound Contracture

Upon completion of this section the reader will be able to:

1. *Define hand rehabilitation as it relates to personnel qualifications and other medical professions and explain its origin.*

2. *Identify the types of patients treated in hand rehabilitation centers and surgical procedures commonly associated with these patients.*

3. *Understand the importance of basing treatment on physiologic timing concepts.*

4. *Recognize the consequences of prolonged edema when left untreated or exacerbated in upper extremity injuries.*

5. *Describe the anatomic and biomechanical foundations for the positions of deformity and antideformity as they relate to the wrist and each digital joint.*

6. *Explain why "stretching" soft tissue can cause additional injury in terms of tissue remodeling concepts.*

7. *List in order of importance and define six criteria for selection of assessment instruments.*

8. *Identify advantages and disadvantages of commonly used hand assessment instruments in the categories of condition, motion, sensibilty, and function.*

9. *Choose four assessment instruments that best meet reliability and validity criteria.*

10. *Interpret basic rehabilitation goals as they relate to patients, physiologic timing, assessment, and treatment techniques.*

Hand rehabilitation is a specialty area in which the surgeon, occupational therapist, and physical therapist work closely together as a team to treat patients whose hands or upper extremities have been debilitated by disease or injury. Because of the hand's delicate and intricate anatomy, complicated kinesiology, and highly refined functional capacity, exacting knowledge of normal and abnormal UE anatomy, physiology, kinesiology, and biomechanics is required of all those involved in the rehabilitation process. Over the years, this need for additional knowledge and expertise has led to the development of hand specialty fields for both therapists and surgeons. Acknowledging that there has been and continues to be considerable controversy in the AOTA regarding establishment of specialty areas (Welles, 1958; American Journal of Occupational Therapy, 1979; Hirama, 1982; Slaymaker, 1986; Heater, 1992), it is not the intent of this section to debate the advantages and disadvantages of specialization but rather to provide a historical perspective for the evolution of hand therapy and to describe current practices in the already established field of hand rehabilitation.

Historical perspective

Hand therapy is a relative newcomer to the rehabilitation scene when compared to the long and respected histories of the occupational therapy and physical therapy professions. Hand surgery as a specialty area emerged in the late 1940s, but therapy was not highly regarded by early hand surgeons. Techniques that had

been effective on larger joints, such as hips and knees, produced disastrous results on the smaller, delicate joints of the hand, creating additional stiffness and scarring to already dysfunctional extremities. Attitudes began to change as therapists better understood hand anatomy, kinesiology, and the body's physiologic response to injury (Fess, 1990a).

By the mid-1960s, the first hand rehabilitation centers in the United States were being developed. The impetus for these centers came from three sources. First, Dr. Paul Brand, a renowned British hand surgeon working in India, trained assistants to provide postoperative therapy. His program was so well regarded that American hand surgeons visited and trained in his clinic. In 1960, Brand came to the United States to receive an honorary award, and during his stay, he discussed his concept of the role of therapists in hand rehabilitation with another award winner, the first Commissioner of the Vocational Rehabilitation Administration. Shortly thereafter, Dr. Earl Peacock, an American hand surgeon who had trained in Dr. Brand's clinic in India, requested funding for a hand rehabilitation center in Chapel Hill, North Carolina. In a quirk of fate, the person responsible for obtaining the requested funds was the same commissioner to whom Dr. Brand had spoken, and the first hand rehabilitation center in the United States was created (Bell-Krotoski, 1989). Although few are aware of the events that preceded the formation of this center, most therapists in the field of hand rehabilitation readily acknowledge Irene Hollis, OTR, FAOTA, the director at Chapel Hill from 1964 to 1978 (I. Hollis, personal communication, January 2, 1992), as the "grandmother" of hand therapy. Hollis's tremendous knowledge and enthusiasm influenced surgeons and therapists alike. In 1967, the first hand rehabilitation symposium was organized at Chapel Hill by Dr. Peacock, Dr. Madden, and Irene Hollis (I. Hollis, personal communication, January 2, 1992). These symposia provided the springboard for the formation of many of the well-established hand centers in the United States.

A second major influence in the initial development of hand rehabilitation centers came from World War II. Many early hand surgeons trained at military installations, such as Fort Sam Houston and Valley Forge, where they worked with military therapists on hand rehabilitation units. A third impetus came from England, where Commander Wynn Parry, a physiatrist, had organized a Royal Air Force hand rehabilitation unit. In 1958, Wynn Parry published the first edition of his book, *Rehabilitation of the Hand,* which is currently in its forth edition (Wynn Parry, 1981).

As surgeons increasingly recognized the value of working closely with therapists to provide preoperative and postoperative therapy to their patients, additional hand rehabilitation centers were established throughout the United States, and hand therapy began to emerge as an accepted specialty area. In 1976, based on their own successful team experience, Dr. James Hunter, Dr. Lawrence Schneider, and Evelyn Mackin, LPT from the Hand Rehabilitation Center in Philadelphia, presented the first of what are now sixteen annual educational meetings on hand rehabilitation. In a rarely encountered format both then and now, surgeons and therapists participate in this annual meeting on an equal basis, sharing knowledge and concerns. The Philadelphia meetings resulted in publication of *Rehabilitation of the Hand,* now in its third edition (Hunter, Schneider, Mackin, & Callahan, 1990). The book includes chapters written by therapists and surgeons. The leadership and steadfast belief in the team concept by Hunter, Schneider, and Mackin has been one of the primary reasons for acceptance and growth of hand rehabilitation as a specialty field.

In 1978, the first annual meeting of the American Society of Hand Therapists (ASHT) was held in Dallas, Texas. This society was formed as the result of the dedication and persistence of six people: four occupational therapists, Judith Bell (Krotoski), Margaret Carter (Wilson), Mary Kasch, and Bonnie Olivett; and two physical therapists, Evelyn Mackin and Karen Prendergast (Lauckhardt) (Bell-Krotoski, 1989; Mackin, 1988). Over the years, ASHT has played a major role in hand rehabilitation education and research (Callahan, 1988) by providing a forum for sharing state-of-the-art theories and techniques. In ASHT, occupational and physical therapists work closely together to advance the level of practice for their patients. A natural outgrowth of ASHT, the first issue of the *Journal of Hand Therapy,* was published in 1987. With emphasis on clinical issues related to hand dysfunction, the journal has international readership and is in its fifth year of publication.

The first Hand Therapy Certification Examination was given in May 1991. "Certification is the process by which a nongovernmental agency or association validates, based on predetermined standards, an individual's qualification and knowledge for practice in a defined area" (Hand Therapy Certification Commission, Inc. [HTCC], 1990, p. 1). The need for certification was identified by ASHT in 1983, and the scope of practice of hand therapy was defined (Chai, Dimick, & Kasch, 1987). In 1989, HTCC was incorporated and became legally separate from ASHT. Test items were written and screened through field testing, and the first certification examination in hand therapy was created. Over 1100 occupational and physical therapists passed the first examination and are designated Certified Hand Therapists (CHTs) (HTCC, 1991). Given on an annual basis, the certification examination legally defines the requirements for qualification as a CHT.

On the international scene, 16 countries, including the United States, belong to the International Federation of Societies of Hand Therapists. Established in 1980 and meeting every 3 years, the International Federation strives to promote hand rehabilitation concepts and educate therapists throughout the world. Thus far, meetings have been held in Rotterdam, Boston, Tokyo, Tel Aviv, and Paris.

Patients and practices

Although hand rehabilitation patients have diversified diagnoses, acute trauma injuries often represent a major proportion of patients treated in a hand center. Fractures, dislocations, tendon lacerations or avulsions, nerve compressions or lacerations, amputations, soft tissue injury, infection, or a combination of any or all of these are common. Chronic injuries are also frequently referred to hand therapy units, including cumulative trauma disorders, such as nerve compression, tendinitis, and other related inflammatory responses that are the result of prolonged extremity use and poor positioning. Additionally, patients who have problems related to specific disease processes, such as rheumatoid arthritis, osteoarthritis, or Dupuytren disease, are candidates for hand rehabilitation endeavors. Although some centers specialize in UE dysfunction resulting from congenital abnormalities or tumors, these diagnoses are less frequently encountered in most hand rehabilitation centers, as are problems related to upper motor neuron lesions and spinal cord injuries.

Therapists specializing in UE dysfunction may be based in general hospitals, privately owned hand centers, or in rehabilitation hospitals (Chai et al., 1987). An interesting trend has been noted with ASHT members. Although most members began their hand specialization careers in hospitals, over the past two decades, many of these therapists have relocated to therapist-owned private practices (Fess, 1990a).

Although some patients are able to achieve their maximal potential with therapy alone, most patients treated in hand rehabilitation centers require surgical intervention at some time during their rehabilitation programs. When surgery is elective, patients are seen both preoperatively and postoperatively, allowing dysfunctional hands to reach maximal preparedness before surgery. If injuries are the result of acute trauma, preoperative therapy is not feasible, and postoperative therapy alone is provided. When wounds have healed from the initial trauma or surgery, it is not unusual for secondary reconstructive surgical procedures to be undertaken. Throughout the entire rehabilitative process, therapists work closely with their patients to help them gain and maintain the function they have achieved through surgery and therapy. Some of the more commonly encountered surgical procedures include open reduction and internal fixation of fractures; repair or grafting of lacerated or avulsed tendon, nerve, or artery; ligament repair or reconstruction; skin grafting; neurovascular flap; debridement; nerve decompression; fasciotomy; fasciectomy; capsulotomy or capsulectomy; synovectomy; arthroplasty; arthrodesis; tendon transfer; amputation; transposition; replantation; and transplantation. In addition to understanding anatomy, physiology, and biomechanics as they relate to UE pathology, it is critical that therapists be thoroughly versed in the intricacies of the surgical procedures themselves and in their specific preoperative and postoperative requirements. Most hand surgeons encourage therapists to observe surgery, especially when it involves patients with whom the therapists are working.

Because of the great complexity of the hand and UE, advanced technical knowledge is required for successful therapeutic intervention. Although generalist therapists are not specifically excluded, some form of postgraduate specialty training in hand rehabilitation is encouraged, if not required, for entry into most hand specialization practices. Training may be obtained on the job, or it may be more formal as in a fellowship or postgraduate degree in hand rehabilitation.

Extremity function and rehabilitation philosophy

Although often taken for granted, the human hand is a wondrous and awe-inspiring mechanism. Through its structure and integrated functional capacity, an almost limitless number of tasks may be accomplished. The entire UE functions as an intercalated, open kinematic chain to which an opposable thumb is attached distally, allowing a single unit to accomplish the work of many through adaptation of segmental posture. The osseous skeletal components of this chain, coupled with smooth, gliding, articular surfaces with taut ligamentous support, permit simultaneous stability and mobility of the extremity. Extrinsic and intrinsic muscles, innervated by peripheral nerves that occur in predictable patterns, provide motor power to the articulated chain and enhance the delicate balance and interplay between strength and precision. Additionally, the normal extremity, which is covered by a flexible, durable, and stain-resistant cutaneous surface, possesses an almost unbelievable ability to perceive even the slightest touch; when necessary, the touch of a hand may substitute for occluded or impaired sight. Further, the only aspects of the body, aside from the face, that are routinely unclothed, hands are used as vehicles of communication at both the conscious and subconscious levels. It is no wonder that debilitation of a hand or UE can lead to serious problems both functionally and psychologically.

The job of the hand rehabilitation team is to restore patients whose hands have become dysfunctional from injury or disease to their maximal rehabilitation potential. This includes consideration of psychological, sociologic, economic, vocational, and avocational ramifications as well as physical factors. Emphasizing close communication among patient, therapist, and surgeon, each member of the team contributes specialized expertise toward achieving predetermined rehabilitative goals. Without close communication between team members, the entire rehabilitation effort is jeopardized.

Occupational therapy provides an excellent background for hand rehabilitation because of its inherent emphasis on functional activity. It is not sufficient simply to restore isolated components of function, such as strength or ROM, to an injured extremity. Instead, in hand rehabilitation, emphasis is placed on extremity use and returning patients to the home and work environments from which they came. Individual goals, such as diminishing edema, controlling pain, and increasing ROM and strength, are always viewed in the context of total patient requirements relating to performance of daily skills.

Physiologic response to injury

Hand therapy involves understanding, use, and manipulation of the body's normal healing processes to attain the best possible rehabilitation outcomes. To be successful, it is critical that all members of the rehabilitation team thoroughly understand the process and timing of the normal physiologic response to injury because this is the foundation on which all therapeutic intervention is based (Madden & Arem, 1981; Peacock, 1984; Strickland, 1987).

In the healing process, injury results in an alteration and replacement of normal structures with scar tissue. Scar in specialized tissues of the hand, such as tendon, bone, and joint, can cause severe impairment of function. Resulting not only from accidental injury, scar is also the sequela of surgical intervention and improper therapeutic techniques (Brand, 1985; Fess & Philips, 1987; Strickland, 1987). Increased scar formation may be caused by greater wound size, contamination, additional injury, and persistent edema.

Inflammation, fibroplasia, maturation, and wound contracture

Scar is formed through a predicable order of events to which treatment is directly correlated. Decisions of whether to rest or stress healing tissue depend on physiologic timing (Brand, 1985;

Strickland, 1987). The normal sequence of tissue healing includes inflammation, fibroplasia, scar maturation, and wound contracture. The *inflammation* phase is characterized by transient vasoconstriction followed by vasodilatation of local small blood vessels and migration of white blood cells. Allowing the removal of dead tissue and foreign bodies by phagocytic cells, the acute inflammatory response generally subsides within several days. During this time, the injured part is usually immobilized to promote healing. In special instances where control of scar is critical, as with tendon gliding, early motion programs may be initiated (Duran, Coleman, Nappi, & Klerekoper, 1990; Kleinert, Kutz, & Cohen, 1975; Evans, 1990). Beginning on the fourth or fifth day and continuing for 2 to 4 weeks, *fibroplasia* involves the synthesis of scar tissue by fibroblasts. As collagen fibers increase, the tensile strength of the wound increases. During this stage, active motion may be initiated, and splints may be used to protect healing structures or to control unbalanced forces of uninjured musculature. Changes in the architecture of the collagen fibers occurs during the *scar maturation* phase (Madden & Arem, 1981). Collagen becomes more organized, and tensile strength continues to increase. Carefully graded, resistive activities may be added to existing active motion exercises, and gentle corrective splinting may be initiated. With age, *wound contracture* occurs, in which the edges of wounds contract, and the area of scar becomes smaller. Although a scar may not completely disappear, the deposition of new collagen and resorption of old collagen is a constant process that continues throughout life. Collagen remodeling occurs in normal tissue as well as in scar tissue, and even longstanding soft tissue contractures may be altered with prolonged gentle stress (see Chapter 9, Section 5A) (Brand, 1985, 1990; Fess & Philips, 1987).

Edema, scar, and deformity

Although it is part of the normal inflammatory response, *edema,* if allowed to persist, will result in marked tissue scarring and fibrosis (Bunnell, 1944; Hunter et al., 1990; Strickland, 1987). Acting as a biologic "glue," the protein-rich edema fluid fills the spaces around ligaments and the soft tissues surrounding tendons and joints. Injured tissues, those immediately adjacent to the injury, and those in general proximity may all become involved as the fluid evolves into collagen, forming scar and limiting both active and passive motion.

To this physiologic transformation of protein into collagen, related mechanical factors that lead to deformity are added. Injury often results in a protective posture of wrist flexion, which, when combined with the presence of dorsal hand edema, places tension on the extrinsic digital extensor tendons, causing a zigzag collapse of the joints distal to the wrist and establishing a predictable *position of deformity* with the wrist in flexion; metacarpophalangeal (MP) joints in hyperextension; interphalangeal (IP) joints in flexion; and the thumb in adduction (see Chapter 9, Section 5A, Figure 9-8).

Additionally, anatomic configuration predisposes joints to specific deformities. The metacarpal head has a palmar protuberance or cam that causes the collateral ligaments to be taut in MP flexion but loose in MP extension (see the discussion of splinting in Chapter 9, Section 5A). If the MP joints are allowed to remain in extension for a prolonged period of time, the collateral ligaments become shortened, and MP joint flexion is mechanically blocked by lack of ligament length. Therefore, the *posi-*

tion of antideformity for the MP joints is flexion, which allows full MP collateral ligament length to be maintained. In contrast, the heads of the phalanges have a constant radius, allowing a consistent tension on the collateral ligaments regardless of joint position. Since the zigzag collapse predisposes the IP joints to flexion contractures, the antideformity position for the IP joints is extension.

The composite antideformity position for the hand and wrist is wrist neutral or extension, MP flexion, IP extension, and thumb abduction (see Chapter 9, Section 5A, Figure 9-11). In this position, the negative influences of poor wrist posture, pressure on extrinsic extensor tendons, zigzag collapse, and joint configuration are abated, and collateral ligament length is maintained. Barring extenuating circumstances, such as the presence of flexor tendon repairs, palmar skin grafts, joint subluxation or dislocation, and so forth, the antideformity position is used when a tendency to develop joint stiffness exists and immobilization of the hand is required.

Scar control

If untreated, the triad of injury, prolonged edema, and prolonged immobilization will result in restrictive scarring. Joint stiffness may result from direct injury or may occur secondarily from injury to adjacent structures. The scar **remodeling** process may be positively influenced by various methods, including edema control techniques; antideformity positioning through pinning or splinting; early passive motion techniques to tendon repairs; active ROM programs; maintenance of uninjured joint motion; pain control; maintenance and corrective splinting; functional hand use; and elimination of hematoma and infection.

When using therapeutic techniques designed to enhance motion, such as active or passive ROM exercises, joint mobilization, and splinting, it is important to understand that too much force too quickly causes microscopic tearing of tissue, and the cycle of scar production begins anew. The concept of "stretching tissue" can be potentially dangerous for two reasons. First, stretch is a temporary elongation of tissue that is not sustained for a sufficient length of time to allow tissue growth; second, stretch often involves forces great enough to cause additional injury to articular surfaces or surrounding structures (Brand, 1985, 1990). Forceful stretch increases scar formation by disrupting tissue and reinitiating the inflammatory response and collagen synthesis. Splinting, the method of choice for increasing passive ROM, is the only technique that is able to apply gentle stress over a period of time of sufficient length to allow collagen remodeling and tissue growth (Brand, 1985, 1990; Fess & Philips, 1987) (see Chapter 9, Section 5A).

Assessment

Working with hand problems requires careful and continuous patient monitoring because changes in extremity status may occur relatively quickly over days or sometimes hours depending on physiologic timing. To keep abreast, treatment programs must be altered, with evaluation measurements providing guidelines for making these modifications. Assessment is critical to the rehabilitation process because without measurement, therapeutic intervention cannot be undertaken.

Objective measurements delineate baseline pathology, help predict rehabilitation potential, and allow ranking of treatment priorities. They also define patient progress, provide data from which subsequent measurements may be compared, and assist in identifying effective treatment techniques. Patient and staff incentive is enhanced through objective measurement, and final functional capacity is defined. Additionally, through analysis, integration, and sharing of data, measurement serves as a vehicle of professional communication that eventually influences the comprehensive body of professional knowledge.

Instrument selection criteria

The accuracy of information gathered through evaluation procedures is directly dependent on the level of sophistication of the instruments used. Because they influence all levels of treatment, the best possible assessment tools must be used when evaluating patients with UE problems. Instruments that measure inaccurately or inconsistently provide diffuse or meaningless data, resulting in needless patient expense and loss of time.

The best tools available meet six selection criteria; the two most important of these are (1) statistical proof of reliability and (2) statistical proof of validity (ASHT, 1981; Currier, 1984; Fess, 1986, 1987 [pp. 103–122], 1988a, 1988b, 1988c, 1990b; Payton, 1984; Rothstein, 1985). Usually defined by correlation coefficients, **instrument reliability** indicates that an instrument measures accurately and consistently within each instrument and between like instruments; for one examiner and for multiple examiners; and for patient-specific populations. Also defined by a correlation coefficient, **instrument validity** means that an instrument appropriately measures the phenomenon for which it was designed (eg, strength, ROM, sensibility). Other instrument criteria include (3) administration and (4) interpretation instructions, (5) equipment standards, and (6) normative data based on large population samples (ASHT, 1981; Fess, 1986, 1990b). Reliability is the first criteria that must be satisfied. Without statistical proof of reliability, the remaining requirements for a test are without foundation, including attempts to show validity or the gathering of norms. If reliability has been demonstrated statistically, validity is the next most important criteria. Normative data for an assessment instrument cannot be collected before statistical establishment of both reliability and validity.

Unfortunately, few available hand assessment instruments meet all the selection criteria outlined above. In fact, most do not satisfy even the most fundamental elements of reliability and validity. Although these criteria are unquestioned requirements in a field such as engineering, their importance is just beginning to be fully recognized in the hand specialty area. Until better instruments are developed, therapists and surgeons must choose those instruments that most closely meet the six criteria. It is also important to become more demanding consumers of commercial evaluation products. Too often, therapists and surgeons are dazzled by "gadget appeal." Just because an instrument is expensive, seems sophisticated, or is computerized does not mean that it meets any of the selection criteria, especially those of reliability or validity. If a vendor cannot demonstrate statistical proof of reliability and validity, then the instrument in question should not be purchased. Poor assessment tools perpetuate misinformation, cause needless expense, and ultimately limit the effectiveness of the entire profession. We, as professionals, must take a stand against the further propagation of poorly documented, inherently faulty evaluation equipment. It harms our patients, and it harms our profession.

Timing and recording

The combination of thorough interview, careful observation, and precise measurement provides a composite picture of the patient and allows members of the rehabilitation team to appropriately design and implement a plan of treatment. Both history and physical examination provide important initial information. An intake history should include specific facts regarding how and when the injury occurred and how the injury is affecting accomplishment of daily living skills, work, and avocational pursuits. Assessment of pain and its perceived level of intensity, paralleled with observation of spontaneous extremity use during the interview, provides insight into the patient's attitude and ability to cope. Cursory examination of the involved extremity with comparison to the uninvolved side determines the focus of more detailed assessment. Discrepancies from normal that include but are not limited to extremity configuration, condition of soft tissue, skeletal stability, sensibility, strength, and dexterity require further investigation and documentation.

Most patients evaluated in a hand rehabilitation center do not need to be given all the available tests. For example, it would be neither practical nor efficacious to test in depth those areas initially deemed to be normal. Hand specialists use a few quick tests for initial triage and add more sophisticated testing procedures as dictated by patient condition. Initial and final evaluations are usually more comprehensive in scope, while intervening evaluations focus on specific problem areas. The frequency of reevaluation sessions depends on the rapidity of change demonstrated by the patient. Although ROM or edema may require daily measurements to reflect changes that are occurring, measurement of sensibility or strength may be appropriate on a weekly, biweekly, or even monthly basis due to the longer time required to effect measurable change. It must be remembered that each patient responds to treatment in a slightly different manner and that individualized monitoring is essential. There is no one formula that works for all patients.

In an age of patient awareness, third-party reimbursement, outcome legislation, and increasing litigation, thorough and complete documentation of patient status and progress is tantamount to professional survival (Fess, 1990a). The astute hand specialist—surgeon or therapist—must be able to prove in measurable terms the results of therapeutic intervention. For example, it is no longer sufficient to note that "the patient is much improved." Instead, one must indicate that "active flexion of the index MP has improved by 30 degrees since (date of last measurement) and is now 10 degrees/75 degrees." Documentation is a major reason why careful selection of assessment instruments is important. Treatment outcomes must be demonstrated numerically. If poor assessment instruments are used as the foundation for therapeutic decisions, results are open to question, and those in charge of directing patient care may be held responsible for less than favorable outcomes.

Assembling a test battery

Currently, a universal assessment instrument for the UE does not exist. Instead, a variety of evaluation tools must be used to measure the full spectrum of hand performance. UE assessment may be divided into four basic categories: (1) condition, (2) motion, (3) sensibility, and (4) function (Fess, 1990b). Since many of the instruments currently used do not meet all the selection criteria, it is helpful to include at least two tests within each category to further verify the data collected. Additionally, both the American Society for Surgery of the Hand (ASSH, 1983) and the American Society of Hand Therapists (ASHT, 1981) have developed clinical assessment recommendations relating to specific instruments and their protocols for use.

Current instruments

It is beyond the scope of this section to provide in-depth instructions for use of each instrument discussed. Instead, instruments are presented briefly, and the reader is referred to basic texts, such as *Rehabilitation of the Hand* evaluation and sensibility chapters (Hunter et al., 1990), and the ASSH (1983) and ASHT (1981) references in this section for additional information.

Condition assessment instruments

Condition assessment instruments noninvasively measure responses of the neurovascular system as it pertains to tissue viability, nutrition, vessel patency, and arterial, venous, or lymphatic flow. Monitoring of extremity volume and cutaneous temperature provides important information about the status of skin, subcutaneous tissues, and neurovascular function, including inflammatory response to injury or disease.

The ***volumeter*** (Figure 18-21) measures hand or extremity mass through the Archimedes principle of water displacement. Proved to be accurate to within 10 mL if the manufacturer's instructions are followed (Waylett-Rendall & Seibly, 1991), the

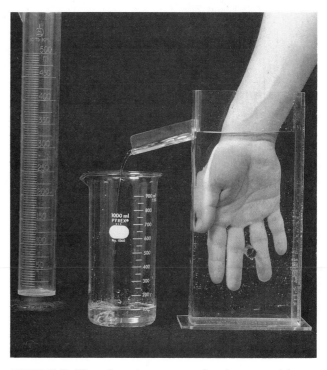

FIGURE 18-21. *The volumeter measures hand mass and is reflective of soft tissue inflammatory response to injury.*

volumeter is the most sensitive instrument available for monitoring inflammatory response, edema, or wasting conditions such as atrophy. Depending on individual circumstances, the volumeter may be contraindicated for patients with open wounds or infections. If the volumeter is used with an infected extremity, it should be sterilized before use with other patients. Closed wounds or presence of percutaneous K wires or sutures usually are not contraindications for use of the volumeter. When uncertainty exists as to whether the volumeter is appropriate, consultation with the referring surgeon is recommended. Normal comparison values may be obtained by measuring the uninvolved extremity.

Circumferential measurements may also be used to monitor extremity mass. Care must be taken to ensure consistent placement of and tension on the tape during subsequent measurements (Figure 18-22). An external caliper is an alternate method of assessing smaller diameter areas. Again, consistent instrument placement and tension are important for maintaining accuracy.

Skin temperature is an accepted method for assessing tissue viability and is often used to monitor replanted parts during early postoperative stages. Normal digital temperature ranges between 30°C and 35°C. If the temperature of a revascularized digit drops below 30°C, it should be reported immediately because it may indicate possible vascular compromise. In nonrevascularized cases, elevated temperatures over digital joints may be indicative of too strenuous exercise or splinting programs that have triggered an acute inflammatory response.

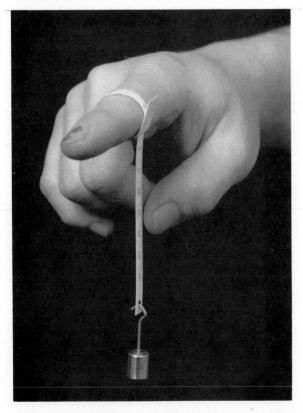

FIGURE 18-22. *Suspension of a weight on the end of a tape measure makes circumferential measurements more accurate and repeatable.*

Motion assessment instruments

Goniometric measurements are used to monitor joint motion and musculotendinous function. Passive ROM measurements demonstrate the ability of a joint to be moved through its normal arc of motion, while active ROM measurements reflect the ability of a muscle or group of muscles to cause joint motion. Limitations in passive ROM may result from pericapsular structures, such as ligaments that have shortened or developed adhesions, or from adhesions or mechanical blockage within the joint itself. When passive joint motion is present but active motion is restricted, the musculotendinous unit may be disrupted, as with a tendon laceration or rupture; or if the musculotendinous unit is intact, adhesions may be limiting normal tendon excursion. Regardless of the etiology, both passive and active joint motion should be evaluated, and in the presence of limitations, goniometric measurements should be recorded.

Total active motion (TAM) and *total passive motion* (TPM) (ASSH, 1983) are composite digital measurements. TAM is computed by adding the active flexion measurements for the MP, proximal interphalangeal (PIP), and distal interphalangeal (DIP) joints of a given digit and subtracting the sum of the extension deficits for the same three joints. TPM is similarly computed, but passive measurements are used in the computations. TAM and TPM are expressed as single numeric values, with normal being 270 degrees for both active and passive composite statements for digital motion.

Torque-angle ROM measurements (Brand, 1985) control the amount of force applied to a joint during evaluation of passive joint motion. When using torque-angle measurements, a consistent amount of weight, say 300 g, is perpendicularly applied at a consistent distance from the axis of a given joint when passive motion is measured with a goniometer (Figure 18-23). The same amount of weight is applied at the same distance for subsequent measurements, eliminating inconsistencies of applied force during passive motion assessment. A second method of torque-angle measurement involves adding progressive increments of weight, for example, 50, 100, 150, 200, and 250 g, to a joint at a constant distance from the axis and measuring the resultant joint angle with a goniometer after each successive addition of weight. The joint measurements are plotted on a graph, and the amount of give in the joint may be visualized (Figure 18-24). Steepness of the plotted curve indicates the variation in passive joint motion as more weight is added, with a vertical curve reflecting little increase of motion with added resistance and a more horizontal curve demonstrating an increase of passive motion as weight is added. A joint with a more horizontal curve has better potential to improve passive motion with therapy because it exhibits more give with progressively increasing resistance.

Isolated muscle strength as determined through manual muscle testing may be used to evaluate peripheral nerve lesions. The two most accepted methods of grading of manual muscle testing include numeric ratings of 0 through 5 as described by Seddon (1975) and the ratings of zero, trace, poor, fair, good, and normal as defined by the Committee on After-Effects, National Foundation for Infantile Paralysis (Kendall, Kendall, & Wadsworth, 1971). Although testing of isolated muscle strength is helpful in delineating baseline pathology or status of regenerating peripheral nerves, it is not appropriate for use with upper motor neuron lesions due to fluctuating muscle tone and altered reflex activity that are often present in conditions such as cerebral palsy or cerebral vascular accidents.

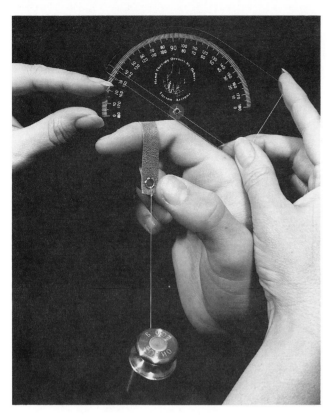

FIGURE 18-23. *Torque-angle measurements quantify the amount of resistance applied during measurement of passive range of motion.*

Sensibility assessment instruments

The two most common sensibility evaluation procedures used in hand rehabilitation are the Semmes-Weinstein Calibrated Monofilament Test (Figure 18-25) and the Two-Point Discrimination

Test (2PD) (Moberg, 1958; Dellon, Curtis, & Edgerton, 1974). Although the 2PD test traditionally has wider hand surgeons, the Semmes-Weinstein calibrated monofilaments are gaining in recognition because they are the only hand-held commercially available sensibility testing instrument that controls the amount of applied stimulus force (Bell-Krotoski & Buford, 1988; Bell-Krotoski, 1990a, 1990b). Control of force is a critical concept in sensibility testing. Monofilaments should never be bounced during application (Bell, personal communication, September 1992). Inconsistency of force application results in poor test reliability, especially when monitoring nerve compression lesions. Through extensive testing, the monofilaments have been shown to have intrainstrument and interinstrument reliability (Bell & Tomancik, 1987) and intrarater and interrater reliability (Griener, Bowen, & Jones, 1989). They also have administration and interpretation guidelines (Bell-Krotoski, 1990b). Once considered controversial, even the most staunch advocates of 2PD now admit that control of force stimulus is fundamental to testing sensibility. Unfortunately, a 2PD instrument that controls force application is not currently available. It is important to understand that this is not a fallacy in the concept of testing ability to distinguish between two points but rather a problem with instrumentation.

Other sensibility tests, such as the Ninhydrin test, the wrinkle test, and the Moberg pick-up test, are used in specialized situations (Moberg, 1958; O'Rain, 1973; Seddon, 1975; Sunderland, 1978; Fess, 1990b). Based on **sudomotor response**, or sympathetic response, the Ninhydrin and wrinkle tests have a narrow window of application that is limited to early, complete transection, peripheral nerve injuries. These tests measure presence of sweat (Ninhydrin) or skin moisture (wrinkle) and are ineffective in distinguishing nerve injury in the presence of an intact or regenerating autonomic nervous system (Onne, 1962; Phelps & Walker, 1977; Fess, 1990b). The Moberg pick-up test involves picking up small common objects and placing them one at a time into a larger container. When vision is occluded, patients with digital impairment of sensibility alter their prehension

FIGURE 18-24. *In this graphic representation of torque-angle measurements using progressively greater increments of weight, joint B exhibits more passive range of motion than joint A. Joint B therefore, may be viewed as having better rehabilitation potential. (From Fess, E. E., Philips, C. A. [1987]: Hand splinting principles and methods. [2nd ed.]. St. Louis: C. V. Mosby Co.)*

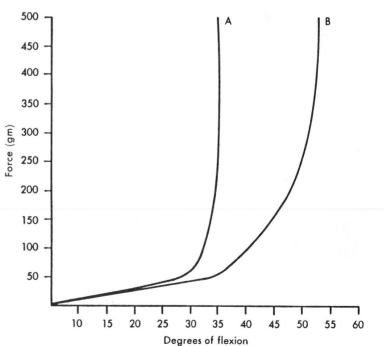

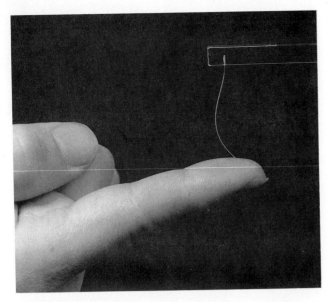

FIGURE 18-25. *The bend of a Semmes-Weinstein monofilament controls the amount of force applied and dampens vibration from the examiner's hand.*

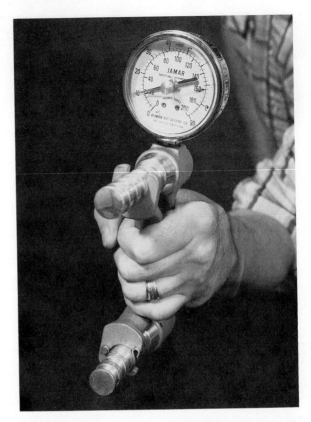

FIGURE 18-26. *When calibrated, the Jamar dynamometer has a high level of instrument reliability. (From Fess, E. E. [1984]: Rehabilitation of the patient with an upper extremity replantation. In J. M. Hunter, L. H. Schneider, E. J. Mackin, A. D. Callahan [Eds],* Rehabilitation of the hand *[2nd ed.]. St. Louis: C. V. Mosby Co.)*

patterns to grasp the test objects with those digits having normal sensation. These tests do not require patient interpretation or verbal response, and as long as they are used within the narrow diagnostic parameter described, they may be helpful when evaluating patients with cognitive or language problems, young children, or those whose motivation may be suspect. It is important to remember, however, that none of the three tests has statistical proof of reliability or validity.

Numerous other sensibility tools and techniques have been advocated by various people. Lacking even the most fundamental elements of statistical reliability and validity, most meet few if any of the selection criteria for an acceptable test instrument.

Function assessment instruments

Hand and UE function requires smooth and complex integration of all systems, including vascular, skeletal, muscular, and neural components. Functional tests range from assessing simple tasks, such as measurement of grip or pinch strength, to assessing complex activities that use tools and require positioning of the entire body.

Grip strength is measured with a commercially available, hand-held hydraulic dynamometer (Figure 18-26) (ASHT, 1981; ASSH, 1983, Fess, 1990b). The Jamar dynamometer has been shown to have high reliability (Mathiowetz, Weber, Volland, & Kashman, 1984; Fess, 1987, 1990c) when calibrated and has specific recommendations for administration and interpretation (ASHT, 1981; ASSH, 1983; Mathiowetz, Rennells, & Donahoe, 1985). Normal grip strengths change with the size of the object grasped, and assessment of grip strength is directly dependent on which Jamar handle position is used. Because normal grip strengths differ between handle positions, it is recommended that grip measurements be taken in the second handle position if only one position is used (ASHT, 1981; ASSH, 1983). Normative data for the Jamar dynamometer has not been thoroughly assessed. Unfortunately, one of the more well-known normative

studies (Kellor, Frost, & Silberg, 1971) did not distinguish between handle positions, resulting in meaningless data to which subsequent patient or normative values cannot be compared. Schmidt and Toews (1970) used one handle position and tested a large population sample, but they altered their Jamar dynamometers slightly with a sand and paint mixture to enhance grip. In addition, although the second handle position was used and recommended protocols were employed, the normative data from Mathiowetz, Kashman, and Volland (1985) are based on a narrow population sample for age, gender, and occupation. Further study based on statistically proven reliable instruments (Fess, 1987) and recommended protocols (ASHT, 1981; ASSH, 1983) is needed. Additionally, maintenance of instrument calibration is critical. It has been found that slightly over half of used dynamometers tested were sufficiently out of calibration to require return to the manufacturer for adjustment (Fess 1987, 1990c).

Pinch strength is measured with a commercially available pinchometer (ASHT, 1981; ASSH, 1983). Three types of pinch are usually evaluated, including lateral, three-jaw-chuck, and tip. Although Mathiowetz and colleagues (1984) studied the pinchometer for reliability and validity, larger and more in-depth studies are needed. This is also true of normative studies (Mathiowetz, Kashman, & Volland, 1985). Interestingly, in a literature review, Casanova and Grunert (1989) found that "thirty-seven distinct pinches were identified although they were referred to by many more terms than this" (1985, p. 231). In response to this diversity of nomenclature, they developed a classification system based on anatomic description that provides an organizational system for identifying two- and three-digit prehension patterns. This is an important step toward standardization of hand rehabilitation terminology.

Standardized dexterity tests, such as the Jebsen Hand Function Test (Jebsen, Taylor, & Triegchmann, 1969), the Minnesota Rate of Manipulation Test, the Purdue Pegboard (Tiffin & Asher, 1948), and the Crawford Small Parts Test are some of the few hand and UE evaluation instruments that meet all six of the instrument selection criteria. When ranked according to level of difficulty, these four tests range from assessing relatively gross hand dexterity to testing very fine coordination that requires manipulation of small tools. Although many evaluation tools on the market purport to be standardized tests of dexterity or coordination, very few, aside from those listed above, satisfy the criteria when examined closely. As with other hand assessment instruments, they often lack the fundamental elements of reliability and validity, although they frequently tout extensive normative data. This, of course, is misleading to say the least. In reality, norms gathered from instruments that measure inaccurately and inconsistently have tremendous potential for error and actually may be harmful when used to implement treatment.

The Minnesota, Purdue, and Crawford tests may be purchased commercially, but the Jebsen is assembled according to guidelines in the original article (Jebsen et al., 1969). As with all standardized tests, equipment criteria must be strictly followed, without alteration. Although the Jebsen test is inexpensive to assemble (Figure 18-27), because the original equipment criteria were conceived over 20 years ago, some of the test items are somewhat difficult to find. In an important study, Rider and Linden (1988) found that substitution of slightly different test items, such as plastic checkers for wooden checkers, statistically alters the test and therefore invalidates it. Also, it is important to present the subtests of standardized tests in the order recommended. To alter the order or omit portions invalidates the test unless each subtest has independent instrumentation criteria, including reliability, validity, and instructions for administration and interpretation.

Other dexterity tests are available, and in a changing market, it is important to compare these tests to the instrument selection criteria. If they meet the criteria, consideration of purchase is appropriate, but if they do not, then the buyer must beware.

Assessment of daily living skills depends on the type and level of injury or the severity of involvement of the disease process. The open kinematic chain configuration of the UE permits great adaptability to limitation, especially when more distal joints are involved. The more proximal the limitation, the more debilitating it becomes. Most hand rehabilitation patients sustain acute traumatic injury with unilateral disability, requiring minimal ADL evaluation and training unless more proximal joints, such as the shoulder or elbow, are involved. Patients with bilateral UE involvement are candidates for considerable ADL intervention, especially when proximal joints are limited. Because a standardized universal test is not available, impairment of daily living skills is determined through interviews, observations (Figure 18-28), and when necessary, site visits.

Return-to-work evaluations are based on a combination of hand assessment instruments, standardized dexterity tests, observational tests, knowledge of the specific work situation, site visits, insight into patients' motivational and psychological orientation, and understanding of UE anatomy, kinesiology, physiology, and biomechanics (Baxter-Petralia, Bruening, & Blackmore, 1990). Patient programs are specifically tailored to meet individual needs (Figure 18-29), since few rigid protocols for therapy exist in this area. Most large hand rehabilitation centers have specialized work hardening and return-to-work programs, allowing consistent, high-quality treatment from the initial injury through discharge to patients' own environments (Bear-Lehman & McCormick, 1985). Employers, rehabilitation nurses, and vocational counselors are usually involved in the back-to-work process, and if returning to the original job is not feasible, other alternatives are explored until satisfactory placement is achieved (Figure 18-30). For more detailed information, the reader is referred to the Physical Capacity Evaluation and to the Worker and Performer in a Hand Rehabilitation Setting sections of *Rehabilitation of the Hand* (3rd ed.) (Hunter et al., 1990, pp. 1155–1224).

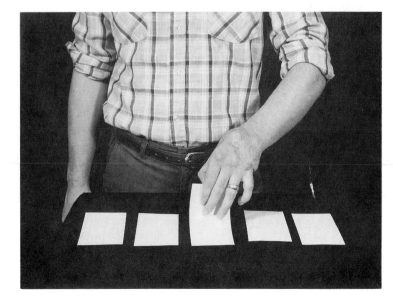

FIGURE 18-27. *The Jebsen dexterity test consists of seven subtests that measure different aspects of hand function. (From Fess, E. E. [1984]: Rehabilitation of the patient with an upper extremity replantation. In J. M. Hunter, L. H. Schneider, E. J. Mackin, A. D. Callahan [Eds], Rehabilitation of the hand [2nd ed.].* St. Louis: C. V. Mosby Co.)

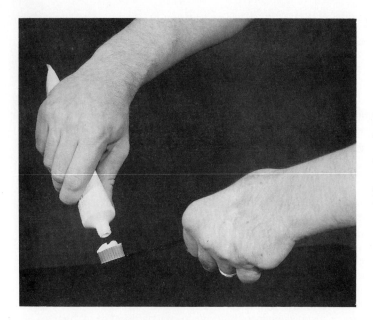

FIGURE 18-28. *Daily living skills requiring bilateral hand use may be difficult for a person who has sustained a hand injury. (From Fess, E. E. [1984]: Rehabilitation of the patient with an upper extremity replantation. In J. M. Hunter, L. H. Schneider, E. J. Mackin, A. D. Callahan [Eds],* Rehabilitation of the hand [2nd ed.]. *St. Louis: C. V. Mosby Co.)*

Return-to-work assessment tools that meet instrument selection criteria include the standardized dexterity tests discussed above and the Valpar Work Samples, a series of 19 standardized tests that provide information regarding speed of coordination and performance of physical demands, including reaching, handling, manipulating, and feeling. Using normative data to which comparison of patient work performance may be made, some of the Valpar tests are more applicable to hand rehabilitation needs than others. These include the Valpar Upper Extremity Range of Motion Work Sample, the Valpar Whole Body Range of Motion Work Sample, the Valpar Small Tools Mechanical Work Sample, and the Valpar Simulated Assembly Work Sample. Other instruments that are often associated with return-to-work programs include computerized work simulators. Surprisingly, to date, none of these simulators have statistical proof of reliability or validity, although they are sold as "assessment" instruments. Although these work simulators make excellent therapeutic tools, they should not be relied on to provide accurate or consistent evaluation data until further studies are conducted regarding their reliability and validity.

Four instruments

Excluding the standardized tests of dexterity and the Valpar Work Samples, only four hand assessment instruments meet even the fundamental criteria of reliability and validity. They include the volumeter, goniometer, Semmes-Weinstein monofilaments, and the Jamar dynamometer. In addition to reliability and validity, some administration and interpretation guidelines, equipment criteria, and normative data are available or are being developed for all four instruments. Although further study is needed, these four instruments are the best evaluation tools available to hand rehabilitation specialists at this time. It is interesting to note that none of the four is computerized, and in comparison with many of the high-technology gadgets on the market, they are relatively inexpensive. Together, these instruments provide accurate and trustworthy data for the total spectrum of UE evaluation areas, including condition (volumeter), motion (goniometer), sensibility (monofilaments), and function (Jamar dynamometer). The quality of assessment tools is the foundation on which therapeutic intervention is built, and in an age of outcomes management (Fess, 1990a), with the ugly specter of litigation ever-present, it is ludicrous not to use these four tools to their fullest extent. For the time, they represent the means of professional excellence and professional survival.

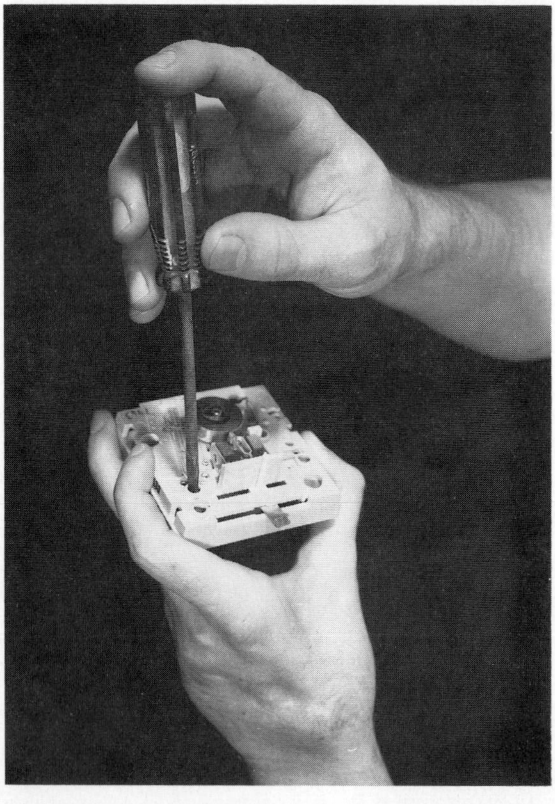

FIGURE 18-29. *Work assessment reflects individual patient requirements. (From Fess, E. E. [1984]: Rehabilitation of the patient with an upper extremity replantation. In J. M. Hunter, L. H. Schneider, E. J. Mackin, A. D. Callahan [Eds],* Rehabilitation of the hand [2nd ed.]. *St. Louis: C. V. Mosby Co.)*

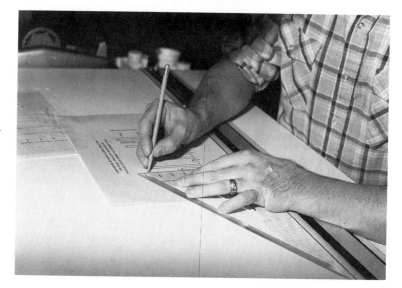

FIGURE 18-30. *Unable to accomplish his original job, this patient received specialized drafting training and returned to productive employment. (From Fess, E. E. [1984]: Rehabilitation of the patient with an upper extremity replantation. In J. M. Hunter, L. H. Schneider, E. J. Mackin, A. D. Callahan [Eds], Rehabilitation of the hand [2nd ed.]. St. Louis: C. V. Mosby Co.)*

Rehabilitation goals

Certain goals are fundamental to all hand rehabilitation endeavors, and when combined with knowledge of anatomy, kinesiology, biomechanics, and physiologic timing, they provide guidelines for treatment. Understanding physiologic timing is especially important. In the early days of hand rehabilitation, specific treatment protocols for therapy had not been developed. Therapists had to understand how basic physiologic timing interfaced with each diagnostic category and surgical procedure. They also had to be able to understand and deal with slight variations individual to each patient. Now there are specific treatment protocols for almost every diagnosis and procedure imaginable. Although this is helpful in that therapists are not constantly "reinventing the wheel," there is the potential danger that the underlying rationale for the protocols may be lost. There comes a time when it is neither possible nor efficacious to remember every detail and intricacy of every protocol written. Also, reliance on protocols without understanding of the foundation from which they were developed leads to rigidity of approach to treatment, reduces those who insist on strict adherence to technicians, and limits the rehabilitation potential of patients (Figure 18-31).

The basic process of physiologic response to injury does not change. It may be slightly altered or prolonged for various reasons, but the chemical and cellular activity remain constant within a relative time frame. Understanding this phenomenon provides continuity and structure to treatment regardless of diagnosis or surgical procedure.

Reduce or control edema

Edema control is an early priority in the rehabilitation process. A normal response to injury, edema is part of the inflammatory and early fibroplasia stages of wound healing. When left untreated or aggravated by contamination or additional injury, the presence of edema may be prolonged, leading to excessive scar formation, limitation of function, and often, increased pain. Postoperative dressings are bulky and compressive in design, and elevation of the extremity is stressed to control edema. During the early

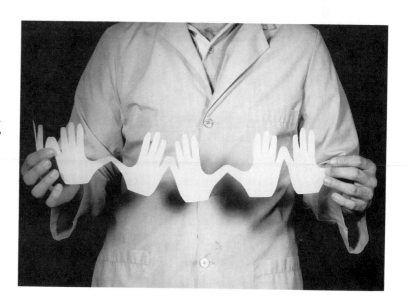

FIGURE 18-31. *A cookbook approach to hand rehabilitation patients leads to less than satisfactory results and should be studiously avoided. (From Fess, E. E. [1990]: Fourth Nathalie Barr lecture.* Journal of Hand Therapy, 3, *1.)*

postoperative days, it is not unusual for operated extremities in their bulky dressings to be attached to intravenous poles or over-bed traction systems to ensure extremity elevation. To be effective, the hand must be above the wrist, the wrist above the elbow, and the elbow above the level of the heart. Patients are taught to avoid positions in which the injured extremity is dependent. This can be especially problematic during times of sleep. Active motion is also helpful in decreasing edema. The natural pumping action generated by volitional muscle contraction serves as a mechanism to move edema fluid away from the periphery and toward the heart. Although it may not be indicated for some specific healing tissues, active motion may be initiated at non-immobilized joints within hours to a few days after surgery.

Once the bulky dressings are removed and superficial skin closure is present, edema may be monitored with a volumeter. Occasionally, hands may be so edematous that they do not fit into the volumeter; external hardware may be too bulky; or infection may preclude volumeter use. In these cases, circumferential measurements are helpful in measuring extremity mass. Reduction in edema usually is apparent within a few days, and at 2 weeks after injury or surgery, much of the edema is gone. Increases in edema or prolonged persistence should be monitored carefully, and all members of the team should be made aware of the problem.

Techniques and modalities, such as massage, string wrapping, intermittent pressure machines, and continuous passive motion machines have been advocated for decreasing edema. Although these represent traditional therapeutic approaches, there are no prospective statistically significant studies that prove that these methods produce lasting reduction of edema. Use of any of the above techniques or modalities should be accompanied by pre- and posttreatment volumetric measurements to ensure that microscopic injury to tissue is not occurring (Fess, 1990a). Posttreatment measurements should be timed to identify those changes in volume that are only temporary.

Maintain or increase motion

Maintenance or enhancement of joint ROM is another priority in hand rehabilitation. Because the structures of the hand are so delicate, interdependent, and enclosed within a small area, maintenance of normal glide and excursion of mobile structures is critical to achieving optimal hand and extremity function. With skeletal stability a requisite, active ROM cannot occur without the presence of equal or better passive joint motion. Depending on the circumstances, skin closure is preferable but not mandatory to initiating motion programs. In the past, surgeons and therapists delayed initiation of motion until soft tissue healing had occurred, but they discovered that by the time this took place, the repaired structures and those surrounding them were mired in scar, and motion was limited.

Because protein-rich edema fluid acts as a biologic glue, early motion is emphasized by most hand rehabilitation specialists. During the inflammatory and fibroplasia stages (1 to 3 days to 4 weeks), active and passive motion of uninvolved joints is encouraged to limit adhesion formation to adjacent noninjured structures. Early passive motion programs may also be started to provide controlled glide to healing structures, such as tendon (Duran et al., 1990; Evans, 1990; Kleinert et al., 1975). Splinting to maintain or increase passive motion of uninvolved joints may also be carried out so long as it does not stress repaired struc-

tures. This is a time in which the cellular predecessors to collagen are being deposited in the wound; the transformation from fibrin to collagen is occurring; and wound **tensile strength** is beginning to increase. It is also a time of undesirable adhesion formation to surrounding structures. It is important to know the philosophy of the referring physician before initiating treatment. Although few will argue with early active and passive motion for uninvolved joints, some surgeons are not advocates of early passive motion to repaired structures. A word of caution: the timing of initiation of motion programs with patients who have undergone extensive revascularization procedures, such as replantation or transplantation, should be carefully coordinated with the surgeon in charge. Motion begun too early may jeopardize the viability of the revascularized part.

In general, by the third to fourth postoperative week, depending on the type of tissue repaired, tensile strength to the wound has increased sufficiently to allow gentle, protected active motion of repaired structures. If circumstances are questionable, however, as with a problematic tendon repair in an early passive motion program, initiation of active motion may be delayed until the fifth week. Active and passive motion to uninvolved joints, of course, continues; but because the acute inflammatory process has subsided, chances of developing adhesions to noninvolved structures is considerably diminished.

Tensile strength of repaired structures has increased sufficiently by the sixth postoperative week to permit more vigorous active motion, and splinting that minimally stresses healing tissue may be carefully initiated.

Changes in passive and active joint motion are monitored with goniometric measurements. These measurements provide precise information on which treatment program modifications are made. The first 6 to 8 weeks after injury or surgical intervention represent a golden period in which the reparative process progresses quickly, requiring close monitoring of change and decisive updating of therapeutic endeavors. Torpid or inconsistent monitoring at this critical time results in irrevocable loss of opportunity to use and manipulate the early remodeling process.

Techniques and modalities that assist in maintaining or improving active and passive ROM include active exercise, extremity use within parameters of the healing tissues, and splinting. Since tensile strength of a wound progresses from none to the ability to withstand minimal stress during the first 6 to 8 weeks, activities that provide even small amounts of resistance should be used with caution. Biofeedback is useful in helping patients identify muscle groups and their actions, and if pain is problematic (it often is not), transcutaneous electrical nerve stimulation (TENS) may be helpful. As with any pain modifier, if TENS is used, patients should be weaned from it as soon as possible, reducing patient expense and diminishing modality dependency. Although continuous passive motion (CPM) and functional electrical stimulation (FES) are advocated by some hand rehabilitation specialists, there are no prospective, statistically significant studies that show that these modalities effect permanent motion improvement. Thermal modalities used to effect motion have the potential to seriously increase edema, especially during this physiologically fragile time. Additionally, the long-range effects of using heat to increase tissue elasticity have not been proved. The concern that stretching heated tissues may cause microscopic tearing is real. If heat is used, careful, long-term monitoring of edema levels both before and after application must be done to ensure that further damage is not occurring.

Maintain or increase function

By the eighth postoperative week, wound tensile strength has increased considerably, and graded resistive activities may be added to the treatment program. Functional use of the hand, starting with light activities and adding resistance gradually, is encouraged. Barring extenuating circumstances, full use of the extremity usually is permitted by the 12th week. The scar remodeling process continues, and the ability to effect changes in motion is somewhat less than it was during the early stages of wound healing but better than it will be at 1 year or more. At this point, it is often easier to improve passive motion of stiff joints through the application of prolonged gentle force by splinting than it is to increase the tendon glide required in active motion. After several months, if motion continues to be limited and this interferes with extremity use, additional surgery may be considered, and if carried out, the entire physiologic process of wound healing begins anew. If active and passive motion are not limited, or if limitations do not significantly impede function, strengthening, endurance, and work hardening programs may be progressively implemented.

Goniometric measurements continue as the cornerstone for monitoring changes in joint ROM and dynamometer readings, which were previously contraindicated due to stress on healing tissues, are added to assess strength progress. Dexterity testing and return-to-work evaluations are incorporated as patient progress permits.

Use of techniques and modalities remain similar to those employed previously except resistive exercises and graded functional activities are added to improve strength, endurance, and dexterity. If either TENS or FES was used earlier, it probably is discontinued by this time. In unusual circumstances, if pain sufficient to warrant TENS use into the 12th postoperative week is present, something may be askew, and the pain control program should be reevaluated. The previous concerns regarding heat modalities remain. Although the internal environment of the wound is now less susceptible to the effects of increased blood flow, potentials for increased edema and microscopic tearing of tissues continue to be concerns.

Occasionally, highly motivated patients overexercise or increase the tension of their splints, causing redness and localized swelling around joints. Indicative of tissue injury, this inflammatory response should be heeded, and the causative activity or tension immediately discontinued. Therapists may also be too enthusiastic in their efforts to improve motion or strength, resulting in a similar localized inflammatory response that, if allowed to persist or become worse, may lead to a stiff hand syndrome.

Maintain or enhance sensibility

Although they have distinctly different meanings, the terms **sensibility** and sensation frequently are confused or used interchangeably. Sensibility is the "capacity to receive and respond to stimuli," whereas sensation is "a feeling or awareness . . . resulting from the stimulation of sensory receptors" (Taber, 1989, p. S25). In testing situations patients, are asked to receive and respond to stimuli, not just receive.

The ability to perceive external stimuli through touch is critical to UE function. Moberg (1966) noted that without sensation, the hand is blind. Hand function of patients using visual cues may seem normal to an observer, but when vision is occluded, patients with impaired or absent sensation adapt their functional patterns to use those portions of the extremity that have normal sensation. Additionally, anesthetic or poorly innervated digits or hands are at risk for acute and chronic injury because patients simply are not aware when physical contact with noxious elements of the environment occurs or when excessive pressure is used to grasp and manipulate objects.

After transection and subsequent Wallerian degeneration, and depending on the extent of damage and the extent of repair, peripheral nerve regenerates at a rate of about 2 cm per month, assuming all goes well (Seddon, 1975; Sunderland, 1978). Unlike transection injuries, nerve continuity is maintained in compression problems, and spontaneous recovery may occur or surgical intervention may be necessary. Sensory disruption may result from direct injury to nerve, or it may be secondary to inflammation of adjacent structures. Monitoring sensibility and educating patients about their disabilities are important aspects of hand rehabilitation.

Although therapy cannot speed the reparative process, it can assist in eliminating or controlling those factors that may impede return of function, such as excessive edema, contamination, poor extremity posture, or overuse. Careful monitoring of sensibility is important throughout treatment, from establishment of baseline parameters to the time of discharge. Because of their ability to control stimulus force, the Semmes-Weinstein monofilaments are the instruments of choice for assessing nerve compression problems or regenerating nerves. Nerve function in transition can be unpredictable and vulnerable to even small changes in the internal or external environments. Any decrease in function should be documented and reported to the referring physician as soon as possible.

Sensory reeducation programs retrain the brain to interpret and recognize altered sensation patterns that result from peripheral nerve injury (Dellon, 1981; Wynn Parry, 1981; Callahan, 1990). Although children generally have good prognoses for return of normal nerve function, adults frequently exhibit poor to fair sensory recovery. Therapy for those patients who require assistance in adapting to their altered sensation involves teaching compensatory extremity use if protective sensation is absent and teaching recognition of new or altered sensory input patterns if sensibility is testable with the 4.31 Semmes-Weinstein monofilament or lighter (Callahan, 1990). Touch localization and texture and shape discrimination activities are used in the retraining process.

Control or decrease pain

From initial contact, whether in the emergency room, physician's office, or therapy clinic, all members of the rehabilitation team strive to control and diminish pain experienced by patients. Pain, a normal response to injury, diminishes in intensity with time, and most patients are able to adapt to early, more acute pain of injury or surgical intervention with the help of prescribed analgesics. After a few days to a week or so, as the acute pain subsides, patients need less and less pharmaceutical assistance until none is required. A subjective response, perception of pain is different from person to person. These normal variations make identification of pathologic pain difficult for the hand rehabilitation team members. When pain does not follow a normal diminishing pattern, it must be taken very seriously. It is important to identify and treat the source of pain, not the symptomatology exhibited. Prolonged, increasing, or inappropriately intense pain may be indicative of physical pathology, such as ischemia or neuroma, or it may be the start of a chronic pain syndrome, such as reflex sympathetic dystrophy. Either way, it needs to be dealt with quickly and effectively before irreversible damage is done if the cause is physical, or before it can magnify into a full-blown chronic pain syndrome.

Reduction of edema, eradication of infection, elimination of further additional trauma, and initiation of active motion are some of the most effective means of diminishing pain. If edema is allowed to persist; if the inflammatory response is prolonged by the presence of foreign material or bacteria; if additional injury is caused by too forceful therapy; or if the extremity is guarded in an immobile and dependent posture, pain may become uncontrollable. Once this happens, it is almost impossible to reverse. Experienced hand specialists are constantly on the alert for potential pain problems. They understand and recognize normal pain thresholds and work within them, always striving to avoid tipping the delicate balance between acute and chronic pain.

Subjective pain is difficult to evaluate. Commonly used, **pain analog scales** are simple to administer and have been found to be accurate indicators of pain intensity. On lines divided into equal increments, patients are instructed to locate on a scale of 1 to 10, or on a no-pain to as-intense-as-it-can-be continuum, the level of their pain (Michlovitz & Wolf 1986). This type of assessment provides insight into patients' perceptions and coping abilities.

Techniques and modalities, aside from those discussed earlier in this section, include use of TENS, massage, and desensitization programs (Figure 18-32). Because pain itself is so difficult to assess, it is also difficult to evaluate the effects of treatment on pain. Each patient must be considered on an individual basis, with adaptation of therapy as needed. There appear to be no universal, definitive answers to the treatment of pain problems at this time.

Maintain or improve physical daily living skills; return to work

As noted previously, many hand rehabilitation patients with unilateral involvement require little assistance with personal self-care skills. When proximal joints or bilateral involvement is present, however, assessment and training in self-care skills usually are necessary.

In contrast, returning to work may be problematic for a patient with limitation of a single distal joint if the patient's particular job requires use of the disabled joint. Identification of potential return-to-work problems begins when taking the initial history, and with reassessment, it becomes a continuous process throughout the duration of the rehabilitation program. Returning patients to the environments from which they came, be they student, homemaker, banker, or farmer, is the ultimate goal in hand rehabilitation. All therapeutic intervention, surgical or therapeutic, is carried out with this in mind.

Patients often are hesitant to use their injured extremities, and if injury is job-related, they are reluctant to return to their places of work. Acknowledging that this may be problematic from the onset, patients are encouraged to return to work as soon as possible. Ideally, with the cooperation of their employers, patients may be given alternative assignments that allow them to be in the work environment within a few days to a few weeks after injury. As their physical status improves, they may be shifted to jobs that allow protected use of involved extremities, eventually returning to their original jobs or to jobs of equal status if the requirements of the original jobs are physically impossible. This is the perfect scenario, and it does happen on occasion. Clinically, however, the whole continuum from best to worst is encountered. Some patients are highly motivated and have supportive employers; others could care less, and their employers do not want them back; and most patients fall between these extremes. Each patient must be considered independently. "Cookbook" approaches are ineffective and, in the long run, expensive to patients and to society.

Splinting

Splinting is an integral part of hand rehabilitation. Individually designed and fitted, splints may be used to support or immobilize healing tissues; to correct or prevent deformity; to assist motion; or to serve as a basis of attachment for self-help devices. If exercise is viewed as the warp of the fabric of hand rehabilitation techniques, splinting provides the weft. It is the careful balancing between the two that leads to successful therapeutic intervention. Splints provide one aspect of treatment that no other technique or modality can accomplish. They may be used to hold or stress soft tissues over a long period of time, therefore effecting collagen remodeling. Although motion and functional use of the extremity effects active ROM, splinting is the only method for increasing passive motion without creating disruption of tissue and initiating the inflammatory process anew. There is no substitute for carefully planned and executed splinting programs. The reader is referred to Chapter 9, Section 5A for a detailed explanation of splinting nomenclature, principles, fabrication, and uses.

Modalities

In the past few years, the use of thermal and electrical modalities by occupational therapists has resulted in much controversy between leaders of AOTA. After much debate, AOTA stated:

> [P]hysical agent modalities may be used by occupational therapy practitioners when used as an adjunct to/or in preparation for purposeful activity to enhance occupational performance and when applied by a practitioner who has documented evidence of possessing the theoretical background and technical skills for safe and competent integration of the modality into an occupational therapy intervention plan. (1991, p. 1075)

The AOTA Commission on Practice, at the direction of the Representative Assembly, published a Physical Agent Modalities Draft Position Paper (AOTA, 1992) to further define modality use by occupational therapists.

It is not within the scope of this section to argue whether or not occupational therapists should use physical agent modalities. Because they are employed by some occupational therapists

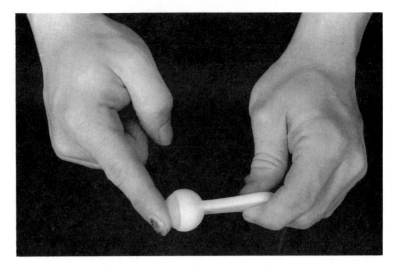

FIGURE 18-32. *Desensitization techniques use progressively graded stimuli to diminish inaccurate noxious or painful perceptions of normally occurring tactile stimuli in hand-injured patients.*

working in hand rehabilitation centers, modality use has been described briefly in relation to the physiologic wound healing process.

Conclusion

Hand rehabilitation is a viable and exciting specialty field that has contributed significantly to the treatment of UE dysfunction resulting from disease or injury. In just 30 years, the art of therapy is well on its way to becoming the science of therapy. Although many techniques and procedures need further study, important advances have been made by therapists actively engaged in the practice of hand rehabilitation.

References

American Journal of Occupational Therapy [Specialization issue]. (1979). *33*, 15–49.

American Occupational Therapy Association (1991). Official: AOTA statement on physical agent modalities. *American Journal of Occupational Therapy, 45*, 1075.

American Occupational Therapy Association, Commission on Practice (1992). Physical agent modalities draft paper. *Occupational Therapy Week, 5*, 6–7.

American Society for Surgery of the Hand (1983). Clinical assessment recommendations (pp. 106–112). In *The Hand*. New York: Churchill Livingstone.

American Society of Hand Therapists (1981). Fess, E., & Moran, C. (Eds.), *Clinical assessment recommendations*. Garner, NC: The Society.

Baxter-Petralia, P., Bruening, L., & Blackmore, S. (1990). Physical capacity evaluation (pp. 93–108). In Hunter, J. M., Schneider, L. H., Mackin, E. J., & Callahan, A. D. (Eds.), *Rehabilitation of the hand* (3rd ed.). St. Louis: C. V. Mosby.

Bear-Lehman, J., & McCormick, E. (1985). The expanding role of occupational therapy in the treatment of industrial hand injuries. *Occupational Therapy Health Care, 2*, 79–87.

Bell, J., & Tomancik, E. (1987). Repeatability of testing with Semmes-Weinstein monofilaments. *Journal of Hand Surgery, 12A*, 155–163.

Bell-Krotoski, J. (1989). Hands, research, and success. *Journal of Hand Therapy, 2*, 5–11.

Bell-Krotoski, J. (1990a). Sensibility testing: state of the art (pp. 575–584). In Hunter, J. M., Schneider, L. H., Mackin, E. J., & Callahan, A. D. (Eds.), *Rehabilitation of the hand* (3rd ed.). St. Louis: C. V. Mosby.

Bell-Krotoski, J. (1990b). Light touch-deep pressure testing using Semmes-Weinstein monofilaments. In Hunter, J. M., Schneider, L. H., Mackin, E. J., & Callahan, A. D. (Eds.), *Rehabilitation of the hand* (3rd ed.). St. Louis: C. V. Mosby.

Bell-Krotoski, J., & Buford, W. (1988). The force/time relationship of clinically used sensory testing instruments. *Journal of Hand Therapy, 1*, 76–85.

Brand, P. W. (1985). *Clinical mechanics of the hand*. St. Louis: C. V. Mosby.

Brand, P. W. (1990). The forces of dynamic splinting: Ten questions before applying a dynamic splint to the hand (pp. 1095–1100). In Hunter, J. M., Schneider, L. H., Mackin, E. J., & Callahan, A. D. (Eds.), *Rehabilitation of the hand* (3rd ed.). St. Louis: C. V. Mosby.

Bunnell, S. (1944). *Surgery of the hand* (pp. 198–203). Philadelphia: J. B. Lippincott.

Callahan, A. D. (1988). Hand rehabilitation and the American Society of Hand Therapists: A decade of progress. *Journal of Hand Therapy, 1*, 53–57.

Callahan, A. D. (1990). Methods of compensation and reeducation for sensory dysfunction (pp. 611–621). In Hunter, J. M., Schneider, L. H., Mackin, E. J., & Callahan, A. D. (Eds.), *Rehabilitation of the hand* (3rd ed.). St. Louis: C. V. Mosby.

Casanova, J. S., & Grunert, B. K. (1989). Adult prehension: Patterns and nomenclature for pinches. *Journal of Hand Therapy, 2*, 231–244.

Chai, S. H., Dimick, M. P., & Kasch, M. C. (1987). A role delineation study of hand therapy. *Journal of Hand Therapy, 1*, 7–16.

Currier, D. P. (1984). *Elements of research in physical therapy* (pp. 145–174). Baltimore: Williams & Wilkins.

Dellon, L., Curtis, R., & Edgerton (1974). Reeducation of sensation in the hand after nerve injury and repair. *Plastic and Reconstructive Surgery, 53*, 297–306.

Dellon, L. (1981). *Evaluation of sensibility and re-education of sensation in the hand*. Baltimore: Williams & Wilkins.

Duran, R. J., Coleman, C. R., Nappi, J. F., & Klerekoper, L. A. (1990). Management of flexor tendon lacerations in zone two using controlled passive motion postoperatively (pp. 410–413). In Hunter, J. M., Schneider, L. H., Mackin, E. J., & Callahan, A. D. (Eds.), *Rehabilitation of the hand* (3rd ed.). St. Louis: C. V. Mosby.

Evans, R. B. (1990). Therapeutic management of extensor tendon injuries (pp. 492–511). In Hunter, J. M., Schneider, L. H., Mackin, E. M., & Callahan, A. D. (Eds.), *Rehabilitation of the hand* (3rd ed.). St. Louis: C. V. Mosby.

Fess, E. E. (1986). Editorial: The need for reliability and validity in hand assessment instruments. *Journal of Hand Surgery, 11A,* 621–623.

Fess, E. E. (1987). A method for checking Jamar dynamometer calibration. *Journal of Hand Therapy, 1,* 28–32.

Fess, E. E. (1988a). Using research terminology correctly: Reliability. *Journal of Hand Therapy, 1,* 109.

Fess, E. E. (1988b). Using research terminology correctly: Validity. *Journal of Hand Therapy, 1,* 148.

Fess, E. E. (1988c). Reply to letter to the editor. *Journal of Hand Therapy, 1,* 219–220.

Fess, E. E. (1990a). Hands, changes, quality, and survival. *Journal of Hand Therapy, 3,* 1–6.

Fess, E. E. (1990b). Documentation: Essential elements of an upper extremity assessment battery (pp. 53–81). In Hunter, J. M., Schneider, L. H., Mackin, E. M., & Callahan, A. D. (Eds.), *Rehabilitation of the hand* (3rd ed.). St. Louis: C. V. Mosby.

Fess, E. E. (1990c). Reliability of new and used Jamar dynamometers under laboratory conditions. In Proceedings of the American Society of Hand Therapists 12th Annual Meeting. *Journal of Hand Therapy, 3,* 36–37.

Fess, E. E., & Philips, C. A. (1987). *Hand splinting principles and methods.* St. Louis: C. V. Mosby.

Griener, J., Bowen, L., & Jones, S. (1990). Threshold of sensation: Inter-rater reliability and establishment of normal using the Semmes-Weinstein monofilaments. In Proceedings of the American Society of Hand Therapists 12th Annual Meeting. *Journal of Hand Therapy, 3,* 36–37.

Hand Therapy Certification Commission (1990). *Hand therapy certification examination: 1991 handbook and application for candidates.* Garner, NC: Hand Therapy Certification Commission, Inc.

Hand Therapy Certification Commission (1991). Hand therapy certification list. *Journal of Hand Therapy, 4,* 133–140.

Heater, S. L. (1992). Specialization or uniformity within the profession. *American Journal of Occupational Therapy, 46,* 172–173.

Hirama, H. (1982). Toward specialization. *American Journal of Occupational Therapy, 36,* 601–602.

Hunter, J. M., Schneider, L. H., Mackin, E. J., & Callahan, A. D. (Eds.). (1990). *Rehabilitation of the hand* (3rd ed.). St. Louis: C. V. Mosby.

Jebsen, R., Taylor, N., Triegchmann, R. (1969). An objective and standardized test of hand function. *Archives of Physical Medicine and Rehabilitation, 50,* 311–319.

Kellor, M., Frost, J., Silberg, N. (1971). Hand strength and dexterity. *American Journal of Occupational Therapy, 25,* 77–83.

Kendall, H., Kendall, F., & Wadsworth, G. (1971). *Muscle testing and function.* Baltimore: Williams & Wilkins.

Kleinrt, H. E., Kutz, J. E., & Cohen, M. J. (1975). Primary repair of zone two flexor tendon lacerations (pp. 91–104). In American Academy of Orthopaedic Surgeons, *Symposium on tendon surgery in the hand.* St. Louis: C. V. Mosby.

Mackin, E. J. (1988). Building a legacy through mentorship. *Journal of Hand Therapy, 1,* 105–108.

Madden, J. W., & Arem, A. (1981). Wound healing: Biologic and clinical features. In J. Sabiston (Ed.), *Davis-Christopher textbook of surgery* (12th ed.) (pp. 265–286). Philadelphia: W. B. Saunders.

Mathiowetz, V., Kashman, N., Volland, G. (1985). Grip and pinch strength: Normative data for adults. *Archives of Physical Medicine and Rehabilitation, 66,* 69–74.

Mathiowetz, V., Rennells, M., & Donahoe, L. (1985). Effect of elbow position on grip and pinch strength. *Journal of Hand Surgery, 10A,* 694–696.

Mathiowetz, V., Weber, K., Volland, G., & Kashman, N. (1984). Reliability and validity of grip and pinch strength evaluations. *Journal of Hand Surgery, 9A,* 222–226.

Michlovitz, S., & Wolf, S. (1986). *Thermal Agents in Rehabilitation* (pp. 38–41). Philadelphia: F. A. Davis Co.

Moberg, E. (1958). Objective methods of determining the functional value of sensibility in the hand. *Journal of Bone and Joint Surgery, 40B,* 454–461.

Moberg, E. (1966). Methods for examining sensibility in the hand. In J. Flynn, (Ed.), *Hand surgery* (1st ed.) (pp. 435–439). Baltimore: Williams & Wilkins.

Onne, L. (1962). Recovery of sensibility and sudomotor activity in the hand after severe injury. *Acta Chirurgica Scandinavica* [Suppl], *1,* 300–307.

O'Rain, S. (1973). New and simple test for nerve function in the hand. *British Medical Journal, 3,* 615–618.

Payton, O. D. (1984). *Research: The validation of clinical practice* (pp. 111–123). Philadelphia: F. A. Davis.

Peacock, E. E. (1984). *Wound repair* (3rd ed.). Philadelphia: W. B. Saunders.

Phelps, P., & Walker, E. (1977). Comparison of the finger wrinkling test results to established sensory tests in peripheral nerve injury. *American Journal of Occupational Therapy, 31,* 565–572.

Rider, B., & Linden, C. (1988). Comparison of standardized and nonstandardized administration of the Jebsen hand function test. *Journal of Hand Therapy, 1,* 121–123.

Rothstein, J. M. (1985). Measurement and clinical practice: Theory and application. In Rothstein, J. M. (Ed.), *Measurement in physical therapy* (pp. 1–46). New York: Churchill Livingstone.

Schmidt, R., & Toews, J. (1970). Grip strength as measured by the Jamar dynamometer. *Archives of Physical Medicine and Rehabilitation, 51,* 321–327.

Seddon, H. (1975). *Surgical disorders of peripheral nerves* (2nd ed.). New York: Churchill Livingstone.

Slaymaker, J. H. (1986). A holistic approach to specialization. *American Journal of Occupational Therapy, 40,* 117–121.

Strickland, J. W. (1987). Biologic basis for hand splinting. In Fess, E. E., & Philips, C., *Hand splinting principles and methods* (2nd ed.) (pp. 43–70). St. Louis: C. V. Mosby.

Sunderland, S. (1978). *Nerves and nerve injuries* (2nd ed.). New York: Churchill Livingstone.

Taber, C. W. (1989). *Taber's cyclopedic medical dictionary* (16th ed.). Philadelphia: F. A. Davis.

Tiffin, J., & Asher, E. (1948). The Purdue pegboard: Norms and studies of reliability and validity. *Journal of Applied Psychology, 32,* 234–241.

Waylett-Rendall, J., & Seibly, D. S. (1991). A study of the accuracy of a commercially available volumeter. *Journal of Hand Therapy, 4,* 10–13.

Welles, C. (1958). DaVinci is dead. The case for specialization. *American Journal of Occupational Therapy, 12,* 289–290.

Wynn Parry, C. B. (1981). *Rehabilitation of the hand* (4th ed.). Boston: Butterworths.

Additional Resources

Crawford Small Parts Dexterity Test, The Psychological Corporation, 304 E. 45th Street, New York, NY.

Minnesota Rate of Manipulation Test, Lafayette Instrument Company, Sagamore and North Ninth Street, Lafayette, IN.

Valpar Component Work Samples Series, 3801 East 34th Street, Suite 105, Tucson, AZ.

SECTION 5

Burn rehabilitation

CHERYL J. LEMAN

LEARNING OBJECTIVES

Upon completion of this section the reader will be able to:

1. *List the treatment goals for the three phases of burn recovery.*

2. *Identify the criteria used to classify burns as minor or severe.*

3. *Discuss the importance of therapeutic positioning for the burn patient and give one example.*

4. *Discuss the importance of scar management to the rehabilitation of the burn patient and give one example of a technique used to prevent or minimize scarring.*

5. *Describe the role of occupational therapy in burn management.*

Since the early 1970s, significant advances in burn care have improved burn survival and overall morbidity. Progressive surgical management and wound care, critical care monitoring, nutritional support, and early, comprehensive rehabilitation are just a few examples of the advances that have contributed to improved burn injury outcomes. These advances have expanded the focus of burn care professionals to include the quality of life after a burn injury. A comprehensive team approach to patient care is needed, however, to effectively address the medical, functional, and psychosocial problems associated with burn recovery.

The burn team concept must start on the day of admission to the hospital and continue throughout wound maturation to ensure successful outcomes (Petro & Salisbury, 1986; Stern & Davey, 1985). Although the burn team now consists of physicians, nurses, occupational and physical therapists, nutritionists, social workers, and other health care professionals, this has not always been the case. The role of occupational therapists in burn treatment probably gained initial recognition from the early work of Dr. Duane Larson and Barbara Willis Galstaun, OTR, at the Galveston Shrine Burn Institute. Their findings on the effects of pressure, stretch, and splints on burn scars is the basis for a number of the treatment techniques used today (Larson, Abston, Evans, Dobrovsky, & Linares, 1971; Willis, 1970). In addition to burn scar control, self-care independence and return to work or school have become primary goals of therapy. To effectively address these goals, occupational therapists must understand the functions of the skin, results of different surgical treatments and wound care techniques used in burn care, and scar pathophysiology.

The skin

The skin is the largest organ in the body. Its structure and appendages provide an extensive, complex, physical barrier for protection from environmental stresses. Included in its functions are thermoregulation; sensation; prevention of water loss; protection from chemical and bacterial invasion, ultraviolet rays, and mechanical trauma; and provision of form and shape to body areas. When the skin is damaged, myriad systemic, physiologic, and functional problems can occur.

Skin is made up of two distinct layers: the epidermis and dermis. The epidermal cells originate in the basal layer and undergo a process of keratinization as they migrate to the surface to form a protective barrier of keratin. Other cells in the epidermis are Langerhans cells, Merkel cells, and melanocytes. Although the full role of Langerhans and Merkel cells is not understood, melanocytes produce melanin to provide protection from the ultraviolet rays of the sun (Johnson, 1987a).

The dermis is made up of vascular connective tissue. Epidermal cells lining the hair follicles and sweat glands (or epidermal appendages) serve as a source of epithelium for healing wounds (Solem, 1984). Cells in the dermis, called fibroblasts, produce elastic fibers and collagen. Interlacing collagen fibers interspersed with elastic fibers give the skin strength and elasticity. Sebaceous glands, another epidermal appendage, are found in most areas, except where there is no hair. Secretion from sebaceous glands, sebum, moves toward the surface and has been proposed to enhance barrier properties by moisturizing the skin (Johnson, 1987a).

Burn classification

Burn classification is based on the cause of injury, depth of injury, the percentage of body surface area involved, location of the burn on the patient, and age of the patient.

Depth

The depth of the burn is estimated from clinical observation of the appearance, sensitivity, and pliability of the wound (Wachtel, 1985). Traditionally, burns were classified as first-, second-, and third degree; today, they are described as superficial, partial-thickness, or full-thickness wounds.

First-degree, or *superficial*, burns involve only the outer layers of the epidermis. The skin is red but never blisters. These burns are painful but heal uneventfully in 4 to 8 days. A sunburn is a good example of a superficial burn.

Second-degree, or *partial-thickness*, burns can be superficial or deep. Superficial partial-thickness wounds involve only the epidermis and generally blister. When a blister is removed, the wound is erythematous, weeping, and painful. *Superficial partial-thickness* wounds generally heal in 10 days to 2 weeks with minimal permanent changes. *Deep partial-thickness* burns involve the epidermis and varying depths of the dermis. Hair follicles, sweat glands, and sebaceous glands are spared to some extent. These wounds are either hemorrhagic or waxy white in appearance. They are generally soft, dry, edematous, and occasionally insensate, with pain increasing as wound healing occurs. Sometimes a deep partial-thickness wound can convert to full thickness by bacterial proliferation and infection. Deep partial-thickness wounds require more than 3 weeks to heal and nearly always result in some amount of scar or poor skin quality. Treatment with skin grafts is generally used in areas in which function can be affected.

Third-degree, or *full-thickness*, burns involve the epidermis, dermis, and the epidermal appendages. Full-thickness burns are dry, tan or deep red in color, with thrombosed vessels visible. The skin is cold, hard, and insensate. Edema is present due to capillary damage causing fluid shifts from the intravascular to the extravascular space. Movement is generally restricted because of edema, eschar tightness, and wound inelasticity. Surgical treatment with skin grafts is needed to achieve timely wound closure. Scar and disfigurement are frequently the outcome.

Body surface area involved

The extent of the burn is classified as a percentage of the total body surface area (TBSA) involved. Two methods for estimating burn size are the rule of nines and the Lund and Browder chart. The rule of nines is simple and quick but relatively inaccurate. It divides the body surface into areas comprising 9%, or multiples of 9%, with the perineum making up the final 1%. The head and neck is 9%, each UE is 9%, each leg is 18%, and the front and back of the trunk are each 18%. This method is modified for children up to 1 year of age, with the head and neck being 18% and each LE 14%. The percentages for the head and neck and LE are gradually modified from ages 1 to 10 years.

The Lund and Browder chart provides a more accurate estimation of the TBSA (Lund & Browder, 1944; Solem, 1984; Wachtel, 1985). This chart assigns a percentage of surface area for more specific body segments by equating proportions of each segment to the TBSA. An example of body segments is the division of the arm into the upper arm, forearm, and hand. (Due to the chart's detail, the reader is referred to the following references to gain an understanding of it: Lund & Browder, 1944; Solem, 1984.) A patient's palm print, excluding the fingers, is about 1% of the TBSA, and may be used as a quick estimate of burn surface area involvement.

Location of the burn

The percentage of TBSA involved and the depth of the burn are generally used to classify injuries as either minor or severe. Involvement of specific body areas is also used in determining minor or severe burn injuries, even if the percentage of surface area involved is limited. Partial- or full-thickness burns of the hands, face, or perineum are frequently considered severe burns (Wachtel, 1985). For example, burns of the face, eyes, and neck may cause respiratory compromise, restrict the person's vision and ability to eat, and can result in significant cosmetic and functional impairment. Bilateral hand burns initially limit self-care abilities but also can result in long-term functional disability. A 5% full-thickness burn can be a severe burn injury if it involves deeper structures that may limit recovery of normal function, such as tendon and joint involvement on the lower leg. A partial-thickness burn injury covering greater than 20% TBSA is considered a severe burn at many burn centers.

Age of the patient

Age is an important variable in hospital course and prognosis (Wachtel, 1985). A traditional but crude method for determining survival potential is to add the age of the patient to the percentage of TBSA and then to subtract this number from 100 to determine the estimated survival (percent). This equation has become inaccurate with the advances in burn care; and age, burn size, severity of injury, and severity of associated problems, such as an inhalation injury, are all considered in predicting prognosis.

Mechanisms and incidence of burn injuries

The annual incidence of burn-related injuries in the United States is estimated at 2.5 million, of which over 70,000 require hospitalization (M. Jordan, personal communication, July 1991).

Burns and fire-related injuries are the third leading cause of accidental death in the United States. Despite extensive burn prevention programs, home-related accidents account for 66% of all burn injuries (Feller & Jones, 1984).

The severity of a burn injury depends on the area exposed and the duration and intensity of thermal exposure. Therefore, the mechanism of the burn injury should be identified immediately. Superficial partial-thickness burns typically occur after a brief contact with hot liquids or flames. Deep partial-thickness burns are caused by longer exposure to intense heat, such as with hot water immersion scalds or contact of flaming materials with the skin. Full-thickness burns result from longer exposure to flames, prolonged immersion scalds, contact with hot oil, tar, or chemical agents, and electrical contact.

In 1988, the American Burn Association's Committee on Organization and Delivery of Burn Care surveyed burn care facilities in the United States to identify the predominate causes of burn injury. The results of this survey indicated that about 55% of all burns treated were the result of flame or flash exposure. Hot liquids and immersion scalds accounted for 35% of the injuries. Electrical contact and chemical burns were each about 5% of all admissions (M. Lewis & M. Jordan, personal communication, August 1991).

Fluid resuscitation and burn wound care

A burn injury causes translocation of body fluids. With large burn injuries, burn shock can occur due to extensive intravascular fluid loss that causes decreased plasma volume, blood volume, and cardiac output. If fluid resuscitation is inadequate or the patient does not respond to the resuscitative efforts, acute renal failure and death ensue (Hartford, 1984). Several formulas are available for calculating fluid requirements for burn patients; however, the specifics regarding the type of fluid, hourly rate, and amount used are determined by the individual physician's philosophy.

After fluid resuscitation has been started, attention is directed to wound care. Various topical agents are available to treat burn injuries. Their purpose is to delay colonization and reduce bacterial counts on or in the wounds (Hartford, 1984). Silver sulfadiazine, silver nitrate soaks, and Sulfamylon are just a few examples. Although all burn wounds are generally treated with some type of topical antibacterial agent, they do not substitute for surgical treatment if the need is indicated. When the depth and extent of the wound are known to require 3 or more weeks for healing, surgery is generally needed to decrease burn morbidity and mortality (Hartford, 1984).

Surgical treatment for burn wounds consists of excision (removal) of the burned tissue (*eschar*) and placement of skin grafts. Transplantation of the person's own skin from one site to another is referred to as an ***autograft***. Microvascular skin flaps are used when the wound is limited in size but the defect is so deep that tendon survival or graft adherence is doubtful. When adequate autograft is not available because of the extent of body surface area involvement, or when wound depth is such that graft take is questionable, a biologic dressing is frequently used.

Biologic dressings, either viable or nonviable, can be used as a temporary wound covering (Hartford, 1984). The proposed benefits of biologic dressings are that they reduce fluid loss, decrease pain, inhibit bacterial growth, and protect the wound until autografting is possible. Examples of biologic dressings are *homografts*, which are made from processed cadaver skin; *xenografts*, which are made from processed pig skin; synthetic products such as Biobrane, a nylon-silicone mesh coated with collagen; or artificial skin substitutes (Hartford, 1984).

Hypertrophic scars

Burn scar and contracture are common sequelae after a burn injury, with collagen being their primary structural component. The quality of burn wound maturation can be affected by numerous factors, some of which can occur during the early phases of burn care. A significant determinant in potential for scar development is the time required to achieve wound closure. Bacterial infection in a burn wound can increase the inflammatory response and delay healing. Spontaneous healing of full-thickness burns can be a timely process that contributes to collagen overgrowth. The potential for burn scar contracture can be minimized by strict adherence to infection control procedures and the use of topical antibiotics, scrupulous cleansing of the burn wound, and early surgical burn wound repair (Rivers, 1984). Despite these procedures and surgical interventions, scarring continues to be a major deterrent in recovery of function after a major burn injury.

Race, age, anatomic location, and depth of the burn wound can influence scar formation. ***Hypertrophic scars*** can develop anytime from 4 to 8 weeks after wound closure and are initially thick, rigid, and hyperemic in surface appearance. Their func-

tional or cosmetic significance varies with the anatomic location of the wound. Hypertrophic scars that cross joints can limit ROM and function by contracture or skin shortening over the joint. If left untreated, shortening of the muscle and fibrous contracture of the joint capsule eventually occur. Scars on the face can distort facial features while also limiting function (Abston, 1987).

Biologic research studies of burn wound scars have increased our understanding of hypertrophic scars but have not found a cure. Linares, Kischer, and Dobrkovsky (1972) described stages of development for burn scars. Histologically, immature hypertrophic scars have increased vascularity, fibroblasts, myofibroblasts, and whorls or nodules of collagen, whereas the collagen in nonhypertrophic scars is oriented in parallel bands. As the hypertrophic scar matures, capillaries, fibroblasts, and myofibroblasts decrease significantly, and the collagen is arranged in parallel bands. The time required for hypertrophic and nonhypertrophic scars to mature differs markedly: nonhypertrophic scars mature in 5 to 8 weeks, while hypertrophic scars take up to 1 or 2 years to mature.

Baur, Barrett, and Brown (1979) examined hypertrophic scars using electron microscopy. They identified four cell types: fibroblast, myofibroblast, fibroclast, and myofibroclast. In hypertrophic scars, the myofibroblasts and myofibroclasts contained intracellular contractile bundles of collagen.

Biochemical research of hypertrophic scars, mature scars, and normal dermis have revealed increased synthesis of collagen and connective tissue in the hypertrophic scars (Abston, 1987). These studies imply that this increased synthesis continues for at least 2 years after wound closure. With maturation, the hypertrophic scar softens, thins, and flattens, with collagen synthesis and degradation becoming balanced. The process of collagen degradation in hypertrophic scar is still not fully understood.

Phases of recovery

Burn care techniques and the focus of the burn team change with the phase of recovery. There are essentially three phases of burn recovery: the ***acute care phase***, the ***surgical and postoperative phase***, and the ***rehabilitation phase***. Whether the patient goes through all three phases depends on the depth and extent of the burn injury.

The acute care phase consists of fluid resuscitation, patient stabilization, and initial wound care procedures. With superficial or partial-thickness wounds that heal without surgery, the acute care phase is also considered the period from the date of injury until epithelial healing (Rivers, 1987). When the wounds are superficial, this is the only phase the patient experiences. When the wounds are partial thickness in depth, do not require surgery, but take 2 to 3 weeks to heal, the patient may also require treatment that is associated with the rehabilitation phase.

After acute resuscitation of major burn injuries, the second phase is the surgical and postoperative phase. During this phase, the patient undergoes multiple surgical procedures and immobilization periods. This is also the period when infections and other medical complications can occur.

The third phase is the rehabilitation phase. This phase starts with wound closure and continues through wound maturation. After severe burn injuries, therapy assumes the primary role during the rehabilitation phase.

Treatment goals related to phases of recovery

For many occupational therapists working in burn care, occupational therapy is synonymous with burn rehabilitation. Burn care is one area in which the occupational therapist must constantly integrate and use both physical and psychosocial treatment skills. This is easily understood considering the physical and cosmetic disability that is often the sequela of a burn injury. Due to the multitude of problems associated with a severe burn, burn care is most effective when a team approach is used.

Although specific rehabilitation goals may be the primary responsibility of certain burn team members, everyone is focused on the same outcome. Therefore, the burn rehabilitation goals that follow are also goals of the occupational therapist. In the following sections, there may be overlap of other disciplines with occupational therapy, and the goals will be referred to as rehabilitation goals.

Acute care phase

During the acute care phase, the focus of the burn team is directed to wound care. When the wounds are superficial, the goal of rehabilitation therapy is to prevent loss of strength and endurance by promoting normal function. Skin care education is needed to limit the itching and dryness frequently experienced with epithelial healing.

When burn wounds are partial thickness or full thickness, the acute care rehabilitation goals are to:

- Control edema
- Prevent loss of joint mobility
- Prevent loss of functional strength and endurance
- Promote self-care skills
- Provide orientation activities and stimulation
- Begin patient and family education about rehabilitation

Surgical and postoperative phase

During the surgical phase of care, patients are frequently immobilized in different positions for varying amounts of time. Immobilization is necessary to prevent displacement of skin grafts during their vascularization. The position and length of time of immobilization vary with the body area treated, the depth of the excision, the type of surgical procedure performed, and the physician's preference. The range of time for postoperative immobilization is generally 3 to 7 days.

During this phase, occupational therapy goals are to:

- Design splints and implement positioning techniques for immobilization in consultation with the surgeon
- Provide appropriate sensory stimulation to prevent disorientation
- Provide adaptive devices to increase self-care skills when appropriate

Other rehabilitation goals at this time are to:

- Continue patient and family education
- Prevent thrombophlebitis, skin tightness, and disuse atrophy of areas not immobilized by implementing a controlled exercise plan for areas proximal and distal to the grafted site

Rehabilitation phase

The rehabilitation phase starts as wound closure is being achieved. A patient with a severe burn can enter this phase before all wounds are healed. Many times, a patient with a severe burn injury needs one or two more surgical procedures or has certain small areas still requiring topical antibiotics upon entering the rehabilitation phase.

The rehabilitation phase is the most challenging of all for burn patients and their families. It is the period when burn scar and contracture can occur, and the patient must assume responsibility for self-care. The need for care does not end when the patient is discharged from the hospital; it continues until wound maturation is complete. This is difficult for some patients because they usually view hospital discharge as the end of the discomfort, pain, and burn care.

Although burn wound maturation is described as taking up to a year after injury, every patient is different. The time needed for wound maturation can sometimes be as much as 2 years, but wound maturation can also occur in less than 1 year (Rivers & Fisher, 1990). Patient compliance with treatment and patience on the part of the therapist and patient are important for dealing with the problems encountered during this phase.

The goals of therapy are to:

- Promote or improve joint mobility or flexibility
- Encourage return of normal strength and endurance
- Emphasize or teach normal self-care skills
- Stimulate reacquisition of social and vocational skills
- Fit splints, compression and vascular garments, and pressure adapters for edema and scar maturation control when needed
- Teach home care activities, including exercises and positioning techniques
- Teach skin and scar care techniques
- Implement a plan for resumption of school, work, and recreational activities

The goals listed above are extensive but so are the potentially disabling effects of burn wound maturation. Although there are many techniques available to control burn scar maturation, every patient has different needs and reactions. The functional complications that can occur as a result of scar tightness vary depending on the location and size of the burn, patient compliance with treatment, and time after injury.

Treatment process

Positioning, splinting, ADL, exercise, skin and scar care, and return to work or school conditioning activities are some of the responsibilities of the occupational therapist. Although basic splint designs, specific resting positions for burned body areas, and exercise techniques frequently are taught as the standard for burn rehabilitation, every treatment plan should be developed by determining the specific needs of each patient. To do this, the occupational therapist must continually assess the patient's function, wound status, and psychological adaptation throughout the treatment process. It must be remembered that every patient is unique, with his or her own problems and specific needs, and that no two wounds are the same.

Assessment procedures and treatment techniques used

vary with the phase of recovery. A burn injury can cause myriad problems, and not all burn patients will progress through recovery at the same pace or level of function. Therefore, assessment and treatments are discussed separately here. The integration of specific procedures depends on the patient's needs and function at the time.

Assessment

When a patient with a severe burn injury is admitted to the hospital, a multitude of procedures must be done, and many personnel need to see the patient. Initially, lines for intravenous fluids are put in place, and the wounds are cleansed and dressed with a topical agent. When possible, the occupational therapist should try to view the patient's wounds during these initial procedures to determine areas of involvement that may require positioning splints. This is generally done before a complete assessment is performed.

Portions of the initial therapy evaluation can be done when the patient is in hydrotherapy (Covey, 1987). The therapist should view the wounds to determine the extent and depth of the burn injury, noting any critical areas involved. If the patient is cognitive and cooperative, the therapist should ask the patient to perform functional motions. Although it is easier for some patients to move without their dressings, active ROM should also be assessed when dressings are in place.

Function of the body areas involved is the primary concern; however, it is important to establish a baseline of overall function at the beginning of the treatment process. A complete ROM and strength evaluation should be part of every initial assessment. Goniometer measurements over dressings are possible by making allowances for the thickness of the dressings. Active ROM of uninvolved areas should also be documented. Although it is difficult to objectively assess strength at this time because of edema and pain, it should be noted whether the patient can move each joint through a full ROM against gravity. If the hand is not involved, or if the burn is only a superficial partial-thickness burn with minimal surface area involvement, and no edema is present, hand dynamometer and pinch gauge measurements should be obtained.

The patient's preinjury level of function should be obtained through interview with the patient. When this is not possible, or when the patient is intubated for an inhalation injury, it should be obtained from a close family member as soon as possible. Hand dominance, self-care function, job title and a basic description of work skills, educational level achieved, personality traits, and recreational activities should be determined. Only after this information is obtained can an individualized treatment plan be developed.

Range of motion, strength, endurance, and function must be assessed at frequent intervals during hospitalization and after hospital discharge. This is necessary to identify specific problem areas and decreases in function that commonly occur. Although changes in function are generally attributed to the scarring associated with burn wound healing, hospitalization and the metabolic effects of a burn injury also contribute to decreases in strength, endurance, and functional activities performance. In addition to the physical components of function, skin and scar status, sensation, emotional responses, and coping skills should be monitored. The patient's understanding of recovery needs, compliance, and ability to assume responsibility for long-term care are important considerations in the assessment process for determining treatment needs.

Patient and family education

Education about burn care is important in helping the patient and family cope with the multiple facets of burn care. This education must start at the beginning of the recovery process to ensure the patient and family's understanding of the long-term needs associated with burn recovery. Pain, immobilization, and lengthy hospitalizations can alter the thought processes of a burn patient. Seeing the appearance of his or her wounds at varying stages of recovery can be disconcerting. A burn team member saying that the wound looks good may mean nothing to the patient if the patient does not understand that it is only a phase in the healing process. Experience has proved that patients can cope more easily with the constant changes that occur if they are taught what to expect.

Family education and understanding occurs at a slower pace than that of the patient. The patient is constantly seeing the members of the burn team, whereas the family may only speak to a burn team member for a few minutes during visiting hours. Convening family groups that discuss various burn care topics is one way to augment learning. The most important concept for home care education is for every family member to learn that the patient will require support to function independently. For example, helping the patient to eat or dress, if the family has been told not to, may only prolong the recovery process.

Although education is the responsibility of each team member, occupational therapy program effectiveness is contingent on the knowledge and understanding that the patient acquires. Functional recovery after a burn injury is a dynamic process, considering the scarring and deconditioning that can occur with hospitalization and bed rest. Since burn recovery is a painful process, it is important that patients become actively involved with their rehabilitation program at the beginning. The patient should be taught pain and stress management techniques early since motivation and compliance with therapy treatments are essential for a successful outcome (Giuliani & Perry, 1985). For patients to assume responsibility for their long-term recovery, they must understand the purpose of specific treatments, potential outcomes if treatment is avoided, the time required for recovery, pain management techniques, and methods for assessing scar maturation.

Positioning

Positioning techniques were first developed for the acute phase of burn care. It was taught that the position of comfort is the position of contracture (Larson et al., 1971). Early implementation of positioning for burn patients is still taught today, but the objectives have changed with reference to the stages of burn recovery.

To understand and effectively use positioning techniques, one must understand the problem. In response to pain, the burn patient frequently assumes a protective posture. This posture generally consists of adduction and flexion of the upper extremities, flexion of the hips and knees, and plantar flexion of the ankles. Hand burn pain causes patients to hold their hands in a dysfunctional position, and certain resting positions are also contraindicated with burn injuries. For example, use of a pillow when there are neck burns and resting with the head of the bed in an upright position when there are trunk burns contribute to inappropriate posturing. If the burn patient is allowed to maintain these positions as wound healing progresses, contractures can develop that limit function. In general, therapeutic burn positioning entails encouraging some degree of extension of all involved areas when resting.

The purposes for therapeutic positioning of burn patients are to:

- Aid in edema control and reduction
- Maintain normal muscle length when resting
- Ensure wound coverage immediately after placement of skin grafts
- Limit the degree of scar contracture
- Teach patients methods for combating the skin tightness that affects function

During the acute phase of care, the main purpose for positioning is to limit edema formation (Pullium, 1984). Although there is an initial diffuse capillary leak with a severe burn, the severity or impact of distal extremity edema formation can be limited with elevation of the limb at or slightly above heart level. For hand and arm burns, this can be done using pillows. In these cases, extension of the elbows is important to prevent restriction of venous return. When there are leg and foot burns, the foot of the bed can be raised. Caution should be taken to not flex the hips more than 30 degrees when the legs and hips are burned and to keep the knees extended. With face burns, raising the head of the bed at least 30 degrees is helpful.

As wound closure begins and progresses, attention should be directed to more proximal positioning concerns. When the axillae and anterior trunk are involved, the arms should be abducted to 90 degrees using armboards attached to the side of the bed or overhead suspension (Cooper & Paul, 1988). Blanket rolls placed along the upper trunk also promote shoulder abduction. If any portion of the neck is involved, the patient should not use a pillow for head support. A small towel roll behind the neck aids in proper positioning of the head and neck. When the legs are involved, the hips should be maintained in neutral with slight abduction, and the knees should be extended when resting.

Postoperative immobilization positions may entail many of the techniques already described but may also be specific for the type of procedure used or area treated. When a skin graft is used for wound coverage, the body area or joint treated is usually held in some degree of extension or abduction (Figure 18-33). When a skin flap is performed, positioning specifics change. For example, when an axillary advancement flap is performed, the shoulder is generally positioned in 40 to 45 degrees of abduction instead of the traditional 90 degrees of abduction. This is to prevent stress on the suture lines. Knowledge of the surgical procedure performed and determination of potential postoperative complications, such as suture-line stress or graft shifting, enable the therapist to institute effective positioning techniques.

It is often difficult for patients to maintain specific positions when resting at home. When ineffective posturing occurs, functionally limiting contractures can develop. In these cases, splints should be used for positioning when the patient is discharged from the hospital. Teaching the patient effective ways to rest and stretch are also treatment components. For example, when neck and trunk scars are maturing, the patient should be taught activity adaptations, such as watching television from a prone position and not reclining on a soft couch.

Exercise

Active exercise is an important component of every burn treatment program. The sequelae of burn scar contracture and the deconditioning effects of hospitalization result in the need for exercise after a burn injury. Many factors can influence the therapist's ability to engage a burn victim in an exercise program. Burn wound pain, edema, effects of postoperative immobilization, and patient's lack of understanding about the importance of exercise are just a few examples why patients evade exercise sessions during the early stages of burn recovery. Although patients tend to avoid movement in general, when they do move, it is adapted, slow, and labored. As burn wound closure is achieved, scar tightness, hypersensitivity, pain and discomfort experienced with stretching scars, the patient's adjustment to the injury, and a generalized feeling of fatigue can limit a burn patient's willingness or ability to exercise. During this period,

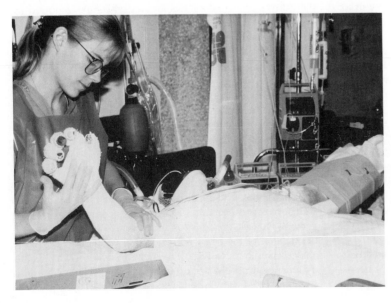

FIGURE 18-33. *Armboards used for shoulder positioning in bed. During postoperative immobilization, active and active-assistive exercises of joints distal to the grafted site are performed with therapist supervision.*

motions can sometimes be like a robot, with fluidity of movement absent; spontaneity is missing, with normal motions altered; and joint ROM is limited. If allowed to persist, functional limitations can develop.

Although activity and active exercise are needed for muscle strength and endurance, continuous passive motion (CPM) devices can be used as an adjunct to the exercise regime (Covey, Dutcher, Marvin, & Heimbach, 1988.) CPM devices are beneficial when the patient's active motion is limited secondary to pain, edema, or anxiety (Covey, 1988). When used, a CPM device takes the body part through a slow, continuous ROM for an extended period. The end points for the motion can be preset and gradually adjusted to increase ROM during the treatment session. Although the therapist must monitor the patient's response when initially using the device, a CPM device can be used as an extension of treatment when the therapist is not available. It is especially appropriate for use when the patient is resting.

The goals of exercise with burn patients are to:

- Preserve normal joint ROM
- Minimize the risk of thromboembolism
- Assist in edema reduction
- Assist in preventing pulmonary complications
- Increase or maintain strength and endurance
- Provide stretch to healing tissues
- Preserve or improve coordination and dexterity
- Promote normal performance of functional activities

Exercise protocols used during acute burn care are not unique for the injury. They are basically active, active-assistive, or passive, depending on the patient's condition. Emphasizing full joint ROM is important to preserve joint and muscle function. Daily evaluation of the patient's status and identifying changes needed in the exercise plan should be done to prevent complications such as graft shearing or exposed tendon rupture.

Increasing strength and endurance should also be a goal of the exercise program. Free weights using the Delorem method or electronically controlled dynamometers are examples of strengthening techniques. Using a bicycle ergometer for endurance is also appropriate in burn rehabilitation. Although exercise tolerance in the hypermetabolic patient is a concern, there are methods for assessing exercise response. Monitoring pulse rate, blood pressure, and respirations are just a few of the techniques that should be used in grading exercises (Johnson, 1987b).

Stretching exercises are frequently performed before exercise or sports to prevent injury. This is also important for exercising during burn recovery. Before stretching, a lubricating cream should be massaged into the maturing tissues. This is done to prevent skin rupturing due to dryness and scar rigidity. Slow, sustained stretches are then performed before active exercise. When stretching, the patient should try to gradually increase ROM through slow, controlled repetitions of the motion. Once stretching is complete, the active resistive exercises are performed.

Complex motions and resistive exercises should be used during the rehabilitation phase of recovery. Flexibility exercises, or combined joint movements, are complex motions. Although a burn scar can limit motion of the joint it crosses, it can also affect those proximal and distal to it. Therefore, it is important to provide exercises that require concurrent joint motions. For example, an exercise program for a UE burn may emphasize elbow function but should also incorporate coordinated movements of the shoulder, elbow, and hand. In designing an individualized exercise plan, it is important to analyze the total effect of the scar while also considering the functional and vocational needs of the patient.

Exercise is an important component of every burn rehabilitation program. Grading exercise frequency, intensity, and duration is necessary to successfully regain or improve the patient's strength, flexibility, and endurance. Active ROM exercises and activity can improve a burn patient's function for the moment; however, strength and endurance are needed to sustain activity throughout the day.

Activities of daily living

As soon as acute resuscitation is completed, the patient begins eating. Although dressings and edema may alter eating skills performance, the patient should try to eat independently. Adapting utensils to increase independence is sometimes needed; however, it should be clear that the adaptations are only temporary with most burn injuries. This is an important point to teach the patient, family, and nursing staff. Wrapping adhesive tape or foam on utensil handles and providing large-handled cups are two temporary methods for improving grasp. Extension of utensils and extended straws should be avoided to promote more normal ROM. It should be remembered that performance of ADL is one of best methods for achieving active ROM. Therefore, adaptive devices should be removed as soon as possible to avoid dependence on them.

Patients usually receive hydrotherapy on a daily basis as part of wound care. Nurses cleanse the wounds, but patient participation in bathing and grooming should be encouraged. Although it is difficult for patients to reach all body areas in a hydrotherapy tub, getting involved in bathing is a beginning point for wound healing education, fostering independence in self-care. Overall, providing support for some level of ADL function during this early phase of care can aid the patient's perception of recovery status, emphasize abilities, and provide a means for independent self-care education.

As wound closure is achieved and the patient nears discharge from the hospital, stressing normal independent self-care is extremely important. Independence in bathing, grooming, eating, and dressing skills should be emphasized. Bathing and grooming should be performed in a bathroom with appliances similar to those used at home as much as possible. Often, the patient or family thinks that they should change the style of clothing the patient wore before injury. Practicing dressing skills with clothes from home is also necessary to avoid home adaptation once discharged from the hospital. With major burn injuries, adaptations may be needed to encourage self-care independence. Before teaching adaptive self-care, self-care skills should be assessed, noting when scar stretching is needed to regain function, instead of providing permanent adaptation.

Experience has shown that many patients fear hot water, especially if they were injured in the shower or bath tub. Methods to test water temperatures and safe temperatures at which to set the thermostat of their hot water tank should be taught as part of self-care education. Cooking is another activity that many patients avoid once they are home because of their fear of heat or the fact that they were injured while cooking. Cooking activities in the clinic should be organized in an effort to decrease fears and teach safe cooking procedures that can be used at home.

Skin and scar care education should include home wound care, skin lubrication, and independent donning of compression and external vascular support garments. Family members must learn that assisting the patient in ADL will only prolong the recovery process. Showing patience and providing support to the patient are the family's most important roles. Patient awareness and understanding of the time it may take to perform certain ADL activities, developing patience, and allowing time to perform tasks independently are important components of ADL education.

Splints

The use of certain splints in burn care varies with the phase of wound healing but, more important, with the philosophy of the burn center. Traditionally, splints were used during acute care to assist in positioning. There was a splint for almost every area burned. They were usually worn all the time but were taken off for meals, dressing changes, and exercise. Today, splints are not used as consistently during acute care as they were in the past. When a splint is used in acute care, it is generally static in design and is used at night or for short periods, with activity and exercise emphasized during the day.

The primary splint still used in acute burn care is the burn hand splint. The time of application differs, with many therapists waiting until after the first 48 to 72 hours after injury to apply the hand splint (Miles & Grigsby, 1990). This is because the extreme fluid shifts that occur during acute resuscitation can greatly affect splint fit. The purposes of the burn hand splint are to prevent ligamentous stress at the interphalangeal joints, to assist in edema reduction, and to allow flow to the intrinsic muscles of the hands by emphasizing the distal transverse arch of the hand. In other words, it is designed to prevent the burn claw deformity, which is flexion of the wrist, hyperextension of the metacarpophalangeal joints, and flexion of the interphalangeal joints.

The burn hand splint differs from other hand splints by the position of its components. Usually made out of a low-temperature thermoplastic material, the splint positions the wrist in about 30 to 35 degrees of extension, the metacarpophalangeal joints are flexed to 70 degrees, the interphalangeal joints are held in extension, and the thumb is abducted (Figure 18-34). These positions vary with the surface area burned, with the preceding design being used for dorsal hand burns. When there are circumferential hand burns, the positions can be modified. If a hand splint is used during acute care, it is generally applied using disposable elastic wraps. Straps are not used because of infection control concerns and the possibility of distal edema.

Except for the hand, positioning techniques are frequently used in place of splints during acute care. If a splint is used, it is usually a conformer splint that has total contact with the surface area being treated and generally places the body area in an extended position (Helm et al., 1983). Frequent assessment of fit and readjustments are needed with these types of splint to accommodate fluid volume changes in the extremity and variations in dressing bulk.

A conforming positioning splint may be needed after operation when skin grafts are applied. Due to the bulk of the postoperative dressing, plaster strips are frequently used for splinting during operation. Most postoperative splints hold the joint or limb in extension, with the exception of a foot splint, which positions the ankle in dorsiflexion, and the airplane splint, which positions the shoulder in about 90 degrees of abduction (Figure 18-35).

Although static splints are frequently needed during burn wound maturation, every effort should be made to support function rather than restrict it. Low-temperature thermoplastic dynamic splints are usually more appropriate when scar contracture is present. The purpose of a dynamic splint is to assist or regain function or to provide slow dynamic stretch to contracting tissues. When fabricating and fitting a dynamic splint, caution must be taken to prevent the splint components from exerting ligamentous stress, friction, or joint compressive forces. There are a few commercially available dynamic splints for elbows, knees, and ankles, but these should be used with caution. Whenever a commercial splint is used, frequent assessment of fit is necessary to prevent edema, to accommodate volume changes in the extremity, and to avoid joint compressive forces.

Plaster casts can be used for positioning or to correct contractures during the recovery process. Advantages of plaster casting are the low cost of materials and the characteristics of circumferential and conforming contact when appropriately applied. Serial casting and a dynamic plaster casting technique have

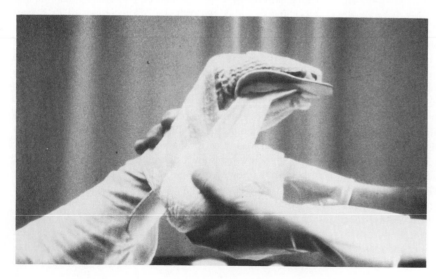

FIGURE 18-34. *Gauze and elastic wraps are used to maintain hand position on a burn hand splint.*

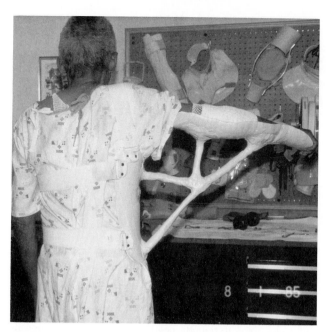

FIGURE 18-35. *An airplane splint allows mobility while maintaining the shoulder in 90 degrees of abduction.*

both been described for treatment of scar contractures of the hand, wrist, elbow, knee, and ankle (Bennett, Helm, Purdue, & Hunt, 1989; Jordan, Lewis, Wiegand, & Lemand, 1984). The dynamic plaster casting technique consists of applying a conforming cast, with the contracture being stretched. The cast is left intact for 24 to 48 hours. It is then cut on the contracture side, and a transverse wedge is removed on the opposite side, leaving the cast intact on both sides of the wedge as hinges. The contracture is then stretched an average of 15 to 20 degrees using the cast as lever arms. The cast defect is then replastered, and the cast is left in place for another 24 to 48 hours (Jordan, Lewis, Wiegand, Lemand, 1984). This process can be done sequentially until the contracture is resolved. Once casting is discontinued, a conforming night splint should be used for positioning.

In many instances, it is difficult to discuss burn splinting as a separate treatment entity without including scar management principles. Traditionally, acute burn splints were frequently described as prevention of scar contracture; however, this complication in burn recovery does not begin until wound closure is being achieved and burn scar maturation begins. Splints such as the total contact transparent face mask and neck splints are more appropriately presented as methods of scar management, when positioning techniques are used acutely. Regardless of how a splint is presented, splint design should be specific for the particular problem. Knowledge of basic splinting principles; frequent assessment of patient function, needs, skin condition, and splint fit; and design creativity are necessary for any successful splint program.

Scar management

Mechanical pressure has long been advocated as a way to influence scarring and has been used as treatment for or prevention of hypertrophic scars. As a scar develops, it becomes hyperemic (red), raised, and rigid (Johnson, 1984). Kischer, Sheltar, and

Sheltar (1975) found that scars treated with compression did not have the whorls or nodules of collagen and that the diameter of collagen filaments was increased compared with untreated hypertrophic scars. Parks, Evans, and Larson (1978) reported that a constant pressure of greater than 25 mmHg (capillary pressure) produced rearrangement of collagen bundles.

Effective scar management is the long-term goal of the entire burn team. Rehabilitation treatments emphasize activity, stretch, and exercise as methods to combat contracture development. Long-term scar care includes the use of splints and compression or external vascular support garments (Figure 18-36).

Coordination and integration of scar treatment activities is important. When developing a scar treatment plan, the patient's daily activities and responsibilities must be considered. This is necessary to ensure that independent function and normal activity are part of the plan since scar maturation may take up to a year after injury. Patient compliance, motivation, and patience are also necessary for treatment success.

The purpose of using elastic compression garments and splints on maturing burn wounds is to apply perpendicular pressure that approximates capillary pressure (Rivers, 1984). No pressure appliance or garment is perfect, however, and frequent reassessment is needed to ensure appropriate pressure and fit. Whenever possible, function should be maintained while the patient is wearing a garment or splint. Providing for normal motions while maintaining adequate scar control and coverage is difficult. Creativity, skill, perseverance, and always questioning what else can be done are needed qualities for the occupational therapist.

Numerous established techniques are available for applying compression to healing and maturing wounds. A custom-fitted external compression or vascular support garment is frequently the choice for long-term care; however, numerous pressure dressings and techniques are available for use early during

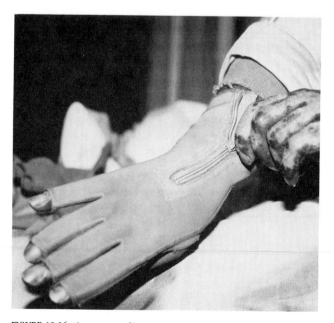

FIGURE 18-36. *A custom-fitted external compression/vascular support glove is worn 23 hours a day to minimize scarring, edema, and vascular pooling. Open fingertips in gloves can improve fingertip prehension and sensation.*

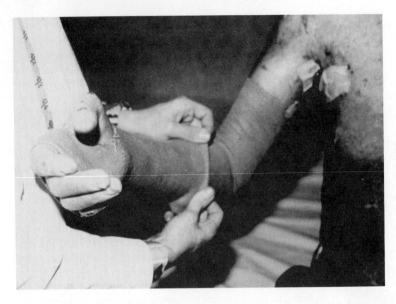

FIGURE 18-37. *Tubular elastic dressings are used for skin conditioning on the extremities. The hand or foot must be included in the dressing to prevent distal swelling.*

wound healing. Although scar contracture generally does not occur until after wound closure, some compression techniques are applied early to:

- Control edema
- Minimize vascular and lymphatic pooling in the extremities
- Condition the new skin for the shear force demands of commercial garments (Bruster & Pullium, 1983)
- Begin skin desensitization and sensory reeducation
- Teach independent dressing or garment-donning skills
- Provide timely compression therapy education

Graded compression therapy is part of basic burn care. During acute care, external support is needed on UE and LE burns when they are in a dependent position. Elastic wraps applied over gauze dressings in a figure-eight fashion are the primary treatment choice in most burn centers. They are also considered the first stage of graded pressure therapy.

As the wounds heal and dressing needs diminish, compression therapy can be progressed to using tubular elastic dressings that are pulled on. Elastinet and Tubigrip, available in rolls of various circumferences, are frequently used for intermediate compression therapy on the extremities (Kealey, Jensen, Laubenthal, Lewis, 1990) (Figure 18-37). Interim pressure on the hand can be accomplished by progressing to an intermediate Spandex glove that is made by the therapist (Bruster & Pullium, 1983), by using manufactured presized gloves, or by applying a total-contact Coban wrap (Figure 18-38). The purposes for using interim pressure must be considered when deciding which method to use. Skin condition, the need to decrease edema, and the patient's functional abilities and understanding are just a few of the points that must be considered. The overall goal is to prepare the patient, both physically and psychologically, for custom-fitted vascular support or burn compression garments.

Although custom garments are made from sequential measurements of the patient, actual garment fit is not perfect. To be effective, the elastic garment must exert equal pressure over the entire area. This is not always possible because of body contours, bony prominences, and postural adjustments by the patient. When the garment does not fit consistently, pressure adapters or inserts under the garment are needed to distribute pressure

uniformly. Areas frequently needing inserts are the superior anterior chest, breast areas on women, web spaces on the hand, anterior surface of the toes, the upper and lower lip areas, and nasolabial folds on the face. Inserts are also needed to prevent garment overlap and folding in the antecubital areas of the elbows, posterior aspect of the knees, axillary folds, and anterior aspect of the ankle.

Pressure inserts were originally made from thermoplastics, but problems of skin maceration under the inserts were common. Today, thermoplastics are only used for fairly large surface areas where positioning is also needed, like the anterior chest, or areas where there is minimal motion, such as between the breasts. Most inserts are now made from more flexible materials, such as Plastazote, silicone gel, Otoform K, Aliplast, silicone elastomer, or a closed cell foam (Malick & Carr, 1980; Miles &

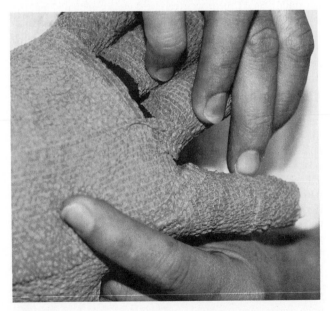

FIGURE 18-38. *Coban wraps are used to minimize edema and to prepare the hand for a custom-fitted glove. A strip placed dorsal to volar provides web-space control.*

Grisby, 1990; Parks, Evans, & Larson, 1978; Perkins, Davey, & Wallis, 1983). Friction or skin maceration are not common with these materials because they are flexible. The material chosen depends on the function of the area being treated. If the insert is needed to provide gentle positioning at rest, along with being flexible to allow some motion, Otoform K, Aliplast, or silicone elastomer can be used (Malick & Carr, 1980). When flexibility and pressure distribution in smaller areas are the primary needs, Plastazote, silicone gel, or a closed cell foam is used. Many of the materials for pressure inserts are subject to tearing and eventual compression; therefore, frequent assessment and replacement are necessary. The patient's ability to place the insert in the correct position under the garment must also be addressed.

Despite advances in scar control using garments and inserts, splints may still be needed for certain body areas. There are also areas where effective pressure distribution is not possible with elastic garments. The neck, face, and mouth are good examples of areas where an alternate method for pressure therapy is needed.

Preventing scar contracture of the neck is difficult due to neck mobility, ineffectiveness of elastic garments, and dysfunctional postural adjustments that the patient may make in response to scar tightness and discomfort. Scar involvement of the neck region can extend from the face to the superior aspect of the chest, causing distortion of the lower face and lip commissures, eversion of the lower lip, limited neck rotation and extension, and shoulder protraction (Figure 18-39).

Early splint designs for neck contracture prevention consisted of a total-contact neck conformer made from a thermoplas-

tic material (Willis, 1970). Problems encountered with this neck conformer are mandibular retraction, minimal to no neck rotation allowed, and decreased surface contact with neck motion. An advancement of this splint design is a rigid, total-contact, transparent chin and neck orthosis (Rivers, 1987) (Figure 18-40). Fabricating a transparent plastic splint is an involved process but allows more precise alterations and assessment of fit compared with thermoplastic materials. An alternate splint design is the triple-component neck splint, which consists of a chin cup, chin strap, and modified neck conformer (Leman & Lowery, 1986). It is basically a two-piece neck conformer with an elastic chin strap. Its design allows neck rotation and some extension and flexion, preserves the cervicomental angle of the chin, and provides compression to supraclavicular scar.

Burn scar contracture of the perioral facial region may lead to cosmetic and functional impairment. Microstomia, or contracture of the oral commissures, can affect eating skills, oral hygiene, dental care, facial expression, and sometimes speech. Due to the structure of the perioral region and the need for stretching pressure when scar is developing, elastic garments are ineffective. A microstomia-prevention appliance is commercially available for preventing or decreasing microstomia during wound healing (Heinle, Kealey, Cram, & Hartford, 1987). The commercial microstomia-prevention appliance is effective in preserving the horizontal width and can be adapted to increase vertical stretching by molding a piece of thermoplastic to its acrylic sections. Problems with this approach are distortion of the tis-

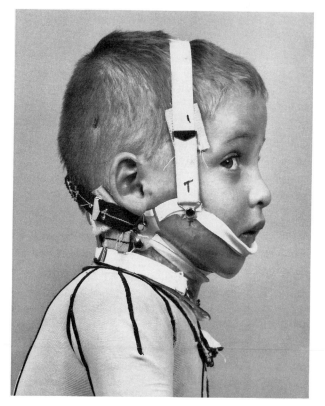

FIGURE 18-39. *Scar contracture of the neck. When the scar shortens by contraction, the chin shelf and cervicomental angle are lost, and range of motion is restricted.*

FIGURE 18-40. *A profile of a transparent chin and neck orthosis worn with a presized external vascular support garment.* (*Photo courtesy of Elizabeth Rivers, OTR, Burn Rehabilitation Specialist, Ramsy Burn Center, St. Paul, MN.*)

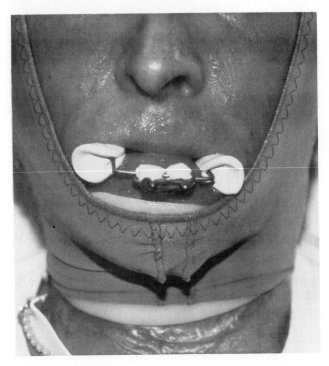

FIGURE 18-41. *A therapist-made microstomia-prevention splint. A thermoplastic chin cup, worn under the elastic chin strap, is molded to the patient to preserve the cervicomental angle and chin shelf.*

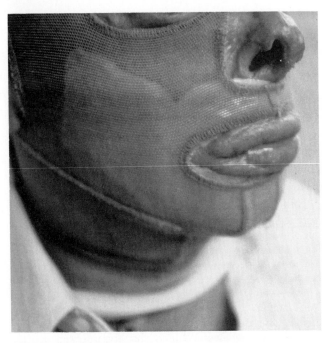

FIGURE 18-42. *Elastomer insert worn under an external compression and vascular support face mask distributes pressure more uniformly.*

sues surrounding the oral commissures and potential pressure sores of the oral mucosa. A modified microstomia-prevention splint, constructed by the therapist, has been reported (Fowler & Pegg, 1986) (Figure 18-41). The advantage of this design is its flexibility in allowing modification of the splint's commissures without adding additional material.

In the face, it is difficult to exert adequate pressure to all involved areas using elastic garments. This is due to its multiple contour changes and soft tissue planes. Facial pressure devices include elastomer inserts under elastic garments, low-temperature thermoplastic masks, and total-contact, transparent face orthoses (Covey, Prestigiacomo, & Engrav, 1987; Gallagher, Goldfarb, Slater, & Rogoski-Grassi, 1990) (Figure 18-42). Rivers, Strate, and Solem (1979) described the five-step process of making a transparent facial orthosis: (1) taking a negative impression of the patient, (2) making a positive plaster cast of the impression, (3) heating and stretching the plastic over the cast, (4) finishing the edges, (5) and fitting it to the patient. Elastic straps are used to hold the mask in place (Figure 18-43). The advantages of a transparent mask are that more precise alterations are possible, the amount of scar contact can be easily assessed, and facial contours can be emphasized. Many patients prefer the transparent mask because it is simple to don and doff, is less obtrusive, and the hair can be uncovered, allowing some identity.

As previously stated, consideration must be given to the patient's daily activity schedule and responsibilities when designing the scar treatment plan. Preserving as much independent function as possible is important for the patient to begin early reintegration into the home environment during recovery. Scar management is a long-term process requiring frequent assess-

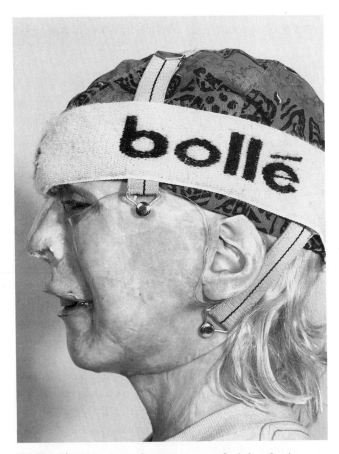

FIGURE 18-43. *Side view of a transparent facial orthosis. Headbands are frequently used for forehead scar control. (Photo courtesy of Elizabeth Rivers, OTR, Burn Rehabilitation Specialist, Ramsey Burn Center, St. Paul, MN.)*

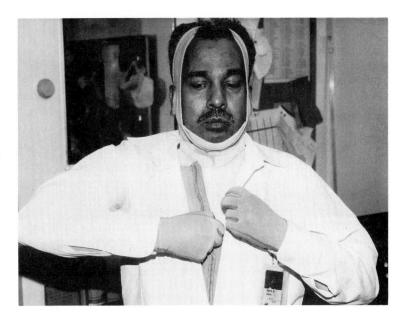

FIGURE 18-44. *A patient independently donning a triple-component neck splint and external compression/vascular support garment.*

ment and adjustment of garment and splint fit. Increasing the person's ability to don and doff garments and splints is an important objective in design selection (Figure 18-44). In most cases, success is dependent on the person's compliance and ability to assume responsibility for self-care.

Skin care

Whether or not scar contracture develops during burn wound maturation, the new skin (epithelium) will never look or react to exposure or contact like it did before injury. Common problems include edematous, insensate or hypersensitive, dry, and unusually fragile skin (Figure 18-45). Newly healed skin is also vulnerable to exposure to ultraviolet light, extremes of temperature, and chemical irritation (Rivers & Fisher, 1990). Because of changes in elasticity, shear tolerance, sensation, and pigmentation, **skin care** and conditioning should be part of self-care education in every burn treatment plan.

Before discharge from the hospital, the patient should learn how and when to lubricate the skin. This is necessary because most deep partial-thickness and full-thickness burns frequently

damage epidermal appendages that contribute to the skin's moisture balance. Lubrication should be done everyday after bathing and at intervals during the day when the skin feels exceptionally dry, tight, or itchy. Massage, using a nonwater-based cream, should always precede stretching exercises to prevent the dry skin from rupturing (Miles & Grisby, 1990).

Improving skin tolerance and sensitivity to friction or trauma is also part of skin care. Scratching, rubbing, bumping into something, and the shearing forces of custom-made, external vascular support garments can cause blisters. Patients should be taught not to be alarmed when blisters occur and to leave small blisters intact. If the blister is large, it should be drained, and mercurochrome and dry gauze should be applied. Spenco dermal pads, other gel pads, or extra linings in garments over areas prone to trauma, such as the knees, can be used for prevention of trauma (Rivers, 1987). Interim pressure dressings and presized garments, massage, exercise and activity while wearing interim garments, and desensitization activities are also effective in increasing skin tolerance and decreasing sensitivity.

Injured skin is more sensitive to temperature differences and exposure to ultraviolet light. Significant sun exposure can

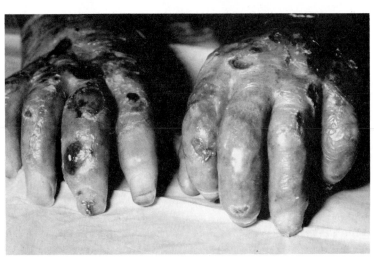

FIGURE 18-45. *Burn wounds that heal without surgery are frequently edematous, fragile, and prone to blistering. Skin conditioning and intermediate garments are used to prevent this type of problem.*

alter the pigment that is regenerating. Skin protection using a 15-rated paraaminobenzoic acid should be recommended (Rivers, 1984). Sunscreens should be applied anytime a patient is in the sun, even if simply riding in a car. Wearing wide-brim hats is recommended for any one with maturing face and neck burns.

Heat is a problem because of alteration in sweating, whereas frostbite in colder temperatures can be an issue with insensate skin. Education about proper clothing to prevent exposure is also important.

Return to work

Burn rehabilitation treatments and work skills training have many similarities. Often identified as work tolerances, strength, endurance, and flexibility are also treatment goals of burn rehabilitation (Leman, 1987). The basic difference between the two therapies is the patient's initial level of function. Physical demands of jobs, such as reaching, stooping, pulling, lifting, and manipulating, are also components of many functional activities. Since the emphasis of burn rehabilitation is on functional recovery, many of the activities and exercises used can have dual purposes—both functional and work-related (Figure 18-46).

Identifying and integrating certain job skills in the acute care treatment plan can decrease the potential for loss of skills and also foster the patient's realization that he or she is going to be okay. Returning to work before scar maturation is complete can also help in preserving function and improving the patient's self-concept. This is only possible, however, after reintegration into the family and socialization concerns are resolved.

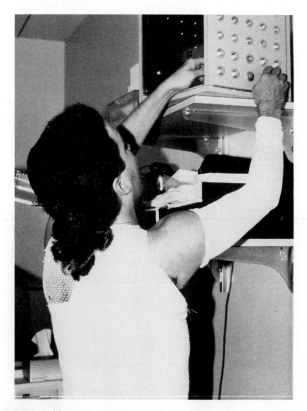

FIGURE 18-46. *Work samples such as the Valpar Small Tools Work Sample can be used to simulate both functional motions and work skills during acute care.*

Preparing a burn patient for return to work does not have to be a long-term process if treatment plans incorporate both job demands and basic functional needs. To do this, a job description should be included in the activity needs analysis. If the patient was injured on the job or is lacking confidence in his or her abilities, many psychosocial issues may emerge when discussing return to work. Fear, anger, and pain are just a few of the issues that may need to be addressed. The person may not feel capable of performing the job again, may be anxious about being injured again, or may be self-conscious about appearance. One technique for job desensitization is to have the patient go to the workplace and observe the job to discuss concerns during therapy. Group sessions that include both inpatients and outpatients have also had positive results in resolving return to work issues (Leman, 1987).

Burn-related programs

Numerous special programs can be organized to increase awareness and prevention of burn injuries and to improve socialization and reintegration of burn patients into the community. These include burn camps for recovering burned children, puppet shows that teach fire safety and burn care, fire prevention, and school reentry programs (Haney, Seh, & Krob, 1988; Meyer, Barnett, & Gross, 1987; Morrison, Herath, & Chase, 1988; Rosenstein, 1986, 1987; Varas, Carbone, & Hammond, 1988). For adults, there are usually local recovered burn groups or hospital-based burn support groups. Burn care professionals' participation in regional health fairs and fire station's open house programs also help improve public awareness of burn injuries.

The occupational therapist's participation in any of these programs depends on community need, financing, and the therapist's time availability. Although prevention of disability after burn injury is the primary focus of occupational therapy, public education and burn injury prevention should be a goal of all burn team members (Schmeer, Stern, & Monafo, 1988; Victor, Lawrence, Munster, & Horn, 1988).

Summary

Advances in burn care have improved burn injury outcomes. Today, most patients recovering from a burn injury can expect to return to a near-normal life, including return to school or work early during the recovery process. To achieve this goal, a team approach to patient care is necessary.

The occupational therapist is an integral member of the burn care team. Through the use of splints, positioning techniques, exercise, ADL, skin conditioning activities, patient education, and external compression and vascular support garments, treatments support recovery of functional skills. Assessment of patient needs and function throughout recovery is essential for effective treatment programming and progression of activities. Patient compliance and motivation are also essential for successful outcome.

Numerous burn-related programs are available for burn patients, the public, and health care professionals. School reentry programs, burn camps, and recovered burn groups are just a few of those programs for recovering burn patients. For health care professionals, the American Burn Association, a national organization, is dedicated to burn rehabilitation, education, research, and burn prevention.

References

Abston, S. (1987). Scar reaction after thermal injury and prevention of scars and contractures. In J. Boswick (Ed.), *The art and science of burn care* (pp. 359–371). Rockville, MD: Aspen.

Baur, P., Barrett, G., & Brown, M. (1979). Ultrastructural evidence of the presence of "fibroclasts" and "myofibroclasts" in wound healing tissue. *Journal of Trauma, 19,* 744–756.

Bennett, G., Helm, P., Purdue, G., & Hunt, J. (1989). Serial casting: A method for treating burn contractures. *Journal of Burn Care and Rehabilitation, 10*(6), 543–545.

Bruster, J., & Pullium, G. (1983). Gradient pressure. *American Journal of Occupational Therapy, 37,* 485–488.

Cooper, S., & Paul, E. (1988). An effective method of positioning the burn patient. *Journal of Burn Care and Rehabilitation, 9*(3), 288–289.

Covey, M. (1987). Occupational therapy. In J. Boswick (Ed.), *The art and science of burn care* (pp. 285–298). Rockville, MD: Aspen.

Covey, M., Prestigiacomo, M., & Engrav, L. (1987). Management of face burns. *Topics in Acute Care and Trauma Rehabilitation, 1*(4), 40–49.

Covey, M. (1988). Application of CPM devices with burn patients. *Journal of Burn Care and Rehabilitation, 9*(5), 496–497.

Covey, M., Dutcher, K., Marvin, J., & Heimbach, D. (1988). Efficacy of continuous passive motion (CPM) devices with hand burns. *Journal of Burn Care and Rehabilitation, 9,* 397–400.

Feller, I., & Jones, C. (1984). Introduction—Statement of the problem. In S. Fisher, & P. Helm (Eds.), *Comprehensive rehabilitation of burns* (pp. 1–8). Baltimore: Williams & Wilkins.

Fowler, D., & Pegg, S. (1986). Modified microstomia prevention splint. *Burns, 12,* 371–373.

Gallagher, J., Goldfarb, I., Slater, H., & Rogoski-Grassi, M. (1990). Survey of treatment modalities for the prevention of hypertrophic facial scars. *Journal of Burn Care and Rehabilitation, 11,* 118–120.

Giuliani, C., & Perry, G. (1985). Factors to consider in the rehabilitation aspect of burn care. *Physical Therapy, 65*(5), 619–623.

Haney, A., Seh, D., & Krob, M. J. (1988). Fire prevention for teenage mothers enrolled in high school. *Journal of Burn Care and Rehabilitation, 9*(6), 648–649.

Hartford, C. (1984). Surgical management. In S. Fisher, & P. Helm (Eds.), *Comprehensive rehabilitation of burns* (pp. 28–63). Baltimore: Williams & Wilkins.

Heinle, J., Kealey, G., Cram, A., & Hartford, C. (1987). The microstomia prevention appliance: 14 years of clinical experience. *Journal of Burn Care and Rehabilitation, 9*(1), 90–91.

Helm, P., Kevorkian, G., Lushbaugh, M., Pullium, G., Head, M., & Cromes, F. (1983). Burn injury: Rehabilitation management in 1982. *Journal of Burn Care and Rehabilitation, 4*(6), 411–422.

Johnson, C. (1984). Physical therapists as scar modifiers. *Physical Therapy, 64*(9), 1381–1387.

Johnson, C. (1987a). Wound healing and scar formation. *Topics in Acute Care and Trauma Rehabilitation, 1*(4), 1–14.

Johnson, C. (1987b). The role of physical therapy. In J. Boswick (Ed.), *The art and science of burn care* (pp. 299–306). Rockville, MD: Aspen.

Jordan, M. J., Lewis, M., Wiegand, L. & Leman, C. (1984). Dynamic plaster casting for burn scar contracture. Proceedings of the American Burn Association 16th Annual Meeting, 1984.

Kealey, G., Jensen, K., Laubenthal, K., & Lewis, R. (1990). Prospective randomized comparison of two types of pressure therapy garments. *Journal of Burn Care and Rehabilitation, 11,* 334–346.

Kischer, C., Sheltar, M., & Sheltar, C. (1975). Alteration of hypertrophic scars induced by mechanical pressure. *Archives of Dermatology, 111,* 60–64.

Larson, D., Abston, S., Evans, E., Dobrkovsky, M., & Linares, H. (1971). Techniques for decreasing scar formation and contracture in the burned patient. *Journal of Trauma, 11,* 807–822.

Leman, C. (1987). An approach to work hardening in burn rehabilitation. *Topics in Acute Care and Trauma Rehabilitation, 1*(4), 62–73.

Leman, C., & Lowery, C. (1986). The triple-component neck splint. *Journal of Burn Care and Rehabilitation, 7,* 357–361.

Linares, H., Kischer, K., & Dobrkovsky, M. (1972). The histiotypic organization of the hypertrophic scar in humans. *Journal of Investigational Dermatology, 59,* 323–331.

Lund, C., & Browder, N. (1944). The estimation of area of burns. *Surgical Gynecology and Obstetrics, 79,* 352–355.

Malick, M., & Carr, J. (1980). Flexible elastomer molds in burn scar control. *American Journal of Occupational Therapy, 34*(9), 603–608.

Meyer, D., Barnett, P., & Gross, J. (1987). A school re-entry program for burned children. Part II: Physical therapy contribution to an existing school re-entry program. *Journal of Burn Care and Rehabilitation, 8*(4), 322–324.

Miles, W., Grigsby, L. (1990). Remodeling of scar tissue in the burned hand. In J. Hunter, L. Schneider, E. Mackin, & A. Callahan (Eds.), *Rehabilitation of the hand: Surgery and therapy* (3rd ed.) (pp. 841–857). St. Louis, C. V. Mosby.

Morrison, M., Herath, K., & Chase, C. (1988). Puppets for prevention: Playing safe is playing smart. *Journal of Burn Care and Rehabilitation, 9*(6), 650–651.

Parks, D., Evans, E., & Larson, D. (1978). Prevention and correction of deformity after severe burns. *Surgical Clinics in North America, 58*(6), 1279–1289.

Perkins, K., Davey, R., & Wallis, K. (1983). Silicone gel: A new treatment for burn scar contracture. *Burns, 9,* 201–204.

Petro, J., & Salisbury, R. (1986). Rehabilitation of the burn patient. *Clinics in Plastic Surgery, 13*(1), 145–149.

Pullium, G. (1984). Splinting and positioning. In S. Fisher, & P. Helm (Eds.), *Comprehensive rehabilitation of burns* (pp. 64–95). Baltimore: Williams & Wilkins.

Rivers, E., Strate, R., & Solem, L. (1979). The transparent face mask. *American Journal of Occupational Therapy, 33,* 108–113.

Rivers, E. (1984). Management of hypertrophic scars. In S. Fisher, & P. Helm (Eds.), *Comprehensive rehabilitation of burns* (pp. 177–217). Baltimore: Williams & Wilkins.

Rivers, E. (1987). Rehabilitation management of the burn patient. *Advances in Clinical Rehabilitation, 1,* 177–214.

Rivers, E., & Fisher, S. (1990). Rehabilitation for burn patients. In F. Kottke, & J. Lehmann (Eds.), *Krusen's handbook of physical medicine and rehabilitation* (pp. 1070–1100), Philadelphia: W. B. Saunders.

Rosenstein, D. (1986). Camp celebrate: A therapeutic weekend camping program for pediatric burn patients. *Journal of Burn Care and Rehabilitation, 7*(5), 434–436.

Rosenstein, D. (1987). A school re-entry program for burned children. Part I: Development and implementation of a school re-entry program. *Journal of Burn Care and Rehabilitation, 8*(4), 319–322.

Schmeer, S., Stern, N., & Monafo, W. (1988). An outreach burn prevention program for home care patents. *Journal of Burn Care and Rehabilitation, 9*(6), 645–647.

Solem, L. (1984). Classification. In S. Fisher, & P. Helm (Eds.), *Comprehensive rehabilitation of burns* (pp. 9–15). Baltimore: Williams & Wilkins.

Stern, L., & Davey, R. (1985). A teach approach with severely burned children in a multidisciplinary rehabilitation setting. *Burns, 11*(4), 281–284.

Varas, R., Carbone, R., & Hammond, J. (1988). A one-hour burn prevention program for grade school children: Its approach and success. *Journal of Burn Care and Rehabilitation, 9*(1), 69–71.

Victor, J., Lawrence, P., Munster, A., & Horn, S. (1988). A statewide targeted burn prevention program. *Journal of Burn Care and Rehabilitation, 9*(4), 425–429.

Wachtel, T. (1985). Epidemiology, classification, initial care, and administrative considerations for critically burned patients. In T. Wachtel (Ed.), *Critical care clinics* (pp. 3–26). Philadelphia: W. B. Saunders.

Willis, B. (1970). The use of orthoplast isoprene splints in the treatment of the acutely burned child. *American Journal of Occupational Therapy, 24*(3), 187–191.

Bibliography

Apfel, L. (1984). Occupational therapy techniques for the patient with thermal injuries of the head and neck. In T. Wachtel, & D. Frank (Eds), *Burns of the head and neck* (vol. 29). Philadelphia: W. B. Saunders, p. 133.

Covey, M. (Ed.). (1987). *Topics in acute care and trauma rehabilitation, 1*(4). Frederick, MD: Aspen.

Falkel, J., Richard, R., & Staley, M. (Eds.). (1992). *Understanding the application of burn care and rehabilitation: Principles and practice for the treating therapist.* Philadelphia: F. A. Davis.

Fisher, S., & Helm, P. (Eds.). (1984). *Comprehensive rehabilitation of burns.* Baltimore: Williams & Wilkins.

Leman, C. (1992). Splints and accessories following burn reconstruction. In R. Salisbury (Ed.), *Clinics in plastic surgery.* Philadelphia: W. B. Saunders.

Questad, K., Patterson, D., Boltwood, M., Heimbach, D., Dutcher, K., de Lateur, B., Marvin, J., & Covey, M. (1988). Relating mental health and physical function at discharge to rehabilitation status at three months postburn. *Journal of Burn Care and Rehabilitation, 9*(1), 87–89.

Richards, R., Miller, S., & Staley, M. (1990). The physiologic response of a patient with critical burns to continuous passive motion. *Journal of Burn Care and Rehabilitation, 11*(6), 554–556.

Salisbury, R., Reeves, S., & Wright, P. (1990). Acute care and rehabilitation of the burned hand. In J. Hunter, L. Schneider, E. Mackin, & A. Callahan (Eds.), *Rehabilitation of the hand: Surgery and therapy* (3rd ed.) (pp. 831–840). St. Louis: C. V. Mosby.

Ward, R. (1991). Pressure therapy for the control of hypertrophic scar formation after burn injury. *Journal of Burn Care and Rehabilitation, 12*(3), 257–261.

Ward, R., Saffle, J., Schnebly, A., & Hayes-Lundy, C. (1989). Sensory loss over grafted areas in patients with burns. *Journal of Burn Care and Rehabilitation, 10*(6), 536–538.

SECTION 6

Sensory loss: Deafness and blindness

JANE E. JOHNSTON ALLINDER

KEY TERMS

American Sign Language

Audiogram

Braille

Central Visual Acuity

Conductive Hearing Loss

Fingerspelling

Legally Blind

Sensorineural Hearing Loss

Teletypewriter

LEARNING OBJECTIVES

Upon completion of this section the reader will be able to:

1. *Describe the role that the senses play in a person's life and in the process of rehabilitation.*

2. *Define the terms deaf, blind, and deaf–blind.*

3. *Explain the basic anatomy and physiology of the working senses.*

4. *Refute common misconceptions about deafness and blindness.*

5. *Describe the emotional, physical, and psychosocial needs of the deaf and blind communities.*

6. *Describe some of the technology that can aid a person with a sensory loss.*

The unique senses of sight and sound

Although each of the five human senses seems unique, such as the smell of burning wood seemingly unrelated to a beautiful sunset or the sound of a violin, a complex union of anatomy and physiology links them all. Each sense receives information from the external world by means of nerve cells, called *receptors*, that lie on or just beneath the surface of the human body. In turn, each of these sets of sensors is linked by a network of nerves to a specific part of the brain designed to receive and interpret this vast diversity of information. The receptors for each of the senses are stimulated by a particular kind of energy—mechanical energy for touch and hearing, chemical energy for smell and taste, radiant energy for sight (Murphy, 1982). By a process called *transduction*, the specific receptors for each sense converts that energy received into a code of electrical impulses. Through this transduced form of energy, a kind of internal physiologic Morse code, all sensory information travels along the nerve pathways to the brain. Because all these senses are basic to survival, and all contribute to the quality of one's life, the loss or impairment of any is potentially devastating. Even a slight deterioration is a loss. The frost-bitten fingertips that can no longer feel the softness of a kitten's fur also lose their ability to locate a key in the bottom of a cluttered bag. Understanding the senses, protecting them, and easing or remedying their disorders contributes to good health care.

Each of our five senses, their abilities and their contributions to human existence, is amazing in its own right. The senses of hearing and sight, however, require complex accessories that enable the receptors to work: in the ear, tubes, membranes, and an intricate sculpture of bones; in the eye, optical focusing mechanisms, muscles, and transformable parts. On the other hand, the more primitive senses of touch, taste, and smell, which sample the world's textures, fragrances, and flavors, do so directly through the nerve endings, without the need for such "middlemen."

Along with the need for additional anatomic hardware for sight and hearing, these two senses have a greater risk for injury and impairment, increasing the challenge for professionals in the health care fields.

Vision, visual impairments, and blindness

The human eye is a dual organ—two eyes working together to transmit visual information to the brain. Although it is certainly possible to see with only one eye, it takes two normally functioning eyes to achieve normal vision.

With so much delicate machinery operating within the eye's structures, as well as the decoding process of the brain to make vision meaningful, it is something of a miracle that human eyes are not completely troubled by impairment and disorder. In fact, during a lifetime of constant use, most people experience only occasional eye irritation or minor infection and some degree of focusing error, which is easily corrected. For those who do experience visual impairment, the effects can greatly impact their daily functioning.

The term blind is not synonymous with *totally blind*. When a person is classified as being totally blind, it means he or she has no light perception, or is unable to distinguish light from darkness. Blindness is generally defined as central visual acuity for distant vision of 20/200 or less in the better eye, with best correction, or central visual acuity for more than 20/200 if there is a field deficit in which the peripheral field has contracted to such an extent that the widest diameter of visual field subtends an angular distance no greater than 20 degrees. To give a comparative interpretation of these numbers, a measure of 20/200 visual acuity means that a person can see at a distance no greater than 20 feet what a normally sighted person can see at 200 feet (Taylor, 1975). In other words, an object that a normal eye can see 200 feet away must be brought to a distance of 20 feet to be recognized by the eye with a visual acuity of only 20/200.

This measuring system is done by use of a Snellen chart on which letters of varying sizes are printed. The term **central visual acuity** means that the eye should be focused on the object when the distances are measured. The measurements must be taken with the best possible corrective lens (glasses), and the vision in the better eye determines the degree of sight. Therefore, a person who has lost sight completely in one eye, but retains vision better than 20/200 in the other eye, is not considered legally blind (Table 18-2).

A defect in the field of vision is more difficult to measure. Normally, an eye, when focused on an object, takes in a significant amount of the surrounding area above, below, and to the left and right. This ability in the normal sighted eye encompasses an area of 60 to 70 degrees beyond the central focus. If this area, called the *field of vision*, contracts so that the angle is only 20 degrees, severely limiting the peripheral range of vision, the person is considered **legally blind**.

TABLE 18-2. *Central Visual Acuity for Distance and Corresponding Percentage of Visual Efficiency*

Snellen Measure of Central Visual Acuity	Percentage of Visual Efficiency
20/20	100
20/40	85
20/50	75
20/80	60
20/100	50
20/200	20

This definition does not include the important factor of *near vision*, also called reading vision, which is relevant to an person's functioning. Near vision is also measured in terms of visual efficiency using another type of Snellen chart (Lowenfield, 1973). This measurement is based on a normal acuity at a distance of 14 inches. Some people who have visual acuity of 20/200 or less have comparatively good near vision and may be able to read even ordinary print, particularly if they use good reading glasses.

Therefore, the definition of blindness must include a wide range of visual ability. It must account for those who are totally blind, those who can function with near vision, and those whose visual field appears to be looking through a tunnel.

Current statistics show that about 500,000 people are legally blind in the United States. Of these, over 75% have some remaining vision (Sardegna & Paul, 1991). The classification of legally blind is an important one since benefits such as tax deductions, Medicare programs, reduced rates for utilities, and financial aid are available to those who qualify.

A person whose visual ability exceeds the measure of legally blind but whose lack of visual skills, even with correction, interfere with the performance of daily activities is referred to as having *low vision*, being *visually impaired*, or being *partially sighted*. According to the American Foundation for the Blind, there are over 11 million people in the United States who have below normal vision, even with correction. Of these, almost 1.5 million can be classified as having low vision. Although these people do not receive the same services as those classified as legally blind, they still may have as significant a need for assistance with daily living.

The cause of blindness is not always known. The scientific community, however, is becoming more adept in diagnosing and, in some cases, preventing blindness. According to the National Society to Prevent Blindness, the four leading causes of existing blindness in the United States are: glaucoma, age-related maculopathy, senile cataract, and optic nerve atrophy. Retinitis pigmentosa is a leading cause of blindness in those aged 20 to 64 years. Among new cases of blindness, the four major causes are, in order of prevalence: age-related maculopathy, glaucoma, diabetic retinopathy, and senile cataract. These are responsible for nearly half of all new cases of blindness (Sardegna & Paul, 1991).

Hearing, hearing impairments, and deafness

Although the eye is wonderfully versatile in its complex parts and functions, the ear is equally or more so. The ear and its functions actually house two senses. A part of the ear's sensors provides the brain with raw material for the sense of hearing, while another part serves as a kind of automatic pilot for the body, monitoring posture, balance, and movement.

Sound is pervasive in our environment. It moves through darkness or light, through objects, and around barriers. Unlike our eyes, which can block out their stimuli by the convenience of eyelids, our ears have no such convenient barrier system. Thus, our sense of hearing is always evaluating our environment.

Just as classifying visual impairments is a multifactored task, so is the challenge to classify hearing impairments. The general public often uses terms such as deaf, hearing impaired, and *hard of hearing*, which give little information about the actual level of functional hearing.

Four factors are significant in understanding hearing loss:

degree of loss, age of onset, cause, and site of lesion. These factors help to determine not only the amount of functional hearing a person has but also the means to help remedy or compensate for the hearing loss.

The degree of hearing loss is determined through various tests, but one standard measure used by audiologists is the pure tone *audiogram*, which measures in decibels (Db) a scale of loudness or intensity. The loss in each ear is measured over a range of frequencies or pitch, and this measurement is recorded in Hertz (Hz). The audiogram then provides a graphic display of the results of the testing.

Normal hearing should be able to detect sounds between 20 to 20,000 Hz at a level of 0 to 25 Db of sound. Hearing level at the 25- to 45-Db level is referred to as a 25- to 45-Db loss and is considered a mild hearing loss. A loss of 45 to 65 Db is classified as a moderate loss, while a loss of 65 to 85 Db is considered severe. A loss of 85 Db or greater is considered to be a profound hearing loss (Figure 18-47). Although the degree of decibel loss is significant, it must also be noted over what frequency range this occurs.

Age of onset is important not only in terms of hearing capabilities but also in terms of language. A person who lost hearing before developing speech is said to be *prelingually deaf*. This person's ability to learn a spoken language clearly is more difficult. Even the child who has some experience with hearing speech, even if only 1 or 2 years, has an advantage over a prelingually deaf child. This is not to say that a prelingually deaf child cannot learn a spoken language; however, it cannot be acquired in the same manner that a postlingually deaf child acquires language.

The cause of the hearing loss and the location of the impairment go hand in hand since the cause of the impairment determines the location and therefore the type of hearing loss. There are two major types of hearing loss. The most common type is a *conductive* hearing loss, which involves damage to the mechanisms that transmit sound energy to the cochlea. A conductive loss may be caused by something as simple as a collection of ear wax that prevents the sound waves from vibrating the eardrums. A conductive loss can also result from fluid in the middle ear, which impedes the normal vibration of the three small bones.

The normal aging process can contribute to several forms of conductive hearing loss. As the eardrum ages, it becomes less pliable and does not vibrate as well as a young, more subtle eardrum. The joints between the bones of the ears can harden with age, interfering with normal sound wave transmission. Chronic middle-ear infection can cause scar tissue to form and immobilize the bony structures. The muscular structures can atrophy as well. The most common form of conductive hearing loss is caused by otosclerosis. This is a condition in which bone deposits form around the stapes, adhering it to the opening of the cochlea, which drastically restricts the normal movement of sound vibrations.

Human speech is produced in the range of 300 to 4000 Hz (Mindel & McCay, 1971). If, for example, a person has a 70-degree loss in the range of 125 to 800 Hz, that person may have some difficulty hearing a very deep male voice but would probably have no problem hearing a woman or a small child talk. Because conductive hearing losses are due to impairments of the movement of the sound energy, they are limited to the location of the outer and middle ear. In this type of hearing loss, the specialized hair cell receptors of the inner ear are intact and able to send the impulses to the brain for decoding. When this function is still intact, sound waves that can be forwarded to the cochlea can be perceived normally. Because this function remains intact, as does the ability to correct or repair some of the physical barriers which impair hearing, the conductive hearing loss is the most correctable form of hearing loss (Smith, 1989).

The second type of hearing loss is the *sensorineural hearing loss*. This form affects the inner ear and the nerve pathways within the brain. Two thirds of all profoundly deaf people have sensorineural hearing loss.

Because we rely on the sensory hair cells of the cochlea to send electrical signals to the brain for its interpretation of sound, these hair cells play a critical role in our ability to hear. These hair cells are housed in the cochlea, a structure the size of a pea. Despite the protective structures of the ear, these sensory hair cells are vulnerable to damage. The typical sounds of our environment are actually a vast array of energy wave lengths, so if all the sensory receptors are not working correctly, we are unable to perceive our environment accurately through sound. Due to the nature of this form of hearing loss, it is also a more prevalent form of prelingual deafness.

Almost any of the common infectious childhood disease, which are generally viral in nature, can affect the inner ear in severe cases. A virus, which is microscopic in size, usually reaches the ear directly from the bloodstream instead of through the cerebrospinal fluid or the cranial cavity (Davis & Silverman, 1978). One particular viral disease, maternal rubella, has been attributed as a major cause of congenital deafness. Rubella, or German measles, for an adult woman is usually a mild infection. It is the developing fetus that is highly vulnerable to this disease, and congenital deafness is only one of the many developmental defects likely to occur. The developing fetus is most vulnerable during the first trimester, and it previously was believed that this is the only time during a woman's pregnancy that the fetus is at risk. It is now evident that the virus

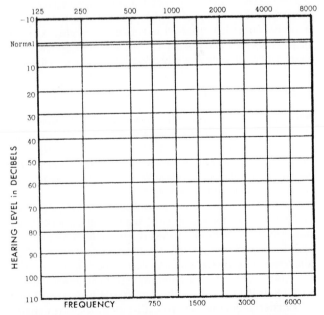

FIGURE 18-47. *The audiogram is one method for measuring the degree of hearing loss. (From Helleberg, M. [1979]. Your hearing loss (p. 69). Chicago: Nelson-Hall Inc.)*

might persist in a woman's body and affect a developing fetus even if she contracted the disease weeks before conception (Davis & Silverman, 1978). The virus acts by destroying the vital sensory receptors. Other viral causes of hearing loss include mumps and viral encephalitis.

Sensorineural hearing loss can be caused by bacterial means as well. The inner ear can be a target for a bacterial infection similar to the infections of the middle ear. This infection, if it reaches the inner ear, can destroy the auditory nerve, rendering sound waves indecipherable. This is not a congenital condition but tends to occur during the first 2 years of life, causing a severe hearing loss. As mentioned previously, this is a critical time for the acquisition of language, and a bout of meningitis during these early years can have a devastating effect on this development.

Certain incompatibilities of parental blood types are responsible for hearing loss. Rhesus factor is one such incompatibility, which can result in the mother's blood destroying the Rh blood cells of the fetus. Consequently, the brain and central nervous system often sustain damage that affects, among other systems, the auditory nerve. Eighty percent of children who survive this blood incompatibility have complete or partial deafness (Tweedie & Shroyer, 1982).

In some cases, the cause of the hearing loss is unknown except that it is genetic, or hereditary in nature. Often, hereditary deafness runs for generations. In many cases, however, the trait was unsuspected. It may be that only after a couple with normal hearing have more than one hearing-impaired child that they learn of a distant relative who was deaf and of their predisposition for deaf offspring. Although most cases of hereditary deafness are not accompanied by other associated disorders, there are some cases in which genetic deafness is one characteristic of a syndrome. Two of the most common syndromes that involve deafness are Waardenburg and Usher syndromes.

In the United States, almost 21 million people (8.8% of the total population) were reported to have a hearing impairment (Hotchkiss, 1989). The most significantly affected age group are those 65 years and older, whose prevalence is seven times that of the age group of 45 years and younger.

Simultaneous deafness and blindness

The simultaneous occurrence of severe visual and hearing impairments is relatively rare. As of 1980, the overall national estimate of the number of deaf–blind people was about 20,000, with 6200 being school aged (Kates & Schein, 1980). Although there is the tendency to broadly categorize a person with both visual and hearing impairments as deaf–blind, this term lacks descriptive accuracy. The total absence of hearing and seeing abilities rarely occurs. Most people considered to be deaf–blind have severe limitations of both sight and hearing but have residual function of one or both senses.

A second misconception with this nomenclature is that the dual impairments are chronologically coordinated. On the contrary, most deaf–blind people tend to have a preceding impairment. Either they are deafened blind people or blind deafened people. The distinction is made by the residual functioning of the two senses and, more important, by the age of onset of each impairment. In general, a deaf person who becomes blind tends to identify with and react as a deaf person. Likewise, blind people who lose their hearing continue to resemble their blind counterparts more than they resemble deaf people in their daily functioning.

As suggested in the preceding sections on visual and hearing impairments, the combined loss of both senses may be caused by hereditary or congenital factors, infection such as rubella, or trauma to the central nervous system, or it may be exacerbated by the natural process of aging. The primary cause of this dual impairment is Usher syndrome, which is hereditary in nature. Usher syndrome is characterized by congenital deafness accompanied by retinitis pigmentosa, a gradual degeneration of the retina, which results in a gradual rather than congenital loss of vision. Usher syndrome is responsible for about 10,000 of the deaf–blind cases in the United States (Sardegna & Paul, 1991).

Although Usher syndrome can be diagnosed by audiometric testing and the detection of retinal changes, little is known about the cause of the syndrome. What is known is that it is a recessively inherited disorder that requires both the mother and father to contribute the necessary genes. Even when this pairing does not occur, the genetic trait can be passed on to future generations. Although there is no cure for Usher syndrome and no method for determining a gene carrier at present, genetic counseling may be beneficial in prevention of the disease.

Occupational therapy services for the blind and deaf

Both vision and hearing are *distance* or *distant* senses—primary channels by which most people gather information and receive pleasure from the environment without making physical contact with it. The *near senses* of touch, movement, taste, and smell are also important; information transmitted by tactile, kinesthetic-proprioceptive, gustatory, and olfactory channels requires either direct contact or, in the case of olfaction, closer range. Particularly during infancy and early childhood, the individual seeks to touch, manipulate, taste, and smell himself or herself and the surroundings as well as to look and listen. Vision and hearing become increasingly sophisticated and reliable in the course of normal development. The match between near and distant sensory data gathered and integrated during early exploration and manipulation of the world gradually enables the child to identify human and nonhuman sounds, objects, senses, and events through visual and auditory information. The contributions of visual and acoustic senses are understandably great both in the development and continuation of communication skill; perceptual-motor ability, including purposeful manipulation and mobility within one's environments; psychosocial function; and cognitive capability. This should not imply that a blind or deaf person cannot develop and use all residual and intact senses to their full extent, only that acquisition of such skills present challenges to the individuals, their families, and the professional people who work with them.

Prevalence within the field

Respondents to the AOTA 1990 Member Data Survey indicated the three most frequent health problems of their patients. Of the members who responded, 0.1% of the registered occupational therapists listed the most frequent health problem seen among their cases to be a hearing deficit, while 0.3% of the certified occupational therapy assistants documented this impairment as the most frequent. Similarly, the response was a small percentage for visual impairments listed as the most frequent health problem. Of the registered occupational therapists who responded, only 0.3% indicated that patients with visual impairments were most frequently treated, while 0% of the certified occupational therapy assistants declared this to be the prevalent health disorder (AOTA, 1990).

Because the survey asked only for the most frequently seen problem, it is not unlikely that the incidence of visual and hearing handicap was low. It is also natural to assume that many more occupational therapists deal with cases of hearing or visual loss either as the primary impairment or accompanying other health problems.

Of those members whose clients' primary health impairment is a hearing or a visual deficit, it is likely that they are therapists working in residential schools for the deaf or blind, public schools that have special programs for the visually or hearing impaired, rehabilitation service centers for the blind, and nursing homes.

No members indicated that simultaneous deafness and blindness was the most frequent health impairment among clients. Whether this was due to its possible inclusion in the category of "other" or whether no therapists see this problem as most prevalent is unknown. It is more likely that this type of impairment is seen only in unique situations and therefore is not listed in this manner.

Considerations when working with the blind

When working with a person with a visual impairment, there are some obvious challenges that one might need to face. Included in these might be issues of orientation and mobility, accessibility, and communication and correspondence.

Orientation and mobility, or the ability to navigate safely, independently, and confidently in the environment, is a high-priority skill for visually impaired people. There are various means by which a visually impaired person can deal with mobility. The best avenue must be determined based on each person's needs, abilities, and environment. Some of the skills taught in training programs include sensory training, concept development and motor skills, long-cane skills, moving with sighted guides, and moving with guide dogs. Sensory training includes learning how to use and sharpen the senses, including residual vision to the maximal capability. The senses are used to determine landmarks, orient to surroundings, and maneuver safely within an environment. Concept development includes learning spatial concepts and understanding fundamental structures, such as compass direction, building layout, or the design of a city block (Sardegna & Paul, 1991). Concept development training is especially important for people with congenital blindness. Motor skills include proper posture, body movement, and coordination. These skills can be developed through exercise, games, and dance. Long-cane skills are taught after the above-listed skills and other fundamental skills are mastered. Training involves the correct grip, movement of the cane, and use of the cane while walking to identify and maneuver obstacles. The purpose of the cane is to alert the user not only to obstacles but also to changes in the terrain. The cane is for use only on the walking surface and cannot alert the user to obstacles overhead. Although the use of a sighted human guide is the least independent, it is sometimes

the most practical form of travel. Because this method is more prevalent with the deaf–blind, it will be described further in that section. Guide dogs are specially trained to provide protection, travel, and companionship. Because of restrictions and limitations on both the dogs and their user, only about 1% of blind people use guide dogs (Sardegna & Paul, 1991). Those who do use guide dogs are put through the training along with the dog to learn how to give directions, understand the signals the dogs give back, and work with the dog to learn to deal with the distractions of the everyday environment.

The blind person's *accessibility* to the environment is often inadequate, possibly because their needs are misunderstood. Accessibility needs relate to features such as entrances, walkways, doors, floors, stairs, lighting, signs and signals, and tactile cuing. Standards for accessibility suggest that entrances that lead to a lobby or public space include a vertical means of access, such as a ramp or stairs. Standard curb cuts or ramps need to be provided at all street crossings and should not create a hazard for pedestrians. Standard doorways must provide adequate openings to allow for two people or one person and a dog. Doorway thresholds need to have no more than a 1/4-inch rise that is marked by a visual and textural cue. Automatic doors should have a sensing device to keep it open until the doorway has been completely cleared. Other recommendations include the use of adequate markings for signs, obstacles, entrances, exits, stairs, ramps, elevators, doorways, and restrooms. Suggestions for these markings or labels include improved lighting, use of contrasting colors, use of textures and other tactile auditory signals, standardized placements of common facilities, and braille markers.

One of the most common methods blind people use to *communicate and correspond* is through the **Braille** system. This is a tactile system that consists of raised dots. The dot system is based on a configuration of six dots, which, when used individually or in combinations, can represent each letter of the alphabet and form punctuation as well as 189 contractions and standard abbreviations. Braille is embossed onto thick paper and is read with the fingertips of one or both hands. An average Braille reader using both hands can achieve a speed of 200 or more words per minute (Sardegna & Paul, 1991). Information can be recorded in Braille similarly to the way a spoken language is recorded in printed form. Braille can be recorded manually using a stylus and a manual slate. The slate provides a boundary for each space, which the user follows tactually. Within each space, the user forms the necessary configuration of dots in the same manner we use specific configurations of lines to form printed letters. Braille can also be recorded faster and more conveniently by the use or a Braille writer, which is similar to a regular typewriter. The Braille writer has dot placement keys, one for each of the possible placements in a set, and a space key. Keys are pressed singularly or in simultaneous combination to achieve the desired dot pattern. Braille writers are available in both manual and electric models (Lowenfeld, 1971). Braille is not used by all blind people.

Some people have adequate visual function to enable them to read and write with the use of a visual aid, such as a magnifier. Others with less functional vision may decide not to use this system due to physical problems that make Braille reading and writing difficult or impossible. For those who have some remaining functional sight, there are also communication aids that assist in reading and writing. A script writing guide is one example

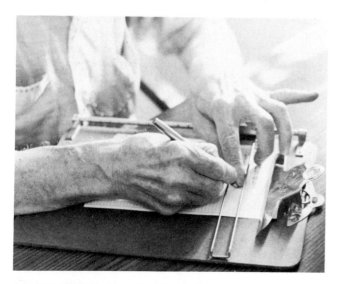

FIGURE 18-48. *With the aid of the Marks Writing Guide plus his own kinesthetic, tactile, and visual memory abilities, the blind man prepares a grocery list. (Photo courtesy of Ann Wade.)*

(Figure 18-48). This is a template, usually oriented horizontally, with an opening that corresponds to one line on a page. The device is then lowered to correspond with each line as the writer moves down the page. Templates and stencils are also used to provide a tactile cue to orient to the writing surface. These can be custom-ordered to meet specific needs or can be obtained for standard sizes, such as for envelopes or for check writing. Bold-lined paper is specially lined writing paper that has dark, heavier lines in place of the standard blue lines. The bold lines may be all that a low-vision person needs to write independently. These people also benefit from books printed in large print, which are now available through libraries and bookstores. Magnification aids make ordinary-sized print readable for some visually impaired people.

Technology for the blind

Technology affects us all daily, so much so that we take for granted many of the time-saving, convenience items we use. As our understanding of special needs populations increases, so does our understanding of technologic accomplishments. Some of these accomplishments have been made in the field of visual impairments.

Because occupational therapy is a field of health care professionals whose focus is on independent living skills, the advances in household and health aids are of special interest. Household aids include cooking devices, such as a liquid level indicator. This device hooks over the lip of a container, such as a cup, bowl, or pan, and signals through beep or vibrations when the liquid nears the top. Raised, large-print telephone dials and one-button automatic dialing systems are available. Other household aids that aid in independence include sewing machine magnifiers, self-threading needles, and Braille clothing tags. Adaptive aids that provide a voice reading can also be obtained, including talking scales, clocks, timers, and watches (Figure 18-49). Tools, including rulers, yardsticks, and tape measures, are available with tactile markings. Even saw guides, drill guides, and calipers

that have raised markings for specific degrees are available. Meters used to detect light, flames, metal objects, and electrical currents are available that alert the user with an audible signal (Sardegna & Paul, 1991). Household items are also available to provide a safe environment. Knife-slicing guides and elbow-length oven mitts are two examples.

Many visual impairments are associated with other medical conditions, and it is important to be aware of health aids for safety and independence. Devices for monitoring temperature, blood pressure, pulse, and glucose level are marked in Braille or give a synthetic voice reading. Pill-splitters can divide pills into halves, and measurement guides are available for measuring liquid medications. Many syringes are marked with large print, and diabetes-related devices can measure insulin and serve as needle guides.

Avocational activities that are a part of daily living need consideration as well. The large-print materials that were discussed as part of communication needs are also applicable to avocational needs. Talking books or books on cassettes make written material accessible. Books, journals, and magazines can be recorded on audiotape on a variety of instruments for the consumer. Television is even becoming an aid for low-vision reading. Closed-circuit television consists of a video camera that focuses on printed material or distant objects, such as a blackboard, and electronically magnifies the object up to 60 times its original size. The user can scan the material with either black print on a white background or vice versa.

As computers become a way of life for many people, they have an impact on the world of visual impairment. Many visually

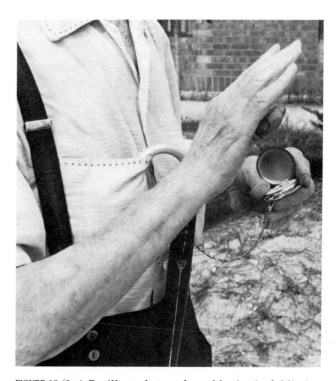

FIGURE 18-49. *A Braille pocketwatch enables its deaf–blind owner to perceive tactually that the time is 4:05. (In this photo, the owner is conveying the "four" to another person.) Note that the cane has been hooked in the chest pocket to free hands and yet make retrieval certain. (Photo courtesy of Ann Wade.)*

impaired people, even those who are unable to read printed material, have keyboarding skills for communication with the sighted world. There are word processing programs that use magnification or voice-activated readings to assist with the input process. Magic Slate is one program that aids low-vision people through 2-inch lettering that appears on the screen. Keytalk is a voice-activated program. As the user types the information, it is read back by synthetic voice at the letter, word, and sentence level. In terms of using a computer, input is not the major obstacle. The question for most blind people is how to get the information out. Three methods discussed previously apply here as well: Braille, magnification, and voice synthesizers.

Computer programs are available that instruct voice synthesizers to read the computer screen in its entirety or just selected parts. Audio signals are included to indicate features such as capitalization and punctuation. There are also proofreading features that perform similarly to the Keytalk program previously described. These systems are useful for programs such as writing and word processing due to their fairly consistent linear forms. Graphics programs, such as accounting programs, are able to use this system, but is more time-consuming. The format for this type of information frequently changes, and the entire screen must be read to obtain one piece of information.

For those who need hard copies of computer information, there are some programs that print out the written information in Braille using a standard, letter-quality printer. The platen is replaced by a soft rubber one, and the period key is used alone to print the text backwards, in Braille. When removed from the printer, the back side of the sheet can be read (McWilliams, 1984).

Low-vision people sometimes prefer reading from a computer screen over reading printed material because the light comes from the letters on the screen instead of reflecting off them, as is the case with words on paper. In addition, the contrast and brightness on the screen can be adjusted for maximal visibility. There are also programs that enlarge the print seen on the screen. It is also helpful to replace the normal 12-inch video monitor with a 25-inch monitor. This gives a full-sized screen display in large letters (see Chapter 9, Section 6).

Considerations when working with the deaf

Described as an invisible handicap, deafness has become increasingly more visible within the last 10 years. Efforts have been made not only to bring the needs of the deaf to the forefront but also to remove the stigma that has been historically associated with it. This will serve to improve the psychosocial image of the deaf community, allowing them to be more assertive in pursuing their right to available services.

For many deaf people, the inability to hear is the least handicapping part of their deafness. This is not to minimize the hearing loss they experience but rather to put it into perspective. The isolation they encounter from being cut off from the rest of the world is far more disabling emotionally, socially, physically, and cognitively.

One immediate consideration when working with the deaf population has to be communication. It is an apparent reality that deaf people do not access services due to communications barriers. Eliminating our egocentric ideals about our own spoken language can be the first step to bringing down this barrier.

What do we mean by communication anyway? Is it speech

and hearing, language, verbal or nonverbal? When speaking in terms of the deaf community, communication has been historically defined within the constraints of two modes: the oral–aural mode and the visual–gestural mode. The oral–aural approach to language, also referred to as *oralism,* is one that puts high priority on spoken language skills. Oral training emphasizes skills such as use of residual hearing, speech training, and speech reading. As mentioned in the previous section on deafness, most deaf people have some residual hearing. The goal within this approach to language is to enhance what hearing a person has and to improve its accuracy to make it function as normally as possible. Amplification is a major step toward accomplishing this goal.

Different types of hearing aids meet the different needs of consumers. Hearing aids must be prescribed and fitted by trained professionals to ensure proper amplification. Most hearing aids work basically the same way: a battery-powered microphone picks up sound waves from the air and changes them into electrical energy. This amplified energy is then sent through a receiver and is converted back to sound and directed into the ear by a fitted ear mold. The function of the hearing aid is to boost the sound wave energy through the mechanical mechanisms within the ear so that it can successfully activate the sensory neurons that send the sound impulse to the brain for processing. Since the mechanical structures of the hearing process are functions of the outer and middle ear, amplification through hearing aids can benefit hearing loss stemming from these areas, or conductive hearing loss. Amplification does not have a significant affect on sensorineural hearing loss, however. Because this deficit has more to do with neurologic damage and the inability of the impulses to travel the neural pathways to the brain, bombardment of sound energy into the ear is nonproductive. Although amplification does not make sound intelligible, as in normal hearing, it can help to heighten the deaf person's awareness of the environment.

This heightened awareness is also attempted by means of auditory training. Auditory training involves normal environmental sounds and teaches the deaf person to identify and remember distinct characteristics of each. Although a deaf person may not be able to understand speech, he or she may be able to learn to discern a human's voice from a dog's bark, for example.

Speech reading, also called lip reading, is an approach to understanding spoken language, primarily from the visual cues of the speaker. Speech reading is a much more accurate term for this enormously complicated task since only a small percentage of speech is actually visible on the lips. Other necessary cues must be perceived from the speaker's tongue, eyes, and neck and facial muscles. In speech reading, not only are the visual and auditory senses of the speaker provided to the reader, the reader's proprioceptive and kinesthetic senses also are important. Because so much of what is said is not visible, a speech reader must be able to fill in the gaps for what is not seen or heard. The speech reader can assist in this process by using the sensations imagined or actually felt in his or her own speech muscles while watching the speaker. Many speech readers silently imitate the movements of the speaker while watching the speaker talk to help translate the visual image into a recognizable motor image (Davis & Silverman, 1978).

When we think of speech and speech training we generally assume it is the instruction of articulation. Almost everyone can picture the small child sitting with a lighted candle, practicing the "pah" sound of the letter "p," which when articulated correctly, will extinguish the flame. Although this is an important aspect of speech, it is by far not the only one. *Articulation* is the formation of individual speech sounds by shaping the flow of breath from the larynx out through the mouth. *Voice* is another important component of speech and is produced by respiration, phonation, and resonation. These occur simultaneously to produce changes in pitch, loudness, and quality of voice (Davis & Silverman, 1978). Because these are characteristics of speech that we tend to monitor by what sounds appropriate, they are difficult to learn. This explains the common tendencies of a deaf person's voice to be monotonous, abnormally high or low in pitch, or an inappropriate volume. Articulation and voice, when working together, make up a third component of speech, *rhythm*. Rhythm includes the features of accent, emphasis, intonation, phrasing, and rate (Davis & Silverman). These are all characteristics that we acquire effortlessly in our native language but can render a deaf person incomprehensible.

Although almost all deaf people have had some oral training, many do not use it as their primary mode of communication. Instead, they use a form of visual–gestural or manual communication. This includes the use of gestures, manual codes, and sign language.

Because many deaf people come from families of normal-hearing members, the use of gestures is often started early to communicate basic needs and commands. These gestures, sometimes general in nature, when specific to something within the family are often referred to as *home signs*. Although a deaf person might be fluent in sign language, if the person he or she is trying to communicate with is not, gestures might be the most appropriate means.

Manual codes are systems that attempt to represent a spoken language manually. Examples of these include signed English and cued speech. It is important to understand that these are not true languages. Signed English attempts to use signs to represent all parts of spoken English, including plurals, possessives, contractions, prefixes, and suffixes. Cued speech is a system of hand markers on or about the face to provide speech cues to a speech reader. Manual codes typically do not achieve the results they strive for partly because the users do not follow the rigorous set of rules consistently; also, since the nature of the English language is spoken, it cannot be reproduced within the limits of a manual code.

American Sign Language (ASL), however, is a true language. It meets all the requirements of the definition of a language, including its own complete grammatical structure, syntax, semantics, and set of rules that the user must follow to ensure understanding. ASL uses an ever-expanding vocabulary of signs as well as fingerspelling and nonmanual grammatical markers. Each sign is executed by a specific hand shape, movement, orientation of the palm and site of contact on the body. ***Fingerspelling*** is the use of a set of 26 single hand shapes that correspond to the 26 letters of the alphabet. Fingerspelling is used most often for proper names or when a specific term is used that does not already have a corresponding sign. Nonmanual grammatical markers are as important in ASL as tone, pitch, and intonation are in spoken English. They provide information vital to the meaning of the message, such as mood, intent, and even punctuation.

Although the two forms of communication are distinctly different, they have one thing in common, which is of interest to those professionals working with them: the use of interpreters. An interpreter's primary function is to aid in communication between deaf and hearing consumers. The interpreter is responsible for accurately conveying the message from one consumer to the other without becoming involved. This is not to say that the interpreter is robot-like but rather that the presence of the interpreter should not bias the interaction.

Technology for the deaf

The deaf community is already becoming accustomed to the daily uses of technology for independence. Whereas technology for the blind often uses sound, technological aids in the deaf world use the sense of sight. Light is a common visual cue that can be found in the deaf person's environment as a substitute for sound. Lights wired to conventional doorbells or pressure-sensitive devices that flash in response to a knock on the door alert the deaf person of a visitor. Similarly, a flashing light installed by the bed and attached to the alarm clock lets the deaf person know it is time to get up. Lights are also used to signify a ringing telephone.

The telephone has been accessible to the deaf community since the invention of the **teletypewriter** by Robert Weitbrecht in 1964 (Gannon, 1981). In its original form, the teletypewriter was a large machine with a typewriter keyboard. Typing out a message was done manually and when connected by telephone could be used to send messages by calling another teletypewriter. Today, teletypewriters are small enough to fit in a briefcase and are able to send messages along electrical screens. The teletypewriter is now available with a built-in answering machine that leaves printed messages.

Of all the devices used today, the one that provides the most accessibility to daily living is closed-caption television. Closed captioning is a process whereby the dialogue of the program is printed within the transmission. For those who have a closed-caption machine, this printed dialogue can be accessed. It comes across the bottom of the screen as it is being spoken. For those who do not access the transmission, the print is not visible, nor does it disrupt the program. When President George Bush signed the Americans with Disabilities Act in July 1990, he enacted a law that required all televisions manufactured after the year 1993 to include closed captioning. The cost of this additional mechanism is nominal compared with the cost of a television's normal sound mechanism.

Considerations when working with the deaf–blind

The deaf–blind person can benefit from many of the same strategies as the blind or deaf person when residual senses continue to have functional abilities. When this is no longer the case, creativity becomes a necessary characteristic in dealing with common obstacles.

Communication is one such obstacle. Because of the various options, it is important to find out how the deaf–blind person prefers to communicate. For the deaf–blind person who already knows sign language, this often continues to be the preferred mode of communication (Figure 18-50). When the deaf–blind person is the speaker, the signing takes place normally, including the nonmanual grammatical features. When the deaf–blind person is the "listener," the sense that receives the message is often

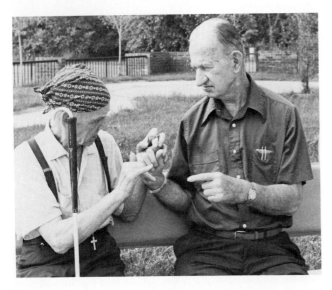

FIGURE 18-50. *The deaf–blind person is receiving his companion's fingerspelling tactually with his left hand while fingerspelling with his own right hand. (Photo courtesy of Ann Wade.)*

the tactile sense rather than the visual. The most common way for this to occur is for the deaf–blind person to rest one or both hands lightly over the speaker's hands and receive the input of the hand shapes, movement, and palm orientation necessary to comprehension. Fingerspelling is also perceived this way, which seems an amazing accomplishment for those who have tried it.

Another form of tactile communication may be more appropriate for those with stronger oral skills. This method is called the *Tadoma method* and requires even closer contact with the speaker. The deaf–blind person places his or her hand on the face of the speaker with the thumb gently touching the lips with the other fingers spread over the cheek, jaw and throat. As speech is produced, the deaf–blind person is able to feel the muscular movement of the face and throat as well as the vibrations of the nasal areas to understand the speech patterns.

Mobility for the deaf–blind person also involves direct body contact when using the services of a sighted human guide (Figure 18-51). This method involves the deaf–blind person holding onto the sighted person's arm just above the elbow. This enables the deaf–blind person to remain one step back and slightly behind the sighted guide, providing protection to the deaf–blind person's body. The sighted guide can give cues by moving his or her arm or by changes in step to alert the deaf–blind person to obstacles, such as stairs, ramps, doors, elevators, and curbs. Obstacles such as stairs and moving in and out of cars require special care and skills, which is why special training is necessary not only for the guide but also for the deaf–blind consumer.

Technology for the deaf–blind

For many deaf–blind people, the tactile sense becomes a dominant one for perceiving the environment, both inside and outside the home. Where lights are typically used to alert a deaf person of ringing telephones and doorbells, a deaf–blind person's home can have similarly functional cues. One such method is the use of strategically placed, low frequency fans. The fans

generate a sensation that the deaf–blind person learns to detect and understand. The placement of the fans and the direction of the air flow can indicate to the deaf–blind person whether, for example, the doorbell or the telephone is ringing.

Vibration is another commonly used tactile source of information. A flat, vibrating pad placed under the pillow can be connected to the clock to act as an alarm. Advances are also being made with mobility aids using this mode. Long-cane techniques for the blind normally provide many auditory cues to the user about the terrain. Electronic canes are being developed to provide vibratory input to aid in mobility.

As important as communication is for the deaf and the blind, it is equally so for the deaf–blind. Even the telephone has become an everyday household appliance. The Telebraille is a device that can be attached to a person's teletypewriter to con-

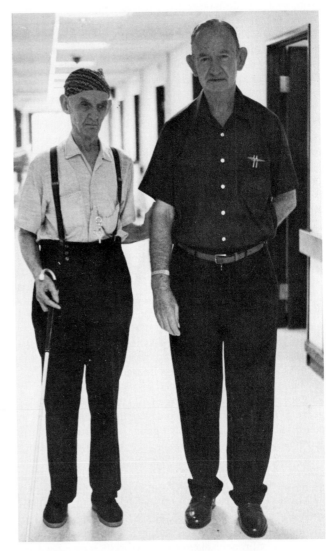

FIGURE 18-51. *When he and his companion begin to move, the blind gentleman will drop back a half step, maintaining grasp at or just above his companion's elbow. White cane technique is adequate for navigating the hall independently in spite of obstacles, but a crowded lobby and walking outdoors are more comfortably managed with a sighted guide. (Photo courtesy of Ann Wade.)*

vert the printed message into Braille (Kates & Schein, 1980; Sardegna & Paul, 1991). The deaf–blind person then sends a response back by typing the Braille message, which is converted back to a normal printed form and sent by the teletypewriter. With Telebraille, it is possible for the deaf–blind person to speak with anyone who has a teletypewriter.

Summary

The senses of sight and hearing are miraculous in their functions and their contribution to human existence. Even when these senses are impaired or absent, however, people can enjoy an independent and stimulating life. The occupational therapist, working with the fundamental tools of the profession and with advances in technology, can aid in increasing the independence and quality of life for those who live with sensory loss. For the occupational therapist working with this population, it is important to be informed about sensory deficits, not only to determine the best treatment program but also to assist the client in building a therapeutic relationship. Through this positive relationship, meeting the challenges of sensory loss can be a positive and beneficial experience for both parties.

References

American Occupational Therapy Association. (1990). *1990 Member data survey summary report.* Rockville, MD: AOTA.

Davis, H., & Silverman, S. (1978). *Hearing and deafness* (3rd ed.). New York: Holt, Reinhart and Winston.

Eden, J. (1978). *The eye book.* New York: Viking.

Gannon, J. (1981). *Deaf heritage: A narrative history of deaf America.* Silver Spring, MD: National Association of the Deaf.

Hotchkiss, D. (1989). *Demographic aspects of hearing impairment: Questions and answers* (2nd ed.). Washington DC: Gallaudet University.

Kates, L., & Schein, J. (1980). *A complete guide to communication with deaf-blind persons.* Silver Spring, MD: National Association of the Deaf.

Lowenfeld, B. (1971). *Our blind children: Growing and learning with them* (3rd ed.). Springfield, IL: Charles C. Thomas.

Lowenfeld, B. (1973). *The visually handicapped child in school.* New York: John Day.

McWilliams, P. (1984). *Personal computers and the disabled.* Garden City, NY: Quantum Press.

Mindel, E., & McCay, V. (1971). *They grow in silence: The deaf child and his family.* Silver Springs, MD: National Association of the Deaf.

Murphy, W. (1982). *Touch, taste, smell, sight, and hearing.* Morristown, NJ: Silver Burdett.

Sardegna, J., & Paul, T. (1991). *The encyclopedia of blindness and vision impairment.* New York: Facts on File.

Smith, J. (1989). *Senses and sensibilities.* New York: John Wiley and Sons.

Taylor, B. (1975). *Blind pre-school.* Colorado Springs, CO: SPED Publications.

Tweedie, D., & Shroyer, E. (Eds.). (1982). *The multihandicapped hearing impaired.* Washington DC: Gallaudet College Press.

Bibliography

American Occupational Therapy Association. (1980). *Hearing impaired/visual impaired.* Rockville, MD: AOTA.

Chaney, E. (1990). *The eyes have it.* York Beach, ME: Samuel Weiser.

Cherow, E. (Ed.). (1985). *Hearing impaired children and youth with developmental disabilities.* Washington DC: Gallaudet College Press.

Deafness Research and Training Center. (1973). *Electronic communication With deaf and deaf-blind persons.* New York: New York University.

Doyle, P., Goodman, J., Grotsky, J., & Mann, L. (1979). *Helping the severely handicapped child.* New York: Thomas Y. Crowell.

Furth, H. (1973). *Deafness and learning: A psychosocial approach.* Belmont, CA: Wadsworth, 1973.

Gallaudet College Department of Sociology Social Work Program. (1975). *An orientation to deafness for social workers: Papers from the workshop.* Washington DC: Gallaudet College.

Gearheart, B., & Weishahn, M. (1976). *The handicapped child in the regular classroom.* St. Louis: C. V. Mosby.

Gonzalez-Crussi, F. (1989). *The five senses.* San Diego: Harcourt Brace Jovanovich.

Heller, B., & Watson, B. (Eds.). (1983). *Mental health and deafness strategic perspectives.* Silver Springs, MD: American Deafness and Rehabilitation Association.

McCrone, W., Beachm R,, & Zieziula, F. (Eds.). (1983). *Networking and deafness.* Silver Springs, MD: American Deafness and Rehabilitation Association.

Naiman, D. (1980). *Education for severely handicapped hearing impaired students.* Silver Springs, MD: National Association of the Deaf.

National Association for Hearing and Speech Action. (1986). *Directory of assistive listening devices.* Rockville, MD: Author

Owellette, S., & Lloyd, G. (Eds.). (1980). *Independent living skills for the severely handicapped deaf person preparing to enter gainful employment.* Silver Springs, MD: American Deafness and Rehabilitation Association.

Ritter, A., & Hopkins, K. (1985). *A deafness collection: Selected and annotated.* Rochester, NY: National Technical Institute for the Deaf at Rochester Institute of Technology.

Schubert, E. (1980). *Hearing: Its function and dysfunction.* New York: Springer-Verlag.

Spencer, M. (1960). *Blind children in family and community.* Minneapolis: University of Minnesota Press.

Stahlecker, T., Glass, L., & Machalow, S. (Eds.). (1985). *State of the art: Research priorities in deaf-blindness.* San Francisco: Center on Mental Health and Deafness.

Tweedie, D., & Shroyer, E. (Eds.). (1982). *The multihandicapped hearing impaired.* Washington DC: Gallaudet College Press.

Vail, D. (1950). *The truth about your eyes.* New York: Farrar, Straus.

Ward, B. (1977). *The ear and hearing.* New York: Franklin Watts.

Watson, D., Anderson, G., Marut, P., Owellette, S., & Ford, N. (1983). *Vocational evaluation of hearing-impaired persons: Research and practice,* Little Rock: Arkansas Rehabilitation Research and Training Center on Deafness and Hearing Impairment.

Watson, D., Anderson, G., Owellette, S., Ford, N., & Marut, P. (Eds.). (1983). *Adjustment services for hearing-impaired persons: Research and practice.* Little Rock: Arkansas Rehabilitation Research and Training Center on Deafness and Hearing Impairment.

Watson, D., Barrett, S., & Brown, R. (Eds.). (1983). *A model service delivery system for deaf-blind persons.* Little Rock: Arkansas Rehabilitation Research and Training Center on Deafness and Hearing Impairment.

SECTION 7

HIV infection and AIDS

MICHAEL PIZZI

LEARNING OBJECTIVES

Upon completion of this section the reader will be able to:

1. *Describe the spectrum of HIV disease and its impact on occupational behaviors of men, women, and children.*

2. *Describe the themes of occupational science that underlie practice in occupational therapy related to patients with HIV and AIDS.*

3. *Define the physical, psychosocial, and environmental needs of people with HIV infection and AIDS.*

4. *Explain the assessment process and assess people with HIV infection and AIDS with an understanding of the unique occupational needs of this population.*

5. *Develop appropriate treatment plans, goals, and strategies for people with HIV infection and AIDS.*

Human immunodeficiency virus (HIV) infection and **acquired immunodeficiency syndrome** (AIDS) are considered in the United States to be social as well as medical diseases. In addition to the millions of people infected, there are millions more *affected*—those who are somehow linked, directly or indirectly, with a person with HIV infection.

This section explores the epidemiology and virology of HIV; the physical, psychosocial and environmental aspects of the disease; occupational therapy theory in relation to HIV and AIDS; and occupational therapy assessment and treatment. Women, adolescents, and children with HIV and AIDS are also discussed separately because they reflect the growing population of those infected and affected. This section deals primarily with adults with HIV infection type 1 and AIDS.

HIV infection and AIDS

In 1982, the *Morbidity and Mortality Weekly Report* (Centers for Disease Control, 1982) reported that five gay men from New York and California had been diagnosed with Kaposi sarcoma, a cancer traditionally seen in older men of Mediterranean origin, and *Pneumocystis* pneumonia, commonly seen in severely impaired cancer patients. Within a brief period of time, intravenous drug users and hemophiliacs were becoming infected. In the same year, children experiencing the same cluster of symptoms and similar features were observed.

Human immunodeficiency virus is transmitted by several routes: through unprotected sexual intercourse with an infected person (primarily anal and vaginal), by exposure to contaminated blood (either through shared injection equipment associated with intravenous drug use or transfusion), and from mother to fetus. Once acquired, HIV lives in the body for life. Despite the often seemingly healthy appearance of an infected person who is asymptomatic, an infected person is always contagious and can spread the virus only through one of the three transmission routes described.

Human immunodeficiency virus is a retrovirus. Retroviruses are prevalent in many animals and have only recently been described in humans. The backward flow of information from RNA to DNA—the reverse of most genetic message movement—gives the virus its family name. Reverse transcriptase, an enzyme in the body, makes the reverse movement possible.

The primary targets of HIV are the T4 cells, also known as CD4 cells.

CD4 cells perform a multitude of essential functions in the immune system. They specifically recognize and proliferate in response to antigens (foreign molecules) that they encounter in the body, at the same time releasing a variety of proteins known as lymphokines that regulate other immune system cells. Upon signaling by CD4 cells, cells known as B lymphocytes, recognizing antigens, secrete specific antibodies to neutralize or eliminate antigenic bacteria and viruses as they travel through body fluids between cells. Similarly, following recognition of antigens and signaling from CD4 cells, some CD8 cells called cytotoxic T cells become activated to kill cells infected with intracellular pathogens; others called suppressor T cells dampen an ongoing immune response. Furthermore, CD4 cells are known to modulate the activities of immune system cells known as natural killer cells and macrophages, which are involved in responses to infection and perhaps to incipient malignancies. (Institute of Medicine, 1988, p. 43)

The codiscoverers of the virus, Gallo and Montagnier (1988), believed that the virus had existed in small, isolated groups in people in central Africa or elsewhere for years. Because these groups had little contact with the outside world, HIV stayed within the groups. As the way of life changed in central Africa, however, the pattern of transmission most likely was affected. Migration from remote areas to urban centers increased, sexual mores changed, and blood transfusions became more common. "Once a pool of infected people had been established, transport networks and the generalized exchange of blood products would have carried it to every corner of the world" (Gallo & Montagnier, 1988, p. 47).

It is estimated that there are 1 to 1.5 million infected people in the United States and 10 million around the world, with over 80% still asymptomatic and unaware of their seropositive status.

The latency period (time from initial infection to symptoms) can be anywhere from 7 to 12 years in adults. This varies because of personal health histories, number of exposures to the virus, and other factors (Miller, Turner, & Moses, 1990).

Stages of HIV infection

Four stages of HIV infection were classified by the Centers for Disease Control. These stages were developed early in the epidemic for purposes of tracking the natural history of the epidemic. Before any of the stages, there is a group of people known as the *worried well.* These are people who may engage in high-risk behaviors (behaviors that put them at risk for HIV infection) and suffer from anxiety. Some may be infected yet not symptomatic.

In stage 1, the person experiences symptoms of an acute nature, often within 3 weeks of infection. This stage is characterized by fever, lymphadenopathy (swollen lymph glands), fatigue and other mononucleosis-like symptoms, and less commonly, aseptic meningitis or rash. This stage is often associated with seroconversion (appearance of antibodies to HIV). Stage 2 is the period after initial infection and is the asymptomatic period. People can be asymptomatic for months to several years. In stage 3, the person has the symptom of lymphadenopathy. A number of people with HIV with no other symptoms have persistent generalized lymphadenopathy. In stage 4, HIV-infected people with clinical symptoms can be divided into several groups based on type and severity of symptoms. Some may have constitutional symptoms, such as fever, weight loss, and diarrhea, which are persistent and are not related to anything else except HIV. Other people suffer from neurologic manifestations, such as cognitive, affective, and sensory changes due to dementia, myelopathy, and peripheral neuropathies, which are a direct result of HIV disease. Others may have classic opportunistic infections, such as Kaposi sarcoma or *Pneumocystic carinii* pneumonia, that are diagnostic of AIDS (Report of the Presidential Commission on HIV, 1988). For a more complete listing of signs and symptoms of HIV sensory and neurologic sequelae, refer to Galantino (1992).

Physical considerations

People with the HIV virus who are asymptomatic may, over time, develop fatigue, shortness of breath, visual impairments, peripheral and central nervous system damage, various forms of cancer, opportunistic infections, cardiac problems, and the wasting syndrome (DeVita, Hellman, & Rosenberg, 1988). Physical pain is often noted, especially in people with peripheral nervous system damage. Postural changes can occur secondary to wasting syndrome and severe weight loss, which can also result in physical pain (Galantino, Mukand, & Freed, 1991). Neuropathies are common and are evident in both the upper and lower extremities. Central nervous system damage results in dementia, spinal cord dysfunction, and stroke. People with central and peripheral nervous system damage show evidence of gait, balance, and general mobility problems as well as changes in muscle tone. ROM, strength, coordination, and sensation can be affected, resulting in mild to severe changes in function.

The continuum of function and dysfunction is unique for each person with HIV. Often, physical problems impede function in self-care, work, and leisure activities. Daily occupational routines are impaired due to the progressive and variable nature of the disease. For example, tasks that normally required 45 minutes to complete may now take 2 hours with intermittent rests due to pain and fatigue. Physical problems must be fully assessed for their effect on occupational roles (Galantino & Pizzi, 1991).

Psychosocial considerations

Human immunodeficiency virus is a disease that is often viewed as a "death sentence." People with HIV can easily become immobilized by the diagnosis alone. Depression, anxiety, guilt, and preoccupation with illness and imminent death are characteristic. People with HIV are often angry at the disease, at the discrimination that usually accompanies it, at the prospect of a lonely and painful death, at the lack of treatments, at medical staff, and at themselves (U. S. Department of Health and Human Services, 1986).

Anxiety may be manifested as tension, stress, tachycardia, agitation, insomnia, anorexia, and panic attacks. Denial may alternate with realistic concerns or hypochondria. People with HIV may interpret any new symptom as bringing them closer to death. This can perpetuate an already maladaptive cycle of behavior. In most cases, there are neuropsychiatric symptoms, such as forgetfulness, lack of concentration, apathy, withdrawal, and decreased alertness. In the later stages of the illness, there may be severe confusion and disorientation (DeVita et al., 1988; Navis, Jordan, & Price, 1986).

Physical disfigurement caused by AIDS often leads to problems with self-image. Physical disfigurement and neuropsychiatric dysfunction may result in limited social and occupational activity. There may exist a poor sense of control over the environment and a perception of loss of mastery of the self. People with HIV often state that the disease controls their lives, contributing to a sense of helplessness and hopelessness. This sense may result in decreased function and a loss of favored activities. A sense of the future is threatened, and occupational goals need to be prioritized and redefined in light of the disease process. The meaningfulness of activity is often critically analyzed by the person with HIV. In these areas of goal planning and activity analysis, the occupational therapist can offer unique skills to people with HIV (Pizzi, Mukand, & Freed, 1991).

People with HIV who have high standards of performance, organize time rigidly, have difficulty identifying other interests to replace work, or are compulsive workers at risk for psychosocial dysfunction (Pizzi, 1988; Pizzi et al., 1991). Adaptation of life roles is needed. Grief and bereavement issues related to the loss of a variety of roles should be examined by the occupational therapist in conjunction with other team members.

Environmental considerations

The social, physical, cultural, and even economic environments of people with HIV must be considered. Most people with HIV have already been stigmatized by society. Gay or bisexual men and intravenous drug users comprise most of people with HIV and have had to contend with discrimination. The occupational therapist must be aware of the perceived stigma felt by people with HIV and provide a safe and comfortable therapeutic milieu.

Family members must often cope with a relative who reveals HIV seropositivity and, at the same time, that he or she is gay, bisexual, or an intravenous drug user. This can lead to alienation by the family, leaving the person without a support system. Also, the significant other (spouse, lover, roommate) of the person with HIV may leave the situation for any number of reasons (eg, guilt, fear of the disease process, fear of also being infected, or perceived inability to care for the infected person). Health care providers may have value systems that differ from those of the person with HIV or may suffer from irrational fear of HIV itself. The occupational therapist must be aware of these possibilities as they affect the occupational therapy process and the patient's functioning.

People with symptomatic HIV may have difficulty negotiating physical environments. Fatigue, shortness of breath, and central and peripheral nervous system damage may affect mobility in the community, at work, or at home. Visual and sensory problems may also make it difficult to negotiate physical environments.

Economic loss experienced by the inability to work can dramatically affect interactions with the physical and social environments. The loss may be so profound that the person with HIV may need to find alternative housing or may even become a homeless person. Loss of friends, in part due to the inability to keep up financially (for movies, going out to dinner, leisure trips), will alter socialization; fears of future losses can prevent making new friends. The occupational therapist must consider the economic situation of the patient before making treatment recommendations, particularly if the patient must purchase adaptive equipment and materials to maintain productivity (Pizzi et al., 1991; Pizzi, 1991).

Occupational therapy intervention

It is essential that occupational therapists start from an ***occupational science*** perspective to guide practice with clinical research in HIV disease. (See Chapter 3 for an overview of occupational science.) Several themes of occupational science that guide occupational therapy practice for people with HIV and AIDS can be described as symbolism, control, temporal rhythms, wellness through occupation, occupational role, and environment (Clark & Jackson, 1990).

Symbolism refers to meaningfulness of occupations to a person within the sociocultural and historical context of that person's life. Symbolic meaning varies among people. Examples include having a favorite stuffed animal in bed when one is 35 and terminal that provides security and comfort after years of suffering discrimination, or making craft objects and wrapping them for the child that a parent-to-be living with AIDS might never see.

Control relates to the ability to have and maintain control over one's life, purposefulness, and productive living. "The capacity to exercise control over one's life is a variable that fluctuates from one person to the next. It must be seen as an extension of earlier life experiences" (Pizzi, 1984, p. 253). People with HIV and AIDS often feel that all control has been taken away and that life and one's subsequent productive actions are dictated by the virus harbored in one's body. Mastering and controlling one's destiny and productive pursuits is vital for people with HIV and

AIDS throughout the disease process (Clark & Jackson, 1990; Pizzi, 1990b; Schindler, 1988).

Temporal rhythms relate to the organization of time and occupations. Priority occupations are identified and pursued, and the occupational therapist assists with developing adaptive strategies to maintain one's natural temporal rhythms (Pizzi, 1988, 1989a, 1990b). Futuristic treatment planning is suggested to diminish possibilities of psychosocial dysfunction related to loss of roles, skills, and habits throughout disease progression (Pizzi, 1990b).

Wellness through occupation occurs when people are engaged in productive and meaningful occupations of their choice that are within the sociocultural context of their lives. Many people with HIV are between the ages of 20 and 60 years, which are the productive, working years. One of the most stressful losses a person incurs while living with HIV is the loss of the worker role. In one study, changes in work situation were viewed as highly stressful by 60% of respondents (Pizzi, unpublished). Stress has been shown to contribute to immunosuppression (Jemmott & Locke, 1984; Solomon, Temoshak, O'Leary, & Zich, 1987; Ironson et al., 1990). Wellness can be fostered in occupational therapy through adaptation of chosen roles, habits, and skills for people with HIV and AIDS, thereby also fostering a stronger and more competent immune system (Clark & Jackson, 1990; Pizzi, unpublished).

Occupational roles are defined as "the part enacted by the individual which enables him or her to fulfill self and social expectations as a player, student, worker, homemaker or retiree" (Yerxa et al., 1989, p. 16). Over time, engagement in occupational roles shifts in levels of productivity and function, and role changes occur for both the patient and caregivers. Role transitions need to be made, and often, caregivers must undertake certain role functions formerly occupied by the patient as the patient increasingly has difficulty performing tasks. Loss of roles such as friend, worker, and player can result in maladaptive occupational behaviors. Clark and Jackson (1990) state that "eventually 'work' might become executing the process of dying in such a way so that preemptory concerns are addressed, obligations are met, and a shortened life is experienced to its fullest" (p. 81). In an adaptive way, even the sick role known to Western medicinal clinicians can be transformed to a productive and valued role for the patient and caregivers.

Environment is an essential theme to consider and is vital to holistic assessment and treatment of people with HIV and AIDS. It encompasses the physical, social, and cultural aspects of daily living. For people with HIV and AIDS, it is essential to provide safe, comfortable, and secure environments so they can engage in productive and meaningful occupations for as long as possible. Occupational therapy's historical roots are in "moral treatment," and social environments resembled family units that were supportive and nonjudgmental about functional abilities. Approaches of caregivers were kind, considerate, and emphasized strong therapeutic relationships and positive outcomes no matter the diagnosis or stage of illness. It is essential that these same types of approaches be used by occupational therapists for people with HIV and AIDS. Respect for and knowledge of cultural diversity and religious and spiritual beliefs and values also influences therapeutic outcomes. Finally, physical environments need to be created and adapted for accessibility, safety, comfort, and to facilitate productive living.

Occupational therapy assessment

An assessment battery for adults with HIV and AIDS was proposed by Pizzi (1990b) to holistically examine function. For many people with HIV and AIDS, however, time constraints can limit the extent to which the battery can be administered. The Pizzi Assessment of Productive Living (PAPL) for Adults with HIV Infection and AIDS was developed in consideration of limited time and endurance of many patients and to holistically assess all domains of function and occupational behaviors (see the display on pages 720 and 721).

Before assessment, it is vital that the occupational therapist be aware of the stage of illness and extraordinary precautions needed (eg, mask because patient has tuberculosis that is transmitted by air). Also, if the therapist has a slight cough, sneezing, or other symptom of an illness, it is vital to assess one's own likelihood of transmission to the patient and to take precautions when treating immunosuppressed patients. The occupational therapist may be the first health care person to touch, hold, or work nonjudgmentally with a person with HIV infection or AIDS, and the therapist should acknowledge the positive impact of this human contact on patient care.

The PAPL has several sections: demographics, physical assessment, ADL, work and leisure, time organization, environment, psychosocial function, and occupational questions. Therapists need to assess the extent to which patients can tolerate the assessment, and they may have to administer the assessment over time. In the demographics section, it is important to know the stage of illness because that can help with future treatment planning. The identified caregiver and the people living with the patient may not be the same, and this data can assist when working with social environment and social skills. Past medical history is important because people with HIV may have had numerous complications due to the disease as well as numerous hospitalizations, times of inactivity, and role changes. In addition, they may have had to cope with different medical systems and repeated discrimination. It is also vital to note medications, life-sustaining drugs, and their side effects since they enhance or impede occupational behaviors and performance (Table 18-3).

The physical assessment is a general assessment of physical function and underlying neurologic, musculoskeletal, and cognitive processes. It is important to note side effects of drug interventions as well as past medical history whereby function had already been compromised.

Activities of daily living, work, and leisure are primary areas of occupations engaged in by most people. It is important to note physical and psychosocial variables that impact on these areas and that may limit or enhance performance. In ADL, both personal and instrumental areas need to be addressed. If a person is independent in personal ADL but cannot shop or do laundry due to fatigue or generalized weakness, these may be areas for intervention and for involvement of community support networks.

Given that most people with HIV or AIDS are between 20 and 60 years of age, they often are gainfully employed and may be having work adjustment problems. Therapists fully assess work as a productive occupation as well as the need to adapt skills, habits, or environments to maintain the worker role. If the person is not working but work normally is a primary role for the person, it is important to note physical, psychosocial, and environmental reasons for not working.

Leisure and play need to be addressed in terms of types of occupations (sedentary versus active), environments in which they occur, and how often they occur. Adaptation in any of these areas, as needed, can lead to enhanced productivity.

For ADL, work, and leisure, therapists need to assess the level of importance and meaningfulness of any of these activities and the level of independence the patient may choose. For example, if the occupational therapist knows that adaptive equipment can facilitate independence in bathing but that both the patient and the caregiver choose to have the caregiver bathe the patient, then this may not be an area for occupational therapy intervention in terms of facilitating independence.

Daily routine assessment helps the therapist, patient, and caregiver determine any changes that have occurred since diagnosis in the patient's normal routine. Information about level of flexibility in how the patient organizes time and activity is vital because, over time, HIV alters performance and the amount of time any chosen occupation takes to perform. It is also important to note if the patient performs occupations better at certain times of day.

Assessment of the patient's physical, social, and cultural environment helps to determine the extent to which it impedes or enhances function and productivity. The physical environment is assessed for accessibility and safety. The social environment is assessed for level of support to patient, role stress, caregiver burden, and occupations engaged in with the patient that may have been altered due to HIV. Cultural considerations enhance the occupational therapy process by examining cultural beliefs, values, and rituals and incorporating those as much as possible in the occupational therapy program.

Stressors for people with HIV are unique and need to be acknowledged by the occupational therapist because they affect occupational behaviors. These stressors can include not working, performing daily tasks, or engaging in meaningful leisure occupations and extend through perceived discrimination, loss of medical insurance, and having a life-threatening illness. Other stressors with which the patient must cope can include numerous daily losses of function, support systems, and friends to the same disease (Faulstich, 1987; Kiecolt-Glaser & Glaser, 1988; Servellen, Lewis, & Leake, 1990; Kassel, 1991; Pizzi, unpublished). It was previously noted that stress is a cofactor regarding immunosuppression and HIV. Occupational therapists need to recognize the stress management techniques that the patient currently uses so that these can be incorporated into the occupational therapy plan of treatment.

Finally, occupational questions can glean information about the patient's sense of accomplishment and completion, locus of control, meaningfulness of occupations, and any other issues the patient wishes to share. These can provide initial rapport building and can help demonstrate the therapist's care and concern for important and valued areas of concern to the patient.

Other assessment tools are used by occupational therapists to supplement the PAPL, many of which are also used in hospice care (see Chapter 30). These include the ADL Checklist for People with Chronic or Terminal Illness and the Hospice Assessment of Occupational Function (see Chapter 30); the Role Checklist (Oakley, Kielhofner, Barris, & Reichler, 1986); the Level of Interest in Particular Activities (Scaffa, 1981); the Social Environment Interview (Pizzi, 1989b); and specific work assessments (see Chapter 8, Section 2).

PIZZI ASSESSMENT OF PRODUCTIVE LIVING FOR ADULTS WITH HIV INFECTION AND AIDS

Demographics

Name _____ Age _____ Sex _____
Lives with (relationship) _____
Identified caregiver _____
Race _____ Culture _____ Religion _____ Practicing? _____
Primary occupational roles _____
Primary diagnosis _____
Secondary diagnosis _____
Stage of HIV _____
Past medical history _____
Medications _____

Activities of Daily Living (use ADL performance assessment)

Are you doing these now? _____
Do you perform homemaking tasks? _____
(For areas of difficulty) Would you like to be able to do these again like you did before? Which ones? _____

Work

Job _____ When last worked _____
Describe type of activity _____
Work environment _____
If not working, would you like to be able to? _____
Do you miss being productive? _____

Play/Leisure

Types of activities engaged in _____
_____
Are you doing these now? _____
If not, would you like to? _____ Which ones? _____
Would you like to try other things as well? _____
Is it important to be independent in daily living activities? _____

Physical Function

Active/passive range of motion:
Strength:
Sensation:
Coordination (gross and fine motor/dexterity):
Visual–perceptual:
Hearing:
Balance (sit and stand):
Ambulation/transfers/mobility:
Activity tolerance/endurance:
Physical pain:
    Location: _____
    Does it interfere with doing important activities? _____
Sexual function:

Cognition

(attention span, problem solving, memory, orientation, judgment, reasoning, decision making, safety awareness)

(continued)

PIZZI ASSESSMENT OF PRODUCTIVE LIVING FOR ADULTS WITH HIV INFECTION AND AIDS (*continued*)

Time Organization

Former daily routine (before diagnosis) _____
Has this changed since diagnosis? _____ If so, how? _____
Are there certain times of day that are better for you to carry out daily living tasks?
Do you consider yourself regimented or flexible in organizing time and activity? _____
What would you change, if anything, in how your day is set up? _____

Body Image/Self-Image

In the last 6 months, has there been a recent change in your physical appearance? ___
How do you feel about this? _____

Social Environment

(describe support available and used by patient)

Physical Environment

(describe environments where patient performs daily tasks and level of support or
     impediment for function)

Stressors

What are some things, people, or situations that are or were stressful?
What are some ways you manage stress?

Situational Coping

How do you feel you are dealing with:
a. your diagnosis
b. changes in your ability to do things important to you
c. other psychosocial observations

Occupational Questions

What do you consider to be important to you right now?
Do you feel you can do things important to you now? In the future?
Do you deal well with change?
What are some of your hopes, dreams, aspirations? What are some of your goals?
Have these changed since you were diagnosed? _____ How? _____
Do you feel in control of your life at this time?
What do you wish to accomplish with the rest of your life?
Plan:
Short-term goals:
Long-term goals:
Frequency:
Duration:
Therapist:

Copyright 1991 by Michael Pizzi, MS, OTR/L, CHES. Adapted with permission.

Treatment

The major focus of occupational therapy treatment of adults with
HIV and AIDS is to restore and maintain functional performance
of self-chosen occupations that enhance competent performance of valued occupational roles. The common primary treatment focuses on adaptation and occupation to revitalize the
human spirit and to restore order and control. Data from the

PAPL and other assessments provide necessary information to
plan specific, individualized treatment.

There are several considerations for therapists when developing treatment plans and goals due to the many unique
features of HIV:

1. Any treatment may indicate necessity for universal precautions. Check with your department and hospital policies and
   primarily use common sense.

TABLE 18-3. *Agents for the Treatment of HIV Infection Antiviral*

Agent	Purpose	Effect
Antiviral		
AL721	Alters outer envelope of HIV	Little objective evidence has supported this agent's use
	Inhibits infectivity of HIV by preventing attachment of virus	Available over the counter
Azidothymidine (AZT); zidovudine (zdv); Retrovir	Antiviral	Toxicity: bone marrow
	Thymidine nucleoside analog	Blood transfusions may be needed for anemias
	Inhibits HIV replication	
Axidouridine (AzdU)	Similar to AZT	In phase 1 study
		Less toxic than AZT
Dideoxycytidine (DdC)	Cytidine nucleoside analog	Inhibits reverse transcriptase
		Toxicity: peripheral neuropathy; rash; stomatitis; fever
Dideoxyinosine Videx (Ddl)	Dideoxynucleoside agent	Inhibits reverse transcriptase
		Toxicity: peripheral neuropathy; acute pancreatitis
Dextran sulfate	Treatment for hyperlipidemia	Anticoagulant
	Interferes with the ability of HIV infected cells to form giant cells	Questionable antiviral activity, still under study
Peptide T	Mimics the HIV envelope protein, gp 120	Blocks CD4 receptor on T-helper cells
	Little toxicity	
Ribavirin	Antiviral	Under investigation
Immunomodulator		
Alpha-interferon	Antiviral	Inhibits transcription of viral messenger RNA and protein synthesis
	Antineoplastic	
	Immunomodulator	
	Treatment of HIV and Kaposi sarcoma	
Ampligen	Antiviral	Mismatched, double-stranded RNA that has viral activity against HIV
	Still under investigation	
Beta-interferon	Antiviral	Protein produced with recombinant technology
	Antineoplastic	
	Immunomodulator	
CD4	Soluble CD4 binds to the gp 120 receptor of HIV	Synthetic mimic of the CD4 molecule
	Blocks the ability to infect or destroy T4-helper cells	Studies at San Francisco General Hospital and the National Cancer Institute
Erythropoietin (EPO)	Stimulates bone marrow to produce viable erythroid precursors and red blood cells	Efficacious for the patient with anemia (Hct < 30)
Imuthiol (DTC)	Immune stimulator	Induces the liver to produce a substance, hepatosin, which is a thymic hormone
	Increases CD4 cells	
	Still under investigation	Antiabuse properties
Interleukin-2 (IL-2)	Glycoprotein by stimulated T-helper lymphocytes	Undergoing trials with antiviral agents
IMREG-1	Enhances production of IL-2 and gamma-interferon	Under investigation
Isoprinosine	Synthetic immunomodulator	Under investigation
Lentinan	Stimulates production of lymphokines	May be synergistic with AZT
	Enhances cell-mediated immunity	Under study at San Francisco General Hospital
Trichosanthin (Compound Q)	Selected inhibitory activity against HIV	Isolated from the Chinese cucumber root
		Under investigation

2. Subtle cognitive and physical status changes can occur rapidly, and reassessment is indicated each visit (although not formally). This is also true for hospice patients.

3. Most adults with HIV have experienced perceived or real discrimination. Having a nonjudgmental, open, caring and honest attitude and approach can make the difference in a therapy program.

4. There are more unique psychosocial aspects of HIV rehabilitation than in most other physical or psychosocial cases. Many people with HIV have lost numerous friends to the same disease for which they are receiving therapy; have undergone losses of work and family due to discrimination, rejection, or physical inabilities; and may have lost life partners to the same disease. All these losses, for many patients, occur before the age of 40. Women with HIV suffer similar losses, cope with poverty and homelessness, and are often underrecognized in this epidemic.

5. There is no known cure or vaccine for HIV to date, although the research is promising. This is a major consideration as a stressor of daily living.

6. Most patients with symptomatic HIV and AIDS have an altered worker role. Specific treatments regarding alternatives to work and productive living are necessary if work is a valued role. Physical as well as psychosocial work assessments for holistic work hardening programming is vital.

7. Fatigue and generalized weakness and deconditioning are primary physical manifestations of HIV. Energy conservation, work simplification, and occupational adaptations are used to enhance productivity.

8. Adaptive equipment and positioning are used to assist in return to independent performance of ADL, work, and leisure tasks. Often, people with HIV may reject such equipment even though it can benefit them. This rejection signals the rejection of the sick role and sometimes denial of being less able. This must be respected until the time when the person chooses, if at all, to use the equipment.

9. Habit training and adaptation of routine of daily living are essential treatments and include performance of favored occupations, with respect to physical and cognitive status; level at which the patient feels comfortable adapting routines; and times of day, environments, and with whom the patient chooses to perform occupations. Patients must be given choice of scheduling within their own normal routines and not those routines that fit the health care professional's schedule. Since HIV is progressive, adapting routines and occupations within those routines is vital to assist in maintenance of competence, mastery, and facilitation of positive feelings of self-worth and self-esteem.

10. Control and choices of daily living options must be provided as much as possible. Often, people with HIV feel a sense of loss of control as the virus slowly invades body systems and manifests itself in further occupational dysfunctions. Provision of occupations that promote occupational choice and provide a sense of control are essential concepts to consider in treatment.

11. Short-term and long-term goals may change and need to be readily adaptable.

12. Alternative options need to be considered in the array of treatments traditionally used by occupational therapists. These can include progressive relaxation, biofeedback, prayer, therapeutic touch, Chinese medicine techniques, myofascial release and craniosacral therapy, imagery, and visualization. Therapists need to know about current treatment methods employed by patients and not to judge those treatments but to be aware of their potential to harm or empower and heal. A person's belief system is the most powerful healing technique that can be used.

13. Proper nutrition is vital for people with HIV and can be incorporated into the occupational therapy program. "The therapist, in collaboration with the nutritionist, can develop strategies to meet the needs of a sound nutritional program in concert with activity level; enhance fatigue tolerance, and emphasize the importance of a wellness program" (Galantino & Pizzi 1991, p. 167).

Numerous and diverse treatment programs are evident in the literature. Treatment also helps the patient to resume chosen and valued occupational roles as independently as possible for as long as possible. Stress management and psychosocial treatments focused on self-empowerment, motivation, developing competence in occupational tasks and coping skills to prevent maladaption, as well as treatment sessions on nutrition and safer sex are emphasized for people who are HIV-positive but asymptomatic (Denton, 1987; Schindler, 1988; Pizzi, 1988, 1989a, 1990b; Gutterman, 1990). Exercise programming and aerobic training are also viewed as therapeutic strategies to enhance immunocompetence, diminish stress, and develop a positive sense of wellness (Galantino & Levy, 1988; Spence, Galantino, Mossberg, & Zimmerman, 1990; LaPerriere et al., 1990).

For people who are more symptomatic, strategies of energy conservation, adaptive equipment, neurodevelopmental treatment for those with neurologic damage, cognitive retraining and compensatory techniques, caregiver education, health promotion and wellness strategies to enhance immunocompetence and physical and psychosocial well-being, and adaptive strategies for environments, skills, and routines of daily living are emphasized (Denton, 1987; Pizzi, 1988, 1989a, 1990b; Pizzi et al., 1991; Gutterman, 1990; Weinstein, 1990). Pain management is also necessary at this stage for many patients. Myofascial release, craniosacral therapy, acupressure, biofeedback, imagery and visualization, and adaptations of skills and environments to facilitate productivity have been used with great success (Galantino & Pizzi 1991; Galantino et al., 1991; Pizzi et al., 1991). All psychosocial strategies used in the initial stage of HIV are also used throughout the disease process, adapted to physical and cognitive changes.

For people with AIDS, all of the above can apply, with modifications as needed. In the later stages of illness, therapists may also deal more extensively with grief, loss, and bereavement issues. Caregivers may need social support and assistance in making role transitions and activity and occupational routine modifications. Projects that symbolize completion of a life and immortality and occupations that may be spiritual in nature are indicated in this stage. It is also vital that therapists constantly examine proper positioning and comfort of patients for all occupational tasks, including sleep.

Throughout the occupational therapy treatment process, it is important to assess the levels at which caregivers wish to be involved and are capable of being involved. Therapists must be keenly aware of the time when caregivers wish to withdraw or need respite from involvement. Teaching caregivers hands-on techniques and developing adaptive strategies for coparticipation in previously shared activities can help make role transitions easier and maintain continuity of relationships.

Women with HIV and AIDS

The epidemiologic data show that women are the fastest growing group of people with AIDS in the United States. Particularly at risk are minority women and women who are directly (through their own intravenous drug use) or indirectly (through their sexual partners' intravenous drug use) at risk because of drug-related exposure to the virus (Miller et al., 1990). Many women are at risk for HIV because they are injecting drugs with shared needles; are partners of people who inject drugs, trade sex for drugs, and engage in unprotected sexual intercourse; have received infected blood or blood products; or engage in unprotected sex with men who have become infected through exposure to contaminated blood.

Some of the most startling statistics include the following:

- Among women diagnosed with AIDS, 53% use injectable drugs and another 20% have male partners who inject drugs (NOVA Research Company, 1990)
- In 1981, cases of AIDS attributable to heterosexual transmissions and intravenous drug use constituted 0.5% and 11%, respectively, of all reported cases; by 1989, these rates increased to 5% and 23.2% (Miller et al., 1990)
- The proportion of all cases reported among women has grown from about 6% in 1982 to about 10% in 1989 in the United States (Stoneburner, Chiasson, Weisfuse, & Thomas, 1990)
- Most women with AIDS (79%) are within childbearing years, from 13 to 39 years old (Wofsy, 1987)
- AIDS case data and neonatal seroprevalence rates reflect the differential risk of AIDS among minority women. Black women account for 51.7% of all AIDS cases diagnosed among women; and Hispanic women account for an additional 20%; however, blacks and Hispanics constitute only 11% and 8% of the U. S. population, respectively (U.S. Bureau of the Census, 1987)

The day to day reality of women living with AIDS is inseparable from the myriad of occupational roles such as worker, mother, family provider, spouse, or health care provider to children and partners with AIDS. Many women with AIDS simultaneously suffer from addictions and are from the most economically and educationally disadvantaged segment of our society. In short, to understand a woman with AIDS, one must understand the developmental, social, economic and cultural matrix of her life (Wood & Aull, 1990, pp. 153–154)

Women with HIV and AIDS undergo tremendous occupational challenges. They often must balance roles, attempt to gain access to adequate health care (often for themselves and their children, who may be HIV-infected), and cope with stigma, discrimination, and numerous losses. These losses include loss of function and favored roles; children, friends and partners dying from AIDS complications; and loss of dignity, control, self-esteem, and self-respect.

Occupational therapy interventions for women with HIV and AIDS include assessment using the PAPL and other recommended assessment tools suggested in this section. Based on assessment data, the occupational therapist can then design a program structure to meet occupational needs. The program must be holistic in scope and consider the sociocultural and historical context of the woman's life to develop appropriate treatment. Specific treatment approaches can incorporate individual or group therapy and can include developing or recreating role performance with respect to self-identified and valued occupational roles; developing occupation-centered routines and time management to enhance productive living and alternatives to substance abuse (this can be done in conjunction with or after substance abuse treatment); developing self-esteem, self-worth, and self-empowerment in women who must also cope with poverty, abuse, and homelessness; adapting roles, skills, and environments secondary to cognitive and physical limitations throughout the disease process; and providing parenting skills training and nutrition and meal planning training when appropriate (Pizzi, 1989a; Pizzi et al., 1991; Wood & Aull, 1990; Pizzi, 1992).

Children and adolescents with HIV and AIDS

Infants and children (0 to 12 years as defined by the Centers for Disease Control) and adolescents (13 to 19 years) are a rapidly growing group of people with HIV and AIDS.

In the United States, pediatric AIDS is 2% of all reported cases, whereas in developing nations pediatric AIDS may constitute 15–20% of all of the total AIDS cases. In the United States, the number of pediatric AIDS cases reported in 1989 represents an estimated 38% increase over 1988. This is similar to the 36% increase in cases attributable to heterosexual transmission. It is estimated that by 1992 more then 250,000 infants will have been infected in Africa alone. The HIV seroprevalence in women of childbearing age has already been reported as 2.3% in New York City and 13.5% in Kampala, Uganda. These data suggest that AIDS is an infection that will involve children of every nation of the world, and the occurrence of pediatric infection parallels heterosexual transmission (Koop, 1991, p. vii)

Since 1982, when children with HIV were first recognized, there has been a steady increase in the number of AIDS cases in adolescents comparable to that of adults and children. Fifty-three percent of cases have been reported by only five states and Puerto Rico. Older adolescents, males, and racial and ethnic minorities predominate among adolescents, with 75% of the cases reported occurring in 17- to 19-year-olds (Miller et al., 1990; Gayle & D'Angelo, 1991). The latency period of 5 to 10 years is a primary reason for the high proportion of AIDS cases in 20- to 29-year-olds.

Modes of transmission

It is estimated that there are 10,000 to 20,000 cases of HIV-infected children in the United States, most of whom are asymptomatic. Infants and children primarily acquire HIV perinatally, with 80% being 1 to 12 years of age (Institute of Medicine, 1988). Other modes include blood product transfusion and treatment for hemophilia and sexual abuse. Adolescents acquire HIV through treatment for hemophilia and coagulation disorders, unprotected sexual contact, intravenous drug use, or blood transfusion. In young adolescents, 91% of cases are due to HIV infection through blood transfusion and treatment for hemophilia. Behavior-related exposure (sexual contact or intravenous drug use) increases with age, from 9% for 13- to 14-year-olds to 24% for 15- to 16-year-olds to 69% for 17- to 19-year-olds. Over 90% of cases of AIDS in young adults aged 20 to 24 years are attributed to behavior-related exposure (Gayle & D'Angelo, 1991).

Cultural differences also play a major role in the epidemic. Fifty-three percent of the cases of HIV in white adolescents are attributed to transfusion-related exposure for treatment for hemophilia, while 63% of black adolescents are exposed through unprotected sexual contact, and 57% of Hispanics are exposed through intravenous drug use and unprotected sexual contact (Miller et al., 1990; Gayle & D'Angelo, 1991).

Medical clinical manifestations

Children with HIV present a spectrum of clinical manifestations. They may range from being asymptomatic to being critically or terminally ill. Scott (1987) and Oleske (1987) describe a range of clinical manifestations (see the display below).

The time from infection to overt AIDS is shorter in children than in adults and is shorter in children infected perinatally than in those infected through transfusion (Rogers, Thomas, & Starcher, 1987). Perinatally infected children have a median age at diagnosis of 9 months, whereas children with transfusion-acquired HIV have a median age at diagnosis of 17 months (Rogers et al., 1987).

Falloon, Eddy, Roper, and Pizzo (1988) describe several nonspecific manifestations (eg, weight loss, low birth weight or failure to thrive, diarrhea, hepatosplenomegaly, dermatitis, fevers), bacterial infections (eg, sepsis, pneumonia, meningitis), and opportunistic infections (eg, *Pneumocystis* pneumonia, disseminated cytomegalovirus, *Candida* infection, disseminated *Mycobacterium avium-intracellulare*).

The most common neurologic manifestation in children with HIV is encephalopathy. Encephalopathy can be the primary manifestation in children, resulting in developmental delay or in a deterioration of motor skills and cognitive function (Belman, Ultmann, & Houroupian, 1985; Rubinstein, 1986; Diamond, 1989; Brouwers, Belman, & Epstein, 1991). Neurologic abnormalities such as paresis, pyramidal tract signs, ataxia, abnormal tone or pseudobulbar palsy and microcephaly have been described

(Rubinstein, 1986; Epstein, Sharer, & Oleske, 1986). Computed tomographic scans have shown cerebral atrophy and ventricular enlargement, calcification in the basal ganglia, and frontal white matter (Belman et al., 1985; Epstein et al., 1986).

Clinical manifestations in adolescents closely parallel those in adults because their immune systems have already developed.

Occupational therapy assessment and treatment

Holistic functional assessment of children and adolescents with HIV and AIDS must be undertaken. Typical assessment includes chart review; clinical observations; history taking; developmental, play, and ADL assessments; standardized testing; and caregiver interviews. Neurodevelopmental assessment is a major part of the overall assessment of children with HIV, particularly for children 5 years of age and younger. A holistic assessment includes psychosocial, emotional, and environmental (social, physical, and cultural) domains of function. These domains, in concert with the physical domain, include the skills of play and self-care (Pizzi & Hinds-Harris, 1990).

In the population of children and adolescents with HIV and AIDS, important and different issues arise regarding intervention. Noteworthy are the issues of regression in skill performance, cultural considerations, caregivers who may also be coping with their own HIV disease, stigma, and environmental issues (most children and adolescents with HIV are poor urban dwellers with few community resources) (Pizzi, 1989b). Children with HIV may never achieve normal developmental milestones, or they may develop slowly or experience loss of function. Occupation and adaptation through positioning, adaptive equipment, play interventions, and neurodevelopmental treatment facilitate enhancement of function. Intervention with children with HIV must always include the family system and caregiver education (Pizzi, 1989b 1989c; Pizzi & Hinds-Harris, 1990; Anderson, Hinojosa, Bedell, & Kaplan, 1990).

Adolescents require special considerations of their developmental stage. This is the time for exploration with sexual identity and drug use, the two major modes for transmission of HIV among adolescents. Tremendous efforts by occupational therapists can be directed at individual and group treatments regarding issues of self-esteem, exploration of occupational choices, and leisure or alternative recreational choices. Facilitating meaningful occupational performance and adaptive occupational behaviors is the cornerstone to functional treatment in adolescent HIV management. Psychosocial treatments can also include educational efforts aimed at prevention, particularly regarding safer sex practices and alternatives to drug use, as well as situational coping around issues of loss, grief, and terminal care. Treatments in the physical domain include adaptation of physical environments, mobility, cognitive training, energy conservation, habit retraining, self-care training, and use of physical disability principles found elsewhere in this text. Assisting adolescents in resuming or developing occupational roles is an essential task of occupational therapists.

Traditional occupational therapy assessment and treatment for infants, children, and adolescents can be used, but the unique considerations already outlined must be undertaken for this population. A child with central nervous system damage with HIV cannot be viewed the same as one with central nervous system damage due to a head injury and cannot be evaluated and treated the same. Holistic assessment and treatment must be viewed

---

SYNDROMES AND NEUROLOGIC FINDINGS IN CHILDREN WITH HIV

- Wasting syndrome
- Lymphoid interstitial pneumonitis
- Recurrent bacterial infections
- Lymphadenopathy syndrome
- Cardiomyopathy
- Hepatitis
- Renal disease
- Developmental delay; loss of developmental milestones
- Chronic encephalopathy
- Seizure disorders
- Motor dysfunction
- Microcephaly
- Abnormal computed tomographic scan findings: cortical atrophy, calcifications

UNIVERSAL INFECTION CONTROL GUIDELINES

The increasing prevalence of HIV increases the risk that health care workers will be exposed to blood from patients infected with HIV, especially when blood and body fluid precautions are not followed for all patients. Thus, this document emphasizes the need for health care workers to consider all patients as potentially infected with HIV and/or other blood-borne pathogens and to adhere rigorously to infection control precautions for minimizing the risk of exposure to blood and body fluids of all patients.

The recommendations contained in this document consolidate and update Centers for Disease Control (CDC) recommendations published earlier for preventing HIV transmission in health care settings; precautions for clinical and laboratory staffs and precautions for health care workers and allied professionals; recommendations for preventing HIV transmission in the work place and during invasive procedures; VXK for preventing possible transmission of HIV from tears; and recommendations for providing dialysis treatment for HIV-infected patients. The recommendations contained in this document have been developed for use in health care settings and emphasize the need to treat blood and other body fluids from all patients as potentially infective. These same prudent precautions also should be taken in other settings in which people may be exposed to blood or other body fluids.

Universal Precautions

Since medical history and examination cannot reliably identify all patients with HIV or other blood-borne pathogens, blood and body fluid precautions should be consistently used for all patients. This approach, previously recommended by CDC, and referred to as *universal blood and body fluid precautions* or *universal precautions* should be used in the care of all patients, especially those in emergency care settings in which the risk of blood exposure is increased and the infection status of the patient is usually unknown.

1. All health care workers should routinely use appropriate barrier precautions to prevent skin and mucous membrane exposure when contact with blood or other body fluids of any patient is anticipated. Gloves should be worn for touching blood and body fluids, mucous membranes, or nonintact skin of all patients, for handling items or surfaces soiled with blood or body fluids, and for performing venipuncture and other vascular access procedures. Gloves should be changed after contact with each patient. Mask and protective eyewear or face shield should be worn during procedures that are likely to generate droplets of blood or other body fluids to prevent exposure of mucous membranes of the mouth, nose, and eyes. Gowns or aprons should be worn during procedures that are likely to generate splashes of blood or other body fluids.

2. Hands and other skin surfaces should be washed immediately and thoroughly if contaminated with blood or other body fluids. Hands should be washed immediately after gloves are removed.

3. All health care workers should take precautions to prevent injuries caused by needles, scalpels, and other sharp instruments or devices during procedures, when cleaning used instruments; during disposal of used needles; and when handling sharp instruments after procedures. To prevent needlestick injuries, needles should not be recapped, purposely bent or broken by hand, removed from disposable syringes, or otherwise manipulated by hand. After they are used, disposable syringes and needles, scalpel blades, and other sharp items should be placed in puncture-resistant containers for disposal; the puncture-resistant containers should be located as close as practical to the use area. Large-bore, reusable needles should be placed in a puncture-resistant container for transport to the reprocessing area.

4. Although saliva has not been implicated in HIV transmission, to minimize the need for emergency mouth-to-mouth resuscitation, mouthpieces, resuscitation bags, or other ventilation devices should be available for use in areas in which the need for resuscitation is predictable.

5. Health care workers who have exudative lesions or weeping dermatitis should refrain from all direct patient care and from handling patient care equipment until the condition resolves.

(continued)

UNIVERSAL INFECTION CONTROL GUIDELINES (*continued*)

6. Pregnant health care workers are not known to be at greater risk for contracting HIV infection than health care workers who are not pregnant; however, if a health care worker develops HIV infection during pregnancy, the infant is at risk for infection resulting from perinatal transmission. Because of the risk, pregnant health care workers should be especially familiar with and strictly adhere to precautions to minimize the risk of HIV transmission.

Implementation of universal blood and body fluid precautions for all patients eliminates the need for use of the isolation category of "Blood and Body-Fluid Precautions" previously recommended by CDC for patients known or suspected to be infected with blood-borne pathogens. Isolation precautions (eg, enteric, "AFB") should be used as necessary if associated conditions, such as infectious diarrhea or tuberculosis, are diagnosed or suspected.

Environmental Consideration for HIV Transmission

No environmentally mediated mode of HIV transmission has been documented. Nevertheless, the precautions described below should be taken routinely in the care of all patients.

Sterilization and Disinfection

Standard sterilization and disinfection procedures for patient care equipment currently recommended for use in a variety of health care settings—including hospitals, medical and dental clinics and offices, hemodialysis centers, emergency care facilities, and long-term nursing care facilities—are adequate to sterilize or disinfect instruments, devices, or other items contaminated with blood or other body fluids from people infected with HIV.

Instruments or devices that enter sterile tissue or the vascular system of any patient or through which blood flows should be sterilized before reuse. Devices or items that contact intact mucous membranes should be sterilized or receive high-level disinfection, a procedure that kills vegetative organisms and viruses but not necessarily large numbers of bacterial spores. Chemical germicides that are registered with the U. S. Environmental Protection Agency as "sterilants" may be used either for sterilization or for high-level disinfection, depending on contact time.

Adapted from "Recommendations for Prevention of HIV Transmission in Health Care Settings" by Centers for Disease Control, August 21, 1987, Morbidity and Mortality Weekly Report, 36(25).

---

from a sociocultural context and within the context of unique and diverse family systems.

Universal precautions and infection control

The Centers for Disease Control developed recommendations for infection control regarding transmission of HIV. These universal precautions are recommended to prevent transmission to all who come in contact with someone with HIV. Universal precautions are *guidelines* and are used when the possibility exists that people caring for those with HIV or AIDS may come in contact with patients' body fluids. These fluids include blood, semen, vaginal secretions, cerebrospinal fluid, synovial fluid, pleural fluid, peritoneal fluid, pericardial fluid, and amniotic fluid. "General infection control practices to prevent gross microbial contamination of hands (eg, hand washing) should further minimize the risk, if any, for HIV transmission from body fluids and materials not covered under universal precautions" (Villarino, Beck-Sague, & Jarvis, 1991, p. 378–9). For more complete and concise infection control procedures, refer to the display.

Summary

It is vital that occupational therapists holistically assess people with HIV and AIDS and include physical, psychosocial, and environmental aspects of living and their impacts on occupational behaviors. Because there are many unique features to HIV rehabilitation, it takes a transformation of our knowledge base in occupation and adaptation, combined with social and medical knowledge of HIV infection, to assess and treat appropriately people with HIV and AIDS and their caregivers. In HIV and AIDS rehabilitation, transformation occurs through nonjudgmental, ethical, and authentic caregiving (Pizzi, 1990a).

References

Anderson, J., Hinojosa, J., Bedell, G., & Kaplan, M. T. (1990). Occupational therapy for children with perinatal HIV infection. *American Journal of Occupational Therapy, 44*(3), 249–255.

Belman, A., Ultmann, M. H., & Houroupian, D. (1985). Neurological complications in infants and children with acquired immunodeficiency syndrome. *Annals of Neurology, 18,* 560–566.

Brouwers, P., Belman, A., & Epstein, L. G. (1991). Central nervous system involvement: Manifestations and evaluation. In P. Pizzo and C. Wilfert

(Eds.), *Pediatric AIDS: The challenge of HIV infection in infants, children and adolescents* (pp. 318–335). Baltimore: Williams & Wilkins.

Centers for Disease Control. (1982). Explained immunodeficiency and opportunistic infections in infants—New York, New Jersey, California. *Morbidity and Mortality Weekly Report, 31,* 665–667.

Clark, F., & Jackson, J. (1990). The application of the occupational science negative heuristic in the treatment of persons with human immunodeficiency infection. *Occupational Therapy in Health Care, 6*(4), 69–91.

Denton, R. (1987). AIDS: Guidelines for occupational therapy intervention. *American Journal of Occupational Therapy, 41,* 427–432.

DeVita, V. T., Hellman, S., & Rosenberg, S. A. (Eds.) (1988). *AIDS: Etiology, diagnosis, treatment and prevention* (2nd ed.). Philadelphia: J. B. Lippincott.

Diamond, G. W. (1989). Developmental problems in children with HIV infection. *Mental Retardation, 27*(4), 213–217.

Epstein, L., Sharer, L. R., & Oleske, J. M. (1986). Neurological manifestations of HIV infection in children. *Pediatrics, 78,* 678–687.

Falloon, J., Eddy, J., Roper, M., & Pizzo, P. (1988). AIDS in the pediatric population. In V. DeVita, S. Hellman, & T. Rosenberg (Eds.), *AIDS: Etiology, diagnosis, treatment and prevention* (2nd ed.) (pp. 339–351). Philadelphia: J. B. Lippincott.

Faulstich, M. E. (1987). Psychiatric aspects of AIDS. *American Journal of Psychiatry, 144*(5), 551–555.

Galantino, M. L. (Ed.). (1992). *Clinical assessment and treatment of HIV: Rehabilitation of the chronic illness.* Thorofare, NJ: Slack.

Galantino, M. L., & Levy, J. (1988). HIV infection: Neurological implications for rehabilitation. *Clinical Management in Physical Therapy, 8*(1), 6–13.

Galantino, M. L., Mukand, J., & Freed, M. M. (1991). Physical therapy management of patients with HIV infection. In J. Mukand (Ed.), *Rehabilitation for patients with HIV disease* (pp. 257–282). New York: McGraw-Hill.

Galantino, M. L., & Pizzi, M. (1991). Occupational and physical therapy for persons with HIV disease and their caregivers. *Journal of Home Health Care Practice, 3*(3), 46–57.

Gallo, R. C., & Montagnier, L. (1988, October). AIDS in 1988. *Scientific American,* 40–48.

Gayle, H. D., & D'Angelo, L. J. (1991). The epidemiology of AIDS and HIV infection in adolescents. In P. Pizzo and C. Wilfert (Eds.), *Pediatric AIDS: The challenge of HIV infection in infants, children and adolescents* (pp. 38–50). Baltimore: Williams & Wilkins.

Gutterman, L. (1990). A day treatment program for persons with AIDS. *American Journal of Occupational Therapy, 44*(3), 234–237.

Institute of Medicine (1988). *Confronting AIDS: Directions for public health, health care and research.* Washington, DC: National Academy Press.

Ironson, G., LaPerriere, A., Antoni, M., O'Hearn, P., Schneiderman, N., Klimas, N., & Fletcher, M. A. (1990). Changes in immune and psychological measures as a function of anticipation and reaction to news of HIV-1 antibody status. *Psychosomatic Medicine, 52,* 247–270.

Jemmott, J. B., & Locke, S. E (1984). Psychosocial factors, immunologic mediation and human susceptibility to infectious diseases: How much do we know? *Psychological Bulletin, 95*(10), 78–108.

Kassel, P. E. (1991). Psychological and neuropsychological dimensions of HIV illness. In J. Mukand (Ed.), *Rehabilitation for patients with HIV disease* (pp. 217–240). New York: McGraw-Hill.

Kiecolt-Glaser, J. K., & Glaser, R. (1988). Psychological influences on immunity. *American Psychologist, 43,* 892–898

Koop, C. E. (1991). Forward. In P. Pizzo and C. Wilfert (Eds.), *Pediatric AIDS: The challenge of HIV infection in infants, children and adolescents* (pp. vii–viii). Baltimore: Williams & Wilkins.

LaPerriere, A. R., Antoni, M. H., Schneiderman N., Ironson, G., Klimas, N., Caralis, P., & Fletcher, M. A. (1990). Exercise intervention attenuates emotional distress and natural killer cell decrements following noti-

fication of positive serologic staus for HIV-1. *Biofeedback and Self-Regulation, 15*(3), 229–242.

Miller, H. G., Turner, C. F., & Moses, L. E. (Eds.) (1990). *AIDS: The second decade.* Washington, DC: National Academy Press.

Navis, D. A., Jordon, B. D., & Price, R. W. (1986). The AIDS dementia complex I: Clinical features. *Annals in Neurology 19,* 517–524.

NOVA Research Company (1990). *Aids prevention model: Reaching women at risk.* Bethesda, MD: Author

Oakley, F., Kielhofner, G., Barris, R., & Reichler, R. K. (1986). The Role Checklist: Development and empirical assessment of reliability. *Occupational Therapy Journal of Research, 6,* 157–170.

Oleske, J. M. (1987). Natural history of HIV infection II. In *Report of the Surgeon General's workshop on children with HIV infection and their families.* Washington, DC: U.S. Department of Health and Human Services.

Pizzi, M. (1984). Occupational therapy in hospice care. *American Journal of Occupational Therapy, 38*(4), 252–257.

Pizzi, M. (1988, August 18). Challenge of treating AIDS patients includes helping them lead functional lives. *Occupational Therapy Week, 31,* 6–7.

Pizzi, M. (1989a). Occupational therapy: Creating possibilities for adults with HIV infection, ARC and AIDS. *AIDS Patient Care, 3,* 18–23.

Pizzi, M. (1989b). Occupational therapy: Creating possibilities for children with HIV infection, ARC and AIDS. *AIDS Patient Care, 3*(6), 31–36.

Pizzi, M. (1989c, November 23). Pediatric AIDS: Occupational therapy assessment and treatment. *Occupational Therapy Week,* 6–7, 10.

Pizzi, M. (1990a). Nationally speaking—The transformation of HIV infection and AIDS in occupational therapy: Beginning the conversation. *American Journal of Occupational Therapy, 44*(3), 1–5.

Pizzi, M. (1990b). The Model of Human Occupation and adults with HIV infection and AIDS. *American Journal of Occupational Therapy, 44* (3), 42–49.

Pizzi, M. (1991a). Adaptive human performance and HIV infection: Considerations for therapists. In M. L. Galantino (Ed.), *Clinical assessment and treatment in HIV: Rehabilitation of a chronic illness.* Thorofare, NJ: Slack.

Pizzi, M. (1991b). *Stress and HIV infection.* Unpublished manuscript.

Pizzi, M. (1992). Women, HIV infection and AIDS: Tapestries of life, death, and empowerment. *American Journal of Occupational Therapy, 46*(11).

Pizzi, M., & Hinds-Harris, M. (1990). Infants and children with HIV infection: Perspectives in occupational and physical therapy. In M. Pizzi, & J. Johnson (Eds.), *Productive living strategies for people with AIDS.* New York: Haworth Press.

Pizzi, M., Mukand, J., & Freed, M. (1991). HIV infection and occupational therapy. In J. Mukand (Ed.), *Rehabilitation for patients with HIV disease* (pp. 283–326). New York: McGraw-Hill.

Report of the Presidential Commission on the Human Immunodeficiency Virus (1988). Washington, DC: United States Government Printing Office.

Rogers, M. F., Thomas, P. A., & Starcher, E. T. (1987). Acquired immunodeficiency syndrome in children: Report of the Centers for Disease Control national surveillance, 1982–1985. *Pediatrics, 79,* 1008.

Rubinstein, A. (1986). Pediatric AIDS. *Current Problems in Pediatrics, 16,* 361.

Scaffa, M. (1981). *Temporal adaptation and alcoholism.* Unpublished master's thesis. Virginia Commonwealth University, Richmond, VA.

Schindler, V. (1988). Psychosocial occupational therapy intervention with AIDS patients. *American Journal of Occupational Therapy, 42,* 507–512.

Scott, G. (1987). Natural history of HIV infection in children. In *Report of the Surgeon General's workshop on children with HIV infection and their families.* Washington, DC: United States Department of Health and Human Services.

Servellen, G., Lewis, C. E., & Leake, B. (1990). The stresses of hospitalization among AIDS patients on integrated and special care units. *International Journal of Nursing Studies, 27*(3), 235–247.

Solomon, G. F., Temoshak, L., O'Leary, A., & Zich, J. (1987). An intensive psychoimmunologic study of long surviving persons with AIDS. *Annals of the New York Academy of Science, 496,* 647–655.

Spence, D. W., Galantino, M. L., Mossberg, K. A., & Zimmerman, S. O. (1990). Progressive resistance exercise: Effect on muscle function and anthropometry of a select AIDS population. *Archives of Physical Medicine and Rehabilitation, 71,* 644–648.

Solomon, G. F., Temoshak, L., O'Leary, A., & Zich, J. (1987). An intensive psychoimmunologic study of long surviving persons with AIDS. *Annals of the New York Academy of Science, 496,* 647–655.

Stoneburner, R. L., Chiasson, M. A., Weisfuse, I. B., & Thomas, P. A. (1990). The epidemic of AIDS and HIV-1 infection among heterosexuals in New York City. *AIDS, 4,* 99–106.

U. S. Bureau of the Census (1987). *Statistical abstract of the United States: 1988* (108th ed.). Washington, DC: National Academy Press.

U. S. Department of Health and Human Services (1986). *Coping with AIDS.* Washington, DC: U. S. Government Printing

Villarino, M. E., Beck-Sague, C., & Jarvis, W. R. (1991). AIDS, infection control, and employee health: Considerations in rehabilitation medicine. In J. Mukand (Ed.), *Rehabilitation for patients with HIV disease,* pp. 371–392. New York: McGraw-Hill.

Weinstein, B. (1990). Assessing the impact of HIV disease. *American Journal of Occupational Therapy, 44*(3), 220–226.

Wood, W., & Aull, M. R. (1990). Women and AIDS: Implications for occupational therapists. In M. Pizzi, & J. Johnson (Eds.), *Productive living strategies for people with AIDS* (pp. 151–160). New York: Harrington Park Press.

Wofsy, C. (1987). Human immunodeficiency virus infection in women. *Journal of the American Medical Association, 257,* 2074–2076.

Yerxa, E. J., Clark, F., Frank, G., Jackson, J., Parnam, D., Pierce, D., Stein, C., & Zemke, R. (1989). An introduction to occupational science: A foundation for occupational therapy in the 21st century. *Occupational Therapy in Health Care, 6*(4), 1–17.

UNIT VIII

Implementation of occupational therapy in geriatrics

CHAPTER 19

Aging and health

BETTY RISTEEN HASSELKUS

LEARNING OBJECTIVES

Upon completion of this chapter the reader will be able to:

1. *Know basic statistics such as rates of growth and life expectancies of the older population in the United States.*
2. *Understand the health context of old age including the nature of illness and relevant social issues.*
3. *Be able to discuss biologic and psychosocial theories of aging and relevant physical and psychological aspects of aging.*
4. *Demonstrate an understanding of professional and family caregiving for older persons.*
5. *Be able to name and describe settings of care for older persons and recent shifts in care patterns.*

The title of this chapter appears to be an oxymoron, that is, a combination of incongruous or self-contradictory words such as "jumbo shrimp." In other words, are aging and health incongruous and self-contradictory, and do they constitute another oxymoron? We all know older persons who are experiencing significant health problems and who have had to make major adaptations in old age to maintain their accustomed lifestyles and activities. Yet we also know older persons who are healthy, who are carrying on their usual daily routines, and who lead lives very much as they always have.

This chapter explores the mysterious process known in Western society as aging—the theories of aging, age-related changes, illnesses of aging, and health care systems for long-term care settings. The focus will be on the unique health context of aging as revealed in the "complex intermingling of wellness, acute illness, and chronic illness, which are superimposed on normal age-related changes" (Hasselkus & Kiernat, 1989, p. 77). The translation of these phenomena and the understanding of them in the practice of occupational therapy in geriatrics are described in Chapter 20.

Geriatrics, gerontology, and occupational therapy

Gerontology is the study of aging per se. Gerontology encompasses the development of theories of aging, research on the social and physical aspects typical of aging, and practice issues that address these age-related phenomena. *Geriatrics* is the study of health and medical care in old age. Research on diseases that occur in old age, medical care practices, and health care services systems are examples of geriatric issues.

Both gerontology and geriatrics are terms used in the profession of occupational therapy. In addition, a term borrowed from nursing, *gerontic*, is sometimes used to describe occupational therapy with older clients (Davis, 1988). Because of the focus on everyday life tasks within a health care context, occupational therapists often find themselves acting as a bridge between the medical and life worlds of the clients with whom they work. It has been suggested that the term "gerontic" effectively represents that bridge. Although the differences among these terms may seem subtle at first glance, it is not unusual for an occupational therapist to voice a strong preference for one or the other term as an expression of his or her beliefs about the nature of the profession of occupational therapy.

Although health care professionals have always treated patients of all ages, geriatrics as a specialty within health care is a recent phenomenon. As recently at 1985, only 10% of medical schools in the United States reported requiring geriatrics in their curricula (Estes & Binney, 1989). Resistance to the development of geriatrics as a medical specialty stemmed from at least two primary sources: (1) the belief that human development is a phenomenon that occurs only between conception and puberty, that is, that development stops after maturity is reached (therefore the health care needs of older persons would be the same as those of other adults), and (2) the negative stereotypes that health care in old age is uninteresting, unchallenging, and less worthy of our attention and resources.

In occupational therapy, the Gerontology Special Interest Section of the American Occupational Therapy Association (AOTA) was created in 1976. To our profession's credit, gerontology was one of the charter special interest sections in the AOTA and it continues to maintain a strong presence within the profession. The recognition of geriatrics as an area of specialization within health care is based on the argument that older persons have special health problems and circumstances that need to be considered in their health care and that special training is needed to adequately and appropriately meet these needs. As Lewis (1990) stated,

> One of the questions most frequently asked by rehabilitation professionals is, "What's so different about treating the older person? A hip is a hip. . . . " Although it is true that a hip is a hip, if you can expand your focus and look at the whole picture—the person, the support system, his or her living environment, and history—you will have a much better idea of the needs of that particular hip. (p. 1)

The following case study is used in this chapter and Chapter 20 to illustrate important and relevant issues about aging, health, and occupational therapy.

CASE STUDY

G.P. is an 86-year-old man whose wife died 3 years ago. He had been living alone in an apartment on the west side of town until his daughter felt that a move was necessary because of his deteriorating physical health and increasing confusion and forgetfulness. At that point, he moved in with his daughter on the far east side.

G.P.'s health problems are congestive heart failure, chronic pulmonary disease, impaired vision, and impaired hearing. He ambulates with a cane but is unsteady on his feet, and he has experienced fairly frequent falls and periods of dizziness.

G.P.'s confusion has increased since the move to the daughter's house: he got lost one day in the front yard; he could not remember who his daughter was on one occasion; he got up in the middle of the night several times and rummaged through drawers and closets and cupboards; he poured milk into an empty pepper shaker one day and drank it; and he poured salt on his cereal, then accused his daughter of putting pieces of broken glass in the cereal.

G.P. sits most of the day and listens to his radio (his daughter has a full-time job). He talks about wanting to fly to Florida for the winter.

Burgeoning of the older population

In the case study, 86-year-old G.P. is a member of an age group sometimes referred to as the "oldest old." People who are 80 years of age and older constitute the most rapidly growing proportion of the total population, now totaling more than 6 million in the United States (Torrey, Kinsella, & Taeuber, 1987). The number of those over 85 years old increased by 60% between 1970 and 1980 and is projected to continue at slightly more than that rate until the year 2000 (Soldo, 1980). People over age 65 constitute 12% of the population in the United States. This is almost twice the percentage that was present in the population of 50 years ago, and it is projected to rise to 20% by the year 2025 (Torrey et al., 1987).

In the United States, life expectancy at birth for white males is 71.8 years and for white females is 78.7 years (National Center for Health Statistics, 1987). G.P. has lived beyond the norm. Statistics for other races are lower, for example, 65.6 years for African American men and 73.7 years for African American women. As people age past these at-birth life expectancies (as G.P. has done), new expectancy curves are calculated. Therefore, G.P. now has a life expectancy of 90.1 years, or 5.1 years beyond the age of 85. As a corollary, G.P. is also in a minority as a surviving spouse. Eighty percent of all older persons who live alone are women. Since women live longer, they are far more likely than men to be widowed and to live on into older age alone.

G.P. is in the majority, however, in that he lives in the community and not in an institution. It is a myth that most older persons are in institutions; in fact, most older persons (95%) live in the community (Palmore, 1976) and those who need support rely on family members for their care. Of all health care for people in old age—formal and informal—estimates for the amount provided by family **caregivers** are as high as 80% (Shanas, 1979). Most adult informal caregivers are women, and most of these women caregivers are daughters (with wives running a close second) (Stone, Cafferata, & Sangl, 1986). So it is not unusual for G.P.'s daughter to have agreed to have her father move in with her and to provide his needs for care.

Health context of old age

What makes G.P.'s **health context** different from a young adult or a middle-aged male? Is health different in old age? Health in old age is different from health at other life stages in at least five significant ways.

First, in older age, disease and illness, if present, are superimposed on normal age-related changes. It becomes extremely important to differentiate between illness and age-related changes, since one process is pathologic and the other is not. One demands treatment, and the other does not.

Second, health in older age is likely to be dominated by chronic rather than acute needs. Even acute needs tend to be exacerbations of chronic disease such as the need for hip replacement after long-term degenerative joint disease or the need for bypass surgery after long-term coronary artery disease. Generally, however, the health concerns of older persons are problems associated with day-to-day management of chronic disease and its impact on independence in activities of daily living (Davis, 1986). The emphasis is on living with a health problem, not on finding its cure.

Third, an older person rarely has a *single* health problem.

> Geriatric patients tend to be characterized by multiple problems in multiple areas of life. Physical health problems may be accompanied by mental health problems, and these may be compounded by social issues such as isolation, financial insecurity, and the inability to live independently. (Kiernat, 1991, p. 7)

Health problems in old age are anything but simple and uninteresting. They are complex and challenging, requiring broad and exceptional skills from the health professional who chooses the geriatric field of practice.

The above quotation from Kiernat leads us to the fourth difference—that older persons live in a different social context. For example, they live in a different economic context, they experience changes in roles (an older person's work role is different from a younger person's work role), and changes in social connections and networks. Loss of a spouse and addition of a grandchild are both examples of the latter. Neighborhood transitions such as the loss of a neighborhood friend through death, the closing of a corner grocery store, and the deterioration over time of a familiar neighborhood environment are other examples of changes.

Finally, older persons live in a societal context that is different from that of other age groups. In Western society, many stereotypes of old age exist. The term for such stereotyping on the basis of age is **ageism**, and it is more often negative than positive (Butler, 1969). Examples of such labeling are easy to recall: "rigid," "narrow-minded," "forgetful," and "sick," to name a few. Negative ageism can affect health care, often creating a climate of false debility, frailty, and dependency in the older clients of health professionals. The thoroughness and vigor of an assessment and treatment process are related to age, with evidence suggesting that older persons tend to receive less energetic workups and treatment (Barta Kvitek, Shaver, Blood, & Shepard 1986; Crane, 1975). Marshall (1981) has called this an "undue tendency toward therapeutic inactivity" (p. 111).

Health is different in old age. The traditional focus of medical care on symptom-oriented treatment is obviously inadequate for geriatric medical care. The health of older persons exists within the developmental and social context of their lives, just as is true for people of *all* ages. For example, G.P., at 86 years of age, has health problems superimposed on age-related problems (eg, his hearing problem may be the result of neural aging or it may be a treatable condition), multiple chronic problems (congestive heart failure, chronic pulmonary disease, vision and hearing impairments), a social context of change in networks and relationships (widowhood, move to daughter's house), and vulnerability to society's ageism (the confusion and forgetfulness may be typical of old age or may merit a thorough work-up). It takes special knowledge and training to work with older persons to assist them to adapt to the challenges of the many interrelated variables of "health and aging"—not an oxymoron but perhaps a conundrum. The challenge of geriatrics lies in balancing the many factors that make up health in old age and painstakingly sorting out treatable from nontreatable, physical from psychosocial, and adaptive from maladaptive conditions.

The aging process

Distinguishing between normal aging processes and disease processes is no easy task. Further confusion is generated by **age-related diseases**, that is, those diseases that usually occur in older populations and accompany the aging process. Normal age changes may be defined as changes that seem universal, progressive, and irreversible, such as graying of hair and the need for reading glasses. What about aches and pains and joint stiffness at age 70? Are these normal age changes or do they indicate the presence of disease? What about forgetfulness and confusion at age 86? Are these normal age changes or manifestations of disease?

Figure 19-1 is a reproduction of a road sign depicting elderly persons. It is universal in its ability to convey meaning. The words under the picture aren't needed. We use the following clues to come to this conclusion:

1. The figures in the picture appear to be having difficulty getting around and to be moving slowly.
2. The posture and body alignment of the figures seem typical of older people, for example, flexed hips and knees.
3. The figures seem unsteady, vulnerable to falling; the man uses a cane and the woman takes the man's arm for support.

We know by the visible, outward signs that these people are old, but we don't know whether they are ill or have a disease. Aging and illness are not the same. Figure 19-1 is intended to represent signs of universal age changes.

Errors concerning normal aging and disease-related processes can be made in either of two directions (Dye & Sassenrath,

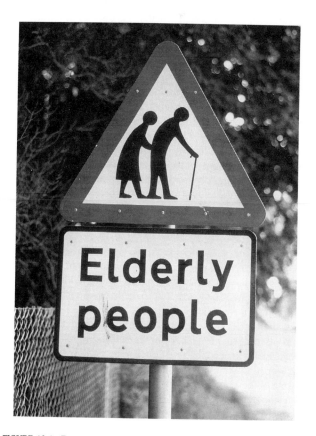

FIGURE 19-1. *Road sign in Sussex, England.*

1979). First, a problem may be incorrectly identified as a disease when in fact it is the result of normal aging. This kind of error can lead to needless expenditures of time and energy on the part of both the health professional and the older person, and it may cause stress and frustration from expectations for improvement that can never be realized. An example is interpreting a rise in blood pressure as a symptom of disease when in fact blood pressure shows a certain amount of normal increase with aging.

The second error is that of incorrectly considering disease processes as signs of normal aging. For obvious reasons, this can be a serious error, since a condition may be overlooked that might be treatable. An example of a quote from a physician's hospital discharge note for an 83-year-old patient illustrates this kind of error. "It is felt that the patient's organic brain syndrome is mild, especially considering his age." This physician is saying that the patient's forgetfulness and confusion are normal and to be expected and that the patient is doing pretty well considering his age. This 83-year-old man may in fact have a condition that is treatable, an illness that is not normal aging at all. This example also illustrates ageism in health care and negative stereotyping based on age; the resulting treatment approach certainly represents "therapeutic inactivity."

The boundaries between disease and normal aging are not always easy to discern. The difference between pneumonia and age-related decreased vital lung capacity is generally clear-cut and readily distinguishable; pneumonia, however, is not a chronic, age-related disease. On the other hand, it is known that with normal aging, the lens of the eye thickens, hardens, and becomes more opaque. For some, this opacity may be severe enough that it becomes a "condition" and is called a *cataract* (Hooyman & Kiyak, 1991). Almost 50% of all persons aged 75 to 85 have a cataract in one or both eyes; this is an age-related condition. It can be asked whether cataract is an exaggerated state of a normal aging process? Where does normal aging end and disease begin?

Biologic theories of aging

Biologic theories of aging attempt to explain the underlying mechanisms for the normal changes that occur in the body over the life span. These theories focus on cellular changes. They attempt to sort out intrinsic primary mechanisms of aging from secondary events, the triggering mechanisms of aging from the results. The "aging program" hypothesis draws on the assumption that the genetic information contained in the genes on the chromosomes in each cell nucleus of the body orchestrates the aging process, just as it orchestrates other developmental processes (Von Hahn, 1973).

The work of Hayflick (1965, 1980) provided strong support for this theory. The phenomena he demonstrated included evidence that normal human cells have a limited ability to divide in cell culture; in other words, human cells, in essence, have a finite life span, approaching 50 doublings (the Hayflick limit) before they die. Hayflick also noticed that certain intracellular changes take place during the latter phases of the cell, such as reduced DNA levels that lead to the ultimate reduction of enzymes necessary for cellular function. Thus, the limited doublings may be the result of the cumulative effects of primary changes within the cell, and the eventual loss of cells in the organs and tissues of the body may be what we think of as the aging process (Campanelli, 1990). The theory of aging seems to be supported by the tendency for longevity to run in families. Additionally, there appears to be a maximum life span for humans that has not changed for centuries.

An alternative biologic theory states that the primary aging event is not preprogrammed but is governed by laws of chance (Von Hahn, 1973). This is the ***error accumulation theory***, and it is based on the assertion that the adaptive capacities and repair mechanisms of human cells are susceptible to errors. If these errors occur in the systems of the cell that controls protein synthesis or cell chromosome replication, the errors can become rapidly magnified and lead to *error-catastrophe*, or death of the cell (Orgel, 1963).

Other cellular theories of aging are the cross-linkage theory (Bjorksten, 1974), the free radical theory (Harman, 1969), and the autoimmune theory (Ram, 1967). All these theories are based on evidence of cellular changes in older age that result in such phenomena as loss of elasticity and flexibility of tissue, loss of immune system efficacy, damaged membrane functions, and accumulation of aging pigments. Hayflick (1983) has suggested that genetic explanations may yet be the trigger for these changes. And finally, Bortz (1989) has recently stated succinctly, if bluntly, that aging is entropy. That is, aging simply reflects the principle of physics in which, over time, all ordered matter spreads out and becomes diffused into disorder (not unlike the "big bang theory" of the universe).

Physical aspects of aging

The biologic processes that accompany aging, triggered by the theoretical cellular mechanisms just described, are commonly referred to as *senescence*. Texts on geriatrics usually describe the biologic aspects of aging by providing an inventory of the body's organ systems and the details of each system's response to aging. Each system—the skin, sensory organs, nervous system, gastrointestinal system, musculoskeletal system, pulmonary system, cardiovascular, and so on—demonstrates changes with aging that are usually described as decremental or deteriorative in nature. Loss of cells, decreases in functional rates such as glomerular filtration and neural conduction, decreased elasticity of tissues, increased fibrous tissue deposition, and cell atrophy all are conventional descriptors of these changes (Levenson, 1985; Reichel, 1983). Physical aspects of the aging organ systems are also described in functional terms (Ellis, 1991; Levenson, 1985). Functions such as smell, balance, hearing, cognitive responsivity, sexual arousal, and urinary continence are discussed in relation to changes brought about by aging; these changes, too, are usually described as deteriorative.

Levenson (1985) cautions, however, against assuming that structure and function go hand in hand. Many organs have far more structural units than are needed and adequate function can be maintained even in the face of anatomic abnormality or loss of cellular substance. "Though many structural changes take place in various organ systems as we age, function is not necessarily adversely affected because of this enormous functional reserve capacity" (Levenson, 1985, p. 54). For example, although skin changes represent probably the most visible evidence of aging, no correlation exists between skin changes and longevity. The skin continues to adequately serve its function of protection for the other body systems and exchange of heat and moisture throughout life.

Thus, it may be presumptuous to assume that the biologic

changes of aging are "deteriorative." That *changes* occur is not disputed, but loss of cells does not necessarily mean loss of function, and change does not necessarily mean deterioration. It is simply a new state of being.

Psychosocial theories of aging

Psychosocial theories of aging represent an attempt to explain normal psychological processes of aging. It is striking that these theories, arising out of the fields of psychology and sociology, draw heavily on the very essence of occupational therapy for their own core meanings. That is, at the heart of many of these theories is the concept of activity as a reflection of developmental change—activity or *in*activity as the key to "successful" aging.

Two opposing psychosocial theories of aging are the disengagement theory (Cumming & Henry, 1961) and the activity theory (Lemon, Bengston, & Peterson, 1972). The **disengagement theory of aging** has been modified, but its original stance was to claim that successful aging was the result of an older person's gradual withdrawal or disengagement from society, a process that was accompanied by a parallel disengagement of society from the older person. These processes were conceptualized as normal and adaptive, leading to the ultimate and final disengagement—death. More recently, it has been proposed that if disengagement occurs in old age, it is not necessarily adaptive but is more likely the end result of failing health and depression or a person's new awareness of finitude (Sill, 1980).

The **activity theory of aging** claims that successful aging depends on the older person being able to maintain as much as possible the activity levels of earlier adulthood (Lemon et al., 1972). If change occurs, the adaptive response is to restore the previous equilibrium. To continue to take part in the same activities that were participated in during middle age is the essence of a happy and satisfying older age. At the very least, a good substitute for earlier activities (walking instead of jogging) must be found to prevent decreased life satisfaction during aging.

A more complex psychosocial theory is found in the **continuity theory of aging**. Continuity is defined as a "grand adaptive strategy" that draws on an older person's individual history of preferences and past experiences (Atchley, 1989, p. 183). Continuity of a person's outer life and inner psyche is maintained in old age by linking changes brought about by aging to prior familiar strategies, building on the person's past experiences, and retaining the stability of the person's inner being. The person maintains both his or her external behavioral continuity and internal psychological continuity. The continuity theory "allows change to be integrated into one's prior history without necessarily causing upheaval or disequilibrium" (Atchley, 1989, p. 183). In other words, the changes that evolve with aging are incorporated into a person's life experience in a way that preserves the person's "self."

Psychological (versus psychosocial) theories of aging also contribute to our understanding of the aging process. Erikson's (1963) **stages of personality and ego development** describe the life span process of personality development, culminating in the resolution of ego integrity versus despair in old age. To gain the stage of integrity means that one accepts one's "one and only life cycle as something that had to be and that, by necessity, permitted of no substitutions" (Erikson, 1963, p. 168). With this acceptance of one's life as the ultimate life, death loses its terror. The hierarchic development of the ego through Erik-

son's eight stages represents both the inner drive of the individual and the supportive forces of society.

Another psychological theory worth noting is Maslow's (1954) **hierarchy of human needs**. This is the well-known pyramid of needs, supported at the bottom by the fulfillment of physiologic/survival needs and culminating at the top with the attainment of self-esteem and self-actualization. It can be readily acknowledged that in old age, changes in energy, strength, sensory acuities, and social context may shift the older person's motivational level back to Belongingness and to the meeting of safety and physiologic needs.

Psychosocial aspects of aging

Do the above-mentioned psychosocial and psychological theories of aging lead to certain recognizable psychosocial patterns of behavior and personality in old age? Are these patterns adaptive or maladaptive?

A recurring theme in the gerontology literature is the belief that as people age, they do not become more and more alike but more and more different.

> A long life brings with it an accumulation of distinctive and unique experiences. Seven, eight, or nine decades of living often etch a deeper individuality than what one encounters among those who have been living for only two or three decades. (Kastenbaum, 1985, p. 69)

Thus, we must approach with caution the concept of generalized patterns of personality and psychosocial function in old age.

Studies of activity in old age yield support for any or all the psychosocial theories of aging presented here, depending on the author's or reader's way of interpreting the findings. Nystrom's study (1974) on activity patterns among the elderly attempted to examine both the external behavioral components of activity and the internal meaning of activity. In this way, it reflected the principles of the continuity theory of aging. The activities most represented in this sample of older persons were television viewing, visiting with friends, working on small handcrafts, and reading. These passive activities carried out near home could be interpreted as evidence of disengagement. These pastimes can also be interpreted as efforts to remain active, however, with the substitution of more sedentary activities for the strenuous ones of the past. Other studies provide evidence that satisfaction in old age is achieved not so much by the frequency and variety of activities in which an older person engages, but by the opportunity to engage in *valued* activities of whatever form (Ray, 1979).

Cognition and intellect represent areas of psychological function in which generalizations and stereotyping are rampant and certain patterns of decline are presumed to be a part of aging. In reality, research findings have shown that *speed* of performance declines with aging (the older person takes *longer* to answer questions) and it is important to distinguish between the decline in speed and in overall intellectual functioning (Birren, Butter, Greenhouse, Sokoloff, & Yarrow, 1963). The older person is definitely at a disadvantage in situations of timed pressure determined by external circumstances (a timed questionnaire). Verbal intellectual abilities, however, are generally retained and learning continues.

In the complex domain of memory, the operation of the memory system itself has been differentiated from recall of specific information (Salthouse, 1982). These metamemory processes of the memory system appear to remain largely intact at all ages. It has been demonstrated by some that older persons experience difficulties in what is known as *secondary memory*, that is, retention of items that have been recently learned, whereas memory for items of the remote past remains intact (Botwinick & Storandt, 1974). These conclusions are based on mixed findings from studies that have methodologic problems, however, and Salthouse (1982) concludes that it is impossible at this point to reach any conclusions about the influence of age on memory for remote information. It seems that the recognition of individualization in old age and significant differences among older persons is especially important in intellectual areas of function, and we should resist the tendency to assume the presence of intellectual decline on the basis of age alone.

Another area of psychosocial function is what Kastenbaum refers to as "adaptive uses of the past" (1985, p. 75). Processes such as life review, validation, boundary setting, ritual perpetuation of the past, and replaying are strategies by which older persons use the past to help cope with the present and future. In boundary setting, for example, the older person uses the past as a standard of comparison in determining the boundaries of their life in the present: "Does my neighborhood still exist for me, even though I now live in a nursing home?" In the strategy of replaying, the older person selects a few past memories to replay, perhaps in an effort to avoid the unacceptable reality of the future: "Remember the time we. . . . "

Although there may be no denying that deficits in psychosocial functioning occur with aging, Kastenbaum (1985) cautions us to also recognize the compensatory strategies that older persons use successfully and the potential recuperative and coping resources that can be fostered. In addition, conditions such as depression and dementia must be recognized as *not* normal or expected deficits but as indications of abnormalities in psychosocial functioning in old age that need to be assessed for treatability.

As may be seen, the psychosocial and psychological theories of aging do not play themselves out very readily in actual patterns of behavior in old age. At best, they provide broad theoretical guidelines for ways to examine and interpret psychosocial aspects of the aging person's life. In our case example, G.P.'s restricted life experience could be interpreted as adaptive disengagement; alternatively, his efforts to feed himself and move around the house and yard could be interpreted as an attempt to maintain his previous level of activity; finally, the same activities could be viewed as filling the need for continuity in his life. The mystery of what is and is not adaptive aging is not easy to solve, because tremendous variation in all aspects of aging exists among older persons.

Chronic and acute illness

At least 80% of persons age 65 or over have at least one chronic health condition (National Center for Health Statistics, 1982). The most common causes of morbidity are arthritis, hypertension, hearing impairments, and heart disease. Heart disease, cancer, and strokes are the leading causes of death among persons 65 years or older. **Chronic illnesses** are characterized by long-term duration (usually lifelong), often have no known cause, are generally progressive and lead to irreversible changes, and re-

quire symptomatic (not curative) treatment aimed at control and rehabilitation.

Only a small proportion (4%) of persons aged 65 or older are severely disabled. The extent of disability increases with age, with those aged 85 or older being four to six times more likely than those aged 65 to 74 to be disabled and to require assistance in daily activities. "Chronic conditions have replaced acute diseases as a major health risk for older people and have increased the need for long-term care services" (Hooyman & Kiyak, 1991, p. 148).

The incidence of acute illness decreases with age, although the acute conditions that do occur are more debilitating for older persons than for younger persons. People aged 65 or over account for 42% of all hospital days in any given year and almost twice as many physician visits (American Association of Retired Persons, 1987). Not the least of the risks associated with acute illness are the physiologic complications of bed rest.

The bed remains the focus of the acute care setting (on entry to a hospital, a patient is immediately assigned to a bed); yet the elderly are particularly vulnerable to the adverse consequences of bedrest (Harper & Lyles, 1988). For the older person, rapid loss of muscle strength (as much as 5% per day), decreased bone density, susceptibility to pressure sores, and temporary periods of confusion can result from even a relatively short period of bed rest. For some people, health and aging are self-contradictory, mutually exclusive terms.

Scott-Maxwell has stated, "The crucial task of age is balance . . . " (1968, p. 36). The bodies and social circumstances of the elderly no longer have much reserve capacity to call upon when out-of-the-ordinary physical or life situational demands arise. Maintaining a balance in daily life by avoiding excessive demands on their physical and social systems is essential in old age. Often we as professionals try to increase an older person's reserve so that the system doesn't go into crisis so easily and the crucial balance can be maintained even with fluctuating demands.

For example, the amount of cardiac reserve (capacity of the heart to respond to greater physical demands such as strenuous exercise) of a normal 20-year-old athlete will be decreased when he or she reaches age 80. This decrease is the result of at least three processes:

1. The aging process itself in which there is a normal decrease in the heart's ability to respond to increased demands in the environment
2. Deconditioning secondary to a sedentary lifestyle or lack of exercise, which further encroaches on the cardiac reserve capacity
3. Heart disease, such as the damage due to heart attack or atherosclerotic disease, which may significantly reduce the reserve capacity of the heart (Irwin & Zadai, 1990).

All three processes may leave an older person in a state of precarious balance, able to maintain that crucial equilibrium of everyday living only by avoiding situations that demand cardiac reserve. Obviously, one way an occupational therapist can help a person to increase his or her remaining reserve capacity is by instituting a reconditioning program. Disease control is another way to help stabilize the amount of remaining reserve.

Other kinds of losses of reserve are represented in the social context of older persons' lives. The inability to drive or to walk more than one or two blocks at a time eliminates options for getting around in the community for tasks such as grocery shopping. Riding with a neighbor may be the only option that remains; that is, the neighbor is the only "reserve" to help accomplish this life demand. If the neighbor dies or moves away, the older person faces a crisis and loses the balance of his or her life. If we provide other options such as home-delivered meals, grocery store delivery, or special transportation services, however, we have once more increased the person's "reserve capacity," and he or she is better able to handle a variety of life's demands without losing the critical balance.

Who are the caregivers of the elderly?

As previously stated, most caregiving for older persons is carried out by family caregivers (Figure 19-2). It is estimated that 80% of all health care for older persons in the United States is provided by family members (Shanas, 1979). It is a myth that most older persons are in nursing homes being cared for by professionals; most older persons who need care are in the community being cared for by family members or other lay caregivers.

In the literature, lay caregivers are referred to as *informal caregivers* and professionals are referred to as *formal caregivers*. It might be assumed that most lay caregivers are getting help from professionals as they carry out the caregiving responsibilities. That assumption is another myth. Data show that only 10% of all informal caregivers use formal services to supplement their caregiving (Stone et al., 1986). Yet the strain and burden of family caregiving have been well researched (Cantor, 1983; Crossman, London, & Barry, 1981; George & Gwyther, 1986).

Informal caregiving tasks may include personal care assistance (bathing, toileting, shaving), administering medication, household chore assistance, community errands such as grocery shopping and medical appointments, and financial management. Responsibilities also are likely to include worries and concerns such as safety in the home, planning for an uncertain future, and acting as a liaison with medical personnel and service agencies. Both the division of tasks themselves (Clark & Rakowski, 1983) and the relationships between lay and formal caregivers (Hasselkus, 1988) have been studied and are of continued research interest.

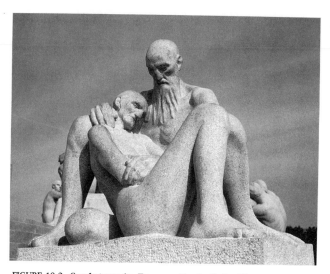

FIGURE 19-2. *Sculpture in Frogner Park, Oslo, Norway.*

Among formal health professionals, a gradual trend toward increased interest and specialization in geriatrics is occurring. In the profession of occupational therapy, the 1990 AOTA Member Survey reported that over 28% of all registered occupational therapists (OTRs) list 65 years or older as the primary age range of their patients/clients. Thirty-seven percent of all certified occupational therapy assistants (COTAs) work with clients in this older age range. Thus, about one third of all occupational therapy personnel work primarily with older adults. These figures are in contrast to the 1986 Member Survey data, which reported 16% of OTRs and 22% of COTAs working primarily with clients 65 years old or older. The demand for therapists and other personnel in this area of health care service, which is already high, is expected to skyrocket in the next three decades as the baby boomer generation reaches its peak number during the year 2025.

Where are older persons cared for?

Obviously, one location of care for older persons is acute care settings. Statistics from the 1986 National Health Survey on use of short-stay hospitals clearly indicate three facts: (1) the rate of hospital days per year for persons 65 years of age or older is greater than for all younger aged persons; (2) the rate of hospital days increases linearly with aging, that is, as age increases, the rate of hospital days increases; and (3) for each age group *except* the oldest, there is a decided reduction in rate from 1965 to 1986, reflecting the general trend in our health care system toward shorter hospitalizations. The older age group shows only a small proportional reduction in rate, and in the Northeast section of the United States, the older age group shows an actual small *increase*.

At present, the newly instituted (1984) Medicare Prospective Payment System (PPS) is affecting these hospital-stay statistics. The PPS relies on diagnostic-related groups (DRGs)—a listing of diagnoses (eg, hip fracture, heart failure), with each diagnosis assigned an expected length of hospital stay for which Medicare coverage is guaranteed. Costs for hospital stays beyond the stated guidelines may have to be assumed by the hospital itself, the patient's supplemental insurance, or private resources. Earlier hospital discharge is one ramification of this new prospective payment system.

Shifts in location of health care for older persons, resulting from the PPS, have already been documented. A dramatic intensification of nursing care in skilled nursing facilities was demonstrated in a pre-DRG/post-DRG study by Harron and Schaeffer (1986). These authors state that "elderly persons are being discharged from the acute-care facility sooner, and are entering the skilled nursing facility with more severe problems than previously were seen in most nursing homes" (p. 31). The implications of this for professionals is the need for personnel in these settings who are skilled in acute care procedures and rehabilitative techniques. Nursing homes have long been considered the flagship setting for formal long-term care. In recent years, the role of the nursing home in the care of older persons has shifted toward rehabilitation and discharge back to the community as well as long-term lifelong health maintenance.

Another arena of health care for older persons is adult day care (National Institute on Adult Daycare, 1984; Neustadt, 1985). This concept of community care evolved during the 1980s and has become an important component in the continuum of long-term care offered to older persons. The purposes of day care programs include the provision of respite to family members, the restoration or rehabilitation of the older person to his or her highest level of function, and the provision of socialization and meaningful activity. Hundreds of adult day care centers now exist within the United States. In 1989, Wood published a study that included data on the impact of DRGs on the adult day care system. Findings were parallel with those of the nursing home study cited above, that is, that the population of adult day care clients post-DRG was more disabled than pre-DRG and required more intensive care for longer periods of time (Wood, 1989).

Home health care is the third major arena of long-term care for older persons. According to health statistics reported in 1983 (National Center for Health Statistics, 1983), almost five million adults living in the community needed the help of another person to carry out their daily activities. Almost 3 million of these adults were 65 years of age or older. As might be expected, the rate of requiring help increased substantially with age, with 5% of those in the 65- to 75-year-old age group needing home help compared with 38% of those in the 85 and older age group. Although about 25% of these adults required nursing or medical care, the largest needs were in basic self-care areas such as needs for help with walking, going outside, bathing, and dressing.

More recently, home health agencies have experienced a shift toward "more acute high-tech care; more skilled nursing; and more antibiotic intravenous therapy," since the advent of the Medicare Prospective Payment System (Wood & Estes, 1990, p. 841). It seems evident that the impact of both the growth of the older population and the trend toward earlier hospital discharges is resulting in an increased demand for home health services and a shift in those services toward care of "sicker" clients.

Summary

Persons 65 years of age or older constitute an ever-increasing proportion of the population in the United States. A variety of biologic and psychosocial theories of aging have been proposed to help explain the process of aging. The context of health in old age is one of multiple chronic illnesses superimposed on normal age changes, all occurring within a unique social and societal environment. The oldest population, those 85 years old and over, are at the highest risk for disability and need for long-term care. Health professionals and family members who care for older persons need to work together to share the responsibilities of caregiving. Institutional and community health care options will be increasingly important to meet the future demand for services.

References

American Association of Retired Persons. (1987). *A profile of older Americans: 1987*. P.O. Box 2240, Long Beach, CA 90801.

Atchley, R. C. (1989). A continuity theory of normal aging. *Gerontologist, 29*, 183–190.

Barta Kvitek, S., Shaver, B., Blood, H., & Shepard, K. (1986). Age bias: Physical therapists and older patients. *Journal of Gerontology, 41*, 706–709.

Birren, J. E., Butler, R. N., Greenhouse, S. W., Sokoloff, L., & Yarrow, M. R. (1963). *Human aging: A biological and behavioral study*. Washington, DC: U.S. Government Printing Office.

Bjorksten, J. (1974). Crosslinkage and the aging process. In M. Rockstein (Ed.), *Theoretical aspects of aging* (pp. 43–59). New York: Academic Press.

Bortz, W. M. (1989). Redefining human aging. *Journal of the American Geriatrics Society, 37*, 1092–1096

Botwinick, J., & Storandt, M. (1974). *Memory, related functions and age*. Springfield, IL: Charles C Thomas.

Butler, R. N. (1969). Age-ism: Another form of bigotry. *Gerontologist, 9*, 243–246.

Campanelli, L. C. (1990). Theories of aging. In C. B. Lewis (Ed.), *Aging: The health care challenge* (2nd ed., pp. 7–21). Philadelphia: F. A. Davis.

Cantor, M. (1983). Strain among caregivers: A study of experience in the United States. *Gerontologist, 23*, 597–603.

Clark, N. M., & Rakowski, W. (1983). Family caregivers of older adults: Improving helping skills. *Gerontologist, 23*, 637–642.

Crane, D. (1975). *The sanctity of social life: Physicians' treatment of critically ill patients*. New York: Russell Sage Foundation.

Crossman, L., London, C., & Barry, C. (1981). Older women caring for disabled spouses: A model for supportive services. *Gerontologist, 21*, 464–470.

Cumming, E., & Henry, W. E. (1961). *Growing old: The process of disengagement*. New York: Basic Books.

Davis, L. J. (1986). Introduction. In L. J. Davis & M. Kirkland (Eds.), *Role of occupational therapy with the elderly* (pp. 1–5). Rockville, MD: American Occupational Therapy Association.

Davis, L. J. (1988). Gerontology. In H. L. Hopkins & H. D. Smith (Eds.), *Willard and Spackman's occupational therapy* (7th ed., pp. 742–755). Philadelphia: J. B. Lippincott.

Department of Health and Human Services. (1988). *Utilization of short-stay hospitals, U.S. 1986 Annual Summary*. DHHS Publication No. (PHS) 88–1757. Hyattsville, MD: National Center for Health Statistics.

Dye, C. J., & Sassenrath, D. (1979). Identification of normal aging and disease-related processes by health care professionals. *Journal of the American Geriatrics Society, 27*, 472–475.

Ellis, N. B. (1991). Aging, functional change, and adaptation. In J. Kiernat (Ed.), *Occupational therapy and the older adult* (pp. 26–42). Gaithersburg, MD: Aspen Publications.

Erikson, E. H. (1963). *Childhood and society*. New York: W. W. Norton & Co.

Estes, C. L., & Binney, E. A. (1989). The biomedicalization of aging: Dangers and dilemmas. *Gerontologist, 29*, 587–596.

George, L. K., & Gwyther, L. P. (1986). Caregiver well-being. A multi-dimensional examination of family caregivers of demented adults. *Gerontologist, 26*, 253–259.

Harman, D. (1969). Prolongation of life: Role of free radical reaction in aging. *Journal of the American Geriatrics Society, 17*, 721–735.

Harper, C. M., & Lyles, Y. M. (1988). Physiology and complications of bed rest. *Journal of the American Geriatrics Society, 36*, 1047–1054.

Harron, J., & Schaeffer, J. (1986). DRGs and the intensity of skilled nursing. *Geriatric Nursing*, January/February, 31–33.

Hasselkus, B. R. (1988). Meaning in family caregiving: Perspectives on caregiver/professional relationships. *Gerontologist, 28*, 686–691.

Hasselkus, B. R., & Kiernat, J. (1989). Not by age alone: Gerontology as a specialty in occupational therapy. *American Journal of Occupational Therapy, 43*, 77–79.

Hayflick. L. (1965). The limited in vitro lifetime of human diploid cell strains. *Experimental Cell Research, 37*, 614–636.

Hayflick, L. (1980). The role of cell biology in aging research and education. *Gerontology and Geriatrics Education, 1*(2), 149–152.

Hayflick. L. (1983). Theories of aging. In R. Cape, R. Coe & M. Rodstein (Eds.), *Fundamentals of geriatric medicine* (pp. 43–50). New York: Raven Press.

Hooyman, N. R., & Kiyak, H. A. (1991). *Social gerontology: A multidisciplinary perspective* (2nd ed.). Boston: Allyn & Bacon.

Irwin, S. C., & Zadai, C. C. (1990). Cardiopulmonary rehabilitation of the geriatric patient. In C. B. Lewis (Ed.), *Aging: The health care challenge* (pp. 181–211). Philadelphia: F. A. Davis.

Kastenbaum, R. (1985). Psychological aspects. In G. H. Maguire (Ed.), *Care of the elderly: A health team approach* (pp. 69–79). Boston: Little, Brown & Co.

Kiernat, J. (1991). The rewards and challenges of working with older adults. In J. Kiernat (Ed.), *Occupational therapy and the older adult* (pp. 2–10). Gaithersburg, MD: Aspen Publications.

Lemon, B. W., Bengston, V. L., & Peterson, J. A. (1972). An exploration of the activity theory of aging: Activity types and life satisfaction among in-movers to a retirement community. *Journal of Gerontology, 27,* 511–523.

Levenson, S. A. (1985). Physical aspects and problems. In G. H. Maguire (Ed.), *Care of the elderly: A health team approach* (pp. 95–112). Boston: Little, Brown & Co.

Lewis, C. B. (1990). Introduction. In C. B. Lewis (Ed.), *Aging: The health care challenge* (2nd ed., pp. 1–4). Philadelphia: F. A. Davis.

Marshall, V. W. (1981). Physician characteristics and relationships with older patients. In M. R. Haug (Ed.), *Elderly patients and their doctors* (pp. 94–118). New York: Springer.

Maslow, A. (1954). *Motivation and personality.* New York: Harper & Row.

National Center for Health Statistics. (1982). Current estimates from the National Health Interview Survey: U.S. 1981. *National Health Survey,* Series 10, #141:DHHS Publication #82–1569.

National Center for Health Statistics (B. Feller, Ed.). (1983). Americans needing help to function at home. *Advance data from Vital and Health Statistics,* No. 92. Hyattsville, MD: Public Health Service.

National Center for Health Statistics (R. J. Havlik, et al., Eds.). Health Statistics on Older Persons, United States, 1986. *Vital and Health Statistics,* Series 3, No. 25, DHHS Pub. No. (PHS) 87–1409. Public Health Service. Washington, DC: U.S. Government Printing Office, June 1987.

National Institute on Adult Daycare. (1984). *Standard for adult daycare.* Washington, DC: National Council on the Aging.

Neustadt, L. E. (1985). Adult daycare: A model for changing times. *Physical & Occupational Therapy in Geriatrics, 4*(1), 53–66.

Nystrom, E. (1974). Activity patterns and leisure concepts among the elderly. *American Journal of Occupational Therapy, 28,* 337–345.

Orgel, L. E. (1963). The maintenance of the accuracy of protein synthesis and its relevance to ageing. *Proceedings of the National Academy of Science, 49,* 517–521.

Palmore, E. (1976). Total chance of institutionalization among the aged. *Gerontologist, 16,* 504–507.

Ram, J. S. (1967). Aging and immunological phenomena: A review. *Journal of Gerontology, 22,* 92–107.

Ray, R. O. (1979). Life satisfaction and activity involvement: Implications for leisure service. *Journal of Leisure Research, 11,* 112–119.

Reichel, W. (1983). *Clinical aspects of aging.* Baltimore: Williams & Wilkins.

Salthouse, T. A. (1982). *Adult cognition. An experimental psychology of human aging.* New York: Springer-Verlag.

Scott-Maxwell, F. (1968) *The measure of my days.* New York: Penguin Books.

Shanas, E. (1979). The family as a social support system in old age. *Gerontologist, 19,* 169–174.

Sill, J. S. (1980). Disengagement reconsidered: Awareness of finitude. *Gerontologist, 20,* 457–462.

Soldo, B. (1980). *American's elderly in the 1980's, 35*(4). Washington, DC: Population Reference Bureau.

Stone, R., Cafferata, G. L., & Sangl, J. (1986). *Caregivers of the frail elderly: A national profile.* Rockville, MD: National Center for Health Services Research.

Torrey, B. B., Kinsella, K. G., & Taeuber, C. M. (1987). *An aging world.* Washington, DC: Bureau of the Census.

Wood, J. B. (1989). The emergence of adult day care centers as post-acute care agencies. *Journal of Aging and Health, 1,* 521–539.

Wood, J. B., & Estes, C. L. (1990). The impact of DRGs on community-based service providers: Implications for the elderly. *American Journal of Public Health, 80,* 840–843.

Von Hahn, H. P. (1973). Primary causes of ageing: A brief review of some modern theories and concepts. *Mechanisms of Ageing and Development, 2,* 245–250.

Bibliography

Biegel, D. E., & Blum, A. (Eds.). (1990). *Aging and caregiving. Theory, research, and policy.* Newbury Park, CA: Sage Publications.

Binstock, R. H., & Shanas, E. (Eds.), (1985). *Handbook of aging and the social sciences* (2nd ed.). New York: Van Nostrand Reinhold.

Birren, J. E., & Schaie, K. W. (Eds.). (1985). *Handbook of the psychology of aging* (2nd ed.). New York: Van Nostrand Reinhold.

Cohen, U., & Weisman, G. (1991). *Holding on to home: Designing environments for people with dementia.* Baltimore: The Johns Hopkins University Press.

Finch, C. E., & Schneider, E. L. (Eds.). (1985). *Handbook of the biology of aging* (2nd ed.). New York: Van Nostrand Reinhold.

Gubrium, J. F. (1990). *The mosaic of care. Frail elderly and their families in the real world.* New York: Springer.

Gubrium, J. F., & Sankar, A. (1990). *The home care experience. Ethnography and policy.* Newbury Park, CA: Sage Publications.

Kane, R. A., & Caplan, A. L. (Eds.). (1990). *Everyday ethics. Resolving dilemmas in nursing home life.* New York: Springer.

Kaufman, S. R. (1986). *The ageless self. Sources of meaning in late life.* Madison, WI: University of Wisconsin Press.

CHAPTER 20

Functional disability and older adults

BETTY RISTEEN HASSELKUS

LEARNING OBJECTIVES

Upon completion of this chapter the reader will be able to:

1. *Understand the components of building therapeutic relationships with older clients.*
2. *Be familiar with basic concepts of assessment of functional performance and the choice of assessment instruments.*
3. *Recognize the contribution of both individual competence and environmental factors to functional performance.*
4. *Understand and describe a variety of assessment tools used by occupational therapists in geriatrics.*
5. *Name and give examples of three treatment approaches in geriatric occupational therapy.*

Occupational therapy (OT) is the therapeutic use of self-care, work, and leisure activities to increase independent function, enhance development, and prevent disability. The focus of the profession is on functional performance in daily activities. This is also the focus of gerontology and geriatric health care. In their seminal text on assessment and the elderly, Kane and Kane (1981) stated,

> ... measures of functional status that examine the ability to function independently despite disease, physical and mental disability, and social deprivation are the most useful overall indicators to assist those who care for the elderly. (p. 1)

Thus, occupational therapists should feel right at home in geriatrics.

During the first two decades after World War II, occupational therapy drew heavily on the medical model of service (medical rehabilitation of disabled veterans). The model of practice has broadened in more recent years to include many components that are not strictly medical. As Kiernat (1991b) has stated,

> ... the occupational therapist serving older adults must have advanced knowledge of physical rehabilitation and behavioral health and be a specialist in independent living and the repertoire of community agencies and social support services. (p. 7)

In tracing the historical development of occupational and physical therapy in geriatric rehabilitation, five themes of therapeutic practice in geriatrics emerge:

1. The *medical–physiologic approach*—physician-directed treatment, a professional health team, and (often) institutional location of care
2. *Focus on function*—the consideration of health in old age within the context of functional ability rather than the context of disease, with the environment as a key factor
3. The *promotion of self-care*—the maintenance of control and self-directedness in late life via a partnership relationship between professional and client
4. The *family* context—use of a family-oriented approach to health care for elderly people

5. *Rehabilitation in the community*—the development of independent living situations and supportive services in the community for older people (Hasselkus, 1989).

This chapter focuses on occupational therapy practice with older adults, thus adding specialized knowledge to the more general geriatrics background provided in Chapter 19. The continuum of function/dysfunction in geriatrics draws heavily on the concept of activity and functional performance in everyday life. Assessments tend to focus on the individual *and* the environment, and more often than not, change is sought in the environment to facilitate maximum daily function. This chapter reviews the nature of the relationship between occupational therapists and their clients in geriatrics, geriatric assessment tools used in occupational therapy, and treatment areas in OT including prevention, accommodation, and restoration.

Therapeutic relationships with older clients

How do we begin to establish rapport and a therapeutic relationship with G.P., whose case was presented on page 734 of Chapter 19? What are the important and unique features of relationships between professionals and older persons?

A **therapeutic relationship** is one that promotes the cure or management of disease and ill health. The giving and receiving of help are at the core of this relationship. Peloquin (1990) stated, "The therapeutic relationship promoted in occupational therapy has been an evolving blend of competence and caring" (p. 13).

In occupational therapy, we seek to establish therapeutic relationships with our clients to facilitate functional performance. For example, based on the problems outlined in the previous case example, a therapist might try to work with G.P. to enhance safe mobility within the house and yard, to facilitate food preparation and performance in other kitchen tasks, to promote independence in self-care, and to assist in the development of meaningful use of time. Whether or not these goals are set and attained depends heavily on the quality and character of the therapeutic relationship.

Age biases

Remember the "undue tendency toward therapeutic inactivity" cited in the previous chapter (Marshall, 1981, p. 111), that is, the tendency to set lower goals and undertake less aggressive therapy with older people based on negative ageist attitudes? In such instances, the therapist's own view of the situation (eg, G.P. is frail and not too much can be done to improve this function) can lead to erroneous presumptions about the need to limit goals and treatment approaches. Older people are particularly likely to find such attitudes in professionals with whom they work and are particularly affected by these attitudes; therefore, these attitudes and their potential impact on therapeutic activity must be guarded against.

In a study of **age bias** among physical therapists, Barta Kvitek et al. (1986) measured goal-setting aggressiveness and found significant differences between goal setting for older patients compared with goal setting for young patients based on age alone. In their study, they provided the same patient case

example to two groups of therapists with one difference—the patient's age was given as 28 years for one group of therapists and as 78 years for the other group. The findings revealed significant differences between the groups on aggressiveness of goal setting in six of nine treatment areas (ambulation assistance, ambulation endurance, use and type of prosthesis, general rehabilitation, return to work, and return to living situation), with the therapists setting less aggressive goals for the older patient. The authors concluded,

> . . .therapists may assume that old people as a group are less capable physically and, therefore, automatically set lower goals for them . . . if a therapist sets a lower than justifiable goal for an old patient, the patient may not achieve his or her maximum physical potential. (Barta Kvitek et al., 1986, p. 709)

Although no study of age bias among occupational therapists has been found in the literature, there is no reason to suppose that, if such a study were conducted, findings would be different from those found in the physical therapy study. Ageism is a pervasive phenomenon, which demands that we each search within ourselves to clarify our own attitudes and strive to change those that inappropriately shape our therapeutic practice.

Creating dependencies

Ironically, health professionals, in their zeal to be helpful to their clients and to respond to their clients' needs, can unwittingly *cause* dependencies. As occupational therapists, with our focus on maximizing a person's functional independence, such dependencies are certainly the exact opposite of what we hope to be our mission. Yet studies in nursing homes provide strong evidence of staff patterns of overhelping in their daily interactions with persons who live there. The aura of frailty and debility that accompanies older persons, especially those in institutional settings, makes them particularly vulnerable to assumptions of incompetence and of needing help.

In her nursing home research, Baltes (1988) described three kinds of **dependency**: (1) dependency due to true physical and mental incompetence; (2) dependency due to selective optimization; that is, the older person selects to be dependent in one area of daily life (such as getting dressed), so that he or she may be *in*dependent in another area (such as having enough energy to independently use a wheelchair to get to a morning activity); and (3) dependency due to social stereotyping and underestimation of competence. The third type of dependency results in patterns of **overhelping**. Baltes called such overcare by staff "dependence-supportive behavior" (p. 314) and described the vicious cycle of dependent behavior followed by dependence-supportive behavior (staff helping) followed by more dependent behavior that was observed in the nursing home residents and staff. Occupational therapists may play a vital role in sensitizing institutional staff about negative stereotypes of older people and their competencies; careful assessments of true competencies by an occupational therapist can be provided to document instances of overhelp.

In our case example, G.P.'s daughter could easily fall into an overhelping pattern of doing all her father's daily self-care. It would be faster and would ensure acceptable results and perhaps be safer. However, certain areas of self-care may be entirely within G.P.'s range of remaining abilities and for the daughter to take over in *all* self-care activities is an example of overhelping. A vicious cycle of accelerated decline by G.P. would likely result. Thus, family members, as well as health professionals, must also resist this tendency to overhelp. Occupational therapists may teach family members about rehabilitation philosophies and help family caregivers to determine the best routines and techniques to use in their own personal home contexts (Hasselkus, 1988).

Communicating with older persons

Two major age-related changes that occur in most elderly persons contribute significantly to making it difficult to communicate with them: changes in vision and changes in hearing (Falconer, 1985/86; Jacobs et al., 1983). If a person can't see you very well and can't hear you very well, most of the sensory cues that convey interest (an alert look in your eye, eye contact, body at attention), respect, affection, warmth, concern, confidence, and so on, may never be perceived. Difficulties with communication naturally also mean difficulties with establishing therapeutic relationships, since the latter is very dependent on the smooth functioning of the former. The professional must work very hard to communicate clearly and to somehow use other sensory channels to convey therapeutic meanings.

G.P. has markedly impaired vision and hearing. An occupational therapist seeking to communicate as effectively as possible with this client could do the following:

I. To compensate for vision impairment
   A. Wear bright-colored clothing. Most visually impaired people can see *something*, and bright colors may enable G.P. to keep track of where you are in the room and help him to find your face when you are speaking together at close range.
   B. Do not sit with your back to a window or other bright light as you are talking to G.P. If the light comes from behind you, your face will appear dark and any **communication cues** that G.P. could possibly pick up from your facial features (smile, look of puzzlement) are lost. Sit with the light on your face, if possible.
   C. Avoid anything that might distort or hide your facial features such as gum chewing, long hair, or a hand in front of your mouth. These suggestions are related to the point made above—it is important to keep your face visible to maximize the communication cues that G.P. can use. Sit close together during an interview to further enhance your communication.
   D. Use touch (appropriately) to get G.P.'s attention before you speak. A light touch on the hand or arm can signal to an older person to ignore other distractions and focus on you.

II. To compensate for hearing impairment
   A. Many of the previous suggestions also apply to communication with a person who is hearing-impaired, that is, keep your face in the light and visible, and sit close together. If there is no vision impairment, eye contact can be used as well as touch to gain the person's attention before speaking.
   B. Lowering the pitch of your voice is often helpful; the hearing loss of old age affects higher voice sounds. Speaking louder and louder does not usually help.
   C. Use key words to start a topic rather than long, complex phrases; when repeating, use different words and rephrasing rather than repeating the same words over and over.
   D. Enhance your communication with nonverbal cues such as facial expressions, body language, and gestures.
   E. Many older persons have better hearing in one ear than the other; ascertain this and speak toward the ear that hears best.

Therapeutic strategies

A number of other strategies are useful in helping to establish a therapeutic relationship with an older client. One strategy is to think about the relationship as a partnership with the older person. In a partnership, people share their views of the situation, they share control and authority, and they share responsibilities for problems and solutions (Kleinman, 1988; Schön, 1987). It is generally agreed that when people have long-term, chronic health problems, a partnership approach to health care, rather than an authoritarian approach of telling people what to do, is most appropriate. The goals of health care are not to cure but to help the client achieve independence in the day-to-day management of chronic problems.

A partnership relationship may depend on active promotion of participation of the client in the therapeutic process. In other words, an older client may *expect* to be told what to do, and yet we believe it is far better in the long run that he or she learn to act and make health judgments independently. An occupational therapist may need to facilitate this active participation through strategies such as patient education (Hasselkus, 1983, 1986) and special interviewing techniques (Hasselkus, 1990; Kleinman, 1988; Payton et al., 1990).

A final strategy for establishing therapeutic relationships with older clients is for the occupational therapist to sensitize him- or herself to the unique cultural context of the particular client. "Culture largely determines why people suffer from what they do, and why treatment follows a particular course and not another" (Logan & Hunt, 1978, p. xiii). The age biases described earlier in this chapter are part of our culture. So, too, are such patterns of behavior as how close together we stand when we are conversing, how much eye contact we expect during communication, our beliefs about the causes and treatments of illness, our values related to individualism or group welfare, gender appropriateness of behaviors, and the formality or informality of our interactions with one another.

Ethnicity (racial, religious, national, or linguistic identity) is one aspect of culture. It has been argued that the importance of ethnicity increases with aging and that it serves to provide a sense of integration for the older person in the face of alienating forces in society (Barney, 1991). Sensitivity to the ethnicity of older clients, such as those who are African American, Hispanic, Appalachian, Native American, and Jewish, has been sparsely addressed in our literature (Barney, 1991; Blakeney, 1989; McCree, 1989; Neustadt, 1982). Nevertheless, as Barney (1991) has stated,

> ... culturally sensitive approaches can promote effective service provision, but more important, ... this sensitivity can make the critical difference between whether services are accepted or refused by the client. (p. 586)

Summary of therapeutic relationships

In summation, therapeutic relationships between occupational therapists and older clients are embedded in societal beliefs such as age biases, age-related patterns of helping, and age-specific communication variables due to sensory impairments. Strategies to overcome inherent barriers to therapy include sensitization to the cultural context of both the therapist and the client, modified communication techniques to compensate for impaired vision and hearing, and the active promotion of care partnerships between the therapist and the older person.

Geriatric assessment in occupational therapy

In 1983, Katz and his associates developed a new measure of life expectancy that combined mortality and disability. They called this index a *measure of active life expectancy* (ALE), defined as that period of life free of disability in activities of daily living (Katz et al., 1983). The ALE measure reflects the belief that death and disease are not the only criteria for assessing the health of people in old age and that functional status represents an important part of the definition of quality of life in old age (Branch et al., 1991). For example, although the average remaining life expectancy for 65-year-old white men in the United States is 14.6 years (National Center for Health Statistics, 1987), the average *active* life expectancy for this same group is 13 years (Branch et al., 1991). In other words, independent 65-year-old white men in the United States can expect on average 1.6 years of dependency before they die.

G.P., by the definition of dependency offered by Katz et al. (1983), may or may not have entered his years of dependency, that is, his years of *in*active life expectancy. The responsibility of the occupational therapist is to determine whether he is dependent in one or more activities of daily living (ADL) such as bathing, dressing, transferring from bed to chair, and eating. Since functional status can improve, stabilize, and decline, it is the further responsibility of the occupational therapist to determine potential for change and the treatment means to bring that about.

The next section will concentrate on occupational therapy assessments to determine areas of performance dysfunction in older people, and the subsequent section of this chapter will examine treatment approaches.

As in any area of occupational therapy practice, **geriatric assessments** take both standardized and nonstandardized forms. The purpose of the assessment should be the determining factor in what specific assessment is used by a therapist. A narrative interview assessment may be the best tool to use for individualized treatment planning; a brief standardized screening tool may be best for an efficient initial assessment to identify problem areas; a moderately detailed standardized tool may be the choice for repeated monitoring of patient status over time.

The focus of geriatric assessment on functional performance is different from a focus on components of performance such as joint range of motion or grip strength. Obviously, such components of performance may be important objects of assessment in certain older persons, but generally the emphasis in geriatrics is at the functional performance level. Component measurements tend to be more appropriate and useful in acute illness situations, and, as stated earlier, the illness processes of aging tend to be chronic. In addition, because functional performance is *behavior* and because behavior is the outcome of the interaction of the person and the *environment*, as occupational therapists, we also assess the environment (Lawton & Nahemow, 1973; Lewin, 1936). Some geriatric assessments try to assess both the functional performance of the person and the environment of the person; others are specific to one or the other.

Functional performance assessment

A multitude of **functional performance** assessments are available in the literature. See Law and Letts (1989) and Kane and Kane (1981) for comprehensive reviews of tools currently used in practice. As early as 1969, Lawton and Brody published standardized scales to measure daily functional abilities in older people, and the terminology they used has been widely adopted by gerontology practitioners and researchers. Briefly, Lawton and Brody separated everyday activities into two categories—self-maintaining activities of daily living (ADL) and instrumental activities of daily living (IADL). ADL included the basic self-care activities such as bathing, dressing, and toileting. IADL included what were considered hierarchically more complex tasks such as using the telephone, making meals, and managing medications (Lawton & Brody, 1969).

Lawton and Brody's scales were among the first to address daily living tasks that are associated with community living. Before this, and even for some time thereafter, many "geriatric" scales that claimed to measure function were appropriate only for older people in institutions. For example, included on one scale were items such as "Patient helps out on the ward" or "The patient is objectionable to other patients" (Meer & Baker, 1966). Obviously, such items would not be appropriate or relevant to an older person living at home; also, many tasks important to living at home were missing from the assessment.

Some early scales included questions that were vulnerable to excesses of subjectivity in their grading. The PULSES scale developed by Moskowitz and McCann (1957) included several items with grading based solely on the examiner's perception of what was appropriate for an old person; for example, grading on mental and emotional status included one option that stated, "No deviations considering the age of the individual." Obviously, what one examiner might consider usual and expected for a person of a specific age may be vastly different from that of another examiner. It is evident that early geriatric scales of function reflected common myths and stereotypes of aging.

In an earlier paper, I described the use of the Barthel Self-Care Index (Mahoney & Barthel, 1965) with geriatric outpatients (Hasselkus, 1982). In choosing this scale for use with a population of community-living older clients, the following factors were considered:

1. Does the content of the scale include all items deemed important to the self-care function of this group of clients?
2. Are the scale items appropriate for community-living clients? Can it be administered in the client's home environment?
3. Is the weighting of the items (how much each one counts toward the total score) appropriate to these clients and their life context?

4. Is the scale manageable in length and complexity so that it lends itself to regular and repeated administration, and, at the same time, is it sensitive enough to reflect change over time?

5. Is the scale easily interpretable by other team members? In other words, will it help team communication or generate confusion?

6. Is the scale valid and reliable as documented in previous research?

The occupational therapist must ask these kinds of questions before selecting a tool for clinical use. The items on the Barthel Self-Care Index and their scoring categories are shown in Table 20-1; a specific protocol describing the meaning of each score is part of the assessment. A tool such as the Barthel Self-Care Index is useful clinically to gather quantitative data for describing the needs of a patient population, to help establish the need for community supports or institutional living, and to document change in functional status over time.

The Barthel Self-Care Index is an example of a moderately sensitive screening tool; a therapist would likely want to follow up on identified problem areas with a more detailed assessment. For example, a finding on the Barthel screening that the client is partially dependent in dressing would lead to planning a therapy session to thoroughly evaluate the client's dressing skills, possibly including an assessment of types of clothing worn, accessible or inaccessible clothing storage, fastenings used, specific causes of difficulties (limited range of motion), available help, and so on. Of course, the therapist should also ascertain the client's perspective on the problem; after all, the client may feel that he or she has worked out a reasonable and satisfactory arrangement of assistance that enables him or her to get on with the day without undue energy expenditure on one activity. On the basis of such a detailed assessment, treatment planning could then be instituted.

Specialized in-depth assessments are available to occupational therapists in many deficit areas. One such tool, the Functional Low Vision Assessment, can be used to gather detailed information about an older person's visual status plus the impact of that status on his or her activities of daily living (McGrath, 1983). The former section of the assessment includes such items as color identification and visual field deficits; the latter includes assessment of abilities to read medication labels, read stove dials, write checks, and so on.

The Functional Low Vision Assessment is a tool that measures IADL, in this instance, as they relate to vision impairments. Another IADL tool in the literature is the ALSAR or Assessment of Living Skills and Resources (Williams et al., 1991). With strong occupational therapy involvement in its development, the ALSAR combines 11 IADL tasks with the client's available resources to determine levels of risk for the older person. For example, a skill level in meal preparation may be low (patient can neither prepare nor independently procure own meals), but the resource level may be high (resources enable meal preparation on a consistent basis and include . . .). With such a combination, the patient's risk level would be determined by combining the skill level and the resources scores (in this case, 2 plus 0) to yield a risk score. In the example, a risk score of 2 indicates a moderate risk in the area of meal preparation. This seems logical because the client cannot prepare or procure meals and has made very satisfactory arrangements for meal preparation by other means, but is at some risk because these arrangements involve total dependence on other resources and could be subject to sudden change. In cooperation with the client, total risks and priorities are reviewed and a plan of care is developed to reflect agreed-on priorities.

A few assessment tools attempt to combine many aspects of basic ADL skills with IADL skills to provide a multidimensional functional assessment tool. Two such early tools were the Older American Resources and Services (OARS) (Pfeiffer, 1975) and the Geriatric Functional Rating Scale (Grauer & Birnbom, 1975). The latter tool included the following interesting group of categories: physical condition, mental condition, functional abilities, support from the community, living quarters, relatives and friends, and financial situation. On the basis of "minus" scores in the first two categories (physical and mental deficits) and "plus" scores in the other categories (social resources), a total score was computed and tested for its predictive power regarding the type of living situation needed by the individual. Low scores, of course, predicted the need for institutionalization and high scores predicted independent living potential. The in-between scores, however, were less powerful and included a mix of dependent and independent living outcomes. This scale, in many ways, was a precursor to the ALSAR, providing an innovative combination of deficits and resources to assist in making independent living decisions.

Very recently, as a result of 1987 legislation (Omnibus Budget Reconciliation Act, 1987), the federal government has added new assessment requirements for nursing homes that use federal third-party payors (Medicaid or Medicare). The new resident assessment system includes a Minimum Data Set (MDS) and Resident Assessment Protocols (RAPs)—the former a lengthy comprehensive screening tool and the latter in-depth follow-up assessments for use in treatment planning. Items on the MDS range from eating patterns to ADL self-performance to disease diagnoses to activity pursuits. The tool is meant to be more reflective of quality of life concerns than previous, more medically oriented admission assessments. Many categories on the MDS, such as activity pursuits and ADL self-performance, certainly indicate the need for an occupational therapist to be in-

TABLE 20-1. *Barthel Self-Care Index*

Self-Care Task	Score
Feeding	0–5–10
Transfer skills	0–5–10–15
Personal hygiene	0–5
Toileting	0–5–10
Bathing	0–5
Ambulation (wheelchair)	0–(5)–10–15
Stairs	0–5–10
Dressing	0–5–10
Continence/bowel	0–5–10
Continence/bladder	0–5–10
Total (range)	0–100*

* 0, dependent in all self-care tasks; 100, independent in all self-care tasks.
(Adapted from Mahoney, F., & Barthel, D. (1965). Functional evaluations: The Barthel Index. Maryland State Medical Journal, 14, 61–65.)

volved in the admission assessment process. This is a new component of long-term care to which occupational therapy has much to contribute.

Environmental assessments

The **environment** is composed of all the people, physical objects, and cultural conditions that surround a person. Many theories of human behavior and human development incorporate the environment in their models (Barris et al., 1985; Cooper et al., 1991; Lawton & Nahemow, 1973; Lewin, 1936). Basically, the theories state that the behavior and development of human beings are the result of an interaction between the person and the environment. Under optimal conditions, the interaction represents a match between the person and the environment, leading to behavior that is efficient and competent. Under less than optimal conditions, when the person and the environment are mismatched, the resulting behavior can be a struggle or can result in failure.

In Lawton and Nahemow's terms (1973), a *person–environment match* is present when the person's level of competence matches the demands of the environment. For example, a person–environment match occurs when a college student achieves a satisfactory grade in a college course; the demands of the course (environment) are a "match" with the competence of the student. In a mismatch, the course demands could be too high (leading to failure) or too low (leading to boredom).

An extension of the theory of environmental demands is the *environmental docility theory*. This theory holds that the lower the person's competence, the greater the reliance of that person on the environment for support. In other words, a person who has lowered competence because of a disability or frailty can match only with those environments that have certain kinds of supports. Any environment that is different would not support adequate behavior. Two examples are (1) an older person with a physical disability who uses a walker can match only with an environment that has ramps, wide doorways, and so on; (2) an older person who has dementia can match only with an environment that is familiar and not complex. Otherwise, each will experience struggle and failure. Alternatively, persons who do not have a mobility problem or dementia can function adequately in a wide range of environments; that is, they can match with a variety of environments.

Occupational therapists who work with the elderly assess the older person's environment as well as his or her functional performance to evaluate the match between environment and person. Bringing about changes in the environment may bring about a match, thus supporting a return to competent behavior by the client.

Some of the assessment tools discussed in the previous section include elements of the environment, for example, the living quarters item in the Geriatric Functional Rating Scale (Grauer & Birnbom, 1975). These elements represent early recognition of the importance of the environment to the behavior of individuals. However, assessment of the environment is not nearly as well developed as assessment of the individual's functional performance. Kiernat (1982) called the environment a "hidden modality" and urged therapists to give the environment "special attention when attempting to change the behavior of older clients" (p. 3). Cooper et al. (1991), too, cited the paucity of occupational therapy literature that addresses the environment.

Because the demands for accessible environments are increasing, particularly to enable elderly and disabled persons to remain in the community, increased occupational therapy input will be required in the future. (p. 349)

At this point in time, occupational therapy assessments of the environment tend to address the physical features of the environment such as accessibility and design, and the focus has been on the assessment of private residences (Hasselkus & Kiernat, 1973; Malik, 1988; Cooper et al., 1991). Room-by-room checklists are used to assess safety, access, ease and range of maneuverability, and types of function (Trombly & Versluys, 1989). Environmental factors that affect an older person's risk of falling in the home have been identified (Tinetti & Speechley, 1989), and a home hazards checklist has been published that includes such environmental factors as lighting, furniture features, handrail positioning, and condition of carpeting (Tideiksaar, 1986).

In addition to physical characteristics, Levine (1988) and Kiernat (1982) both cite the importance of the cultural and psychosocial aspects of the environment as they relate to behavior. These aspects include such qualities as privacy, territoriality, identity, and continuity. Probably the most comprehensive review and discussion of the environment and aging is by Christenson (1990). Christenson reviews the many attributes of the environment and addresses in depth the issues of environmental compensation for sensory changes, promoting independence in the home, and redesigning of the long-term care facility. An occupational therapist by background, Christenson is a consultant to architects and developers of residential housing and care facilities, blending her expertise in human performance factors with specialized knowledge in the designed environment. Christenson, too, concludes that the environment is an underused modality in therapeutic interventions.

The importance of the environment is often overlooked, perhaps, because of the obvious nature of the interplay between behavior and environment. . . . Because activity and environment cannot be separated, the environment for the elderly must be designed in such a way that optimum functioning can take place. (Christenson, 1990, p. 31)

In the case study of G.P., it is highly probable that G.P.'s new environment is contributing to his problems with function. Thus, the occupational therapist should assess not only this older man's functional performance (using a tool such as the Barthel Self-care Index followed by in-depth assessments in specific problem areas) but also his home environment. G.P.'s competency is compromised by his impaired vision and hearing, plus his mobility problems and cardiopulmonary disease. It is likely that the unfamiliarity of both the physical environment and the daily routine are exerting overwhelming demands on G.P., and the result is behavior and function that represent a struggle and even failure (lost in the front yard; could not remember who his daughter was). At the same time, the unfamiliarity of the new home has also *removed* sources of stimulation from G.P.'s daily routine. Familiarity with his previous home and neighborhood had enabled him to engage in a variety of activities throughout the day that are now beyond his capabilities. As a result, he sits by the radio and is bored. An assessment of G.P.'s new home environment and daily routine is a starting point for identifying problem areas and potential strategies for change to bring about a better match between G.P. and his environment.

Occupational therapy treatment in geriatrics

As Davis has said, "sorting out the functional problems of the older adult is a complex challenge" (1988, p. 749). Geriatric occupational therapy is usually linked to services of other health care professionals or community service providers. Within the profession itself, registered occupational therapists often work together with certified occupational therapy assistants (COTAs) to plan and carry out programs for older clients. Geriatric practice includes the following three treatment approaches:

1. *Prevention approach*—the maintenance of current health status and the prevention of decline or injury
2. *Accommodation approach*—the use of compensatory strategies to help older persons live with a disability
3. *Restoration approach*—the use of rehabilitative techniques to help older persons regain maximum function

Prevention

Occupational therapy aimed at prevention uses two primary treatment approaches: accident prevention and activity promotion. For accident prevention, many environmental considerations are of prime importance. Accident prevention in the home is one objective of treatment and the home hazard checklist referred to previously could be a basis for such treatment planning (Tideiksaar, 1986). Occupational therapists may work with carpenters or may have the skills themselves, to measure for and install handrails and grab bars on stairways and in bathrooms (Figure 20-1) (Hasselkus, 1985). Home modifications specific to persons with dementia have been outlined, such as keeping medications locked up and storing cleaning compounds in inac-

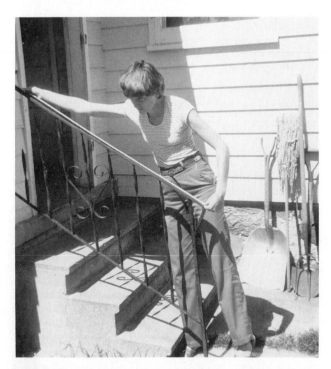

FIGURE 20-1. *Occupational therapist takes measurements to install new sturdy railings beside steps.*

cessible cupboards (Kern, 1986). Devising memory strategies for medication management is another example of therapy that aims at prevention and safety (Hasselkus & Bauwens, 1982). Therapists have been involved in the development of public education programs on home adaptation (Hasselkus & Kiernat, 1973). A slide/tape presentation on accident prevention and older people broadly addresses safety in many areas of daily activity within the home and community (Kiernat, 1977).

Activity promotion is a preventative approach based on the basic occupational therapy belief that activity *per se* is healthful and its converse belief that inactivity often leads to dissatisfaction with life and the loss of a sense of well-being. "Our daily activities are health maintaining in that they provide the mental and physical challenge to keep our body and mind adequately stimulated" (Crepeau, 1986, p. 5). Activity levels may become impaired for any number of reasons—health problems, age changes, institutionalization, societal attitudes. Therapeutic planning may be helpful in sustaining or reengaging a person in meaningful activity.

Activity programming that seeks to establish for an individual a healthful balance of work and play activities is important both in the community and in the institution. If life changes occur too rapidly or are severely disruptive to the balanced daily routine of a person's life, a negative cycle of impaired activity may result. An example of preventing such a negative cycle in the community would be assisting an older person to prepare for the life change of retirement, with its accompanying dramatic shift toward additional large blocks of leisure time and loss of work time (Cantor, 1981).

Another life change in older age may be a move to a supported living environment or to a long-term care facility. Such a relocation is inherently disruptive to usual activities and routines (Hasselkus, 1978); an occupational therapist can prevent or minimize relocation stress by incorporating preventive measures in the situation such as providing the older person with choices whenever possible, including him or her in decision making during the process, and providing familiarity of physical environment and routine in the new environment.

A special developmental activity of old age may be what Kastenbaum refers to as "adaptive uses of the past" (1985, p. 75). These are activities such as life review by which an older person uses memories of the past to adapt to the present situation. Therapists may at times appropriately stimulate memory activities to help sustain an older person's health and well-being in the present (Friedlob & Kelly, 1984; Merriam & Cross, 1981). Reminiscing activities may, of course, occur spontaneously, but they may also be purposefully planned for individuals or groups around themes such as pets, schooldays, a county fair, clothes, holiday traditions, and music. Kits of materials to stimulate memories are also available (Bi-Folkal Productions, Inc., 809 Williamson Street, Madison, WI 53703).

How does preventive treatment fit into the case example scenario of G.P.? It is obviously too late for some kinds of prevention: the relocation has already occurred, and the health problems are already fairly advanced. However, there is certainly the need to prevent further problems. Thus, given G.P.'s vision and mobility problems, the occupational therapist would help plan and install safety features in the home to minimize the probability of falls and injuries. Grab bars and a bath bench for bathing, sturdy handrails by the steps, good lighting throughout the house, bright-colored tape to mark the bottom step on the stairway (Figure 20-2) and enlarged markings on the stove dials are all possible recommendations. Close discussion with G.P. and his daughter about areas of risk in the house and potential remedies would be important, as would inclusion of both people in the decision making regarding recommended changes.

Additionally, an interview with G.P. regarding his past interests and daily routines might be helpful for finding ways to incorporate familiar activities into his present situation, thus preventing further decline in his skills and activity level. It seems likely that prolonged inactivity (listening to the radio all day long) will only lead to further deconditioning, boredom, frustration, and loss of a sense of competency. Again, close consultation with G.P. and his daughter will maximize the potential for successfully reinstating previous interests and daily habits.

Accommodation

Many of the safety recommendations made by an occupational therapist both prevent injury and accommodate an existing disability. By accommodation we mean modification of the older person's environment to enable him or her to carry out ADL as independently as possible. So, for example, installing grab bars near the bathtub may prevent falls and injury, but it may also enable a person to independently transfer in and out of the tub instead of relying on assistance from another person.

The principle of accommodation extends broadly into many facets of independent living. Enlarged numbers on a telephone may enable a person to use the telephone independently. Built-up handles on eating utensils may make it possible for a person to self-feed. A wedge seat cushion or raised platform may enable a person to get in and out of a chair without assistance (Figure 20-3) (Olin, 1982). On a larger scale, different types of adapted housing such as group homes or specially designed units for persons with dementia accommodate disabilities, always striving to permit the older person to live as independently as possible

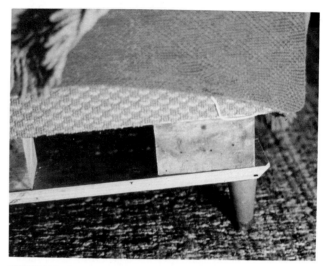

FIGURE 20-3. *Raised platform under chair.*

(Coons & Weaverdyck, 1986; Hasselkus, 1977). It is probably obvious that the essence of accommodation is the modification of the environment so that it matches and supports the person's competencies, reflecting the theory of environmental docility already referred to in this chapter.

The psychosocial environment may also be accommodated to support function. Occupational therapists and COTAs have been involved in the development of support groups for older persons and their families in the community (Curley, 1987; Gessert, 1987). Support groups can offer a number of services to participants including respite from caregiving, opportunities to share expertise and problem solving, emotional support, and information giving. Support groups with an educational format are reviewed by Hasselkus and Kiernat (1991); such groups may address memory changes, vision impairments, home safety, surviving the loss of a spouse, staying active, spiritual growth, and so on.

A special type of psychosocial support may be facilitated by a therapist or COTA in a long-term care facility by the provision of group programs that foster the development of *community* (Kiernat, 1991a). Community is the antithesis of isolation. Community is belonging and connectedness. It encompasses shared symbols, shared contacts, interdependence, and work for the good of the whole. Community combats a sense of disenfranchisement and alienation expressed by so many nursing home residents. The use of activities to foster community development might include planning communal work (making a quilt for a raffle, creating and tending an herb garden for use in the facility kitchen, building birdhouses for installation outside the facility windows), forming facility-wide groups and events (a choir or kitchen band), or promoting helping relationships among the facility residents (a sighted resident assisting a blind resident) (Kiernat, 1991a).

Many service agencies in the larger community can assist the older person and his or her family as they try to live with a disability. Older adult day care services offer respite care and social stimulation for older persons in the community; sometimes the availability of such programs enables the older person to avoid institutionalization (Aronson, 1976; Neustadt, 1985). Other community services such as Meals-on-Wheels, adapted

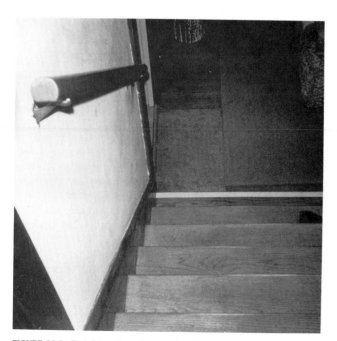

FIGURE 20-2. *Bright-colored tape is placed on bottom step for older client with visual impairment.*

transportation, talking books, and home health aides all help older persons accommodate their life to their disability without unduly sacrificing the quality of their daily existence. Occupational therapists in geriatrics need to at least be informed about these services so that appropriate referrals can be made. In some instances, for example, in adult day care, therapists themselves provide direct services (see Chapter 26).

Another aspect of accommodation is the adaptation of techniques during everyday living to accommodate a specific disability. Therapeutic treatment approaches such as joint protection techniques for persons with arthritis and work simplification for those with heart disease or pulmonary disease are examples of such adapted techniques (Trombly, 1989a, 1989b).

For G.P., the occupational therapist might recommend the use of a number of accommodations in his daily routine and living environment (in addition to the safety features in the home already discussed). Any proposed daily activities need to be planned to accommodate G.P.'s vision and hearing impairments; telephone amplifiers and dials with large numbers may be considered so that he could safely communicate with his daughter (and vice versa) during the day. Perhaps a friendly reassurance call scheduled every day from a volunteer agency or church group could be successfully implemented, providing a safety check as well as a social activity for G.P. Attendance at an older adult day care program might be recommended, perhaps for 2 days a week to provide a safe and stimulating environment for G.P. during the day. Confusion might be mitigated by putting large-print labels on drawers and storage areas so that G.P. could better learn and remember where his belongings are located. A distinctive "marker" such as a sundial or birdhouse might be positioned in the front yard to help G.P. orient to his surroundings. All these are examples of therapeutic accommodations that potentially help to bring about a match between G.P.'s competencies and his environment.

One final area of accommodation is important to recognize—the therapeutic accommodation that is appropriate for the dying person (Tigges & Marcil, 1988). A review of the dying person's occupational history can lead to the therapist's understanding of the activities and roles that the person has had to give up, those that are still important to the person, and those that may still be part of the person's remaining life. For the elderly dying person, opportunities to continue to be a mother, a friend, a grandmother, a helper, a comforter, and so on, all can be facilitated by an insightful geriatric occupational therapist, whether that therapist is working in home health care, acute hospital care, a long-term care facility, or hospice care.

Restoration

Restorative care is remedial care that seeks to restore the older person to former levels of function following an acute illness or traumatic injury. If G.P. fell and sustained a hip fracture, he would need a postfracture period of rehabilitative therapy to restore his function as best as possible to its former level. Because of G.P.'s age, his rehabilitative course of treatment would not be the same as that for a younger person with a similar fracture. G.P. would lose function faster during the period of trauma (quickly diminished strength due to bed rest, probable confusion due to anesthetic and other medications, the stress of relocation, and the impaired vision and hearing) and would recover more slowly postsurgery.

An occupational therapist working with G.P. in this hypo-thetic situation would work closely with the hospital team to carry out restorative programming. Strengthening, endurance building, and gait training followed by functional training in dressing and other self-care activities would be part of the program. Cooperative and coordinated efforts by the physician, nursing staff, health aides, physical therapist, and social worker would be important to bring about a return to functional independence and ultimate discharge back to living with the daughter. If full restoration of function is not possible, further *accommodation* of the home environment may be indicated (eg, a ramp to replace the outside steps).

With the current trend toward shorter hospital stays (see Chapter 19), older persons often are discharged from the hospital to nursing homes for rehabilitative care before returning to their community homes. Extended recovery from a cerebrovascular accident, amputation, joint replacement, myocardial infarction, congestive heart failure, and other acute conditions often takes place in a long-term care facility. As a consequence, occupational therapists in long-term care have focused more and more on restorative programming in preparation for discharge back to the community. Self-care, meal preparation, home maintenance, independent medication management, and mobility within the home and community are key issues in therapy. A similar shift toward rehabilitative therapy has occurred in home health care, also because of the earlier hospital discharge trends.

Restorative programming may be aimed at mental reconditioning as well as physical reconditioning (Docherty, 1986; Smith, 1986). In programming for older persons who are depressed, rehabilitative goals focus on helping the person restore and build social relationships and gain the motivation to return to former levels of independence (Docherty, 1986, p. 72). The general overall plan of a rehabilitative program with depressed older persons may follow a sequence from individual treatment, to group therapy, to self-help groups. Docherty (1986) quoted one participant in such a program as saying,

> The group is my lifeline. . . . We exchange needs and views and rejoice when things go well and try to help when they go ill. It all helps to restore one's confidence and makes life worth living. (1986, p. 76)

Summary

Occupational therapy for older adults is a rapidly growing area of practice that encompasses acute care, long-term care, adult day care, and home health care. Geriatric occupational therapists use their training in physical and psychosocial dysfunction to assess and plan therapy for elderly persons. Both the competencies of the older person and the person's environment are therapeutic concerns. With a focus on independent living and functional performance, the therapist must draw on a wide spectrum of skills to address the often complex and interrelated aspects of the older person's health situation. As in all other areas of practice, the occupational therapist's work with older persons may be for them the key that makes life worth living.

References

Aronson, R. (1976). The role of an occupational therapist in a geriatric day hospital setting. *American Journal of Occupational Therapy, 30,* 290–293.

Baltes, M. M. (1988). The etiology and maintenance of dependency in the elderly: Three phases of operant research. *Behavior Therapy, 19,* 301–319.

Barney, K. F. (1991). From Ellis Island to assisted living: Meeting the needs of older adults from diverse cultures. *American Journal of Occupational Therapy, 45,* 586–593.

Barris, R., Kielhofner, G., Levine, R., & Neville, A. (1985). Occupation as interaction with the environment. In G. Kielhofner (Ed.), *A model of human occupation: Theory and application* (pp. 42–62). Baltimore: Williams & Wilkins.

Barta Kvitek, S. D., Shaver, B. J., Blood, H., & Shepard, K. F. (1986). Age bias: Physical therapists and older patients. *Journal of Gerontology, 41,* 706–709.

Blakeney, A. B. (1989, June). Providing services to the elderly in Appalachia. *AOTA Gerontology Special Interest Section Newsletter, 12*(2), 2–3.

Branch, L. G., Guralnik, J. M., Foley, D. J., Kohout, F. J., Wetle, T. T., Ostfield, A., & Katz, S. (1991). Active life expectancy for 10,000 Caucasian men and women in three communities. *Journal of Gerontology: Medical Sciences, 46,* M145–150.

Cantor, S. G. (1981). Occupational therapists as members of pre-retirement resource teams. *American Journal of Occupational Therapy, 35,* 638–643.

Christenson, M. A. (1990). Aging in the designed environment. *Physical & Occupational Therapy in Geriatrics,* Special issues 8, (3/4).

Coons, D. H., & Weaverdyck, S. E. (1986). Wesley Hall: A residential unit for persons with Alzheimer's disease and related disorders. *Physical & Occupational Therapy in Geriatrics, 4*(3), 29–53.

Cooper, B. A., Cohen. U., & Hasselkus, B. R. (1991). Barrier-free design: A review and critique of the occupational therapy perspective. *American Journal of Occupational Therapy, 45,* 344–351.

Crepeau, E. L. (1986). *Activity programming for the elderly.* Boston: Little, Brown & Co.

Curley, J. (1987). Care for the caregiver: A support group for caregivers of persons with Alzheimer's disease. *AOTA Gerontology Special Interest Section Newsletter, 10*(4), 4,8.

Davis, L. J. (1988). Gerontology. In H. L. Hopkins & H. D. Smith (Eds.), *Willard and Spackman's Occupational Therapy* (7th ed., pp. 742–755). Philadelphia: J. B. Lippincott.

Docherty, F. (1986). Steps in the progressive treatment of depression in the elderly. *Physical & Occupational Therapy in Geriatrics, 5*(1), 59–76.

Falconer, J. (1985/86). Aging and hearing. *Physical & Occupational Therapy in Geriatrics, 4*(2), 3–20.

Friedlob, S. A., & Kelly, J. J. (1984). Reminiscing groups in board-and-care homes. In I. Burnside (Ed.), *Working with the elderly. Group process and techniques* (2nd ed., pp. 308–337). Monterey, CA: Wadsworth Health Sciences.

Gessert, V. G. (1987). Living room: A support group for families with aging relatives. *AOTA Gerontology Special Interest Section Newsletter, 10*(4), 1–3.

Grauer, H., & Birnbom, F. (1975). A geriatric functional rating scale to determine the need for institutional care. *Journal of the American Geriatrics Society, 23,* 472–476.

Hasselkus, B. R. (1977). A small group home for the elderly. *American Journal of Occupational Therapy, 31,* 525–529.

Hasselkus, B. R. (1978). Relocation stress and the elderly. *American Journal of Occupational Therapy, 32,* 631–638.

Hasselkus, B. R. (1982). Barthel Self-Care Index and geriatric home care patients. *Physical & Occupational Therapy in Geriatrics, 1,* 11–22.

Hasselkus, B. R. (1983). Patient education and the elderly. *Physical & Occupational Therapy in Geriatrics, 2*(3), 55–70.

Hasselkus, B. R. (1985). The occupational therapist. In G. H. Maguire (Ed.), *Care of the elderly: A health team approach* (pp. 145–158). Boston: Little Brown & Co.

Hasselkus, B. R. (1986). Patient education. In L. Davis & M. Kirkland (Eds.), *The role of occupational therapy and the elderly* (pp. 367–372). Rockville, MD: American Occupational Therapy Association.

Hasselkus, B. R. (1988). Meaning in family caregiving: Perspectives on caregiver/professional relationships. *Gerontologist, 28,* 686–691.

Hasselkus, B. R. (1989). Occupational and physical therapy in geriatric rehabilitation. *Physical & Occupational Therapy in Geriatrics, 7*(3), 3–20.

Hasselkus, B. R. (1990). Ethnographic interviewing: A tool for practice with family caregivers for the elderly. *Occupational Therapy Practice, 2,* 9–16.

Hasselkus, B. R., & Bauwens, S. F. (1982). Occupational therapy and pharmacy: Adapting drug regimens for older people. *AOTA Gerontology Special Interest Section Newsletter, 5*(4), 1–2.

Hasselkus, B. R., & Kiernat, J. M. (1973). Independent living for the elderly. *American Journal of Occupational Therapy, 27,* 181–188.

Hasselkus, B. R., & Kiernat, J. M. (1991). Education for empowerment. In J. Kiernat (Ed.), *Occupational therapy and the older adult* (pp. 61–74). Gaithersburg, MD: Aspen Publications.

Jacobs, P. L., VanZandt, S., & Stinnett, N. (1983). Working towards independence for the elderly visually impaired. *Physical & Occupational Therapy in Geriatrics, 2*(3), 39–53.

Kane, R. A., & Kane, R. L. (1981). *Assessing the elderly. A practical guide to measurement.* Lexington, MA: D. C. Heath and Co.

Kastenbaum, R. (1985). Psychological aspects. In G. H. Maguire (Ed.), *Care of the elderly: A health team approach* (pp. 69–79). Boston: Little, Brown & Co.

Katz, S., et al. (1983). Active life expectancy. *New England Journal of Medicine, 309,* 1218–1224.

Kern, T. (1986). Safety first: Modifying and adapting the environment for the patient with Alzheimer's disease. *AOTA Gerontology Special Interest Section Newsletter, 9*(3), 4–5.

Kiernat, J. M. (1977). *Accident prevention and the elderly.* Slide tape presentation available for loan from Middleton Health Sciences Library, 1305 Linden Drive, University of Wisconsin–Madison, Madison, WI 53706.

Kiernat, J. M. (1982). Environment: The hidden modality. *Physical & Occupational Therapy in Geriatrics, 2*(1), 3–12.

Kiernat, J. M. (1991a). Community building as a basis for activity programs. In J. M. Kiernat (Ed.), *Occupational therapy and the older adult* (pp. 275–284). Gaithersburg, M.D: Aspen Publications.

Kiernat, J. M. (1991b). The rewards and challenges of working with older adults. In J. M. Kiernat (Ed.), *Occupational therapy and the older adult* (pp. 2–10). Gaithersburg, MD: Aspen Publications.

Kleinman, A. (1988). *The illness narratives.* New York: Basic Books.

Law, M., & Letts, L. (1989). A critical review of scales of activities of daily living. *American Journal of Occupational Therapy, 43,* 522–528.

Lawton, M. P., & Brody, E. (1969). Assessment of older people: Self-maintaining and instrumental activities of daily living. *Gerontologist, 9,* 179–186.

Lawton, M. P., & Nahemow, L. (1973). Ecology and the aging process. In C. Eisdorfer & M. P. Lawton (Eds.), *Psychology of adult development and aging* (pp. 619–674). Washington, DC: American Psychological Association.

Levine, R. E. (1988). Community home health care. In H. L. Hopkins & H. D. Smith (Eds.), *Willard and Spackman's Occupational Therapy* (7th ed., pp. 756–780). New York: J. B. Lippincott.

Lewin, K. (1936). *Principles of topographical and vector psychology.* New York: McGraw-Hill.

Logan, M. H., & Hunt, E. E. (1978). *Health and the human condition.* North Scituate, MA: Duxbury Press.

Mahoney, F., & Barthel, D. (1965) Functional evaluations: The Barthel Index. *Maryland State Medical Journal, 14,* 61–65.

Malik, M. (1988). Activities of daily living and homemaking. In H. L. Hopkins & H. D. Smith (Eds.), *Willard and Spackman's Occupational Therapy* (7th ed., pp. 258–271). New York: J. B. Lippincott.

Marshall, V. W. (1981). Physician characteristics and relationships with older patients. In M. R. Haug (Ed.), *Elderly patients and their doctors* (pp. 94–118). New York: Springer.

McCree, S. (1989, September). Sensitivity to the black elderly client. *AOTA Gerontology Special Interest Section Newsletter, 12*(3), 1–2.

McGrath, L. (1983). Functional low vision assessment. *Physical & Occupational Therapy in Geriatrics, 3*, 55–61.

Meer, B., & Baker, J. (1966). The Stockton geriatric rating scale. *Journal of Gerontology, 21*, 392–403.

Merriam, S. B., & Cross, L. H. (1981). Aging, reminiscence and life satisfaction. *Activities, Adaptations and Aging, 2*, 39–50.

Moskowitz, E., & McCann, C. (1957). Classification of disability in the chronically ill and aging. *Journal of Chronic Disease, 5*, 342–346

National Center for Health Statistics (R. J. Havlik, B. M. Liu, M. G. Kovar, et al., Health Statistics on Older Persons, United States, 1986. *Vital and Health Statistics*, Series 3, No. 25, DHHS Pub. No. (PHS) 87–1409. Public Health Service. Washington, DC: U.S. Government Printing Office, June 1987.

Neustadt, L. E. (1982). Developing a program for Jewish residents in non-Jewish nursing homes. *Physical & Occupational Therapy in Geriatrics, 2*(1), 13–23.

Neustadt, L. E., (1985). Adult day care: A model for changing times. *Physical & Occupational Therapy in Geriatrics, 4*(1), 53–66.

Olin, D. W. (1982). Evaluation for furniture riser modifications. *Physical & Occupational Therapy in Geriatrics, 1*(4), 55–58.

Omnibus Budget Reconciliation Act of 1987 (Public Law 100–203).

Payton, O. D., Nelson, C. E., & Ozer, M. N. (1990). *Patient participation in program planning: A manual for therapists.* Philadelphia: F. A. Davis.

Peloquin, S. M. (1990). The patient-therapist relationship in occupational therapy: Understanding visions and images. *American Journal of Occupational Therapy, 44*, 13–21.

Pfeiffer, E. (1975). *OARS multidimensional functional assessment questionnaire.* Durham, NC: Duke University Center for the Study of Aging and Human Development.

Schön, D. A. (1987). *Educating the reflective practitioner.* San Francisco: Jossey-Bass.

Smith, H. (1986). Mastery and achievement: Guidelines using clinical problem solving with depressed elderly clients. *Physical & Occupational Therapy in Geriatrics, 5*(1), 35–46.

Tideiksaar, R. (1986). Preventing falls: Home hazard checklists to help older patients protect themselves. *Geriatrics, 41*(5), 26–28.

Tigges, K. N., & Marcil, W. M. (1988). *Terminal and life-threatening illness: An occupational behavior perspective.* Thorofare, NJ: Slack.

Tinetti, M. E., & Speechley, M. (1989). Prevention of falls among the elderly. *New England Journal of Medicine, 320*, 1055–1059.

Trombly, C. A. (1989a). Arthritis. In C. A. Trombly (Ed.), *Occupational therapy for physical dysfunction* (pp. 543–554). Baltimore: Williams & Wilkins.

Trombly, C. A. (1989b). Cardiopulmonary rehabilitation. In C. A. Trombly (Ed.), *Occupational therapy for physical dysfunction* (pp. 581–603). Baltimore: Williams & Wilkins.

Trombly, C. A., & Versluys, H. P. (1989). Environmental evaluation and community reintegration. In C. A. Trombly (Ed.), *Occupational therapy for physical dysfunction* (pp. 427–440). Baltimore: Williams & Wilkins.

Williams, J. H., Drinka, T. J., Greenberg, J. R., Farrell-Holtan, J., Euhardy, R., & Schram, M. (1991). Development and testing of the assessment of living skills and resources (ALSAR) in elderly community-dwelling veterans. *Gerontologist, 31*, 84–91.

Bibliography

Brever, J. (1982). *A handbook of assistive devices for the handicapped elderly: New help for independent living.* New York: Haworth Press.

Brody, S. J., & Ruff, G. E. (Eds.). (1986). *Aging and rehabilitation: Advances in the state of the art.* New York: Springer.

Burnside, I. (Ed.). (1984). *Working with the elderly. Group process & techniques* (2nd ed.). Monterey, CA: Wadsworth Health Sciences.

Butler, R. N., & Lewis, M. I. (1982). *Aging and mental health: Positive psychosocial and biomedical approaches* (3rd ed.). St. Louis: C. V. Mosby.

Davis, L. J., & Kirkland, M. (Eds.). (1986). *Role of occupational therapy with the elderly.* Rockville, MD: American Occupational Therapy Association.

Dychtwald, K. (1986). *Wellness and health promotion for the elderly.* Rockville, MD: Aspen Publications.

Ernst, N. S., & Glazer-Waldman, J. R. (Eds.). (1983). *The aged patient: A sourcebook for the allied health professional.* Chicago: Year Book Medical Publishers.

Helm, M. (1987). *Occupational therapy with the elderly.* New York: Churchill Livingstone.

Kiernat, J. M. (Ed.). (1991). *Occupational therapy and the older adult. A clinical manual.* Gaithersburg, MD: Aspen Publications.

Lewis, C. B. (Ed.). (1990). *Aging: The health care challenge* (2nd ed.) Philadelphia: F. A. Davis.

Lewis, S. C. (1989). *Elder care in occupational therapy.* Thorofare, NJ: Slack.

Mace, N. L., & Rabins, P. V. (1981). *The 36-hour day.* Baltimore: Johns Hopkins University Press.

Maguire, G. H. (Ed.). (1985). *Care of the elderly: A health team approach.* Boston: Little, Brown & Co.

Tigges, K. N., & Marcil, W. M. (1988). *Terminal and life-threatening illness. An occupational behavior perspective.* Thorofare, NJ: Slack.

CHAPTER 21

Geriatric psychiatry

JOAN C. ROGERS

LEARNING OBJECTIVES

Upon completion of this chapter reader will be able to:

1. *Delineate the characteristics of occupational therapy practice in geriatric psychiatry.*
2. *Outline the purposes of conducting an occupational therapy assessment in geriatric psychiatry.*
3. *Describe the content and outcomes of the occupational therapy assessment.*
4. *Describe skill-based, habit-based, and environmentally based occupational therapy interventions.*

Unique features of geriatric psychiatry

Creation of a subspecialty of psychiatry in geriatrics implies that it has key features that distinguish it from adult psychiatry. Among the most distinctive features is the need to differentiate pathologic changes from normal age-associated changes (Sadavoy, Lazarus, & Jarvik, 1991).

Psychiatry deals with abnormalities in cognition, judgment, motivation, affect, personality, impulse control, and vegetative functions. Some of these behaviors are known to change throughout adulthood, whereas the life course of others is still being explored. The risk of failing to distinguish normal from abnormal changes is twofold. If normal changes are regarded as pathologic, the meaning of declining function is exaggerated. For example, the declines observed on intelligence tests in the performance of novel, speeded, perceptual–motor tasks may be interpreted as indicative of dementia (Spar & La Rue, 1990). Conversely, if pathologic changes are regarded as normal, clinical symptoms are overlooked and hence go untreated. For instance, when confusion is viewed as a concomitant of aging, treatable causes of confusion, like urinary tract infections or drug toxicity, are ignored. Determining whether changes in behavior and function are normal or abnormal requires a thorough understanding of normal age-associated changes and of pathology.

A second conspicuous feature of geriatric psychiatry is use of the biopsychosocial approach. There is a keen recognition of the interaction among biologic, psychological, and social factors in producing health in late life (Cohen, 1990). Physical impairments like hearing loss have been associated with late life paranoid disorders (Cohen, 1990; Cooper, Garside, & Kay, 1976). Similarly, psychiatric symptoms like anxiety have been related to gastrointestinal problems (Cohen, 1990). Bereavement, especially loss of a spouse, is a prognosticator of depression, and there is a high incidence of depression in the physically ill elderly (Clayton, Halikas, & Maurice, 1972; Cohen, 1990). Interactions among the biologic, psychological, and social domains of human functioning support a comprehensive medical, social, and functional assessment in geriatric psychiatry in addition to a thorough psychiatric workup.

A third feature of geriatric psychiatry is the need to adjust psychiatric interventions to take into account normal age-associated changes. This is best illustrated in regard to psychopharmacology. With age, the absorption, distribution, metabolism, and excretion of psychotropic drugs is slowed (Salzman, 1987; Young & Meyers, 1991). Hence, these medications take longer to take effect and remain longer in the body. As a consequence, the elderly are more likely to experience adverse drug reactions. An equivalent dose of medication produces a greater effect in an older adult than in a younger adult. To adjust for altered drug activity, starting, therapeutic, and maintenance dosages of psychotropic medications for the elderly are about one third to one half of those given to younger adults (Salzman, 1987). Medications may also be administered less frequently.

Just as multiple pathology is a hallmark of geriatric medicine, so, too, is it a hallmark of geriatric psychiatry (Kane, Ouslander, & Abrass, 1989). It is rare to find an elderly patient whose sole diagnosis is depression. The patient who has one or several physical health problems coexisting with depression is more common. Depression may also coexist with dementia. In managing any one health problem, other psychiatric and medical problems must be simultaneously taken into account, so that the resolution or alleviation of one problem does not create or exacerbate others.

For example, when a patient's cardiac status is severely compromised, special precautions may need to be taken when electroconvulsive therapy (ECT) is administered (Hays, 1991). Similarly, tricyclic antidepressant medications may complicate the treatment of cardiovascular disorders by precipitating hypertension, orthostatic hypotension, tachycardia, or palpitations.

A discussion of the unique features of geriatric psychiatry would be incomplete without recognition of the differential presentation of some psychiatric disorders in late life. For example, older patients with depression are more likely to complain about somatic problems but less likely to express guilt or feelings of worthlessness than younger patients (Dovenmuehle, Reckless, & Newman, 1970; Small, Komanduri, Gitlin, & Jarvik, 1986). They also tend to deny feeling depressed, although they may admit to losing interest in usual activities (Lesse, 1974). During a depressive episode, older patients are more likely to experience weight loss (Blazer, Hughes, & George, 1987), reduced energy, difficulty concentrating, and memory impairment (Spar & La Rue, 1990).

A particularly difficult problem arises when both depression and dementia are present, because the psychiatrist must ascertain whether depression is causing the dementia, which is known as *pseudodementia* (or preferably *the dementia syndrome of depression*), or whether dementia coexists with depression. Unlike dementia, the dementia syndrome of depression has a distinct onset and symptoms progress rapidly. Patients complain about difficulties in cognition and often give "I don't know" responses to questions. Their performance on cognitive tests is inconsistent rather than uniformly low. They do not exhibit the bizarre behaviors that are typical of patients with organic dementia, like eating plant leaves or donning socks over shoes (Spar & La Rue, 1990).

Finally, geriatric psychiatry is characterized by a **coordination of care**. Coordination is manifested through (1) coordination of multidisciplinary services, (2) coordination of inpatient and outpatient services, and (3) coordination of informal and formal services.

Multidisciplinary services

Core members of the geriatric psychiatric team are the psychiatrist, primary care physician or physician's assistant, nurse, social worker, occupational therapist, and activities professional. The psychiatrist conducts the psychiatric evaluation, renders the psychiatric diagnosis, and designs and coordinates the overall care plan. The primary care physician or physician's assistant obtains the medical history, performs the physical examination, implements and coordinates the care for active medical problems, and advises the team about medical precautions. The nurse assesses nursing needs, administers medications, and documents patients' daily behavior. The social worker conducts the social history, evaluates social and financial resources, counsels patients and their caregivers, and manages the discharge plan. The occupational therapist assesses functional status (occupational performance) and designs interventions to protect patients' strengths and reduce their incapacities. The occupational therapist may also be responsible for planning and implementing a varied program of therapeutic activities. This responsibility may be shared with other activities professionals such as recreational, art, and dance therapists. Services from nutritionists, pharmacists, neuropsychologists, and physical therapists, are often added to the team or made readily available through consultation.

Inpatient and outpatient services

Geriatric psychiatry spans a continuum of services that includes acute care units, outpatient clinics, day programs, and long-term care facilities, including state hospitals and nursing homes (Curlik, Frazier, & Katz, 1991; Steingart, 1991; Tourigny-Rivard, 1991). Mention should also be made of consultation liaison services for elderly patients needing psychiatric assessment or treatment who are hospitalized on medical–surgical units (Folks & Kinney, 1991). Coordination of care aims at facilitating movement from one mode of service delivery to another as well as returning patients to community living as expeditiously as possible.

Formal and informal services

With advancing age, the older person's likelihood of disability increases. Psychiatric illness may further hinder independent functioning. Social support in the form of aid and caring relationships is provided by informal and formal services (Phillips, 1991). Informal services emerge from bonds of affection and obligation and are provided by family members, friends, neighbors, and church associates (Phillips, 1991). Multiple formal services have been devised to augment informal services in maintaining older adults in their own homes in the community. Formal services are provided by institutions, government agencies, and private organizations (Phillips, 1991). These include home nursing and rehabilitative services, personal care assistance, transportation services, Meals-on-Wheels, nutritional sites, chore workers, friendly visitors, activity programs, and adult day care centers. When the need for services exceeds that which can be provided in the home, a supervised living situation, such as a personal care home, may provide the range of care required. In coordinating care, informal and formal services are combined to yield a plan that is responsive to both the patient's and the patient's caregiver's needs and resources.

The population served

Currently, about 21% of the population of the United States is 55 years or older, and 12% is 65 or older. It is projected that by 2030, one in three Americans will be at least 55 years old, and one in five at least 65. Persons aged 85 and older account for the fastest growing segment of the population. In 1980 an estimated 2.2 million people were 85 years or older; the number is projected to climb to 16 million by 2050 (U.S. Senate, 1987–1988).

Older adults with mental disorders constitute a significant subgroup of the elderly population. Overall, it is estimated that 15% to 25% of older adults have significant mental health problems (U.S. Senate, 1987–1988). About 12% of older adults living in the community have mental disorders (Regier et al, 1988). Of those elderly hospitalized for medical conditions, about 40% to 50% are estimated to experience psychiatric conditions (Rapp, Parisi, & Walsh, 1988; Small & Fawzy, 1988). In long-term care settings, between 70% and 94% of residents have been found to have mental disorders (Rovner, Kafonek, Filipp, Lucas, & Folstein, 1986; U.S. Senate, 1987–1988).

Although older adults experience the same mental health disorders as younger adults, certain conditions are of particular concern in late life because of their increased incidence or the high rate of associated morbidity. Older adults are at greater risk for dementia than younger adults. It is estimated that about 7.5% of the elderly suffer from dementia and most of these reside in the community (Gurland & Cross, 1982). Less than 1% of those 65 years of age are estimated to have dementia but the percentage climbs to more than 15% for those over 85 years of age (Katzman, 1986). Alzheimer's disease is the leading cause of dementia and the life expectancy for older adults with Alzheimer's disease is about 8 years from the time of onset (Katzman, 1986; Kokmen, Offord, & Okazaki, 1987).

The percentage of elderly who meet the strict diagnostic criteria for major depression or dysthymic disorder is low, about 2% to 4% (Myers et al., 1984). However, the estimates increase to between 10% and 15% when all older adults with clinically significant depressive symptoms are included (Blazer, Hughes, & George, 1987; Gurland, Copeland, Kuriansky, Kelleher, Sharpe, & Dean, 1983). Depression accounts for nearly 50% of admissions to psychiatric hospitals and about 25% of the elderly in medical hospitals have diagnosable mood disorders (Rapp, Parisi, & Walsh, 1988; Small & Fawzy, 1988). Older men with depression are at high risk for suicide (Manton, Blazer, & Woodbury, 1987; Stenbeck, 1980).

Anxiety disorders occur in about 4% of the elderly population, alcohol and drug dependence in about 1% to 2%, and schizophrenia and paranoid states in less than 0.5% (Bland, Newman, & Om, 1988; Kramer, German, Anthony, Von Korff, & Skinner, 1985; Turnbull & Turnbull, 1985). A high proportion of patients in state psychiatric hospitals have schizophrenia, and most have been admitted early in life (Goodman & Siegel, 1986).

Implications for occupational therapy

The unique characteristics of geriatric psychiatry and of the older population experiencing psychiatric illness have several critical implications for the practice of occupational therapy. First, occupational therapists working with older adults encounter patients with psychiatric disorders whether or not they are employed in a mental health setting. A high concentration of older patients with mental health problems are found in hospitals, rehabilitation units, long-term care facilities, and community agencies. Therapists must be skilled in recognizing psychiatric disorders so that they can initiate referrals to psychiatrists. They must be equally skilled in devising intervention plans that simultaneously take into account the medical and psychiatric conditions of patients.

Second, the occupational therapist must be prepared to treat a caseload composed primarily of patients with dementia or depression. Patients with dementia have task performance problems attributable to skill deficits. Because of cognitive impairments, they no longer know how to do tasks. They have difficulty initiating tasks at the appropriate time, locating objects required to do a task, sequencing the steps involved in task completion, attending to a task, and executing required actions. Memory loss, attention deficit, apraxia, and perseveration serve to disrupt task performance. Behavioral complications such as wandering, agitation, aggression, screaming, paranoia, and delusions may further depress function. In contrast to patients with dementia, patients with depression have task performance problems attributable to habit deficits. These patients typically know how to do tasks; however, since they lack the will or motivation to do them, their daily living routines are disrupted. Symptoms of depression such as inattention, indecision, decreased concentration, disinterest, lack of energy, impaired problem solving, psychomotor retardation, a tendency to focus on the present, apathy, a lowering of personal standards for task performance, and an indifference to the expectations of others contribute to habit deficits. The occupational therapist working in geriatric psychiatry must be skilled in distinguishing performance dysfunctions arising from skill and habit deficits and in implementing appropriate intervention.

Third, occupational therapists working in geriatric psychiatry must be prepared to assess and treat task performance dysfunctions caused by physical impairments as well as *cognitive* and *affective impairments*. To be able to complete tasks, patients must have the cognitive capability to plan an activity, the motor capability to carry out the plan, and the affective capability to want to do the activity. The cumulative effects of aging and physical and mental illness can disrupt cognitive, motor, or affective capability. The biopsychosocial model is implemented in geriatric practice and the traditional separation of physical disabilities and mental health practice is not applicable. For example, in geriatric psychiatry the occupational therapy assessment must be carried out so that task performance dysfunctions due to cognitive, motor, and affective impairments can be detected. The mere donning of a shirt and slacks is not an adequate test of dressing skills for these patients because this procedure emphasizes the motor components of dressing. The cognitive components, involved in selecting clothing and sequencing the donning of undergarments and street clothes, are neglected. By asking patients to "dress so that you can go outdoors for a walk," the complete range of motor and cognitive components of dressing can be evaluated.

Occupational therapy intervention in geriatric psychiatry involves a similar recognition of biopsychosocial factors. For example, the therapist may need to teach depressed (biopsychological factor) older patients, who also have hip fractures (biologic factor), how to use a walker so that they can get to group activities (social factor). Learning how to use the walker may be complicated by decreased concentration (cognitive [psychological] factor) and motivation (affective [psychological] factor).

Fourth, in geriatric psychiatry, occupational therapy focuses on task performance as opposed to the components of task performance. Task performance involves the skillful conduct of mobility, personal self-care, home management, leisure, and work tasks. The components of task performance are the cognitive (memory), motor (strength), and affective (interest) factors that enable task performance. Occupational therapy intervention stresses skill training and maintenance of mobility, personal self-care, and leisure tasks; home management and work tasks are included if appropriate. Skills are maintained through the practice of daily living habits. Deficiencies in the components of task performance are identified and treated within the context of skill and habit training.

The focus on daily living skills and habits (occupational performance) in geriatric practice is supported from two perspectives. One perspective emerges from the finding that training in the components of occupational performance does not necessarily result in improvements in occupational performance (McCue, Rogers, & Goldstein, 1990). For example, although a memory training program may improve a patient's ability to remember a list of groceries, it may not improve his or her ability to shop for groceries. The second viewpoint rests on the argument that older adults are motivated to learn tasks that they perceive as relevant to their daily lives. Whereas the connection between independent living and shopping for the food to cook for the evening meal is obvious, the connection between independent living and memorizing a grocery list is obscure and lacks the same motivational power. The older adults' needs for independence, safety, stimulation, and self-esteem are addressed through task performance (Trace & Howell, 1991).

Fifth, caregiver training is an integral part of occupational therapy programming in geriatric psychiatry. Although an older adult's chances of becoming institutionalized increase with age, most elderly persons continue to live in the community (Glick, 1979). However, community residence and functional independence are not synonymous. About 20% of the population aged 65 or older has difficulty performing at least one mobility, personal self-care, or home management task. Of those 85 and older, about 57% have difficulty with daily living tasks (National Center for Health Statistics, 1983). Family members provide most of the care needed by these persons (Bengston & Treas, 1980). The primary caregiver is usually a spouse if the marriage is still intact and if the spouse is able to give the care needed. If the spouse is not able to provide the assistance or is unavailable, caregiving responsibilities generally fall to a daughter, daughter-in-law, or granddaughter (Horowitz, 1985). Teaching caregivers effective strategies and techniques for managing task performance dysfunctions and disruptive behaviors can alleviate the stress of caregiving.

Occupational therapy process

Purposes of occupational therapy assessment

Data from the occupational therapy assessment may serve several purposes. In conducting the assessment, the occupational therapist must attend to the reason for which a patient was referred. The occupational therapy assessment may be more or less extensive, depending on the reason or reasons for referral. The following are the most common reasons for conducting an assessment:

- To screen for disability
- To describe functional status
- To provide data for planning occupational therapy intervention
- To assist in determining competence for independent living
- To monitor the effects of psychiatric modalities
- To evaluate the need for physical restraints

Screening for disability

The purpose of screening is to identify patients who have or are at risk for developing disabilities. *Disabilities* are dysfunctions in task performance. *Screening* is a case-finding procedure aimed at identifying patients who need more extensive, in-depth assessment. Patients are screened for disabilities on admission for psychiatric care and periodically thereafter (eg, every 6 months). Referrals are sought for patients in need of further assessment. Because screening is applied to a large number of patients, it is desirable to have screening procedures that are brief and easy to administer. At the same time, the procedures must be highly sensitive so that patients needing functional status assessment are not overlooked. For example, screening for cognitive impairment might include evaluations of money management and cooking because these tasks are known to be among the first to be affected by declines in cognition (Fortinsky & Hathaway, 1988).

Describing functional status

Assessment may be undertaken to provide a description of a patient's functional status, usually in terms of tasks that are done independently and dependently. The baseline functional status provides a standard against which the outcomes of intervention are evaluated. Intervention may be psychiatric, medical, or rehabilitative or any combination of these methods. Examining the effects of intervention on functional status provides an index of the impact of this intervention on daily life. The desired outcome is an improvement in functional status or, minimally, no decline in functional status. Descriptive data are also of value if no intervention is undertaken. Sequential measures of functional status may be compared with the baseline measure to ascertain the natural course of a disease process on functional status. Measures of the tasks that exhibit change in the absence of intervention and the rate at which change takes place are needed to evaluate whether intervention retards deterioration or expedites improvement. Individual patient data may be aggregated to provide group descriptions of functional status. Group portraits of the kinds and extent of disabilities typically seen in occupational therapy provide the foundation for program planning and evaluation. For example, a high incidence of task dysfunctions in grooming and meal planning addresses a need for structured programs in these life skills. The effectiveness of the newly introduced life skills programs can be evaluated by comparing the results of these programs with those obtained before their advent.

Planning intervention

A major reason for undertaking the occupational therapy assessment is to plan an individualized intervention program to maintain, restore, or improve a patient's functional status or to prevent or retard functional decline. An occupational therapy assessment undertaken to plan intervention goes beyond that required to describe functional status. In addition to ascertaining the level of independence of task performance, the occupational therapist must also ascertain the patient's potential for improving or restoring functional status and the means through which this change can be accomplished. This requires the therapist to evaluate a patient's capacity for learning or, minimally, for responding as intended to environmental modifications. In other words, it is not sufficient for a therapist to ascertain whether a patient is dependent in the task of bathing. The therapist must also ascertain whether the patient is capable of moving from a dependent to a more independent status in bathing. A bathtub transfer bench enabled Mrs. X to overcome her fear of falling in the bathtub; hence, she was able to resume bathing. When the same intervention was used with Mrs. Y, however, her concern about slipping was transferred from the bathtub bottom to the chair, and she remained dependent in bathing.

Determining competence to live independently

Deficits in mobility, personal self-care, and home management tasks place older patients at risk for continuing to live independently in the community. One use of functional status data is to assist in making decisions about community residence or placement in supervised settings. The implications of disability for community living must be interpreted in the light of the services that can be provided by family members and friends as well as those that can be purchased from formal geriatric services. For example, cooking is a critical skill for independent living. If a patient is unable to cook or cannot cook safely, this disability alone can pose a salient risk for independently living. However, if a spouse or adult child (*informal supports*) or Meals-on-Wheels (*formal support*) provides food on a daily basis, the patient's need to cook is met. Conversely, if neither informal nor formal supports were available to the patient, the need to cook would be unmet and would constitute a threat to survival.

When independent living is no longer feasible, functional status data are used to determine the specific type of supervised living situation that is needed. *Personal care homes* (provide board and care) provide room, meals, assistance with personal self-care, and protective oversight. *Congregate housing facilities* offer central dining, transportation, and social and recreational programs in the overall context of independent living. In a shared housing arrangement, two or more unrelated persons live together and share space, expenses, and responsibilities. Nursing home care is reserved for those who require extended nursing services. Patients who exhibit behaviors that place themselves or others at risk are transferred to state hospitals.

Monitoring effects of psychiatric modalities

The psychiatric modalities of pharmacology, ECT, and psychotherapy are initiated to relieve psychiatric symptoms such as anxiety, agitation, insomnia, depression, and paranoia. During the course of psychiatric treatment, periodic reevaluations of functional status are undertaken to ascertain whether relief of these symptoms is accompanied by improvements in activities of daily living. For example, it is necessary to note whether, as patients become less depressed, they also take better care of their personal appearance and socialize more. Functional status assessment done for monitoring purposes is scheduled to coincide with the course of psychiatric treatment, such as before and after ECT or before nortriptyline (antidepressant medication) is given and after therapeutic level has been reached. Functional status may also be monitored to ascertain any adverse effects of

psychopharmacology or ECT. Because many psychotropic medications affect motor control, daily testing of functional mobility and dexterity may be indicated.

Determining need for physical restraints

Historically, physical restraints have been used in psychiatry to manage violent behaviors (Soloff, 1984). Restraint by physical or chemical (medications) means or both has been widespread in the care of geriatric patients (Frengley & Mion, 1986; Zimmer, Watson, & Treat, 1984). Physical restraints include vests, mitts, seatbelts, waist ties, wrist/hand cuffs, wrist/elbow cuffs, laptrays, and geriatric chairs. Restraints are applied to older adults to control disruptive behavior like agitation, restlessness, aggression, combativeness, and wandering; to protect a patient, others, or equipment from harm; and to prevent interference with treatment (eg, removal of nasogastric tubes; Frengley & Mion, 1986). The evidence supporting the effectiveness of restraints for achieving these objectives is sparse. In fact, restraints may exacerbate confusion (Patrick, 1967), increase agitation (Edelson & Lyons, 1985), and fail to prevent accidents (Barbieri, 1983). In addition, restraints predispose patients to the deleterious effects of immobility such as skin breakdown, constipation, and disorientation (Miller, 1975; Rader, Doan, & Schwab, 1985) and have caused death (Dube & Mitchell, 1986). Tranquilizing medications are often used as substitutes for physical restraints.

Growing concern about the abuse of physical and chemical restraints led to passage of the nursing home reform amendments to the Omnibus Budget Reconciliation Act of 1987 (OBRA '87). Accordingly, physical restraints may be used only to "ensure a patient's physical safety and only upon the written order of a doctor that specifies the duration and circumstances under which the restraints are to be used." Restraints are not to be used for discipline or convenience. Residents must be free of unnecessary drugs, and behavioral programming is to be used in lieu of medications whenever possible. The effects of OBRA '87 are being felt in all segments of geriatric care. Functional status assessment to establish the need for restraints focuses on patients' mobility characteristics and their response to activity as a method of behavioral control. The assessment results in recommendations concerning alternatives to the use of restraints, the circumstances under which a restraint may be needed, and the least restrictive type of physical restraint, if one is needed.

Occupational therapy assessment

The occupational therapy assessment focuses on the performance of daily living tasks. Daily living tasks span five major categories—mobility, personal self-care, home management, leisure, and work. All categories may not be appropriate to assess for all patients. Two dimensions of task performance are assessed. The first dimension is skill and involves an evaluation of capability, that is, of what patients are able to do. *Skills* are generally described in terms of the degree of independence, safety, and correctness a patient uses to complete a task. Skill assessment yields both an ability and a disability profile. Tasks that are carried out independently, safely, and acceptably make up the ability profile, whereas those that fail to meet these criteria make up the disability profile. Habits are the second dimension of task performance that is assessed. *Habits* refer to the usual or routine task performance of a patient. Habit assessment yields a description of how frequently patients use their task skills. For example, patients may exhibit the physical skill to walk to the bathroom and use the toilet but may be incontinent habitually because of a failure to anticipate the need to urinate. Together, these two dimensions of task performance provide the comprehensive description of a patient's functional status needed to plan intervention or make recommendations.

The five categories of daily living tasks form a hierarchy. At the lowest end of the hierarchy are mobility tasks. Mobility tasks involve the ability to move the body from one place to another. Functional movements that are commonly assessed are moving in bed from side to side, to the head and foot of the bed, and to a seated position; transferring to and from a bed, chair, toilet, bathtub, and car; coming to and maintaining a standing position; walking on level and inclined surfaces and up and down stairs and turning to reverse direction; reaching overhead; bending; and stooping. The ability to move purposefully from one place to another indoors and outdoors (wayfinding), such as to a bathroom or a pharmacy, is also evaluated. Endurance for standing and walking is also considered since fatigue influences safety and capability. Because mobility tasks are generally less complex than other kinds of tasks, it is advantageous to begin the assessment with the mobility category. In addition to providing a measure of movement capability, functional mobility assessment provides a global impression of the patient's functional status.

Functional mobility assessment is also incorporated into the assessment of personal self-care, home management, leisure, and work tasks. Testing mobility in isolation from more complex tasks yields an index of skill when a patient's attention is on occupation. The two tests may yield different results. Mrs. Frank, for example, bumped into walls and grabbed onto furniture and personnel to maintain her balance when mobility was tested. However, her balance was maintained without incident during dressing, tub bathing, and bed making.

Personal self-care follows mobility in the hierarchy. Personal self-care tasks involve the ability to provide for basic personal needs. Typically, feeding, toileting, bathing, hygiene, grooming, and dressing (less frequently functional communication) are included in this category. These tasks are more complex than mobility tasks because they require a person to control the objects needed to complete tasks in addition to being able to control his or her body in space. For example, in combing hair, object control is reflected in grasping and holding the comb and in transporting it to the head for hair combing. Factors like appetite, weight loss, bladder and bowel incontinence, body odor, and unkempt appearance are incorporated into the assessment strategy to tap the habit dimension of personal self-care tasks.

The third rung of the hierarchy is occupied by home management. Tasks included in this category are associated with human needs for food, clothing, housing, health care, and social interactions. See the display on page 759 for an outline of specific home management tasks typically evaluated. Home management tasks place greater performance demands on older adults than do self-care tasks because they require control of a greater number of objects, some of which are technologically sophisticated. The sequence of steps needed to complete home management tasks is also more lengthy and the risks associated with task dysfunctions, such as financial mismanagement tasks, are pivotal to the determination of competence to live independently. Factors such as spoiled food in the refrigerator, untidy rooms, garbage accumulation, and soiled appliances reflect habit patterns.

Work is on the highest step of the hierarchy. Intrinsically,

work tasks may be no more complex than home management tasks; however, the need to meet externally imposed performance standards and time schedules increases their complexity. Because most patients seen in geriatric psychiatry have retired from their positions, work assessment is relatively infrequent. Occasionally, functional status assessment centers on a patient's continued ability to work and is often triggered by tardiness, absence from work, increased accidents or near-accidents, and inefficiency. *Work assessment* is individualized and entails an evaluation of a patient's fitness for doing the assigned job, the need to adapt the assigned job, or the need to transfer to a less responsible or less physically or mentally demanding job.

Because of the creative, exploratory, challenging, and recreational nature of leisure tasks, leisure is sometimes placed at the highest position in the hierarchy (Lawton, 1972). *Leisure activities*, however, may be readily graded in terms of the motor, cognitive, emotional, and social demands that they place on patients. Artwork may involve reproducing the detail of a landscape or creating an abstract image. Playing solitaire is less demanding than responding to the game requirements and social interactions of a four-handed rummy game. Bowling with lightweight balls and pins in a nursing home activity lounge is less demanding than using regulation equipment in a bowling alley. Because of the adaptability of leisure tasks, they may be placed on any rung of the hierarchical scheme, depending on how they are structured. Like work, the occupational therapy assessment of leisure competence is individualized. It involves an appraisal of leisure interests, skills, and participation, in addition to the specific activities used to satisfy leisure needs. In view of the decreasing emphasis on work in late life, leisure involvement assumes a critical role in giving structure and meaning to the postretirement years. Indeed, leisure is generally the vehicle for maintaining physical, mental, and social acuity.

In addition to assessing each of the five categories of daily living tasks separately, attention is also directed to the organizational skills used by patients to integrate daily living tasks into habits that result in an effective lifestyle. Patients with depression, for example, can generally demonstrate home management skills but are unable to plan or adhere to a daily schedule that supports task participation in a timely manner. Other patients allocate an inordinate amount of time to one task category such as personal self-care, leaving insufficient time for other kinds of tasks like taking care of the home. The evaluation of daily living habits is usually approached through occupational role assessment (Jackoway, Rogers, & Snow, 1987).

Data about task performance are gathered by asking questions (interviews, questionnaires) or by actually observing task performance (in the patient's natural living situation or controlled conditions in occupational therapy). Asking questions is the most practical method for obtaining data about daily living habits, because it is difficult to observe patients frequently enough to ascertain their activity patterns. Observation is the preferred method for appraising skill (Rogers, 1986). While observing patients perform tasks, the therapist has the opportunity to assess performance qualitatively as well as quantitatively (eg, level of independence). *Qualitative accounts of task performance* may include but not be limited to the following: psychomotor agitation, psychomotor retardation, tremor, trembling, perseveration, lethargy, impulsiveness, somatic complaints, and manifestations of hallucinatory or paranoid behavior. Observations such as these are invaluable for treatment planning.

HOME MANAGEMENT

Advanced Mobility

- enter and exit one's home, including manipulating locks and doors
- walk carrying a weight (e.g., take out the garbage, carry a package)
- climb a foot stool or ladder (e.g., to change a light bulb in a ceiling fixture)
- move around the community (e.g., using car, bus, taxi)

Advanced Personal Self-Care

- manage medications, including opening containers and adhering to a schedule
- use the telephone to obtain information, make appointments, and summon help in an emergency

Light Housekeeping

- shop for food and clothing (e.g., may be done over the telephone)
- plan and prepare hot and cold foods, including using range, oven and microwave
- wash and dry dishes
- care for clothing: in washing, drying, ironing, and mending clothes
- dust furniture
- vacuum/sweep floors
- make a bed
- perform minor home repairs (eg, fix flashlight)
- rake leaves
- water lawn

Heavy Housekeeping

- change bed linens
- clean household items (eg, bathtub, refrigerator, toilet)
- wash floors, windows, or walls
- perform major home maintenance tasks or repairs (eg, putting up storm windows)
- shovel snow
- mow the lawn
- weed

Financial Management

- exchange money for purchases
- pay bills
- write checks (or money orders) and balance checkbook

Functional diagnosis

Data from the occupational therapy assessment is summarized in a series of problem statements that make up the *functional* or *occupational therapy diagnosis* (Rogers & Holm, 1991b). These statements indicate the tasks that are dysfunctional and the hypothesized reason or reasons for the dysfunction. One example of a functional diagnosis is a dressing dysfunction due to an inability to locate clothing and to sequence the steps involved in donning and doffing clothing. Patients with cognitive impairment secondary to Alzheimer's type dementia often exhibit this behavior. Another example of a functional diagnosis is dressing dysfunction due to (a) a lack of motivation as indicated by an unkempt appearance and (b) restricted range of motion of the right hip. In this case, the inability to dress appropriately appears to stem from an affective impairment, like that associated with depression, but it is also complicated by a physical impairment. Both impairments must be taken into account in planning inter-

vention; otherwise, the desired outcome—dressing—will not occur.

These examples illustrate the importance of the qualitative observations of task performance. The observations furnish the cues that serve as a basis for inferences about the etiology of task dysfunctions. In turn, the etiology provides the cues for planning interventions.

Occupational therapy intervention

Skill-based intervention

Skill is the ability to perform a task proficiently. Geriatric psychiatric patients experience skill deficits when a skill becomes impaired due to illness or age-related processes, becomes atrophied due to disuse, or is disrupted due to environmental changes. Skill deficits also occur when patients need or desire to perform tasks that they have never learned (Rogers & Holm, 1991a). Regardless of the cause of skill deficit, intervention involves skill learning (Poole, 1991; Rogers & Holm, 1991a). Skill learning includes knowing about a task and knowing how to perform a task. Skill-based intervention has six components: imparting knowledge, establishing a relevant learning environment, supervising practice, promoting self-assessment, designing opportunities for skill generalization, and integrating skills into daily living habits (Rogers & Holm, 1991a).

The knowledge aspect of skill learning, the "knowing about a task," can be managed in formal or informal teaching sessions aimed at conveying information about task requirements. For example, a patient might be told that a walker is moved forward and set down on the floor before one steps into it. The process of using the walker might then be demonstrated. Similarly, patients may be educated through a group discussion about the value of activity participation for the relief of feelings of grief, boredom, or depression. Included in the knowledge component of skill acquisition is information about the subtasks involved in the task, the sequencing and timing of these subtasks, the rhythm of decisions and movement, and the desired outcome.

After patients understand what is expected to start, sustain, and stop a task, the emphasis of intervention switches from learning about a task to learning how to perform it. The goal of learning about the walker is to be able to use the walker, independently, safely, and correctly. The goal of learning about the relationship between activity participation and feelings is to be able to use productive activity to manage negative affect. These goals are achieved through supervised practice of the respective task in a controlled, structured environment. During practice, patients repeat tasks until a level of proficiency is achieved, which is functional and usable in daily life. Supervision is provided to maximize the likelihood that the task is learned correctly. Supervision focuses on alerting patients to cues that facilitate task performance and giving feedback about the quality of performance (correctness of action) and quality of outcome (correctness of goal). Patients are encouraged to evaluate their own task performance to facilitate internalization of performance standards.

The occupational therapist assumes responsibility for establishing an environment that is conducive to learning. This involves beginning skill acquisition at a level that is within the patient's capability and gradually increasing task demands so that the goal is eventually reached. Achieving the goal of using a walker to support functional activities in the home may be preceded by walking 2 feet on a level surface and gradually progressing to 25 feet. During the course of progression, patients are challenged to maneuver their way between furniture, to maintain correct performance while being distracted by people talking to them, to step over obstacles (eg, door thresholds), and to walk on a variety of walking surfaces (concrete, carpet).

In activity–affect training, patients might initially participate in a common activity of short duration. Gradually, the choice and duration of activity are increased. Activity involvement is followed by an exploration on a group and then individual basis of the feelings associated with the specific task as well as the contrast between productive and idle time. Intervention aims at approximating as closely as possible the conditions under which the task is to be performed in real life. To promote generalization to a variety of community settings, various practice materials are used so that patients become familiar with the full array of task requirements. A unique set of learning conditions may need to be designed for each patient.

After a skill is acquired, it must be integrated into a patient's daily living habits. Use of the walker in the home may require a rearrangement of furniture or caregiver cooperation in carrying the walker upstairs and downstairs. Patients may need to be accompanied to the senior center and introduced to members who have interests similar to theirs so that their increased activity participation can be sustained. Skill maintenance is achieved through frequent use of tasks.

Habit-based interventions

A **habit deficit** is a cessation or disruption of daily living routines (Rogers & Holm, 1991a). Habit deficits occur when daily living routines are disorganized, imbalanced, inflexible, or socially inappropriate. If an older adult's daily life has an identifiable structure that is ineffective for meeting the person's needs, daily living habits are disorganized. Habits are imbalanced when the number, diversity, type, and pacing of activities are restricted; they are inflexible when the person is unable to vary routines to accommodate unforeseen or changing circumstances. Habits characterized by a disregard for normative standards of behavior, such as cleanliness and functional independence, are socially inappropriate (Rogers & Holm, 1991a).

Task skills are the building blocks for habit formation. In habit deficits, individual task skills remain intact. The older adult can demonstrate the capacity to cook, sew, and do the laundry. Dysfunction lies in the inability to coordinate or link tasks together into a daily living routine that fosters the timely completion of obligatory tasks and provides time for discretionary activities. Because habits involve larger and more complex units of behavior than skills, habit acquisition is more difficult than skill acquisition. **Habit training** has four key stages: maintaining mobility and personal self-care routines; engaging in meaningful activity; initiating and sustaining activity; and reconstituting the habits relevant for the living situation. The goal is to approximate successively the complexity and rhythm of daily life that is required for the living situation, whether in the community or in a restricted setting.

In the first stage of habit training, routines are set up to support the performance of mobility and personal self-care tasks. Initially, the occupational therapist may plan these routines. This includes scheduling the times that tasks are to occur, setting time limits for completing tasks, establishing performance standards, and monitoring task performance. Gradually, patients take more responsibility for managing mobility and personal self-care tasks.

For example, after admission to the hospital, Mr. Jones was awakened by the occupational therapist at 7:00 AM and reminded to get washed and dressed. Later, he was given an alarm clock and instructed to get up in time to wash and dress before breakfast, which is served at 8:15 AM.

After a structure is given for mobility and self-care tasks, engagement in other meaningful activities is introduced. The objective is to engage patients in a limited number of carefully selected, time-limited tasks. Tasks are selected that are consistent with a patient's skill level and interests (Zgola, 1987; 1990a). Training emphasizes "within task" and "between task" organization and planning. Mr. Jones might be taught how to fold and hang his clothing so that he does not have to waste time looking for items or wear wrinkled clothing. He might also be reminded to drop off his laundry on the way to breakfast. After task involvement, the patient and the occupational therapist jointly evaluate the overall quality of task performance. Objective elements (quantity of work, quality of work) are evaluated as well as subjective elements (perceptions, feelings). The occupational therapist provides matter-of-fact feedback to patients and lends an overall positive tone to their self-assessments (Rogers & Holm, 1991a).

After the initial scheduling and diversification of tasks, additional tasks are added and incorporated into the daily living routine. The specific tasks to be added are determined by the patient's discharge living situation. If after discharge, Mr. Jones is expected to fix his own breakfast, then preparing breakfast might be the next task added to his schedule. As each task is added, an assessment is made of the organizational skills that patients use for executing the task and the most advantageous place for fitting the task into the daily, weekly, or monthly schedule. In scheduling tasks, provision is made for fatigue through rest breaks and by interspersing tasks with a heavy physical or mental load with tasks with a lighter physical or mental load. Gradually, a schedule is drawn up that is optimal for each patient and fosters a sense of self-control.

In the final stage of habit training, the focus is on daily life as it transpires in the living environment, whether this is a private home, personal care home, intermediate care facility, foster home, nursing home, or state hospital. The objective is to resume or assume an activity level that provides an optimal balance of mobility, personal self-care, and leisure involvement and affords the patient a measure of life satisfaction. If appropriate, work tasks are included in the time management plan. Training at this stage highlights transferring task performance from the controlled setting of occupational therapy to the real life setting. Patients are expected to take more responsibility for the planning and organizational aspects of task performance. Time management training includes accounting for all obligatory tasks, allowing for discretionary tasks, and managing unexpected events.

Before discharge, Mr. Jones worked out a time management plan that included, among other things, weekly trips to the laundromat and grocery store and daily visits to the local senior center. During the 4 weeks after discharge, Mr. Jones called the therapist weekly to resolve problems with his schedule and discuss his sense of personal control and the pleasure and frustration arising from his use of time. At Mr. Jones' first outpatient appointment, his overall activity plan was reviewed and found to be functional and operational, and he was discharged from occupational therapy.

Environmentally based interventions

The capacity to perform tasks is determined by factors internal and external to older adults. The internal factors are referred to as *competence;* the external factors are referred to as *task demands* (Lawton, 1972). When a patient's competence cannot be improved or has already been improved maximally, task demands can often be reduced to enable greater participation. Environmentally based interventions are used to support functional competence, provide appropriate stimulation, and pro-

mote safety (Hiatt, 1990; Paire & Karney, 1984; Rogers, 1989; Rogers, Marcus, & Snow, 1987; Zgola, 1990b). The challenge to the occupational therapist is to match the task demands to the patient's competence so that function can be improved or maintained.

Environmentally based interventions involve manipulation of built-in structures, objects, time, or persons (Rogers, 1989). Typically, environmental elements are used to promote task performance; however, in the care of older adults the need to preclude task performance may assume equal importance. For older adults with physical impairments, built-in structural adaptations, like wheelchair ramps or chair glides, facilitate mobility. For older adults with cognitive impairments, actual physical movement may pose no problem. In fact, the environment may need to be secured to curtail wandering into spaces that pose danger, such as the garage, where power tools are stored or "outside" of the personal care home.

Objects like furniture, appliances, tools, and gadgets can also be used to promote or hinder task performance (Fernie & Fernie, 1990; Zgola, 1990b). Assistive technology devices, such as reachers and utensils with built-up handles, compensate for physical impairments like lack of joint range of motion and grip strength, respectively. Similarly, "smart appliances," which know when to turn themselves on and off substitute for attention and memory deficits. For many persons with cognitive impairments, the mere provision of task objects is sufficient to elicit the object-related task. A patient may shave when handed a razor or comb hair when given a comb. The converse is also true: failing to provide task objects is as effective a strategy for inhibiting task performance as providing locks and bolts is for preventing access to potentially dangerous objects, such as matches and cleaning fluids.

Tasks take place in time as well as space, and time can be managed in a way that makes environmental demands more predictable. Toileting schedules may be devised to prevent incontinence. Recreational activities may be scheduled to encourage activity participation. Scheduling as a behavioral management strategy is particularly helpful for older adults with affective disorders, because they usually have difficulty deciding what to do, when to do it, or whether to do it at all. Doing routine tasks at the same time each day is also recommended for patients with cognitive impairments. This is one means of reducing the catastrophic reactions that are often exhibited when routines are broken and task demands become unclear (Mace, 1990).

People also influence task performance. Caregiving skills that make an impact on task performance range from directing attention to giving verbal cues, modeling task performance, providing task objects, developing schedules, and giving physical help. As with each of the other environmental elements, caregivers may encourage ("pick up the spoon") or discourage ("don't throw food on the floor") certain actions in their attempts to assist patients. Occupational therapists need to work with caregivers so that their attitudes and skills are compatible with the patient's level of competence.

The net effect of environmental demands on older adults is to furnish the optimal amount of stimulation for mental, physical, and emotional well-being or to understimulate or overstimulate, both of which negatively influence task performance (Hall, 1988; Lawton, 1989). Thus, the overall plan of care must be periodically reevaluated so that the patient's competence is challenged but not exceeded.

Use of restraints

The need for physical and chemical restraints to control behavior can often be reduced through participation in orienting and stimulating activities in a safe and functional environment. At admission to an acute psychiatric unit, Mrs. Bena was restrained in a posey vest because of an unstable gait, a history of falls with injury, and an inability to remember to walk only with assistance. Occupational therapy intervention was multifaceted. Mrs. Bena was given a sign with large letters reminding her to call the nurse when she wanted to walk; she was to be walked once each hour by the certified occupational therapy assistant using the Swedish walker. Between walks she was seated at a work table and the following were available to her: a simple puzzle, large-print playing cards, a tape recorder with music tapes, magazines, and napkins to fold for the dinner meal. The milieu therapist was instructed to initiate task involvement if Mrs. Bena did not do this on her own. With the institution of this program the posey vest restraint was no longer needed.

In the event that a physical restraint is needed, the occupational therapist recommends the least restrictive device. The device must be of the proper size and fit and allow patients to maintain optimal postural alignment (Bower, 1991). While in restraints patients should be observed frequently. Physical restraints should be released at least every 2 hours, and activities for active range of motion should be engaged in for 10 to 20 minutes. Often the behavioral control that is needed can be accomplished with restraint alternatives. For instance, a cushion that slants slightly toward the back of a chair (hip flexion cushion) makes it difficult to get up without assistance and is often sufficient to control unsupervised walking. Door buzzers and bed check alarms can be used to alert staff of behaviors that require supervision (Bower, 1991). The continuing need for restraints or restraint alternatives should be reviewed often and removed as soon as possible.

Summary

Geriatric psychiatry has several features that distinguish it from adult psychiatry. In assessing symptoms, normal age-associated changes in biologic, psychological, and social functions must be differentiated from pathologic changes so that normal changes are not diagnosed as abnormal and pathologic changes are not perceived as normal. It should also be recognized that some of the characteristics of psychiatric disorders may be different in older adults than in younger adults, although both groups experience the same range of disorders. In geriatric psychiatry, a comprehensive medical, social, functional, and psychiatric assessment is supported by the interaction of biopsychosocial factors in producing health and illness in late life. Normal age-associated changes must be considered during treatment as well as diagnosis. In addition, psychiatric intervention must take into account coexisting psychiatric and medical problems. Finally, optimal patient care emerges from the coordination of multidisciplinary services, inpatient and outpatient services, and formal and informal services. These features shape the context for the practice of geropsychiatric occupational therapy.

Regardless of the setting in which occupational therapy is practiced, therapists working with older adults are likely to encounter a significant subgroup of older patients with mental health problems. Hence, the need for knowledge about geriatric psychiatry is not confined to therapists employed in psychiatry. Because a high proportion of the geropsychiatric population suffers from depression or dementia, therapists must be highly skilled in distinguishing task dysfunctions due to skill and habit deficits and in planning and implementing appropriate interventions. Occupational therapy assessment and intervention focus on the performance of mobility, personal self-care, home management, leisure, and work tasks. The components of these tasks, such as visual–spatial deficits and memory problems, are treated within the context of these daily living tasks. Successful task performance requires motor, cognitive, and affective abilities. Therapists working with older adults must be prepared to treat disabilities emerging from physical impairments as well as cognitive and affective ones, since disease-related and age-related changes often result in multiple types of impairments. In view of the high level of functional dependence of older adults, caregivers should be included in occupational therapy to enable optimal task performance after discharge.

References

Barbieri, E. (1983). Patient falls are not patient accidents. *Journal of Gerontological Nursing, 9*, 165–173.

Bengston, V. L., & Treas, J. (1980). The changing family context of mental health. In J. Birren & R. B. Sloan (Eds.), *Handbook of aging and mental health* (pp. 400–428). Englewood Cliffs, NJ: Prentice-Hall.

Bland, R. C., Newman, S. C., & Orn, H. (1988). Prevalence of psychiatric disorders in the elderly in Edmonton. *Acta Psychiatrica* Scandinavica, 77(Suppl 338), 57–63.

Blazer, D., Hughes, D. C., & George, L. K. (1987). The epidemiology of depression in an elderly community population. *Gerontologist, 27*, 281–287.

Bower, H. T. (1991). The alternatives to restraints. *Journal of Gerontological Nursing, 17*, 18–26.

Clayton, P. J., Halikas, J. A., & Maurice W. (1972). The depression of widowhood. *British Journal of Psychiatry, 120*, 71–78.

Cohen, C. (1991). Integrated community services. Introduction. In J. Sadavoy, L. W. Lazarus, & L. F. Jarvik (Eds.), *Comprehensive review of geriatric psychiatry* (pp. 613–634). Washington, DC: American Psychiatric Press.

Cohen, G. D. (1990). Normal changes and patterns of psychiatric disease. In W. B. Abrahms & R. Berkow (Eds.), *The Merck manual of geriatrics*, (pp. 995–1004). Rathway, NJ: Merck, Sharpe & Dohme Research Laboratories.

Cooper, A. F., Garside, R. F., & Kay, D. W. K. (1976). A comparison of deaf and non-deaf patients with paranoid and affective psychosis. *British Journal of Psychiatry, 129*, 532–538.

Curlik, S. M., Frazier, D. F., & Katz, I. R. (1991). Psychiatric aspects of long-term care. In J. Sadavoy, L. W. Lazarus & L. F. Jarvik (Eds.), *Comprehensive review of geriatric psychiatry* (pp. 547–564). Washington, DC: American Psychiatric Press.

Dovenmuehle, R. H., Reckless, J. B., & Newman, G. (1970). Depressive reactions in the elderly. In E. Palmore (Ed.), *Normal aging* (pp. 90–97). Durham, NC: Duke University Press.

Dube, A. H., & Mitchell, E. K. (1986). Accidental strangulation from vest restraints. *Journal of the American Medical Association, 256*, 2725–2726.

Edelson, J. S., & Lyons, W. H. (1985). *Institutional care of the mentally impaired elderly*. New York: Van Nostrand Reinhold.

Fernie, G., & Fernie, B. (1990). Technological innovations for individuals with Alzheimer's disease. *American Journal of Alzheimer's Care and Related Disorders and Research, 5*, 9–14.

Folks, D. G., & Kinney, F. C. (1991). Consultation-liaison is the general hospital. In J. Sadavoy, L. W. Lazarus & L. F. Jarvik (Eds.), *Comprehensive review of geriatric psychiatry* (pp. 565–581). Washington, DC: American Psychiatric Press.

Fortinsky, R., & Hathaway, T. J. (1988). The appropriateness of boarding home care for persons with Alzheimer's disease. *American Journal of Alzheimer's Care and Related Disorders and Research, 3,* 37–44.

Frengley, J. D., & Mion, L. C. (1986). Incidence of physical restraints on acute general medical wards. *Journal of the American Geriatrics Society, 34,* 565–568.

Glick, P. C. (1979). The future marital status and living arrangements of the elderly. *Gerontologist, 19,* 301–309.

Goodman, A., & Siegel, C. (1986). Elderly schizophrenic inpatients in the wake of deinstitutionalization. *American Journal of Psychiatry, 143,* 204–207.

Gurland, B. J., Copeland J., Kuriansky J., Kelleher, M., Sharpe, L., & Dean, L. L. (1983). *The mind and mood of aging.* New York: Haworth Press.

Gurland, B. J., & Cross, P. S. (1982). Epidemiology of psychopathology in old age: Some clinical implications. *Psychiatric Clinics of North America, 5,* 11–26.

Hall, G. R. (1988). Care of the patient with Alzheimer's disease living at home. *Nursing Clinics of North America, 23,* 31–46.

Hays, D. P. (1991). Electroconvulsive therapy. In J. Sadavoy, L. W. Lazarus & L. F. Jarvik (Eds.), *Comprehensive review of geriatric psychiatry* (pp. 469–485). Washington, DC: American Psychiatric Press.

Hiatt, L. G. (1990). Design of the home environment for the cognitively impaired person. In N. L. Mace (Ed.), *Dementia care: Patient, family, and community* (pp. 231–242). Baltimore: Johns Hopkins University Press.

Horowitz, A. (1985). Sons and daughters as caregivers to older parents: Differences in role performances and consequences. *Gerontologist, 25,* 612–617.

Jackoway, I. S., Rogers, J. C., & Snow, T. L. (1987). The role change assessment: An interview tool for evaluating older adults. *Occupational Therapy in Mental Health, 7,* 17–37.

Kane, R. L., Ouslander, J. G., & Abrass, I. B. (1989). *Essentials of Clinical Geriatrics* (2nd ed.). New York: McGraw-Hill.

Katzman, R. (1986). Alzheimer's disease. *New England Journal of Medicine, 4,* 964–972.

Kokmen, E., Offord, K. P., & Okazaki, H. (1987). A clinical and autopsy study of dementia in Olmstead County, Minnesota, 1980–1981. *Neurology, 37,* 427–430.

Kramer, M., German, P. S., Anthony, J. C., Von Korff, M., & Skinner, E. A. (1985). Patterns of mental disorders among the elderly residents of eastern Baltimore. *Journal of the American Geriatrics Society, 33,* 236–245.

Lawton, M. P. (1972). Assessing the competence of older people. In D. P. Kent, R. Kastenbaum & S. Sherwood (Eds.), *Research planning and action for the elderly: The power and potential of social science* (pp. 122–143). New York: Behavioral Publications.

Lawton, M. P. (1989). Environmental proactivity and affect in older people. In S. Spacapan & S. Oskamp (Eds.), *The social psychology of aging* (pp. 135–163). Newbury Park, CA: Sage Publications.

Lesse, S. (1974). *Masked depression.* New York: Raven Press.

Mace, N. L. (1990). The management of problem behaviors. In N. L. Mace (Ed.), *Dementia care: Patient family, and community* (pp. 74–112). Baltimore: Johns Hopkins University Press.

Manton, K. G., Blazer, D. M., & Woodbury, M. A. (1987). Suicide in middle age and later life: Sex and specific life tables and cohort analysis. *Journal of Gerontology, 42,* 219–227.

McCue, M., Rogers, J. C., & Goldstein, G. (1990). Relationship between neuropsychological and functional assessment in elderly neuropsychiatric patients. *Rehabilitation Psychology, 35,* 91–99.

Miller, M. (1975). Iatrogenic and nursigenic effects of prolonged immobilization of the ill aged. *Journal of the American Geriatrics Society, 23,* 360–369.

Myers, J. K., Weissman, M. M., Tischler, G. L., Holzer, C. E., Leaf, P. J.,

Orvaschel, H., Anthony, J. C., Boyd, J. H., Burke, J. D., Kramer, M., & Stoltzman, R. (1984). Six-month prevalence of psychiatric disorders in three communities, 1980 to 1982. *Archives of General Psychiatry, 41,* 959–967.

National Center for Health Statistics (B. Feller). (1983, September). Americans needing help to function at home. *Advance Data from Vital and Health Statistics,* No. 92. DHHS Pub. No. (PHS) 83–1250. Public Health Service, Hyattsville, MD.

Omnibus Budget Reconciliation Act of 1987 (Public Law 100–203)

Paire, J. A., & Karney, R. J. (1984). The effectiveness of sensory stimulation for geropsychiatric inpatients. *American Journal of Occupational Therapy, 8,* 505–509.

Patrick, M. L. (1967). Care of the confused elderly. *American Journal of Nursing, 67,* 2536–2539.

Phillips, L. R. (1991). Social support of the older client. In W. C. Chenitz. J. T. Stone & S. A. Salisbury (Eds.), *Clinical gerontological nursing: A guide to advanced practice* (pp. 535–545). Philadelphia: W. B. Saunders.

Poole, J. L. (1991). Application of motor learning principles in occupational therapy. *American Journal of Occupational Therapy, 45,* 531–537.

Rader, J., Doan, J., & Schwab, M. (1985). How to decrease wandering behavior, a form of agenda behavior. *Geriatric Nursing, 6,* 196–199.

Rapp, S. R., Parisi, S. A., & Walsh, D. A. (1988). Psychological dysfunction and physical health among elderly medical inpatients. *Journal of Consulting and Clinical Psychology, 56,* 851–855.

Regier, D. A., Boyd, J. H., Burke, J. D., Rae, D. S., Myers, J. K., Kramer, M., Robins, L. N., George, L. K., Karno, M., & Locke, B. Z. (1988). One month prevalence of mental disorders in the United States. *Archives of General Psychiatry, 45,* 977–986.

Rogers, J. C. (1986). Occupational therapy assessment for older adults with depression: Asking the right questions. *Physical and Occupational Therapy in Geriatrics, 5,* 13–33.

Rogers, J. C. (1989). The occupational therapy home assessment: The home as a therapeutic environment. *Journal of Home Health Care Practice, 2,* 73–81.

Rogers, J. C., & Holm, M. B. (1991a). Teaching older adults with depression. *Topics in Geriatric Rehabilitation, 4,* 27–44.

Rogers, J. C., & Holm, M. B. (1991b). Occupational therapy diagnostic reasoning: A component of clinical reasoning. *American Journal of Occupational Therapy, 45,* 1045–1053.

Rogers, J. C., Marcus, C. L., & Snow, T. L. (1987). Maude: A case of sensory deprivation. *American Journal of Occupational Therapy, 41,* 673–676.

Rovner, B. W., Kafonek, S., Filipp, L., Lucas, M. J. & Folstein, M. F. (1986). Prevalence of mental illness in a community nursing home. *American Journal of Psychiatry, 143,* 1446–1449.

Sadavoy, J., Lazarus, L. W., & Jarvik, L. F. (1991). Introduction. In J. Sadavoy, L. W. Lazarus & L. F. Jarvik (Eds.), *Comprehensive review of geriatric psychiatry* (pp. 3–24). Washington, DC: American Psychiatric Press.

Salzman, C. (1987). Geriatric psychopharmacology. *Journal of Geriatric Psychiatry, 20,* 11–27.

Small, G. W., & Fawzy, F. I. (1988). Psychiatric consultation for the medically ill elderly in the general hospital: Need for a collaborative model of care. *Psychosomatics, 29,* 94–103.

Small, G. W., Komanduri, R., Gitlin, M., & Jarvik, L. F. (1986). The influence of age on guilt expression in major depression. *International Journal of Geriatric Psychiatry, 1,* 121–126.

Soloff, P. H. (1984). Historical notes on seclusion and restraint. In K. Tardiff (Ed.), *The psychiatric uses of seclusion and restraint* (pp. 1–9). Washington, DC: American Psychiatric Press.

Spar, J. E., & La Rue, A. (1990). *Concise guide to geriatric psychiatry.* Washington, DC: American Psychiatric Press.

Steingart, A. (1991). Day programs. In J. Sadavoy, L. W. Lazarus & L. F. Jarvik (Eds.), *Comprehensive review of geriatric psychiatry* (pp. 603–611). Washington, DC: American Psychiatric Press.

Stenbeck, A. (1980). Depression and suicidal behavior in old age. In J. E.

Birren & R. B. Sloan (Eds.), *Handbook of mental health and aging* (pp. 616–652). Englewood Cliffs, NJ: Prentice-Hall.

Tourigny-Rivard, M. (1991). Acute care inpatient treatment. In J. Sadavoy, L. W. Lazarus & L. F. Jarvik (Eds.), *Comprehensive review of geriatric psychiatry* (pp. 583–602). Washington, DC: American Psychiatric Press.

Trace, S., & Howell, T. (1991). Occupational therapy in geriatric mental health. *American Journal of Occupational Therapy, 45,* 833–838.

Turnbull, J. M., & Turnbull, S. K. (1985). Management of specific anxiety disorders in the elderly. *Geriatrics, 40,* 75–82.

U.S. Senate Special Committee on Aging. *Aging America—trends and projections.* Washington, DC: U.S. Department of Health and Human Services, 1987–1988.

Young, R. C., & Meyers, B. S. (1991). Psychopharmacology. In J. Sadavoy, L. W. Lazarus & L. F. Jarvik (Eds.), *Comprehensive review of geriatric psychiatry* (pp. 435–467). Washington, DC: American Psychiatric Press.

Zgola, J. M. (1987). *Doing things: A guide to programming activities for persons with Alzheimer's disease and related disorders.* Baltimore: Johns Hopkins University Press.

Zgola, J. M. (1990a). Therapeutic activity. In N. L. Mace (Ed.), *Dementia care: Patient, family, and community* (pp. 148–172). Baltimore: Johns Hopkins University Press.

Zgola, J. (1990b). Alzheimer's disease and the home: Issues in environmental design. *American Journal of Alzheimer's Care and Related Disorders and Research, 5,* 15–22.

Zimmer, J. G., Watson, N., & Treat, A. (1984). Behavioral problems among patients in skilled nursing facilities. *American Journal of Public Health, 74,* 1118–1121.

CHAPTER 22

Elder abuse

ELLEN DUNLEAVEY TAIRA

KEY TERMS

Active Neglect

Financial or Material
  Abuse

Natural Monitors

Passive Neglect

Physical Abuse

Psychological Abuse

LEARNING OBJECTIVES

Upon completion of this chapter the reader will be able to:

1. *Identify the five most common types of abuse found among the elderly.*
2. *Recognize the relationship between deteriorating functional status and the potential for abuse and neglect.*
3. *Incorporate preventive strategies in the treatment plan.*

The notion that families or others might neglect or harm an older relative or elderly care recipient is relatively recent. Early studies by Hickey and Douglass (1981a) surveyed community practitioners and professionals most likely to come in contact with vulnerable adults. Lawyers, policemen, social workers, health professionals, members of the clergy, coroners, and aging network personnel were asked to focus on issues related to their perceptions of the cause of mistreatment, the process of identifying and reporting the problem, and their personal and professional experience with instances of mistreatment. Their findings indicated that of the 223 persons surveyed more than 60% had observed or suspected physical abuse to an older person in the course of their work. Virtually all the respondents were aware of some type of neglect (Hickey & Douglass, 1981b).

Advocates for the elderly received the news that caregivers were mistreating older persons with shock and disbelief. While working as a long-term care specialist, I convened the first-ever workshop on elder abuse in Hawaii. No one in attendance expected the outpouring of stories from caregivers and law enforcement specialists that were reported. The following is an example.

> A 79-year-old widow who was living on the benefits of a substantial trust was unexpectedly visited in her very remote residence by a conscientious bank employee who was astonished to find her tied in her wheelchair and being fed only minimal food rations by her well-paid caretaker who had been retained by the trust. As is usually the case, this "nurse" had proper credentials and was quite charming; otherwise, the bank would not have hired him.

Stories similar to this are not uncommon. One thing that was lacking in this scenario was any sort of routine surveillance. Surveillance is particularly problematic in rural areas, where there are few naturally occurring monitors such as neighbors, handymen, and service persons, who could provide a form of oversight in an urban or suburban setting.

Natural monitors of the welfare of children such as teachers and emergency room staff are alerted to notice children in danger of neglect or abuse since there has been considerable media attention to cases of suspected child abuse. Mandatory reporting of suspected child abuse is federal law and is now required in every state (Quinn & Tomita, 1985). It may be well to remember that the suggestion that relatives might be physically abusing children was first considered in the United States in the latter part of this century.

Historical context

Traditionally, children and wives were considered chattel; parents and spouses were within their rights to expect obedience and well-prescribed behavior. Fairy tales with cruel parents like Hansel and Gretel's parents were probably based on historical data. Our tendency to romanticize the role of an older relative in centuries past may not be accurate.

Myths referring to earlier, more idyllic periods when the oldest family members were revered and respected for their wisdom and kindness have fallen prey to more realistic views that take literature and historical documents into account. In the pre-industrial era, disagreements over property inheritances created serious family tensions. In the Western tradition, the common occurrence of late marriages was frequently the result of an adult postponing marriage until a parent dies. Since ownership of the land was usually delayed until the death of the parent, there was considerable relief when parental control of financial resources was ended (Pillemer & Wolf, 1986). The temptation to hasten a parent's demise was present.

Those few parents who did grow old were just as likely to be subjected to the vicissitudes of their adult children as they would be today. An example of elder abuse from literature is King Lear, who abdicated his throne and divided his kingdom among his daughters in exchange for their care. He had treated his daughters badly and was in turn mistreated by them.

Magnitude of the problem

As the number of very old persons living at home continues to rise, the potential for neglect as well as mistreatment increases proportionately. The Senate Select Committee on Aging held extensive hearings in 1981 and concluded that elder abuse is only slightly less common than child abuse. Estimates are that at least 1 of every 25 elderly persons is a victim of abuse (Quinn & Tomita, 1985).

Elder abuse is now considered another aspect of domestic violence. Whether it is a new problem or an age-old issue is open to debate. What is certain is the vastly increasing number of persons over 75 who are becoming dependent on middle-aged children for financial, social, and psychological support, and for physical assistance.

The 1982 Long Term Care Survey sheds light on the enormous role of the family in providing informal care to their relatives (Doty, 1986). Despite the fact that 20% of all persons over 65 are functionally disabled—that is, they require some assistance in personal care or instrumental activities of daily living (IADL) such as shopping, laundry, and money management—only one in five of these functionally impaired persons is cared for in nursing facilities. Most of the others "rely on a combination of family care and paid help. Only a small minority (5 percent in the Long Term Care Survey) receive all their care from paid providers" (Doty, 1986, p. 35; United States Department of Health and Human Services, 1990).

These statistics contrast with images of families abandoning relatives in institutions and explain to some extent the rising concern over abused and neglected elderly. As the level of disability increases, older persons become more vulnerable to mistreatment. The more traditional forms of neglect are generally related to personal care: inadequate bathing, soiled underwear, and withholding food or liquid.

Kinds of abuse and neglect

Although opinions differ on what constitutes abuse of the elderly, it is generally agreed that elderly mistreatment can be divided into five distinct types.

Physical abuse is defined as causing physical pain or injury such as slapping, bruising, cutting, molesting, burning, and restraining.

Psychological abuse is defined as mental anguish, such as verbal taunting, threatening, and name calling.

Material abuse is "the illegal or improper exploitation and/or use of funds or other resources."

Neglect can be divided into two categories:

Active neglect, "refusal or failure to fulfill a caretaking obligation, including a conscious and intentional attempt to inflict physical or emotional distress" (Wolf & Pillemer, 1989, p. 18)

Passive neglect, "refusal or failure to fulfill a caretaking obligation excluding a conscious and intentional attempt to inflict physical or emotional distress" (Wolf & Pillemer, 1989, p. 18)

Neglect is far more prevalent than abuse and the more likely arena wherein the occupational therapist would be involved. Cases of neglect seem to be concentrated among the oldest and most dependent elderly who are more apt to be cognitively and physically impaired. Generally, neglect is the result of stress and burden, and abuse is more typically caused by interpersonal pathology between victim and perpetrator. Material exploitation is most often explained by the financial needs of the perpetrator (Pillemer & Wolf, 1986).

Financial or material abuse is frequently a concern if the older person has some mental impairment and is not aware of the status of his or her bank account. A person who thinks that it is 1960 and John F. Kennedy is President can also be convinced that you can buy a week's worth of groceries for $20.00.

Role of the occupational therapist

In their exhaustive analysis of data from four sites, Wolf and Pillemer (1989) found that activities of daily living played a crucial role in cases of active and passive neglect. Persons who were dependent for personal care and selected IADL were much more likely to be neglected. Not providing care, whether life-threatening (food and water) or potentially harmful (not changing diapers), is a form of neglect, physical abuse, and psychological abuse and can be classified as withholding of personal care, which is an area of urgent concern for rehabilitation specialists (Quinn & Tomita, 1985).

As health care delivery continues to move away from expensive institution-based models and more toward community care, it will be the increasing responsibility of home care providers to be alert to potential cases of abuse and neglect. Occupational therapists are essential to the provision of home care and often have lengthy and intimate contact with the functionally impaired older person. This puts the therapist in an opportune position to identify and aid the abused, provide support to the abuser, and aid in prevention (Holland, Kasraian, & Leonardelli, 1987).

Because of the crucial role of the occupational therapist in promoting self-care independence, a strong focus on activities of daily living is needed. The tendency to give only brief attention to self-care when there is paid help or informal support can only perpetrate the neglect syndrome. Training in the essential self-care skills of transfers, toileting, mobility, and home management tasks should be the primary goal in home care treatment.

Similarly, the selection of wheelchairs and other aids that can be easily maneuvered around doorways and in the kitchen and bathroom maximizes independence of the mobility-impaired person and reduces the need for costly paid help or stressed unpaid help. Very small gains in functional levels can sometimes translate into enormous benefits for caregivers.

As an example, a 75-year-old man with Alzheimer's disease lived with his 70-year-old wife on a reduced income; they were not eligible for paid help. When his ability to toilet himself independently began to deteriorate, the man's wife was referred to a therapist who worked as a consultant to her Alzheimer's support group. The occupational therapy evaluation revealed a man who could locate the bathroom without difficulty but began having accidents because of his inability to unzip his trousers. A simple familiar adaptation (a safety pin hooked to the zipper pull) provided the independence necessary for this man to stay alone for a few hours and allowed his wife to find essential respite by helping out at her church.

Summary

Awareness of abuse and neglect has been thrust on us because of the rapidly escalating numbers of persons over 75 years whose disabilities multiply with age and who have middle-aged and older children. Despite an emphasis on wellness and health programs, a general deterioration in function is a fact of aging.

The purpose of this chapter was to briefly review the literature on elder abuse and neglect, explore current research on the causes of abuse and neglect, and to highlight the important role of the occupational therapist in prevention. For the more prevalent problem of neglect, increased functional limitations only serve to add to the stress and burden of caregivers. Occupational therapy treatment should focus on self-care and training of caregivers to reduce dependency and prevent unnecessary or premature loss of function.

References

Doty, P. (1986). Family care of the elderly: The role of public policy. *The Milbank Quarterly, 64*(1), 34–75.

Hickey, T., & Douglass, R. L. (1981a). Mistreatment of the elderly in the domestic setting: An exploratory study. *American Journal of Public Health, 71*(5), 500–507.

Hickey, T., & Douglass, R. L. (1981b). Neglect and abuse of older family members: Professionals' perspectives and case experiences. *Gerontologist, 21*(2), 171–176.

Holland, L., Kasraian, K., & Leonardelli, C. (1987). Elder abuse: An analysis of the current problem and potential role of the rehabilitation professional. *Physical and Occupational Therapy in Geriatrics, 5*(3), 41–50.

Pillemer, K., & Wolf, R. (1986). *Elder abuse: Conflict in the family*. Dover, MA: Auburn House.

Quinn, M. J., & Tomita, S. (1985). *Elder abuse and neglect*. New York: Springer.

United States Department of Health and Human Services. (1990). *Functional status of the noninstitutionalized elderly: Estimates of ADL and IADL difficulties*. Rockville MD: DHHS Publication No. (PHS) 90–3462.

Wolf, R., & Pillemer, K. (1989). *Helping elderly victims*. New York: Columbia University Press.

UNIT IX

Environments for practice

CHAPTER 23

Acute care occupational therapy

MARTY TORRANCE

LEARNING OBJECTIVES

Upon completion of this chapter the reader will be able to:

1. *List three ways acute care occupational therapy differs from occupational therapy in long-term hospitals, rehabilitation centers, and nursing homes.*

2. *Discuss the interrelationship between psychosocial factors and functional outcome.*

3. *Develop an occupational therapy treatment plan for a patient suffering from intensive care unit (ICU) psychosis.*

4. *Discuss the occupational therapist's role in the treatment of cancer patients.*

5. *List and discuss five components of cardiac rehabilitation for which occupational therapy may be responsible.*

6. *List ways in which occupational therapy can increase a transplant patient's endurance and activity level; brainstorm and list corresponding modalities to accomplish this.*

7. *Discuss occupational therapy's role in the treatment of dysphagic patients.*

Occupational therapists working in an acute care, general hospital setting need to be knowledgeable about a wide range of diagnoses, medical procedures, occupational therapy interventions, and community resources. Patients seen in this setting are acutely ill and may have a multitude of medical problems.

Many patients seen in a general hospital are discussed in other sections of this book, such as those with cerebrovascular accident, arthritis, AIDS, and spinal cord injury. This chapter focuses on occupational therapy assessment and intervention in the acute care setting, as well as other commonly seen diagnoses.

Acute care hospitals

General acute care hospitals serve all ages from birth to death and often serve as an entry point into the health care system. Acute care hospitals provide diagnostic, medical, and surgical intervention for patients who have acute, transient problems or those with an episodic exacerbation of a chronic illness.

The provision of health care has changed dramatically in the past 5 years, and nowhere has this change been more evident than in the acute care hospital. With the implementation of diagnostic-related groups (DRGs) and insurance regulations, there has been a concerted effort to control health care costs, thus making an impact on the types of patients admitted to the general hospital. Patients are now having diagnostic testing on an outpatient basis, more surgeries are performed on an outpatient basis, and only those patients who are seriously and acutely ill are admitted for exacerbations of chronic illness. Hospitalization periods are shorter; the length of stay for the acute care hospital is 7.2 days. It is anticipated that the length of stay will continue to decrease (American Hospital Association, 1991). This short length of hospital stay has profound implications for the acute care occupational therapist. Short-term hospitalizations mandate prioritization of evaluation and treatment, flexibility and adaptation of the therapist, and thorough discharge planning, all of which are discussed in depth later in this chapter.

The constraints of time and resources in the acute care setting often require prioritization of patients, as do natural fluctuations in case loads and inpatient census. In the competitive health care environment, where staff shortages are now common and practically routine, it is essential to develop a policy and philosophy that will allow acute care therapists to establish a logical prioritization system. One such philosophy of acute care is "the belief that the ability to perform basic self-care is intimately connected with recovery from illness and essential for successful timely discharge" (Rausch & Melvin, 1986, p. 319). On the basis of this philosophy, Rausch and Melvin classified the types of acute care patients referred to occupational therapists as one possible method of determining the allocation of both staff and resources:

1. The single-episode or injury population, for example, patients admitted for total hip replacement or hand injury. These patients typically have a short hospitalization with a predictable course of treatment.
2. Patients in the acute phase of long-term rehabilitation, such as those with head trauma, cerebral vascular accident, or spinal cord injury. The length of hospitalization for these patients is more variable, and patients often have life-threatening medical complications.
3. Chronically ill patients admitted for an acute exacerbation, surgical procedure, or concomitant disease. This group includes persons with diabetes, arthritis, cardiac conditions, neurologic diseases, or cancer. The length of hospital stay is unpredictable and patients may require a period of complete bed rest.
4. Patients admitted for invasive diagnostic testing or regulation of medications. Typical diagnoses in this group are acute back injury, poorly controlled diabetes, and Parkinson's disease. The course of hospitalization typically is brief and relatively predictable, and it may include activity restrictions due to diagnostic testing.

These categories allow patient classification, which may help to determine the importance of a given occupational therapy intervention.

In addition, the occupational therapist may function in a consultant's role, completing a brief assessment and providing recommendations for further care. It is stressed that these categories are not meant to be all-inclusive or restrictive but to provide useful guidelines for the acute care occupational therapist.

Psychosocial coping

The acute care hospital is often a frightening and bewildering environment, especially to a patient and family who are facing serious illness. Often the setting is hectic and chaotic, and because of the presence of "high tech" medical intervention, the psychological needs of the patient may be overlooked. In addition, the patient may be newly diagnosed and thus just beginning to adjust to an acquired illness or accident.

It is essential that an occupational therapist working in the acute care environment develop strong interpersonal and therapeutic skills. It is the occupational therapist who can provide the patient and his or her family with the psychological support needed to develop positive coping mechanisms.

Patients who are hospitalized may be devastated by the overwhelming losses facing them: health, life, security, occupation, and social changes. A working model that was developed at Indiana University Medical Center looks at how psychosocial aspects can either positively or negatively affect the rehabilitation and functional outcome of the patient. Psychosocial aspects include premorbid personality, control issues and how one responds to control, distorted self-image, previously used coping mechanisms, age tasks, role reversal, socioeconomic class, support systems, culture, secondary gains derived from illness, societal reactions, and the therapist–patient relationship. All these factors have a direct impact on the patient's motivation, which in turn affects rehabilitation outcome. A strong set of psychosocial components positively affects motivation, thus having a positive affect on outcome. However, when psychosocial components are not well developed or are negative in nature, there may be a subsequent negative impact on motivation and a decrease in functional outcome (Figure 23-1).

In addition, one coping factor may be so overwhelming that it negates the other aspects. For example, a patient may have absolutely no support systems yet have such a driving, inherent will to get better that the negative aspects are minimized.

Some areas of the psychosocial arena cannot be changed (eg, premorbid personality, culture, societal reaction); however, it is important for the occupational therapist to develop a therapeutic relationship with the patient to enhance and to help develop strengths in the psychosocial arena. Alternative support systems and additional coping mechanisms may be developed to further increase motivation and thus positively affect the rehabilitation outcome.

Assessment

Assessment in acute care is a challenge because there is limited time to complete assessment and develop a treatment plan. Patients often have a multitude of diagnostic tests as well as additional services that are being provided to the patient, such as respiratory care, social services, speech pathology, physical therapy, and occupational therapy. It thus becomes extremely important that assessment is completed in a short time to maximize the time for treatment. In an ideal setting, it is imperative to have objective, standardized testing to delineate a patient's strengths and weaknesses. In acute care this is often not feasible due to time limitations, however; thus, subjective, observational data assume greater importance and are relied on to a great extent. For this reason, it is found that assessment and treatment may occur simultaneously and provide assessment data as well as intervention.

Demographic information

The demographic factors considered should include personal information: name, address, telephone number, date of birth, age, and sex. The date of admission to the hospital, referral date, date first seen by the occupational therapist, and the name of the physician who referred the patient to occupational therapy

FIGURE 23-1. *The effect of psychosocial factors on motivation and rehabilitation outcome.*

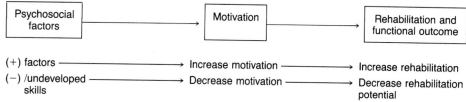

should be recorded. The type of insurance coverage is important for both billing and planning for occupational therapy intervention. For example, certain insurance coverage requires prior approval for occupational therapy services. Other data include the diagnosis being addressed in occupational therapy and additional diagnoses that may affect the patient's life, the date of onset, present problems and symptoms, medications, precautions, complications, and other pertinent medical history. The family situation including marital status, family members at or near the home, and people who are with the patient during the day and night need documentation. A brief description of the home should be included, such as whether it is an urban or a rural setting, the type of structure, and the number of stairs the patient normally uses within the home.

Independent living and daily living skills

During the initial assessment, the current self-care status should be documented. It should be noted whether the patient is independent, requires assistance of a person or adaptive equipment, or is dependent in any given task. The areas that should be considered are grooming and hygiene, eating, dressing, homecare responsibilities, leisure activities, and functional mobility within the home and in the community. Safety of the patient in all the above-mentioned areas is essential to the well-being of the patient and must be considered first and foremost.

It is also important to note the patient's activity of daily living (ADL) status before admission. If discrepancies are found between what the patient was previously able to perform and the current status, it is necessary to document the potential for return to the patient's premorbid/prehospitalization level of functioning.

There is some evidence that professionals and perhaps even patients tend to overestimate the ability to perform ADL (Spiegel, Hirshfield, & Spiegel, 1985). Although patients may appear capable of performing certain tasks, therapists should know whether these tasks are actually being performed at home or in the hospital.

Documentation of family involvement is an important aspect of the patient's daily living assessment. The amount and appropriateness of the assistance provided should be noted, as well as how both the patient and the family feel about the assistance. If assistance will be needed after hospitalization and these needs cannot be satisfied by the family or adaptive equipment, social services should be consulted.

Work

Data should be gathered regarding the patient's former and present occupations. Specific education and training, as well as job requirements and responsibilities, should also be documented. Any potential need for occupational change should be

noted by the acute care therapist; such situations usually necessitate referral for later intervention.

Sensorimotor skills and performance components

Reflex integration, range of motion and muscle strength, gross and fine motor coordination, sensation, endurance, and abnormal positioning all should be evaluated as appropriate for the individual patient. It is important to remember that formalized testing in the acute care setting may be difficult due to the patient's medical equipment and precautions; it is thus necessary to adapt even though specific guidelines for testing may not be observed. If testing is done with adaptations, it is important to note these in documentation.

Cognitive skills and performance components

This assessment should include orientation, cognition, ability to follow commands, perceptual–motor skills, and conceptualization.

Psychosocial skills and performance components

As discussed earlier, healthy psychosocial coping mechanisms in the acutely ill patient are essential to adaptation and return to a healthy lifestyle. It is thus important to gather information during the assessment on the patient's self-concept and self-identity, situational coping, and available support systems.

Therapeutic adaptation

The use of prosthetic or orthotic devices should be recorded. The occupational therapist should ask and record whether the patient has any adaptive equipment and whether it is used regularly. The appropriateness of fit of these devices should be checked, so that modifications can be made, if indicated.

Therapist's impression

Before treatment goals can be developed, the therapist must take into consideration the potential benefit of treatment, the presumed reliability of the patient's responses, and the motivation of the patient to participate in the occupational therapy program.

Patient goals

The therapist should document the patient's short-term and long-term goals that have been determined with patient input. The therapist should note the patient's understanding of the disability or disease, responses to a brief description of the occupational therapy program, and the attitude of the patient toward the program.

Occupational therapy program plan

In summation, the treatment plan should reflect the assessment information, therapist impressions, and subsequent goals. In addition, the plan should indicate the need for further evaluation, follow-up or referral considerations, estimated duration of treatment, and potential of the patient to reach stated goals.

Discharge planning and home assessment

Discharge planning should begin immediately after referral to ensure continuity of care and also to ensure that all the patient's needs will be met after discharge. Discharge planning will vary with the patient's functional ability. Some patients may need only a home program so that they may continue occupational therapy independently. Patients who need more structured intervention may benefit from outpatient treatment or admission to a rehabilitation hospital. Others, however, may not be able to return to the same level of functioning as they had at admission, and plans must be formulated to assist the patient and family to develop alternate plans. Some patients may have adequate support systems in place so that they may return home with assistance; others may need more help than family and friends can provide. In such cases, contract nursing services may be available to provide needed services (home health aide, nursing, physical therapist, occupational therapist), whereas at other times placement in a retirement community or nursing home may be needed. Consultation with the patient, family, and all services working with the patient is essential before the final decision regarding discharge and placement can be made. Social services then initiates all paperwork and related documentation for discharge. Occupational therapy provides continuity of care forms to the referring agency.

In some community hospitals, if there is a question of a patient returning to their home environment, a ***home assessment*** may be performed. Areas to be addressed in the home assessment include safety in all self-care tasks, mobility in the home, ability to negotiate stairs, performance of necessary homemaking tasks (cooking, and so on), needed durable medical equipment, and the ability to manipulate the environment (light switches, phone, and so on). Evaluation forms are available that provide structure and areas to be evaluated and are helpful to use while doing a home assessment (see Chapter 8, Section 2A).

Special treatment procedures

Intensive care unit

It is common for occupational therapists to provide services to patients in ***intensive care units*** (ICUs) of general hospitals. To develop an occupational therapy program on a given ICU, the therapist must know the purpose of the unit and work supportively with the physician and nursing teams. Any occupational therapy program represents a coordinated effort that considers the patient's medical needs, nursing procedures, respiratory care, and physical therapy programs. It is important to note that patients in ICU are critically ill and are often in a battle for survival. Although occupational therapy is essential, especially to

help promote recovery and minimize residual deficits, it may not be the primary focus since the patient is involved in many medical and nursing procedures.

The ICU is an equipment-laden environment that provides constant monitoring of patients' vital signs. It is of the utmost importance for therapists to have a thorough knowledge of where invasive lines go, what they do, what problems they can cause, and what precautions they warrant (Table 23-1) (Affleck, Bianchi, Cleckly, et al., 1984).

Many patients in the ICU are on a ventilator with numerous monitors that affect their response to the environment. Patients may be ventilated via nasotracheal, endotracheal, or tracheostomy intubation, all of which may impede the patient's ability to communicate. Some patients are pharmacologically sedated, whereas others may be comatose. The effects of constant monitoring with complete disruption of daily life routines, together with the fear, depression, and pain of being ill, can also lead a patient to a state of generalized disorientation. Intensive care psychosis is a diagnosis often applied to patients exhibiting acute agitation, which can manifest from mild confusion to advanced delirium. Patients who have sustained severe trauma, prolonged surgical procedures, and lengthy anesthesia have a greater tendency to develop this diagnosis. The common features of this ICU syndrome consist of clouding of the consciousness, decreased ability to maintain attention, orientation difficulties, memory problems, and labile affect. Patients may display symptoms of altered time perception, lack of emotion, feelings of surrealism, a sense of detachment, loss of control, revival of memories, and a sense of ineffability (Civetta, Taylor, & Kirby, 1989). In addition, physical movement may be hampered due to the disease process (eg, cerebrovascular accident) or activity restrictions.

All patients referred to occupational therapy who are in the ICU should be evaluated and treated in the following areas: orientation and cognition, physical and motor skills, splinting, endurance and activity tolerance, and activities of daily living.

Orientation and cognition

Occupational therapy programs in the ICU can alleviate some of the problems of isolation and sensory deprivation by providing gradual application of specific stimuli to increase arousal and awareness. Early research has shown that vestibular input and upright positioning can help increase alertness; therefore, it is advantageous to get a patient in the sitting position as soon as medically feasible to increase eye opening, head control, purposeful use of upper extremities, and awareness of the environment (Dale, 1991). The occupational therapist should use orientation techniques for patients who are confused; these may include provision of a calendar, digital clock to differentiate between night and day, cognitive games, daily schedule, and use of family history and other methods to help orient the patient. Activities of daily living programs can help restore a sense of daily routine and personal independence. Relaxation techniques can be incorporated with reality orientation programs to provide organized, patterned stimulation and to develop an increased sense of personal control (Affleck et al., 1984). It is also extremely helpful to give the patient choices as often as possible, and as much as their orientation allows, to enhance some feelings of control. These choices may be as simple as deciding which

TABLE 23-1. *Common Life Support and Monitoring Lines*

Line/Catheter	Location	Purpose	Precautions	Implications
CVP	Threaded through superior vena cava into right atrium	Monitors right side of the heart filling pressures; used to introduce drugs	Line is sutured in; do not pull; normal CVP is 9–12 mm Hg	Should not restrict ROM at head, shoulder, or scapula; should not restrict activity
Arterial line	Usually in radial or femoral artery; can also be in artery in the foot (dorsum pedis)	When continuous monitoring of blood pressure is indicated or when frequent blood gas measurements are required	Inserted into artery; looks like an IV but is not; usually sutured in. Do not pull; immobilize wrist, no movement to dislodge line; normal MAP is 70–90 mm HG; transducer must be at level of patient's heart for accurate reading	Know patient's normal MAP and monitor with any change in activity; notify nurse of any change
Swan–Ganz catheter	Threaded into the superior vena cava into right ventricle; pulmonary valve catheter tip rests in pulmonary artery	Indirectly monitors function of the left side of the heart; can also obtain CVP and cardiac output readings; used following open heart surgery, trauma, heart failure	Line is sutured in; do not pull; usually, patients with this line are in serious condition; check activity orders closely; nurse monitors PAWP.	Specific activity order with specific parameters for each patient's MAP from physician; watch pulmonary artery pressure wave for damping with activity
Central line	Most frequently in subclavian vein	To administer very high concentration of calories, often following extensive surgery or trauma when oral or NG intake is inadequate	Line is usually sutured in; do not pull.	Usually, activity is indicated secondary to high-calorie intake; line should not restrict mobility or ROM
Neurologic monitors		Monitors ICP following surgery or trauma	Head of bed is usually limited to no more 30°	Usually on bed rest; check with physician
Examples:				
IVC	IVC tip rests in the ventricle of the brain		Normal ICP ≤15 mm Hg	
Subarachnoid bolt, Richmond bolt	Subarachnoid space-CSF in contact with column of H_2O to measure pressure			
Chest tube	Usually through intercostal or subcostal space into pleural space	Drains fluid from chest cavity and restores normal pressure relationships within pleural space	Usually sutured in; do not pull	Avoid tension, torque, or kinking

CSF, cerebrospinal fluid; CVP, central venous pressure; ICP, intracranial pressure; IVC, intraventricular catheter; MAP, mean arterial pressure; NG, nasogastric; OTR, occupational therapist, registered; PAWP, pulmonary artery wedge pressure; ROM, range of motion.

(Modified from Affleck, A. T., Lieberman, S., Polon, J., & Rohrkemper, K. (1986). Providing occupational therapy in an intensive care unit. American Journal of Occupational Therapy, 40, 325.)

modality to use in treatment, selecting the time of day to be seen by the occupational therapist, or deciding when to take rest breaks. Patients who are unable to communicate verbally should be provided with communication boards to facilitate communication, as well as a speech pathologist to consult with the patient and provide augmentative communication devices as needed.

Physical and motor skills

As indicated, patients may not have complete movement, and assessment must be done for limited range, strength, sensation, and coordination. Treatment should address those areas where deficits exist and may include passive range of motion, active or active assistive range of motion, proper positioning to prevent deformity, strengthening, and coordination programs. Patients with decreased trunk stability need to also focus on mobility exercises of rolling and sitting.

Splinting

All patients who have been on or are presently on prolonged bed rest, have the potential to develop contractures. Decreased mobility of ankles and resting in a dependent position can lead to plantar flexion contractures. Dorsiflexion splints are indicated for these patients to maintain a neutral position and prevent deformity. Likewise, patients may need proper hand positioning to prevent deformity. Assessment may indicate the need for resting pan splints, safe position splints, or hand cones.

Endurance and activity tolerance

Patients who have been on extended bed rest will have very low endurance, low sitting tolerance, and generalized weakness—effects that can be reversed through therapy. Activities such as bed mobility, sitting on the side of the bed, transfer training, graded self-care, and strengthening programs all can be initiated in the ICU environment when the patient is medically ready and the physician approves. These activities can be graded in terms of length of treatment time, amount and speed of active movement, level of assistance given, adaptive aids, and position and postural support.

Activities of daily living

Depending on the patient's medical status and orientation, the patient may be performing some simple self-care activities. It is difficult for many patients to be completely independent even in sponge bathing in the ICU due to the numerous lines and monitors to which the patient is attached. However, it is important for the patient to perform portions of his or her own care as soon as possible. This may involve simple activities such as face washing, trunk washing, mouth care, or brushing hair. An occupational therapist may need to work with the patient to perform ADL in the morning and address additional rehabilitation goals during a separate treatment session.

Because of the nature of the ICU, close teamwork is necessary to provide patients with a daily schedule that can balance rest, mobilization, and functional recovery directly and effectively. Activities are appropriate to use in the ICU, because they can help in orientation, physical functioning, and development of sense of control. It is essential to provide emotional support to the patient and family during this stressful period.

Examples of treatment programs

This section addresses specific diagnostic categories frequently seen in the acute care, general hospital setting. Symptomatology is briefly discussed, and the role of the occupational therapist with each specific category is presented. Many of the orthopedic, neurologic, and cardiopulmonary conditions seen by the occupational therapist are covered in other sections of this book.

Cancer

The term "cancer" refers collectively to all malignant tumors. *Malignancy* implies the ability of the tumor, or neoplasm, to invade and destroy adjacent structures and to spread to distant sites (metastasis). Tumors are classified according to their histogenesis; tumors of mesenchymal origin are called *sarcomas*, whereas tumors of epithelial origin are called *carcinomas*. Classification and terminology are important because they convey the specific clinical significance—the likely behavior—of a given neoplasm (Robbins, & Angell, 1971). The location, rate of growth, spread, and amount of interference with normal function determine the pathologic effects of a tumor.

Cancer affects a wide variety of organs; incidence varies with age, sex, and site. Prognosis varies according to the type of cancer and according to the stage at which the cancer was diagnosed. Etiology of cancer has not been determined, but several factors have been identified that favor its development, including heredity, hormonal states, and exposure to carcinogens. Blood diseases, such as the lymphomas and leukemias are also considered by lay persons to be cancer of the blood. Subsequent complications and chemotherapy can also be debilitating.

The means of slowing, arresting, or curing the disease are surgery, chemotherapy, radiation, and, more recently, bone marrow transplantation. Any of these treatment regimens can result in amputation, seriously altered ways of functioning, changes in self-image, adjustment of lifestyle, and varying states of well-being. Survival time is increased since early detection and improved treatment methods allow control of the disease for longer periods of time. For some patients, cancer becomes a chronic disease requiring long-term monitoring and treatment. As in other chronic diseases, rehabilitation can maintain optimum function in the cancer patient and improve the quality of the person's life.

Rehabilitation

In general, the goals for cancer rehabilitation may be divided into four categories (Dietz, 1981). The *preventive* category involves treatment in anticipation of potential disability to decrease its severity or shorten its duration. In the *restorative* category are programs for the patient who can be expected to return to premorbid status without significant handicap. The *supportive* category is defined by controlled disease or handicap that will persist, in which much disability can be eliminated by training or treatment. The last category is *palliative*, in which increasing disability from progressive disease is present but in which appropriate rehabilitation can prevent complications such as decubitus ulcers, contractures, problems of personal hygiene, and emotional deterioration due to inactivity and depression.

Rehabilitation of cancer patients differs from standard rehabilitation in several important ways. The single most important factor is that cancer rehabilitation is an ongoing process that does not wait for the patient to be medically stable. Therapists must develop a philosophy of treatment that enables them to cope with the realities of the situation (Bierenger, 1981):

1. Occupational therapy may be started before the long-term results of the patient's medical treatment are known.
2. Patients may be discharged before rehabilitation is complete.
3. Much treatment is done at the bedside, which limits activities.
4. Evaluation is brief and ongoing rather than complete.
5. Rehabilitation sessions are often interrupted by treatment or diagnostic procedures.
6. Side effects of treatment may prevent occupational therapy treatment.
7. Rehabilitation may not be foremost in the mind of the patient.

The task of the occupational therapist is to trigger useful coping mechanisms, to teach adaptation and compensation, to help the patient regard problems as challenges, and to foster creativity and flexibility. Interventions may be psychosocial support, physical restoration, training in the use of adaptive equipment, design and construction of orthotic devices, retraining in activities of daily living, teaching of satisfying leisure activities, and family support and teaching. The physical restoration measures necessary to rehabilitate the residual problems of the disease or its treatment follow the usual principles of functional occupational therapy. However, the patient may deteriorate in other areas because of disease progression during or after the rehabilitation therapy.

The psychosocial aspects of the patient's treatment are as

important as the physical restoration measures. Although occupational therapy may be limited and intermittent, an effective therapeutic relationship between patient and therapist early in the disease will make it easier to reinstitute treatment as new problems occur. With each successive rehospitalization, the patient and family may lose more of their hope for recovery. Feelings of helplessness and loss of control and relinquishment of their social roles of wage earner, homemaker, or parent may occur. Occupational therapy can be instrumental in reestablishing the patient's area of control by helping him or her to identify attainable short-term and long-term goals.

Radical mastectomy patients

Occupational therapy services for women who have undergone radical mastectomies are designed to help prevent problems of decreased shoulder range of motion (pain, edema, weakness), to provide education through discussion, and to demonstrate available adaptive equipment such as bras, prostheses, and clothing. The therapist should explain which activities are contraindicated postoperatively while providing therapeutic activities. Instruction in the principles of work simplification and energy conservation may be helpful.

Surgeons vary in their referral patterns, but physical activity and exercise are usually not initiated until 3 or 4 days postoperatively. It is important for therapists to consult with the surgeon to establish the specific rehabilitation program and rate of progression for each patient. The specific objectives must take into consideration that particular patient's premorbid condition and activity level in addition to any postoperative complications such as shoulder–hand syndrome.

In coordination with the social services or rehabilitation psychology departments, psychological support for the individual and her family should be offered to facilitate acceptance of her condition. After discharge from the hospital, the patient may be seen for review and reinforcement of instructions presented during hospitalization. Outpatient treatment may be done in groups to facilitate mutual support in conjunction with physical rehabilitation. (If appropriate, referral should be made to community agencies such as the Reach for Recovery Program of the American Cancer Society.)

The dying patient

People dying from cancer may experience physical isolation, an actual withdrawal by family and medical personnel. Even with the greater awareness of this problem and a subsequent increased sensitivity, it still may occur. It is not uncommon for patients, their families, and the medical staff to experience feelings of denial, avoidance, and anxiety. The therapist who works with the dying patient must be secure in his or her attitude toward death and dying. The therapist must be able to listen, hear, understand, be sensitive, and be able to respond verbally and nonverbally to spoken and unspoken requests. The ability to recognize when a patient needs you and the willingness to give the time, regardless of personal or professional schedule, are essential.

Occupational therapy is unique in that the patient's physical, psychosocial, and occupational performance needs are assessed and incorporated into treatment. The occupational therapist can provide meaningful, purposeful activity to help the patient main-

tain occupational function and preserve dignity, self-respect, and self-esteem (Pizzi, 1986). The patient should ultimately determine the quality of life and the occupational roles he or she wishes to maintain. Activities that promote a feeling of self-worth and productivity may be used to facilitate the adaptive process. Frequent reevaluation is necessary due to the continuing deterioration of the patient's condition, so that priority setting and goals may be adjusted accordingly.

Cardiac disease

Cardiac disease is discussed in Chapter 18, Section 2; however, this disease should be mentioned here, since acute care occupational therapists perform a primary role in cardiac rehabilitation while a patient is hospitalized in a general hospital. Patients seen in the acute phases of cardiac involvement have had myocardial infarction, coronary artery bypass grafts, valve replacements, and congestive heart failure.

Most frequently, occupational therapists are on a cardiac rehabilitation team, including a nursing coordinator, physical therapist, exercise physiologist, social worker, and dietitian. It is essential for the occupational therapist to work in conjunction with the team and be constantly aware of the patient's medical status and how the patient performs in the other disciplines. Therapists who want to specialize in cardiac rehabilitation should acquire more knowledge of cardiovascular physiology, management of heart disease, electrocardiographic interpretation, and exercise physiology.

Depending on the facility and the region of the country, different rehabilitation professionals may perform the same role in different programs. Thus, the occupational therapists's role may vary widely. He or she may provide one or more of the following components of the program in the acute care setting (Killeen, 1986):

1. Progressive activity and exercise—to assess and help the patient to develop tolerance for activity.
2. Work-equivalent activity—to teach the patient about the energy cost of activity and to promote a vocational interest.
3. Activities of daily living evaluation and training—to assess cardiac response to these activities and to make appropriate recommendations.
4. Work simplification training—to promote maximum independence in patients whose cardiac reserve is impaired and for postoperative recuperation.
5. Patient education about activity and exercise—to educate regarding precautions (limitations in lifting and driving due to precautions related to healing of the sternum and postsurgical intervention of bypass graft/valve replacement).
6. Psychosocial support—to assist the patient to cope with the event and to make lifestyle changes.
7. Leisure counseling—to assist the patient in emotional adjustment and stress management.
8. Stress management training.
9. Education about cardiac risk factors.

The role of the acute care occupational therapist may be varied as indicated, but it is the primary starting point for those who have cardiac involvement. This material is a brief synopsis; for complete details of cardiopulmonary programming see Chapter 18, Section 2.

Diabetes mellitus

Diabetes mellitus is a disorder of the metabolism of insulin. In type I diabetes, an insulin deficiency is present, and most affected persons require insulin injections to survive. Type I diabetes, also referred to as *insulin-dependent diabetes mellitus* (IDDM), is usually of sudden onset and most commonly appears in childhood and adolescence. Hence, it is sometimes called juvenile or juvenile-onset diabetes. Type II diabetes is characterized by the presence of some insulin in the blood levels. The insulin level may be normal, elevated, or depressed, and the response to the insulin is abnormal. Type II diabetes, or *non-insulin-dependent diabetes mellitus* (NIDDM), has a gradual onset and may appear at any age, although most frequently in persons over age 40. It often is associated with obesity. Decreasing insulin requirements by diet or weight loss or stimulation of insulin production with oral medication may be sufficient to control type II diabetes; however, the administration of insulin may be necessary in some cases.

In diabetes mellitus, a balance must be achieved between available insulin, intake of food, and consumption of energy in activities. Longstanding diabetes may lead to decreased vision from retinal vessel disease, kidney lesions and renal failure, neuropathies, arteriosclerosis, and peripheral vascular disease, resulting in gangrene or amputation.

Occupational therapy has four potential objectives for persons with diabetes: (1) providing regulated activity to assist in insulin regulation, (2) providing an environment in which the patient can demonstrate knowledge of diet regulations through meal planning and preparation, (3) evaluating and teaching compensatory skills when the patient has complications that result in visual loss, sensory loss, or amputation, and (4) providing psychological support. The pervasiveness of the treatment regimen can produce feeling of depression, anger, and dependency, and the patient may demonstrate manipulative behaviors. Patients may feel overwhelmed and the occupational therapist should allow them to make as many choices as possible with the therapy session to facilitate the patient's feelings of control.

Renal disease

Chronic renal failure (CRF) is a condition in which the kidneys fail to function as a result of progressive destruction of the *nephrons*, the functional units of the kidney. Filtration, secretion, and reabsorption take place in the nephrons, whereas the kidney regulates the volume and chemical composition of blood and extracellular fluid. When CRF occurs, the kidney is unable to perform its normal functions. Metabolic end products such as urea build up in the bloodstream, producing uremia. The clinical manifestations of uremia vary with the medical condition of the patient and may include gastrointestinal upset, decreased mental concentration, apathy, lethargy, confusion and increased irritability, peripheral neuropathy, dermatologic changes, generalized itching of the skin, anemia, weakness, and changes in cardiovascular function (Chyatte, 1979).

Medical treatment of chronic renal failure consists of hemodialysis, peritoneal dialysis, or kidney transplantation. Hemodialysis uses a blood circuit to a machine called a *hemodialyzer*. The most common vascular access is an internal arteriovenous fistula, which is an anastomosis created surgically between an artery and a vein. The radial artery and cephalic vein in the upper extremity are most often used. When a patient cannot tolerate hemodialysis, when the patient prefers another method of treatment, or while the patient is waiting for a permanent hemodialysis vascular access, *continuous ambulatory peritoneal dialysis* (CAPD) may be used. This type of dialysis involves the surgical placement of a catheter into the abdominal cavity, where the peritoneum acts as a semipermeable membrane. Bags of dialyzate are then run through the body, cleansing and purifying the body of waste products.

Patients on CAPD or hemodialysis may develop disuse atrophy, distal edema, and contractures. Many of these patients have concomitant disease processes, putting them at additional risk for development of complications. Diabetes is a common cause of CRF and thus many renal patients present with diabetic complications: retinopathy, neuropathies, and peripheral vascular disease.

Occupational therapy for the renal patient should include assessment and treatment in the following areas: physical and motor skills, splinting, endurance and activity tolerance, activities of daily living, and psychological support.

Physical and motor skills

Range of motion, strength, and coordination need to be evaluated in the renal patient. Deficits are often seen in all these areas, with long-term renal disease and hemodialysis causing such problems. A strengthening program to combat disuse of all proximal and distal musculature should be initiated. Such a program could include exercises (with dowel rod, theraband, theraputty), as well as activities to promote the same. Exercise/activity programs also serve to increase vascular flow. Coordination deficits may also be noted with the renal patient, and coordination exercises and activities are prescribed.

Splinting

Renal patients who develop complications with their access sites may be at risk for hand deformity. It is important for the occupational therapist to be aware of such possibilities and for the subsequent need for splinting. Safe position splints are often fabricated to prevent deformity, but the occupational therapist should consult with the physician regarding the splint, its relationship to the access site, and any precautions that need to be followed. It is also important to remember that renal patients may have neuropathies and decreased sensation, so it is essential that they visually check their skin for reddened areas indicating the need for splint modifications.

Endurance and activity tolerance

Renal patients may demonstrate a significantly impaired activity tolerance, which many report is worse on hemodialysis days. A structured program can increase endurance by gradually increasing time spent in treatment, number of repetitions, and difficulty of task. Instruction in work simplification and energy conservation is also appropriate to increase functional status despite low tolerance. Occupational therapy needs to treat the patient around their dialysis schedule, which may interfere with the ability to see the patient on a daily basis due to extreme postdialysis fatigue.

Activities of daily living

A complete and thorough assessment must address patient's needs while hospitalized and after discharge. Equipment assessment should include the need for all durable medical equipment (bedside commode, tub transfer bench, grab bars, wheelchair), as well as small ADL equipment (reacher, hand-held shower, coordination needs). Assessment of leisure activities should be done and alternative avocational interests investigated.

Psychological support

The psychological reactions of renal patients are similar to those of patients with other chronic diseases. Feelings of helplessness and depression are common. Lack of motivation toward rehabilitation may be encountered, particularly when uremia is exhibited as decreased mental concentration, apathy, and lethargy. Patients with end-stage renal disease must tolerate considerable life restrictions: dependency on and proximity to the hemodialysis machine and multiple dietary and fluid restrictions. It is important for the occupational therapist to take all these factors into consideration while planning an effective treatment program.

Transplantation

The most famous 13th century legend of **transplantation** is the medieval myth in which Sts. Damian and Cosmas transplanted the leg of a Moor to a dying patient, and the patient was saved. Fascination with transplantation has continued with what is perhaps that earliest recording of a transplant. The first reported bone transplant was done in 1682, the first skin transplant in 1881, and the first kidney transplant in the goat model in 1902. It was not until 1954 that the first human kidney transplant was performed on twins, with the recipient living with normal kidney function for 7 years posttransplant (Norris & House, 1991; Surman, 1989). During the following years, the first successful transplants of other organs were performed: liver/lung (1963) and pancreas/heart (1967). Despite these first successes, transplantation of the liver, heart, and pancreas was principally a laboratory event in the 1960s; yet renal transplantation was gaining clinical acceptance and becoming an alternative to dialysis. Relatively poor results in transplantation of the liver and heart led to surgical moratoria in the 1970s (Surman, 1989).

Technical advances in surgery and new immunosuppression regimens have led to improved outcomes for organ transplantation. Currently, about 75% of liver transplant recipients, 75% to 80% of heart transplant recipients, and over 90% of kidney transplant recipients are alive at 1 year (Surman, 1989). Organ transplantation has become a viable option for end-stage organ failure. Currently, there are 21,000 Americans waiting for organs; of those, about 17,500 need kidneys, 1700 need hearts, 1000 need livers, 250 need combined heart and lungs, 400 need a pancreas, and another 100 are waiting for a single- or double-lung transplant (Norris & House, 1991).

It is common that large, acute care hospitals have transplant units. Occupational therapists thus can play an active role in the rehabilitation of transplant patients. It is important to note that roles may vary in different settings, and occupational therapy may not be involved in all types of transplants. Transplantation has given thousands a second chance at life, and occupational therapy needs to keep abreast of the changes in the field of transplantation and be ready to meet the needs of transplant patients.

Each type of transplant will be briefly presented, with the occupational therapy intervention for them discussed.

Renal

Renal transplants can be performed from a living related donor (LRD) or a cadaveric donor; the LRD transplants have greater success rates. The transplanted kidney is placed retroperitoneally in the right or left iliac fossa. The patient's native kidney is left in place unless it is a source of infection or uncontrolled high blood pressure. Immunosuppression begins immediately to help control rejection. Occupational therapy for the renal transplant patient is mainly dependent on pretransplant status and need for intervention. The patient with recent renal failure probably has fewer problems than the patient who has been on dialysis for several years. If dialysis has been brief and concomitant disease is absent, residual deficits are uncommon. Currently the length of stay after renal transplantation is 7 to 10 days, and in many cases the patients do not need occupational therapy. If pretransplant problems are still occurring, occupational therapy can address those specific problems as needed, including but not limited to range of motion, strength, endurance, and ADL performance.

Liver

The liver performs many complex functions, including vascular, secretory, metabolic, and storage functions. When pathology of the liver occurs, many symptoms are manifest: peripheral edema, ascites, pleural effusions, impaired immune system, severe hypoglycemia, amenorrhea, abnormal body hair distribution, scaly skin, hepatic encepalopathy, jaundice, and nutritional problems (Norris & House, 1991). With liver transplantation, the native liver is removed and the donor liver is put in its place.

The first human liver transplant was performed in 1963, and over the next 17 years, the 1-year survival rate for liver transplantation in the United States was about 28%. Cyclosporine was introduced in 1981 as a more effective immunosuppressive agent, and along with better candidate selection and management, survival rate has soared, making liver transplantation more actively sought by those with end-stage liver failure.

Occupational therapy can play an aggressive role in the life of the liver transplant patient. Many of these patients are extremely ill and have multiple complications. While the liver transplant patient is hospitalized in the ICU, thorough assessment and treatment are indicated (see previous discussion on ICU intervention). It is important to remember that this patient may have been suffering from hepatic encepalopathy preoperatively and may thus still have such symptoms as confusion and agitation, and possibly ICU psychosis. After the liver transplant patient has been moved from the ICU, more aggressive rehabilitation can begin. The following areas need to be addressed when working with a liver transplant patient: orientation and cognition, physical and motor skills, endurance and activity tolerance, and activities of daily living.

Orientation and cognition

After any initial problems are cleared, orientation and cognition usually are not problems.

Physical and motor skills

Liver transplant patients seen in occupational therapy routinely have limitations in strength, with many being in the poor ranges of manual muscle testing. Hand strength is decreased as well, with changes seen in both grip and pinch. An exercise/activity program is indicated, with upgrading of the program carried out as needed.

Endurance/activity tolerance

Along with the decreased strength, liver transplant patients usually are extremely limited in endurance; many are able to tolerate only 15 minutes, with rest breaks, of minimal activity when treatment is initiated. It is most helpful to get these patients to the clinic, where a broader range of activities may be performed and with the transportation also serving as a means of increasing endurance. Endurance can be improved by previously mentioned methods: by increasing time of treatment, difficulty, and repetitions of task.

Activities of daily living

Liver transplant patients can resume their own self-care as soon as medically feasible and as soon as they are able to perform safely around their drains, lines, and so on. The patients will not resume tub bathing or showering for an extended period of time; therefore, showering equipment is not needed at this time. Occasionally, if patients have suffered multiple complications and are still impaired, a toilet safety frame or bedside commode may be warranted. Instruction is also reviewed regarding lifelong restrictions (eg, no contact sports).

Heart

After the surgical moratorium in the 1970s, a cautious resurgence of heart transplants was beginning by 1977. In the past decade, improvements in drug therapies, development of the endomyocardial biopsy technique, and better understanding of the rejection process have helped to improve survival rate. In 1987, 1512 heart transplants were done in the United States (Monaco, 1990).

Anything that interferes with the normal function of the heart can precipitate cardiac disease. Weakening of the cardiac muscle because of excessive stretching (dilatation) or thinning (as in an aneurysm), scarring of the muscle wall, inflammation (myocarditis), or anoxia-induced cell death after infarction may prevent normal contraction and pumping. The result of any of these problems is the inability of the heart to perform sufficiently as a pump, with a lowered cardiac output and stagnation or backup of blood. Patients in heart failure thus usually complain of profound fatigue, shortness of breath, and pedal edema due to the poor blood flow to the brain and extremities. They may also complain of mood swings, poor memory, abdominal enlargement (ascites), and loss of weight and abdominal pain (intestinal

ischemia). As the heart attempts to compensate, tachycardia and dysrhythmias may occur (Monaco, 1990).

Heart transplants are unique in that they are considered only after all other medical and surgical options are exhausted. In an orthotopic heart transplant procedure, the recipient's anterior atria and ventricles are completely replaced (Monaco, 1990).

Occupational therapy may vary widely for each cardiac transplant patient. In some instances, the patient is hospitalized while awaiting a donor heart. Because this time can be lengthy and indefinite, the occupational therapist can use a structured activity program to appropriately manage stress, minimize depression, and decrease anxiety. This has been shown, according to patient report, to significantly assist during the waiting period. After the transplant, the patient most often feels relief of all the aforementioned symptoms, since a functioning, healthy heart is now in place. In some facilities, the patient is actively involved in the cardiac rehabilitation program to facilitate exercise and activity tolerance. In other facilities, occupational therapy may not be involved postoperatively, because the patient's return to function is dependent on his or her tolerance and because posttransplant function is greatly enhanced.

Pancreas

Pancreatic transplantation has lagged behind the other organ transplantations because of the relatively poor technical success rate, limited ability to detect early rejection, and lack of convincing evidence that successful pancreas transplantation prevents the ongoing progression of secondary symptoms related to diabetes mellitus (Alexander, 1990). There is current debate regarding the best method of pancreatic transplantation—whole-organ transplantation, transplantation of segment, or transplantation only of the islets of Langerhans. Pancreatic transplant may also occur simultaneously with renal transplantation.

Occupational therapy has been most active in dealing with the pancreas population pretransplant because of the multitude of problems and complications that may occur with diabetes and mandate occupational therapy intervention.

Dysphagia

Swallowing impairment (**dysphagia**) often results from mechanical deficits (from radical neck/mouth surgery for carcinoma, laryngectomy, long-term tracheostomy), from myopathies/myotonias (polymyositis, myasthenia gravis), neuromuscular esophageal disorders (scleroderma, Raynaud's phenomenon), acquired central disorders (cerebrovascular accident, Parkinson's disease), and acquired peripheral disorders (X nerve involvement; Groher, 1984). As indicated, the list of disease processes that can make an impact on swallowing is extensive; thus, it is essential that swallowing not be overlooked. The occupational therapist must be knowledgeable about the anatomy and neurophysiology of swallowing, including specific volitional and reflexive components.

The occupational therapist is a team member in the swallowing team that consists of the medical staff, nurse, speech pathologist, and dietitian. Once again, as with other programs, the role of the occupational therapist and the other health professionals may vary, depending on the facility. The goal of the entire team is to make the patient as functional and as safe as possible with oral intake. All team members may gather parts of the following information based on their role in the team.

Assessment

History with subjective description of the problem; influence of solid, semisolid, or liquid foods; and specific information regarding nasal regurgitation, mouth odor, aspiration, reflux, pain, weight loss, and pneumonia all need to be documented. Physical/ bedside evaluation includes mental status, weight, muscles of facial expression, muscles of mastication, pathologic reflexes, oral mucosa, dentition, pharyngeal palate, and tongue. To assess what occurs with swallowing beyond the oral phase of the swallow, it is important to perform a videofluoroscopy, which is a radiographic study that allows visualization of the pharyngeal and esophageal phases of the swallow (Groher, 1984). The barium swallow helps to document aspiration, which is the major cause of morbidity and mortality in patients with swallowing dysfunction (Zimmerman & Oder, 1981). It may also be found that the patient is not able to tolerate oral intake because of the severe risk of aspiration, and oral feeding may not be recommended. As indicated, assessment of the dysphagic patient is complex, and no one team member can be expected to gather all the necessary information. Therefore, teamwork is critical.

Prerequisites for treatment

There are several prerequisites to implementing a swallowing program. First, the patient must be mentally alert and able to follow instructions and carry them over from day to day, as well as to concentrate on the task well enough to support a reflex behavior. Second, the physiologic potential to swallow must be determined. Last, a gag reflex must be present. If a patient has little or no gag reflex unilaterally or bilaterally, a stimulation program needs to be initiated before food is introduced. In addition, tongue mobility and good laryngeal closure should be established through tongue exercises and stimulation.

Treatment program

A swallowing program has three basic components: (1) exercises to improve strength, coordination, and range of motion; (2) verbal coaching to bring swallowing under volitional control; and (3) graduated feeding. Exercises to strengthen the mechanical swallowing abilities include those for tongue lateralization, elevation, and retraction, strengthening the cheeks and lips, chewing, swallowing, and strengthening the gag reflex. An example of such an exercise is to inhale through a straw to pick up small pieces of paper to increase lip closure. For children, a washcloth over the fingers creates a "bunny" and can facilitate lip closure by instructing the child not to let the "bunny" in the mouth.

When the patient is ready to attempt oral feeding, several factors must be considered in the diet selection, such as other methods by which the patient may be receiving nutrition or hydration, the evaluation results, and the patient's food preferences. Specific foods are selected to provide maximum sensory feedback to enhance the volitional and reflexive components. Common practice in the general hospital is a dietary progression from clear liquids to thick liquids, purées, and soft solids. Unfor-

tunately, patients with swallowing dysfunction have difficulty with this sequence. Liquids provide poor sensory stimulation and present the greatest difficulty (Surman, 1989). Puréed or minced foods provide good sensory stimulation within the mouth and are easier to swallow, but they may not have an aroma and may taste bitter. Sweet foods decrease saliva, while the casein in milk products thickens mucus secretions, thereby decreasing sensation and making control of secretions more difficult. Sour food facilitates swallowing. Bland and unattractive foods should be avoided. Sticky foods, dry substances, and boluses that fall apart should be avoided (Surman, 1989). Food items that have proved to be effective are mildly sweet and salty foods, gelatin, eggs, and soft vegetables (peas, carrots, beans) (Surman, 1989).

While motor deficits are being treated, the therapist may be teaching the patient new compensatory techniques to enhance the swallowing procedure and decrease aspiration. These techniques may be the epiglottic swallow, turning the head to one side, and methods for moving the bolus of food. Adaptive equipment may also be beneficial (utensils, cups, and so on).

Positioning during the swallowing program is important to decrease the chances of aspiration. The patient should sit in a chair at 90 degrees with the neck slightly flexed. If the therapist is spoon feeding the patient, the utensil should be placed at or below chin level to encourage neck flexion. The food should be placed in the mouth at the point where the patient will receive the most sensory feedback from the taste, pressure, and temperature of the food. Placement of the food on the back of the tongue may be helpful with patients who have decreased tongue mobility. Pauses between swallows allow the patient to rest, because swallow efficiency decreases with fatigue. The therapist should inspect the mouth periodically to make sure all food has been swallowed. Small portions of food given five or six times per day are preferable to larger portions three times a day.

After eating, the patient should continue to sit up for a period of time (1 hour, if tolerated). The therapist should instruct the nursing staff and family in the swallowing program, including ways to advance the diet so that the program can be continued until independence is reached.

As the reader can probably ascertain, treatment of the dysphagic patient can be challenging and difficult. It is essential to have proper knowledge of the anatomy and physiology of the swallow, as well as advanced training in the performance and assessment of radiographic studies.

Summary

Solutions to the variety of problems that an occupational therapist may encounter in a general hospital are limited only by the therapist's creativity, knowledge, and adaptability. Despite a move toward shorter hospitalizations and alternative health care settings, hospitals have a wide range of resources and can effectively provide occupational therapy intervention to a wide range of acutely ill patients. According to the results of a 1985 American Occupational Therapy Association survey, since the initiation of Medicare's prospective payment system, early referrals to occupational therapy and referrals from ICU have increased significantly so that evaluation and treatment can begin early (Gray, 1985). There has also been a greater intensity of services, that is, more occupational therapy treatment over a shorter period. The role of the occupational therapist in an acute care setting is primarily one of assessment, provision of efficient prioritized treatment, and participation in discharge planning, including provision of a home program, recommendations for outpatient therapy, home health referral, or referral to other facilities offering traditional rehabilitation services. To have a good occupational therapy department in an acute care setting, therapists must not only keep up on current medical treatment but must be able to apply their skills in an efficient and cost-effective manner.

Appreciation is extended to Judy Feinberg, PhD, OTR, for allowing me to revise her previous work, and to the staff at Indiana University Medical Center for sharing their expertise in acute care occupational therapy: Becky Barton, MS, OTR, Lucinda Dale, MS, OTR, Karen Dezelan, OTR, Nancy Connett, COTA, and Maureen Hays, OTR.

References

Affleck, A. T., Bianchi, E., Cleckly, M., et al. (1984). Stress management as a component of occupational therapy in acute care settings. *Occupational Therapy Health Care, 1*(3), 22.

Affleck, A. T., Lieberman, S., Polon, J., & Rohrkemper, D. (1986). Providing occupational therapy in an intensive care unit. *American Journal of Occupational Therapy, 40,* 323.

Alexander, J. W. (1990). The cutting edge: A look to the future in transplantation. *Transplantation, 49*(2), 237.

American Hospital Association. (1991). Chigago: Personal communication.

Bierenger, A. (1981). Cancer and impaired independence. In B. C. Abreu (Ed.), *Physical disabilities manual.* New York: Raven Press.

Chyatte, S. (Ed.). (1979). *Rehabilitation in chronic renal failure.* Baltimore: Williams & Wilkins.

Civetta, J. M., Taylor, R. W., & Kirby, R. R. (1989). *Introduction to critical care.* Philadelphia: J. B. Lippincott.

Dale, L. (1991). *Vestibular input to the non-alert patient.* Personal communication.

Dietz, J. H., Jr. (1981). *Rehabilitation oncology.* New York: John Wiley & Sons

Gray, M. S. (1985). Occupational therapy use rises under PPS. *Hospitals, 59*(11), 60.

Groher, M. E. (Ed.). (1984). Dysphagia: Diagnosis and management. Boston: Butterworth & Co.

Killeen, K. (1986). I'm glad you asked. *Occupational Therapy News, 40*(10), 15.

Monaco, A. P. (1990). Transplantation: The state of the art. *Transplantation Proceedings, 22*(3), 896.

Norris, M. K., & House, M. A. (1991). *Organ and tissue transplantation nursing care from procurement through rehabilitation.* Philadelphia: F. A. Davis.

Pizzi, M. A. (1986). Occupational therapy in hospice care. *American Journal of Occupational Therapy, 38,* 252.

Rausch, G., & Melvin, J. L. (1986). A new era in acute care. *American Journal of Occupational Therapy, 40,* 319.

Robbins, S. L., & Angell, M. (1971). *Basic pathology.* Philadelphia: W. B. Saunders.

Spiegel, J. S., Hirshfield, M. S., & Spiegel, T. M. (1985). Evaluating self-care activities: Comparison of a self-reported questionnaire with an occupational therapist interview. *British Journal of Rheumatology, 24,* 357.

Surman, O. S. (1989). Psychiatric aspects of organ transplantation. *American Journal of Psychiatry, 146,* 8, 972.

Zimmerman, J. E, & Oder, L. A. (1981). Swallowing dysfunction in acutely ill patients. *Physical Therapy, 61,* 1755.

Bibliography

Assessment

Cautela, J. R. (1981). *Organic dysfunction survey schedules.* Champaign, IL: Research Press.

Kottke, F. J., Stillwell, G. K., & Lehmann, J. F. (1982). *Krusen's Handbook of physical medicine and rehabilitation* (3rd ed.) Philadelphia: W. B. Saunders.

Psychosocial skills

Stearns, A. K. (1984). *Living through personal crisis.* Chicago: Thomas More Press.

Cancer

Day, S. B. (Ed.). (1986). *Cancer, stress, and death.* New York: Plenum Press.

Dudgeon, B. J., DeLias, J. A., & Miller, R. M. (1980). Head and neck cancer: A rehabilitation approach. *American Journal of Occupational Therapy, 34,* 243.

Grabois, M. (1985). Physical rehabilitation following mastectomy. *Texas Medicine, 34,* 100.

May, H. J. (1980). Psychosexual sequelas to mastectomy: Implications for therapeutic and rehabilitative intervention. *Journal of Rehabilitation, 46,* 29.

Mehls, J. D. (1983). Occupational therapy as a component of cancer rehabilitation. *Progress in Clinical and Biological Research, 121,* 231.

Heart disease

Atwood, J. A., & Nielson, D. H. (1985). Scope of cardiac rehabilitation. *Physical Therapy, 65,* 1812.

Harrington, K. A., Smith, K. H., Schumacher, M., et al. (1981). Cardiac rehabilitation: Evaluation and intervention less than 6 weeks after myocardial infarction. *Archives of Physical Medicine and Rehabilitation, 62,* 151.

Wenger, N. K., & Hellerstein, H. K. (1984). *Rehabilitation of the coronary patient* (2nd ed.). New York: John Wiley & Sons.

Diabetes mellitus

Cyrus, J. (1986). Role of exercise in management of diabetes. *Journal of the Kentucky Medical Association, 84*(4).

Dysphagia

Gallender, D. (1979). *Eating handicaps: Illustrated techniques for feeding disorders.* Springfield, IL: Charles C Thomas.

Logemann, J. (1983). *Evaluation and treatment of swallowing disorders.* San Diego: College-Hill Press.

Mody, M., & Nagai, J. (1990). A multidisciplinary approach to the development of competency standards and appropriate allocation for patients with dysphagia. *American Journal of Occupational Therapy, 44*(4), 369.

General medicine

Steinber, F. U. (1980). *The immobilized patient: Functional pathology and management.* New York: Plenum Press.

General practice

Baum, C. M. (1980). Occupation therapists put care in the health system. *American Journal of Occupational Therapy, 34,* 505.

Bell, E. (1985). The changing faces of practice. *American Journal of Occupational Therapy, 39,* 637.

Florian, V., & Sacks, D. (1985). Reasons for patient referral to occupational therapy units by health care professionals. *Journal of Allied Health, 14,* 317.

Schwartz, K. B. (1984). Balancing objectives of efficient and effective occupational therapy practice. *American Journal of Occupational Therapy, 38,* 198.

Renal disease

Carney, R. M., McKevitt, P. M., Goldberg, A. P., et al. (1983). Psychological effects of exercise training in hemodialysis patients. *Nephron, 33,* 179.

Kutner, N. G., & Cardenas, D. D. (1981). Rehabilitation status of chronic renal disease patients undergoing dialysis: Variations by age category. *Archives of Physical Medicine and Rehabilitation, 62,* 626.

Victor-Gittleman, B. (1981). The role of the occupational therapist in the rehabilitation of end-stage renal disease patients. *Dialysis and Transplantation, 10,* 738.

Transplantation

Ball, P. (1986). Pancreatic transplantation. AORN Journal, *43,* 632.

Kuchler, T., Kober B., et al. (1991). Quality of life after liver transplantation: Can a psychosocial support program contribute? *Transplantation Proceedings, 21*(1), 1541.

Pereyra, L. H. (Ed.). (1987). *Complications of organ transplantation.* New York: Dekker.

CHAPTER 24

Rehabilitation centers

SHARON INTAGLIATA

LEARNING OBJECTIVES

Upon completion of this chapter the reader will be able to:

1. *Develop an appreciation for the dynamic and multi-faceted nature of the rehabilitation process.*
2. *Be able to describe the benefits of a team approach to service delivery and recognize the unique role that occupational therapists play within this context, while acknowledging opportunities for collaboration with other professionals.*
3. *Be able to describe the typical diagnoses and characteristics of patients treated within a rehabilitation setting.*
4. *Develop an understanding of the factors that have influenced recent changes in admission and discharge patterns and the development of alternative care options.*

History, perspective, and functions

Definitions

Impairment—any loss or abnormality of psychological, physiologic, or anatomic structure or function (World Health Organization, 1980).

Disability—any restriction or lack resulting from an impairment of ability to perform an activity in the manner or within the range considered normal for humans.

Handicap—a disadvantage for a given person, resulting from an impairment or disability, which limits or prevents the fulfillment of a role that is normal (depending on age, sex, social and cultural factors) for that person.

Rehabilitation is a relatively new concept in the history of medicine. In fact, the rehabilitation field did not come of age until during and after World War II (1939 to 1945). Disabled soldiers returning home from the two World Wars and persons disabled as a result of the polio epidemic of the 1940s presented new medical challenges that demanded novel approaches and resulted in the development of rehabilitation methods and technologies. By the 1950s allied health disciplines had developed their own professional identities and unique clinical intervention strategies. During this decade rehabilitation centers began to be built.

Howard A. Rusk of New York University was one of the early visionaries instrumental in the development of rehabilitation centers. He recognized that persons with severe physical disabilities have problems in many areas cutting across the biomedical, psychological, vocational, and social domains. He believed that these problems could best be addressed by placing experts who were knowledgeable in all of these different areas into one place. During this time the United States was experiencing a period of prosperity and optimism that followed World War II. An attitude of good will to disadvantaged people was in the air. Rusk's approach was extremely successful and served as a model for service delivery in the United States as well as other countries throughout the world (Diller, 1990). Other early leaders in the field of rehabilitation are Frank H. Krusen of the Mayo Clinic and Miland E. Knapp of the University of Minnesota (Egli et al., 1991).

The mission of a comprehensive rehabilitation center is to offer an intensive interdisciplinary rehabilitation environment that will enable persons to return to their highest level of independent functioning in the least amount of time possible. In addition to patient care, most rehabilitation centers are committed to education, research, and advocacy for persons with disabilities. At teaching institutions the development of rehabilitation professionals through student training programs as well as staff development and continuing education efforts are always a priority. Centers have also accepted the responsibility of advancing the field of rehabilitation through research efforts aimed at scientific validation of rehabilitation techniques and the discovery of new methodologies. Finally, rehabilitation centers have taken a leadership role in advocating for equal opportunity and full participation of persons with disabilities in community living through public relations activities as well as involvement in the legislative arena.

Conceptualizing disability

The significance of disability is felt at an individual, organizational, and societal level. During the last 20 years, many different authors have expressed a need for a consistent terminology and an accepted classification system to accurately describe the progressive consequences of disease or injury. Topliss (1978) pointed out that it was inappropriate to classify people with disabilities by diagnostic categories according to the traditional medical model because the degree of disability rather than the disease affects the person's capacity for normal living, whether in the sphere of personal care, employment, family relationships, social activities, or leisure. Although acknowledging the dangers of the labeling process, Hobbs and associates found that within the field of special education, categorization was necessary to get help for a child, to write legislation, to appropriate funds, to design service programs, to evaluate outcomes, to conduct research, and even to communicate about the problems of the exceptional child (Hobbs, 1975). These reasons are valid in the field of rehabilitation as well.

Many different groups have attempted to define the dimensions of disability to meet their own unique information needs. In the United States, the Commission of Chronic Illness and agencies concerned with providing public compensation and insurance benefits have been instrumental in driving early attempts to conceptualize and classify disability. The most frequently cited conceptual model and classification system was developed by the World Health Organization (WHO) International Classification of Impairments, Disabilities and Handicaps (ICIDH). The authors of this internationally recognized system use the terms impairment, disability, and handicap (defined at beginning of chapter) to describe the disablement process. Although a stepwise progression from one stage to another may be assumed, the authors of this model stress that a variety of personal, social and environmental factors can influence the progression of a chronic condition along the continuum. These terms are helpful in conceptualizing the context of the health experiences that lie behind them.

Nagi (1991) presented the "functional limitations" framework to describe the disablement process that has also received widespread attention (Duckworth, 1984). Finally, the Committee on a National Agenda for Prevention of Disabilities (CNAPD) has recently developed a new model of disability that builds on the previous work of the WHO and Nagi (Pope & Tarlov, 1991). This model is worthy of mention here because it uses current terminology (avoiding the use of the term "handicap," which has negative connotations) and incorporates findings from contemporary research. This model emphasizes the impact that biologic, environmental, and behavioral risk factors as well as components of quality of life such as intellectual capacity and socioeconomic resources have on the ultimate functional status of the individual. The model presented by this committee (CNAPD) is especially helpful in understanding that disability is the result of a complex interactive process, which involves numerous internal as well as external variables. In this model, *disability* is defined as the gap between a person's capabilities and the demands of their environment (Pope & Tarlov, 1991).

Goals and philosophy

The American National Council on Rehabilitation has defined the task of rehabilitation as that of restoring persons to "the fullest physical, mental, social, vocational and economic usefulness of which they are capable" (Duckworth, 1984). Rehabilitation professionals are committed to enhancing the quality of life for persons with severe disabilities by assisting them in achieving the highest degree of independence possible in view of their limitations. Comprehensive rehabilitation of persons with severe physical disabilities presents a complex and difficult challenge because virtually all aspects of a patient's life are affected.

Marceline Jacques (1970) first described the "holistic" approach used in rehabilitation due to the multifaceted needs encountered. She emphasized that professionals must be prepared to work with the whole person because it is impossible to divide a person into their physical, mental, psychological, social, and economic parts. She also encouraged clinicians to use a holistic perspective in understanding that the process of human development is dynamic, with each of its continuing stages affecting the next. Therefore, she emphasized the need for professionals to study a person's history and identify constructive patterns that they have used in the past to help them meet their current and future challenges. Finally, Jacques emphasized the importance of a holistic approach in recognizing that human problems tend to cluster together. Hence, disability does not usually appear as a single problem. The highest incidence of disability occurs among the financially disadvantaged, who are, as a group, also undereducated and underemployed. Poverty, unhealthy environments, family deterioration, substance abuse, and crime all have been linked with the occurrence of disability. Therefore, an understanding of these interacting factors is needed to determine the most effective interventions (Wright, 1980).

Team approach and organization

Because of the broad spectrum of problems encountered, treatment of patients with long-term disabilities is generally organized around the **team approach**. As you can see from the display on page 786, a variety of organized professions have arisen to meet the need for specialized knowledge regarding

REHABILITATION PROFESSIONALS

Audiologist—specializes in diagnosis and treatment of hearing impairments; is able to identify specific types of hearing loss and recommend hearing aids and other assistive devices to enhance residual hearing loss

Chaplain—focuses on the religious and spiritual needs of patients; provides non-denominational individual and family counseling, as well as special weekly and holiday services

Occupational therapist—identifies performance strengths and deficits taking into consideration patient interests and life roles, and provides therapeutic activities to enhance performance in self-care, work, and leisure tasks

Orthotist—designs and fabricates braces to help stabilize a weakened body part, assist or limit certain motions of a joint, or help prevent future deformities of the body

Physiatrist—specializes in the practice of physical medicine and rehabilitation, which is one of medicine's most comprehensive and multifaceted modes of treatment (focus is on function of patient rather than nature of the disease)

Physical therapist—evaluates the patient's musculoskeletal and cardiopulmonary status. Treatment may include exercise, activity, and/or modalities for the purpose of decreasing pain and/or increasing soft tissue flexibility, strength, and endurance.

Prosthetist—designs and fabricates artificial limbs with special attention to enhancing proper fit, function, and appearance.

Psychologist—provides neuropsychological and behavioral assessments; provides individual, marital, and group psychotherapy and acts as consultant to the team and family members on behavioral or adjustment issues

Recreational therapist—provides services that include leisure education and skill building; uses social and recreational activities to aid in adjustment to disability and participation in community activities

Rehabilitation engineer—provides technical expertise in recommendation of commercial products and the modification of existing devices or the design and fabrication of custom equipment or adjusted environments

Rehabilitation nurse—administers medication and instructs patients and family members in care management, which may include hydration and elimination, skin management, safety, and health maintenance regimens

Respiratory therapist—provides oxygen assessment programs, breathing exercises, and bronchial hygiene treatments as well as patient and family education

Social worker—assists patient and families to achieve a maximal level of social and emotional functioning; provides patient and family counseling, discharge planning, and education on entitlements and other available resources; assists in identifying transportations and attendant care resources

Vocational counselors—provides diagnostic evaluation of transferable skills, achievement levels, aptitudes, and interests to determine employability and job placement potential; works with employers to facilitate successful work placements

---

discrete aspects of human behavior. Input from consumers has also emphasized the importance of including the patient and family members as well as representatives of the insurance industry in the team process, whenever possible. The advantage of the team approach is that recommendations and treatment interventions can be developed based on a variety of different perspectives. The patient and family members provide important input, and their acceptance of team recommendations or participation in the treatment process ultimately determines the success of the program. Therefore, their involvement in the process is crucial at all stages.

The professionals involved in the team for a particular patient varies based on the patient's needs. In a medical setting, all disciplines operate under a physician's order. The team may minimally consist of a doctor, nurse, and therapist or maximally involve all disciplines represented in the display.

For most patients occupational therapy, physical therapy,

social work, and speech therapy are standard. Other disciplines may be called in as needed at various points in the patient's stay.

Although each discipline has a unique focus of treatment, there are also many areas of overlap; for example, occupational therapists may work closely with psychologists and speech pathologists in developing programs for cognitive retraining that will be applied across disciplines. Occupational therapists may work with orthotists in developing definitive positioning equipment for upper extremities, with rehabilitation engineers and physical therapists in seating and positioning programs that focus on designing customized wheelchairs, and with speech pathologists in developing access methods that enable the patient to use augmentative communication equipment.

Coordination of the multitude of available professional resources at the rehabilitation center demands skillful leadership. Three different leadership patterns have been successfully used. In the first pattern, a physiatrist or other knowledgeable physician is the head of the team. This leadership pattern has been used most frequently in the past and is in keeping with the traditional lines of authority in the medical model. A second type of team leadership involves putting another rehabilitation professional in a coordinator or manager position, which requires that professional to provide the team leadership. The "case management" approach is a third and more recent approach to team leadership. In this model, team members accept responsibility for the coordination responsibilities for specifically assigned patients. Advantages and disadvantages accompany each of the leadership models. Some facilities have developed approaches that combine the various models. Success of any model depends on having clear lines of authority as well as a skillful person in the leadership position.

Teams may also be organized around a multidisciplinary, an interdisciplinary, or a transdisciplinary philosophy. In the multidisciplinary approach, members work side by side and each discipline has a clearly defined role with specific areas of responsibility. Assessment, planning, and treatment take place independently. In an interdisciplinary team, members work together, often sharing roles. Areas of responsibility are determined around individual cases. Members of different disciplines often evaluate, plan, and treat together. In a transdisciplinary team, members assimilate knowledge from other professions, traditional role borders are crossed, and skills used by other fields are incorporated into one's own practice. A single professional is generally responsible for the coordination and delivery of care but must rely heavily on consultation and support from other disciplines to ensure appropriate interventions (Holman et al., 1978). The transdisciplinary model is the most nontraditional model and often uses a case management approach to providing team leadership.

Historically, teams have been expected to handle patients with a variety of different diagnoses and levels of functional abilities. This generalized approach to rehabilitation has kept physician and therapist case loads diverse and tended to promote the development of well-rounded and flexible rehabilitation professionals. More recently, teams have become more focused on the treatment of one particular diagnosis (spinal cord injury, head injury, cerebrovascular accident) or functional level within a diagnosis (high-level head injury). This programmatic approach is popular owing to the specialized knowledge and technology that are currently available and to increased competition being experienced in the field. This approach is often attractive to experienced staff who are ready to develop advanced competencies in a focused area of treatment. As consumers have become more selective in choosing treatment programs, centers have found that the specialized programmatic approach has been successful in attracting patients to their facilities. The availability of a highly specialized staff is also helpful in promoting the center's education and research efforts.

Treatment programs

Rehabilitation treatment can be applied at any of the stages along the continuum of disablement, generally the earlier the better. Treatment programs begin with an assessment of functional abilities and limitations. Intervention strategies are highly individualized according to the patient's unique needs and life roles. Efforts may be directed toward restoring function through thera-

peutic exercise and activity or toward capitalizing on the person's residual capacities by using assistive technology (any item, piece of equipment, or product—whether acquired commercially, modified, or customized—that is used to increase, maintain, or improve functional capabilities of persons with disabilities) or adapted environments (widening entrances, providing a ramp, and so on). Emphasis is always placed on the prevention of further limitations and the development of secondary conditions that could decrease health and functional status (the development of pressure sores for a spinal-cord–injured person or the development of joint contractures in a patient with brain injury).

Registered occupational therapists (OTRs) and certified occupational therapy assistants (COTAs) are primarily interested in the development of daily living skills. *Activities of daily living* (ADL) refers to basic self-care activities such as toileting, grooming, eating, dressing, functional mobility, and communication. *Instrumental activities of daily living* (IADL) refers to preparing meals, shopping, using the phone, doing laundry, and other activities involved in living independently. These activities are the primary treatment media for OTRs and COTAs.

Owing to the personal nature of ADL, most treatment in this area is provided individually. Therapists also often function as consultants to nursing staff in the area of ADL. Treatment for IADL is often provided in group settings. Meal preparation and community reentry groups provide an arena for patients to practice building skills while socially interacting with other patients with similar problems. The camaraderie and support that can develop among patients being treated at the center can have tremendous therapeutic value. Therefore, skillful use of group process is an important treatment strategy for the therapist.

Exempt status

In a 1983 survey, it was found that the costs of about 50% of all patients admitted for rehabilitation were paid for by Medicare (National Association of Rehabilitation Facilities, 1985). In a more recent study, 62% of a sample population of rehabilitation patients were covered by Medicare (McGinnis et al., 1988). As the population continues to age, this trend is increasing. Medical rehabilitation facilities are currently exempt from the prospective payment system mandated for acute care inpatient hospital services under the 1983 Amendments to the Social Security Act for three reasons: (1) their patients' diagnoses did not conform to the diagnosis-related groupings (DRGs) established for acute care centers; (2) the mix of services provided differed significantly from those of acute care facilities; and (3) the data used to develop DRGs contained little, if any, input from the field of medical rehabilitation (Ernst & Whinney, 1983).

Gornick and Hall (1988) have provided the following summary of the conditions for Medicare reimbursement of intensive rehabilitation care. Instead of being reimbursed using the DRG system, rehabilitation and other specialty hospitals are reimbursed on a cost-based system subject to limits imposed by the Tax Equity and Fiscal Responsibility Act (TEFRA) of 1982. The Health Care Financing Administration (HCFA) requires all rehabilitation facilities to apply annually for the exemption from DRGs. To be eligible for Medicare payment, services must be reasonable and necessary with respect to efficacy, duration, frequency, and amount. Medicare also requires that it must be reasonable and necessary to furnish the care on an inpatient hospital basis rather than on an outpatient basis or in a less care-intensive facility such as a skilled nursing home.

To qualify for an exemption from the Prospective Payment System (PPS) system, these authors also state that a hospital specializing in rehabilitation must demonstrate that it is primarily engaged in providing intensive rehabilitation services, with 75% of their patients falling into 10 specific diagnoses: stroke, spinal cord injury, congenital deformities, amputations, multiple trauma, hip fracture, brain injury, polyarthritis, neurologic disorders, and burns. In addition, the patient must require the following:

Twenty-four-hour availability of a physician with special training or experience in rehabilitation and frequent (every 2 to 3 days) direct, and medically necessary physician involvement.

Twenty-four-hour availability of a registered nurse with special training or experience in rehabilitation.

At least 3 hours per day of physical and/or occupational therapy in addition to other required therapies or services (speech therapy, social services, psychological services, prosthetic–orthotic services).

Care from a multidisciplinary team, minimally including a physician, rehabilitation nurse, and therapist.

A coordinated program of care, including team conferences held at least once every 2 weeks to determine appropriateness of continuing care.

Admission and discharge patterns

Most rehabilitation patients are initially admitted to an acute care hospital, where their medical conditions are diagnosed and stabilized. In a study by the American Hospital Association (AHA) reported by Solnik (1987), it was found that of the patients who entered rehabilitation units, 81% came from hospitals, 49% from within the same hospital, and 32% from other hospitals. According to Solnik (1987), about 72% of rehabilitation patients were discharged from inpatient rehabilitation facilities to their homes, 12% to acute care hospitals, 11% to nursing homes, and 4% to other facilities (eg, residential care facilities); 1% were discharged due to death or unknown reason.

Acute care hospitals, which, as discussed earlier, must now comply with DRGs, have powerful financial incentives to transfer patients earlier and more frequently to rehabilitation facilities. Under the PPS, those hospitals are reimbursed a set amount per length of stay (LOS) per diagnosis. If the LOS is shortened for acute care hospitals, costs are generally less per case discharged. Therefore, patients are entering rehabilitation centers much sooner and often more medically compromised than ever before. It is not uncommon for rehabilitation care to be interrupted by a readmission to an acute care hospital because of either a reoccurrence of the original problem or a secondary problem or complication.

Also, there is evidence that LOS in rehabilitation centers is decreasing. An American Hospital Association survey found that average LOS for hospital-based rehabilitation was 34 days in 1980 (Muller et al., 1983). A follow-up survey found that LOS had decreased to 25.6 days in 1984 and to 24.8 days in 1985 (McCormick, 1987). This phenomenon is primarily due to pressure from third-party payors. Payors are motivated to get the most services for their beneficiaries for the least cost. Therefore, appropriate placement of patients has become a very significant concern.

Growing demand

Rehabilitation has continued to prosper in the restructuring of health care services that has taken place during recent years. Surveys conducted by the American Hospital Association have shown that the number of rehabilitation hospitals and units have more than doubled from 395 in 1980 to 738 in 1987. In contrast to the number of acute care beds, which decreased during this period, the number of rehabilitation beds increased from 14,674 in 1980 to 24,267 in 1987. Total inpatient revenue from rehabilitation hospitals, units, and programs was more than $1 billion in 1986 (Keith, 1991). Three major causes have precipitated the greater demand for rehabilitation services: (1) the greater number of persons with disabilities (created by increased life expectancies and improved medical technology); (2) medical rehabilitation facilities' current exemptions from Medicare's PPS; and (3) the growing awareness of the efficacy of medical rehabilitation (McGinnis et al., 1988).

Alternative care options

Health care providers have been responsive to the challenges of heightened competition within the rehabilitation industry and the concern for cost containment by developing a wide variety of alternative care options. These options include subacute rehabilitation units for patients who are leaving an acute hospital and are too medically fragile or unable to benefit from an intensive rehabilitation program for a variety of other reasons. Skilled nursing facilities (SNF) are expanding their therapy staffs to effectively manage their residents' needs for geriatric rehabilitation. In addition to these options, home health services and outpatient programs (ambulatory care) designed to meet the needs of all age groups and diagnoses are currently available. All these options are significantly less costly than an inpatient hospitalization.

A more recent concept is the day hospital or community reentry program, which provides specialized treatment to a specific population, that is, patients with traumatic brain injuries or general rehabilitation services compared with patients with a variety of different diagnoses and degrees of functional limitations. Work hardening clinics have recently been recognized by the Commission on Accreditation of Rehabilitation Facilities (CARF), and on-site occupational health clinics are being supported by industry. Finally, entrepreneurial professionals have ventured away from hospital settings and developed their own private practice clinics.

These are exciting times for rehabilitation professionals. With all these options currently available and with many new developments on the horizon, the demand for occupational therapy services seems almost limitless. Although opportunities abound, this dramatically expanded continuum of care creates new challenges as well. It is becoming more and more common for patients to receive rehabilitation services in a variety of different settings from a variety of different professionals. Therefore, skills in effective discharge planning and interagency coordination of care are becoming essential for all occupational therapists.

Summary

The rehabilitation center provides a rich environment for OTRs and COTAs to learn and apply the full range of skills relevant to occupational therapy practice. These settings also offer the opportunity to be involved in continuing education and research projects. Patients in these settings generally present significant challenges due to the severe nature of their limitations. Occupational therapists are able to work as an integral part of an interdisciplinary team approach in the delivery of comprehensive patient care.

Opportunities in rehabilitation are unlimited because the field is experiencing significant growth due to increased demand for service caused by the aging of the population and by technologic advancement in life-saving techniques. Therapists can still practice in general rehabilitation programs, which provide services to patients with a variety of different diagnoses and functional limitations. However, the trend is toward programs that provide a specialized approach designed to meet the needs of a particular population. Therapists play a very important role in their patients' lives in the rehabilitation setting. Being able to make a direct impact on the recovery process and to see the results of treatment firsthand are truly exciting and rewarding experiences.

Reference

Brown, S. C. (1991). Conceptualizing and defining disability. In S. Thompson-Hoffman & I. F. Storck (Eds.), *Disability in the United States: A portrait from national data* (pp. 1–14). New York: Springer.

Catalogue of Services. (1991). *The Rehabilitation Institute of Chicago.* Chicago.

Diller, L. (1990). Fostering the interdisciplinary team, fostering research in a society of transition. *Archives of Physical Medicine and Rehabilitation, 71,* 275–278.

Duckworth, D. (1984). The need for a standard terminology and classification of disablement. In C. V. Granger & G. E. Gresham (Eds.), *Functional assessment in rehabilitation medicine* (pp. 1–13). Baltimore: Williams & Wilkins.

Egli, H. J., Strakal, G., & Long, M. (1991). Rehab team functioning. *Rehab Management,* June/July, 47–107.

Ernst & Whinney. (1983). *Medicare prospective payment system: Implementing regulations—implications for hospitals.* E & W Pub. No. J58475.

Fuhrer, M. J. (1987). Overview of outcome analysis in rehabilitation. In M. J. Fuhrer (Ed.), *Rehabilitation outcomes: Analysis and measurements* (pp. 1–3). Baltimore: Paul H. Brooks.

Gornick, M., & Hall, M. J. (1988, December 27). Trends in medicare use of post-hospital care. *Health Care Financing Review,* 38.

Hobbs (Ed.). (1975). *The future of children: Categories, labels and their consequences.* London: Jossey-Bass.

Holman, V. A., McCarlin, R. E., & Schiefelbusch, R. L. (Eds.). (1987). *Early intervention: A team approach.* Baltimore: University Park Press.

Jacques, M. E., (1970). *Rehabilitation counseling: Scope and services.* Boston: Houghton Mifflin.

Keith, R. A. (1991). The comprehensive treatment team in rehabilitation. *Archives of Physical Medicine and Rehabilitation, 72,* 269–274.

McCormick, B. (1987, August 17). AHA survey shows greater competition among rehab providers. *American Hospital Association News,* 6.

McGinnis, G. E., Osberg, J. S., Seward, M. L., Campion, E. W., Branch, L. G., & DeJong, G. (1988). Total charges for inpatient medical rehabilitation. *Health Care Financing Review, 9,* 31–39.

Muller, R., Nuzum, F. J., & Mathews, D. (1983). Inpatient medical rehabilitation: Results of the 1981 survey of hospitals and units. *Archives of physical Medicine and Rehabilitation, 64,* 354–8.

Nagi, S. Z. (1991). Disability concepts revisited: Implications for prevention. In A. M. Pope & A. R. Tarlov (Eds.), *Disability in America: Toward a national agenda for prevention* (pp. 309–327). Washington, DC: National Academy Press.

National Association of Rehabilitation Facilities. (1985). *NARF Position paper on prospective payment system for inpatient medical rehabilitation services and a study regarding prospective payment system for inpatient medical rehabilitation services: Final report.* Washington, DC: Author.

Pope, A. M., & Tarlov, A. R. (Eds.). (1991). *Disability in America: Toward a national agenda for prevention.* Washington, DC: National Academy Press.

Solnik, S. (1987). Rehabilitation programs face increasing competition. *Trustee, 40,* 12–14.

Topliss, E. (1978). The disabled. In P. Breasley & E. Topliss (Eds.), *The social context of health care.* London: Martin Robertson and Basil Blackwell.

World Health Organization. (1980). *International classification of impairment, disabilities and handicaps.* Geneva: World Health Organization.

Wright, G. N. (1980). Human philosophy. In G. W. Wright (Ed.), *Total rehabilitation* (pp. 10–18). Boston: Little, Brown & Co.

CHAPTER 25

Occupational therapy in the school system

NANCY ALLEN KAUFFMAN

KEY TERMS

Cascade System
Criterion-Referenced Tests
Due Process
Extended School Year
    Programs (Related to
    Regression and
    Recoupment)
Individualized Educational
    Program (IEP)

Individual Family Service
    Program (IFSP)
Individual Transition
    Plan (ITP)
Interdisciplinary
    (Multidisciplinary) Team
Learning Stations
Normalization
Related Service

LEARNING OBJECTIVES

Upon completion of this chapter the reader will be able to:

1. *Identify legislative changes leading to current due process provisions for the handicapped.*
2. *Identify steps that lead to the completion of an individualized educational plan (IEP) and school/class placement decisions for students with special needs.*
3. *Review the considerations of the Americans with Disabilites ACT (ADA) that are most likely to have an impact on the school setting.*
4. *Identify a variety of models of service delivery for occupational therapy in schools and the rationale for choosing integrative or segregated educational and therapeutic programming for the student with a handicap.*
5. *Describe the information about a student's learning style that is likely to be indentified by the occupational therapy assessment procedures, including clinical observation.*
6. *Review developmental considerations and curriculum material for the school setting to be included by the occupational therapist in programming for the school child.*

The role of student dominates a large percentage of the child's time in the developmental years. The occupational therapist's task in the school setting is to facilitate competencies that will help the child benefit from the total educational experience.

Private schools for the handicapped were the first educational programs to hire occupational therapists. By the early 1970s, therapists were being hired by public schools as well, to treat children who previously had been excluded from public education such as the severely mentally retarded and physically handicapped. By the 1980s, the behaviorally and emotionally disturbed, the moderately retarded and learning disabled, and the severely sensory-impaired were also included in some school therapists' case loads.

In 1980, the American Occupational Therapy Association (AOTA) passed the first Standards of Practice for Occupational Therapy in Schools and in 1981 prepared the first version of the position paper, "The role of occupational therapy as an education related service." The World Federation of Occupational Therapists documented occupational therapists' growing involvement in educational settings abroad (Flynn, 1980).

The AOTA developed a comprehensive program in every state to train occupational therapists to work in schools (Gilfoyle, 1980). The AOTA also developed a self-study course for school therapists (Royeen 1991) and workshops to train therapists in the family-centered approach for working with the youngest handicapped children affected by federal education legislation (Hanft, 1989). Optional master's degree training for therapists interested in school employment became available in 1986, and by 1987 the Council on Practice developed a document to help define the roles and responsibilities of the COTA in the public school setting.

By 1992, a second self-study course was being developed to focus on classroom application, and AOTA was considering the formation of a Special Interest Section to meet the special needs of school system practitioners (eg, case load size, role differentiation, pay parity, supervision). With the passage of federal legislation mandating appropriate personnel in every school district receiving federal funds, parent advocate groups became effective in creating occupational therapy positions in many states. In the 1990 Member Data Survey, AOTA documented that 18.6% of registered occupational therapists (OTR) and 17% of certified occupational therapy assistants (COTA) were primarily employed in school systems (I. Silvergleit, 1991)

Legislation

In the early 1970s, a legislative trend at the state level initiated educational rights for the retarded and other handicapped persons. Section 504 of the Federal Rehabilitation Act of 1973 was intended to eliminate discrimination against handicapped citizens.

Public law 94–142

In 1975, the federal government responded further to state legislative changes by passing the Education of the Handicapped Act, P. L. 94–142, requiring free and "appropriate" public education for all handicapped children even to age 21, if necessary. Education in its broadest sense was intended. The changes had a dramatic effect on occupational therapy, which was specifically

included as a ***related service*** (along with transportation, speech, and physical therapy) necessary to help a child benefit from or gain access to the educational program.

One emphasis of the law was the "mainstreaming" of as many handicapped children as possible into regular education classes, a concept commensurate with the normalization concept developed during the preceding decades. ***Normalization*** recommends conditions for the handicapped as close as feasible to the mainstream of society. The ***Cascade System*** (Figure 25-1) is a theoretical prototype used in many states as a conceptual framework for providing educational services for the handicapped. Children are placed in "the least-restrictive alternative," (the class that best fits their needs and is as close as possible to the everyday classroom). Also called the *inverted pyramid*, this system assumes that the greatest number of handicapped children can be absorbed into mainstream education, thus allowing financial resources to be directed to the most handicapped. Ideally, support from counseling, educational, and therapeutic services is provided as needed to facilitate each transition, which is made as soon as educationally feasible. By 1986, in keeping with the least restrictive placement policy, 93% of handicapped children were served in settings that included their nonhandicapped peers.

P. L. 99–457 was passed in 1986 as an amendment to P. L. 94–142. The new law provided the same special education and related services to handicapped preschoolers as to school-aged children, with emphasis on training family involvement in furthering the child's development and on interagency service delivery combining health, education, and social services. Programs for handicapped 3- to 5-year- olds were required first. By

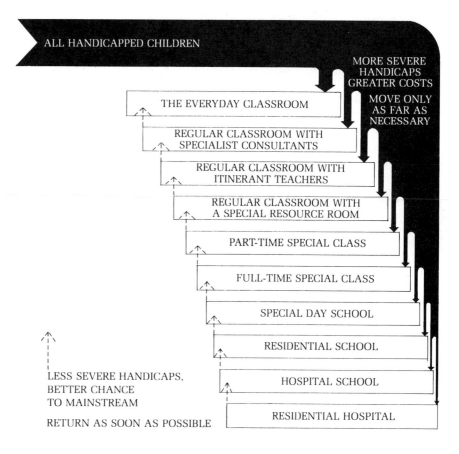

FIGURE 25-1. *The Cascade System.* (One Out of Ten: School Planning for the Handicapped, *p. 7, 1974. Educational Facilities Laboratories, New York.*)

the 1991 to 1992 school year, districts were required to provide "early intervention services" to handicapped children from birth to 3 years and to include occupational therapy as a primary early intervention service, independent of medical, health, and special education services (Dunn, 1989; Mancuso et al., 1990; Manes, 1985; AOTA, 1986).

Due process

Parents or guardians have the legal right to examine all school records. They also participate with professionals in making educational placement decisions and in developing written diagnostic–prescriptive plans. These are called an *individualized educational program* (IEP) for school-aged children (must be revised annually) and an *individualized family service plan* (IFSP) for younger children (must be reviewed every 6 months). Adolescents approaching graduation may have an *individual transition plan* (ITP), which focuses on preparation for vocational or educational programming immediately after high school.

Parents may bring trained advocates to help them understand and protect the rights of their child at meetings of interdisciplinary teams that create these decisions and documents. The parents are entitled to *due process* of the law in safeguarding their child's rights. They may bring legal counsel and other professionals before an impartial Fair Hearing Officer of the state to question school decisions. Therapists must be prepared to present testimony at due process hearings and to be cross-examined by lawyers representing the parent and the school district (see the display).

The law requires public participation in the development of educational policies, and occupational therapists have presented testimony at state public hearings and federal House and Senate subcommittee hearings. They also participate in state task forces for determining the role of occupational therapists within school systems and in interagency coordinating councils of parents and

providers of early intervention services for preschoolers (Rourk, 1985).

CASE STUDY

Dick and Mary Abrams finished breakfast Thursday morning and packed Philip, his bookbag, and his wheelchair in their green station wagon. At the school they waved their son off to Miss Amberly's classroom and headed for the principal's office. A few days before, Dick had taken advantage of his family's legal right to examine Philip's school records in preparation for today's interdisciplinary (or multidisciplinary) team conference for writing Philip's IEP.

Formal testing had been done recently and would be discussed at the meeting. The Abrams had noticed that the 2-year legal deadline for completing Philip's reevaluation was approaching, and the written permission form had arrived by mail a few weeks before the testing was scheduled. They received a copy of the interdisciplinary committee's evaluation findings last week.

A few minutes later the advocate for Philip (Ms. Wells) arrived, as requested. Ms. Wells, a parent of a handicapped child herself, is specifically trained to know the family's legal rights as well as to help them understand educational terms and their choices for classroom placement options. The school's coordinator of special education services was awaiting the start of the meeting as well, and Philip's occupational, physical, and speech therapists had sent to the meeting written long-term goals and short-term behavioral objectives that could be included. Dick and Mary also brought their own goals and objectives that they are hoping to have included in the IEP. Miss Amberly, Philip's teacher, came in to add her input to the IEP developed by the team members that day.

TIPS TO HELP REDUCE ANXIETY IN PREPARING TESTIMONY FOR A DUE PROCESS HEARING

Rely on the high standards of documentation you have maintained. (They will help prove your testimony.)

Organize your testimony carefully. Include treatment goals, objectives, and progress measured by pre- and post-testing.

Informally review your testimony with a co-professional who has testified or with a due process lawyer.

Read Bateman (1981) or other introductory due process information.

Have in hand records that might help you document answers to questions posed during cross-examination.

Project confidence and self-assurance but not presumptuousness.

Use clear communication without therapy jargon. State observations and behaviors, not hypotheses (about causes of deficits).

Answer questions as asked by the lawyers. Do not say more than asked.

Discussion

The Abrams knew they were entitled to due process of the law to safeguard their son's rights, but they never felt it necessary to take legal action because they disagreed with the school's decision or with the carrying out of an IEP such as the one the team established at the above-mentioned meeting. In addition, they knew they could have requested Philip's psychological, educational, or therapy testing to be done free of charge through the public school system even if Philip had been in a private special education placement.

The Abrams also had taken advantage of their right to participate in the interdisciplinary evaluation when Philip was younger, and Philip's earliest educational settings included them along with Philip. The whole family had learned to carry out stimulation of Philip's growth and development right in the middle of home and family life in ways consistent with the preschool's handling and management techniques.

In Philip's preschool programs for handicapped children, his federally mandated individualized family service plan (IFSP) was revised every 6 months instead of every 12 months as required for the IEP. His formal reevaluation was done every year instead of every 2 years. The Abrams had played an important role in establishing the educational goals for the IFSP and had felt it necessary at that time to insist that Philip's occupational therapist be present at the meeting.

Additional legislative and judicial changes

By 1981, many states had adopted statutes requiring **extended school year (ESY) programs.** These special education programs are required if regression in skills after an extended vacation is expected to be excessive, and recoupment or regaining of the lost abilities is expected to be unduly slow, especially in self-care skills. The ESY programs take place during the summer or on weekends for children who have certain severe handicapping conditions.

In June 1982, the Supreme Court ruled that although public education must "benefit" handicapped children, the school districts were not obliged to provide *all* services such children need (Greenhouse, 1982; Rehnquist, 1982). The federal government provided states with block grants (unrestricted federal funds) to enhance the development of programs for handicapped infants and toddlers, thus reducing society's lifetime educational costs for each child and minimizing the likelihood of later institutionalization. Later, Congress clarified that schools are allowed to access Medicaid to pay for certain health services that have been written into a child's IEP or IFSP (Chandler, 1990). Some schools began (with parents' permission) to bill private health insurance for related services. In the early 1990s, funding shifted to local school districts in many states and existing programs and services experienced major cutbacks and, in some cases, extinction.

Child abuse legislation that affects occupational therapy personnel has been in place in most states since at least the 1970s. In 1990, a primary focus of the Eighth International Congress on Child Abuse and Neglect in Germany was on such problems within institutions (Child Protection Congress, 1990). In many states, therapists and school personnel *must* report suspected child abuse (or cause it to be reported) to law enforcement officials. In addition, many states require therapists and teachers applying for positions in public or private educational and day care programs to undergo criminal and child abuse history checks through their state police.

The passage of the Americans with Disabilities Act (ADA) in 1990 alerted school therapists to renew their efforts to promote barrier-free environments in public places (including schools), transportation, and telecommunication relay services.

Team approach

Position of occupational therapy

It is important to understand the role of the occupational therapist within the particular local school system by first studying the state and local hierarchy of administration and service delivery. Does the therapist fit into the health chain of command or that of education? How are therapy services provided locally and statewide? How effective is the state Interagency Coordinating Council (with its representatives from agencies, parent groups, providers, and educators) in coordinating a comprehensive system of services for handicapped preschoolers? Are local parents strong advocates in favor of occupational therapy?

The occupational therapist functions often as a member of the local school system interdisciplinary committee, which makes decisions about academic needs and about placement of children in programs at various levels of the Cascade System.

These decisions are based on such things as developmental level, adaptive ability, academic performance, social maturity, and behavior, in addition to IQ. Learning style is also an important consideration. The primary cause of the child's learning problem determines placement; if a secondary problem such as emotional overlay has developed, appropriate education emphasizing treatment of the primary problem often eliminates it.

Gilfoyle (1980) and Kielhofner and Knight (1989) emphasize the importance of knowing how to participate effectively in the group decision-making process. Communication skills should enhance understanding by other members of the team, and jargon specific to occupational therapy should be avoided. Hypotheses regarding causes of deficits in observable behavior should be clearly stated as such. It is important for therapists to become familiar with tests frequently used by each team member; this allows better interpretation of results. A task analysis, after observation of pertinent tests being administered, is one effective method.

The role of members who usually serve on the interdisciplinary committee within school systems is described later in this chapter. Others who may serve as committee members or who may provide consultation are medical, neurologic, psychiatric, and optometric personnel. If necessary, a person familiar with the student's cultural or language background should be added to the team. Important team members who do not serve on interdisciplinary committees are teachers of art, music, and physical education. These teachers may have been specially trained to work with handicapped children. The child, classroom aide, and volunteer also play important roles in the team effort.

The COTA carries out treatment programs under the supervision of the OTR. Although the school principal may be responsible for *administrative* supervision of the COTA (payroll, vacations, working hours), an OTR provides *professional* supervision (case load determination, daily schedule, treatment activities; Wendt, 1984).

Interdisciplinary team members

Members of the interdisciplinary committee assist in formulating decisions on appropriate placement and educational programming for children. Decisions cannot be made on the basis of any one test or any one professional's viewpoint.

School professionals

School principals, program directors, and directors of special education are committee members who interpret local administrative policies in special education.

Counselor

The counselor reports about the child's family milieu and the school placement options and services available in the community.

Parent

The parent, as the primary caregiver for the child, helps set goals commensurate with family expectations. With the help of their trained advocate or lawyer, parents may initiate suggestions regarding educational placement and programming or, through team meetings, may be better prepared to give informed consent. For preschoolers, the family's strengths and needs are a major consideration in establishing intervention strategies, which may include parental training and counseling (Manes, 1985).

Psychologist

The psychologist reports mental age or IQ scores, cognitive and adaptive functioning, and sometimes social and emotional information resulting from projective tests. Consideration of scores and quality of performance on tests and subtests given by the psychologist may give diagnostic information that can reduce the amount of time spent in evaluation by the therapist. Figure 25-2 and the display on page 795 provide information to help with interpretation of subtest scores from two psychological tests. A breakdown of subtest scores may have to be specifically requested.

Educational evaluator

An educational evaluator is a specially trained teacher who reports results of tests of academic, developmental, and readiness levels in number concepts as well as the sequence of listening, speaking, reading, and, finally, writing. The evaluator may report on perceptual, language, and motor performance if these areas are not tested by other services. This professional is particularly crucial if a child is thought to have a learning disability (with or without other handicapping conditions).

Special education teacher

After the parent, the teacher probably has the most consistent contact with the handicapped child. This classroom teacher makes recommendations about everyday social maturity and behavior as well as academic, perceptual, and language performance of children in the classroom. The resource room teacher sees mildly handicapped children for a portion of each day to work on specific deficit areas.

Physical therapist

The physical therapist reports on quality of movement, reflex development, equilibrium reaction, gait, and gross motor development.

Speech and language clinician

The speech and language clinician reports test results of the child's receptive language (comprehension or decoding of what is heard) and expressive language (encoding through the use of linguistic symbols). For both expressive and receptive language,

THE TESTS	Spatial	Quantitative	Sequencing	Perceptual organization	Conceptualization and verbal comprehension	Ability to concentrate: Distractibility	Visual motor integration: Fine motor	Verbal expression
● VERBAL SCALE Information					✓			✓
Similarities					✓			✓
Arithmetic		✓			✓	✓		
Vocabulary					✓			✓
Comprehension					✓			✓
Digit Span		✓	✓			✓		
● PERFORMANCE SCALE Picture Completion	✓					✓		
Picture Arrangement			✓		✓			
Block Design	✓			✓				
Object Assembly	✓			✓			✓	
Coding	✓		✓				✓	
Mazes	✓						✓	

FIGURE 25-2. *Content of test items of the Wechsler Intelligence Scale for Children (WISC-R). (Modified from Waugh, K.W., & Bush, W.J. [1971]. Diagnosing learning disorders. Columbus, OH: Charles Merrill.)*

SUBTESTS OF THE KAUFFMAN ASSESSMENT BATTERY FOR CHILDREN (K-ABC)

Intellectual Functioning

Sequential Processing Scale
    Hand movements ....Copying a movement series
    Number recall..Digit repetition
    Work order ....Touching objects in sequence named
Simultaneous Processing Scale
    Magic window.....................Identifying picture moving behind screen
    Face recognition ....Selecting from group photograph
    Gestalt closure ....Naming partially completed inkblot drawing
    Triangles...........................Assembling to match pattern
    Matrix analogies ....Completing visual analogies
    Spatial memory...............................Recalling picture placement
    Photo series.................................Sequencing photographs

Acquired Knowledge

Achievement Scale
    Expressive vocabulary ....Naming object photograph
    Faces and places ....Recognizing and naming pictures
    Arithmetic.................................School math abilities
    Riddles ....Inferring concept when told its characteristics
    Reading/decoding ....Recognizing letters and words
    Reading/understanding ....Following commands

(*Modified from American Guidance Service.* [*1985*]. Important advances in individually administered measures of intelligence, achievement and adaptive behavior. *Circle Pines, MN.*)

---

consideration is given to the child's use of sounds (phonology), meaning (semantics or vocabulary and concepts), and grammar (syntax and morphology). Integration (inner associative language processing such as categorization and understanding of analogies) is also considered, as well as retention (memory) and such perceptual problems as auditory discrimination and speed of verbal response. Articulation is also reported.

Occupational therapist

Examples of developmental areas in which the occupational therapist reports quality and level of functioning are movement, visual perception, visual–motor integration, independent living skills, and play. Other important considerations reported by the therapist are architectural planning, positioning for seatwork, assistive devices for functional skills such as eating and writing, and work-related programming (even from the earliest grade school years).

    Team members should make every effort to maintain close professional involvement with parents through telephone or personal contact, written test results or progress notes, and team meetings. Parents may appreciate suggestions of reading publications such as *The Exceptional Parent* magazine (Schleifer) and books written for parents, or of joining such national organizations as the Association for Children with Learning Disabilities (ACLD), Association of Retarded Citizens (ARC), Council of Exceptional Children (CEC), and Children with Attention Deficit Disorder (CHADD).

Assessment

Evaluation of handicapped children in the areas just mentioned provides the basis for planning treatment. The occupational therapist can, and should, also help the educational team identify learning style elements that affect particular students' abilities to process, integrate, and recall information.

1. Does the student learn best from auditory, visual, tactile, or kinesthetic sensory input, or from a combination of these? (Learning style does not necessarily correlate with discrimination ability.)
2. Does the student use an analytic or global approach to problem solving or new learning?
3. What aspects of the environment are most favorable for this student's learning? Consider architectural barriers; time of day; amount and quality of light, temperature, and background sounds; firm or soft sitting or reclining surface; firmly structured or mildly or warmly cluttered room?
4. What people-related aspects work best for a particular child: one-to-one or small group instruction and therapy, self-generated exploring, working with younger or older children?
5. How do similar and dissimilar factors make an impact? Should the handwriting instructor present "e" or "h" next after "c" to minimize this child's apraxia?
6. For each child consider cycle of medication effectiveness, types of rewards that motivate, and abilities to persist, struc-

ture, and take responsibility (Carbo, 1987; Guild & Garger, 1985).

Howard Gardner, an American authority on creativity, identifies several different areas of intelligence that occur in different degrees in different people and at varying levels within each person: spatial, logical/mathematical, self-knowledge, music, verbal, interpersonal, and body/kinesthetic. Which of these areas makes a positive impact and which makes a negative impact on each child's functioning in school, home, and therapy (Gardner, 1983)?

In keeping with the Americans with Disabilities Act, school therapists must also take notice of their students' accessibility to school buildings, transportation vehicles, public telephones, (including locations and communication devices for the speech and hearing impaired), and of the sizes of desks and chairs. Therapists may need to point out to school administrators when physical barriers could or do already inhibit students. The National Easter Seal Society (1991) publishes an "ADA Checklist" (Americans with Disabilities Act: An Easy Checklist, publication E-69) to help people comply with the Americans with Disabilities Act regarding public access to buildings and transportation.

Screening

The goal of screening is to identify mildly impaired children who need help without interfering in the lives of those who have only a temporary developmental delay. Early detection of children with attention-deficit disorder, mild mental retardation, or mild emotional disturbances helps prevent secondary emotional overlay resulting from learning failure in later grades. It also provides intervention procedures at a critical time in the child's life when they will be most helpful. Occupational therapists may play a key role in district-wide and local school methods for finding such children and planning suitable programs for them.

In one school district, teachers identified young children with suspected problems by color-coded name tags while occupational therapists led the whole class through informal screening tasks. The therapists observed especially carefully the children whose colored tag suggested the likelihood and severity of subtle problems in motor skills, perception, or sensory-based poor behavior. Classroom recommendations for training of problem children were made, and a small percentage of children was recommended for further standardized testing.

Another school district sent a team of medical and educational personnel to individually observe and screen a few problem children identified by each teacher. Recommendations were made to the teacher and parents for managing the specific educational and behavioral problems. Later, the team returned and used additional test measures for the one or two children who, in spite of several months of maturation and special teaching techniques, still had the greatest problems.

The School District of Philadelphia developed a 5-page, easily understood learning disabilities checklist to be marked by classroom teachers for each of their kindergarten or first-grade students (Cornman, 1975). It eliminated the need for screening by specialists, and contained sections on behavior, motor coordination, orientation, visual–motor integration, and language.

Using the Child Development Chart (Table 25-1), an occupational therapist can quickly determine the normal age at which children acquire some commonly tested abilities. The chart reads developmentally from the top to the bottom. It also reads across from left to right, as some developmental sequences on the right side of the chart may be interrupted because of deficits in developmental sequences on the left side. For example, equilibrium (in the fourth column) may not be developing properly because of poorly inhibited reflexes (first column). Body scheme and eye–hand coordination (3rd and 7th columns) may be negatively affected by poor sensory development, which appears in an earlier column. Inadequate development of language (last column) in some cases is a reflection of poorly integrated visual perception or sensory information. The use of the chart is intended to promote continual awareness in the mind of the therapist of the many different goals established for each child and their interrelationship. Also, the chart can be helpful in talking with parents, recommending developmental activities, or making general judgments about children's performance levels.

Testing

After such screening methods as those just described or after the direct referral of educational or medical personnel, therapists can further evaluate children showing evidence of dysfunction. They may use informal functional assessments based largely on clinical impressions (Dunn, 1981); or, they may use standardized tests, which compare a child's performance with that of many other children (eg, the Miller Assessment for Preschoolers, 1982). Some standardized instruments may be used in shortened form as screening tools (eg, Bruininks-Oseretsky Test of Motor Proficiency [1978]). Standardized test administration methods must be followed exactly and may require special training, such as with the Sensory Integration and Praxis Tests (Ayres, 1984).

In addition to clinical impressions and standardized tests, the therapist may use criterion-referenced tests, some of which have instructional activities suggested to remediate each test item or section in which the child needs additional help. **Criterion-referenced tests**, now widely used to establish goals and objectives, evaluate performance on specifically described skills or knowledge without comparisons among individuals as in standardized testing. Skills are listed approximately in the order in which they are normally acquired. Specific skills on the test that have not yet been acquired are trained for, and the criterion of the test is 100% mastery. An example of a criterion-referenced test is the Portage Guide to Early Education: Checklist (Bluma et al., 1985).

Other chapters in this textbook suggest appropriate assessment tools for various types of handicaps found in children of all ages. They describe methods of testing range of motion, muscle strength, sensation, motor skills, sensory integration, cognition, developmental reflexes and reactions, eating, writing, activities of daily living, and prevocational and vocational skills. In addition, assessments are included for cerebral palsy (see Chapter 13, Section 2) and hand rehabilitation (see Chapter 18, Section 4). Lerner et al. (1987), and King-Thomas and Hacker (1987) give thorough bibliographies of published screening and evaluation tools for children.

Lists of tests for screening and evaluating learning-impaired children are available from federally funded area learning resource centers and local centers, sometimes called Special Educational Instructional Materials Centers (SEIMC). These centers, which are in many locations around the country, also have samples and lists of educational curriculum materials. *The Mental Measurements Yearbook*, published every several years by the Buros Institute of Mental Measurements, is an important reference that groups tests by topic and includes several critiques of each one by authorities in the field (Connoley & Kramer, 1989).

When screening and testing children, constellations in the results of all testing must be considered rather than single low scores. Even normal children may fail in some aspect of motor, sensory, or psychosocial functioning. Plan goals and make recommendations that are relevant to the child's *educational* problem or ability to reach full potential. All the testing methods described are only as valuable as the program planning that results.

Program planning and documentation

After using assessment procedures, the occupational therapist documents the results in writing. Information related to the client's personal data and history as well as the referral is included. Therapists should include skill/performance in independent living, sensorimotor areas, cognition, psychosocial areas, therapeutic adaptation, and prevention. In addition to this initial evaluation report, the therapist keeps daily progress records of treatment programs and of recommendations to or from teachers, administrators, parents, and volunteers. Once or twice a year, therapists send descriptive reports home and write formal progress notes that are added to the child's school records.

Specific documentation of planned treatment is required by law, although school personnel are not held accountable for children's progress. The occupational therapist's testing, treatment, and consultative information and recommendations are often written into the student's IEP (or IFSP for preschoolers). These documents include a statement of present educational levels, annual or semiannual long-term goals relevant to education for achieving potential (a general statement of treatment intent), and short-term objectives. The latter are written in behaviorally observable (not theoretical) terms and include the conditions under which they will take place, terminal behavior, a measurable criterion level, and expected completion date (Figure 25-3).

Figures 25-4 and 25-5, adapted from Llorens and Seig (1975), show a method of organizing treatment goals for whole classes or small groups of young children. Such an evaluation record provides a visual chart of assets and deficits. The therapist administers only those evaluation procedures most suitable to the age and capability of the child. Clusters of low scores suggest treatment goals. Listing them on such an evaluation record helps point out remedial needs of the individual or group.

Test results of 5½-year-old Richard, a student with attention-deficit disorder, are recorded in Figure 25-4 as an example of the use of this evaluation record. A diagnostic–prescriptive program for improving motor and perceptual functioning might be correlated as follows:

Through sensory integrative techniques, the occupational therapist would use vestibular and tactile stimulation and developmental activities to enhance motor planning, body scheme, reflex development, ocular control, and visual perception. The need to follow three auditory sequential directions using a scooter board could frequently be included in the activities. The physical education teacher could emphasize prone extension and supine flexion along with games involving moving specific body parts. The classroom aide, volunteer, or resource room teacher could supervise Richard's copying of specifically selected inch cube and pegboard designs to help fine motor and prereading perceptual skills. Independent work may include worksheets or computer games emphasizing embedded geometric shapes and alphabet letters for visual figure–ground discrimination. The parents could be providing daily tactile stimulation and discrimination at home.

Such a complete program could be organized by the therapist or planned and agreed on by all the professionals at a team meeting. The language therapist emphasizes Richard's associative language processing and the speed with which he makes oral responses. Awareness of the language problems helps all members of the team understand his learning style better.

The columns listed in Figure 25-4 are examples of test results or developmental activities that could be listed. Other standardized or observational score items can be substituted; for example, pertinent subtests of the WISC-R or K-ABC psychological tests.

Figure 25-5 shows a similar group evaluation record designed for younger or more handicapped children. Rather than listing standardized tests, space is left under each heading for listing skills or clinical observations indicating strengths or deficits of each child. Red pencil hachures can be used to mark columns indicating current treatment objectives, as they do in Figure 25-4.

Interpreting performance

Testing and treatment of the youngster in the special education setting may be complicated by undetected deficits in visual, auditory, or tactile acuity. On the other hand, a child may hear well and express well verbally but may have a severe impairment in auditory reception. In that case, automatic or learned reliance on visual cues may cause misinterpretation by the child unless gestural cues and body language accurately convey the therapist's intent. Instructions for tactile testing, for example, may need to be demonstrated to be understood. In that case, the written report must reflect the deviation from standardized instructions and the possible educational significance of the language processing confusion.

In addition, "Do this [demonstration], this [gesture], and this after you roll to the ladder," may be an impossible activity for the child who cannot remember the sequence of three visual stimuli or who does not understand the temporal concept "after." It is important to know a child's sensory, language processing, and cognitive deficits as well as to task analyze testing and treatment requirements to understand the full impact of a child's performance.

Implementing the program

The therapist is encouraged to update treatment skills often but to avoid applying one treatment method exclusively or following a bandwagon approach to solving children's problems. Community resources must be well known and commonly used, partic-

(*Text continues on page 802*)

TABLE 25-1. *Child Development Chart*

	General Reflex Development	Sensory Development	Body Scheme	Equilibrium
0–3 mo	• 0–2 mo. Phasic/movement spinal cord reflexes predominate. Limbs coordinated in total flexion or extension • 0–6 mo. Static, brain-stem–mediated reflexes are present. Stimulation of labyrinths or neck muscle feedback changes distribution of muscle tone throughout body.	• 1–4 wk. Differentiates: tactile (touch, pressure); temp. (hot, cold); taste (sweet, sour, salty, bitter); vision (see Visual Perception column) • Also experiences vestibular input, internal chemical changes, audition	• 1 mo. Mass motor activity reaction to stimuli • 3 mo. Plays regarding hands	• 2 mo. Prone, head and chest up to 45° recurrently • Head bobs when sitting, back rounded
3 mo to 1 yr	• 4–15 mo. Midbrain-mediated reactions in all-fours position help child right self, turn over, assume crawl and sit positions. Maximum concerted effort 10–12 mo. • 6 mo. Equilibrium reactions under cortical control begin to gradually modify, inhibit, and dominate righting reactions if muscle tone is normal. Results in standing, walking, well-coordinated person	• 3 mo. Tickle reaction	• 4–6 mo. Plays with hands and feet in supine. Hands come together in play • 5–6 mo. Pats mirror image • 7–8 mo. Plays peek-a-boo	• 3 mo. Prone, supports weight on forearms • 5 mo. Pull to sit; no head lag • 6–8 mo. Sits, head erect • 7–9 mo. 4-point kneel; rocks back and forth
1–2 yr			• 12–18 mo. Points to 2 of own body parts	• 12–13 mo. Kneels/stands • 14 mo. Stands • 14–18 mo. Walks; feet wide apart, arms in primary balance role usually at or above shoulder height • 17 mo. Stoops to pick up toy without losing balance
2 yr			• Identifies 2 body parts from picture • Touches tummy, cheek, arm, leg, mouth, hair	• Up and down stairs independently, 2 steps per tread, holding on • 2½ yr. Jumps, 2-foot take off; tiptoes briefly • Runs; walks sideways and backwards • Kicks ball on request

Bilateral Integration	Visual Perception	Eye–Hand Coordination	Language
• 1–4 wk. Asymmetric postures predominate	• 3–4 wk. At 10″ discriminates ⅛″ stripes from plain surface	• 0–4 wk. Reflexive grasp; no eye–hand coordination. Touch tells when to grasp.	• 1 mo. Responds to sound; undifferentiated crying
• 2 mo. Supine, can hold head in midline and extremities symmetric	• 1–2 mo. Discriminates stylized face from oval pattern; also color	• 1–4½ mo. Fixates on light monocularly	• 2 mo. Single vowel sounds; coos
• 2 mo. Eyes begin to follow past midline.	• 2 mo. Visual size and near distance constancy developing; unable to apply them simultaneously	• 2 mo. Prone, head and chest up for forward vision	• 3 mo. Vocalizes pleasure in response to social stimuli; vocal noises resemble speech.
	• 2 mo. Recognizes visual cliff	• 3 mo. Eye follows across midline and past 90°	• 2 mo. Discriminates intonations and 2 voices
		• 3 mo. Plays regarding hands	
• 4–6 mo. Hands together in play	• 6–7 mo. Discriminates + ○ □ △. 3-dimensional discrim. easier than 2-dimensional	• 4 mo. Rotates head to inspect surroundings	• 3 mo. Chuckles
• 6 mo. Symmetric arm use and postures predominate	• 8–24 mo. Convergence to 2″ from nose; divergence to 20″; primitive depth perception	• 4–6 mo. Visually pursues lost toy	• 4 mo. Turns to noise and voice
• 7 mo. Transfers toy from 1 hand to other; hands cross midline	• 9 mo. Recognizes danger of visual cliff	• 6 mo. Eye–hand coordination begins	• 6 mo. Distinguishes angry/friendly voices
• 7–8 mo. Creeps amphibian; tactile stimulation to abdomen		• 6 mo. Palmar grasp	• 6 mo. Intonational jargon
• 7–8 mo. Bunny hops		• 6 mo. Reaches with fully extended elbow	• 9 mo. Comprehends a few gestures, intonations, "no-no," "hot." Echolalia
• 7–9 mo. 4-point crawl; homolateral, then heterolateral		• 10 mo. Crude release; pokes finger in holes	• 10 mo. Word-like syllables: ma-ma-ma, da-da-da. Comprehends, waves bye-bye
		• 10 mo. Instinctive grasp integrated with vision	
		• 10 mo. 3-jaw chuck grasp, wrist and fingers appropriately extended	
• 11–12 mo. Cruises sideways, holding furniture	• 15 mo. Looks selectively at pictures in book	• Imitates scribble	• 12 mo. First word, usually a noun
• Creeps up stairs	• 21 mo. Aligns 3 blocks for train	• 12 mo. Neat pincer grasp; supinated grasp developing, wrist extended	• Action response to commands
• 15 mo. Creeps down stairs	• Object permanence	• 13 mo. Good release	• 1–5 word vocabulary
• 15 mo. Holds object with hand, manipulating it with other		• Tower of 2 cubes	
		• 15 mo. Places objects into and out of containers	
		• Spontaneous scribble	
		• 18 mo. Turns pages, 2 or 3 at a time	• 1-word sentences
		• Uses spoon, cup well	• Can mentally perform behavior before physically performing
		• 21 mo. Puts large pegs in pegboard	• Produces all vowel sounds
			• 1½ yr. Extension of word meanings; overgeneralizations
			• 50-word vocabulary, mostly nouns
• Rhythmic bounce, sway, nod, swings arms	• Enjoys watching moving objects	• Hand preference beginning	• 2-word sentences that are functionally complete
	• Simultaneous visual size and distance constancy developing	• Tower of 6–7 cubes	• Imitates absent models; pretends; reconstructs memories
	• 20/70 visual acuity	• Strings large beads	• Knows "in" and "under"
	• Points to pictures of familiar objects	• Throws	• Knows "I," "you," "me," "mine"
	• 2½ yr. Adds chimney to 3-cube train □ ☐☐☐	• Imitates /	• 2½ yr. Telegraphic speech
	• Begins matching colors	• 2½ yr. Imitates —, ○	• 3-word sentences
		• Copies /	
		• Pours well, glass to glass	
		• Digital pronate crayon grasp	

(continued)

TABLE 25-1. *Child Development Chart* (*continued*)

	General Reflex Development	Sensory Development	Body Scheme	Equilibrium
3 yr		• Vision occluded, matches grossly different textures, *eg*, sandpaper and satin	• Knows front, back, side of self; also chin, neck, forearm	• Jumps from 12″ height, feet together or 1 foot lead • Upstairs 1 foot per tread, no support; down 2 steps per tread, no support • Hops 1 foot 2, 3 times • Climbs 3 rungs • Squats • 3½ yr. Tandem walks 10 ft
4 yr		• Names heavier of 2 weights • Discriminates different scents • Compares different textures; *eg*, soft, smooth	• Draws man with head and legs	• Stands on 1 foot 4 sec. Broad jumps... • standing: 8–10″ • running: 23–33″
5 yr	• Primitive reflexes inhibited or dominated. In supine and all-fours child can turn head side-to-side, up, down without elbows, shoulders, or knees changing angle • Can flex in supine and extend in prone position for 10 sec • Sits and stands symmetrically from supine with only slight body rotation	Vision occluded... • Discriminates ○□☆ blocks (stereognosis) • Points to touched finger ½ times • Points to within 3″ of stimulus spot on arm • Points to hand and/or cheek touched singly or simultaneously	• Copies Simon Says postures • Draws 6-part unmistakable man with body • Points front, back, near, up, down, with eyes closed • Can clench and bare teeth • Aware of, but confuses left and right • In pictures identifies object that is beside, between, in middle, in front of	• Down stairs, alternating feet, no support • Stands 1 foot 6–8 sec. • Balances on tiptoe, ⅓ trials • Running broad jump 28–35″ • Jumps 10″ high hurdle • Begins balance beam backwards • Tries roller skates, jump rope, stilts
6 yr				• Jumps over rope 20 cm high • Standing broad jump 3 ft
7 yr	• Arises from supine to standing in 1–1.5 sec	• Vision occluded, can reproduce– × ○ drawn on back of hand ½ trials	• Good jumping jacks • Can knit eyebrows • 7½ yr. Stabilizes arms and trunk against much resistance • Knows left and right on self	• Stands on 1 foot, eyes closed, 3 sec • Can hop and jump accurately into small squares • Walks 2″ wide balance beam

Bilateral Integration	Visual Perception	Eye–Hand Coordination	Language
• Walks swinging arm with opposite leg, arms free of shoulder ht. balance position • Pedals tricycle • Weight shift in throwing; no step into	• Tends to react to entire stimulus rather than label separate parts, especially if unfamiliar • Picks longer line 3 of 3 times • Imitates cube bridge ⬚ • 3½ yr. Recognizes 2 colors named	• 10 pellets into bottle in 30 sec. • Tower of 9–10 cubes • Copies —, ○ • Simian pencil grasp (fist clenched) • Turns doorknob, forearm rotation • Unbuttons accessible buttons • May shift handedness • Catches large ball, arms extended • 3½ yr. Imitates ×	• Has adult grammatical structure. Complete simple active sentences • Uses sentences to tell understandable stories • 3½ yr. Speech disfluency • "Why" questions • Names 1 color
• Runs with good arm–leg coordination • Up and down stairs 1 foot per tread • Gallops • 4½ yr. Skips, 1 foot only (lame duck skip)	• With increasing age tends to differentiate stimuli in environment, esp. when specific language labels applied to them • Slowing down of rapid visual acuity development since birth • Matches shapes (same color and size) • Can find simple familiar overlapping outline figures • Builds 6-block pyramid • 4½ yr. Copies gate ⬚◇⬚	• Follows moving object smoothly with eyes ↔ ↕ ↘ ↗ ↻ • Crude static tripod pencil grasp • Copies + • Imitates ⬚ • 10 pellets into bottle in 25 sec. • Bounces ball awkwardly • Tries to cut on straight line	• Transforms kernel sentences • 4-word sentences, some complex or compound • Intuitive thought begins less concreteness • Little word analysis; deals with whole sentences • Counts 3 objects, though imperfectly • Uses slang; understands syntax, grammatical contrasts beyond production ability • Repeats 3 digits • 4½ yr. Names primary colors; perceives differences in concrete events
• Mimics pointing to ipsi- or contralateral ear or eye ²⁄₃ trials • Can reproduce simple rhythmic clapping • Marches in time to music	• 20/30 visual acuity • Difficulty with orientation. Can detect ↕ reversals easier than ↔ reversals after instruction • Difficulty performing closure necessary to distinguish incomplete ○⬚⬚ • Simultaneous size constancy and form discrim. developing • Imitates 10-block pyramid • 5½ yr. Begins to mentally rotate simple shapes for solving puzzles	• Copies / ⬚ \ × • Imitates △ • Sequential finger opposition (1, 2, 3, 4) with visual regard and minor associative movements. Slow • Throws 16″ playground ball 10–11 feet. Catches bounced large playground ball • Dynamic tripod pencil grasp, metacarpal phalangeal joint stabilized	• Embeds phrases, clauses in sentences • Develops percepts of number, speed, time, space • Inner logic and imaginative thinking • Categorizes by likeness and difference • Marked increase in vocab. comprehension (not use) • Repeats 4 digits • 5½ yr. Mean length of response, 4.9 words
• Skips alternately • Throws, stepping with foot opposite throwing arm	• Begins to identify imbedded familiar outline figures • Recalls 3½ of the 9 Bender-Gestalt figures • May still reverse some letters or numbers	• Copies △ ✗ • Ties shoelaces • Learns to write manuscript alphabet. Neat with effort • 6½ yr. Hand dominance established	• Command every form of sentence structure • Mean sentence length rapidly increasing; now 6.5 words • Asks for and attempts to verbalize explanations, causal relationships
• Can tap floor alternately with feet	• 20/20 visual acuity • b-d, p-q confusions resolved • Builds 6-block pyramid from memory	• Grips pencil tightly, often close to tip. Pressure may be heavy • Good sequential finger opposition (1, 2, 3, 4) • Drops 20 coins, one at a time, into open box in 16 sec.	• Good speech melody and facial/hand gestures • Good inner language • True communication; shares ideas • Mean length of response, 7.2 words

(continued)

TABLE 25-1.   *Child Development Chart (continued)*

	General Reflex Development	Sensory Development	Body Scheme	Equilibrium
8 yr			• Eyes closed, points right and left • Can wrinkle forehead	• Crouches on tiptoes without falling ⅓ trials
9 yr			• 9½ yr. Discriminates left and right on facing person	• Runs 16–17 ft./sec. • Jumps over rope 15″ high ⅔ trials • Jumps, clapping hands 3 times, ⅓ trials
10–12 yr				• 10 yr. Hops 50 ft on 1 foot in 5–6 sec • 11 yr. Standing broad jump 4½–5 ft • 12 yr. Standing high jump 3 ft

Items closer to top of each column suggest remedial sequences for problems observed closer to bottom of column. Items in left hand columns suggest possible causes of problems in certain columns further to the right.

Age norms are approximate. Authors vary. Children vary. Development does not really occur in separate rows and columns. All parts of the nervous system influence each other.

Other important areas that may be observed or evaluated by the therapist include (but are not limited to) reflex development, play (see Chapter 8, Section 3), social skills, more specific temporal, spatial, and Gestalt concepts relevant to learning styles, and the ideational concepts of imagination and creativity.

ularly for the youngest children. Mothers, fathers, and other family members should be included in a collaborative, enabling, empowering relationship with the therapist whenever possible through (1) regular or occasional meetings, (2) telephone conversations, (3) an informal communication notebook that carries messages, plans, and requests to and from families, and (4) formal progress reports. Family-centered service for the youngest children is the law.

OTRs and COTAs must be prepared to provide programs for a wide variety of handicapping conditions (see appropriate treatment sections of this textbook). The age of students served runs the gamut from infant stimulation and preschool programs through the grade school years to secondary education programs and vocational training for special education students to age 21, including "transition planning" from school to adult life. For mainstream classes, the therapist may be called on to suggest classroom or home activities to help the handicapped child who is being integrated or the nonspecial education student who manifests mild motor or perceptual difficulties.

Occupational therapy treatment is intended to allow the child to be able to direct cognitive skills toward the academic task at hand rather than toward execution of balance, motor planning, fine manipulation, and so forth. Therapy prepares the preschool and school-aged child to learn; however, it does not result in increased academic performance for school children unless accompanied by an appropriate academic program. The therapist should avoid removing a child from the classroom unless direct therapy is clearly warranted and ongoing assessment indicates progress is being made.

Models of service delivery

Some therapists are employed by public or private schools, whereas other organizations such as preschools or day care centers contract for occupational therapy services through private therapists' consortiums, public health departments, or hospitals. (Carr [1989] is among those who have observed that when contract therapists provide only treatment, and evaluation is

Bilateral Integration	Visual Perception	Eye–Hand Coordination	Language
		• Accurately taps swinging suspended ball $^2/_5$ tries	• Repeats 5 digits
		• 7½ yr. Copies ◇ ◇	• 80% know comparative relationships (*eg*, bigger than)
• Good 2–2, 2–1, 1–2 hop	• Identifies heavily embedded familiar figures	• Laces 8 beads in 20 sec	• Skilled use of grammatical rules
• Can run into moving jump rope but cannot alter step	• Notices and labels component parts of stimulus more than does younger child	• Places 10 pairs of matchsticks in box in 16 sec	• Acceptable articulation
	• Capable of attending to both whole and part	• Writes manuscript to compose original ideas	
	• Closure figure recognized and seen as incomplete	• Learns cursive writing for direct copying	
	• Notices wholes and parts simultaneously in figures composed of familiar objects		• 80% know passive relationships (*eg*, person was hit by)
		• Writes cursive to compose original ideas	• 75% know familial relationships (*eg*, "your mother's father")
	• 11 yr and over. Recalls 5½–6 of the 9 Bender-Gestalt figures	• 10 yr. Draws 3-dimensional geometric figures:	
		• 10 yr. Judges and intercepts pathways of small balls thrown from a distance	
		• 12 yr. Linear perspective seen in drawings	
		• Anticipates locomotor and manual responses to rapidly moving objects; *eg*, where to catch ball whose complete trajectory is not observable	

(*Developed from Ayres, Banus, Berry, Bobath, Bruininks, Cattell, Colarusso & Hammill, Cratty, Dale, Denhoff, Erhardt, Fantz, Fiorentino, Frostig, Gardner, Gesell & Armatruda, Gilfoyle & Grady, Gibson, Hull & Hull, Kephart, Llorens, Miller, Moore, Norton, Oseretsky, Pearlson, Piaget, Wiig & Semel.*)

done by a therapist from elsewhere to prevent a self-perpetuating treatment plan, the amount of direct occupational therapy service drops.) Private practitioners employed by parents of school-aged clients may interact with school personnel through team meetings, telephone consultation, or other collaboration.

Occupational therapy personnel may provide direct service, including individual or small group treatment or whole class demonstration. Direct service might occur in clients' homes (for the very young) or in one or several educational centers (sometimes including itinerant service, in which therapy equipment may need to be transported from school to school in the therapist's car.

Therapists are learning to be assertive and creative in finding space for hands-on therapy. Therapists at one school in Washington, DC use a trailer that is permanently set up outside the school for individual therapy before, during, and after school hours. In New Orleans, some therapists use a traveling "Therapy Express," which is a converted school bus (Fox, 1990).

The trend has changed from pulling both preschool- and school-aged children out of the classroom for service, however. Integrative rather than segregated or isolated educational programming by occupational therapists is now preferred in most cases, servicing single children or groups right in the classroom or home. There the teacher, aide, or parent can observe and learn, and the therapist can more accurately assess the child's functioning in a real-life situation (Sternat et al., 1980). Some therapists in Philadelphia and Minnesota extol the virtues of using natural environments as teaching settings and provide therapy, not only in classrooms and homes, but also on the playground and stairs, in buses and malls, and beside the coat cubbies (Mastrangelo & Colan, 1990).

A trend also exists toward placing handicapped preschoolers and school-aged children into regular classrooms (mainstreaming) to the fullest extent possible, using a practice of accommodation rather than referral. Some parents view this as more of an attempt to cut costs than to provide services and they resist the trend in due process hearings.

(*Text continues on page 807*)

Individualized Educational Program Plan (I.E.P.)
(abbreviated version)

Name___ Richard (R.)_____   Date of Birth_____
Address _____   Today's Date _____
School_____ Grade/Program_____   I.E.P. Review Date _____

	Date started	Frequency or % of time	Expected duration of services
Primary assignment Integration into regular education (opportunities for child to participate with mainstream children during school hours.) Related Services (e.g., transportation, O.T., P.T., speech, audiology, psychology, counseling, social work, etc.)		(e.g. 20% of each school day) (e.g. 30 minutes 2 times per week)	

Reason for assignment _____

Administrative person responsible for program _____

I.E.P. Planning Meeting Participants_____   _____

_____   _____

Present Educational Levels	Curricular Area	Assessment Procedure	Date	Program Planner
(Results of testing: clinical impressions, standardized tests, criterion referenced measures, etc.)		(tests used)		

Curricular Area (e.g. (1) gross motor)   Annual Goal (e.g. (1) improve balance)

   (e.g. (2) fine motor)   (e.g. (2) improve eye–hand coordination)

Short Term Objectives	Criteria for Successful Performance
(e.g. (1) (R.) will complete desk-top activities without leaning his chest on desk........................	.......for 15 minutes on three successive days)
(e.g. (2) With a ½-inch diameter pencil (R.) will maintain correct pencil grip while copying ◯,▢, & △	.....with shapes clearly discernible.)

FIGURE 25-3. *Sample individualized educational program plan (IEP).*

Head-ings	Column items	Test results			
	Classroom #				
	Age	5½			
	I.Q.	83 ok			
	Behavior	ok			
Reflex development	ATNR	ok			
	Prone Ext. (Kep)	↗ (hatched)			
	Supine Flex.	↗ (hatched)			
	Cocontract'n	→			
	Postrot. Nystag. (SIPT)	+.2			
	Sitt'g Blance				
	Forw'd Bal. Beam (Kep)	okokok			
	Sideway Bl. Bm. (Kep)				
	Backw'd Bl. Bm. (Kep)				
	Stand'g/Walk'g Bal. (SIPT)	+.1 -.2			
	Static Bal. (Dev)	ok			
Bilateral integration	STNR creep (Bndr)	ok			
	Midline Xing (SC)	→			
	Bilat. Mot. Cord. (SIPT)				
	Dbl. Circles (Kep)				
	Skip (Kep)				
	2-2, 1 hop (Kep)				
	Hand Dominance	R	R		
	Eye Foot Dominance	R	L		
Body scheme and tactile discrim.	Postural Prax. (SIPT)	-2.d (hatched)			
	Sequ. Prax. (SIPT)	(hatched)			
	Perc. Mot. (Dev)				
	Sequ. Mot. (Dev)				
	Point Body Parts	↗ (hatched)			
	Angls in Snow (Kep)				
	Kinesthesia (SIPT)	(hatched)			
	Man. Form. (SIPT)	(hatched)			
	Fing. Identif. (SIPT)	-.9.			
	Graphesthesia (SIPT)	(hatched)			
	Loclz'n Tac. Stim. (SIPT)	(hatched)			
	Dbl. Tact. Stim. (SC)	(hatched)			
	Tactile Dfsivenes (SC)	ok			

CLASS DAYS: _____

TIME: _____ TO _____

Name: Richard

FIGURE 25-4. Evaluation record for the mildly neurologically impaired.

Code for standardized tests indicated in parenthesis:

Kep — Kephart's Purdue Perceptual Motor Survey
SIPT — Sensory Integration and Praxis Tests
Dev — Devereux Test of Extremity Coordination
Beery — Beery–Buktenica Test of Visual Motor Integration
MVPT— Motor Free Test of Visual Perception
SC — Southern Calif. Sensory Integration Test
TVPS — Test of Visual–Perceptual Skills (Gardner)

Blank score indicates item not tested because (a) it was not age appropriate, or (b) new insight into deficit areas would not result.

Category		Item	(Test)	Richard			
Language		Oral Praxis	(SIPT)				
		Speed of Auditry Process'g		→			
		Sound-symbol assoc.					
		Word finding (naming)		→			
		Auditory Discrim.		ok ok			
		Integrative (Associative)		→			
		Expressive		ok ok ok			
		Receptive					
Memory	Aud	Sequ. of 3 audit. direct'ns		→			
		Repeat 3 wrds or #'s		37%			
	Vis'l	Vis. Sequ. Mem.	(TVPS)	73%			
		Vis. Memory	(TVPS)	37%			
		Sequ. of 3 vis. instructns		ok ok			
		Sequence of 4 color beads					
Vis. discrim. whole/part		Vis. Fig. Grnd.	(TVPS)	→			
		Fig. Grnd.	(SIPT)	→			
		Perceptual Quotnt	(TVPS)	76%			
		Perceptual Quotnt	(MVPT)	70%			
Spatial orientatn		R-L. Discrim.	(SC)				
		Reading L. to R. direct.					
		Reversals: letter—word					
		Space Visualiz.	(SIPT)	-7 -7			
		Vis.—Spat'l Relat.	(TVPS)	ok -9			
		Envirnmtal Disorientation					
Fine motor		Ocular Converg.	(Kep)	→			
		Ocular Pursuit	(Kep)	→			
		Ocular Fixation		ok			
		Constr. Praxis	(SIPT)				
		Sequent. Fing. Tip Touch		→			
		Handwriting		→			
		Pencil Grip		→			
		Design Copy	(SIPT)				
		Vis. Mot. Integr.	(Beery)				
		(non-domin.)	(SIPT)				
		Mot. Acc. (domin.)	(SIPT)	-2			

After testing use soft pencil to fill in scores on pages 1 and 2 only for those items tested. Then with soft red pencil make hatch marks in boxes of pertinent low scores indicating current treatment objectives. Use the Evaluation Record to see goals common to the whole group, to zero in on particular children's deficits when part of the group is suddenly absent, and for ready reference when talking with parents and teachers. Erase and change scores often as children show progress.

FIGURE 25-4. (continued)

Class	Gross motor and reflexes		Equilibrium		Bilateral integration	Domin: Hand	Body scheme	Tactile and sensory	Self help	Social emotional
Names ↓		PRNT	Dynamic	Static		Eye				
		L				Foot				
		R								

	Eye/hand coordination			Perception		Memory and speed of processing	Language	Cognitive adaptive	Age
	VMI	Dexterity	Ocular motility	Spatial orientation	Visual discrimination and figure ground				I.Q.

FIGURE 25-5. *Evaluation record for young or moderately to severely handicapped children.*

Tracking (monitoring) may accompany the therapist's hands-on intervention for some children, including personal or telephone contact for receiving regular feedback and updating of recommendations suggested to parents, aides, or teachers (such as classroom, physical education, art, or vocational teachers). Other therapists have assumed a consultation model (Table 25-2). Registered occupational therapists may devote consider- able time to the supervising of COTAs, volunteers, and others who help plan or carry out treatment.

The method for service delivery should be chosen primarily according to the age and needs of the child, not the schedule constraints of the therapy personnel or the budget of the school district. Normalization is the goal, that is, to help the student feel most like a "regular" child and later adult.

TABLE 25-2. *The Do's and Don't's of Consultancy*

Do	Do Not
Keep record of consultancy contacts.	
Recognize you hold an equal position with consultee socially, emotionally, administratively.	Try to assume authority or take responsibility (which would be supervision, not consultation).
Evaluate needs.	
Promote learning by consultee *and* yourself.	Act patronizing, benign, or aloof.
Impart specialized knowledge; find solutions jointly. (Share responsibility for problem solving with the consultee.)	Make unilateral decisions.
Suggest changes that are palatable and realistic.	Expect consultee to modify behavior to please you.
Enhance creative, self-directed implementing of your suggestion.	Teach.
Listen; expect 2-way communication.	Ignore feedback.
Be task-oriented; delegate treatment.	Be patient- or student-oriented or provide hands-on treatment.
Recognize you are dealing with a whole social system.	Be an *advisor* who does not become involved with the social system but supervises, dictates authority.
Be nonthreatening in your approach.	Try to upstage the consultee or compete for attention from shared supervisors.
Consider *who* asked you to consult, and *why*.	Fail to obtain and maintain sanction of people who opposed your appointment.
Solve a problem or crisis. Recognize your involvement is likely to be temporary. Consultee may terminate your relationship at any time.	Plan to stay in this position indefinitely.
Recognize that a consultant's role may not establish deep personal relationships and provide deep personal gratification.	

(*Adapted from Leopold, R. [1966]. The techniques of consultation: Some thoughts for the occupational therapist. Presentation before Eastern Pennsylvania Occupational Therapy Association, Norristown, PA.*)

Direct treatment

The goal of occupational therapy evaluation and treatment in the school setting is to promote educational goals and move a child toward achieving full potential. Since the school is not a rehabilitation setting, providing medical services is not a goal. For example, functional life skills (focusing on accomplishments) rather than entirely developmental goals (based on normal cognitive and physical development) now form the bases for educational programming for many retarded students.

Emotional and social considerations

Emotional and social factors as well as physical needs should be considered during treatment. Play, the primary occupation of the child, is an important consideration in program planning. Activities should be fun and should foster in the child a positive self-image. As one therapist said, "every pediatric occupational therapy treatment program should include play, pleasure, and success." Clark, Mailloux, and Parham (1981) point out that play is intrinsically motivating, and self-direction by the child should have a major role in therapy, accompanied by the artful vigilance of the observant therapist. These authors point out that therapy is an art that is best carried out within a healthy helping relationship that values the child as an important contributor to the process. On the other hand, the child must not be permitted to misbehave, control, or misuse activities to the detriment of his or her own progress or that of classmates.

Behavior management

Attention deficits and hyperactivity often cause behavior management problems and inaccurate interpretation of performance capability, particularly for therapists working with several developmentally impaired children at once. Helping a child to manage his or her own behavior may be one goal of therapy. In addition, it is important for children to leave therapy quietly controlled and ready to resume classroom, desk work, preschool, or family activities without disruption.

The occupational therapist may use such techniques as slow rocking, firm pressure on the skin, neutral warmth, and slow rotation for certain conditions associated with overactive behavior. Medications prescribed by the child's physicians may be helpful if the cause of the hyperactivity is organic, particularly in the presence of poor impulse control and short attention span. The central nervous system stimulant methylphenidate (Ritalin) is effective in about 75% of cases, whereas dextroamphetamine (Dexedrine) is a good second choice. The effectiveness of these medications may be due to the release of the neurotransmitters norepinephrine and dopamine at some synapses. Other medications for attention-deficit disorder (ADD), clonidine (Catapres) and desipramine (Norpramin), have similar effects (Casey, 1989).

In a few cases the tranquilizers chlorpromazine (Thorazine) and thioridazine (Mellaril) may help reduce anxiety. The use of medication should be accompanied by special education, environmental control, and sometimes counseling.

Inattention or hyperactivity may be psychogenic, for example, due to either an emotional overlay secondary to a learning or physical problem, or an inconsistent child-rearing approach. In this case, the child is physically able to control his behavior but is preconditioned not to do so.

Management of inattentive behavior requires firmness, structure, and environmental controls. Reducing distractions, defining performance expectations clearly, and giving clear warnings of impending minor changes are helpful. Keeping an accurate daily record of the types and forerunners of inappropriate behavior in the home and classroom helps determine the cause of hyperactivity and the effectiveness of intervention procedures.

Behavior modification is currently widely used in the fields of education and psychology. It is a particularly useful method of managing hyperactive behavior of psychogenic origin and of bringing about improvement in specific behaviors. Performance is assessed first, and terminal goals or "behavioral objectives" are established. Positive rewards or reinforcements that are important to the child are determined so that they may be given after completion of each small step toward the goal. Negative or incorrect behaviors or performance are usually ignored and are rarely negatively reinforced by scolding or criticism. Primitive rewards are often edible. Interim rewards, such as paper tokens that can be traded in for treats or privileges, are more therapeutically desirable, and social rewards such as a handshake or a smile are the highest level. The frequency of rewarding is decreased as the child's performance improves.

During group therapy or classroom demonstration, mildly impaired school-aged children—even the very hyperactive—learn to sit quietly on their special spots waiting for the next activity to begin when they know the star they then receive can later be exchanged for free play time. They understand when newly performed activities are listed on an "I can do" sheet to take home. On individually written self-paced activity sheets, each step leading to correct pencil use or finding one's way around the school building, for example, can be checked off as it is mastered.

Consistency of expectations and rewards is important, especially when working with a group. Motivating and allowing a child to make the decision to cooperate has more positive results than trying to force conforming behavior. Having a child help establish his or her own goals often fosters cooperative behavior.

In a difficult-to-control group, it may be necessary to plan the same activities for all the children. In that case, formal structure or calming activities, at least at the beginning and end of the session, may be necessary to establish control.

This finely delineated sequence of steps might be helpful when working with more than one or two students simultaneously:

1. Have equipment ready and highly motivating activities planned (some will have been selected by the students).
2. Position children with enough space between them to perform the task.
3. Gain the undivided attention of the group.
4. Introduce equipment and wait until reaction subsides.
5. Briefly and clearly explain the task using three or fewer sequential directions.
6. Demonstrate.
7. Gain undivided attention.
8. Have one or all children demonstrate verbally or physically that they understood directions.
9. Gain undivided attention.
10. Signal start of task.
11. Continually reward appropriate performance verbally or with a pat, handshake, star, privilege, or other reward.
12. Conclude task specifically by change in positioning of children or equipment or by some other specific means. Avoid the temptation of rushing into a new activity before the children have had time to "change gears."

Learning stations

The experienced therapist may wish to make efficient use of time with a well-controlled group of mildly impaired children by using "*learning stations*" or "circuit training." At several positions around the room, equipment or activities are placed for use by one or two children. It is important for each unsupervised activity to provide its own feedback so the child knows whether it was performed correctly. ("Did the beanbags go in the can?" "Did you catch the ball?") Children change stations at their own volition, or as "the gong sounds," or as the therapist directs. With this method, all children are therapeutically engaged with activities or equipment that can be used by only one or two children at a time. The therapist stays with the station that is least safe or that needs to have feedback provided. Also, each child can be directed only to those particular stations within his or her treatment program. Classroom and physical education teachers are often experts in using this method and can be helpful models.

Curriculum materials

Curriculum materials written by occupational therapists and suitable for sharing with colleagues from other professions are beginning to emerge. Therapy or demonstration group activity suggestions for young school-aged children are available in Bissell et al. (1988) and Young (1988). Abrams and Kauffman (1990) provide activity suggestions intended for sharing with teachers of individual preschoolers or groups of preschoolers. The activities emphasize the use of toys, sensory integration, motor development, perception, and socialization. VORT Corporation is a publisher of curriculum materials (originally intended for educators of preschool and younger children), which can be suitably adapted by the occupational therapist (Santa Cruz County Office of Education, 1987). VORT also publishes helpful *Parent's Helper* books for sharing with individuals and groups of parents of children ages 1 to 5 and 5 to 10 (Shephard, 1981a, 1981b).

School occupational therapists are often called on by teachers and parents to offer advice, consultation, or direct therapy to improve handwriting. Considerable literature is developing in the field of occupational therapy to support therapists seeking such information (Benbow, 1989; Exner, 1986; Kauffman, 1990; Oliver, 1990; Schnick & Henderson, 1990). Program Planning Guidelines for treatment of mildly impaired early grade-school–aged children can be found on pages 728 to 739 of the 7th edition of this text.

Expanding the occupational therapist's role

In addition to seeking expertise in treating or consulting for various handicapping conditions, the therapist and occupational therapy assistant explore novel roles when appropriate. One therapist in a private high school for the learning disabled and language impaired expanded her role as prevocational therapist to include writing a textbook on work-related school programs, developing curriculum materials to promote work-related habits in the early elementary school years, fund-raising for high school job training equipment, proposal writing to apply for grants, and public relations (Balmuth, 1985; Jacobs, 1985). Another therapist designed a school's aquatics program to include functional learning experiences as well as basic swim instruction and increased adult supervision by importing a group of occupational therapy students to work as aides (Lottes & LaVesser, 1986).

Therapists seek opportunities to serve on committees to develop federal, state, and local policies and personnel standards for school programs for the handicapped.

Collaboration with other disciplines and membership on school curriculum development committees are also encouraged. On such committees therapists point out to others the unique contributions they are qualified to make within the total educational program while remaining open to opportunities for role release exchange with other educational professionals. *Role release* for the therapist involves encouraging classroom and other faculty members to carry out appropriate therapeutic activities, sometimes in conjunction with achieving IEP objectives. It helps the therapy become an integral rather than a peripheral part of the learning process. Occupational therapists may also carry out activities of speech, educational, or other professions in conjunction with their own therapeutic program (Brashear & Berger, 1987; Lyon & Lyon, 1980).

As increasing numbers of therapists become involved with funding and billing concerns, new funding approaches may make possible therapy positions not otherwise financially feasible in schools. For fee-for-service therapists, Medicaid or private insurance may cover not only direct therapy, but sometimes consultative or monitoring services in addition or instead, if either is deemed in the best interest of the child's total educational program. Billing and coding procedures must be employed (see Practice Management Information Corporation, 1991), and therapists must find out for each student whether such funding is available. In some cases documentation of "medical necessity" is required to receive third-party funding.

The well-prepared therapist keeps abreast of relevant books (Dunn, 1984, 1988, Muhlenhaupt, 1985) and journals (Blackman; Campbell; Kratoville; Maher; Senf and Wilhelm; Wiederholt) and publications of the American Occupational Therapy Association (1988, 1989, 1990, 1991). The therapist also acquires information regarding the organizational and legal idiosyncrasies of educational systems. Increasing involvement and professional contributions by therapists in local chapters, national conventions, and journal or newsletter publications of parent and professional organizations for individual handicapping conditions help to highlight for others the expanding role of the school therapist.

Research is an increasingly important role that school system occupational therapists must seek to validate the efficiency of occupational therapy as a service. The value of occupational therapy for helping children (especially for helping them achieve educational goals) is a controversial issue among some educators and physicians. Strongly worded adverse opinions have been published by Accardo (1980), Lehrer (1981), Sieben (1977), Silver (1975), and others (see also Hammill & Bartel, 1975). Carefully designed research studies must be shared with other therapists to broaden the profession's understanding of

treatment results. In addition, results shared with other medical and educational professionals and with parent organizations will open the door for wider acceptance of occupational therapy as an important contribution to the educational progress of the handicapped child.

References

Abrams, B., & Kauffman, N. (1990). *Toys and early childhood development: Selected guidelines for infants, toddlers, and preschoolers.* West Nyack, NY: Simon & Schuster.

Accardo, P. J. (1980). *A neurodevelopmental perspective on specific learning disabilities.* Baltimore: University Park Press.

American Guidance Service. (1985). *Important advances individually administered measures of intelligence, achievement and adaptive behavior.* Circle Pines, MN: Author.

American Occupational Therapy Association. (1988). *American Journal of Occupational Therapy, 42*(11 issue on occupational therapy in schools).

American Occupational Therapy Association. (1989). *Guidelines for occupational therapy services in early intervention.* Rockville, MD: Author.

American Occupational Therapy Association. (1990). *OT Week, 4*(36 issue on occupational in schools).

American Occupational Therapy Association. (1991). *Guidelines for occupational therapy in the school system* (2nd ed.). Rockville, MD: Author.

Ayres, A. J. (1984). *Sensory integration and praxis tests.* Los Angeles: Western Psychological Services.

Balmuth, D. (1985). A therapist with a working philosophy: Karen Jacobs. *Occupational Therapy News, 39*(5), 1.

Bateman, B. (1981). *So you're going to a hearing: Preparing for a Public Law 94–142 due process hearing.* Champaign, IL: Research Press.

Benbow, M. (1989). *Loops and other groups. A kinesthetic writing system.* Randolph, NJ: Occupational Therapy Ideas, Inc., 111 Shady Lane.

Bissell, J., Fisher J., Owens, C., & Polcyn, P. (1988). *Sensory motor handbook: A guide for implementing and modifying activities in the classroom.* Torrance, CA: Sensory Integration International.

Blackman, J. A. (Ed.). *Infants and young children.* Frederick, MD: Aspen Publishers.

Bluma, S., Schearer, M., Frohman, A., & Hilliard, J. (1985). *Portage guide to early education: Checklist.* Portage, WI: Portage Project CESA 12.

Brashear, R. N., & Berger, P. N. (1987). Interdisciplinary collaboration in a school sensory integration program. *Sensory Integration Special Interest Section Newsletter, 10*(1), 1–2.

Bruininks, R. (1978). *Bruininks-Oseretsky Test of Motor Proficiency.* Circle Pines, MN: American Guidance Service.

Campbell, S. K., & Wilhelm, I. J. (Eds.). *Physical and occupational therapy in pediatrics.* 10 Alice Street, Binghamton, NY, 13904: The Haworth Press.

Carbo, M. (1987). Matching reading styles: Correcting ineffective instruction. In *Educational Leadership,* October, p. 57.

Carr, S. H. (1989). Public school practice is alive and well. *Occupational Therapy Forum,* February 27, 1989.

Casey, T. (1989). *Clinical response to medications for attention deficit disorder.* Rosemont, PA (Prepared public address. Copies available from the author of this chapter).

Chandler, B. (1990). Fee-for-service: A new reality. *OT Week, 4*(36), 9.

Child Protection Congress. (1990). *OT Week, 4*(27).

Clark, F., Mailloux, Z., & Parham, D. (1981). *The art of therapy.* Pasadena CA: Sensory Integration International.

Connoley, J. C., & Kramer, J. J. (Eds.). (1989). *Mental measurements yearbook* (10th ed.). Lincoln, NB: University of Nebraska Press.

Cornman Diagnostic Center learning disabilities checklist for kindergarten and 1st grade (2nd ed.). (1975). Philadelphia: The School

District of Philadelphia (out of print; available from the author of this chapter).

Davidson, J. E. (1980). Ways in which occupational therapy involves the community in treatment. *World Federation of Occupational Therapists Bulletin, 5,* 18–20.

Dunn, W. (1981). *A guide to testing clinical observations in kindergarteners.* Rockville, MD: American Occupational Therapy Association Products.

Dunn, W. (1984). *Initiating occupational therapy programs within the school system: A guide for occupational therapists and public school administrators.* Chicago, IL: Slack.

Dunn, W. (1988). *Pediatric management in occupational therapy: Decision making toward the service delivery process.* Chicago, IL: Slack.

Dunn, W. (1989). Occupational therapy in early intervention: New perspectives create greater possibilities. *American Journal of Occupational Therapy, 43,* 717–721.

Exner, C. (Ed.). (1986, September). *Developmental Disabilities Special Interest Section Newsletter, 9*(3 entire issue on handwriting).

Flynn, S. (1980). Pediatric care in occupational therapy in Ireland. *World Federation of Occupational Therapists Bulletin, 5,* 9–13.

Fox, S. (1990) Therapy express: Schools solve space crunch. *Advance for Occupational Therapists, 6*(20), 1–2

Gardner, H. (1983). *Frames of mind.* New York: Basic Books.

Gilfoyle, E. M. (1980). *Training: Occupational therapy educational management in schools.* OSERS Grant #G007801499. Rockville MD: American Occupational Therapy Association.

Greenhouse, L. (1982). Schools backed on limiting aid to handicapped. *New York Times,* June, 29, p. 1.

Guild, P. B., & Garger, S. (1985). *Marching to different drummers.* Alexandria, VA: Association for Supervision and Curriculum Development.

Hammill, D. D. (1975). Thoughts to consider before beginning a visual perception program. In D. D. Hammill & N. R. Bartel (Eds.), *Teaching children with learning and behavior* problems. Boston: Allyn & Bacon.

Hanft, B. E. (Ed.). (1989). *Family centered care: An early intervention resource manual.* Rockville: American Occupational Therapy Association.

Jacobs, K. (1985). *Occupational therapy: Work-related programs and assessments.* Boston: Little, Brown, & Co.

Kauffman, N. (1990) *Handwriting hints.* Unpublished curriculum guide. Available from the author of this chapter.

Kielhofner, G., & Knight, H. (1989). In E. J. Brown (Ed.), Survey targets areas of improvement in school-based occupational therapy. *Advance for Occupational Therapists, 5*(39), 1–2.

King-Thomas, L., & Hacker, B. (Eds.). (1987). *Therapist's guide to pediatric assessment.* Boston: Little Brown & Co.

Kratoville, B. L. (Ed.). *Academic therapy.* 20 Commercial Boulevard, Novato CA: Academic Therapy Publications, Inc.

Lehrer, R. J. (1981). An open letter to an occupational therapist. *Journal of Learning Disabilities, 14,* 3–4.

Leopold, R. L. (1966). *The techniques of consultation: Some thoughts for the occupational therapist.* Norristown, PA: Presentation before Eastern Pennsylvania Occupational Therapy Association.

Lerner, J., Mardel-Czudnowski, & Goldenberg, D. (1987). *Special education for the early childhood years* (2nd ed., pp. 302–331). Englewood Cliffs, NJ: Prentice-Hall.

Llorens, L. A., & Seig, K. W. (1975). A profile for managing sensory integrative test data. *American Journal of Occupational Therapy, 29,* 205.

Lottes, L., & LaVesser, P. (1986). Occupational therapists design children's aquatics program. *Occupational Therapy News, 40*(4), 8.

Lyon, S., & Lyon, G. (1980). Team functioning and staff development: A role release approach to providing integrated educational services for severely handicapped students. *Journal of the Association for the Severely Handicapped, 5,* 250–263.

Maher, C. S. (Ed.). *Special services in the schools.* Binghamton, NY: Haworth Press.

Mancuso, E., Rieser, L., & Stotland, J. F. (1990). *The right To special education in Pennsylvania: A guide for parents.* Philadelphia: The Education Law Center.

Manes, J. (1985). Education for handicapped children now includes preschoolers. *The Mental Health Law Project's update on developments in law and policy of concern to mentally disabled children, 5,* 4–5, 1–2.

Mastrangelo, R., & Colan., B. J. (1990). Integrated models use natural environments as teaching settings . . . but redefining roles can be scary. *Advance for Occupational Therapists,* August 27, 1990.

Miller, L. (1982). *Miller Assessment for Preschoolers.* Denver: Kid Technology, Inc.

Muhlenhaupt, M. (1985). *Occupational therapy in New York State public schools: A reference guide for therapists, educators and administrators.* Northport, NY: The Press Room at TMC.

National Easter Seal Society (1991). *Americans with disabilities act: An easy checklist.* Chicago: Author.

Oliver, C. E., (1990). A sensorimotor program for improving writing readiness skills in elementary-age children. *American Journal of Occupational Therapy, 44*(2), 111–116.

Practice Management Information Corporation. (1991). *ICD-9-CM: International classification of diseases* (9th ed., 3rd ed., vols. 1, 2, 3). Clinical Modification. Los Angeles: Author.

President Reagan Signs P.L. 99–457, the Education for Handicapped Amendments of 1986. (1986). *Government and Legal Affairs Division Bulletin.* Rockville, MD: American Occupational Therapy Association.

Rehnquist, W. H. (1982). Excerpts from Justices' opinions in case of a deaf girl and school district. *New York Times,* June 29, p. B4.

Rourk, J. D. (1985). School therapy task force recommends guidelines. *Occupational Therapy News, 39*(11), 5.

Royeen, C. B. (Ed.). (1990). *School based practice for related services.* Rockville: American Occupational Therapy Association.

Santa Cruz County Office of Education. (1987). *Help for special preschoolers: Ages 3 to 6.* Palo Alto, CA: VORT Corporation.

Schleifer, M. (Ed.). *The exceptional parent.* 1170 Commonwealth Aveo, Third Floor, Boston, MA, 02134.

Schnick, C. M., & Henderson, A. (1990). Descriptive analysis of the developmental progression of grip progression for pencil and crayon control in nondysfunctional 3-and 4-year-old children. *American Journal of Occupational Therapy, 44*(10), 893.

Shephard, L. (1981a). *Parent's helper: For parents of children ages 1–5.* Palo Alto, CA: VORT Corporation.

Shephard, L. (1981b). *Parent's helper: For parents of children ages 5–10.* Palo Alto, CA: VORT Corporation.

Sieben, R. L. (1977). Controversial medical treatments of learning disabilities. *Academic Therapy, 13,* 133–147.

Silver, L. B. (1975). Acceptable and controversial approaches to treating the child with learning disabilities. *Pediatrics, 55,* 406.

Sternat, J., Nietupski, J., Lyon, J., Messina, R., & Brown, L. (1980). *Occupational and physical therapy services for severely handicapped students: Integrated vs isolated therapy models.* Federal Contract No. CEC-0-74-7993. Madison, WI: Madison Public Schools.

Waugh, K. W., & Bush, W. J. (1971). *Diagnosing learning disorders.* Columbus, OH: Charles Merrill.

Wendt, W. (1984). I'm glad you asked. *Occupational Therapy Newspaper, 40*(8), 5.

Wiederholt, J. L. (Ed.) *Journal of Learning Disabilities.* 8700 Shoalcreek Blvd., Austin, TX, 78758: Donald D. Hammill Foundation.

Young, S. (1988). *Movement is fun.* Torrance, CA: Sensory Integration International.

CHAPTER 26

Adult day care

LORY P. OSORIO

KEY TERMS

Individual Plan of Care
Medical/Restorative Model
   Centers
Milieu

Occupational Therapy
   Roles
Respite
Social Model Centers

LEARNING OBJECTIVES

Upon completion of this chapter the reader will be able to:

1. *Describe the key elements of a quality adult day care center.*
2. *Discuss the relationship among participant needs, models of care, and services provided.*
3. *Describe the common values of occupational therapy and adult day care.*
4. *Compare and contrast direct and indirect service roles for occupational therapists in restorative and social model centers.*

Adult day care is a new service option for frail and impaired adults and their caregivers. More than 2100 centers nationwide (National Institute on Adult Daycare [NAID], 1990) provide an alternative to in-home and institutional care for those with functional impairments due to dementia, cerebrovascular accident and other neurologic diseases, psychiatric disorders, cardiac and respiratory diseases, and other chronic illnesses. Although most adult day care centers serve older adults, a growing number of specialized centers are available that target younger adults with physical disabilities, the mentally retarded and developmentally disabled, persons with symptomatic human immunodeficiency virus (HIV) infection, those with mental health needs, and other special need groups.

Definition

Adult day care centers provide outpatient services in a congregate or group setting for less than 24 hours a day. Centers are typically open 8 to 12 hours a day to accommodate the needs of working caregivers. Although most centers operate 5 days a week, the trend toward 7-day-per-week service promises more flexibility in scheduling those who attend part-time and more short-term, intermittent care, or ***respite***, options for caregivers; many attend full-time because they function better in the supportive and predictable day care environment.

Whatever the attendance schedule, program participants come to the center on a planned rather than drop-in basis. Although the length of stay varies, involvement in day care for several years is not uncommon, especially when the service is used as an alternative to residential long-term care. Growing corporate interest in adult day care as a support for employees suggests continued expansion of the day care day and week to accommodate various shifts and flexible time schedules.

Adult day care clients are commonly called "participants" to reflect the orientation toward activity and purposefulness that are characteristic of adult day care and to emphasize the healthy aspects of the person whom the program strives to nurture.

Adult day care programs and the daily routine in most centers are organized around purposeful activities, reflecting both the lifelong interests of participants and their continuing need for new experiences, appropriate stimulation, and a sense of community with peers. Small group activities are the norm, with concurrent groups for those with varied abilities and interests. Self-care and professional services are ideally provided in an informal, nonintrusive manner to maintain a homelike, rather than clinical, human and nonhuman environment, or **milieu**.

Although the participant is the primary focus of the adult day care program, services are also provided for caregivers to assist them in their role. Support groups, educational classes, consultation on home care and home safety, counseling, and referral for other services help family members to develop skills and manage the stress of caregiving.

Services provided

The mix of services available in an adult day care center depends on two variables: the model of care that underlies the philosophy and program emphasis of the individual center and the needs of the participants and caregivers. Centers vary considerably in their program emphasis, creating a diversity across centers that is regarded as unique in the long-term care field and a significant contributor to their success in meeting the varied and changing needs of participants (Kelly & Webb, 1989). This diversity can best be conceptualized as a continuum with **social model centers** serving frail or at-risk, but semi-independent participants on one end and **medical/restorative model centers** on the other, serving significantly impaired participants who would likely be in institutional care if not for the adult day care program (Osorio, 1991). Medical/restorative model centers may be called day treatment, day hospital, or medical day care, a reflection of their ability to provide short-term, intensive services to those who need acute or restorative care or both. Depending on the center's position on the social–medical/restorative continuum, the service mix available includes one or more of the following types of care:

1. *Basic*—meals, transportation, recreation, and personal care (dressing, grooming and toileting)
2. *Professional*—nursing, social services, occupational therapy, physical therapy, and speech therapy
3. *Medical*—physical assessment and treatment, dentistry, podiatry, and psychiatry

Basic and professional services are provided in more than 90% of centers, with basic services provided by staff and professional services provided either in-house or by contract (Von Behren, 1988).

Services provided for an individual participant are based on a functional assessment and are developed through an interdisciplinary care planning process that may be well defined and regulated in states where adult day care centers are licensed or certified. Interdisciplinary functioning of staff is one of the key elements of a successful adult day care program, allowing for flexibility and collaboration in meeting participants' complex and interrelated needs (NIAD, 1990). Care plans are commonly problem oriented and cover in detail goals, activities, time frame, and responsible staff. The participant or caregiver or both may be involved in developing the **individual plan of care**. Coordination with other agencies and providers is essential when the adult day care participant is also receiving in-home or outpatient services.

Day care center services are designed to meet one or more of the following goals:

1. Promote the person's maximum level of independence.
2. Maintain the person's present level of functioning as long as possible, preventing or delaying further deterioration.
3. Restore and rehabilitate the person to the highest possible level of functioning.
4. Provide support, respite, and education for families and other caregivers.
5. Foster socialization and peer interaction (National Council on Aging, 1984).

Decisions about whether adult day care is or continues to be an appropriate service are based on whether the person's abilities and needs are congruent with the services available. Because of the congregate nature of adult day care, it is also important to consider how the person makes an impact on the center milieu since the program emphasizes the sense of community that develops when groups of participants work together through purposeful activity to achieve individual goals. Although most day care centers serve participants with diverse abilities and needs, those who are disruptive or who are so impaired that they require constant one-to-one care are generally not seen as appropriate day care clients except in very specialized programs.

Day care and occupational therapy

If the values and approaches of adult day care seem congruent with occupational therapy practice, the similarities are not accidental. Adult day care centers in the United States are modeled on the day hospital movement developed in England in the 1950s when day services were housed in occupational therapy departments and, although multidisciplinary, were heavily influenced by occupational therapists (O'Brien, 1982). Like occupational therapy, adult day care emphasizes individual potential for growth and development, even in the face of disability, as well as a holistic integration of mental, physical, social, emotional, spiritual, and environmental aspects of well-being (National Council on the Aging, 1984). Values underlying the practice of occupational therapy including productivity, self-directedness, active participation, the value of play and leisure, faith in the patient's potential, and concern for his or her essential humanity are prominent in adult day care philosophy and practice as well (Yerxa, 1983).

Roles for occupational therapists

Occupational therapy roles vary according to the emphasis of the day care center and may involve direct services such as evaluation and treatment, or indirect services including consultation and education.

In centers with a restorative emphasis, the occupational therapist or certified occupational therapy assistant (COTA) provides a comprehensive assessment of the participant's cognitive, sensorimotor, and psychosocial skills including functional performance of self-care, work, and leisure roles (American Occupational Therapy Association, 1986b). Assessment should also include a home evaluation and assessment and modification of the day care center to maximize performance and the participant's sense of mastery and control of the environment. Assessment may lead to actual treatment or to design of a structured program to be carried out by center staff (AOTA, 1986a).

In social/supportive centers the emphasis is on maintenance of skills and adaptation to impairment. Group approaches are used to build social relationships and provide opportunities for achievement and success. Occupational therapists can be effective consultants to social model programs in the areas of activity adaptation, environmental design, group process, and training of paraprofessional staff.

Other indirect service roles are center administrator, educator and researcher (AOTA, 1986b), and board member. As center administrator, an occupational therapist can be responsible for all aspects of agency operation. Given the philosophy of adult day care, occupational therapists with management skills are ideally suited for center administrator positions. Educator roles can include such diverse activities as teaching stress management to caregivers, providing in-service education for day care staff, and supervising field work students. Research opportunities abound in day care centers in such areas as evaluating the effectiveness of center services and studying long-term outcomes of the rehabilitation, which frequently precedes adult day care referral. Most adult day care centers have either policy-making or advisory boards in which the perspective of an occupational therapist can be helpful in setting priorities and policy to guide the program. Since board appointments are volunteer positions, they are a logical choice for therapists who work in other settings yet want to support and influence the day care program.

The following case study illustrates the use of occupational therapy in the adult day care setting.

CASE STUDY

Mrs. R. is a 79-year-old retired retail clerk who came to adult day care after a cerebrovascular accident (CVA) with resulting left hemiparesis. She received inpatient rehabilitation at a local hospital and several home health visits from occupational therapy and physical therapy before she was discharged for lack of progress. She lives with her husband who is several years younger and still employed. Two daughters live 3 to 4 hours away. On admission to adult day care, Mrs. R. was semidependent in all activities of daily living (ADL). She was able to feed herself with positioning, much encouragement, and close observation for choking and pocketing food. She was suspicious of most food and had lost more than 10 pounds just before admission. She needed maximal assistance with dressing, bathing, and toileting. Ambulation was with a quad cane, guarding, and verbal coaching. She was depressed, disoriented to time and place, and often thought small children were living out in the yard.

Mrs. R. began attending adult day care 6 days per week to support her husband's continued employment and to provide him with a day of respite. Mrs. R. has blossomed in the day care milieu. She received additional physical therapy from the center's contract therapist and ambulates with more confidence and less confusion, although she still requires her quad cane and staff assistance. The center occupational therapist evaluated her eating skills and developed a program that is carried out by paraprofessional staff. Mrs. R. now feeds herself with minimal encouragement and help.

The center registered nurse monitors her blood pressure and blood glucose levels regularly and administers seven medications throughout the day. Paraprofessional staff members implement a scheduled voiding program and take walks with her at intervals during the day.

Mrs. R.'s mental status has improved significantly with the structured and supportive day care routine. She continues to be disoriented as to time and place but is relaxed and trusting of staff. Mrs. R. frequently expresses her dry sense of humor, joins in physical games such as bilateral ball activities and musical activities, and enjoys the one-to-one companionship of several other women.

Her husband attends the family support group and has received encouragement from staff to ask his daughters for help with doctor's appointments and housework, which has relieved his stress significantly.

Mr. and Mrs. R. and their daughters agree that adult day care has improved the quality of Mrs. R.'s life and that of her family caregivers. She looks forward to the activities, companionship, and support that the center provides, and Mr. R. goes to work knowing she is happy and well cared for.

Summary

Adult day care provides a variety of services for impaired adults in a group setting during the day. Support for caregivers is also an important aspect of center services, since the overall goal of adult day care is to assist the participant to continue living in the community at the highest level of independence possible. Varied roles are available for occupational therapists and certified occupational therapy assistants who share the adult day care philosophy, which values a holistic approach to well-being for those with functional impairment.

Future

Demand for adult day care is likely to grow as the United States population ages and as increasing numbers of younger adults live in the community with significant disability that requires continuing care.

Cost containment efforts will accelerate during the coming decades as growing numbers of dependent adults and a shrinking pool of workers force utilization of labor-efficient, low-cost services. Adult day care is ideally situated for this future scenario with its low technology, high touch, congregate approach.

References

American Occupational Therapy Association. (1986a). Occupational therapy in adult daycare. *American Journal of Occupational Therapy, 40*(12), 814–816.

American Occupational Therapy Association. (1986b). Roles and functions of occupational therapy in adult daycare. *American Journal of Occupational Therapy, 40*(12), 817–821.

Kelly, W., & Webb, L. (1989). The development of adult daycare in America. In L. Cook (Ed.), *Planning and managing adult daycare*. Owings Mills, MD: National Health Publishing.

National Institute on Adult Daycare. (1990). *Standards and guidelines for adult daycare.* Washington, DC: Author.

National Council on the Aging. (1984). *Standards for adult daycare.* Washington, DC: Author.

O'Brien, C. L. (1982). *Adult day care: A practical guide.* Monterey, CA: Jones Bartlett Publishing Co.

Osorio, L. P. (1991). Adult daycare programs. In J. M. Kiernat (Ed.), *Occupational therapy and the older adult* (pp. 241–258). Gaithersburg, MD: Aspen Publications.

Von Behren, R. (1988). *Adult daycare: A program of services for the functionally impaired.* Washington, DC: National Council for the Aging.

Yerxa, E. J. (1983). Audacious values: The energy source for occupational therapy practice. In G. Kielhofner (Ed.), *Health through occupation: Theory and practice in occupational therapy.* Philadelphia: F. A. Davis.

Bibliography

Goldston, S. (1989). *Adult daycare: A basic guide.* Owings Mills, MD: National Health Publishing.

Webb, L. (1989). *Planning and managing adult daycare: Pathways to success.* Owings Mills, MD: National Health Publishing.

Von Behren, R. (1986). *Adult daycare in America: Summary of a national survey.* Washington, DC: National Council on the Aging.

CHAPTER 27

Long-term care

CYNTHIA F. EPSTEIN

KEY TERMS

Consultation

Disease Prevention and
   Health Promotion

Institutional Services

LTC Constituency

LTC Continuum

Macroenvironment

Microenvironment

Multilevel System

Omnibus Budget
   Reconciliation Act
   of 1987

Resident Assessment
   Instrument

Quality of Life

LEARNING OBJECTIVES

Upon completion of this chapter the reader will be able to:

1. *Recognize the varied constituency of the long-term care (LTC) environment.*
2. *Identify the long-term care continuum.*
3. *Describe the range of institutional settings.*
4. *Analyze the macroenvironmental forces impinging on the long-term care facility and its occupational therapy provider.*
5. *Understand the microenvironmental forces that can be joined to empower the resident.*
6. *Identify multilevel opportunities available to occupational therapy within the LTC environment.*

A revolution has taken place in long-term care! Institutional walls are no longer the boundaries and "care" is about health, well-being, and empowerment rather than sickness, depression, and dependency. Public policy, health care advocates, consumers and caregivers, and providers and funders have incorporated occupational therapy's focus on function and its perspective on enablement. A predominant, advocacy-oriented constituency of older consumers and their caregivers has been joined by younger persons with disabilities and those with life-threatening conditions such as AIDS (Born, 1991). In our rapidly evolving, technologically exploding society, this newly forged constituency group seeks expanded options in the long-term care environment.

Long-term care (LTC) is defined as "an array of services needed by individuals who have lost some capacity for independence because of a chronic illness or condition" (Pepper Commission, 1990, p. 90). These persons require some form of assistance with activities of daily living (ADL) and may also need skilled treatment for their conditions. Services may be provided in the person's home (as in home health care), in the community (as in adult day care), or in an institution (a developmental center or nursing home) (Pepper Commission, 1990). A broad and pervasive issue, LTC affects family ties and caregiving; places demands on personal and family resources; requires expanded medical, therapeutic, and social service interventions; and mandates options to help people live in the least restrictive home environment.

Constituency and continuum

Between 9 and 11 million Americans are chronically disabled, according to a recent report (Figures 27-1 and 27-2). Most (over 7 million) are 65 and over. One million children account for a startling one third of those requiring LTC (Pepper Commission, 1990). Until recently, America's health care system did not recognize this broad-ranging **LTC constituency**. The common perception was that consumers of LTC were all older adults, and their health care costs skewed our national budget. Support for

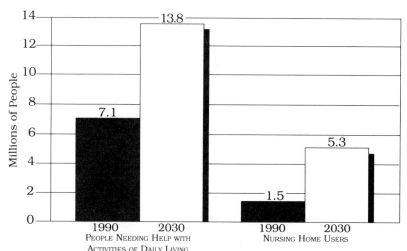

FIGURE 27-1. *Number of elderly needing long-term care, 1990 and 2030. (Copyright by and reprinted with permission of the National Council on the Aging, Inc., 409 Third Street SW, Washington, DC 20024.)*

(From: The Pepper Commission. Data for 1990 from Lewin/ICF estimates using the Brookings/ICF Long-Term Care Financing Model: for 2030. Sheila Zedlewski, et al., (1990). *The Needs of the elderly in the 21st century* Washington DC: The Urban Institute.)

expanding LTC services was viewed with a jaundiced eye, while visions of nursing home scandals and snake pits came to mind. Today, there is growing recognition that health care services and funding strategies must change (Castro, 1991; Estes, 1990; Pepper Commission, 1990). LTC has become an important part of the call for universal health care coverage.

The **LTC continuum** is now recognized as a **multilevel system** that must offer varied options for diverse consumers and their caregivers (National Council on the Aging, 1988). Strategies for **disease prevention and health promotion** have surfaced with increasing regularity (Abdellah, 1988). Estes suggests that "[America's health care system] should provide a full continuum of LTC services, both medically and socially oriented, with a goal of maximizing functional independence and preventing illness and disability" (1990, p. 6).

Demographics of the many populations requiring LTC ser-

vices have been extensively described in other chapters in this text. Each practice environment discussed has linkages to the LTC continuum. Each can be viewed from a health promotion and disease prevention frame of reference, with opportunities for the provision of services at primary, secondary, and tertiary levels of care (Johnson & Jaffe, 1989). Within each level, registered occupational therapists (OTRs) and certified occupational therapy assistants (COTAs) identify and assume varied roles as they work toward maximizing the functional independence of clients and their support networks.

At the tertiary level, the practice environment is institutionally based. This setting is often narrowly defined as a nursing facility. In fact, **institutional services** can include "independent living centers, foster care, board and care, assisted living, residential care facilities, nursing homes, state hospitals, chronic care hospitals and rehabilitation facilities" (Estes, 1990, p. 6).

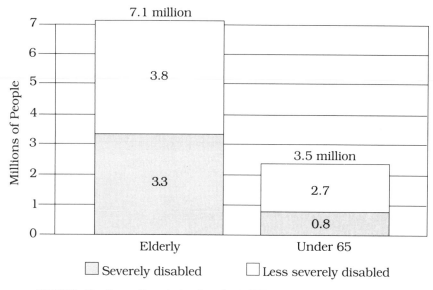

FIGURE 27-2. *People needing long-term care, including the severely disabled, by age. (Copyright by and reprinted with permission of the National Council on the Aging, Inc., 409 Third Street SW, Washington, DC 20024.)*

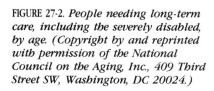

SOURCE: The Pepper Commission, from Lewin/ICF estimates using Brookings/ICF Long-Term Care Financing Model and 1987 National Medical Expenditure Survey.

Within these many environments, occupational therapy practitioners provide medically, socially, and educationally oriented services. Their goal is not only to achieve functional independence for clients or patients but also to prevent illness and disability. To accomplish this, occupational therapy practice roles often include advocacy-oriented and consultative components (Jaffe & Epstein, 1992).

These diverse settings constitute systems within the larger LTC system. Each setting may be analyzed in regard to its ability to facilitate independence and inclusion within the larger community, thus moving people from more restrictive to less restrictive environments and from tertiary to secondary or primary levels of prevention.

To provide services in this multilevel system, occupational therapy practitioners must have a basic understanding of macro- and microenvironmental forces impinging on a given institution. These environments and the forces within them are examined in this chapter. Through this process an expanded conceptual framework will be developed, which includes multiple LTC occupational therapy service delivery models within and outside institutional walls.

The macroenvironment

The **macroenvironment** consists of forces that shape opportunities and pose threats to the specific long-term care system. These forces are demographic, economic, political, technologic, natural, and cultural environments.

Demographic environment

As noted in Chapter 19, the number of older adults has grown at a much faster rate than that of the rest of the population, and future projections estimate that the 32 million adults over 65 in 1990 will double by the year 2030. Those considered to be the *oldest old*—85 and over—may increase fivefold in the same time period. If estimates are correct, 13.8 million older adults will then require LTC, and 40% will reside within institutions (Pepper Commission, 1990). In 1988, 9 of 10 LTC residents were adults 65 and over, and 50% of these were 85 or over. Women account for 75% of the nursing home population. Problems faced by many of these female residents are incontinence, depression, osteoporosis resulting in poor healing after hip fracture, and chronic pain.

Forty-one percent of the nation's severely disabled reside in nursing facilities. Severe disability is defined in terms of ADL function. Those needing personal assistance with at least three out of five self-care ADL, those requiring substantial supervision due to cognitive impairment, and those demonstrating disruptive or dangerous behaviors that impede function are considered severely disabled (Pepper Commission, 1990).

Persons diagnosed with senile dementia of the Alzheimer type (SDAT) are a growing nursing home population. About 2.5% of currently institutionalized elderly are diagnosed with SDAT, and most are over 75 years of age (Baum, 1991).

Other special populations, such as those with traumatic brain injury (TBI), those with AIDS, and children who are dependent on technology to sustain life, are not statistically categorized in the Pepper Commission Report but are acknowledged as growing institutional constituencies.

Occupational therapy personnel are in constant demand to provide services for this expanding population. Recent data indicate that more than 20% of all employed COTAs and 6.4% of all OTRs work in nursing facilities (AOTA Research Information & Evaluation Division, 1991). That is a small percentage working for a large constituency!

Economic environment

Expenditures for LTC have been skewed in favor of those residing in nursing facilities. Although 84% of those requiring LTC services reside in the community, the 16% residing in institutions received 82% of the funds. Of the $43.1 billion spent for nursing home care, almost 50% of the cost was borne by consumers or their families.

Medicaid, a federal-state entitlement program, accounts for 90% of all public spending for nursing home care, whereas Medicare, a federally funded program, constitutes a negligible portion of support (Somers, 1991). In regard to reimbursement for occupational therapy services, Medicare funds constitute our major reimbursement source (Faust & Meaker, 1991). Facilities welcome our services and appreciate their value in regard to improving resident function and expanding staff knowledge.

Reimbursement under Medicare is problem specific and time limited and must meet stringent criteria (Moon-Sperling & Pinson, 1991). **Consultation**, an indirect service, is not reimbursable under Medicare but may be selectively supported through Medicaid. Thirty-one states and the District of Columbia provide Medicaid coverage for occupational therapy services in nursing facilities, according to a 1988 survey (Somers, 1991).

The economic environment must also consider reimbursement through the patient or family. Under Medicare regulations, a coinsurance factor exists, and users of occupational therapy service must be billed for this coinsurance. Prevention has become increasingly important to patients and families, and they may wish to purchase occupational therapy services privately. For example, a patient who is wheelchair bound and at risk for skin breakdown may benefit from an occupational therapy prescription for a supportive and pressure-responsive seating system.

The passage and implementation of the **Omnibus Budget Reconciliation Act of 1987** (OBRA '87) have also had significant economic implications for occupational therapy practice (Health Care Financing Administration, 1989). This law recognizes that in a nursing facility the resident's **quality of life** is of primary importance. It requires assessment of each resident from a functional perspective and identification of interventions to ameliorate dysfunction. During the law's first year of implementation, requests for occupational therapy services escalated. Facilities started to look, through the eyes of the OBRA mandate, at such important quality of life issues as restraints, ADL self-care, cognitive loss and dementia, and rehabilitation potential (Moon-Sperling & Pinson, 1991).

Political environment

The political environment must consider laws, government agencies, and pressure groups that may influence services in long-term care facilities. Occupational therapy practitioners must maintain awareness of law changes that affect LTC, the role played by government and credentialing agencies, and the importance of advocacy groups who work to affect change.

Legislation plays a critical role in LTC, particularly within nursing facilities. From a federal perspective, the OBRA '87 regulations will continue to play a major role in directing service delivery. On a federal–state level, interest has been increasing in Medicaid Waiver Programs. These programs seek to provide broader options that enable states to cover more skilled services so that severely disabled persons may avoid institutionalization (Born, 1991).

OBRA, for example, has implemented a nationwide assessment tool to periodically measure the functional performance of each nursing home resident and to identify problem areas that may be amenable to intervention. Known as the ***Resident Assessment Instrument*** (RAI), its use has created a greater need and demand for occupational therapy services (Morris, Hawes, Murphy, & Nonemaker, 1991).

Nursing homes constitute big business. This law illustrates government response to the concerns of consumers in need of nursing home placement—for either a brief or an undetermined time. Through the RAI, a broad national data base is being developed, giving a more realistic consumer picture. Comprehensive and specific care plans will also be generated, thus protecting the consumer's right to quality care. Society's interests can also be addressed as we plan for more universal health care and use these data to make informed decisions.

Technologic environment

Technology is the wonder child of the health care environment and has made significant contributions to persons with disabilities. In the LTC institutional environment, "high technology" is often called on to sustain life, and "low technology" is called on to help residents increase life functioning.

Occupational therapy LTC practitioners need to keep abreast of both levels of technology as they seek options for their severely disabled patients. As technology advances, not only in the biotechnologic field but in the world of electronics and robotics, institutionalized residents may be candidates for less restrictive living environments in the community.

Natural environment

Ecologists view the natural environment from the perspective of natural resources. In long-term care the natural environment can be considered the space in which the person routinely performs ADL and community living skills. For the older adult, this environment is predominantly their community residence and places of social interaction.

In defining "institutions," we spoke of varied living settings, some more restrictive than others. Occupational therapy practitioners must be aware of these multiple options for institutional living when considering and implementing interventions. Today's supportive living environments offer many opportunities for increased independence. Independent living centers, for example, allow younger disabled persons to reside in their own apartments, with caregiver help on a scheduled basis.

Life care communities offer older adults a range of environments within the same geographic location. Starting out, residents live in a hotel-like setting, which provides one, two, or three meals a day, and other services such as housekeeping, and 24-hour on-call emergency services. An assisted living setting is also part of the life care complex. Here, some personal ADL care and increased nursing supervision are provided. Finally, the life care community provides a full nursing home service for its members when needed.

Spouses, children, and extended families constitute a major aspect of the older adult's natural environment, and studies indicate that the major burden of caregiving falls on their shoulders (Baum, 1991; Pepper Commission, 1990). Families are a vital part of the LTC continuum and they can be the motivating force behind returning the older adult to the community rather than continuing residence within the institution.

Occupational therapy providers can use their knowledge of natural environments to more effectively forecast long-range goals for their patients. Recognizing the power of these environmental forces, the practitioner is able to develop a plan that is responsive to each patient's needs.

Cultural environment

The occupational therapy practitioner must also understand cultural environments existing in the community. Each institution serves a geographic region from which residents and their caregivers are drawn. Cultural influences are reflected in the values, perceptions, preferences, and behaviors of various groups of people within the community. LTC institutions within the same community may tend to draw persons whose cultural heritage is strongly biased in one direction, and the caregiver work force may be coming from a very different cultural background. Unless some commonality of values and beliefs exists between these groups, the chances of establishing a supportive and enabling environment are significantly limited.

Occupational therapy recognizes that culture plays an important role in treatment practice (Hopkins & Tiffany, 1983). In LTC institutional environments, where many older residents have culturally diverse backgrounds, the institution and those within it may be viewed with distrust and apprehension. Awareness of the cultures, traditions, health practices, and languages of resident and caregiver populations will enable practitioners to deliver more effective services (McCormack, Llorens, & Glogoski, 1991)

Using a macroenvironmental perspective, the occupational therapy practitioner enters the ***microenvironment***, the institution, with a broad base of information. This helps further identify concerns within the specific setting.

The microenvironment

Occupational therapy program implementation in any given nursing facility must consider key elements that make an impact on the environment:

- The facility's internal structure
- The structure of the occupational therapy service
- A collaborative environment
- The funding environment
- Publics who have an interest in or impact on service delivery

Facility

Ownership of the facility must be considered. The facility may be sponsored by federal, state, county, or local governments, or it may be a profit-making or nonprofit organization. Most nursing facilities are proprietary or profit-making organizations. Ownership often determines the level of support that occupational therapy can expect for its special projects, such as positioning and seating. For example, wheelchairs, a key factor in out-of-bed seating, are expensive; specialized chairs, even more so. A nonprofit home, which has a wider base of community support, can obtain donations for such equipment more readily than a proprietary home.

Knowledge of the overall *organizational structure* helps build communication, to identify key people within the system, and to develop strategies for team building. In the seating and positioning example, occupational therapy providers might identify the need for a wheelchair management system to ensure appropriate seating of all residents. This would be of particular assistance to the facility considering OBRA regulations, in which restraints are an issue. To plan and carry out such a program, an in-depth understanding of the organizational system is needed.

Occupational therapy

Most often, the occupational therapy service is understaffed and overutilized. Occupational therapists and COTAs are frequently less than full-time and often are "outside contractors." When these circumstances exist, the occupational therapy staff must work even more diligently to obtain system support and carryover for the patient treatment plans and specialized programs that they implement.

Occupational therapy providers must take time to treat the system as well as the patient. Informal lines of communication become an important avenue for gaining support and carryover. A casual discussion at coffee break time regarding the importance of mealtime socialization may help the staff to understand and support placement of a patient in the facility dining room.

For example, an occupational therapist works on self-feeding skills with a patient who had all her meals delivered by tray service to her room. She became more independent, but was afraid to try eating her meals in the dining room. Staff awareness of the importance of socialization would help occupational therapy develop support for the patient's placement in the dining room.

Collaboration

A *collaborative environment* must be developed to ensure a smooth-functioning, goal-oriented team, working toward enablement of each resident. Such collaboration must include the occupational therapy department, other key departments in the facility, the resident, and family.

Two of the facility's largest departments play key roles in occupational therapy service delivery: the nursing and the dietary departments. Occupational therapy's important role in ADL function forges this link. Activities, administration, housekeeping, maintenance, and social services are also necessary components. In the wheelchair example, most of these departments must work together to formulate a facility-wide program. The OTR and COTA can design and adapt each chair. However, unless the nursing department makes sure the wheelchair stays

assigned to the resident, the housekeeping department cleans it without destroying the adaptation, the maintenance staff provides safety checks and needed repairs, the activities department encourages the resident to use it on outings, social service helps involve the family in its purchase, and the administration supports the project with funding, the system will not work (Epstein, 1991).

Residents and families are a critical part of the collaborative team. Whether the resident is a "short stay" and plans to return to a community home, or he or she is a more permanent placement, the team must work diligently to ensure the person's movement from dependence to independence and not the reverse.

Restraints, often imposed on new residents who arrive confused and disoriented from a hospital setting, provide an example of how the facility team can foster dependence. Through more careful functional assessment, as mandated under OBRA, the team, with resident participation, is quickly alerted to potential problems and the need for interdisciplinary care planning.

This same perspective and assessment process are applied to other facility residents, many of whom require special restorative programs designed by occupational therapy. These programs are supportive of the OBRA mandate and include various aspects of ADL, such as mobility, eating, and personal self-care, along with positioning, cooking, and leisure activities. Often these programs are developed by occupational therapy providers using a consultative service delivery model (Epstein, 1991).

Dynamic interaction and open communication among staff, residents, families, and the larger organizational structure create team commitment. Effective teams require members who appreciate each other's roles, the complexity of each person's job assignment, the environmental demands associated within their tasks, and communication to facilitate role clarification and expectations (Maguire, 1985).

Funding

Occupational therapy services may be supported through multiple *funding streams* in varying amounts. As discussed earlier, Medicare pays for a majority of occupational therapy services in most facilities. However, facilities also have options to develop more specialized care units, in which occupational therapy services may be supported as part of the daily bed rate, usually through Medicaid. Such units can be established for Alzheimer's patients, patients with head injuries, patients with AIDS, those with multiple sclerosis, and ventilator-dependent children. In some cases, grant funds may also be obtained to provide new and innovative programs, including participation by occupational therapy.

Funding for consultation, an indirect service, is becoming more important under the OBRA mandate. Administrators may choose to support this with discretionary monies when Medicaid or other funding sources cannot be found. Staff training is a major aspect of consultation service, and funds are often available under this budget to support consultation (Epstein, 1992).

Publics

Each long-term care facility has a group of interested observers or concerned publics. Some visit regularly; others watch from afar. These publics include volunteers; outside service people who make deliveries, repair the telephone, or fix the copy machine; consumer advocates such as the nursing home ombudsman; and regulatory publics such as nursing facility surveyors and those with the Joint Commission on Accreditation of Health Organizations.

Publics provide another perspective and often important support for occupational therapy services. In one facility, a group of enthusiastic volunteers raised enough money to buy 14 wheelchairs for needy residents.

Conclusion

Analysis of both macro- and microenvironments enables occupational therapy practitioners to establish an appropriate service delivery package in a given facility. Using this perspective, services can address facility, patient, family, and occupational therapy needs and wants, and concurrently foster movement toward less restrictive environments. By creatively expanding their influence and services at all levels of long-term care, specifically at the tertiary institutional level, occupational therapists can empower the patient, energize the facility, and optimize their function. To accomplish these objectives, greater emphasis must be placed on consultation, collaboration, and innovation. Medically oriented, direct treatment services must be enhanced through the larger perspectives of consultation and collaborative restorative programming. Reaching beyond the confines of institutional walls, occupational therapy practitioners must continuously seek supportive environments in the larger community, where their patients can reside and occupational therapy can expand its services.

References

Abdellah, F. G., & Moore, S. R. (Eds.). (1988). *Surgeon General's workshop: Health promotion & aging.* Washington, DC: U.S. Department of Health & Human Services, Public Health Services.

AOTA Research Information & Evaluation Division. (1991). 1990 Member data survey: Summary report. *OT Week, 5,* 22.

Baum, C. M. (1991). Addressing the needs of the cognitively impaired elderly from a family policy perspective. *American Journal of Occupational Therapy, 45*(7), 594–605.

Born, B. (1991). Long-term care: A new option for the elderly. *Gerontology Special Interest Section Newsletter, 14*(4), 1–3.

Castro, J. (1991). Call for a cure. Condition: critical. *Time, 138,* November 25, 34–42.

Epstein, C. F. (1991). Specialized restorative programs. In Kiernat, J. M. (Ed.), *Occupational therapy and the older adult: A clinical manual* (pp. 285–300). Gaithersburg, MD: Aspen Publications.

Epstein, C. F. (1992). A systems consultation approach in long-term care. In E. Jaffe & C. Epstein (Eds.), *Occupational therapy consultation: Theory, principles and practice.* St. Louis: Mosby-YearBook.

Estes, C. L. (1990). Long term care *is* mainstream. Why isolate it from acute care? *Perspective on Aging, 19*(4), 4–8.

Faust, L., & Meaker, M. K. (1991). Private practice occupational therapy in the skilled nursing facility: Creative alliance or mutual exploitation? *American Journal of Occupational Therapy, 45*(7), 621–627.

Health Care Financing Administration. (1989). Omnibus Budget Reconciliation Act of 1987 (Public Law 100–203). *54 Federal Register 21,* Washington, DC: Author.

Hopkins, H. L., & Tiffany, E. G. (1983). Occupational therapy—a problem solving process. In H. L. Hopkins & H. D. Smith (Eds.), *Willard and Spackman's Occupational therapy* (6th ed., pp. 89–99). Philadelphia: J. B. Lippincott.

Jaffe, E., & Epstein, C. (Eds.). (1992). *Occupational therapy consultation: Theory, principles and practice.* St. Louis: Mosby-YearBook.

Johnson, J. A., & Jaffe, E. (Eds.). (1989). *Health promotion & preventive programs: Models of occupational therapy practice.* New York: Haworth Press.

Maguire, G. H. (1985). The team approach in action. In Maguire, G. H. (Ed.), *Care of the elderly: A health team approach* (pp. 221–225). Boston: Little, Brown & Co.

McCormack, G. L., Llorens, L. A., & Glogoski, C. (1991). Culturally diverse elders. In J. M. Kiernat (Ed.), *Occupational therapy & the older adult: A clinical manual.* Gaithersburg, MD: Aspen Publications.

Moon-Sperling, T., & Crispen, C. C. (1991). Implications of OBRA '87: Expansion of services and opportunities, *Gerontology Special Interest Newsletter, 14*(3), 1–2.

Morris, J. N., Hawes, C., Murphy, K., & Nonemaker, S. (1991). *Resident assessment instrument: Training manual and resource guide.* Natick, MA: Eliot Press.

National Council on the Aging. (1988). Public policy agenda: Long-term care. *Perspective on Aging, 27*(2), 6–10.

Pepper Commission. (1990). *A call for action: Final report.* (Senate Print #101–114), Washington, DC: U.S. Government Printing Office.

Somers, F. P. (1991). Long-term care & federal policy. *American Journal of Occupational Therapy, 45*(7), 625–635.

CHAPTER 28

Home care and private practice

RUTH E. LEVINE, MARY A. CORCORAN,
and LAURA N. GITLIN

KEY TERMS

Caregiver

Environment

Home Care

Model for Home-Care
  Delivery

Private Practice

Third-Party Reimbursement

LEARNING OBJECTIVES

Upon completion of this chapter the reader will be able to:

1. *Describe the home-care delivery model and identify how it differs from institution-based care.*

2. *Describe a conceptual model for delivering home-care services and incorporate a collaborative approach that includes other team members, the patient, and caregivers.*

3. *Identify components of the home environment that influence patient and caregiver behavior and treatment decisions.*

4. *Compare and contrast home-care and institution-based practices.*

5. *Understand the importance of theory-based practice for home care.*

6. *Identify the influence of caregivers on the home-care delivery process.*

7. *Understand the unique knowledge and skills required for an effective occupational therapy home-care practice.*

8. *List external constraints that affect home-care service delivery.*

Wanted: Experienced OTR with knowledge of physical and psychosocial dysfunction. Must be well-organized person who is able to work without direct supervision. Must have flexible personality and be able to adjust to a variety of social and environmental situations, work collaboratively to identify patient and caregiver goals and values, and instruct both professional and nonprofessional team members as well as patients and their caregivers in activities of daily living and motor skill retraining activities.

Job requires above-average written and verbal communication and driving skills. Salary is competitive. Working hours are flexible.

This job description highlights the elements of home-care practice that make it a unique occupational therapy specialty. Many patients who previously received care as inpatients are now cared for at home. This includes patients who require intravenous solutions, chemotherapy, and respiratory treatment. In fact, home-care practitioners are frequently asked to treat patients in ways that require the use of complex equipment. This change occurred because of the development of Medicare diagnostic-related groups (DRGs), a system that uses statistical averages to determine the reimbursement for a hospital on the basis of a patient's diagnosis and age. Thus, many of the present population of homebound patients are more acutely ill, and the family caregivers are more anxious and taxed.

In addition to the fact that more acutely ill patients are cared for in the home, other factors, such as the family and caregivers, levels of reimbursement, and the influence of the environment, all add to the challenges and joys of delivering home services. Home-care therapists are increasingly aware of the influence of caregivers and the home environment on successful treatment decisions, methods, and outcomes. Caregivers are stressed by the demands of caring for the patient combined with work and normal family activities and the financial burdens of care that are not relieved by reimbursement policies. The home environment is pervasive and influences every treatment decision. It is no wonder that home-care professionals regard the patient, family, caregivers, and environment as interrelated and essential when making treatment decisions.

Home-care services may be defined as "an array of services provided to patients and families in their places of residence or in ambulatory care settings for purposes of preventing disease; promoting, maintaining, or restoring health; or minimizing the effects of disability" (National League of Nursing, 1984, p. 95). **Home care** can be described as a holistic method for providing therapeutic services in the patient's home. A home-care agency offers skilled professional services, such as: nursing; physical, occupational, and speech therapies; medical–social service; laboratory testing; and other services, such as light housekeeping, shopping, and personal care. Also available are counseling, specialized testing, and visits from other health specialists, such as podiatrists, dentists, and respiratory therapists.

This chapter describes the home health care area of occupational therapy practice and its unique features, including the independence of therapists, the variety of home settings, the importance of teaching, the need for autonomy and communication skills, and the physical demands. Recently, many experienced therapists are entering home care after working in an institution. It is an opportunity to have flexible hours and to work independently without the constraints of institution boundaries.

From 1973 to 1986, the number of full-time therapists entering home-care practice increased. This trend is reversing now, and many therapists who enter this specialty work part time. Moreover, home health specialists maintain that many patient needs are unmet because of the shortage of therapists. In 1990, 3.6% of all American Occupational Therapy Association (AOTA) members claimed that a home care agency was their primary place of employment. This number has decreased by 1% since 1986 (Research Information Division, 1986, p.8). On the positive side, the number of certified occupational therapy assistants employed full time in home care has increased slightly from 1.2% in 1986 to 1.5% in 1990 (AOTA, 1991). Therapists who enter home-care practice mention the flexible scheduling, competitive pay, autonomy, work with families, and varied case loads as reasons for their decision to enter the specialty (Bruckner, 1991; Huddeston, 1991; Mastrangelo, 1990). The interest among specialists to form a Special Interest Section under the auspices of the AOTA reflects the growing understanding that home-care practice requires a unique knowledge base, different clinical skills, and the ability to integrate medically based rehabilitation practice with a more community-oriented psychosocial perspective (Steinhauer, 1991).

By working in home care, therapists find that they can augment a full-time position or devote full time to a home-care practice. Fees range from $30 to $60 per visit. A fictitious profile of a person who might enter home care follows.

PROFILE AND CASE STUDY

Stacy Reynolds, OTR, graduated from an entry-level program more than 10 years ago. She liked her job in a rehabilitation center but, although a mother of three children, she wanted to continue her career. Stacy did not feel that full-time, insti-

tution-based practice offered the flexibility in scheduling that her personal life required. Also, she wanted to see patients in their own homes.

For these reasons, Stacy applied for a position with a private practice group where she would receive supervision, realizing she needed to learn more about delivery methods, documentation requirements, and patient and caregiver teaching. The private practice supervisor told Stacy that she would be an asset to the group since Stacy, like many home-care therapists, was an experienced OTR with knowledge of physical and psychosocial dysfunction. The supervisor explained that successful home-care therapists are organized, competent people who create their own schedules, complete their documentation accurately, adjust easily to a variety of social and environmental situations, work independently without direct supervision, and communicate ideas effectively. Because of diverse demands, Stacy would have to be flexible and adjust to a broad range of people, both professional and nonprofessional.

The interviewer asked Stacy about her stamina since home care is demanding on three levels. First, the therapist must demonstrate the ability to transfer and to ambulate patients in less-than-ideal situations. At times, the therapist must teach anxious family members and caregivers to execute difficult techniques. Second, therapists must be able to work and drive in extreme weather conditions, including rain, snow, ice, and hail. Patients may not live in conveniently located, temperature-controlled, accessible homes. Finally, home-care therapists must adjust to different social systems and cultural settings throughout the day as they move in and out of different homes. These shifts require the ability to interact with a variety of people successfully. Stacy asked the supervisor to describe a patient that a member of the group had treated recently.

The supervisor described Mr. H, a 78-year-old African American who was discharged from a 27-day stay in a metropolitan hospital. Mr. H was admitted with a diagnosis of adenocarcinoma of the rectum, chronic obstructive pulmonary disease, a left temporal lobe cerebral vascular accident, glaucoma, anemia, and bladder outlet obstruction. The patient was also diabetic and almost blind. Mr. H underwent a resection with colostomy and was discharged to a home-care team consisting of a nurse, physical and occupational therapists, social worker, and home health aide. The occupational therapy orders were to instruct the patient in activities of daily living and to teach colostomy care.

Mr. H lived with his wife, who was blind and hypertensive, in a modest, two-story house in a densely populated area of the city. The therapist assessed the patient's environment and discovered a number of architectural barriers, such as narrow hallways, steep stairs, a difficult-to-reach bathroom located on the second floor, and a difficult-to-reach kitchen. Mr. and Mrs. H had no relatives or friends well enough to help them. Mr. H had little endurance, was dependent in self-care, and demonstrated perceptual and sensory deficits. He also had little coordination and strength.

The therapist assessed the patient and decided to make the next home visit with the nurse since the patient had so many unmet medical and self-care needs. The nurse and the therapist reviewed general colostomy care with the patient, and the nurse also evaluated the therapist's knowledge regarding the preparation and application of a colostomy bag. Occupational therapy treatment continued for 6 weeks and consisted of upper-extremity resistive exercises, suggestions to ameliorate environmental barriers, and instruction in self-care activities, such as shaving and dressing. Also reviewed were sensory and perceptual activities designed to maximize the patient's ability to identify objects in his paralyzed hand since his vision was so limited. The therapist always included Mrs. H in the therapy sessions to ensure carry-over. Stressed and depressed, Mrs. H had to cope with her own disability as well as that of her husband. The therapist thought carefully about her suggestions, knowing that she could not introduce too many new things to the overburdened wife. She suggested a low-technology adaptation that would permit Mrs. H to draw up her husband's insulin without help, but Mrs. H refused to learn how to use it since she feared that she would hurt her husband. The therapist switched goals and made two suggestions: the use of cushions to improve Mr. H's bed position and the rearrangement of the over-the-bed table and chair to offset a difficult environmental barrier. It should be noted that even this small suggestion was stressful for Mrs. H. Mr. H attained independence in bathing, dressing, and light meal preparation; his incoordination precluded his success in colostomy care. The therapist tried to teach Mrs. H how to perform the colostomy care, and although she gained some proficiency on a model, she refused to attempt actual care on her husband because she feared that she might infect him. The therapist and nurse conferred with the family and decided to decrease other services so that visits for colostomy care could be continued.*

The supervisor explained that the case was illustrative because the patient and his wife had few resources, few family or interpersonal support systems, and multiple medical problems. The home-care team members had to communicate with each other and the family to make the difficult decision regarding Mr. H's continued care. The therapist involved Mrs. H, the primary caregiver, in a collaborative treatment approach that also required close communication with the nurse and home health aide. The entire team encouraged Mr. H to increase his functional abilities. This collaborative approach is mutually satisfying for all the team members. It is important to select culturally appropriate adaptations that reflect patient and caregiver values as much as possible. The supervisor pointed out, however, that the lack of available resources to help community-living, chronically impaired patients remain in their own homes was apparent in this difficult situation. Stacy weighed the demands of the home-care delivery system with her desire to enter this growing area of practice. She decided to join the private practice group and to develop her expertise in home-care delivery.

Overview of home care

Patients are referred to home care by their physicians. The referral may follow a hospitalization, a convalescence in a nursing home, or a stay in a rehabilitation center. In most cases, a

* This patient case study is a fictitious composite developed by Gregory Wilson, OTR/L, Community Occupational Therapy Consultants, Inc., Philadelphia, PA.

nurse visits the patient first and orders the other needed services. When nursing services are not required, a physical therapist or speech pathologist may evaluate the patient and order other needed services.

Occupational therapy is not classified as a primary service, although members of the Legislative and Political Affairs Division of the AOTA have worked to have this regulation changed for over 20 years. This means that the patient must need a nurse or a physical or speech therapist to be eligible for occupational therapy.

The home health team works in conjunction with patients and their families to stabilize health needs and to increase functional abilities. Once a referral for occupational therapy is received, the therapist collaborates with the patient, family, and other team members to promote the patient's independence using functional exercises, sensory retraining, adaptive equipment, perceptual training, and energy conservation techniques. The therapist must consider the patient from a holistic perspective because emotional, social, cultural, and environmental factors have as much influence on the outcome of care as do the medical prognosis and patient's present abilities.

CASE STUDY

Mr. S, a 67-year-old former truck driver, suffered a cerebrovascular accident (CVA) in March 1991. He was rushed to the hospital, where his medical condition was stabilized by medication, rest, remedial diet, and bed exercises. After 1 week, he was transferred to a rehabilitation center. The staff there taught Mr. S to bathe from a basin while in bed, dress if supervised and assisted, eat using adapted equipment, transfer with supervision and assistance, and perform selected joint range of motion exercises with his affected upper extremity. Mrs. S was involved in the rehabilitation program. Mr. S was fitted for a resting hand splint and arm sling. He was sent home with a tub transfer seat, wheelchair, walker, and raised toilet seat.

The rehabilitation center team thought that Mr. S could benefit from additional training; therefore, the physiatrist ordered a home program. Three days before discharge, a hospital social worker referred Mr. S to a home-care agency. The social worker described Mr. S's rehabilitation program and discussed his progress.

A home health agency nurse visited Mr. S on the day that he came home. Mr. S was lying in bed when she arrived. The nurse evaluated his condition, checked on the available medical equipment, and verified the need for other skilled services. She found that Mrs. S seemed anxious and threatened by her new responsibilities. The nursing supervisor referred the case to physical and occupational therapists. The patient's diagnosis, history, and address were given.

The occupational therapist visited the patient 2 days after he came home. The therapist found that Mr. S could eat cut-up food but was dependent on Mrs. S for all other aspects of his daily care. His impulsive behavior, short attention span, and left visual-field cut all limited his performance in daily self-care. The home visiting team continued services for the next 2 months.

The occupational therapist upgraded the therapeutic exercises initiated in the rehabilitation center. Mr. S could use his affected arm to stabilize objects. A complete review of dressing techniques was necessary because Mrs. S initially found it easier to dress her husband. The occupational therapist also taught Mr. S to compensate for his left field cut by using familiar cues from his environment.

After 2 months of training in occupational and physical therapy, Mr. S required minimal assistance to dress, eat, and do light housekeeping. He could ambulate to the front door and go down the front steps if assisted.

In this case, the home-care team reinforced and completed the patient's rehabilitation program. Much therapy was initiated by the rehabilitation hospital staff; however, additional treatment was required to make the patient independent. The home visiting team could adjust Mr. S's program to the needs of his family by using the familiar setting of his home.

Home-care team defined

The *nurse* carries out skilled duties that include supervising medication, giving injections and nutritional advice, giving intravenous medication, caring for wounds and dressings, monitoring vital signs, and teaching and supervising the patient and caretakers regarding daily care. The nurse is usually the coordinator of the patient's care; he or she supervises other nursing personnel, such as home health aides.

The *home health aide* carries out the nursing care plan. Duties include bathing, dressing, and feeding the patient; carrying out or reinforcing therapeutic activities and exercise regimens; maintaining the environment; assisting in the preparation of meals; and providing assistance with ambulation and self-administered medications. The home health aide also offers psychological support.

The *physical therapist* employs physical agents such as heat, light, water, electricity, massage, radiation, and exercise to restore patients to their maximal level of physical function.

The *speech therapist* uses knowledge about speech, hearing, and language to plan and implement a realistic program to increase the patient's communication skills. The patient's emotions affect speech; thus, psychological aspects are an important consideration in speech therapy.

The *occupational therapist* uses specified therapeutic, self-care, homemaking, and creative activities to facilitate or maximize the patient's level of function. Both the psychosocial and the physical aspects of the patient's condition are assessed in terms of the total context for treatment.

The *social worker* uses a problem-solving approach to help patients help themselves. Options and resources are presented to the patient and caretakers in an attempt to maximize the patient's adjustment.

Not all the possible home-care professionals were presented in this section. Others may include a podiatrist, optometrist, dentist, homemaker, dietitian, and home-visiting physician.

Home-bound patients cannot leave their homes without assistance. This is an important classification for **third-party reimbursement** (insurance coverage). *Ambulatory* patients may be asked to travel to outpatient therapy. Most carriers refuse to cover home services if patients can walk out of their house, even if assistance is required. Some third-party carriers consider patients ineligible for homebound services if they can get to their front door. This means that therapists must consider this con-

straint when planning and documenting treatment progress because patients can easily lose their classification as homebound. This issue will be addressed in the Documentation section of this chapter.

Resources are the patient's available human and physical assets. Assets can help to balance the debilitating effects of health problems. Resources can be categorized into human and material classes.

Human resources are **caregivers**—people who assist with the patient's daily care. Caregiver duties include such tasks as preparing meals; caring for the patient's wounds and dressings; offering medication at the appropriate times; bathing the patient; cleaning the surrounding environment; and offering support, encouragement, and entertainment. At times, the caregiver assumes responsibility for the patient's financial obligations. The patient's skills determine the scope of the caregiver's responsibilities and the time required to complete the daily tasks. Human resources are so important that they frequently influence the overall course of the patient's progress.

There are three kinds of human resources. *Primary caregivers* assume full responsibility for all the patient's needs. The amount of effort involved is determined by the extent of the patient's independence. If the patient is dependent in all aspects of self-care, primary care may be equivalent to a full-time job. In many cases, the burdens of patient care are added to the normal responsibilities of the caregiver, so that the caregiver has two jobs. The workload can become emotionally and physically draining. *Secondary caregivers* do not assume total responsibility for the patient's care. However, they frequently perform routine patient care tasks, thereby offering respite to the primary caretaker. *Tertiary caregivers* offer infrequent but welcome assistance. They visit the patient and provide emotional support and social contact. Also important is the periodic help given to the primary and secondary caregiver. Although tertiary caregivers are not available for daily rehabilitation training and personal care, they may perform duties such as shopping for food and medicine, transporting the patient to the doctor, and staying with the patient while the primary caregiver attends to other business.

Material resources consist of the patient's financial assets, including insurance coverage. Insurance coverage may consist of a private or governmental policy. Home care may be covered under Blue Cross, a health maintenance organization (HMO), a private carrier, or a prospective payment organization (PPO). Furniture, equipment, supplies, clothing, medication, safety equipment, and aide services are other material assets that can be purchased if the patient has sufficient funds.

Parameters of home care

Four factors that make home-care delivery different from the care offered in an institution: the unique characteristics of the patient, caregivers, home-care practitioners, and the delivery system.

The patient

The unique characteristics of the home-care patient are determined by factors such as the patient's medical condition, culture, motivation and emotional response to disability, personal competence, and resources.

Medical conditions

Patients recovering from a variety of medical conditions can benefit from home-care services. Most patients are elderly adults who are recovering from fractures, heart or pulmonary diseases, CVA, neurologic disorders, decubitus ulcers, surgical wounds, burns, brain injuries, spinal cord injuries, and arthritis. Younger adults and children with similar medical conditions are also eligible for care.

Patients with acute medical problems should be medically stable before they are admitted to home-care services. Today, patients are discharged from hospitals earlier, and home-care team members are required to treat more acutely ill patients; however, these patients should not require acute care, even though many home-care teams are on call 7 days a week, 24 hours a day. If patients are medically unstable, the physician should be notified and the patient admitted to the hospital if necessary. Terminally ill patients may also be treated at home with the support of a hospice team.

Culture

Culture can be described as a filter through which the practitioner must try to understand the patient's goals, motivation, interests, roles, and habits (Levine, 1987; Levine & Merrill, 1987; Barris, Kielhofner, Levine, & Neville, 1985). Choice of food, dress, activities, language, expression, time use, tool use, roles, and habits all are influenced by culture from early childhood. The child learns these behaviors and choices from parents, family members and friends, significant others, and schoolmates. Culture provides the framework in which ideas for acceptable behaviors are established. By school age, the child is well versed in the norms and values of his or her culture. These basic values often remain stable and unchanged throughout life unless the person decides to devote a considerable amount of energy into self-change. Thus, it is ethnocentric and unrealistic for therapists to plan to significantly alter marital relationships, food preferences, dressing and eating habits, and other basic, culturally derived behaviors in the usual 2 months allowed for treatment. Such change can be initiated but will require considerable thought and commitment from the patient and caregivers. New ideas and suggestions should be described using a communication style familiar and comfortable to both the patient and the caregivers.

Motivation and emotional response to disability

A wide range of motivating sources can be used by an occupational therapist to evoke a patient's active participation in therapy. For instance, therapists frequently support existing sources of motivation such as the positive reinforcement offered by family and friends, customary daily routines, and the familiar environment of the home.

One particularly effective method of motivating a patient or caregiver involves the active engagement of the person in a collaborative relationship. In one study, subjects reported feeling empowered as a result of a collaborative relationship with a home-care therapist (Corcoran & Gitlin, 1991a). Collaboration involves the therapist's use of several therapeutic tools to assist the client to activate personal power not formerly used (Dybwad,

1989; Peloquin, 1990). These tools include client education, sharing perspectives, open communication, mutual respect for skills and knowledge, and support of family values, customs, and beliefs (Bazyk & Trombino, 1990; Hasselkus, 1987, Corcoran & Gitlin, 1991a; Corcoran, 1991a; Corcoran 1991b). Through collaboration, the patient is empowered and motivated to assume responsibility for the management of his or her problems. Therefore, the patient provides the meaning for therapeutic interventions and becomes an integrator of service, not a passive recipient (Bailey, 1989; Hasselkus, 1987). An example of an empowered patient is demonstrated when a suggestion by the occupational therapist is modified by the patient to fit his or her unique situation. In one clinical illustration of empowerment through collaboration, a patient substituted a Victorian bell pull for a rope attached to the door by the therapist for access. This patient, motivated and empowered to shape the intervention, elicited the occupational therapist's suggestion and then modified it to fit her personal vision of her home's decor.

In addition to varying levels of motivation, the home-care therapist's case load represents a range of patient emotional responses to disability. In some instances, the occupational therapist encounters patients who demonstrate remarkable coping skills, resilience, and capacity for adaptation. Other patients welcome stimulation from the outside world and spend a considerable amount of therapy time discussing everything but the therapeutic tasks at hand. Conversely, many patients feel invaded by strangers in their home and respond negatively toward any health care provider who represents the patient's need for formal assistance. Feelings of depression, anger, denial, or grief can create barriers to establishment of an effective therapeutic relationship.

Home-care therapists must respect limits set by the patient and support the patient's efforts to deal with trauma. Goals of therapy include assisting each patient to rediscover and refine his or her unique style of coping and to use it to deal with the disability.

Personal competence

Personal competence refers to the distinctive combination of cognitive, motor, emotional, social, and psychological strengths and weaknesses that each person possesses. Although disability can erode competence in one or several areas, its effects can be offset by strengths in other areas. Home-care therapists can evoke functional independence by recommending techniques that capitalize on the patient's personal competencies while avoiding or remediating weaknesses. In other words, it may be more important for the occupational therapist to know what a patient *can* do than to know what a patient *cannot* do.

Competence combines with characteristics of the environment to produce behavior. For instance, a person with limited competence due to dementia would behave much differently in a quiet environment than in a noisy one. Skilled occupational therapists recognize that both the environment and the patient's level of competence can be modified to promote independence. The challenge for home-care therapists is finding the correct balance between culturally acceptable environmental adaptations and culturally relevant therapeutic occupations. A later section explores the relation between competence and the environment in greater detail.

Resources

Because the home-care patient requires supervision and direct care, available human and material resources become more important. Since patients are being discharged earlier from acute care settings, they require more attention when they arrive home. Family members and caregivers are frequently overwhelmed with the responsibilities of care, and home-care practitioners must be sensitive to stresses caused by these added responsibilities. Therefore, from the start of care, relatives, friends, and neighbors should be encouraged to help with the patient's care. A secondary and tertiary support network can relieve the primary caregivers so they will be able to carry on better. Some tasks that secondary and tertiary caregivers can assume are providing a meal periodically, taking responsibility for the patient's care for a day, shopping for the primary caregiver, and taking the patient to the physician.

In a growing number of cases, the patient has no nearby relatives and no friends. Neighbors may not be close enough to offer emergency help. Isolation is especially problematic in rural towns and farms where children do not live near their parents and friends are inaccessible, deceased, or have moved away. To complicate matters further, there are few agencies or private groups that offer assistance. Private and religious groups sometimes are willing to deliver meals and encourage visits from volunteers who may provide assistance and transportation.

If support networks are lacking, home convalescence can be difficult and awkward. Unfortunately, there are fewer opportunities to substitute institutional care for informal support networks. This is especially true among Medicare and Medicaid patients, who are restricted by constraints on the duration of a patient's stay in an institution.

Therapists must also learn to work collaboratively with the hospital staff as patients who become ill repeatedly are admitted to the institution for a brief period of time, only to be discharged again because of regulations regarding the number of days that the hospital can be reimbursed for care. The patient is discharged, and home-care treatment is resumed, but the disruption becomes another negative factor that must be considered in treatment planning.

The environment

The **environment** is defined broadly as the world around patients and the circumstances or conditions that affect performance. The environment has both human and nonhuman components. The human components include family, friends, peers, neighbors, and colleagues, while nonhuman aspects include anything that is not human, such as animals, possessions, objects, and places (Searles, 1960). Occupational therapists used this concept broadly until Dunning (1972) identified space, people, and tasks as three elements of the environment. Gerontologists describe the environment as multidimensional and complex (Lawton, 1983; Kahana, 1975; Schooler, 1982). Lawton (1983) explored the relationship between external stimulation and individual performance, maintaining that the environment can determine the well-being of the person. Overwhelming stimulation can make someone feel inadequate and discouraged about personal abilities. Kahana's (1975) ideas about the goodness of fit between environmental characteristics and individual needs helps therapists to identify the complexity of the activity process.

Yerxa and Baum (1987) reviewed psychology and gerontology literature and urged occupational therapists to use systems theory to assess the patient's losses, teach compensatory behavior, fit equipment to meet emerging needs, and train caregivers. Kiernat (1987) explained how therapists promote independence by grading environmental stimulation and making the patient feel competent. The ideal environment varies with individual needs; unfortunately, living conditions are rarely ideal for patients.

Home-care therapists use four key concepts identified by gerontology researchers to promote the patient's functional abilities and feelings of efficacy: arousal, press, competence, and adaptation. *Arousal* is defined as the degree to which the internal state of the person is stimulated by the environment. People are constantly seeking a personally satisfying match between environmental stimulation and their own needs. Too little stimulation may result in boredom or lack of motivation to perform self-care tasks. On the other hand, too much arousal may result in anxiety and stress. The occupational therapy process involves the selection of activities and tasks that evoke curiosity and interest within the patient's zone of comfort (Lawton, 1975, 1983). For example, comatose patients are difficult to arouse, but learning-disabled children may be so sensitive to environmental stimulation that they are hyperactive.

Press, the second concept, was defined by Murray (1938) as stimuli possessing some motivating quality that activates an individual need. It refers to the forces in the environment that combine with an individual need to elicit a response. Behavioral choices are shaped by the demands or press of the environment. In a given situation, a person realizes that there are certain behavioral expectations. A patient may not struggle to learn to dress independently after a CVA if his wife insists on doing it for him. The CVA created a decline in competence, and now the environment poses greater press and a barrier to independence.

Competence is the level of ability demonstrated by a person independent of outside factors (Lawton, 1975, p. 15). Consisting of biologic, sensory–perceptual, motor, emotional, and cognitive components, competence is the "theoretical upper limit of capacity of the individual to function in the world" (Lawton, 1975, p. 21). Occupational therapists work to ameliorate the press of the environment so patients perform competently. The feedback from this just-right challenge is expanded to create more exploratory behaviors (Burke, 1977).

Adaptation is the ability to change behavior based on feedback from the environment (Kielhofner, 1985). Patients with decreased functional abilities are more vulnerable to the effects of the environment because they do not possess the energy and skills to change their behavior. The home-care therapist collaborates with the patient and works to develop adaptations—human and nonhuman—that improve the patient's functional abilities (Rogers, 1982).

The caregivers

Because the typical home-care patient of the 1990s needs more supervision and direct care than ever before, available caregivers are important. Despite the fact that more than 80% of all long-term care is provided by friends and family members (Special Committee on Aging, 1987; Pepper Commission, 1990), in-home services cost federal and state governments $7 billion in 1988. Of the 7 million spouses, adult children, and others who provide unpaid assistance to the disabled, 80% spend, on average, 4 hours a day, 7 days a week, at their caregiving tasks. Most caregivers are women (72%), and many are vulnerable themselves in terms of health or income. Most caregivers experience stress from competing demands of family obligation, work conflict, and role overload (Stone, Cafferata, & Sangl, 1987).

The high degree of involvement and commitment demonstrated by most caregivers requires the home-care therapist to use an open systems approach to therapy. In a typical home-care situation, intervention targeted at one part of the system will positively or negatively affect the others. Many factors must be taken into account when suggesting intervention plans and strategies, such as the caregiver's level of competence, attitude toward the patient's disability, and preferred lifestyle.

One particularly important caregiver characteristic to keep in mind when designing treatment is the gender of the caregiver. Men and women define, approach, and implement their caregiving duties in very different ways. Using a task-oriented model found in the workplace, male caregivers concentrate their efforts on systematically and linearly tackling household and caregiving duties (Fitting, Rabins, Lucas, & Eastham, 1986; Bateson, 1991). They are likely to delegate responsibility for housework and physical work to others, usually to women, but are unlikely to join support groups (Corcoran, 1991a; Montgomery & Datwyler, 1990). Women tend to add to their caregiving duties by focusing on the emotional atmosphere of the home, going to great lengths to ensure that the impaired spouse enjoys a sense of well-being (Bearon, 1991; Motenko, 1989; Corcoran, 1991a). Female caregivers are reticent to seek or accept outside assistance, and consequently, they spend more time per week than men in actual caregiving tasks (Sherman, Ward, & LaGory, 1988; Spitze & Logan, 1989; Stone et al., 1987; Young & Kahana, 1989). Not surprisingly, the perceived burdens of caregiving are more pronounced for women than for men, as evidenced by higher rates among women on measures of depression (Pruchno & Resch, 1989), drug use (Clipp & George, 1990), stress (Anthony-Bergstone, Zarit, & Gatz 1988), and burden (Zarit, Todd, & Zarit, 1986).

Home-care therapists must design treatment plans and strategies that flexibly incorporate the unique blend of patient, caregiver, and home environment characteristics. One recent efficacy study revealed that 17 caregivers of demented elderly implemented 17 distinct environmental solutions to caregiving issues. These solutions included the use of graded assistance to the elimination of clutter (Corcoran & Gitlin, 1991b). The range of environmental solutions implemented by caregivers challenges the ability of the home-care therapist to find the just-right combination of strategies for the particular treatment circumstances.

CASE STUDY

Mr. Y decided to retire early to care for his wife, who was experiencing moderate impairment from Alzheimer disease. Mrs. Y was passive and presented few caregiving problems, except for her urinary incontinence. At the time that the home-care therapist made an initial evaluation, Mrs. Y had 15 or more "accidents" per week due to incontinence.

The therapist noted several facts related to Mrs. Y's problem. First, Mrs. Y seemed to be aware of her needs but unable to act on or communicate them. Second, despite the presence of five adults in the household, no one took Mrs. Y to the bathroom on a regular basis. Third, the five caregivers each demonstrated a different response to Mrs. Y's incontinence, ranging from scolding to comforting her. Finally, the therapist noted that Mrs. Y, due to her short-term memory deficit, was apparently unable to associate the commode by her bed with its intended use.

The home-care therapist offered perspectives on Mrs. Y's incontinence and helped Mr. Y to discuss his views about the problem and possible solutions. The therapist helped Mr. Y develop a bathroom schedule and recruit the commitment of the other adults in the household. When the therapist returned the following week, Mr. Y reported that he had modified the plan. He and his daughter had decided to assume responsibility for taking Mrs. Y to the bathroom themselves because they had more patience with her than the others. Mr. Y was delighted to report the success of his just-right plan—his wife had only three accidents in the past week.

The home-care practitioner

The unique characteristics of the home care practitioner are based on the ability to shift social roles, communicate, use available equipment creatively, combat professional isolation, balance teaching with direct care, organize and manage time, adjust to diverse cultural settings, develop a code of ethics, and set continuing education and professional goals.

Shift social roles

The health care practitioner enters the social hierarchy of the patient's family and friends. The therapist is a guest in the patient's house, a visitor in his or her lifespace. The reverse is true with services offered in an institution: the patient enters the institution as a temporary member of the formal social hierarchy.

As a visitor in the patient's world, the practitioner must adjust to values, traditions, communication patterns, and environmental factors. The patient's lifestyle might be unfamiliar, but the practitioner must use verbal, nonverbal, and environmental cues to promote effective interaction. Successful home-care practitioners have the ability to interact in a variety of social systems. Communication skills must promote patient and caregiver cooperation.

Communicate

Home-care therapists must be effective communicators since they interact with many people. Formal and informal interactions having verbal, nonverbal, and written communication patterns are used. Practitioners must relate to family members, caregivers, other professionals, and nonprofessional staff. Thus, the ability to express knowledge in clear, concise language unencumbered by jargon is necessary.

Home-visiting occupational therapists must communicate with colleagues, even though this is time-consuming and requires planning. Telephone conferences and scheduled meetings are the only way that team members can share observations about the patient's progress. Calls can be exchanged at night or during weekends, when there is more time to express different ideas; meetings can be arranged when therapists and nurses are visiting patients in the same neighborhood. It is also essential for therapists to call other professionals before physicians' orders are renewed. The penalty for lack of communication may be an untimely termination of services since the occupational therapist may have a different perspective on the patient's progress than other team members (Trossman, 1984).

Use available equipment creatively

Home-care practitioners cannot rely on the equipment and supplies that are common in most institution-based clinics. Therapists carry a limited supply of evaluation tools and selected activities to promote functional abilities—some TheraBands and hand putty and some simple ADL set-up equipment in their car trunks. The selection of evaluation tools and modalities should be based on the patient's values, goals, interests, roles, habits, skills, and medical condition.

This does not mean that home-care therapists work without the benefit of any equipment. Instead, they adapt objects found in the patient's home. An old sock filled with a soup can and knotted at the top becomes a weight, a rolled washcloth or towel becomes a positioning tool, a chair becomes a bath seat. Home therapists monitor the patient's environment and, through discussion with the patient and caregiver, select appropriate items to use in treatment.

Combat professional isolation

Home-care practice can be a professionally isolating experience unless one deliberately seeks out other occupational therapists. Although there are opportunities to interact with other professionals, such as nurses and physical therapists, opportunities for interactions with other occupational therapists are limited. Therefore, voluntary membership in local, state, and national organizations becomes essential. These organizations have scheduled meetings, continuing education programs, occupational therapy newspapers for communicating ideas, and scholarly and practice-oriented journals. Meetings provide opportunities to discuss treatment ideas and to explore solutions to problems; newspaper articles offer new ideas and opportunities for professional growth; and journal articles validate practice through research.

Balance teaching with direct care

Since home-care practitioners commonly visit the patient only two or three times a week, with each visit averaging 35 to 45 minutes, effective teaching is especially important. Direct, hands-on techniques are required for home-care practice. Of equal importance, however, is the therapist's ability to promote patient and family independence. Effective communication by home-care practitioners encourages carry-over of skills taught during visits. Home-care practitioners realize that teaching skills either make or break the rehabilitation program. Thus, the practitioner must tailor each program to meet the unique needs of a particular family.

Therapists provide direct service and explain how and why a technique or activity is used. This requires knowledge, skills, and attitudinal abilities that make learning meaningful for the patient and the caregivers. As soon as the patient and caregivers become comfortable with the new information, therapists turn control over to the family.

The patient can benefit from a daily treatment regimen if the patient and caregivers are cooperative.

Although therapists feel guilty if they take time to listen to the patient and caregivers, recent research indicates that this is highly valued by occupational therapy patients and their caregivers. Levine and Gitlin (1992) report in a pilot study funded by the American Occupational Therapy Foundation that therapists required at least 3 or 4 hours of visiting to feel that they established sufficient rapport to handle complex issues and goals. Hinajosa (1990) found that the parents of handicapped children valued therapists who took the time to talk to them and offer support, claiming that this was as valuable as technical information and hands-on techniques. Parents and caregivers must be given opportunities to learn and integrate this information with their own ideas if therapy is to have continued impact after discharge.

Hasselkus (1987) found that caregivers initiate therapeutic relationships depending on their comfort level and the therapist's knowledge and skills. As confidence increases, they begin to reverse roles and teach the therapist better ways to accomplish tasks. The therapist must have the ability to encourage this reversal and to recognize when and how to use a variety of teaching techniques.

Another aspect of teaching is the ability to consult with other professional and nonprofessional staff. Home health aides may visit five times a week for 1 or 2 weeks until the family and caregiver network is fully developed. Therapists can train the aide to carry out routine tasks that promote the patient's independence. Visits are decreased as the patient improves. If home health aide services are ordered, then these services must be supervised by the appropriate professional staff; the nurse, the physical therapist, and the occupational therapist must meet with the aide and the patient to evaluate the patient's progress and change the program if warranted. Other professional relationships are discussed later in this chapter.

Organize and manage time

Home-care therapists must be organizers and planners. Tasks must be prioritized and completed in an orderly fashion. Each therapist is responsible for the daily tasks of accepting new referrals, scheduling and making visits, documenting treatment progress, collaborating with other staff, and reporting any unusual situations or circumstances to the patient's nursing supervisor and physician.

Visits must be coordinated so patients are not seen by three people on one day and no one on another day. Therapists usually schedule visits in a selected area on certain days of the week. The selection is based on arrangements with other professional staff. The patient and caregivers may also have preferences for a certain time or day. These choices must also be considered by the home-visiting team.

Home-care therapists are rigidly bound by regulations regarding the timeliness of calls to accept new referrals, the number of days that can lapse between referral and first visit, and the interval between a visit and when the agency receives the progress note. These rules are discussed later in the chapter. Because therapists are commonly reimbursed per visit, it is important to work efficiently so that time is devoted to patient care and not to peripheral concerns.

Adjust to diverse cultural settings

When working in an institution, the staff are part of the permanent social hierarchy, and the patients are visitors. The reverse is true in home care, where the therapist is a guest in the patient's home. Understanding the patient's view of reality is an important first step. This view is based on culture or way of life that is taught during childhood. Therapists must convey their understanding of the patient's values, goals, interests, and emotions gained from cues from the human and nonhuman environments. Home-care therapists learn to adapt their manners to the demands of different social situations. This requires the ability to analyze the meaning of different actions and words regardless of one's own culture.

Develop a code of ethics

Therapists who work without direct supervision need to develop a strong code of ethics. The AOTA has adopted an ethical code that has six principles related to (1) beneficence and autonomy, (2) competence, (3) compliance with laws and regulations, (4) public information, (5) professional relationships, and (6) professional conduct. Therapists should read the *Principles of Occupational Therapy Ethics*, which appear in Appendix A.

Home-visiting professionals represent not only their own profession but in some instances all helping professionals. The unethical conduct of a therapist can create undue suffering for a number of patients and caregivers alike. Examples of such conduct are shortening treatment times even though the patient is capable of participating in longer treatments, evaluating patients and visiting them less frequently because the home is not conveniently situated or the neighborhood is unfamiliar, or offering substandard forms of treatment to minority patients or immigrants from different cultures. If any violation of standards is witnessed, the incident should be discussed with the supervisor or officer of the state association because substandard treatment can only compromise the patient and the profession.

Set continuing educational and professional goals

Home-care practitioners function independently. Although they work on patient-care teams, they rarely work with other occupational therapists. The practitioner's knowledge and skills can become dated by this isolation because there are few opportunities for sharing new treatment ideas and modalities. One way to expand learning is to take advantage of continuing education programs. Advertisements appear in journals, newspapers, and mailings. Participation in local, state, and national organizations also promotes the sharing of ideas. One should never feel that one works alone, separated from new ideas and research. The diverse pressures of home care need to be offset by a conscious decision to seek new ideas to improve one's clinical practice.

Setting yearly goals for continuing education and professional growth and development ensures that one's knowledge and skills are current. Home care is a public arena for practice, and patients are becoming sophisticated and demanding consumers.

How to deliver services

At the heart of home care is the method used to deliver services. This is the hands-on aspect of care that is both exciting and demanding. There are three major components in this how-to section: choosing a theory base, the conceptual model, and a step-by-step guide to home visiting.

Choosing a theory base

The need for a theory base in home-care practice cannot be overemphasized. A theory base is a conceptual model that organizes and guides the therapist to think about complex patient problems in a systematic fashion. This is important because services can become fragmented, and family members, caregivers, and professional colleagues can become confused. A clearly articulated theory or delivery model can explain occupational therapy services to professional and nonprofessional team members. Services that are clearly conceptualized and articulated are also easier to explain to managers and fiscal intermediaries.

A theory base consists of a philosophical base or belief system and a conceptual framework that is used to organize evaluation tools, goal selection, treatment modalities, and quality-assurance practices.

Philosophical base

A philosophical base consists of values that cannot be proved. *Philosophy* is defined as "a study of the processes governing thought and conduct; the general principles or essential elements that produce laws in a field of knowledge" (McKechnie, 1980, p. 1347). The philosophical base of a profession consists of fundamental ideas that govern practice, ideas that are beliefs or values about humankind, suffering, and life (Brameld, 1955). Members of a profession are united by their commitment to the ideas embodied in their philosophical base.

Because the profession of occupational therapy developed as a reaction to the insensitive treatment of the chronically ill in the 1890s, therapists value the "essential humanity of a person in spite of severe and sometimes chronic disease" (Yerxa, 1983, p. 151). Occupational therapists focus on the patient's pathology but also on the capacity of humans to adapt and adjust to internal and external demands (Rogers, 1983; Kielhofner, 1985). Occupational therapists have long demonstrated their belief that people can "do for themselves and take responsibility for their own health" (Yerxa, 1983, p. 151).

Occupational therapists focus on adaptation or what people can do, so this holistic approach requires an understanding of the patient's lifestyle, values, goals, interests, and culture. Yerxa maintains that this view of the patient contrasts with the segmented focus of other hospital-based professionals. At the core of our profession is the belief that a person's active participation in a meaningful activity can promote health and well-being (Yerxa, 1983). Reilly stated this succinctly when she maintained that humans, "through the use of their hands, as they are energized by mind and will, can influence the state of their own health" (1962, p. 8).

Philosophy encourages therapists to critically consider their own treatment, to compare values and beliefs about patient care, and to formulate questions regarding the patient's lifestyle. For example, how do we encourage a person to overcome developmental, traumatic, socioeconomic, and pathologic conditions? A technician can superficially select convenient exercises and crafts, but the therapist searches for activities that reflect the patient's values, goals, and interests. Thus, the philosophical base of occupational therapy practice includes the quest for meaningful existence.

Matching philosophy and values

The first step in establishing a theory-based practice is to explore one's own values. What are values? Rath (cited in Kirschenbaum, 1973) developed criteria that qualify a belief or behavior as a value. The belief or behavior must be: selected from alternatives, prized and cherished, chosen freely after a consideration of the consequences of holding the belief, publicly affirmed, and acted on with some pattern of frequency. Rogers (1969) maintains that there are many definitions to describe values, but he finds the distinctions made by Morris (1956) most useful. Morris identifies three types of values: operative, conceived, and objective. Operative values are preferences that lead to actions that may not involve any cognitive or conceptual thinking. Choices are made and carried out; one object is selected over another. For example, someone may decide to drive to the post office rather than walk. A preference created the tendency to act in one way instead of another. A conceived value requires consideration since it is a preference for a symbolized object or action when the outcome of the choice is anticipated. For example, therapists frequently value independence in self-care, which is a conceived value. An objective value is not necessarily desirable, but it is an objective or ideal. Objective values are "preferable whether or not they are conceived of as desirable." Objective values are not as important since they require less commitment because they are convenient ideas (Morris, 1956, cited in Rogers, 1969, p. 241).

Rogers further explains the importance of operative and conceived values and scarcely discusses objective values since they are not necessarily part of the personal value system. Home-care therapists should identify their operative and conceived values concerning topics such as independence, work, family roles, religion, suffering, death, aging, illness, meaningful activity, and different cultural groups. In other words, a theory-based practice should be based on operative and conceived values rather than on objective values, which are abstract and removed from daily practice.

Engelhardt (1983) discussed conceived values when he urged occupational therapists to balance the technical aspects of occupational therapy with the belief that a patient is a person. The use of activities both as rituals designed to recapture pleasure and as significant experiences for people who are searching for a "sense of place, purpose and function" is an important part of the therapeutic process (Engelhardt, 1983, p. 144). In home care, activities must be meaningful because daily care is delivered by the patient, caregivers, and family members as well as by the therapist. Therefore, activities must reflect patient and caregiver goals, be carried over with relative ease, and maximize the patient's functional abilities.

Therapists who understand their own values can identify disagreements and underlying reasons for the dissimilarities. They can redirect treatment toward the patient's goals, values, interests, and needs.

A common example is a patient who does not want to learn how to dress. There are a number of reasons why this may occur, and the therapist must separate personal values from the needs of the patient. The following vignette is based on a potential values clash.

CASE STUDY

Mrs. K, a 66-year-old obese woman, suffered from arthritis and a recent CVA that resulted in left-sided paralysis with little functional return in the upper extremity. The home-care therapist was referred to maximize the patient's functional status. During the evaluation, the therapist asked Mrs. K about her performance in activities of daily living. The patient, a congenial person, jokingly stated that she alone had raised eight children and felt that some of the eight "could figure out how to take care of me." The therapist tried to convince Mrs. K that dressing would make her feel better. In fact, Mrs. K was enjoying her sick role since she had never taken time to focus on herself.

At first, the therapist began to debate with Mrs. K. the importance of getting dressed. The therapist identified her own objective values regarding the importance of being self-sufficient. She also realized her own conceived values regarding the importance of not depending on others for help. Mrs. K, on the other hand, valued interdependence and felt deserving of the attention and nurturing of her family. Mrs. K decided to concentrate on improving functional movement in her arm before learning how to dress independently. The therapist focused treatment on upper-extremity retraining and noted that Mrs. K requested help with her bathing and dressing activities once her arm regained some movement.

This vignette demonstrates that the patient directs the ultimate focus of care even when these goals are not shared by the therapist.

Conceptual model
Importance of the conceptual model

Conceptual models, or frames of reference, are thought structures used to organize and guide clinical reasoning. Therapists should identify their own values concerning chronic illness, independence, pathology, and activities and then consider a frame of reference or model that best reflects their beliefs. In home care, the conceptual model must be broad enough to encompass the patient's environment, culture, lifestyle, and functional needs. If the base is inclusive, the therapist can rely on the conceptual structure to organize treatment planning.

Model of human occupation

Kielhofner and Burke developed the Model of Human Occupation based on the ideas of Mary Reilly (Kielhofner & Burke, 1980, 1985; Rogers, 1983). Although there are a number of other useful frames of reference that can be applied to home care, the Model of Human Occupation offers a broad organizational framework so that more specific treatment techniques and theories can be systematically applied to the patient's problems. The Model of Human Occupation is based on two major premises: people are open systems that both influence and are influenced by the environment, and the mind and body are interrelated (Kielhofner, 1978; Kielhofner & Burke, 1980). The person can be viewed as an interrelated, three-tiered hierarchy consisting of the volitional, habituation, and performance subsystems (Kielhofner & Burke, 1985). The volitional subsystem consists of values, personal causation, goals, and interests; the habituation subsystem consists of roles and habits; and the performance subsystem consists of skills (Kielhofner & Burke, 1985). Home-care therapists direct attention to the patient's volitional (values, personal causation, goals, and interests) and habituation (habits and roles) subsystems as well as the performance (skills) subsystem. Treatment should include more than deficits; therapists should also consider the functional aspects of the patient (Kielhofner, 1985).

Students interested in acquiring specific information on the application of the Model of Human Occupation should consult the references cited. The text *A Model of Human Occupation: Theory and Application* is designed as an independent learning tool with a self-paced workbook (Kielhofner, 1985). Also useful is the case analysis format developed by Kaplan and Cubie (1982), which is based on a systems perspective. By posing a series of questions, therapists will be able to determine the patient's goals, values, interests, habits, and roles.

Therapists can use the Model of Human Occupation in conjunction with other frames of reference and treatment techniques. For example, a patient with hemiplegia can be treated using the Model of Human Occupation, but specific techniques to treat the upper extremity must be drawn from other frames of reference (Kielhofner, Shephard, & Stabenow, 1985)

Model for home-care delivery

The three phases of the ***Model for Home-Care Delivery*** are: (1) evaluation, (2) treatment and assessment, and (3) discharge. After evaluation, there is a period of treatment and assessment during which relationships and treatment regimes are established. After 6 to 8 weeks, the patient is usually discharged, and the home program is carried on by the family. The phases of the Model for Home-Care Delivery are depicted in Figure 28-1; each represents a stage in treatment:

Assessment

Assessment includes the therapist's preparation for and entry into the new case. The home-care agency receives a referral, and agency personnel intervene and offer direct service. The occupational therapist begins the evaluation phase of care, which includes the referral, rapport building, initial fact gathering (in-

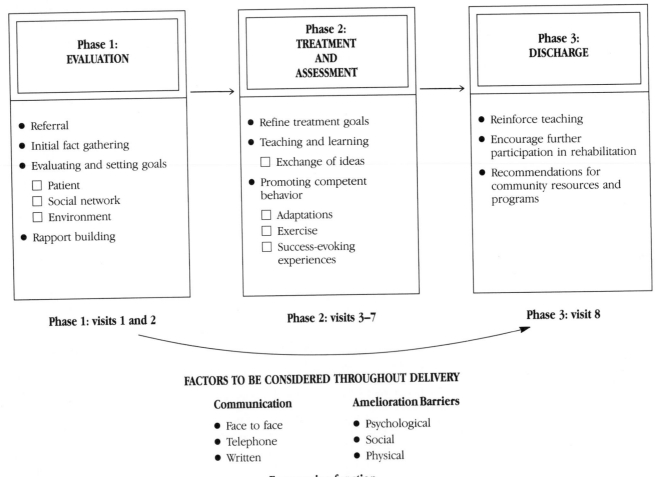

FIGURE 28-1. *Model for Home-Care Delivery.*

cluding human and nonhuman resources), evaluation, goal setting, and role initiation.

Once the therapist enters the patient's home, foremost is the task of building rapport and making the patient and caregivers feel comfortable. Therapists usually try to see as much of the home as possible without appearing to be intrusive or impolite and to meet as many members of the caregiving or social network as possible. This is the initial fact gathering stage, and the therapist uses observation and communication skills to generate treatment hypotheses. Evaluation of the patient's competence—motor, perceptual, cognitive, sensory, social, emotional, and cultural—is initiated. Also important are goals, values, motivation, interests, roles, and habits. The depth and breadth of the primary, secondary, and tertiary caregiver network can help the therapist understand the patient's social network. Both the positive and negative aspects of the environment must be considered since negative factors might create barriers precluding the realization of the patient's goals.

Furthermore, treatment must be offered during these early visits to satisfy the regulations of fiscal intermediaries. An activity, either therapist or patient derived, should be initiated that provides an opportunity to observe the patient's functional abilities. Goals should be set, even though the therapist will continue to gather information that may alter or refine the outcome of treatment. During these early visits, the patient, caregiver, and therapist are establishing roles. Evaluation takes place during the first and second visits.

Assessment and treatment

The second stage of delivery is the time when the bulk of the teaching and learning takes place. There are three phases in this stage: (1) refinement of goal setting, (2) teaching and learning, and (3) promoting patient competence.

As the therapist gets to know the patient and caregivers better, goals are refined to include a more personalized focus. Teaching and learning involve more of an exchange as the therapist presents treatment techniques and adaptations and as the patient and caregiver teach the therapist about their lifestyle and needs. Using graded activities, therapeutic use of self, and ideas derived from the patient and caregiver, the therapist encourages patient motivation. Based on additional information gathered during visits, the therapist continues to modify treatment ideas promoting competent behavior through the use or adaptation of equipment, graded exercises, and introduction of success-evoking experiences that improve functional performance. Treatment and assessment take place during the third to seventh visits.

Discharge

The discharge phase is a time when all the teaching ideas are reinforced. Using memory aids and the social network, therapists encourage continued participation in the rehabilitation process. Recommendations for the use of community resources, outpatient services, and day care facilities are discussed, with materials left for later consideration. The therapist measures the success of intervention by comparing evaluation and discharge performances. Discharge planning begins in the sixth visit, but discharge takes place on the eighth visit.

Three factors must be considered throughout the delivery process: (1) communication, (2) encouraging function, and (3) amelioration of barriers. Communication is the ability to express ideas. It requires observing, listening, and collaborating. Encouraging function requires the use of creative activity analysis and careful selection of choices that promote feelings of competence through deliberate grading and use of parallel choices. See Chapter 9, Section 3 for detailed information on how to use activities in treatment. Finally, the therapist works to ameliorate the deleterious effects of environmental barriers—psychological, social, and physical—that preclude the patient's success in goal attainment.

Step-by-step guide to home visiting

Each phase of the Model for Home-Care Delivery (see Figure 28-1) is given here with information on how to fulfill the tasks.

Phase 1: Evaluation

Referral

The evaluation begins with the referral. Referrals to occupational therapy may be included in the physician's original orders. If not, and if the patient could benefit from occupational therapy, the coordinating nurse contacts the patient's physician, verifies the request, and obtains written occupational therapy orders. Information commonly given in the referral includes the following:

- Patient's location—name, address, telephone number, and zip code
- Patient's date of birth
- Primary and secondary diagnoses and treatment precautions
- Recent hospitalization dates, if applicable
- Physician's name, address, and telephone number
- Primary caregiver's name, address, and telephone number
- Date the agency started care
- Name of the person who opened the case
- Other services the physician ordered
- Frequency of visits if specified
- Physician's specific orders

If the patient was treated in a hospital or rehabilitation facility, the former therapist may be contacted to ensure continuity of the occupational therapy program. The referral must be answered within 48 hours of receipt.

Planning the first visit. After receiving the referral, the therapist prepares for the initial visit, which involves three steps: locating the patient's house, scheduling the visit, and selecting appropriate modalities for the evaluation. Planning maximizes the time spent with the patient and minimizes the time wasted on nonproductive concerns. It is best to make the shortest trips between patients' houses. Using a detailed map makes routing easier.

The new patient must next be contacted by telephone. The occupational therapist should offer an introduction and ask for permission to visit, emphasize the time and day of the visit, verify the address, and discuss directions to the house that will help in avoiding traffic obstacles.

Most therapists carry a bag with evaluation tools and common modalities. The bag may contain a stereognosis testing kit (box of familiar objects), perceptual test materials (formal or informal tests), goniometer, watch with a second hand (for pulse rate measurement), safety pin (to test for neurologic deficits), blindfold (to test for proprioception), and household items (paper towels, soap, crayons, scissors, pens, pencils, and masking tape). Some therapists also carry exercise putty, rubber bands, Theraplast, stacking cones, foam rubber, surgical tubing, and equipment catalogs. Splinting materials, crafts, weights, pulleys, and other equipment may be required later.

Initial fact gathering

Initial visits are crucial to the treatment process. The therapist evaluates the patient's abilities, establishes a baseline for measuring treatment progress, and determines the goals of the program. Also important is the assessment of the entire environment, including the caregiver and resources. Finally, the therapist must determine how to interact effectively within the patient's social system. The therapist takes in as much information as possible.

Six tasks that must be completed during the initial session:

1. Evaluation of the patient's motor, sensory, perceptual, and cognitive abilities
2. Exploration of the patient's present ability to perform life tasks
3. Assessment of human and nonhuman resources
4. Establishment of long- and short-term goals for the occupational therapy program
5. Projection of the time it will take to achieve the goals
6. Consideration of the lifestyle of the patient and caregivers: their values, goals, interests, roles, and habits.

Other objectives of the initial visit are to verify information about the patient's medical history, diagnoses, and treatment precautions and to meet the caregivers.

The therapist must determine the treatment goals and the duration of services during the initial visit. Goals for funding purposes must include independence in self-care and upper-extremity retraining. Most funding sources require evidence of *measurable, practical progress* in a reasonable period of time.

Long-term goals establish the desired outcome of the therapy regime. The success of the patient's progress will be measured in terms of the expected therapy outcome. Short-term goals are the graded steps to attainment of long-term goals. Short-term goals are part of the mastery process.

Evaluating the patient and setting goals

The evaluation form must be completed during the first visit. Read the case study below and develop your own goals and treatment plan. Consider the patient, social network, and environment. Consider the complexity of the patient's home situation. What factors would you consider as most significant? Note how the environment and available human and nonhuman resources influence treatment planning and outcome. Do you agree with the therapist's choice of activities? What factors did the therapist consider in her clinical reasoning process?

CASE STUDY

Mrs. U, an 81-year-old woman with a right above-elbow amputation, right CVA with residual left hemiparesis, and rheumatoid arthritis, lives with her son, daughter-in-law, and granddaughter in a walk-up apartment above a neighborhood tavern. Her son owns the tavern, and the daughter-in-law helps him with cooking and serving and assumes respon-sibility for Mrs. U's care. The granddaughter is mentally retarded and requires supervision and care. Mrs. U has been set up in a rented hospital bed in the living room of the apartment; a commode and wheelchair are also available. The daughter-in-law suffers from cardiac problems and is always guilt-ridden, harried, and stressed. The case was referred to occupational therapy because the patient wanted to learn how to eat independently. Her amputation occurred in 1956. She had no prosthesis but had been totally independent until recently, when she suffered a CVA that abolished isolated movement in her left arm. Tone in the extremity was increased, and sensation was impaired. Mrs. U has good cognitive skills.

Initially, the occupational therapist found Mrs. U totally dependent in all aspects of self-care with the exception of transfers, with which she required moderate assistance. The left upper extremity is spastic, and the elbow usually is held flexed. The therapist and patient agreed that Mrs. U could increase her independence in self-care; this became the long-term goal. They developed the short-term goals of teaching the use of a universal cuff and improving Mrs. U's ability to transfer during self-care activities and to eat independently if set up.†

The therapist taught Mrs. U how to use a universal cuff and sandwich holder and how to exercise her left upper extremity. The therapist worked with the patient to create a built-up work area. The therapist made 16 visits, and the patient achieved the long- and short-term goals.

Rapport building

Rapport building involves time devoted to socializing with the patient and caregivers, listening to their ideas, and observing their lifestyle and values. Using body language that conveys interest and concern, therapists can demonstrate their understanding of the difficulties that are imposed on families when chronic illness disrupts the ebb and flow of home life. During rapport building, therapists work to establish effective relationships, plan treatment, and communicate with the caregivers. The case study offered here demonstrates the importance of evaluation and how nonhuman cues can enhance communication.

CASE STUDY

The occupational therapist walked up a flight of freshly scrubbed marble steps and rang the doorbell of a twin house. Peering through the double glass doors of the glass-enclosed porch, he noted an orderly, modestly furnished porch and living room. Starched, white, ruffled curtains stood out from the window sills. Crocheted doilies adorned the dated, overstuffed sofa and arm chairs. Tiny, delicate china *objets d'art* were displayed on the sofa end tables. The focal point of the living room was a religious statue on an altar. The front windowsill was lined with large potted plants. The potting soil in several pots was decorated with china figurines and large satin bows.

† This case study is a fictitious composite of several patients that was developed by Reneé Baumblatt-Magida, OTR/L, Community Occupational Therapy Consultants, Inc., Philadelphia, PA.

A neatly attired elderly woman hobbled to the door; she seemed hesitant and fearful. The therapist displayed his arm patch and loudly mentioned his name and their earlier telephone call. The woman could see the therapist's name tag. She smiled and opened the door.

The therapist analyzed his observations. Signs indicated that the family did not usually have visitors and that strangers were greeted with suspicion. The orderly rooms implied a formal, respectful demeanor and that a boisterous person might not be well received in this home. He also speculated that changes should be introduced gradually; abrupt decisions should be avoided. The therapist used these cues from the nonhuman environment to enhance the effect of his communication.

A home-care therapist needs to develop the ability to establish a rapport with people in various social systems. Developing this kind of skill depends on making good observations and evaluating what is observed. The therapist must also be aware of his or her own value systems and how they affect the perception of others.

Once communication patterns are established, the therapist may discover information that will affect the outcome of therapy. The therapist addresses the altered goals and changes the treatment plan accordingly.

Phase 2: Treatment and assessment

The treatment regimen can now be given full attention. The program is introduced to the patient and the caregiver. There are three stages in the treatment and assessment phase of the delivery model: (1) treatment goals are refined, (2) teaching and learning fosters the exchange of ideas, and (3) the therapist promotes competent behavior.

Refining treatment goals

As the therapist gains additional insight into the patient's volitional, habilitation, and performance abilities and limitations, goals for treatment are modified. This is an integral part of the therapist's problem-solving skills and clinical reasoning.

Teaching and learning

The heart of the Model of Home-Care Delivery is the exchange of information between the therapist and the patient and caregivers. Teaching methods are described in Chapter 9, Section 3. The therapist must create an atmosphere of shared learning so the patient feels free to take control of the treatment regimen. This requires skillful planning, environmental adaptation, and activity analysis on the part of the therapist.

Promoting competent behavior

Using adaptations, exercise, success-evoking behaviors, and functional skill building, the therapist works with the patient to promote independence.

Adaptations. Adaptations are equipment or tools that ameliorate the press of the environment and improve the patient's performance. Examples are splints, eating utensils, built-up handles, and weights. Rather than order something that the patient will not use, therapists make sure that the adaptation will be accepted. Sometimes incorporation of common items instead of special adaptations are more acceptable. Some examples include the following:

- Weight: place canned goods in a zippered pocketbook or knotted sock
- Stablizer: put a damp cloth under the plate or tray
- Elastic shoe laces: use 1/8-inch elastic cut to shoe lace size
- Skateboard: place a towel under the affected arm; use on a smooth table top
- Bathtub transfer seat: use two chairs, one placed inside and one placed outside the tub

Exercise. Therapeutic exercises to restore sitting balance, re-educate upper-extremity dysfunction, and strengthen movements are discussed in Chapter 18.

Success-evoking experiences. The home setting is an excellent place to demonstrate the value of activities. Therapists devote most of their time to teaching rather than to complex hands-on intervention that cannot be duplicated by caregivers. A carefully selected activity reinforces goals, encourages habit formation, and promotes feelings of competence.

Curiosity about the activity base of occupational therapy has increased. The home setting offers an excellent example of the positive effects that can be derived from goal-directed activities. Few people will work at a task that they neither understand nor find pleasurable, whereas a match between patient needs and an activity can stimulate and motivate the patient.

An easy way to begin the search for a relevant activity is to ask patients about their former lifestyles. What tasks did they perform in their house? How did they manage daily life? Were they interested in any particular activities? A formal activity history might help to organize your thoughts. Another strategy is to ask the patient to describe a typical day.

The occupational therapist tries to find an activity that will motivate the patient. *Motivation* is self-directed behavior that an individual pursues for internal or external reinforcement (Florey, 1969). The individual moves toward a goal. Occupational therapy relies on both extrinsic and intrinsic motivation.

Goal-directed behavior stimulated by rewards outside an organism can be called *extrinsic motivation. Intrinsic motivation*, on the other hand, is dependent on an internal reward system. The person pursues an idea or task to fulfill an inner need. This need is not based on the satisfaction of basic drives, such as hunger, thirst, or libido. "Intrinsic motivation builds toward self-reward in independent action that underlies competent behavior" (Florey, 1969, p. 320) Crucial factors in the environment determine the extent to which a person is motivated by intrinsic rewards.

Successful home-care programs are carried over when the occupational therapist is not present. The choice of activity promotes the patient's goals, ideally generating some intrinsic rewards.

Phase 3: Discharge

The two types of discharge are planned and unplanned. *Planned discharge* takes place after 2 months of treatment. Once the patient's performance in activities of daily living and upper-extremity retraining reaches a plateau, the occupational therapist prepares for discharge. This decision should be discussed with the patient, caregivers, and other home-care team members. If circumstances warrant additional visits, the therapist should contact the case coordinator and discuss the reasons that visits should continue. Occupational therapists can visit a patient even if all other services are discontinued. In cases in which the other team members feel that the patient still has unmet needs, the team can act as the patient's advocate by working with the case coordinator, who can contact the fiscal intermediary and discuss the interpretation of the guidelines. On the other hand, the therapist should remember that fiscal intermediaries will not reimburse agencies for maintenance-level treatment.

If discharge is appropriate, the therapist should devote part of a visit to information on a home program that the patient and caregivers can continue. The therapist should use clear, jargon-free language. When appropriate, diagrams can clarify a point.

These ideas and others can reinforce teaching and improve the impact of the home-care program. Therapists also encourage further participation in rehabilitation activities. Attendance in group or religious activities or social organizations and pursuit of other interests are important to promote functional independence. Finally, the therapist should make recommendations for use of community resources and programs to promote further development and skill acquisition.

Unplanned discharge occurs more frequently than in the past since patients are more acutely ill when they are discharged from hospitals. This means that their medical conditions change rapidly and may necessitate additional inpatient admissions. Communication among the patient, family, caregivers, home health agency, and hospital staff becomes increasingly important.

At present, there are no resources channeled into aftercare. Ideally, each patient would be followed using telephone and brief visits designed to reinforce the rehabilitation program and to offer updated information. Insurance carriers do not recognize the value of aftercare since they are devoting their limited resources to acute patient needs.

Some therapists feel, however, that select cases require aftercare. Using their own time and resources, they telephone the patient, family, and caregivers to see how well they are managing. At times, a strategically planned visit may boost morale and encourage the patient to continue working toward goals. Although this type of follow-up is rare, therapists find that they can help the occasional family cope with emerging needs. This type of maintenance service should be provided as a form of preventive care.

Another aspect of aftercare is a critical evaluation of the occupational therapy services the patient received. Ideally, a questionnaire covering the quality of occupational therapy services should be sent to the patient, family, and caregivers. Outcome studies, whereby the final outcome of the patient's care is weighed against the initial goals, are also important. It is essential that occupational therapists compare the patient's progress with the cost of care. Were resources used wisely?

Factors to be considered throughout treatment

Communication, encouraging function, and ameliorating barriers are three factors that must be considered during every visit.

Communication

In the home setting, there are three basic forms of communication: face-to-face, telephone, and written. Face-to-face communication takes place in the patient's home or in the agency. It

requires observing, listening, and collaborating. This type of interaction may be difficult to arrange because of scheduling conflicts with the patient and other team members. Team goals and roles must be clarified early in the treatment process because confusion could block communication and hamper patient progress.

Telephone communication is a vital component of home care. Calls are made to the patient, caregivers, family members, team members, referring physicians, and referral agency personnel. The call is noted in the patient record with the telephone number. The content of the communication is described in a note. Even busy signals or no responses are noteworthy and must be charted.

Written communication is used to assist the family with items they need to remember or note, to chart the progress of visits and goals for care, and to note the content of conferences and meetings on the patient's progress. The importance of the written record cannot be overemphasized in the home situation. Many fiscal intermediaries have stringent requirements for documentation that must be followed to qualify for reimbursement.

Communication creates a sense of teamwork that is satisfying to the patient, caregivers, and professional and nonprofessional team members. The following quote underscores the effort that every member must invest in developing an effective team.

> It is naive to bring together a highly diverse group of people and expect that, by calling them a team, they will in fact, behave as a team. It is ironic indeed to realize that a football team spends 40 hours a week practicing for those two hours on Sunday afternoon when their teamwork really counts. Teams in organizations seldom spend two hours per year practicing when their ability to function as a team counts 40 hours per week. (Fry, Lech, & Rubin, 1974, p. 56)

Ameliorating architectural barriers

Architectural barriers can impede patient progress, but economic factors limit large-scale changes in many homes and few people have the resources needed to renovate basics such as bathrooms and kitchens. Therefore, the therapist must focus on changes that are desirable and economically feasible since little is gained from dwelling on changes that will never be implemented.

Another less obvious factor is cultural. Although some people enjoy change that will make their daily life easier, others regard new adjustment with discomfort because the daily, smaller energy expenditure attached to the current inconvenience seems more acceptable than the total commitment required for change to occur. Sometimes the only stable part of the patient's world is the unchanging nonhuman environment. The illness may have upset and altered everything else, including roles and relationships. To these patients, investment in the secure and unchanging environment may be more desirable.

The therapist who blindly suggests extensive change in this type of situation may encounter a brittle and resistant response. It seems logical to suggest minor changes, such as moving a bookcase 1 foot to the left to free a passage for wheelchair accessibility; however, the patient may not wish to crowd the picture that hangs next to the bookcase. The nonhuman world may be the last place that remains unscathed by illness (Searles, 1960).

The best approach for the therapist to use cannot be precisely outlined. Patients must be assessed in the context of their nonhuman environments and social interaction patterns. In addition, some ideas for change may be accepted at a later date.

Change was precluded in the next example because of

cultural and economic factors. This family was limited in income and was provincial in outlook. They could not value the suggestions of an outsider. The therapist could raise questions but could never expect to see immediate results. The therapist's role was, at best, that of a catalyst. The only change that was considered was the addition of a snack table to the right side of the refrigerator. Any others would have been too costly. The family seemed to accept the idea, but the item was never purchased. Possibly after the patient was discharged, the family was able to develop its own solution to the problem.

CASE STUDY

The H. family has resided in their small row house for 30 years. The brick house is more than 150 years old; it is situated in a blue-collar residential district in a large metropolitan area.

Mrs. H. is 54 years old. She has a residual left hemiparesis. Her recovery is complete except for a decrease in shoulder function. A perceptual test revealed a possible deficit in visual memory and spatial relations. She can dress independently, although her performance is slow. The occupational therapist has been active with Mrs. H.'s training for 1 month. The long-term goal is to maximize independent functioning. The short-term goal is to help Mrs. H. be independent in the kitchen and increase left upper-extremity function.

The therapist found that Mrs. H. used her disability. She could now garner the sympathy and support of her two teen-aged children. She agreed to try to work in the kitchen only because her children could not cook very well. The biggest problem that hindered progress was the layout of the kitchen and the breakfast room (see floor plan in Figure 28-2). Whenever Mrs. H. wants to take things out of the refrigerator, she has to walk back several feet to place the objects on the table. The food then must be transferred into the pantry. Mrs. H. refused to consider carry-all baskets; she felt that they "looked funny." The therapist suggested that a snack table be placed next to the refrigerator. The patient agreed but never was able to procure the item. The stove is also a problem; it does not have an automatic pilot light. After a few unsuccessful attempts at cooking, Mrs. H. was willing to turn this responsibility over to her oldest daughter. "I guess that she is old enough after all," she said.

The H. family could not afford any extensive changes. Their culture did not support do-it-yourself innovations. The nonhuman environment was one of the few stable things in their lives. There was little energy left to invest in change.

Encouraging function

Throughout treatment, the occupational therapist should emphasize what the patient can do rather than dwell on pathology and loss. Providing an outlet for competent performance requires expert activity analysis and grading. The therapist relies on the patient and caregivers to offer ideas for meaningful activities. Adaptations and work simplification techniques offer other ways to make the patient feel a sense of accomplishment.

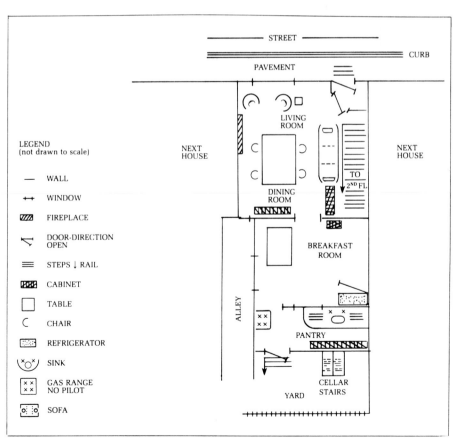

FIGURE 28-2. *Floor plan of the first floor of the H. family's house. The floor plan depicted here is common in a blue-collar neighborhood near the industrial center of a large city. The houses are more than 150 years old. Streets are narrow and barren. Small yards extend for 15 to 20 feet from the back doors. The average income is $35,000 a year for a family of four. This particular neighborhood is close-knit and insular. Relatives live two doors away or around the corner.*

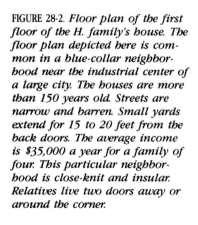

LEGEND
(not drawn to scale)

— WALL

↔ WINDOW

▨ FIREPLACE

⟍ DOOR-DIRECTION OPEN

≡ STEPS ↓ RAIL

▦ CABINET

▢ TABLE

C CHAIR

▦ REFRIGERATOR

⟨×ₒ×⟩ SINK

×× / ×× GAS RANGE NO PILOT

⟨ₒ:ₒ⟩ SOFA

External issues that shape home-care practice

Three external issues shape home-care practice: reimbursement, licensure, and practice groups.

Reimbursement

Reimbursement for home care has been a cause for concern for occupational therapists for over 25 years. Occupational therapy was not considered a primary service when Medicare regulations were originally developed in the mid-1960s. The situation is important and continues to shape home-care practice today; therefore, the next section is presented to focus attention on this aspect of delivery.

Fiscal intermediaries, or insurance companies that pay for health services, determine the amount of cost incurred by the health provider they will reimburse. Their decision is based on the DRG system. DRGs were added to the Medicare legislation as a cost-control method in 1986, and since that time, they have had a profound effect on every aspect of health care delivery. According to the DRG system, reimbursement for service is based on statistical averages of health care costs for the diagnosis being treated. Cost overruns are additional expenses that must be absorbed by the provider. This system has profound implications for home-care practice for two reasons. First, patients are discharged from hospitals "sicker and quicker" in an effort to avoid cost overruns. This trend in earlier discharge from institutional care results in a home-care patient population with acute medical and rehabilitation needs. Second, home health agencies are also anxious to avoid expensive cost overruns and therefore scrutinize the content of each provided service. Thus, the first home visit cannot be devoted entirely to evaluation because each visit must emphasize hands-on treatment of the patient.

Home-care agencies are funded by both public and private sources, including insurance companies, health care corporations, religious groups, charities, endowments, hospitals, and fees collected from patients. In the United States, most home-care programs are funded by Medicare (Scott & Dennis, 1988).

Medicare

Title XVIII of the Social Security Act provides legislation for Medicare funding. Medicare provides medical benefits primarily for older Americans, but people who have been disabled for more than 24 months can also qualify for benefits. Specific requirements are established for all the services that Medicare will fund. Not only do these guidelines influence current practice, they also will affect the future. The importance of Medicare extends beyond funding; it sets national standards for practice. In short, Medicare establishes national priorities regarding the services that will be covered, the quality and nature of those services, and the degree to which the practitioner and the agency will be held accountable for the care they give.

The responsibility for administering the Medicare program was given to the Secretary of Health and Human Services and, within this authority, the Health Care Financing Administration (HCFA). To accomplish this huge task, the United States is divided into HCFA regions, and each regional staff develops agreements with public or private organizations to serve as payment inter-

mediaries. These intermediaries use HCFA guidelines to establish the "services covered, amounts payable, and payments to be paid to beneficiaries and providers such as home health agencies and hospitals" (DePaoli & Zenk-Jones, 1984, p. 739). The intermediary becomes HCFA's representative in the region by supervising and overseeing the disbursement of benefits. In effect, this means that there are differences in the interpretation of the guidelines and regulations among the intermediaries (DePaoli & Zenk-Jones, 1984).

Once a primary service has qualified the patient for home-care benefits, occupational therapy can be ordered. In addition, occupational therapy service can continue after the patient is discharged from the primary, qualifying services. If occupational therapy is the only remaining service provided, the nurse must remain in the open case to supervise the home health aide.

To qualify for home-care services, the patient must be homebound, which means that he or she is unable to walk and get out of the home. The patients also must require skilled levels of care since maintaining function is not covered under the law. Skilled services are nursing and physical and speech therapies.

Medicare requirements for occupational therapy are centered on the expectation that the patient will benefit from the services and make significant practical improvement in functional abilities in a reasonable period of time. If the patient does not make progress, services must be curtailed because the fiscal intermediary may refuse to pay for the service. This action is usually taken retroactively, so therapists must learn to monitor their own cases to prevent costly denials.

At present, Medicare defines occupational therapy as a "medically prescribed treatment concerned with improving, or restoring functions which have been impaired by illness or injury or, where function has been permanently lost or reduced by illness or injury, to improve the individual's ability to perform those tasks required for independent functioning" (U.S. Department of Health and Human Services, 1982, p. 1501). Occupational therapy services may include the following:

- The evaluation and reevaluation as required of a patient's level of function by administering diagnostic and prognostic tests
- The selection and teaching of task-oriented therapeutic activities designed to restore physical function
- The planning, implementing, and supervising of individualized therapeutic activity programs as part of an overall active treatment program for a patient with a diagnosed psychiatric illness
- The planning and implementing of therapeutic tasks and activities to restore sensory-integrative function
- The teaching of compensatory techniques to improve the level of independence in activities of daily living
- The designing, fabricating, and fitting of orthotic and self-help devices
- Vocational and prevocational assessment and training (U.S. Department of Health and Human Services, 1982)

Services must be prescribed by a physician and performed by a qualified occupational therapist or certified occupational therapy assistant who works under the therapist's supervision. The most important clause in the criteria for coverage is that services are considered "reasonable and necessary" only when the patient's condition indicates that there will be a significant practical improvement in the level of function in a reasonable period of time (U.S. Department of Health and Human Services, 1982). Occupational therapy must be goal-directed, purposeful activity that can maximize the patient's level of function in a predetermined period of time.

Medicaid

Medicaid, or Medical Assistance, Title XIX of the Social Security Act, is a program for people who have no other means to pay for medical care. The program is based on a formula for matching federal and state dollars. For example, the state must contribute a percentage of its per capita income to the program. The ratios for the contributions are set by law. Some states do not contribute large sums of money to this program. Their reimbursement rates for home care may cover less than half of the actual cost of the services. If services are rendered, the agency must deal with the resulting deficit. If no alternative income is generated, the agency assets will be eaten away. Usually money from other sources are used to reduce the loss; however, this solution creates a complex and, at times, precarious funding situation. This is one of the reasons for establishment of rigid eligibility criteria. States may also develop their own criteria for eligibility.

Most states are required to provide home health services to Medicaid beneficiaries who are also eligible for skilled nursing care. Occupational therapy coverage varies since it is an optional service under Medicare.

There are strict limitations on the resources available to Medicaid patients. Thus, the nursing supervisor usually works out a rigid schedule of visits so the ceiling is not exceeded (Trossman, 1984). Agencies try to cope with this situation by providing fewer services over a shorter period of time. In rare cases, agencies use private donations to subsidize patients whose benefits have expired. As resources for the poor are stretched further and further, there are fewer sources to tap for providing services for people who have dire needs.

Other sources

Other sources of revenue include third-party carriers, such as private insurance companies. For example, most Blue Cross policies cover limited home-care benefits (Trossman, 1984). Third-party carriers are slowly recognizing the benefits of using home care instead of in-hospital services; however, coverage still differs, even among policies offered by the same carrier. Many prepayment plans—HMOs and PPOs—also cover home-care services.

Many hospitals are developing their own home-care organizations, and the number of privately owned home health agencies grew drastically in the 1980s and decreased in the past few years.

A number of private agencies augment home health services. Funded by private donations and through combinations of federal and state legislation, such as the Older American Act, some of these agencies offer creative solutions for patient problems. Specific services, such as the loan of hospital equipment or home-delivered meals, may be available. Religious groups may also offer patient-visiting services or meal delivery to the chronically disabled.

Another source of referrals and financial support for home care is HMOs. Once federally supported, HMOs are now inde-pendent systems of prepaid group insurance. Each subscriber pays a fee that entitles him or her to receive a wide range of health services. The emphasis in HMOs is on maintenance of health, although complete medical care is provided. HMOs are eligible for a Medicare waiver, which means that they can receive Medicare funds for providing services to older or permanently disabled patients. To receive a Medicare waiver, the HMO must offer subscribers a range of home-care services that include occupational therapy.

The American Occupational Therapy Association has developed a series of workshops and institutes to address reimbursement, documentation, and private practice issues. Several new manuals, such as the *Payment for Occupational Therapy Manual,* have been published and are available from the AOTA Product Division, 1383 Piccard Drive, Rockville, Maryland, 20849-1725.

Documentation

Health care providers sometimes forget that documentation is a form of communication. Home-care delivery is not easy to observe because of the number of patients' residences that are visited. Documentation therefore becomes an important tool to measure the quality of patient care. There is an adage that is frequently repeated by nursing supervisors: "If it isn't written, it hasn't been done." This statement reflects the stringent demands of most fiscal intermediaries. Most fiscal intermediaries demand adherence to their guidelines; if not satisfied, a carrier will refuse to reimburse the agency for the visits. Organized, goal-oriented, concise notes that clearly convey the patient's status to the reviewer are essential. Most fiscal intermediaries demand measurable progress in a reasonable period of time (U.S. Department of Health and Human Services, 1982). There are few funding sources for extended, maintenance-level care.

Most fiscal intermediaries rely on Medicare standards for their reimbursement guidelines. These guidelines determine the thrust of covered services and the diagnoses and care that will be covered. These guidelines establish the narrowest definition for occupational therapy services. Therefore, it seems reasonable to outline this base, although it is hoped that therapists will be able to deliver broader services. In general, Medicare coverage dictates that the patient must be able to improve significantly in a *reasonable* and generally predictable period of time. Claims for reimbursement for custodial care or maintenance are not accepted by Medicare.

On the first visit, the patient must be evaluated, treatment goals must be established, the total number of treatment visits required to attain the goals must be projected, and the patient must be given treatment. The therapist must inform the supervisor about the treatment frequency and plans. The therapist must also fill out a certification form. Every evaluation, certification form, or progress note must demonstrate to a person who is not an occupational therapist how the patient will progress and complete the established goals. Most agencies require a treatment plan for every scheduled visit. If plans change, the therapist must explain why.

The patient's progress is reviewed every 60 days, when a certification and plan of treatment form must be completed. This is the same form that was completed after the evaluation. This justification has three parts: a certification component, a medical and patient information update, and an addendum for additional information. Information commonly given in the recertification includes the following:

- Patient's name and address
- Health insurance number
- Medical record number
- Start-of-care date
- How long treatment can continue
- Name of home health agency
- Principal diagnosis, using code numbers
- Surgical procedure code, if relevant
- Other pertinent diagnoses
- Functional limitations (eg, contracture, endurance, mental, visual, speech) and activities permitted (eg, bed rest, transfer to bed or chair, partial weight-bearing, cane, or no restrictions)
- Safety measures
- Orders for services and treatments, which must specify modality, amount, and frequency
- Medications, including doses, frequency, and route
- Mental status
- Nutritional requirements
- Medical supplies
- Any allergies
- Goals for rehabilitation, patient's potential, and, if pertinent, discharge plans
- Significant clinical findings with a summary from each discipline
- Prognosis
- Attending physician's name and address
- Physician certification regarding need for treatment
- Physician's signature and date signed (U.S. Department of Health and Human Services, 1985)

For reimbursement purposes, home-care therapists must be skilled in focusing on the patient's activities in all notes. Documentation should emphasize the patient's progress toward independent functioning in self-care or a related therapeutic activity. It is important to delineate the relation between the progress and the therapeutic program. The caregiver's participation is crucial; therefore, the degree that the educational aspects of the occupational therapy program involved the caregiver and resulted in increased patient abilities must be documented. Treatment sessions should always include an opportunity for the patient to practice new skills.

Not all programs are governed by Medicare, but the number of older Americans increases daily, and this will influence Medicare services. In 1986, after a number of years of intense lobbying directed by AOTA under the leadership of the Legislative and Political Affairs Division of the Association, two areas of coverage for occupational therapy were added to Medicare: First, occupational therapy services are now covered under Part B, outpatient programming and private practice. Part A covers inpatient, skilled nursing facility, and home health care; and before 1986, part A covered occupational therapy services except when the patient had exhausted his or her need for other services. Occupational therapy services then had to be terminated even if they were needed. Now, occupational therapy can continue, although occupational therapy alone will not qualify as a beneficiary for the home health benefit. Second, private practice in occupational therapy has joined physical therapy as the only nonphysician providers. This means that therapists will be as-

signed a provider number and can bill Medicare directly for services rendered to beneficiaries in the office, skilled nursing facility, home, or any other appropriate setting. There is a $750 limit per beneficiary under this provision, excluding splints.

In some settings, the value of custodial and maintenance services are recognized, and undiagnosed mental illness may also be treated.

The boundaries of Medicare coverage are presented here to establish a base for home-care practice. Services should not be narrowed further. The home-care therapist should define the role of occupational therapy so that the most patients can be reached. If the role were too broadly defined, however, other services could be duplicated, and the unique focus of occupational therapy could be lost. A balanced, well-defined role should be developed and should function within the boundaries of the home-care agency's financial resources.

Licensure

The second issue that affects home-care delivery is that of licensure. Licensure laws protect consumers from unsafe practice in most states. The laws regulate practice and establish guidelines for care. Laws are specific to each state, and the rules and regulations vary. Some states define acceptable modalities, supervision, and continuing education requirements. Home-care practitioners must obey the licensure laws of the state in which they practice. (The state contact person, who can provide details about a specific state's law, can be located through AOTA.)

Practice groups

Occupational therapists who are interested in a ***private practice*** are advised to work for 1 or 2 years in a facility that offers a broad range of learning opportunities under the supervision of an experienced practitioner before entering home care. The more knowledgeable and skilled the practitioner, the more advanced is the level of care offered to patients. The home setting is not an arena to develop basic knowledge and skills because care is isolated from other occupational therapy practitioners.

Some therapists are engaged in private practice. They divide their time among several agencies or settings. These practitioners may also receive private referrals. Payment may be a combination of part-time salary and fees-for-service. A fee-for-service is a lump sum of money paid to the therapist for each visit. The therapist is not a member of the agency; no benefits are paid. Note-writing and travel time is included in the fee. At times, the agency will pay for attendance at staff meetings and conferences.

One advantage of private practice is the freedom that it affords the therapist. Treatment times and hours and patient load and demands can be varied. Practice can be carried out in several specialty areas; programs that could not afford occupational therapy can begin to offer the service. This modest beginning does not put the service in a make-it-or-break-it position. Some therapists combine part-time institutional work with private practice.

Another convenient way to develop part-time occupational therapy is in a group practice, with one therapist acting as coordinator. A registry of local therapists who wish to pursue part-time work is compiled. Once the names are organized, the process is not complex. State laws must be researched for local requirements. This is usually a simple matter for a lawyer to handle. When the group is organized, referrals can be received. Contracts can be signed with several agencies, or single referrals can be accepted. Individual therapists are assigned to a location near their home or work. Referrals are assigned by location. At least one member must be available during the day for telephone calls, referrals, and attendance at meetings.

The benefits of a group practice are numerous. The agency can deal with one coordinator instead of several part-time workers. A broad geographic area can be serviced without wasting time in travel. The group seeks its own members and is better able to evaluate member skills. Service to patients is not interrupted by vacations, illness, and other obligations—the group, not just one person, is responsible for the referrals. The group members benefit because the work is part-time. More therapists can participate in home-care delivery. Agencies with small case loads can still provide occupational therapy services. Therapists can join or leave the group without any major disruption of service. The group name becomes familiar to agencies and community centers, even if individual therapists have to drop out of the group.

The authors extend grateful appreciation to Claire Lozowicki, past-President, Bayard Miller, President, and Phyllis Erlich, Marlene Cohen, and Reneé Baumblatt-Magida, members of Community Occupational Therapy Consultants; to Susan Parker, Supervisor, and Rebecca Austill-Clausen, President, of Austill Aids, who provided critical feedback, case studies, and current practice dilemmas as well as a careful analysis of ideas.

References

American Occupational Therapy Association. (1991). 1990 Member data survey: Summary report. *OT Week*, June 6.

Anthony-Bergstone, C. R., Zarit, S. H., & Gatz, M. (1988). Symptoms of psychological distress among caregivers of dementia patients. *Psychology and Aging, 3*(3), 245–248.

Bailey, D. (1989). Collaborative goal setting with families: Resolving differences in values and priorities for services. In B. E. Hanft (Ed.), *Family-centered care: An early intervention resource manual* (pp. 47–53). Rockville, MD: American Occupational Therapy Association.

Barris, R., Kielhofner, G., Levine, R. E., & Neville, A. M. (1985). Occupation as interaction with the environment. In G. Kielhofner (Ed.), *A Model of Human Occupation: Theory and application* (pp. 42–62). Baltimore: Williams and Wilkins.

Bateson, M. C. (1991). *Composing a life.* New York: Plume Book.

Bazyk, S., & Trombino, B. (1990). Occupational therapy practice: Practice dilemmas. *Occupational Therapy Practice, 2*(1), 84–89.

Bearon, L. B. (1991). No great expectations: The underpinnings of life satisfaction for older women. *Gerontologist, 29*(6), 772–778.

Brameld, T. (1955). *Philosophies of education in a cultural perspective.* New York: Dryeden Press.

Bruckner, B. (1991, August 22). My life is too hectic to work in anything other than home care. *Occupational Therapy Week, 5*(33), 14.

Burke, J. P. (1977). A clinical perspective on motivation: Pawn vs. origin. *Amer Journal of Occupational Therapy, 31*, 254–258.

Clipp, E. C., & George, L. K. (1990). Psychotropic drug use among caregivers of patients with dementia. *Journal of the American Geriatrics Society, 38*, 227–235.

Corcoran, M. A. (1991a). *Gender differences among dementia management plans of spousal caregivers: Implications for occupational therapy. American Journal of Occupational Therapy, 46*(11), in press.

Corcoran, M. A. (1991b). *The nature of collaboration in a therapeutic relationship: Implications for service delivery plans.* Unpublished doctoral paper, City and Regional Planning Department, University of Pennsylvania, Philadelphia.

Corcoran, M. A., & Gitlin, L. N. (1991a). Environmental influences on behavior of the elderly with dementia: Principles for intervention in the home. *Physical and Occupational Therapy in Geriatrics, 4*(3–4), 5–22.

Corcoran, M. A., & Gitlin, L. N. (1991b). *Dementia management: An occupational therapy home-based intervention for caregivers of individuals with dementia. American Journal of Occupational Therapy, 46*(9), 801–808.

DePaoli, T. L., & Zenk-Jones, P. (1984). Medicare reimbursement in home care. *American Journal of Occupational Therapy, 38*, 739–742.

Dunning, H. (1972). Environmental occupational therapy. *American Journal of Occupational Therapy, 26*, 292–298.

Dybwad, G. (1989). Empowerment means power-sharing. In B. E. Hanft (Ed.), *Family-centered care: An early intervention resource manual* (pp. 55–58). Rockville, MD: American Occupational Therapy Association.

Englehardt, T. H. Jr. (1983). Occupational therapists as technologists and custodians of meaning. In G. Kielhofner (Ed.), *Health through occupation: Theory and practice in occupational therapy* (p. 144). Philadelphia: F. A. Davis.

Fitting, M., Rabins, P., Lucas, M. J., & Eastham, J. (1986). Caregivers for dementia patients: A comparison of husbands and wives. *Gerontologist, 26*(3), 248–252.

Florey, L. (1969). Intrinsic motivation: The dynamics of occupational therapy theory. *American Journal of Occupational Therapy, 23*, 319–322.

Fry, R. E., Lech, B. A., & Rubin, I. (1974). Working with the primary care team: The first intervention. In H. Wise, R. Beckhard, & I. Rubin (Eds.), *Making health teams work* (p. 27–59). Cambridge, MA: Ballinger.

Hasselkus, B. R. (1987). *Family caregivers for the elderly at home: An ethnography of meaning and informal learning.* Ann Arbor, MI: University Microfilms International, Dissertation Information Service, Order No. 8713154.

Hinajosa, J. (1990). How mothers of preschool children with cerebral palsy perceive occupational and physical therapists and their influence on family life. *Occupational Therapy Journal of Research, 10*(3), 144–162.

Huddleston, B. E. (1991, August 22). You soon learn that your car becomes your second home. *Occupational Therapy Week, 5*(33), 14–15.

Kahana, E. (1975). A congruence model of person-environment interaction. In P. G. Windley, T. Byerts, & E. G. Ernst (Eds.), *Theoretical development in environment for aging* (pp. 181–214). Washington, DC: Gerontological Society.

Kaplan, K., & Cubie, S. H. (1982). A case analysis method for the Model of Human Occupation. *American Journal of Occupational Therapy, 36*, 645–656.

Kielhofner, G. (1985). Occupational function and dysfunction. In G. Kielhofner (Ed.), *A Model of Human Occupation: theory and application* (pp. 63–75). Baltimore: Williams and Wilkins.

Kielhofner, G. (1978). General systems theory: Implications for theory and action in occupational therapy. *American Journal of Occupational Therapy, 32*(10), 637–645.

Kielhofner, G., & Burke, J. (1980). A Model of Human Occupation: 1. Conceptual framework and content. *American Journal of Occupational Therapy, 34*, 572.

Kielhofner, G., & Burke, J. (1985) Components and determinants of human occupation. In G. Kielhofner (Ed.), *A Model of Human Occupation: Theory and application* (pp. 12–36). Baltimore: Williams and Wilkins.

Kielhofner, G., Shepherd, J., Stabenow, C. A., Bledsoe, N., Furst, G., Green, J., Harlan, B. H., McLellan, C. L., & Owens, J. (1985). Physical disabilities. In G. Kielhofner (Ed.), *A Model of Human Occupation: Theory and application* (pp. 170–247). Baltimore: Williams and Wilkins.

Kiernat, J. M. (1987). Promoting independence and autonomy through environmental approaches. *Topics in Geriatric Rehabilitation, 3*(1), 1–6.

Kirschenbaum, H. (1973). Beyond values clarification. In S. B. Simon, & H. Kirschenbaum (Eds.), *Readings in values clarification* (pp. 92–110). Minneapolis: Winston Press.

Lawton, M. P. (1975). Competence, environmental press and the adaptations of older people. In P. G. Windley, T. O. Byerts, & F. G. Ernst (Eds.), *Theory development in environment and aging* (pp. 33–59). Washington, DC: Gerontological Society.

Lawton, M. P. (1983). Environment and other determinants of well being in older people. *Gerontologist, 23,* 349–357.

Levine, R. E. (1987). Culture: A factor influencing the outcomes of occupational therapy. *Occupational Therapy in Health Care, 4,* 3–16.

Levine, R. E., & Gitlin, L. N. (1992). A model for promoting activity competence in elders. *American Journal of Occupational Therapy,* in press.

Levine, R. E., & Merrill, S. C. (1987). Psychosocial aspects of the environment. *Topics in Geriatric Rehabilitation, 3*(1), 27–33.

Mastrangelo, R. (1990, October 29). Brave new world of home care. *Advance for Occupational Therapists, 6*(44), 1–3.

McKechnie, J. L. (Ed.) (1980). Webster's new twentieth century dictionary of the English language. Williams Collins.

Montgomery, R. V., & Datwyler, M. M. (1990, Summer). Women and men in the caregiving role. *Generations,* 34–38.

Morris, C. W. (1956). *Varieties of human value.* Chicago: University of Chicago Press.

Motenko, A. K. (1989). The frustrations, gratifications, and well-being of dementia caregivers. *Gerontologist, 29*(2), 166–172.

Murray, H. A. (1938). *Explorations in personality.* New York: Oxford University Press.

National League of Nursing (1984). *Administrator's handbook of community health and home care services* (Publ. No. 21-1943) (p. 95). New York: National League of Nursing.

Peloquin, S. M. (1990). The patient-therapist relationship in occupational therapy: Understanding visions and images. *American Journal of Occupational Therapy, 44*(1), 13–21.

Pepper Commission (1990). *A call for action.* Final report by U.S. Bipartisan Commission on Comprehensive Health Care. Washington DC: U.S. Government Printing Office.

Pruchno, R. A., & Resch, N. L. (1989). Husbands and wives as caregivers: Antecedents of depression and burden. *Gerontologist, 29*(2), 159–165.

Reilly, M. (1962). Occupational therapy can be one of the great ideas of 20th century medicine. *American Journal of Occupational Therapy, 16,* 1–9.

Research Information Division (1986, September). Dataline. *Occupational Therapy News, 40,* 8.

Rogers, C. R. (1969). *Freedom to learn.* Columbus, OH: Charles E. Merrill Publishing Company.

Rogers, J. C. (1982). The spirit of independence: The evolution of a philosophy. *American Journal of Occupational Therapy, 36,* 709–715.

Rogers, J. C. (1983) The study of human occupation. In G. Kielhofner (Ed.), *Health through occupation: Theory and practice in occupational therapy* (pp. 93–124). Philadelphia: F. A. Davis.

Schooler, K. K. (1982). Response of the elderly to environment: A stress-theoretical perspective. In M. P. Lawton, P. G. Windley, & T. O. Byerts (Eds.), *Aging and the environment: Theoretical approaches* (pp. 80–96). New York: Springer.

Scott, S. J., & Dennis, D. C. (1988). *Payment for occupational therapy services.* Rockville, MD: American Occupational Therapy Association.

Searles, H. F. (1960). *The nonhuman environment.* New York: International Universities Press.

Sherman, S. R., Ward, R. A., & LaGory, M. (1988). Women as caregivers of the elderly: Instrumental and expressive support. *Social Work, 33,* 164–167.

Special Committee on Aging (1987). *Developments in aging* (Publ. No. 0-291). Washington DC: U.S. Senate Publishing.

Spitze, G., & Logan, J. (1989). Gender differences in family support: Is there a payoff? *Gerontologist, 29*(1), 108–113.

Stone, R., Cafferata, G. L., & Sangl, J. (1987). Caregivers of the frail elderly. A national profile. *Gerontologist, 27*(5), 616–626.

Steinhauer, M. J. (1991, August 22). Committee explores formation of SIS. *Occupational Therapy Week, 5*(33), 15.

Trossman, P. B. (1984). Administrative and professional issues for the occupational therapist in home health care. *American Journal of Occupational Therapy, 38,* 726–733.

U.S. Department of Health and Human Services (1982). Coverage of services: Occupational therapy. In *Medicare Home Health Agency manual* (HCFA Publ. No. 11, Section 205.2, pp. 15.1–15.3). Washington, DC: DHHS.

U.S. Department of Health and Human Services (1985). *Health Care Financing Administration form HCFA-485* (C4) (4–85). Washington, DC: DHHS.

Yerxa, E. J. (1983). Audacious values: The energy source for occupational therapy practice. In G. Kielhofner (Ed.), *Health through occupation: Theory and practice in occupational therapy* (pp. 149–177). Philadelphia: F. A. Davis,

Yerxa, E. J., & Baum, S. (1987). Environmental theories and the older person. *Topics in Geriatric Rehabilitation, 3*(1), 7–18.

Young, R. F., & Kahana, E. (1989). Specifying caregiver outcomes: Gender and relationship aspects of caregiving strain. *Gerontologist, 29*(5), 660–666.

Zarit, S. H., Todd, P. A., & Zarit, J. M. (1986). Subjective burden of husbands and wives as caregivers: A longitudinal study. *Gerontologist, 26*(3), 260–266.

CHAPTER 29

Wellness programs

JERRY A. JOHNSON

LEARNING OBJECTIVES

Upon completion of this chapter the reader will be able to:

1. *Define health, health promotion, and wellness, and describe the ways in which occupational therapy can contribute to health.*
2. *Contrast and compare the concepts of balance and participation that are associated with health to similar concepts associated with occupation.*
3. *Explain the hypothesis that occupation is associated with balance and participation and thus can contribute to health.*
4. *Present the support found in the research literature for the relationship between personal beliefs, choices, decisions, and actions and states of health or disease.*
5. *Explore the differences in illness and disease, and contrast the different interpretations and values placed on both illness and disease by Western medical models and early Hippocratic and Chinese medical models.*
6. *Discuss the link among stress, imbalance, and negative cognition that may lead to lowered immunity and onset of disease.*
7. *Describe the difference between rehabilitation and recomposition of one's life and propose that recomposing one's life may be more beneficial and health-promoting than rehabilitation.*
8. *Discuss the benefits of planning and conducting patient treatment in occupational therapy from the perspective of occupational roles to produce more effective and positive results that contribute to health as well as a return to productive living.*
10. *Promote the value, meaning, and benefits of working collaboratively with patients, within the framework of their occupational roles (past, present, and future) and their visions of the future, to establish goals that have meaning for their lives, to promote self-initiated and purposeful activities within the context of desired occupational roles, and to return control to patients—all of which support health.*

KEY TERMS

Coping	Occupational Behavior
Disease	Occupational Role
Dis-ease	Self-efficacy
Goal-directed Systems	Rules
Goals	Skills
Habits	Stress
Health Promotion	Synchrony
Illness	Value
Meaning	Wellness
Motivation	

Evolution of wellness and health promotion

Wellness is defined as the process of adapting patterns of behavior so that they lead to improved health and heightened life satisfaction (Opatz, 1985). It is a concept that evolved during the mid-1900s as people, especially women and minorities, became disenchanted with medical practices and attitudes. It also became evident during this period that there were links, even though not well understood, that suggested a relation between health and behavior patterns and lifestyles as well as states of mind, thoughts, feelings, self-efficacy, coping strategies, and use of social support (Ader, 1981; Aldwin & Revenson, 1987; Antonovsky & Kats, 1967; Bandura, 1977; Chopra, 1989, 1991;

Csikszentmihalyi, 1990a; Kobasa, 1979; Kobasa, Maddi, & Kahn, 1982; Opatz, 1985; Ornish, 1990; Pearlin, Lieberman, Menaghan, & Mullan, 1981; and Selye, 1936, 1946). Consequently, it is believed that select changes in behavior and lifestyle can influence one's state of health and satisfaction with life.

Health promotion is the process by which one becomes aware of the need for behavioral and lifestyle change and acquires the knowledge and skill to bring about such change. More specifically, health promotion is the systematic effort, by people or organizations, to enhance wellness through education, behavioral change, and cultural support (Opatz, 1985).

Before the early or mid-19th century, health was perceived as an ongoing process involving people and their social networks that was reflected in participation in daily and community activities. *Illness* was viewed as an imbalance or disruption between the person and the surrounding world and was part of the collective experience in particular historical, cultural, and social settings (Berliner & Salmon, 1980). Both health and illness were viewed primarily as an individual responsibility in which the role of the physician was to help the patient and family through difficult times and to encourage people to be responsible for practices that supported their health. The physician–patient relationship was of primary importance in helping patients with problems to bring about changes in their lives that returned them to states of balance or equilibrium.

The belief that health was an individual responsibility was altered in the late 1800s and early 1900s as public health officials became concerned with the relation between environment and prevention of diseases and as medical science, or scientific medicine, evolved. During this period, public health physicians and scientists made an assumption that disease emanated from poverty and filth. This new way of thinking about the probable cause of disease led to improved transportation systems and improved sanitary conditions through the development of centralized water supplies and sewage systems. New systems of transportation made possible the availability in cities of large supplies of fresh food, thereby improving nutrition and reducing the incidence of disease.

Scientific medicine's focus on organic structures and mechanisms and the pathology associated with each made possible the identification of single causes or specific etiologies for individual diseases (Dubos, cited in Jaffe, 1980). The benefits of this approach have been significant. As physicians and medical scientists have studied physiologic changes associated with diseases, they have developed vaccines to prevent serious illness or death, drugs to treat bacterial and viral infections, and techniques and procedures to save, enhance the quality of, and prolong life; and they have identified genetic causes for many conditions that have a serious impact on health, and sometimes life itself, and subsequently found ways to treat many of the genetic defects, thereby reducing the incidence or severity of disabilities associated with them. More specifically, the discovery of penicillin and other antibiotics, the discovery of a vaccine for poliomyelitis, and the almost miraculous advances in microsurgery and organ transplantations led to the growing belief that medicine would provide the "magic bullet" for life's diseases.

The advances associated with scientific medicine resulted in a decline in the death rate (Dubos, cited in Jaffe, 1980). Despite the decline, however, the causes of death in the United States changed significantly between 1900 and 1987. In 1900, infectious diseases (eg, pneumonia, influenza, and tuberculosis) were the leading cause of death. In 1987, chronic diseases were the leading cause of death, with "four of the top chronic diseases (diseases of heart, cancer, stroke and accidents and their adverse affects)" being responsible for 80% of these deaths (U.S. Department of Health and Human Services, 1990, p. 16).

It is relatively clear that the decline in death rates due to infectious diseases was a result of advances in public health (clean water, proper sewage disposal, and improved nutrition) and scientific medicine, particularly the development of antibiotics. On the other hand, whether or not there was a casual or correlational relationship between the increase in chronic diseases and the shift from public health and early medical practice to scientific medicine is not clear. As the emphasis of medicine and the concerns of physicians shifted to scientific medicine and away from the patient–physician relationship, people began to act as if it was no longer necessary to examine their own behaviors, feelings, and family relationships as potential contributing factors to disease. Since they no longer had reason to believe that behavior might be related to disease, it was logical to make the assumption that disease was a result of either genetics or environment, factors about which the person could do little.

Whatever the reasons, there was a reduction in personal responsibility for health and an increasing lack of concern by physicians for complaints for which there was no evidence of physiologic change. The latter resulted in the delineation of illness and disease as two separate phenomena and reinforced separation of mind and body as physicians increasingly limited their attention to diagnosis of physiologic or biologic causes and treatment of disease. These two points are discussed separately.

The period between 1940 and 1980 was a time of considerable sociocultural change and upheaval, which brought about many behavior and lifestyle changes, many of which became acceptable, including the use of tobacco, smoking, alcohol, drugs, and engagement in sexual practices with numerous partners. Other less insidious but potentially harmful lifestyle patterns included lack of exercise, poor diet and nutrition, inadequate dental hygiene, and unsafe home environments. Originally, these behaviors and lifestyle patterns simply reflected lack of personal assumption of responsibility for one's health, whereas now they are known to be associated with chronic diseases such as cancer, stroke, heart disease, alcoholism, drug addiction, emphysema, and AIDS. Chronic, disabling conditions, most frequently associated with addiction, include accidents resulting in traumatic brain injuries and spinal cord injuries.

In other instances, parental behaviors and lifestyle patterns have a direct affect on the health of their children, including those who are still in the womb. Children raised in poverty in older cities may experience brain damage as a result of ingesting lead-based paint. Poor parents or drug-abusing parents tend to underuse medical services (provided they are even available) and consequently may give birth to premature, underweight children, many of whom may experience developmental delays. Children who do not receive vaccinations to protect them from common childhood diseases are at risk for illnesses such as measles and the serious complications associated with them, which can be fatal. Substance-abusing parents may produce drug-addicted babies, many of whom are now believed to have learning disabilities.

In summary, the major causes of death in 1987 involved diseases that are associated with personal choice, decisions, and lifestyles, many of which may be a result of low self-esteem;

hopelessness; lack of goals, purpose, or direction; or the belief, often found among adolescents, that "it won't happen to me." It is believed that most diseases associated with personal behaviors and lifestyle patterns are preventable (U.S. Public Health Service, 1979).

Despite the fact that many major diseases may be preventable, the amount of money spent on prevention is minimal in comparison to costs expended on treatment of disease and accidents. According to a U.S. Public Health Service report, it is estimated that only 1% to 3% of the American health care bill is spent on preventive care. With few exceptions, insurance reimbursement is not available for either illness or preventive care. Health maintenance organizations, however, are more likely to cover preventive services than are traditional insurance policies or preferred provider organizations (Staff, 1991a).

The medical profession has been slow to support preventive actions or behaviors for which people could assume responsibility and that contribute to improved personal health. It also continues to view illness and disease, as well as the mind and body, as separate phenomena. For example, 50% to 80% of visits to physicians are for illnesses that cannot be associated with any physiologic causes. Paradoxically, medical attention is not believed to be justifiable unless evidence is found of structural or biochemical alterations that characterize disease.

The primary focus of medicine has been **disease** syndromes, or diagnosable illnesses, defined as "physical complaints that fit a biological disease classification" (Kimball, 1982, p. 63). This definition limits attention of physicians and scientists to the diagnosis and treatment of disease. Consequently, precursors or markers associated with illness that may suggest risk factors for disease may be ignored or overlooked. Western medical practice does not generally perceive illness as an entity to be recognized or explored.

In Hippocratic and Chinese medical models, illness was believed to be a consequence of mental or spiritual conflict or imbalance and lack of harmony or **synchrony** with one's physical and social environments (Leonard, 1977). It is thus seen as a condition of the total human being and represents inadequate integration or interactions of mind, body, spirit, and environment or loss of flexibility in the system. Poor diet, lack of sleep, inadequate exercise, family disruptions, or social problems could be causes of imbalance.

From the perspective of the Chinese, organisms are self-correcting; consequently, illness is a natural process rather than a defined state. Symptoms of **dis-ease** (defined as sense of unease or discomfort, as contrasted with disease) were thought to serve a valuable purpose by prompting one to examine inner states of being and one's relationship to the larger family and social context (Capra, 1982).

Current Western thought defines illness as a behavioral change resulting in compromised function (Kimball, 1982). Other references, emerging from the study of stress, describe illnesses as more immediate reactions to or eventual consequences of stressful life events, which take from 2 months to 2 years to emerge (Kobasa, 1982). Other words that refer to illness as a reaction to stress include the fight-or-flight syndrome, activation, attempt at adaptation, stress response (Horowitz & Kaltreider, 1980) and strain (Kobasa, 1982).

In summary, the advancement of medicine and medical science has been the forerunner of two pervasive beliefs that have altered perceptions of health and personal responsibility

for maintaining one's health. The first belief is that health care is a right rather than a personal responsibility; therefore, the human body can be treated as a machine (and the mind as a computer) with little concern for its well-being. The second belief is that if one's body breaks or fails, medicine can "fix" it, and insurance will pay for it.

The wellness and holistic health movement that came into prominence in the 1960s and 1970s was a reaction to social forces and medical practices that were perceived as dehumanizing and neglectful, especially of the needs of minorities and women. Even now, recent studies of medical practice continue to show that (1) complaints of women are taken less seriously by physicians than those of men with similar complaints (Bush, Fried, & Barrett-Connor, 1988); (2) women with heart disease are treated less aggressively than are men with heart disease (Ayanian & Epstein, 1991; Steingart et al., 1991); (3) so little is known about women and AIDS that many physicians do not even diagnose their symptoms correctly (Kent, 1991); and (4) depression is twice as prevalent among women as among men (Staff, 1991d). In regard to this last finding, data recently released from the National Study of Medical Care Outcomes reports that mental health specialists tend to overdiagnose depression in women and to underdiagnose it in men (Staff, 1991d).

Because women are more likely than men to seek medical attention, their complaints, which are sometimes symptomatic of illness or dis-ease, are frequently presumed to be psychological and are not taken seriously. Medical neglect of women has recently been addressed by Congress and by the current Surgeon General of the United States, Antonia Novello, who has ordered the National Institutes of Health to include females as subjects in future research studies.

Although medicine and government, respectively, have been slow to endorse or support funding for preventive programs, corporate America, striving to lower medical care costs and lost work time due to illnesses or accidents, has embraced wellness programs. These programs generally emphasize exercise, better nutrition, stress management, and smoking cessation. Cessation of alcohol and substance abuse have been included more recently.

The validity of wellness programs received some support when the death rate from heart attacks dropped suddenly within a relatively short period of time in the 1980s. After a period of puzzlement, accompanied by review of data, this decline was attributed to the positive benefits associated with jogging and improved physical fitness. The acknowledgment of this relation between physical fitness and heart disease had a significant and positive impact on people's attitudes toward wellness and health promotion.

Evaluations of corporate wellness programs demonstrated other advantages, such as financial benefits, particularly in relation to increased productivity and reduction of sick time. These programs also were found to have a positive impact on employee morale, personnel recruitment, and employee retention (Chen, Moon, & Jones, 1982).

In summary, as the wellness movement expanded, people exhibited more interest in exercise, nutrition, and stress management, all of which provide options by which people can assume some degree of responsibility for their own health. New specialties associated with the wellness movement have also evolved, such as exercise physiology, sports nutrition, health psychology, sports gynecology, and sports medicine. Another new discipline, psychoneuroimmunology, has contributed to the growing interest in mind–body relations and their relevance for health and disease. These various disciplines have become well established and are contributing to the body of knowledge about health and the human body.

Most important, recent studies have provided insights into human behavior and health that form a foundation for both treatment programs and behavioral change. These insights suggest that (1) individual health must be considered within the framework of a larger system; (2) health is a reflection of harmony, balance, and flexibility in one's life; (3) stress is a major source of imbalance; and (4) illness may be a natural and creative response to stress and imbalance and thus may lead to healing (Johnson, 1986). Furthermore, chronic disease threatens personal control, reduces self-esteem, limits capacity to carry out various social functions, and creates dependency on medical care (Drory & Florian, 1991). Some of this new research offers support for a number of concepts related to health, many of which are commonly held among occupational therapists and are applicable to occupational therapy.

Research related to wellness and health promotion

A growing body of research literature provides evidence of an association between (1) one's choice of behaviors and lifestyle, state of mind, thoughts, attitudes, beliefs, feelings, access to and use of social support and coping strategies and (2) one's state of health. Each of these factors (individually or in combination) seems to influence whether one is healthy or not. Although the exact relation between these factors and health is not yet fully understood, many researchers have found evidence for a relation in studies of the following associated concepts: chronic disease and reduced personal control, self-esteem, social functioning, and independence (Drory & Florian, 1991); control and health (Folkman, 1984; Folkman & Lazarus, 1988; Kobasa, 1979; Gal & Lazarus, 1975; Langer & Rodin, 1976; Rodin, 1986, 1989; Rodin & Langer, 1977); control, commitment, and challenge and health (Kobasa, 1979); personal beliefs, values, and commitments and health (Lazarus & DeLongis, 1983); coping and health (Folkman, Lazarus, Gruen, & DeLongis, 1986) mastery and health (Folkman et al., 1986; Gal & Lazarus, 1975; Pearlin et al., 1981; Pearlin & Schooler, 1978); goals and health (Csikszentmihalyi, 1990a; Csikszentmihalyi & Larson, 1984; Frankl, 1978); adaptation and health (Selye, 1976); self-efficacy and health (Bandura, 1977; 1982; O'Leary, 1985); stress and health (Fleming, Baum, Davidson, Rectanus, & McArdle, 1987; Pearlin et al., 1981; Vitaliano et al., 1988; Selye, 1980); competence and health (White, 1959); roles and health (Minkler, 1981; Pearlin, 1989; Pearlin & Johnson, 1977; Pearlin et al., 1981; Pearlin & Schooler, 1978; Verbrugge, 1983, 1986); and coping and health (Folkman & Lazarus, 1980; Coyne, Aldwin, & Lazarus, 1981; Aldwin & Revenson, 1987). Although more research is certainly indicated, each of these concepts appears to have a positive relation to health and could well be used more directly in occupational therapy to promote health.

Kobasa (1979) conducted a study of about 500 executives to identify and examine characteristics that might be associated with health. In analyzing her results, Kobasa identified a concept, defined as *hardiness*, that was present among those executives who exhibited good health, as contrasted with those who reported problems with health. Hardiness consists of three characteristics (control, challenge, and commitment), is conceptualized as enhancing resistance to stress, and represents a set of beliefs about self, the world, and their interactions. *Control* refers to the tendency of subjects to believe and act as though they could control external events in their lives. Subjects demonstrated the ability to control their reactions to those events and, in so doing, experienced less negative, or stressful, reactions to them (Kobasa, 1979).

In a somewhat different study of control, Langer and Rodin (1976) found that the perception of control among elderly residents in a nursing home had profound results. Residents were given a choice of caring for a small house plant, and those who chose to provide the care were also asked to make small decisions about their daily routines. At follow-up 1 1/2 years later, those who chose to be responsible for the plants were more cheerful, active, and alert than were those who did not assume these choices and responsibilities. Furthermore, less than half as many of those who chose to make decisions had died as had residents in the other group (Rodin & Langer, 1977; Rodin, 1989).

Subjects in Kobasa's (1979) study sought *challenge*, believed that life changes were positive phenomena rather than threats, and exposed themselves to new, sometimes difficult situations to acquire new coping skills, which enhanced self-efficacy. Finally, the subjects indicated that they had *commitments* reflecting interest and curiosity about life that extended beyond their work to family, community, or church and that added meaning to their lives.

Other authors and scientists have written about the ways in which people open or close the gate to disease through a process, often attributed to "control by the host," which is not yet fully understood. For example, the human body contains bacteria and comes into contact with millions of viruses, allergens, bacteria, and fungi daily. For some 99.99% of the time, these organisms may live harmlessly in the body or enter it without causing sickness. Physical immunity and strong emotional resistance to sickness are credited with the body's ability to keep the gate closed (Chopra, 1991). However, immunity and resistance are known to be affected by smoking, heavy drinking, drug abuse, lack of regular exercise, and poor dietary habits, any or all of which significantly increase one's chances of having cancer, strokes, and heart disease (U.S. Department of Health and Human Services, 1990). Stress is also believed to lower resistance and immunity.

As a consequence of studies resulting in increased awareness of the relation between behavior and health, the belief that genetics is the sole determinant of disease (about which one can do nothing) is being challenged. Furthermore, just as thoughts and behaviors may result in disease, they can also have a positive role in improving health, as illustrated in the following example.

Ornish (1990) conducted a well-publicized study of 40 patients with advanced coronary artery disease and demonstrated that simple yoga exercises, meditation, and a strict low-cholesterol diet could shrink the fatty plaque deposits that progressively blocked coronary arteries. This allowed fresh oxygen to reach patients' hearts, which alleviated their pain and reduced their risks of fatal coronary accidents. This led to the first recognition and acknowledgment by medical scientists that heart disease could be reversed once it had begun (Ornish, 1990; Chopra, 1991). Arterial plaque had previously been believed to be static and consequently unchangeable.

It is also believed that an association exists between human cognition and emotions and health, although the linkages have been more difficult to identify with specificity. Research in the area of ***stress*** and ***coping*** has perhaps led to the most significant understanding of this relation as well as of the relation between stress and disease.

Kimball (1982) proposed that the study of stress and coping suggests the need for a broader perspective of the relation between illness and disease. From this perspective, stress causes a response, identified as a measurable change in the organism's behavior. This change is reflected in social behavior, psychological processes, or biologic response and could be symptomatic of illness. There is no evidence of structural changes indicative of disease in these early stages.

The degree of stress a person experiences is measured by the adequacy of one's response to handle (or cope with) the stressors. If the coping response is optimal, the stressful situation is resolved, and the aroused systems return to a normal baseline. When the coping response is either less than or more than adequate, the response of the aroused systems is aberrant.

Consequently, Kimball (1982) puts forth two proposals. His first proposal is that an inadequate coping response to stress (one that produces identifiable and measurable deviations from optimal social, psychological, or biologic functioning) should be defined as illness. One could have a social illness (eg, drug usage and abuse before addiction occurs or the loneliness phenomenon found among elderly people who visit medical clinics [Hughes, Senay, & Parker, 1972]); a psychological illness (eg, the giving-up, given-up state [Engle and Schmale, 1967] or problems distinct from psychiatric disease); or a biologic illness (usually observed as musculoskeletal or emotional arousal). Examples of a biologic illness might be increased muscle tension resulting in a stiff neck or a headache or elevated blood pressure. These behavioral changes, or symptoms of illness, may serve as markers or risk factors for disease, and earlier attention to their presence might lead to earlier detection of disease, to greater emphasis on health promotion, or to other measures that might prevent either the onset of disease or exacerbation of disease or chronicity.

Kimball's second proposal is that changes in social and psychological behaviors may be precursors to chronicity (defined as fixedness, or irreversibility of behavior) or disease (defined as permanent changes, based on altered biochemical structures or fixed response patterns). When the symptoms of either stress and distress or illness or dis-ease are unrecognized or ignored, they may act as precursors of disease or may exacerbate existing conditions (Brown, 1980; Dohrenwend, Dohrenwend, Dodson, & Shrout, 1984; Drory & Florian, 1991; Fleming et al., 1987; Selye, 1976). The hypothesized process of progression from stress (with perceived inability to cope effectively with the stressor) to disease is described in Figure 29-1.

As noted earlier in this chapter, an increasing body of research literature, often associated with stress, suggests that negative or self-deprecating thoughts, attitudes, states of mind, feelings, and beliefs, often associated with poor coping strategies and inability to develop or use social support systems, may compromise or depress the immune system, thereby putting one at risk for disease. This same process may also negatively affect

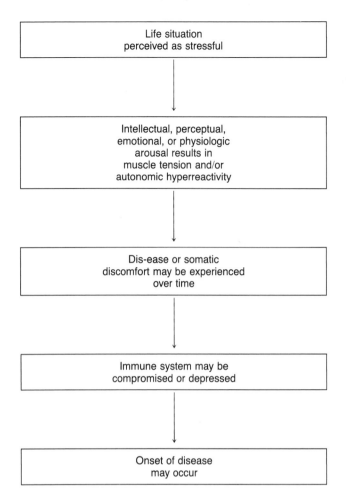

FIGURE 29-1. *Progression from stress to disease.*

recovery from a disease or increase the risk of its exacerbation (Borysenko, 1987; Cohen, Tyrrell, & Smith, 1991; Drory & Florian, 1991; Kobasa, 1979; 1982; Remien, cited in Roan, 1991; Staff, 1991b; Staff, 1991c; Ruberman, Weinblat, Goldberg, & Chaudhary, 1984; Locke & Colligan, 1986; U.S. Public Health Service, 1979; Justice, 1987).

Thus, although Western medical systems may have little to offer people who complain of illnesses, relevant members of the health professions should learn to recognize symptoms of stress and complaints of dis-ease and should address them. Certainly, occupational therapists, who traditionally have been concerned with the totality of human beings, including their biopsychosocial make-up and their remaining competencies, have an ethical responsibility to address stress, poor coping skills, or symptoms of dis-ease because all have the potential to negatively affect a patient's progress in therapy.

Wellness and health promotion in occupational therapy

Many of the principles of occupational therapy assist patients in recomposing their lives, thereby achieving a state of internal and external balance and facilitating their involvement in the fabric of their social networks through participation in daily and community activities. Both balance and participation are widely believed to contribute to or be representative of health.

Reilly (1962, 1966) was one of the first occupational therapists to hypothesize that engagement in an occupation contributes to and influences health. Reilly defined **occupational behavior** as "the entire developmental continuum of play and work" (1969, p. 302) and suggested that occupational therapists are concerned with the developmental continuum of work and play within the context of the particular social role referred to as the **occupational role** (1969).

Yerxa and colleagues (1989) describe occupational role as that part which a person enacts to fulfill self and social expectations as a player, student, worker, homemaker, or retiree. Within the context of occupational roles, occupational behavior refers to one's active engagement in occupation, which includes (1) an act of will, (2) the experience of engagement, and (3) the planning and organization of one's resources (Yerxa et al., 1990). *Occupational therapy* is thus the therapeutic intervention that promotes patient health by enhancing a patient's skills, competence, and satisfaction in the organization and conduct of those daily activities that comprise occupational roles.

Role competence is an important concept for both patients and occupational therapists. For many patients, particularly those with chronic conditions or long-term disabilities as well as those who have had more experience with failure than success, the traditional concept of rehabilitation is insufficient. As defined, *rehabilitation* is the process by which one is returned to the status or functional level one had before an illness or accident.

Today, however, it may be more constructive for many patients to recompose their lives in response to new situations rather than return to their previous pathways or lifestyles. The concept of recomposing one's life was exquisitely described by Bateson (1990), and although her context for recomposing one's life is different from that proposed here, the ideas Bateson proposed lead to balance, represent health, and have significance for people with disabilities. Indeed, if health is perceived as balance and disease as imbalance, to simply allow a patient to return to his or her previous lifestyle without exploration of other options may well mean return to a state of imbalance that promotes neither health nor the healing process.

The value of roles, specifically occupational roles, as the context for planning interventions in occupational therapy is that they are **goal-directed systems**. These systems are composed of rules, habits, and skills that, through the enactment of roles, are directed to a person's self-fulfillment. Consequently, they are identifiable phenomena for study and intervention (Csikszentmihalyi, 1990b).

The act of creating **goals** for oneself is guided by intention and powered by commitment. Once a goal or a set of goals are established, the brain is directed through the reticular-activating system to focus attention on existing skills and resources and to identify the new **habits, rules, skills**, and other resources that must be acquired to attain desired goals.

As new skills, rules, habits, and other resources are developed, **self-efficacy** (the belief that one has the resources to deal with situations or stressors that arise) evolves and provides both feedback about progress and **motivation** to accomplish desired goals. As one nears fulfillment of desired goals, new goals are formulated, and the process is repeated. Ultimately, rewards are associated less with goal achievement per se than with the challenge of learning and acquisition of new skills in pursuit of a goal. Variations of this process have been referred to as *planful competence* or *flow* and are associated with health and a sense of well-being.

The study of flow, or optimal experience, led to identification of those times in life when people report feelings of enjoyment, concentration, and absolute absorption in an activity during which sense of time and emotional problems seem to disappear. During these periods, which are associated most frequently with work and occupation and which can be maintained indefinitely, people report feeling strong, alert, in effortless control, unselfconscious, and as if they are performing at the peak of their abilities (ie, they feel healthy). Learning and challenge are balanced so delicately that each provides motivation and reward (Csikszentmihalyi, 1990a).

Several major findings, or principles, from research associated with stress, coping, and flow that relate to wellness, health promotion, and satisfaction with one's life and that seem to influence one's state of health can be incorporated into most occupational therapy programs. The first principle is that control, or even the perception of control, produces positive results, as illustrated in Langer and Rodin's study (1976; Rodin & Langer, 1977). Establishment of goals is one form of control; another form of control comes from the recognition that one has choice about responses to events that occur in life, even though it may not be possible to control those events.

The second principle is that people can be taught and can learn the rules, habits, and various physical, cognitive, emotional, and social skills and acquire the resources necessary to accomplish goals, primarily through modeling, practice, coaching, and feedback (Bandura, 1974). As these resources are developed or acquired, self-efficacy evolves.

The third principle is that motivation arises from participation in and commitment to roles in one's life that are compelling and have **value**, that have **meaning** for oneself and often for others, and that provide a just-right challenge in that they provide feedback that both motivates and rewards (Csikszentmihalyi, 1990a). The occupational therapist who can wisely incorporate these principles into a therapeutic plan in collaboration with a patient will do much to facilitate the patient's attempts to recompose his or her life and to make a commitment to create and carry out a plan of action to accomplish this.

Occupational roles comprise a large enough area of related and goal-directed, self-initiated and purposeful activities to encompass value, meaning, and commitment, each of which contributes to motivation, acquisition of the rules, habits, and skills to achieve one's desired goals, and ultimately, goal achievement and enhanced self-efficacy. The degree of success one experiences in returning to or assuming highly valued roles may well influence one's continuing recovery or health status.

The rationale for using roles as the context for occupational therapy is that people attach value and symbolic importance to each of their roles (Campbell, 1988). In addition, the choices a person makes in terms of which roles are most important in relation to the amount of time available have social, symbolic, cultural, and spiritual significance (Fraser, 1987). Value is closely related to motivation, and the more highly valued a given role, the more likely it is that a person will make a commitment to become competent in a role held previously or to compose a new role that is perceived as having similar or, in some instances, greater value or meaning.

For example, one perceptive therapist, in talking with a

patient who incurred a traumatic brain injury as a result of drug dealings, reframed his goals by suggesting that the patient was using language that suggested that he wanted to be an executive. This insight was based on the patient's descriptions of the meaning he experienced in his role as a drug dealer. He liked the concept of himself as an executive, and together the patient and therapist developed goals and a plan of treatment that enabled the patient to acquire the knowledge, skills, and behaviors to make specified changes in his life with the potential to open doors of opportunity for the patient to become an executive. As they worked together, the therapist used concepts of executive behavior to provide feedback about the patient's behavior and to illustrate how executives might behave in situations that the patient found to be frustrating. In so doing, the therapist provided a form of modeling for the patient that effectively introduced new behaviors and options associated with a goal that was compelling to the patient.

In essence, the more a person values a given role, the more compelling it is, and the more motivated the person will be to commit to successfully learning the rules, skills, and habits required for role competence. These qualities of motivation and goal-directedness often sustain patients during periods of great frustration. Conversely, the less value a patient associates with a role or task, the more responsibility a therapist has for motivating the patient, and control shifts from the patient to therapist.

Therapeutic interactions between patient and therapist at the level of meaningful occupational roles create an open, direct, collegial, and mutually respectful relationship as therapist and patient collaboratively identify, agree on, and prioritize the problems, goals, and strategies to be addressed in occupational therapy. This level of relationship is different from that in which the therapist presents professional or reimbursement-driven, task-oriented goals for a patient and then attempts to motivate the patient to achieve them.

Occupation (as used in occupational therapy) is derived from the Latin root *occupaio*, which means to seize or take possession. Both occupation and occupaio convey action, employment, and anticipation (Engelhardt, 1977). The nature of the descriptors associated with occupation implies that goals and goal setting are an integral part of occupation.

Goal setting, directed toward something of value, creates *commitment* (defined for this purpose as emotional energy directed to goal achievement and associated with intellectual and physical challenge) and guides progress toward an ongoing process of goal fulfillment and achievement, evaluation, and reformulation of new goals. Increased self-efficacy is an important, and often overlooked, by-product of this entire process, described by Yerxa and colleagues (1990) as taking control of one's life through engagement in occupation.

An inherent component of engagement in occupation for people with disabilities is the creation and implementation of goals and strategies for acquiring the range of physical, cognitive, social, and emotional skills either to recompose one's life or to reengage in meaningful occupational roles. In some instances, the use of environmental adaptations or technology may be necessary to supplement or replace skills and enhance independence and perceptions or experiences of control. These skill areas, when combined with rules and habits, comprise basic biopsychosocial elements, or building blocks, of occupational roles and are integrally related to occupational role fulfillment, to health, and to a holistic approach to treatment.

The current trend in occupational therapy appears gener-

ally to focus most on the physical and cognitive skills of patients, as reflected in the emphasis on function and task performance. Although this may be an efficient approach, the limitations of a primary focus on physical and cognitive skills with limited attention to or exclusion of concerns for emotional expression and social skills should be recognized. For example, two studies have shown that activities associated with self-care and daily living are least valued by patients with physical disabilities (Yerxa & Baum, 1986; Brown, Gordon, & Ragnarsso, 1987). Hawkings (as cited in Sipchen, 1990) also emphasized the importance of a productive existence that involves mental and organizational abilities rather than physical strength and dexterity for people with physical disabilities. These patients recognize that their energy is limited, and they prefer to expend time on activities that are more satisfying (ie, meaningful) and rewarding.

For therapy given within the context of health and wellness and within the sphere of goal-directedness as described here, there is merit to reaching decisions with patients and their families about the extent to which patients must be competent in performing self-care and daily living activities. For some patients, it may be sufficient to know how to instruct others to assist them with these activities rather than having them be fully competent in performing self-care. A shift in priorities could thus free time and energy for learning other skills that may be equally or more necessary for a meaningful life for many patients.

Physical skills enable one to move about in the physical world, and cognitive skills enable one to organize one's life and one's activities in that world. Emotional and social skills are closely related to self-efficacy, motivation, commitment, control, and the ability to be comfortable with oneself and with others. Competence with all four skill areas, as well as with rules and habits, thus becomes a basic constituent of successful occupational role performance, of balance, and of health.

When a patient experiences, and attempts to suppress, normal feelings of grief, loss, anger, sadness, or frustration, many of which arise during the course of therapy as old memories arise or as loss is confronted, less energy and attention are available to do the work required for rehabilitation or recomposition of one's life. The perceptive therapist allows patients to express and explore these feelings during the course of occupational therapy and is sensitive to the needs of some patients to acquire more effective skills for emotional expression as well as social interaction.

The most powerful influence, or determining factor, of patient progress may well be feelings about oneself. These feelings are often based on past experience or perceptions of past experience, and they may constitute the most significant challenge for both patient and therapist, particularly when the perceptions are negative or are based on denial. From the perspective of the therapist who is concerned about prevention, health, and health promotion, addressing and resolving psychosocial issues are equally as important, if not more so, than resolution of physical or cognitive issues primarily because of their impact on a patient's self-perception and on all aspects of role performance.

Most occupational roles require involvement of or interactions with others in at least some of their constituent activities. Both constituent activities and occupational roles become more meaningful when interactions with others are positive and affirming. More specifically, emotional and social skills are requisites for successful occupational role performance.

Exploration of a patient's participation in occupational roles begins in the initial interview between therapist and patient, which may be the most important aspect of treatment. During this interview, the occupational therapist seeks to accomplish several things. First, establishing a level of rapport and trust facilitates openness, frankness, and directness, which allows the patient to discuss and deal with difficult issues that will arise in the course of therapy.

Second, the therapist must establish the domain of concerns to be addressed in occupational therapy, that is, the patient's occupational roles (those previously and currently occupied and those desired) and their value and meaning to the patient, and sometimes to the family. The patient's occupational history may be explored to identify existing competencies (success) or deficiencies in previous occupational roles and their associated skills, rules, and habits, or to identify patterns that may have been dysfunctional or that can now be reinforced to enhance meaning or satisfaction.

Other issues to be explored in the initial interview include stressors associated with occupational roles; level of and availability of coping skills and social support to deal with stressors; the extent of family, environmental, and other external support available to the patient; and the patient's ability to accept and use such support.

Finally, the therapist and patient should explore the patient's perceptions and feelings about the impact of the disease or disability on his or her occupational roles and level of self-efficacy. Therapists interested in prevention may also want to explore the onset and progress of the patient's disease or disability, the quality of the patient's life at the time of onset or exacerbation, and the conditions, stressors, or vulnerabilities associated with either. This area often yields information that can help patients understand when they are most vulnerable and thus when they might be at risk for either another injury or exacerbation of an existing condition. It may also provide valuable information for therapists engaged in health promotion and preventive programs.

The occupational therapist seeks to understand what has meaning in a given patient's life, what the patient wanted for life before the onset of illness or disability, and what continues to be important. Even when meaning is found in dysfunction, it may be possible to attach the identified values to new roles or pathways. Even here, the perceptive therapist and the patient, in collaboration, may find the kernels of a dream, desire, or vision that can be translated into a goal and strategies for its achievement.

If the patient's family is not included in the initial interview, it is often advantageous to talk with family members about their perceptions of the patient's relevant occupational history and patterns, coping skills, stressors, and possibilities. Including family members, when possible, in joint planning sessions with the patient may provide a more realistic framework for treatment and may also facilitate both provision of support by family members and acceptance of that support by the patient.

Based on all the information just described, patient and therapist are in a position to collaborate in developing goals, strategies, and a relevant treatment plan that facilitates rehabilitation or recomposition of the patient's life *and* that enables the patient to engage in a life that is balanced and promotes health. In summary, in developing treatment plans with a patient, occupational therapists must be holistic—that is, equally concerned with physical, cognitive, social, and emotional skills as well as with rules and habits—because all are associated with occupational goals and roles.

From the perspective presented in this chapter, the occupational therapist views a disability within the context of a patient's occupational life, history, and future, not as a separate entity to be treated by the therapist for the purpose of remediating a pathological condition. This approach, designed to restore balance, control, and occupational direction to the patient's life, facilitates the process of rehabilitation or recomposition and promotes health and well-being. Consequently, it is hypothesized that patients may be less prone to other injuries or to exacerbations of disabling conditions.

Summary

The purpose of this chapter is to present the reader with an understanding and appreciation of health, wellness, and health promotion, all of which are associated with and reflected in balance in life and participation in the fabric of family and community activities. Those basic principles of occupational therapy associated with goal-directed, self-initiated, and purposeful activity are also inherently related to health and wellness in that they also contribute to balance and participation in life.

The domain of concern of occupational therapy is most appropriately located within the occupational roles that comprise people's lives. These roles encompass a large enough area of value, meaning, and commitment to provide challenge, enhance motivation, provide feedback about the quality of one's performance, and contribute to development of self-efficacy. Self-efficacy evolves as one develops new skills and an appreciation of the value of rules and acquires habits that save time and energy, thereby contributing to greater satisfaction with one's life and one's contributions to others.

If these principles are used as integral parts of treatment, particularly for people with severe or chronic disabilities, they may contribute to more effective rehabilitation or recomposition of one's life. Consequently, they also may make a valuable contribution in terms of reducing the potential for a second injury or exacerbation of the disease process.

References

Ader, R. (1981). *Psychoneuroimmunology*. New York: Academic Press.

Aldwin, C. M., & Revenson, T. A. (1987). Does coping help? A reexamination of the relation between coping and mental health. *Journal of Personality and Social Psychology, 53*(2), 337–348.

Antonovsky, A., & Kats, R. (1967). The life crisis history as a tool in epidemiological research. *Journal of Health and Social Behavior, 8*, 15–21.

Ayanian, J. Z., & Epstein, A. M. (1991, July 25). Differences in the use of procedures between women and men hospitalized for coronary heart disease. *New England Journal of Medicine, 325*, 221–225.

Bandura, A. (1974). Behavior theory and the models of man. *American Psychologist, 29*, 859–869.

Bandura, A. (1977). Self-efficacy: Toward a unifying theory of behavioral change. *Psychological Review, 84*, 191–215.

Bandura, A. (1982). Self-efficacy mechanism in human agency. *American Psychologist, 37*, 122–247.

Bateson, M. C. (1990). *Composing a life*. New York: Plume.

Berliner, S., & Salmon, J. W. (1980). The holistic alternative to scientific medicine: History vs. analysis. *International Journal of Health Sciences, 10*(2), 133.

Borysenko, J. (1987). *Minding the body, mending the mind*. New York: Addison-Wesley.

Brown, B. (1980). Perspectives on social stress. In H. Selye (Ed.), *Selye's guide to stress research*, Vol. I. New York: Van Nostrand Reinhold.

Brown, M., Gordon, W. A., & Ragnarsso, K. (1987, April). Unhandicapping the disabled: What is possible? *Archives of Physical Medicine and Rehabilitation, 86*, 208.

Bush, T. L., Fried, L. P., & Barrett-Connor, E. (1988). Cholesterol, lipoproteins, and coronary heart disease in women. *Clinical Chemistry, 34*(8B), B60–B70.

Campbell, J. (1988). *The power of myth*. New York: Doubleday.

Capra, F. (1982). *The turning point*. New York: Bantam Books.

Chen, J. R., Moon, S., & Jones, R. M. (1982, June). Establishing priorities in the wellness program. *Occupational Health and Safety, 51*(6), 6–7, 36.

Chopra, D. (1989). *Quantum Healing*. New York: Bantum Books.

Chopra, D. (1991). *Perfect Health*. New York: Harmony Books.

Cohen, S., Tyrrell, D. A. J., & Smith, A. P. (1991, August 29). Psychological stress and the common cold. *New England Journal of Medicine, 325*(9), 606–612.

Coyne, J. C., Aldwin, C., & Lazarus, R. S. (1981). Depression and coping in stressful episodes. *Journal of Abnormal Psychology, 90*(5), 439–447.

Csikszentmihalyi, M. (1990a). *Flow: The optimal psychological experience*. New York: Harper and Row.

Csikszentmihalyi, M. (1990b). Foreword. In J. A. Johnson, & E. J. Yerxa (Eds.), *Occupational science: The foundation for new models of practice*. Binghamton, NY: The Haworth Press.

Csikszentmihalyi, M., & Larson, R. (1984). *Being adolescent: Conflict and growth in the teenage years*. New York: Basic Books.

Dohrenwend, B. S., Dohrenwend, B. P., Dodson, M., & Shrout, P. E. (1984). Symptoms, hassles, social supports, and life events: Problem of confounded measures. *Journal of Abnormal Psychology, 93*(2), 222–230.

Drory, Y., & Florian, V. (1991, April). Long-term psychosocial adjustment to coronary artery disease. *Archives of Physical Medicine and Rehabilitation, 72*, 326–331.

Engelhardt, H. T. (1977). Defining occupational therapy: The meaning of therapy and the virtues of occupation. *American Journal of Occupational Therapy, 31*, 666–672.

Engle, G. L., & Schmale, A. H. (1967). Psychoanalytic theory of psychosomatic disorder: Conversion, specificity, and the disease-onset situation. *Journal of the American Psychoanalytic Association, 15*, 344.

Fleming, I., Baum, A., Davidson, L. M., Rectanus, E., & McArdle, S. (1987). Chronic stress as a factor in physiologic reactivity to challenge. *Health Psychology, 6*(3), 221–237.

Folkman, S. (1984). Personal control and stress and coping processes: A theoretical analysis. *Journal of Personality and Social Psychology, 46*(4), 839–852.

Folkman, S., & Lazarus, R. S. (1980, September). An analysis of coping in a middle-aged community sample. *Journal of Health and Social Behavior, 21*, 219–239.

Folkman, S., & Lazarus, R. S. (1988). The relationship between coping and emotion: Implications for theory and research. *Social Science Medicine, 26*(3), 309–317.

Folkman, S., Lazarus, R. S., Gruen, R. J., & DeLongis, A. (1986). Appraisal, coping, health status, and psychological symptoms. *Journal of Personality and Social Psychology, 50*(1), 571–579.

Frankl, V. E. (1978). *The unheard cry for meaning*. New York: Simon and Schuster.

Fraser, J. T. (1987). *Time, the familiar stranger*. Amherst: University of Massachusetts Press.

Gal, R., & Lazarus, R. S. (1975, December). The role of activity in anticipating and confronting stressful situations. *Journal of Human Stress, 1*(4), 4–20.

Horowitz, M. J., & Kaltreider, N. B. (1980). Brief psychotherapy of stress response syndromes. In T. Karasu, & I. Bellak (Eds.), *Specialized techniques in individual psychotherapy*. New York: Brunner/Mazel.

Hughes, P., Senay, E., & Parker, R. (1972). The medical management of a heroin epidemic. *Archives of General Psychiatry, 27*, 585.

Jaffe, D. T. (1980). *Healing from within*. New York: Alfred A. Knopf.

Johnson, J. A. (1986). *Wellness: A context for living*. Thorofare, NJ: Slack.

Justice, B. (1987). *Who gets sick: How beliefs, moods, and thoughts affect your health*. Los Angeles: Jeremy P. Tarcher.

Kent, M. R. (1991, May 16). Letter to the editor: Women and AIDS. *New England Journal of Medicine, 324*(20), 1442.

Kimball, C. P. (1982). Stress and psychosomatic illness. *Journal of Psychosomatic Research, 26*(1), 63–67.

Kobasa, S. C. (1979). Stressful life events, personality and health: An inquiry into hardiness. *Journal of Personality and Social Psychology, 37*(2), 1–11.

Kobasa, S. C. (1982). Commitment and coping in stress resistance among lawyers. *Journal of Personality and Social Psychology, 42*(4), 707–717.

Kobasa, S. C., Maddi, S. R., & Kahn, S. (1982). Hardiness and health: A prospective study. *Journal of Personality and Social Psychology, 42*, 168–177.

Langer, E. J., & Rodin, J. (1976). The effects of choice and enhanced personal responsibility for the aged: A field experiment in an institutional setting. *Journal of Personality and Social Psychology, 34*(2), 191–198.

Lazarus, R. S., & DeLongis, A. (1983, March). Psychological stress and coping in aging. *American Psychologist, 38*(3), 245–254.

Leonard, G. (1977). The holistic healing revolution. *Journal of Holistic Health, 2*(1).

Locke, S. E., & Colligan, D. (1986). *The healer within: The new medicine of mind and body*. New York: New American Library.

Minkler, M. (1981, June). Research on the health effects of retirement: A uncertain legacy. *Journal of Health and Social Behavior, 22*, 117–130.

O'Leary, A. (1985). Self-efficacy and health. *Behavioral Research Therapy, 23*(4), 437–451.

Opatz, J. P. (1985). *A primer of health promotion*. Washington, DC: Oryn Publishers.

Ornish, D. (1990). *Dr. Dean Ornish's program for reversing heart disease*. New York: Random House.

Pearlin, L. I. (1989, September). The sociological study of stress. *Journal of Health and Social Behavior, 30*, 241–256.

Pearlin, L. I., & Johnson, J. S. (1977, October). Marital status, life-strains and depression. *American Sociological Review, 41*, 704–715.

Pearlin, L. I., Lieberman, M. A., Menaghan, E. G., & Mullan, J. T. (1981). The stress process. *Journal of Health and Social Behavior, 22*(12), 337–356.

Pearlin, L. I., & Schooler, C. (1978, March). The structure of coping. *Journal of Health and Social Behavior, 19*, 2–21.

Reilly, M. (1962). Occupational therapy can be one of the great ideas of 20th century medicine. *American Journal of Occupational Therapy, 16*, 300–308.

Reilly, M. (1966). A psychiatric occupational therapy program as a teaching model. *American Journal of Occupational Therapy, 10*, 60–67.

Reilly, M. (1969). The educational process. *American Journal of Occupational Therapy, 23*, 299–307.

Roan, S. (1991, October 2). Attitude might help some AIDS patients live longer, study says. *The Philadelphia Inquirer*, p. 2-A.

Rodin, J. (1986, September). Aging and health: Effects of the sense of control. *Science, 234*(4781), 1271–1276.

Rodin, J. (1989). *Mindfulness*. New York: Addison-Wesley.

Rodin, J., & Langer, E. J. (1977). Long-term effects of a control-relevant intervention with the institutionalized elderly. *Journal of Personality and Social Psychology, 35*(12), 897–902.

Ruberman, W. M., Weinblat, E., Goldberg, J. D., & Chaudhary, B. S. (1984, August 30). Psychosocial influences on mortality after myocardial infarction. *New England Journal of Medicine, 351*, 552–559.

Selye, H. (1936). A syndrome produced by diverse noxious agents. *Nature, 138*, 32.

Selye, H. (1946). The general adaptation syndrome and the diseases of adaptation. *Journal of Clinical Endocrinology, 6*, 117.

Selye, H. (1976). *Stress in health and disease*. Boston: Butterworths.

Selye, H. (1980). *Selye's guide to stress research*. New York: Van Nostrand Reinhold.

Sipchen, B. (1990, June 6). Simply human. *Los Angeles Times*, p. E1.

Staff. (1991a, May). Are you covered for prevention? *Wellness Letter, 7*(8).

Staff. (1991b, February). Pet owners may be happier and healthier. *Lifetime Health Letter, 3*(2), 7, Houston: The University of Texas Health Science Center at Houston.

Staff. (1991c, February). Keys to losing weight and keeping it off. *Lifetime Health Letter, 3*(2), 2, Houston: The University of Texas Health Science Center at Houston.

Staff. (1991d, December). Personal briefing: Depressing news II. *The Philadelphia Inquirer*, p. 1C.

Steingart, R. M., Packer, M., Hamm, P., Coglianese, M. E., Gersh, B., Geltman, E. M., Sollano, J., Katz, S., Moye, L., Basta, L. L., Lewis, S. J., Gottlieb, S. S., Bernstein, V., McEwan, P., Jacobson, K., Brown, E. J., Kukin, M. L., Kantrowitz, N. E., & Pfeffer, M. A. (1991, July 25). Sex differences in the management of coronary artery disease. *New England Journal of Medicine, 325*, 226–230.

Thoits, P. A. (1987, March). Gender and marital status differences in control and distress: Common stress versus unique stress explanations. *Journal of Health and Social Behavior, 28*, 7–22.

U.S. Department of Health and Human Services, Public Health Service, Office of Disease Prevention and Health Promotion (1990). Prevention '89/'90: Federal programs and progress. Washington, DC: U.S. Government Printing Office.

U.S. Public Health Service. (1979). *Healthy people: The Surgeon General's report on health promotion and disease prevention* (DHEW Publication No. 79-55071). Washington, DC: U.S. Government Printing Office.

Verbrugge, L. M. (1983, March). Multiple roles and physical health of women and men. *Journal of Health and Social Behavior, 24*, 16–30.

Verbrugge, L. M. (1986). Role burdens and physical health of women and men. *Women & Health, 11*(1), 47–77.

Vitaliano, P. P., Maiuro, R. D., Russo, J., Mitchell, E. S., Carr, J. E., & Van Citters, R. L. (1988). A biopsychosocial model of medical student distress. *Journal of Behavioral Medicine, 11*(4), 311–331.

White, R. (1959). Motivation reconsidered: The concept of competence. *Psychological Review, 66*, 297–333.

Yerxa, E. J., & Baum, S. (1986). Engagement in daily occupation and life satisfaction among people with spinal cord injuries. *Occupational Therapy Journal of Research, 6*, 271–283.

Yerxa, E. J., Clark, F., Frank, G., Jackson, J., Parham, D., Pierce, D., Stein, C., & Zemke, R. (1989). An introduction to occupational science: A foundation for occupational therapy in the 21st century. *Occupational Therapy in Health Care, 6*(4), 1–17.

Yerxa, E. J., Clark, F., Frank, Jackson, J., Parham, D., Pierce, D., Stein, C., & Zemke, R. (1990). An introduction to occupational science: A foundation for occupational therapy in the 21st century. In J. A. Johnson, & E. J. Yerxa (Eds.), *Occupational science: The foundation for new models of practice*. Binghamton, NY: The Haworth Press.

CHAPTER 30

Environments of care: Hospice

MICHAEL PIZZI

LEARNING OBJECTIVES

Upon completion of this chapter the reader will be able to:

1. *Describe hospice history and philosophy in relation to occupation and occupational science.*
2. *Describe several themes of occupational science relative to hospice environments of care.*
3. *Explain the assessment process and the Hospice Assessment of Occupational Function.*
4. *Develop treatment programs for hospice patients and their caregivers.*
5. *Explain hospice family systems and the need for treatment of the family as the unit of care.*
6. *Describe characteristics of loss, grief, and bereavement relative to occupational performance.*
7. *Describe the unique occupational needs of the dying child.*

It seems to me that the way to find a philosophy that gives confidence and permits a positive approach to death and dying is to look continuously at the patients; not at their need but at their courage, not at their dependence but at their dignity.

DAME CICELY M. SAUNDERS (1965, p. 70)

Hospice care is defined from the dying person's perspective in terms of individual needs rather than the system of medical knowledge (Agich, 1978). The occupational therapist working with the hospice concept of care transcends the use of a medical model of care. Occupational therapists facilitate engagement in meaningful and productive endeavors within the context of their choices, values, abilities, goals, dreams, aspirations, and hopes. Consideration of the sociocultural, historical, and environmental contexts of life is vital for the occupational therapist to holistically assess and treat the dying with respect.

Capra's (1982) view on the healing of illnesses, especially from a systems view of health and healing, examines the need for a societal and medical change in thinking:

> [M]odern medicine often loses sight of the patient as a human being . . . by reducing health to mechanical functioning. This is perhaps the most serious shortcoming of the biomedical approach. [The phenomenon of healing] cannot be understood in reductionist terms. This applies to the healing of wounds and even more to the healing of illnesses, which generally involve a complex interplay among the physical, psychological, social and environmental aspects of the human condition. (1982, pp. 123–124)

The recent developments to which Capra refers include the development of hospice as an environment for occupational therapy practice. This chapter discusses the history and philosophy of hospice as a concept of care and as an environment in which occupational therapy practice is implemented. Hospice models of care are discussed, and occupational therapy theory, evaluation, and treatment in the context of hospice are presented. Issues of reimbursement and documentation also are addressed.

Hospice history and philosophy

History

The hospice movement was born out of a concern about doing something for dying patients. Western cultures and society believe that people need to have mastery over their environment; in medicine, this includes mastery over disease and thereby death. "Those concerned with palliative care practice from this same Western philosophy of mastery, arguing that symptom control and a concern with physical, psychological, social and spiritual (née cultural) aspects of patient and kin are appropriate areas for action" (Corless, 1983, p. 335).

Hospice dates back to medieval times. Shelters to help the weary traveler and to help the dying were run by religious orders and were widespread throughout Europe. Fabiola, a Roman matron and disciple of St. Jerome, opened a place to give refuge, food, and rest to the healthy traveler and to tend the sick and the dying pilgrim. Monastery-based hospices were established in the 11th century. When monasteries ceased to exist in Britain, the hospice concept gave way to the humanitarian and scientific approaches to health and illness used in medicine today (Corless, 1983).

Hospice concepts were later resurrected in the 17th century by St. Vincent de Paul, a young French priest who founded the Sisters of Charity in Paris. In the early part of the 20th century, hospices again began forming in England. In the early 1950s, at St. Joseph's in London, a young woman named Cicely Saunders, who was a nurse, social worker, doctor, and Christian, developed the technique of pain control and total care for the dying that has become the cornerstone of hospice care all over the world (Corless, 1983). Dr. Saunders later envisioned a center that would be religiously ecumenical and a medical foundation that would combine the best care for its dying patients, with opportunities for teaching in the fields of medicine, nursing, and the allied professions. Dr. Saunders created St. Christopher's Hospice in 1967, which was started with money willed to her by a dying Polish man she helped as a social worker in 1948, who shared her vision.

In the United States, around the turn of the century, Rose Hawthorne Lathrop initiated a program of care for people with cancer by taking them into her home. She later began a domiciliary facility for patients, accepted no compensation from patients or their families, and relied on the community for support. This same tradition extended to the development of hospice care in Connecticut, New Jersey, New York City, Montreal, and Tucson. The first hospice, Hospice, Inc., or the Connecticut Hospice, emphasized home care, with contracts with the Visiting Nurse Association. Volunteers were an integral part of the team and still are regarded as a mainstay of hospice care. An inpatient unit was added, and home care teams throughout Connecticut were established. The Hospice of Marin in California was also a community-based hospice. Free-standing units soon developed in Boonton, New Jersey (Riverside Hospice) and in Tucson, Arizona (Hillhaven Hospice). A hospital consultation model was developed at St. Luke's Hospital in New York City, providing a multi-

disciplinary team to visit patients throughout the hospital (Corless, 1983).

There are currently over 1600 hospices in the United States. The various models of hospice care are clearly delineated in the American Occupational Therapy Association (AOTA) *Guidelines for Occupational Therapy Services in Hospice* (1987).

Philosophy

The philosophy of hospice care is holistic, is health- and occupation-centered, and provides a framework from which hospice occupational therapists can work. The philosophy states,

> Dying is a normal process whether or not resulting from disease. Hospice exists neither to hasten nor to postpone death. Rather, Hospice exists to affirm "life"—by providing support and care for those in the last phases of incurable disease so that they can live as fully and comfortably as possible. Hospice promotes the formation of caring communities that are sensitive to the needs of patients and their families at this time in their lives so that they may be free to obtain that degree of mental and spiritual preparation for death that is satisfactory to them. (National Hospice Organization, 1979)

The standards of hospice care serve as a philosophical basis for evaluating hospice programs. The document contains a definition of a hospice program of care, hospice philosophy, and 22 standards and supporting principles of a hospice program of care. These standards are clear and concise, and therapists working in hospice should be familiar with them as they relate to the occupational therapy process. The standards of care can be found in the AOTA Hospice Guidelines (1987).

Occupational therapy and hospice

The philosophy of hospice—creating a family-centered approach that is life-affirming and through which the dying can live as fully and comfortably as possible—is similar to the philosophy of the founders of occupational therapy and to the profession's historical roots in moral treatment. From the early 1900s, occupational therapy was viewed as a profession with a humanitarian focus, assisting people in rediscovering meaning in their lives through **adaptation** and engagement in self-directed, productive **occupation**. Hospice care is built on much the same principles.

Hospice brings care of the dying out of an institutional setting into a homelike environment, where the dying can be surrounded by their own treasured possessions, friends, family, and significant others. Occupational therapists have always considered the sociocultural and environmental aspects of care and of occupation and adaptation. Hospice environments promote these same concepts.

Hospice teaches basic values of person-centered and family-centered care. These include the following:

1. The basic regard for the recipient of care
2. Acceptance of death as a natural part of living
3. Consideration of the entire family as the unit of care
4. Sustaining the patient at home for as long as possible
5. Helping the patient assume control over his own life
6. Teaching the patient self-care
7. Reduction or removal of pain and other distressing symptoms
8. Total, not fragmented care

9. Comprehensive provision of services by an interdisciplinary team
10. Continuity of services after death (Koff, 1980, pp. 18–19)

Hospice principles, values, and philosophy and occupational therapy easily interface. The terminally ill experience performance deficits in occupation and temporal adaptation; they lose control over being an effective and masterful person in the world; they have problems with the "doing" process; and they experience skill and habit degeneration and thus experience altered meaningfulness of activity and occupational living.

It is vital that we consider and acknowledge our historical roots and use those principles of care in hospice environments and hospice occupational therapy practice. The roots and principles of hospice care enhance the scientific and theoretical basis from which we develop holistic and humanitarian care in occupational therapy for the dying.

When the diagnosis is terminal (usually indicating that the patient has 6 months or less to live), there are fluctuations between occupational function and dysfunction, adaptation and maladaptation. Five stages of dying were identified by Kubler-Ross (1969): denial, anger, bargaining, depression, and acceptance. The terminally ill patient can fluctuate between any of the stages at any given time during the dying process. The terminally ill patient also may fluctuate in occupational behaviors that are adaptive or maladaptive, based on interactions, or lack thereof, with occupations and the human and nonhuman environments.

Occupational therapists have used occupational behavior as the guiding theory for practice. Gammage, McMahon, and Shanahan (1976) examined the roles and functions of occupational therapists and suggest that, relative to terminal care, people must be able to add, modify, or relinquish occupational roles to satisfactorily meet the demands of the environment. Pizzi (1984) supports adaptation and occupation; enhancing the patient's sense of control as the key to quality living; and assisting the dying in making role transitions to effectively and competently interact with the environment. Tigges and Sherman (1983) also support these concepts through the case study of a terminally ill young man, in which they examine the work–play continuum, occupational roles, and occupational choices throughout the dying process. Other therapists advocate examination of open systems approaches, creating environments that support natural and familiar life experiences within the lifestyle of the terminally ill patient, with occupation as the cornerstone to life and living (Flanigan, 1982; Holland, 1984; Holland & Tigges, 1981; Pizzi, 1983, 1986, 1990).

Themes in hospice occupational therapy

In hospice occupational therapy, several themes are relevant to the clinician and researcher: meaningfulness and meaning of occupation, quality of life, temporal adaptation, locus of control, environment, pain and pain control, family systems, adaptation, and death with dignity.

Meaning

Yerxa states that "authentic occupational therapy is based upon a commitment to the client's realization of his own particular meaning." (1967, p. 170). Hospice occupational therapy is re-

plete with symbolism and the enhancement of meaning and meaningfulness of occupation as a life comes to a close. Making a doll for one's grandchild or cooking a significant other's favorite dessert takes on different meaning when viewed in the context of a terminal illness. Meaning is influenced by the sociocultural, historical, and environmental aspects of occupational behavior and needs to be viewed in those contexts.

Quality of life

"Medicine is concerned with preserving life; occupational therapy is concerned with the quality of life preserved, increasing the latitude of choices and the freedom of the individual who is disabled" (Yerxa et al., 1989, p. 8). Medicine cannot cure a person with a terminal illness, but palliation, or care and comfort, are the goals of hospice and therefore the goals of the hospice occupational therapist in enhancing quality of living. **Quality of life** is constantly examined in hospice care, with the occupational therapist facilitating the patient's adaptive responses to life and living while the patient is dying. Adaptation and quality of life are enhanced through engagement in or creation of opportunities for occupation to whatever extent possible for the dying on a physical, social, cultural, emotional, symbolic, sexual, or spiritual level.

Temporal adaptation

Temporal adaptation refers to ways in which humans organize and perceive the use of time and thereby how occupation is engaged in regarding the use of time. It also refers to how one orients oneself in the past, present, or future.

In hospice, the occupational therapist copes with immediacy in creating meaning and engagement in occupation for the terminally ill patient and the significant others. Since the life goals of the terminally ill and affected significant others have been compromised, former goals must be realigned and new goals established and prioritized (Pizzi, 1984).

Locus of control

One of the basic principles of hospice care is to provide choice and control for the terminally ill patient and the significant others on a daily and sometimes hourly basis regarding occupational living. **Locus of control** varies from person to person. People who are dependent all their lives may not wish to be independent at the end of their lives. Control must be viewed as a continuation of earlier life experiences, from a historical context. Occupational therapy facilitates control and mastery over the human and nonhuman environments and enables the terminally ill patient to maximize an independent state of being to the extent the person chooses (Pizzi, 1984).

Environment

Cultural, social, and physical environments must be considered in holistic care of the terminally ill. These environments can impede or enhance occupational living and occupational behaviors and can influence the state of health, level of adaptation to diagnosis, changes in productivity and function, and the occupational therapy process. For example, a patient may not get out of bed unless the spouse is present (social); a patient may not get into a wheelchair to learn alternative mobility patterns in the hospital-based hospice because self-mobilization will not be possible at home after discharge (physical); or a patient may not feed himself or herself unless chopsticks are provided (cultural).

Pain and pain control

Garrett (1978) describes pain in a multidimensional sense: physical, social, psychosocial, and spiritual. *Physical pain* is by far the most debilitating in the experience of most patients. The need for consistent and continuous **pain control** for dying patients is vital so that fears and anxieties about enduring physical pain can be alleviated and the patient can continue with familiar occupational routines and tasks. *Social pain* refers to isolation and abandonment of the patient by significant others, family members, and even health care workers. It also includes a loss of independence in decision making and loss of control in interpersonal communications and in the performance of occupational tasks (Corr & Corr, 1983; Koff, 1980). *Psychological pain* refers to the many fears experienced by dying people. According to Koff (1980) and Corr and Corr (1983), those fears include: the unknown, being alone, the loss of one's body and its identity, loss of ego function and self-control, the process of dying, and that life will have become meaningless. *Spiritual pain* is associated with the religious orientation of dying people and the enigma of the unknown, whether or not one believes in God or another higher power. This is also influenced by one's cultural beliefs.

All these pains, if experienced by the patient, can impede occupational functioning and choices of occupations. Occupational therapists assist with pain management when pain is examined from this multidimensional perspective. It is vital that occupational therapists work as team members in pain control to enhance quality of living.

Family systems and significant others

Koff (1980) states that the way in which every member of the family deals with the dying of one of its community influences the way that person will die and the ability of hospice to have an impact on that death. According to Lidz (1968), the family constitutes the fundamental social unit of virtually every society with respect to four factors: (1) the family forms a group of individuals treated as an entity by society; (2) the family creates a network of kinship systems; (3) the family constitutes an economic unit; and (4) the family provides roles, status, motivation, and incentives that affect relationships between individuals and society.

Hospice recognizes that the family is the unit of care, no matter what is the structure of that unit. A **family system** can include the biologic family, significant others, and friends. Even after a death, hospice offers bereavement services to support the family system. The family system, dependent on level of interactions and the quality and quantity of communications with the dying patient, impedes or enhances a patient's occupational functioning. Patient–family interactions must also be viewed from a sociocultural and historical perspective. Survivors of a death are more likely to develop positive responses toward death and dying if hospice care, including occupational therapy, clearly demonstrates that dying can occur without pain, with dignity, and with the dying person able to maintain contact and control in his or her own life situation.

Adaptation

Dubos (1977) states that "for man, as for other living things, the word 'adaptation' connotes fitness to a particular environment for the possession of attributes, making it possible to function effectively and to reproduce abundantly in this environment" (p. 39). Frank (1991) states that adaptation is a "process of selecting and organizing activities (occupations) to improve life opportunities and enhance quality of life according to the experience of individuals or groups in an ever changing environment" (p. 6).

In hospice, occupational performance and functional status, locus of control, environmental interactions, and temporal dimensions of living are constantly in flux. Adaptive responses of terminally ill people may already be present if they historically adapted to crises. When maladaptation occurs from diagnosis of a terminal illness and throughout the dying process, occupational therapy facilitates adaptive responses by helping the patient create meaning, beauty, and truth in everyday tasks.

Death with dignity

The concept of death with dignity has been a longstanding principle of hospice care. It embraces all the above-mentioned themes of occupational science and occupational behavior. Koff (1980) articulates death with dignity in the following way,

> Enabling a person to die with dignity includes taking whatever measures reduce or eliminate pain and discomfort and always treating the total person, not merely his symptoms. These practices provide security and build trust by focusing on the patient's needs and treating each person as a special and unique being. The dying person is encouraged to express any emotion, without fear of what another may think, and he is helped to die in a way that is appropriate for him, rather than in a way prescribed by others. Permitting death with dignity also means enabling a person and those important to him to practice rituals or to behave in ways keeping with their culture and/or lifestyle. (p. 24)

Occupational therapy assessment

"The door opening interview is a meeting of two people who can communicate without fear or anxiety. The therapist . . . will attempt to let the patient know in his own words or actions that he is not going to run away if the word cancer or dying is mentioned" (Kubler-Ross, 1969, p. 269).

Preparation

Assessment of occupational function and dysfunction and of occupational behaviors is multidimensional and must include physical, biologic, cognitive, sociocultural, and symbolic aspects of daily living. The cultural, social, and physical environments of the terminally ill patient must also be addressed since hospice treats the family as the unit of care.

Assessment begins immediately as the therapist enters the lifespace (human and nonhuman) of the patient. Data gathering occurs through clinical observations, information from charts, other team members, formal assessments, and interviews with family members and significant others. Nonverbal communication must never be underestimated in terms of its impact in hospice care. The therapist represents hope for the patient— hope for a better way to live until death occurs, hope to restore dignity and self-respect, and hope to put meaning back into a life that may have become meaningless. "Occupational therapy is centered on the realization that a person's integrity, equality, purpose, self esteem and mastery and adaptation rest in the ability to be purposefully engaged in regular and familiar life experiences" (Tigges, 1983, p. 162).

In preparation for formal assessment, the therapist must pay attention to any barriers that may interfere with communication and initial rapport. The hospice therapist must be acutely aware of several factors that could influence initial rapport and subsequent assessment. These include the following:

1. The person may feel worthless, not deserving of respect, and that the disease was self-created.
2. Life goals and the temporal dimension of living are altered.
3. Denial may be an adaptive mechanism.
4. The person may be experiencing anticipatory grief or depression and have the attitude that there is no action left to take because another health care professional has given up on a cure.
5. The patient may be in unrelenting pain but putting on his or her best "patient face" to please the therapist.
6. Terminally ill patients often have a heightened sense of how others communicate verbally and nonverbally.

Architectural barriers, such as hospital bed rails, can interfere with establishing rapport. It may be adaptive to have barriers, however, to allow for more comfort, given the patient's culture and lifespace. Social and cultural distance must be respected and acknowledged. The therapist needs to be invited into the world of the patient, including the appropriate time to place a comforting hand.

Formal assessment and screening

Occupational questions can be used to gather initial data on the patient's physical, psychosocial, and environmental aspects of living (Pizzi, Mukand, & Freed, 1991). This may be the only formal part of the assessment process since the patient may be preterminal (very near death) or the patient may not have the necessary time to fill out forms, questionnaires, and a physical assessment. Therapists must respect the unique temporal aspect of most hospice patients, with the ultimate goal of meeting the occupational needs that are of immediate priority to the patient. Clinical observations, data from caregivers and other team members, and chart review can supplement initial occupational therapy data.

Hospice assessment of occupational function

The Hospice Assessment of Occupational Function (HAOF) (see the display on pages 858 and 859) was developed based on an integration of hospice philosophy and practice, occupational therapy history and philosophy, occupational science, and occupational behavior. It is designed to integrate all types of data-gathering procedures, including hands-on assessment, which is a vital part of the occupational therapy process.

Included in the demographics section are the patient's name, birth date, race, culture, religion, diagnosis, medications, identified occupational roles, person to whom diagnosis is communicated, and past medical history. In traditional data gathering, many of these questions are not asked; however, in hospice, many people in the patient's social system, for example, are not aware of the specific diagnosis and prognosis and, by patient or family request, should not be told. Often, the patient is not aware of the diagnosis.

Religious and cultural beliefs must be considered in hospice occupational therapy. As the patient approaches death, it is often noted that the patient wishes to resolve issues in his or her life to have spiritual pain resolved. Clergy are important team members to assist with these issues, and often the occupational therapist is approached with questions regarding the afterlife, God, or a higher power. It is within the value system of the individual therapist to engage in conversation regarding these issues. It is vital that documentation reflect this issue, that the clergy are consulted, and that the therapist maintain the framework of how these issues affect the patient's occupational behaviors, choices, and overall functioning.

Cultural beliefs, especially in hospice and the dying process, are important, given certain cultural rituals that must be considered. Occupations that are culturally focused for the patient and family system can be appropriately defined and implemented, thus maintaining the integrity of the patient's culture.

Sexual orientation, often considered a subculture, is an important part of the person's identity and will have influenced major occupational choices and subsequent occupational behaviors. Therapists need to allow patients the freedom to share this area of their lives. Knowledge in this area for the therapist can enhance the occupational therapy process for the patient and make the patient more comfortable.

The primary caregiver should be identified by the patient and not assumed by the therapist. Often, especially in nontraditional family systems, at the time of death, people in the patient's life become visible after many years of absence or of poor communication. Often, a patients' friend or neighbor is the primary caregiver and not the person the patient lives with or the biologic family.

Past medical history is important because certain occupational areas of living may be disrupted secondary to past medical problems (eg, broken and poorly healed clavicle at 13 years of age limiting current range of motion). Other past emotional, psychological, and physical problems can contribute to present occupational behaviors and adaptive or maladaptive styles of living.

In assessment of activities of daily living (ADL), work, and play and leisure, the HAOF defines five categories for each major area. These need not be formally assessed but can be considered in the context of the relative value each section has to the person's life. These areas are the following:

Interests: what aspects of the occupation are interesting to the patient

Meaningfulness of activity: how important or valuable are the occupations (eg, it is more important to sit up and type on the computer than to bathe or dress independently)

Time organization: how the patient organizes time and participates in the occupation (eg, eats before showering; watches morning news program before going to work)

(*Text continues on page 860*)

HOSPICE ASSESSMENT OF OCCUPATIONAL FUNCTION

Demographics

Today's date _____ Therapist _____
Environment where assessment took place _____
Patient name _____ Birthdate _____
Culture _____ Race _____ Religion _____ Sex _____
Primary caregiver identified by patient _____
Primary diagnosis _____ Secondary diagnosis _____
Medications _____
Primary occupational roles _____
To whom primary diagnosis been communicated _____
Past medical history:

_____
_____
_____

Key

Interests: what parts of the occupation are interesting to do?
Meaningfulness: How important is this occupation? Is independence in this occupation valued by the patient?
Time organization: How does one schedule time in this occupation?
Environment: Where is the occupation performed and with, for, or by whom?

_____
_____

Activities of Daily Living (see also ADL Checklist)

1. Interests:
2. Meaningfulness of activity:
3. Time organization:
4. Social and physical environments in which task occurs:
5. Describe briefly changes since diagnosis:

Work

(Homemaking; child care/parenting/grandparenting; paid employment)
1. Interests and position:
2. Meaningfulness of activity:
3. Time organization:
4. Social and physical environments in which task occurs:
5. Describe briefly changes since diagnosis:

Play and Leisure

1. Interests:
2. Meaningfulness of activity:
3. Time organization:
4. Environments in which task occurs:
5. Describe briefly changes since diagnosis:

Physical Considerations for Function

Active and passive range of motion:
Strength:
Sensation:
Coordination (gross, fine motor, and dexterity):
Visual–perceptual:
Balance (sitting and standing):
Ambulation, transferring and mobility:
Activity tolerance and endurance:

(continued)

HOSPICE ASSESSMENT OF OCCUPATIONAL FUNCTION (*continued*)

Physical pain   Location: _____

In what ways does it interfere with, if at all, doing activities important to the patient?

_____

_____

Cognition

(Attention span, problem solving, memory, orientation, judgment, reasoning, problem solving, decision making, safety awareness)

Stressors

What are some things, people, or situations that are or were stressful for you?
What are some ways you manage stress?

Body Image and Self-Image

Situational Coping

How do you feel you are dealing with:
1.   Your diagnosis
2.   Changes in your ability to do things important to you
3.   Other psychosocial changes

Social Environment

(Significant others and interactions between patient and others)
Who in your life is helpful or supportive since your diagnosis?
Therapist comment:

Physical Environment

As applicable: Home:
                 Community:
                 Church:
                 Other:
Therapist comment:

Occupational Questions

1.   Describe what your day is like from the time you get up until you go to bed.
     Today:
     What was your routine like before your diagnosis, before today?
2.   What do you feel you currently do that is done well and with which you are pleased?
3.   What, if any, are some meaningful or important activities you have given up (forced to or by choice) since diagnosis? What would you choose to be more independent in or do better?
(For questions 4 and 5, ask only when the patient is comfortably open with his or her prognosis.)
4.   If a friend asked how you would like to be remembered as a person:
     a.   What would you say?
     b.   What might you leave for others to remember you by? Is there anything you would like to do, to make, or to tell someone?
5.   What are some of your dreams, hopes and aspirations?
6.   Do you have anything else you would like to share with me at this time?
Occupational Therapy Plan:
Short-term goals:
Long-term goals:
Frequency:
Duration:
Therapist:

Copyright © 1991 by Michael Pizzi, MS, OTR/L, CHES. Adapted with permission.

Environments in which tasks occur: social environment includes the significant others who do occupation for the patient or who support or participate with the patient in that occupation (eg, coworkers at work, husband who feeds wife meals); physical environment is the physical space in which the patient performs occupations (eg, getting dressed supine on bed, or bathing in upstairs bathroom when sleeping downstairs and only when an assistant is present)

Description of occupational changes since diagnosis: in each category, description of changes provides the therapist with a global view of the person in that occupation and possible intervention needs

Physical considerations are important aspects of occupational function and need to be addressed. The physical, biologic, and cognitive systems of humans are phenomena that influence adaptive and maladaptive occupational behaviors. Most important is a general assessment of these areas through activity analysis as well as clinical observations (eg, walking to the living room, dressing, reaching for objects in a cabinet). Formal physical assessments, such as manual muscle tests, goniometric measurements, and hour-long sensory tests, are contraindicated unless for specific rehabilitation outcome measures that are determined by the team. Also, patient perception of these areas in relation to function can assist the therapist in determining patient needs. For example, with lung cancer patients, general strength may be only mildly compromised compared with endurance and activity tolerance. A patient's perception is often one of being weak when it is really an endurance rather than a strength deficiency. A general evaluation of these areas can be performed with more data and frequent reassessment through occupational observations as the therapist implements treatment.

Stressors and situational coping need to be addressed from the perspective of the patient. Many hospice patients cope well with dying, have completed projects, and are living with quality and dignity. An inaccurate assumption by many therapists is that death and the dying process are difficult and painful and that people have a difficult time coping and adapting.

Body image and self-image are often impaired secondary to muscle wasting and atrophy, weight loss, catheters, and continuous infusion pumps attached and implanted into the body. Skin discoloration and various cancers, with resultant radiation damage that can cause permanent scar and tissue damage, contribute to an altered body image. Clinical observations and careful listening to patients can provide evidence for any alteration in body image. Women with breast cancer and subsequent radiation and even mastectomy may have difficulty adapting, especially in relation to career, significant relationships, and other occupational roles. AIDS patients may experience a wasting syndrome and drop from 180 to 140 lb in a few months. Altered body image may also be reflected in maladaptive performance and routine of ADL (eg, patient perception that "I can't wear what I used to, so what's the sense of getting dressed").

Environment is an area that will impede or support occupational behaviors. Occupation is the output of a person's environmental interactions. Thus, to develop or maintain adaptive occupational behaviors, it is necessary that the environment be conducive to facilitating those behaviors. The social environment is comprised of the primary caregiver (if there is one) and significant others (friends, biologic family) and the quality and quantity of interactions of those people with the patient. These

should be described by the patient and assessed by the therapist through clinical observations. For example, an elderly woman, married for 58 years to a physically abusive husband, defined her primary caregiver as her daughter with whom she presently lives after leaving her husband who is in another part of the United States. Another example is that of a wealthy, 34-year-old AIDS patient, whose biologic family visited for the duration of his illness after having barred him from the family since age 17 when he revealed he was gay. His partner of 12 years was identified as the primary caregiver by the patient owing to their significant relationship and the quality of their communications.

The physical environment is the home, community, church, or other physical space with which the patient interacts. Assessment of these areas can be through observation or interview with the patient and caregiver. If patients are to be discharged from a facility (eg, hospital-based hospice to home) therapists can begin to determine the layout of the physical environment of the discharge setting. Therapists must also assess each room with which the patient interacts. For example, if the patient bathes in bed, does the environment facilitate independent performance of task? Are task objects accessible? How are they set up for the patient? The dining room is where the patient eats meals. Are the table and chairs at appropriate heights? Can a wheelchair fit under the table? Are doorways accessible? Is there proper lighting? Assessment of architectural barriers for both current and future performance of occupational tasks is needed to facilitate adaptation throughout the disease process. Finally, brief occupational questions related to temporal aspects of daily living, efficacy, competence and mastery, sense of purpose and meaning, control, and quality of life are a crucial part of hospice occupational therapy assessment. These questions provide opportunities for patients to explore and examine their purpose in life, occupational goals, meaningfulness of activity, and personhood as creators of their own existence. Goal prioritization and restructuring can occur immediately through these general occupational questions. The hospice therapist needs to be centered to elicit authentic responses from patients. The therapist comfort level regarding death and dying will be evident through these questions. These questions also prompt the patient to reminisce and, in that historical context, provide the patient with meaningful, authentic, clear information about the goals and portions of occupational living that need immediate attention.

The method of administration of the HAOF is to first complete an ADL assessment (see the display), which can yield data on performance, some biomedical aspects of living, and environment and psychosocial aspects of ADL. If the patient is extremely short of breath or has a very low activity tolerance, a cointerview with an identified primary caregiver is necessary. The entire HAOF need not be completed in one session, and a focus on ADL, work, play and leisure, and overall productive use of time can be the important assessment tasks initially. Some patients may also have varied psychosocial reactions to assessment, given their physical stage of illness and stage of acceptance of the diagnosis. It is not unusual for hospice patients or caregivers to view hospice personnel as temporary until the patient returns to work or "this thing clears up." This must be respected and documented.

The HAOF is a general hospice occupational therapy assessment. Other assessments that can be administered easily to gather more specific data are the Role Checklist (Oakley, Kielhofner, Barris, & Reichler, 1986), the Level of Interest in Particular Activity Checklist (Scaffa, 1981), the Social Environment Interview (Pizzi, Mukand, & Freed 1991), and an Activities

ACTIVITIES OF DAILY LIVING CHECKLIST FOR PEOPLE WITH CHRONIC OR TERMINAL ILLNESS

Physical task*	I	min A	mod A	max A	Describe Performance
Feeding					
Grooming/hygiene					
Bathing					
Dressing					
Mobility/transfers					
Communication					
Continence					
Homemaking					

Psychosocial consideration (*eg*, chose dependence of caregiver, anger, withdrawal from task performance, patient does not value activity):

Environmental considerations (*eg*, bathes at bedside, wheelchair-bound, uses lap tray to eat in bed):

Biomedical considerations (*eg*, range of motion, strength, endurance):

Adaptive equipment needed:

Other comments:

* I, independent; min A, minimal assistance; mod A, moderate assistance; max A, maximal assistance
Copyright © 1991 by Michael Pizzi, MS, OTR/L, CHES. Adapted with permission.

of Daily Living Checklist for People with Chronic and Terminal Illness (Pizzi, 1990; see the display).

The Role Checklist is easily administered in 10 to 15 minutes and is a patient self-report assessment of the patient's perspective of past, present, and future involvement in specific occupational roles and their significance or value to his or her life. This assessment generates data on immediate role priorities of the terminally ill patient; thus, occupations and adaptations necessary to carry out those roles can be determined easily.

The Level of Interest in Particular Activity Checklist is an interest checklist adapted from the original Interest Checklist developed by Matsutsuyu (1969). This assessment examines the current level of interest in an occupation, identifies the level of interest in the past 10 years and past year, and if the patient currently participates and wishes to participate in an occupation in the future. Patients need to be advised that the checklist is not about performance but interest. Data from this checklist assist hospice therapists in determining immediate areas of intervention to enhance productive use of time and to help the patient adapt from the role of worker to hobbyist.

The Social Environment Interview is based on the hospice principle of treating the family as the unit of care. It is often a health care assumption that when the members of the social system of the patient take care of their own health, then they can better care for the patient. This interview examines the care-giver's life since the patient's diagnosis and identifies occupational problems. Data gathered from the interview can be used by occupational therapists to determine how to help caregivers adapt to changes in their own occupational lives and develop strategies to competently care for their loved one, including redevelopment of previously shared activities.

The Activities of Daily Living Checklist for People with Chronic and Terminal Illness is used with the HAOF as the performance measure of ADL. It incorporates and considers psychosocial, biomedical, and environmental factors that impede and enhance performance. Hospice patients often can physically perform ADL but may be constrained by other factors (eg, depression, the patient will only dress if significant other visits, or the patient will not bathe except in home bathtub). This assessment provides a holistic framework from which to develop treatment strategies in the area of ADL.

Hospice goal planning and treatment

In treatment, adaptation and occupation are the primary tools of the occupational therapist. From assessment, therapists determine occupational needs, goals, and desires of patients and develop appropriate treatment. The founders of occupational therapy used five distinct treatment principles, which are applicable to hospice occupational therapy treatment (Barris, Kiel-hofner, & Watts, 1983):

1. TREATMENT MUST AROUSE INTEREST, COURAGE AND CONFIDENCE. Engaging a terminally ill patient in an occupation that the patient values and in which the patient wishes to become more functional promotes these characteristics of treatment, including the concept of carefully matching occupations with capacities and needs.
2. OCCUPATIONS SHOULD BE APPLIED WITH SYSTEM AND PRECISION.
3. OCCUPATIONS SHOULD BE GRADED ACCORDING TO THE CAPACITY OF THE PATIENT. Careful attention must be paid to mental and physical functioning and to eventual deterioration, both mental and physical, in the latter stages of a terminal illness. Habit training was used to restore basic skills and habits of self care, facilitating a sense of control over the environment. This principle can be applied to terminal care, however plateaus in skill performance may be reached and a deterioration in roles, habits and skills occurs in time. Therefore, occupations must be downgraded and habits and roles adapted to facilitate a sense of competence and control in the ever-changing life situation of the patient.
4. OCCUPATIONAL THERAPY FOCUSES ON THE HEALTH OF PATIENTS RATHER THAN ON PATHOLOGY AND IT EMPHASIZES THE EXPRESSION OF HEALTHY EMOTIONS AND ATTITUDES. Terminal care is involved with death and dying and sometimes only glimmers of life and living shine forth. Occupational therapy emphasizes the life and living aspects by engaging patients in normal life situations and by promoting continuation in occupational roles. Through occupation, an expression of healthy emotions and attitudes prevails.
5. OCCUPATIONAL THERAPY MUST BE A TOTAL PROGRAM OF CARE. This principle advocates a balance in all environments—physical, social and temporal—so that daily life occupations can be pursued with a sense of normalcy. Occupational therapy personnel engaged in terminal care must be aware of that delicate balance and assist patients in planning their life occupations accordingly. (Pizzi, 1984, pp. 244–245).

Creative clinical reasoning is necessary for hospice treatment planning. Unlike the clinical reasoning process that occurs in traditional rehabilitation, hospice clinical reasoning must also incorporate hospice philosophy; death and dying philosophy; and loss, grief, and bereavement issues. To implement successful and meaningful treatment, hospice therapists consider the themes of hospice already discussed, the five basic principles of treatment, principles of occupational behavior, occupational science, and the historical roots of occupational therapy. Together, they form a cohesive and solid focus for sound program design in hospice occupational therapy (Pizzi, 1992).

Occupational therapists are familiar with upgrading occupations and environmental challenges to enhance function and return people to productive living. In the context of hospice, therapists must account for chronically debilitating illnesses in which death is the prognosis. Patients involved with hospice care traditionally have a prognosis of 6 months or less to live. Goals should be short term and measurable (from days to weeks) and should be stated by the patient, with the therapist acting as facilitator by having patients define their lives in view of their choices and interests. "The life situation of the patient, including cultural, educational and socioeconomic facts as well as valued activity, must be taken into account if the patient is to control the situation" (Pizzi, 1984, p. 244).

Family as the unit of care

The family is, in essence, a small group whose structure, functions, and dynamic interactions are aimed at promoting the growth and development of its members, maintaining cohesiveness, and developing and maintaining itself as a viable unit in relation to the society in which it lives. Within a family, certain members have roles that are associated with family functioning.

Although a family's ability to support a dying member should not be minimized, recent perspectives regard the family as the unit facing the disease. The terminal illness of one family member disrupts the lives of the others just as it does the life of the ill person, and it is a threat to the integrity and functioning of the family system. Depending on the family members involved, the patient's roles in the family, and the degree to which the patient's illness prevents performance of those roles, each of the family's functions is likely to become impaired in some way as the family adapts to the patient's impending death.

Often, family members and significant others feel that doing things for the patient is helpful; however, this may have the opposite effect, especially if the patient wishes to be more independent and resents the help being provided. Conversely, family members and significant others may feel inept at handling the crisis situation and may themselves withdraw. "Appropriate recommendations to the family unit and significant others can alleviate stress and help individual members organize their routines and activities to better promote their own health and adaptive ways of living while caring for their dying loved one" (Pizzi, 1984, pp. 245–246).

Loss, grief, and bereavement

Grief is the normal reaction to loss, which is experienced by everyone. Loss is of two types: physical (tangible) and symbolic (psychosocial) (Rando, 1984). For example, losing a favorite piece of jewelry is a physical loss, whereas a symbolic loss may be losing job status or a spouse through divorce. It is common for physical losses also to have symbolic significance.

Rando (1984) states four factors that caregivers should remember when dealing with loss and grief:

1. An illness involves numerous losses that are both physical and symbolic in nature.
2. Each of the specific losses must be identified.
3. Each of these losses prompts and requires its own grief response.
4. The importance of a loss will vary according to its meaning for the specific individual. (p. 18)

Occupational therapists have an obligation to the terminally ill patient and significant others to be acutely aware of specific losses and their significance to the patient. For example, because we can get a quick replacement for a lost toothbrush or comb does not mean that the patient, especially one who is terminally ill, isn't experiencing loss and grief issues, physical and symbolic, related to the object. Consideration of numerous losses—both past and present—and facilitation of resolution of those losses and working through the grieving process with terminally ill patients, through occupation, is a nontraditional role for therapists. Loss and grief alter occupational living and lead to depression and social and physical withdrawal and isolation. The focus must be on helping the person adapt to losses of function, skills, familiar environments and routines, and interpersonal relationships. Through adaptation and occupation, occupational therapy restores meaning and purpose.

Helping significant others and family members with **bereavement**, often including a 1-year follow-up, is an essential component of hospice care. The American Occupational Therapy Task Force on Hospice Care (AOTA, 1987) survey showed that 21% of occupational therapy hospice personnel were involved in bereavement care. Occupational therapists can also help family members and significant others with role transitions (eg, a husband who never learned to cook or pay bills needs to learn home maintenance occupations before his wife dies). Bereavement work can also include helping significant others to develop or restructure routines of daily living. This is a natural part of the occupational therapy process in hospice care and can be viewed by nonhospice therapists as nontraditional. These types of treatments can begin immediately in the occupational therapy process and do not have to occur during traditional bereavement time.

Hospice and the dying child and adolescent

The needs of terminally ill children are vast and unique and unlike those of adults. There are relatively few hospices or hospice programs committed solely to the care of the dying child and the child's family, thus there are a small percentage of pediatric health care professionals caring for dying children.

Dying children experience many losses in all areas of occupational living. Families of these children must cope with devastating changes in family dynamics, role relationships, and occupational routines. The child experiences loss of developmental milestones and changes in function; impairment of exploratory behaviors; incorporation of new activities around the sick role (eg, taking medications, visiting the doctor and hospital); and hidden communication about the disease when families choose not to share. All these occupational changes and losses can adversely affect the child's environmental interactions and play. When this occurs, major occupational dysfunctions can occur, thus creating a more maladaptive cycle of occupational behavior for the child and family system. This can be exacerbated by the child sensing that something is wrong without being directly told and through changes in behaviors of the adults in the child's social environment.

Physical and psychosocial occupational therapy assessments used in pediatrics, along with the Social Environment Interview, can be used while accounting for the above-mentioned considerations. Important to note is that a child's concept of death and dying is different at certain developmental stages and must be considered in assessment and treatment.

Rando (1984) describes several treatment interventions that can be used with dying children and their families:

1. Recognize that children are aware of the seriousness of their condition, although they may not be able to articulate it. Even very young children are capable of reading the cues of concerned, anxious adults.
2. Be honest with children in age-appropriate ways.
3. Remember that ill children and adolescents are working on forming an identity while experiencing a vicious attack on their efforts. Unlike the adult, who already has an identity and oper-

ates from a more secure foundation, the adolescent and child are more insecure and require more structure and support.
4. Recognize that children use three languages for communicating their knowledge of their impending death: plain verbal language, symbolic nonverbal language and symbolic verbal language. Be prepared to listen and respond in all three modalities.
5. Recognize the prevalence of magical thinking in children. Explore with them their understanding of the causality of the illness, its experience and its prognosis. Vigorously correct any misconceptions.
6. Recognize that play is the child's medium and make toys and resources available.
7. Provide challenges as part of treatment intervention, as children and adolescents need them to achieve mastery and competency.
8. Recognize that the child needs to move around, and try to avoid restriction of movement unless absolutely necessary.
9. Assist adolescents in dealing with the acutely painful issues that are a normal part of adolescence. Recognize that these make them particularly vulnerable to the stress of the illness.
10. Remember that adolescents have difficulty communicating with adults in general, and consider this when working with them. There must be a respect for their privacy and their need for honesty and independence.
11. Recognize the issues of sexuality for older children and adolescents who are ill. To deny them their sexuality is to deny them a part of their lives that normally would be a primary concern at this time. (pp. 412–414)

Occupational therapy interventions also include emphasis on developmentally appropriate skills in physical, psychosocial and emotional, and symbolic aspects of living with respect for and consideration of the child's culture, ethnicity, and social and physical environments. Emphasis on play as the primary occupation of children assists children with achievement of age-appropriate developmental skills and helps children adapt to the psychosocial as well as physical changes that occur throughout the dying process. Adaptive equipment and positioning to maintain function and competent occupational behaviors also can provide comfort and diminish physical pain for the terminally ill child. Occupational therapy programming for children needs to involve family members in the treatment process, including siblings, given the physical and psychosocial abilities of family members to participate in the child's care. Families and family members must be individually evaluated, in conjunction with other disciplines, so they can be supported in undertaking whichever roles and activities are the most appropriate for them.

The hospice team

The occupational therapist cannot work alone in developing strategies to maintain occupational function. The occupational therapist is assisted by a wide array of health care professionals that equally impact on a person's life and work in conjunction with meeting physical, psychosocial, emotional, spiritual, sexual, and creative needs of terminally ill patients and their families. These team members include physicians; nurses; social workers; pharmacists; dietitians; physical, speech, and respiratory therapists; chaplains; and volunteers. Each of these disciplines has a unique role in the hospice environment, with each member having equal input into the patient's care. Occupational needs of hospice patients can be identified by any of these disciplines and can request a physician referral for occupational therapy after consulting with the occupational therapist for appropriateness of referral.

Documentation and reimbursement

In 1982, Congress passed legislation to extend Medicare coverage to terminally ill beneficiaries who elected to receive hospice care. Beneficiaries are entitled to Medicare hospice benefits if they are eligible for Medicare Part A and have a prognosis of 6 months or less to live. A statement is signed by the patient transferring from regular Medicare to Hospice Medicare. Medicare hospice beneficiaries may receive hospice care for two periods of 90 days each and one period for 30 days. Conversion back to regular Medicare can occur if the lifetime maximum of 210 days is reached. Conversion back to regular Medicare can occur at any time, if elected by the patient, during the Hospice Medicare benefit period. Eligibility requirements can vary among hospice programs (eg, age or access to primary caregiver).

Occupational therapy is covered under the hospice per diem rate allowed by Medicare. Individual therapists may be employed or contracted by hospices and are paid accordingly. Each Medicare-certified hospice must have an occupational, physical, and speech therapist contracted. Unfortunately, this does not dictate that the therapists must be used. Other insurance companies may reimburse for occupational therapy services in hospice or for terminal care. This must be thoroughly checked before evaluation and treatment. Individual marketing for occupational therapy in hospice is the responsibility of the individual therapist. Possibilities for therapists to cowrite grants for funding of therapy services, develop programs in hospice, or help with fundraising to pay for therapy services also exist.

Documentation for regular Medicare and other insurance reimbursement must reflect progress in patient care, or payment will be denied. Medicare-certified hospice programs require documentation of the treatment session, the patient's response, and any changes that may have occurred since the last visit or last several visits. Functional improvement in each visit is not necessary for reimbursement. Frequency of note writing is dependent on the hospice program and state and federal requirements. For more extensive information regarding hospice documentation and reimbursement issues, the reader is referred to the Health Care Financing Administration ruling on Medicare hospice programs (1983).

References

Agich, G. J. (1978). The ethics of terminal care. *Death Education 2*(1–2), 163–171.

American Occupational Therapy Association (1987). *Guidelines for occupational therapy services in hospice*. Rockville, MD: Author.

Barris, R., Kielhofner, G., & Watts, J. (1983). *Psychosocial occupational therapy: Practice in the pluralistic arena*. Laurel, MD: RAMSCO.

Capra, F. (1982). *The turning point: Science, society and the rising culture*. New York: Bantam.

Corless, I. B. (1983). The hospice movement in North America. In C. A. Corr, & D. M. Corr (Eds.), *Hospice care: Principles and practice* (pp. 335–351). New York: Springer.

Corr, C. A., & Corr D. M. (Eds.). (1983). *Hospice care: Principles and practice*. New York: Springer.

Dubos, R. (1977). Determinants of health and disease. In D. Landy (Ed.), *Culture, disease and healing: Studies in medical anthropology* (pp. 31–41). New York: MacMillan.

Flanigan, K. (1982). The art of the possible . . . Occupational therapy in terminal care. *British Journal of Occupational Therapy, 45*(8), 274–276.

Frank, G. (1991). The concept of adaptation as a foundation for occupational science research. Paper presented at the Third Symposium on Occupational Science, Philadelphia, PA. Unpublished manuscript.

Gammage, S. L., McMahon, P. S., & Shanahan, P. M. (1976). The occupational therapist and terminal illness: Learning to cope with death. *American Journal of Occupational Therapy, 30*, 294–299.

Garrett, D. N. (1978, November/December). The needs of the seriously ill and their families: The haven concept. *Aging*, 12–19.

Health Care Financing Administration (1983, December 16). Medicare program, hospice care: Finale rule. *Federal Register*, 56008–56036.

Holland, A. (1984). Occupational therapy and day care for the terminally ill. *British Journal of Occupational Therapy, 47*(11), 345–348.

Holland, A., & Tigges, K. N. (1981). The hospice movement: A time for professional action and commitment. *British Journal of Occupational Therapy, 44*(12), 373–376.

Koff, T. (Ed.). (1980). *Hospice: A caring community*. Cambridge, MA: Winthrop.

Kubler-Ross, E. (1969). *On death and dying*. New York: MacMillan.

Lidz, T. (1968). *The person: His and her development throughout the life cycle*. New York: Basic Books.

Matsutsuyu, J.S. (1969). The interest checklist. *American Journal of Occupational Therapy, 23*, 323–328.

National Hospice Organization (1979). *Standards of hospice program of care*. Rosslyn, VA: Author

Oakley, F., Kielhofner, G., Barris, R. and Reichler, R.K. (1986). The Role Checklist: Development and empirical assessment of reliability. *Occupational Therapy Journal of a Research, 6*, 157–170. (Can be obtained by writing to Frances Oakley, MS, OTR, National Institute of Health, OT Service, Clinical Center, Building 10, Room 68235, 9000 Rockville Pike, Bethesda, MD, 20892.)

Pizzi, M. (1983). Hospice and the terminally ill geriatric patient. *Physical and Occupational Therapy in Geriatrics 3*(1), 45–54.

Pizzi, M. (1984). Occupational therapy in hospice care. *American Journal of Occupational Therapy, 38*, 252–257.

Pizzi, M. (1986). Care of the terminally ill, Part 1: General principles. In *Role of Occupational Therapy with the Elderly* (pp. 241–249). Rockville, MD: American Occupational Therapy Association.

Pizzi. M. (1990). The transformation of HIV infection and AIDS in occupational therapy: Beginning the conversation. *American Journal of Occupational Therapy, 44*(3), 199–203.

Pizzi, M. Mukand, J. & Freed, M. (1991). HIV infection and occupational therapy. In J. Mukand (Ed.), *Rehabilitation for patients with HIV disease* (pp. 283–326). New York: McGraw-Hill.

Pizzi, M. (1992). Hospice: The creation of meaning for people with life-threatening illness. *Occupational Therapy Practice, 4*(1), 1–7.

Rando, T. A. (1984). *Grief, dying and death: Clinical interventions for caregivers*. Champaign, IL: Research Press.

Saunders, C. (1965). The last stages of life. *American Journal of Nursing, 65*(3), 70–75.

Scaffa, M. (1981) *Temporal adaptation and alcoholism*. Unpublished master's thesis. Virginia Commonwealth University, Richmond, VA.

Tigges, K. N. (1983). Occupational therapy in hospice. In C. A. Corr, & D. M. Corr (Eds.), *Hospice care: Principles and practice* (pp. 160–176). New York: Springer.

Tigges, K. N., & Sherman, L. M. (1983). The treatment of the hospice patient: From occupational history to occupational role. *America Journal of Occupational Therapy, 37*(4), 235–238.

Yerxa, E. J. (1967). 1966 Eleanor Clarke Slagle lecture: Authentic occupational therapy. In *A professional legacy: The Eleanor Clarke Slagle lectures in occupational therapy, 1955–1984* (pp. 155–1730). Rockville, MD: American Occupational Therapy Association.

Yerxa, E. J., Clark, F., Frank, G., Jackson, J., Parham, D., Pierce, D., Stein, C., & Zemke, R. (1989). An introduction to occupational science: A foundation for occupational therapy in the 21st century. *Occupational Therapy in Health Care, 6*(4), 1–17.

UNIT X

Clinical reasoning

CHAPTER 31

Aspects of clinical reasoning in occupational therapy

MAUREEN HAYES FLEMING

KEY TERMS

Clinical Reasoning
Cue
Ethnographic Research
Hypothesis
Hypothesis Generation
Hypothetical Reasoning

Interactive Reasoning
Pattern Recognition
Phenomenologic
  Perspective
Procedural Reasoning

LEARNING OBJECTIVES

Upon completion of this chapter the reader will be able to:

1. *Identify three types of clinical reasoning: interactive reasoning, pattern recognition, and procedural reasoning.*
2. *Identify aspects of domains of occupational therapy professional concerns that influence how therapists think.*
3. *Appreciate the influence that the philosophy of the profession exerts on the day-to-day concerns of practice.*
4. *Describe the importance of taking a phenomenologic approach to understanding patients and their problems.*
5. *Explain the importance of therapeutic interaction.*
6. *Identify some reasoning strategies that guide therapeutic interaction.*
7. *Describe the role of pattern recognition in the process of procedural reasoning.*
8. *Explain the importance of cue identification, hypothesis generation, cue interpretation, and hypothesis evaluation (Elstein, Schulman, & Sprafka, 1978) in procedural reasoning.*
9. *Relate the importance of integrating the procedural and interactive modes of reasoning and treatment.*
10. *Appreciate the complexity of clinical reasoning in occupational therapy.*

Clinical reasoning studies

This discussion is based partly on some of the theories developed as a result of the Clinical Reasoning Study funded by the American Occupational Therapy Association (AOTA) and the American Occupational Therapy Foundation (AOTF) (Gillette & Mattingly, 1987). Other research projects of therapists in similar and in different settings also influenced this discussion. Clinical stories from therapists with a broad range of experience are included as illustrations of many of the concepts presented.

This research is somewhat atypical because both pure and applied research motives guided the work. It is also different from the type of research that many occupational therapists are accustomed to reading about. **Ethnographic research** has many features and qualities that are different from the quantitative research that is more common in occupational therapy research literature. (For a description of the research methodology employed in the AOTA/AOTF study, see Mattingly & Gillette, 1991.)

Two features of the research project are important to note here; both are influenced by a central goal of ethnographic research, which is to understand people as they perceive or understand themselves (Karlsson, 1988). One feature is that the researchers do not start out with a **hypothesis** but rather with an open mind. The other difference is that the principal investigators included the people who were being studied in the discussions of their observations and interpretations that they are making. Thus, the people studied are not subjects, but participants. Since there have been so many people involved in these research projects at a number of levels and in varying degrees of intensity, some of the ideas that are presented here are the product of several minds. The term *we* is often used in this chapter to express the fact that the participants included many people, even though this chapter has a sole author.

Nature of occupational therapy and clinical reasoning

Philosophy and practice

Philosophy guides practice

In observing therapists and listening to their concerns, one is struck by the degree to which the philosophy directs practice. The depth of concern for patients and their functioning and the strength of the values placed on independence and respect for the person strongly influence day-to-day practice. Therefore, philosophy influences reasoning. It is uncommon in our culture to think of philosophy influencing a practice, especially a practice in an environment that is medical and therefore presumed to be scientific. Science is presumed to be value free. Philosophy motivates and guides the humanistic practice of occupational therapy and probably has a great deal of influence on its success, but it is sometimes a source of frustration and confusion for therapists operating in a medical teaching hospital with a hard science orientation. Therapists find it difficult to explain the practice and the importance of the philosophy to the practice. Both Serrett (1985) and Breines (1986) have commented that this tends to lead to a problem in formulating a professional identity.

Values influence practice

Therapists use scientific knowledge and principles when considering the patient's physical problems, but their philosophical stance often influences which functional problems they address. For example, occupational therapists value independence in activities of daily living (ADL) skills. Often, a therapist spends much time and energy helping a person learn to feed himself or herself. Other people might think it simply would be easier to feed the person. Occupational therapists think that the person would feel a greater sense of self-worth and personal dignity if he or she were independent in this area rather than needing to be fed, so the therapist teaches the person this skill (provided that this is what the person wants to do).

In a study conducted to identify values that might influence clinical reasoning among occupational therapists, 18 distinctive value statements were identified; among these were "focusing on the whole person," "respect and empathy," and therapists valuing their own ability to "think both conceptually and specifically" (Fondiller, Rosage, & Neuhaus, 1990, p. 48–49) The profession has a long history of using ethical concerns and particular values to guide practice (Bing, 1986; Engelhardt, 1986; Meyer, 1977; Yerxa, 1979). These values are generally held by occupational therapists regardless of their specialization (Sinnett, 1988). In observing and interpreting the work of the occupational therapists in the various clinical reasoning studies, it was clear that this relation of values to practice is not simply an abstract one. Values play an active role in daily practice.

Ethics influence clinical reasoning

The philosophy and value system of the profession have a strong influence on the practice. Therefore, it is imperative that the therapist be aware of them. This means that therapists must be attentive to ethical concerns at all times. As Joan Rogers (1983) noted in her Eleanor Clarke Slagle lecture:

> The ultimate question we, as clinicians, are challenged to answer is: What, among the many things that could be done for this patient, ought to be done? This is an ethical question. It involves a judgement to which facets contribute but that must be decided by weighing values. A salient criterion of an ethical action is its agreement with the patient's valued goals. The clinical reasoning process terminates in an ethical decision, rather than in a scientific one, and the ethical nature of the goal of clinical reasoning projects itself over the entire sequences. (p. 602)

Including values in our practice is itself a value for the profession. Although this has doubtless improved patient care, it has not been without negative consequences for the profession or for individual therapists (Johnson, 1981; Neuhaus, 1988; Parham, 1987). For example, Fondiller, Rosage, and Neuhaus (1990) comment:

> [T]he American health care system is committed to short hospital stays and increasingly less contact time with patients. Therapists who emphasized the therapeutic relationship, being wholistic in approach and taking the time to obtain a thorough history, find themselves working in a health care system that does not support their values and priorities. (p. 51)

This sort of ethical conflict often influences both *what* therapists think about regarding their patients' problems and *how* they think about resolving those problems. Resolving this sort of conflict is not an easy task for therapists. Therapists employ several different types of reasoning in thinking about the ethical treatment of their patients.

Role of the occupational therapist

Reconstruction

The occupational therapist has a unique and usually not well-understood role. The original Society for the Promotion of Occupational Therapy was formed with the intent of "the advancement of occupation as a therapeutic measure, the study of the effects of occupation on the human being, and the dissemination of scientific knowledge of this subject" (*Constitution of the National Society for the Promotion of Occupational Therapy,* 1917, p. 1.). The Society's intent essentially was to promote research regarding the relation between occupation and health and well being. The founders of the field believed that "[s]ick minds, sick bodies and sick souls may be healed through occupation" (Dunton, 1919, p. 10.). Thus, they concerned themselves with the reconstruction of the physically and mentally disabled. The notion of reconstruction is an interesting one that is no longer part of the explicit theory of the profession but is a strong implicit force underlying practice. Occupational therapists typically work with people who have serious, often permanent, physical injuries. In these situations, the therapist works on reconstruction of the person's ability to function and perform daily life tasks. The therapist and patient essentially reconstruct the person's habit structure, reformulating how the person engages in everyday activities.

At a deeper level, the therapist and patient often work on reconstructing the person's sense of self. The person's life has changed drastically, and the therapist often helps the person envision a new set of life goals and new ways of attaining a satisfying future life. This process is complex, and the reasoning that guides this deeper sort of reconstruction is also complicated. Only a small part of that reconstruction and the reasoning guiding it are discussed in this chapter.

Occupational therapists help people reconstruct ways of accomplishing tasks, of engaging in activities, and of viewing themselves and their lives. Occupation is used as a means to that reconstruction, as an agent or medium to promote change at both a physical and personal level.

Transition from clinic to community

Although occupational therapists often work in hospitals with people who have incurred medical conditions, therapists do not treat the condition per se. Occupational therapists help people to function within the limits of the consequences of their conditions. Therapists help people learn functional activities and skills so that they can leave the hospital and return to life in the community. Thus, an essential role of the occupational therapist is to aid a person in the transition from the hospital or other institutional environment to the usual social environment of the community. Many therapists also assist people who live in the community to function more effectively. For example, large numbers of occupational therapists work with children with special needs who attend public schools. Therapists therefore have a role that includes the notion of transition as well as training. The training role is relatively obvious, but the transition role is more subtle and often more difficult to negotiate.

What occupational therapists think about

Many types of thinking strategies can be used. The subject of the thinking has an influence on the type of thinking strategy a person selects. It is useful to look to studies by other types of clinicians, such as physicians and psychologists, for ideas, research results, and methodology to guide our inquiry. It is not helpful, however, to assume that occupational therapists will or should employ the same thinking strategies used by other clinicians. It is important to recognize that occupational therapy practice has particular aims, goals, and values that influence not only *what* a therapist thinks about but also *how* a therapist thinks. Two distinctive features make occupational therapy different from medicine or other medically related professions: (1) the degree to which the philosophy of the profession influences practice, and (2) the importance of the patient's participation in treatment.

The following six themes in the philosophy of occupational therapy strongly influence the practice and therefore the reasoning of occupational therapists:

1. A focus on future functioning
2. Treating the whole person
3. Individualizing treatment
4. Valuing independence
5. A perception that part of the therapist's role is to teach the patient problem-solving skills
6. Helping a person to regain a sense of self and self-worth

Three of those themes are discussed here.

Focus on functional performance

Diagnosis is often seen as the most critical aspect of decision making in medicine (Kassirer, 1989). History taking is critical to the diagnostic reasoning process. The person's history, including birth, development, habits, environment, and other factors that might contribute to the acquisition of a disease or condition, are important considerations in diagnostic medicine. Diagnosis and history are not the central focus for occupational therapists. Patients come to occupational therapy with a medical diagnosis. The task of the therapist is to know how that diagnostic condition would influence the person's present and future function. Etiology is important, but it is usually in the background rather than the foreground of therapists' minds. Therapists conduct careful evaluations and make precise observations of functional performance. They make accurate predictions of possible gains the person is likely to make in attaining future functional levels. Therapists are concerned about what those gains will mean to the person's future in the community.

History is important to therapists when imagining a person's possible future situation and considering whether the past might influence the potential for actualizing that future. For example, if a person had a history of substance abuse, a therapist might think that the person's ability to live independently would be determined by both the physical gains the person made and the encouragement the family provided to seek treatment for the abuse.

The occupational therapist's primary task is to help the person function in the future. The ability to imagine new ways that a person could function in the future is essential to occupational therapy practice. Therefore, constructing a vision of the future possibilities is an important aspect of clinical reasoning for occupational therapists.

Individualizing treatment

Medical research, like all scientific research, tests theories that can be expressed in general law statements (Bunge, 1967). Medicine, like all applied scientific practices, employs these laws to solve classes of problems. There is a need to know what is generally true, or generally the case. Questions such as, "What are the usual manifestations of this disease?" or "What are generally the results of this treatment?" are answered through scientific medical research.

Therapists have an appreciation for science and medicine. Experienced therapists are familiar with the manifestations, courses, and usual outcomes of a wide range of diseases and disabilities. They work with people with many disabilities and know the limitations that such disabilities generally place on functioning. However, therapists are more often interested in the *particulars* of *this person* than they are in the *generals* of the *condition*. A commonly heard phrase in occupational therapy is, "You have to individualize treatment for each patient."

Individualizing means tailoring the treatment to the particular skills, needs, and interests of each patient. The notion that a treatment may be specific to a particular patient runs counter to the common assumption that all people with a given disease or disability can be treated with the same general solution. Occupational therapists take both the broad approach to the scientific general laws of the disease and the specific approach to the person and combine the two approaches. These two approaches, however, are not usually considered compatible. This presents problems for occupational therapists because they need to use two different styles of thinking to analyze the types of problems they address.

The integration of the dual concerns for the patient and for resolving the physical or functional problem is a common, but not always harmonious, way of thinking about and conducting therapy. Therapists have many procedures, treatment modalities, and strategies that are frequently used with most people who have the same sort of injury. What therapists enjoy most, however, is not the precise application of the correct procedure. Instead, they are interested in finding the best way for this person to attain a goal. Effective occupational therapy depends on knowledge of the general features of the disability but is primarily focused on understanding the particulars of this person. Therefore, reasoning strategies that are sensitive to both the generals and the particulars are employed by occupational therapists.

Treating the whole person

Occupational therapists often comment that they treat the *whole person*. What they mean by this is that they concern themselves with several aspects of the person (the physical, cognitive, psychological, cultural, and so forth) and that they treat the person as a whole, as a real person, and not simply as a collection of functional and dysfunctional parts. For therapists to achieve their goals of helping a person with disabilities to maintain and improve functional performance while tailoring the goals and treatment activities to the person's particular interest and needs, considering the whole person becomes essential. Therapists do not actually treat the whole person so much as they treat the person as a whole. This approach influences the therapist's reasoning. They need to think of several aspects of the person. This means that they must draw on several different bodies of knowledge to analyze and resolve the problems that they address. It is difficult to seek and combine different bodies of knowledge. In addition, various bodies of knowledge are organized differently and require different types of thinking styles to apply that knowledge to a given situation. Particular types of knowledge often require a given form of inquiry for their analysis or application. For example, thinking about the organ systems requires a different body of knowledge and a different style of thinking than does thinking about which cultural factors may influence whether a person will participate in therapy or do a particular activity.

Importance of participation

An early observation by Mattingly was that the "success of occupational therapy treatment is dependent upon the patients' participation, or at the least, cooperation" (1989, p. 135). This need for the patient's cooperation is important to get the patient to go through the (often routine) treatment procedures: range of motion, dressing, memory retraining, kitchen evaluations, and so forth. Participation is even more important for the higher goals of taking charge of oneself through problem solving and assertiveness or regaining a sense of self and self-worth. Occupation is the major treatment medium. Participation and occupation are inseparable. Therapy is not possible without participation.

What is clinical reasoning?

A variety of definitions

Studies of how physicians and psychologists think have been conducted since the early 1950s (Goldberg, 1968). Since that time, however, there has not been a clear and agreed-on definition of exactly what the phenomenon under study is, nor what to call it. Terms used to name this phenomenon range from concrete, definite words like *prediction* (Meehl, 1954) to elusive, subjective sounding terms such as *clinical judgment* (Feinstein, 1967). The phenomenon is variously viewed as the *application of logic* (Cutter, 1979) at one extreme or *wisdom* (Goldberg, 1970) at the other. The designers of the AOTA/AOTF Clinical Reasoning Study (Gillette & Mattingly, 1987) consciously chose not to settle on a definition of clinical reasoning, nor did they wish to limit the study to a particular type or aspect of thinking. We assumed that occupational therapists' clinical activity was guided by thinking. We trusted that therapists' thinking or reasoning strategies could be identified using the careful ethnographic research methods of observing and interpreting their clinical actions and interactions. In conducting the study, Mattingly found that clinical reasoning is "more than the ability to offer explicit reasons and . . . more than the simple application of theory" (1991a, p. 979). Several types of reasoning that therapists used were identified in that and subsequent studies.

Similarities and differences

Like most researchers, we began with a review of the literature. Most clinical reasoning literature at that time reported on studies of physicians or psychologists. In conducting our study, however, we found that clinical reasoning in occupational therapy is only partly analogous to medical problem solving or medical decision making (Fleming, 1991a). In medicine, the primary focus of clinical reasoning is diagnosis, and diagnosis is guided by scientifically derived probabilities (Pauker, Gorry, Kassirer, & Schwartz, 1976). Many researchers in medical decision making assume that **hypothetical reasoning** is a central part of the reasoning strategies that physicians employ.

Medical decision making employs scientific knowledge that seeks to identify the general or usual, such as what is generally or usually the course of a disease. In occupational therapy, therapists are usually aware of the general, but they often focus on what was different or unique about a particular patient. Rather than focusing on generals, they seek particulars. This caused them to use other forms of reasoning in addition to hypothetical reasoning. Occupational therapy is a practical profession, and much of the focus is on concrete action rather than on abstract decision making. Much of the knowledge and reasoning employed to guide action is different from the hypothetical reasoning strategy that the medical decision making literature reports and encourages. Therefore, we use the term **clinical reasoning** to refer to the many types of inquiry that an occupational therapist uses to understand patients and their difficulties. As we use the term here, clinical reasoning includes, but is not limited to, hypothetical reasoning and problem solving. It includes focused inductive or deductive hypothetical reasoning employing scientific knowledge (Cutter, 1979) as well as intuitive reasoning (Hammond, 1988) based on scientific and professional knowledge and the tacit knowledge (Polanyi, 1967) that develops through clinical experience (Dewey, 1915) and interactive reasoning (Fleming, 1989). Clinical reasoning is used as an umbrella term to include all the complex processes that therapists use when thinking about the patient, the disability, the situation, and the personal and cultural meanings that the patient gives to the disability, the situation, and the self.

Different ways of thinking about various aspects of the problem

The goals and nature of the profession require that therapists concern themselves with many facets of a person and that person's functioning. Therefore, therapists are forced to use many ways of thinking to frame, analyze, and influence not just problems, but problem complexes (Schon, 1983). Different aspects of the problem complex tend to trigger the use of different types of thinking strategies (Koestler, 1967). When an occupational therapist is thinking about the person's physical injury, the relevant medical knowledge and hypothetical reasoning strategy are usually employed. But when other aspects of the situation are being considered, other knowledge and forms of reasoning are more useful.

In this chapter, three types of clinical reasoning necessary for beginning practitioners are discussed briefly: *interactive reasoning*, *pattern recognition*, and *procedural reasoning*. The types of reasoning found among experienced or expert clinicians, such as conditional reasoning and narrative reasoning, are discussed elsewhere (Mattingly, 1989, 1991a, 1991b; Fleming 1989, 1991a, 1991b; Mattingly & Fleming, 1992). The philosophy of the profession is deeply embedded in practice. Practice requires the patient's participation. Therefore, interactive reasoning is often more important than procedural reasoning. To highlight that importance, interactive reasoning is addressed first.

Interactive reasoning

Interaction is guided by reasoning

Occupational therapists talk with their patients. Some talk appears to be related to the person's physical problems, but much does not. They converse about weekend activities, hobbies, music, or other common topics. At first glance, this looks like idle chatter; however, talking is an important part of therapy. There are several reasons or purposes for talking. Talking is just one form of interaction that is used to achieve various goals. Formulating these goals requires a thinking process that we call interactive reasoning (Fleming, 1989). Interactive reasoning takes place during face-to-face encounters between therapist and patient. It is a form of reasoning that therapists employ when they want to better understand a patient as a person. The therapist might want to know how the person feels about the treatment at the moment. A therapist may try to understand the person to more finely tailor the treatment to the person's specific needs or preferences. A therapist might want to know the person better to help the person to gain insight into his or her problem.

Phenomenologic perspective

Often, an occupational therapist wants to better understand the experience of the disability from the patient's point of view. This requires taking a particular perspective on the problem. Kleinman (1980) refers to this as taking the *illness perspective* rather than the *disease perspective*. Understanding the illness experience (Kleinman, 1980) is an attempt to understand how the person views the illness and the way the illness changes the persons life and sense of self. The disease perspective means thinking about the disease as the important entity rather than thinking about the person who is experiencing the influences and consequences of the disease.

Knowing the patient as a person is what Sacks (1983) refers to as understanding "this patient." The terms *illness experience* and *this patient*, then, refer to ways in which practitioners take the **phenomenologic perspective** (Kestenbaum, 1982). Taking the phenomenologic perspective means attempting to understand people from their own points of view, to see people as they see themselves. It is also an attempt to understand the meanings people make of themselves, their lives, families, and environments. Phenomenology is concerned with how meanings are made and with how they are embodied in everyday habits and activities (Kockelmans, 1967). This clearly is a different point of view than the disease perspective, whereby the person is viewed as a patient, a container for a particular disease or disability (Foucault, 1973).

Occupational therapists often believe that therapy will not be effective if the therapist does not understand the patient as a person. Therapists use interactive reasoning and other forms of reasoning to achieve this phenomenologic understanding of the people who are their patients. The following excerpt from a clinical story illustrates the phenomenologic perspective. Ellen, a therapist with 15 years of experience in pediatrics, had just taken a new job as a home health agency therapist visiting adult patients when the story took place. This was a different role for Ellen, and she was not accustomed to the patient population. Here she recounts her first meeting with a client named Mac.

CASE STUDY

Taking the Phenomenologic Perspective

Mac is 24 years old. He is clean-cut and handsome, with the healthful look of a tennis player or weekend sailor. He warmly introduced himself and invited me to sit down in the living room. He wheeled his sport wheelchair into the living room area and attempted a rather sloppy transfer with a midway effort to demonstrate his emerging ability to stand independently. I noted and commented on the chair's homemade foot supports, and we engaged in a conversation about his ingenuity (he had devised these) and his interest in aesthetics and design. I looked at the magazines and books around the room, and this led to further discussion of his commitment to the environment, to health, and to his pursuit of a life that would meld his interests and commitments. Feeling internally pressured to be a good occupational therapist, I took the first opportunity to change the subject to his reason for referral—work with his hands. His spinal cord injury, it appeared, and he concurred, was at the C5–C6 level and was quite "incomplete." He proudly told of continuing to see changes of his regaining strength and function now, almost 2 years since his accident. Eventually he showed me his hands. To look at Mac, his physical body appears unimpaired; and without the cue of the wheelchair, on seeing him sitting still, it would be hard to guess what his disability is. He prides himself on that. He explained that he works hard to maintain his upper body strength—going to the gym or pool daily and wearing loose but stylish clothing to appear as "normal" as possible. His hands, however, looked much like those typical of a person with a cervical spinal cord injury.

Mac had been rehabilitated at University Hospital in Boston and was pleased with his services and experience there. We talked about the fact that I had worked there in college and compared notes about the facility. However, Mac now wanted the tenodesis contractures that had been encouraged to develop at University reversed so that he could "shake hands like a regular person." I took strength and range of motion measurements, attending carefully to his reports of new movements and to his questions and hopefulness about further recovery. I asked what services he had had since leaving University Hospital—had he had an exercise program, splints, hand therapy? It took a while, but he eventually left the room and came back with a bag full of finger splints from a local hospital outpatient department. He could not recall how to use them and admitted to not following through on the therapy but said he was now interested in addressing improvement of his hand status and function.

We reviewed his daily routine. He required little or no assistance for most personal care. He had, and used, a variety of adaptive equipment. His housemate did the shopping, most of the cooking and cleaning, and some personal care in exchange for free rent. They appeared to be friends. After Mac's accident and rehabilitation, he had finished college and had an impressive educational performance record, including fluency in French and a year of study at the Sorbonne in Paris. We talked about his family and friends.

It was clear that Mac had adjusted well overall, but his life was now rather routine—self-care, exercise or therapy, and social activities. It occurred to me then, but I chose not to act on it, that perhaps he was looking for meaning, for direction in his life, and that his hands, unable to reach out as he perceived they should, were symbolic of this search.

This is an example of how the therapist engaged in an interaction with a person, let him tell his story, and truly listened to what he had to say about himself. Ellen listened for the meanings that Mac had made about himself, his condition, and what his future might hold. While reading the story, one can easily imagine the therapist conversing with this personable young man. One senses both Ellen's awkwardness in not knowing just what her role is, and conversely, her confidence in her interpersonal skills. Ellen thought she should address Mac's physical problem like a "good occupational therapist" but was continually drawn back to a discussion about Mac and how he sees himself and his life. Ellen attends to Mac in a way that makes him comfortable and lets him know that he really is being not only listened to but also understood. This sort of understanding—understanding the person's attempt to make meaning in life—is typical of the phenomenologic approach but not easy to attain.

Reasons for interactive reasoning

Several people have analyzed various videotapes made during the Clinical Reasoning Study and have examined different aspects of interactive reasoning. Interactive reasoning appears to be employed for at least eight fairly distinct reasons or purposes. These are:

1. To engage the person in the treatment session; Mattingly (1989) identified six such strategies
2. To use humor to relieve tension (Siegler, 1987)
3. To know the person as a person (Cohn, 1989)
4. To understand the disability from the patient's point of view (Mattingly, 1989)
5. To finely match the treatment goals and strategies to this particular person, with this disability, and this experience of it; therapists call this "individualizing" (Fleming, 1989)
6. To communicate a sense of acceptance, trust, or hope to the patient (Langthaler, 1990)
7. To construct a shared language of actions and meanings (Crepeau, 1991)
8. To determine whether the treatment session is going well (Fleming, 1989)

Therapists have several different purposes in mind for using interaction. It appears that there are different reasoning strategies that are employed to implement the goals, or reasons, listed above. For example, in trying to understand the person as a person, therapists' reasoning looks like what Belenky, Clinchy, Goldberger, and Tarule describe as "connected knowing" (1986, p. 101), which those authors link to empathy. In trying to understand the disability from the patient's point of view, they use a phenomenologic approach similar to that advocated by Paget (1988). Their interaction with patients produces an understanding of the person as a person within a culturally constructed point of view as they share a *reciprocity of motives* (Schutz, 1975).

Interactive strategies identified by Mattingly

Mattingly's (1989) strategies indicate that therapists have several ways of engaging the patient in treatment. Some of these require complex interpretations of subtle interactive cues to be effective. Mattingly noticed that the success of occupational therapy practice is dependent on the patient participating in treatment. So many of the strategies that Mattingly observed therapists using were employed specifically to enlist patients' cooperation and participation in treatment. Some of these strategies were: doing with, offering choices, individualizing treatment, telling stories, and joint problem solving. These strategies create and enforce a reciprocity of motives (Shutz, 1975) because the therapist and the patient are participating in the treatment together, are making decisions together, and are both active participants in the therapeutic process. Thus, the patient is helped toward a goal, and the therapist is able to be helpful to the patient's progress in rehabilitation.

Categories of interaction identified by Langthaler

Langthaler (1990) identified nine categories of interaction that therapists used, including "body orientation, activity, eye movements and direct verbal cue" (p. 38). First, Langthaler developed interactive categories: verbal behavior, nonverbal behavior, and activity, and then further divided these. For example, verbal behavior was divided into direct verbal cues and voice elements. Next, Langthaler identified 23 attributes within these categories, including "generalize, interpret, share meanings, attending support" (p. 99). She analyzed a videotaped treatment session and found that the therapist used literally dozens of interactive behaviors, such as facial expressions and words of encouragement, in each 3-minute segment of tape analyzed.

Therapists used these behaviors to convey numerous messages, such as support, encouragement, challenge, and reassurance. In using interactive strategies, therapists appear to be partly influenced by psychoanalytic theorists, such as Carl Rogers (1961), and by occupational therapy theorists, such as Fidler and Fidler (1963) and Mosey (1970). The reasoning style they used appeared to be closely linked to a form of social reasoning, which Gardner (1985) hypothesizes is mediated by personal intelligence. Gardner postulates two interpersonal intelligences. One is "the capacity to access one's own feeling life"; the other is the "ability to notice and make distinctions among other individuals, in particular among their moods, temperaments, motivations and intentions" (1985, p. 239).

When therapists used the strategies that Langthaler identified, it appeared that they were trying to understand the person's moods and feelings and then adjust their own behavior to influence either the mood or the behavior of the patient. Some of these strategies were fairly obvious, such as support or encouragement, but others were quite subtle, such as "matching the behavior to convey the message" or "increasing or decreasing stimuli to support the message" (Langthaler, 1990, p. 44). Langthaler attributed the success of such strategies to the therapist's ability to develop trust, convey a sense of empathy, and have a solid sense of self. These are characteristics that people typically attribute to the mature person.

The following is a short excerpt from Langthaler's analysis of a session between a therapist, Liz, and her patient, Peter:

> *Support:* Like questioning, supporting can have different meanings. For example, L:"O.K. I'll hold it." (L indicating that she will hold the wheelchair). L clearly and precisely announces the action, by which she will support P and help him perform.
>
> When she says, "Yea, that's why it is so hard to pick things up," L is reasoning.
>
> She wants P to understand that a quadriplegic patient with his condition will have difficulty performing this movement. By evaluating and assessing a movement she supports P.
>
> L: "This is kind of heavy." L is comforting P when he is not successful in picking up the key.
>
> Her verbal support conveys her empathy.

Langthaler's work gives us an indication of the great number of behaviors and meanings that comprise part of the therapist's interactive skill. It also indicates what an enormously complex task therapeutic interaction must be. Further analysis of therapists' interactions may yield an understanding of the clinical reasoning that must underlie the process of selecting, monitoring, and evaluating these interactive skills.

Pattern recognition and clinical reasoning

Pattern recognition: A type of problem solving

Newel and Simon identified three types of problem solving: "recognition, hypothesis generation, and heuristic search" (1972, pp. 94–96). Recognition, sometimes called pattern recog-

nition (Coughlin & Patel, 1987), is a commonly used problem-solving strategy employed by many types of practitioners (Schon, 1983). It is especially useful in the problem identification phase of problem solving. Pattern recognition is based on the ability to observe and interpret cues. *Cues* are aspects of the situation that one observes and interprets as potentially significant to understanding the person or object of inquiry. Simply put, pattern recognition is the ability to observe a phenomenon, identify significant characteristics (cues), determine whether there is a relation among the cues, and compare the present observations to a previously learned category or type. The following sequence is often offered as a diagrammatic illustration of the events in pattern recognition:

Observe—Identify Cues—Determine Pattern—Compare To Type

Many cues, however, can be part of more than one pattern. Therefore, a therapist usually does not follow this sequence literally but rather imagines several possible configurations of the cues, then mentally arranges them into several possible patterns. Next, the therapist compares and contrasts these to a variety of learned types, or *templates* (Hammond, 1988). The therapist also may seek additional cues or drop some cues from consideration, rendering them irrelevant. Thus, a therapist actually conducts the pattern recognition form of reasoning in a less linear and more complex way, shifting attention among sets of cues and potential patterns until the best fit between possible patterns and learned templates is perceived.

Experienced clinicians often recognize familiar patterns instantly. They do not have to subject the pattern to any particular analytic skill or process of inquiry. For example, a pediatric therapist instantly recognizes a child's posture and movement patterns as spastic cerebral palsy. The therapist needs only a quick glance at the child to recognize the pattern. Usually, this sort of pattern is recognized as a whole and not as a combination of individual cues.

Other patterns may be recognized, but some analysis or interpretation is required. This involves consideration of the cues in relation to a known pattern or type of physiognomy or behavior. For example, a therapist may observe a person behaving in an unusual or socially inappropriate manner. The therapist would not necessarily be able to tell immediately whether the behavior was a result of a psychotic process, confusion, or apraxia. A therapist gave an example of this from her experience: "I was doing an ADL evaluation with a woman who had been newly admitted. She was slow, but doing okay. Then she took her hairbrush and raised it off the tray and put it in her mouth. I didn't know what to think of this. Then I saw the look of righteous indignation on her face. She was more surprised at this behavior than I was. Then I realized this must be apraxia. She had motor planning problems."

Pattern recognition is important for all practitioners because it makes practice more efficient. If a professional can quickly recognize a problem or a condition, then he or she can move into deeper levels of analysis more quickly and on to the problem resolution or treatment phase. There is evidence that physician's expertise in pattern recognition is strongly related to diagnostic accuracy (Papa, Shores, & Mayer, 1990). Much of the academic portion of the education of health professionals is aimed at describing these patterns, usually called *clinical conditions*, to students. Much of clinical education helps the student to recognize these patterns in real patients (Cohn, 1989).

As useful as pattern recognition is, it is also important to know that this is not simply an automatic process. The ability to recognize many patterns of cues and behaviors quickly becomes part of the proficient therapist's fund of tacit knowledge (Polanyi, 1967). Practitioners need to both trust and question their pattern recognition skills. Therapists need to be attentive to many features of their patients' concerns and to continue to learn to recognize new, more subtle, and more complex cues and patterns throughout their lifetime of practice.

Below are two examples of pattern recognition. In the first case study, the therapist, Marie, is simply communicating some of the behavior patterns of a child with cerebral palsy with whom she worked in a public school setting. These patterns are so familiar to her (and, she expects, to the occupational therapists who would read her story) that they are simply taken for granted in her narration of the story.

CASE STUDY

Using Pattern Recognition

I usually arrive at Jackie's classroom as he is finishing math. I greet him where he is seated in his electric wheelchair with his aide nearby. Once he spots me, he often goes into a total extensor pattern. He usually does this when he is interrupted or excited, and he begins to maneuver his chair erratically, upsetting the group around him. Sometimes he giggles and screeches (overflow), and by now the entire room has been disturbed and the teacher looks perplexed. As the school year passed, Jackie's movements became slightly less erratic, and he was able to leave the classroom with less fanfare. Jackie knew that once he was in the corridor, he was responsible for good, safe driving. Typically, he did not demonstrate the head and upper-extremity control needed for lengthy trips in the chair. Extensor and reflexive patterns often interfered. A crowded hallway continued to be a disaster for most of the year. Increased muscle tone, reflexes, and so forth often made wheelchair operation difficult. After direction, and sometimes redirection, Jackie slowly made his way through the hall. I was often witness to some of his best driving performances because he knew it was what I was watching for. In the hallway, we often encountered a variety of circumstances, such as kids stopping to pat Jackie on the head or touch his wheelchair or ask me a question about him.

This example is simply an introduction to a clinical story that Marie wrote. As a means of introducing the reader to the child, Marie notes eight patterns that are typical of children with cerebral palsy: extensor pattern, overflow, erratic movements, limited head control, limited use of upper extremity, reflex patterns, increased muscle tone, and distractibility. These are mentioned not as a description of the clinical condition but rather to paint a picture for the reader and other occupational therapists of the child and the events in the day that the child and the therapist shared. They provide us here with an illustration of pattern recognition. They also illustrate how much pattern recognition is a part of therapists' everyday working knowledge, or tacit knowledge. This is an example of the sort of pattern that can be taught fairly easily. Classroom descriptions in a clinical conditions course and brief observation or videotape would probably serve to introduce the student to the pattern. Other patterns are

more subtle and require lengthy descriptions or more direct experience.

Possible problems with pattern recognition

Pattern recognition is useful when it leads the practitioner quickly into the problem and saves time in an initial search. It is a deterrent when it limits or precludes further inquiry. Here is an example of an occupational therapist who first worked for about 5 years in a general hospital in California and then moved across the country and took a new job in the psychiatric unit of a community hospital in a town near Boston. Sonja tells a story about a patient whose diagnosis was major depression.

CASE STUDY

Continuing to Search for Patterns

An elderly, widowed, white man was admitted with the diagnosis of major depression. His concerned children brought him to the psychiatric unit because they were afraid that he might commit suicide because he had become so listless and wished to die. In the past, he had taken great pride in caring for his home and cooking meals for his girlfriend. For no apparent reason, he had become more depressed and sedentary, with a loss of interest for all previous activities. Now, most of his days were spent in a recliner chair. Both he and his children were completely overwhelmed by his current useless state.

I first met this patient in the hallway. He stood alone in the unit crossroad between the dining area and the nurses station. He was well dressed and groomed with the exception of noticeable dandruff. Lunch was over so all the other patients had left the area. Meal times are short because patients usually retreat to the safety of their rooms before treatment groups begin again.

I introduced myself by name and extended my hand to him. He hesitated for a few seconds while looking into my eyes then firmly shook my hand and pleaded for help to return home. His anxious voice did not match with the flat, almost masklike affect. This odd combination of anxiety and a blank facial expression reminded me of a previous home health patient of mine. We walked to the interview room together. His slow, stop-and-start shuffling gait clearly did not seem like psychomotor retardation from an affective disorder. Some side effects of antipsychotic medication can mimic Parkinson-like symptoms in some patients, but this was the first psychiatric hospitalization for this man. He had never taken antipsychotics. Even before we reached the interview room, I suspected that this man might have more than just major depression.

When I asked about his self-care and home management he said, "I felt tired all the time. Lately I don't seem to have the motivation to do anything at all. It seems that I'm taking the corners more slowly. . . . Maybe I'm getting too old."

He was a good historian, clearly describing symptoms of depression with a passive wish to die. He was depressed about his increased difficulty to be productive. Therefore, he had lost motivation to work. Losses in some form often precipitate prolonged grief reactions and a major depressive episode. In this case, it appeared that his loss was the ease of movement.

Immediately after the interview, I recommended a referral for neurology, which later confirmed that he had Parkinson disease.

In this story, Sonja recognizes cues and patterns that make her question the diagnosis of major depression. She also sees patterns, such as the anxious voice, that are in conflict with the assumption that this is depression. She notes that he has a "slow, stop-and-start shuffling gait." Although psychomotor problems such as slow gait can accompany depression, Sonja notes that the quality of his gait is not like the quality of the gait patterns of other depressed patients whom she has known. She sees this and other patterns of behavior that remind her of patterns that she has seen in patients with Parkinson disease. Sonja then returns to the notion of depression and reasons that possibly this man's depression is related to his diminished energy and motor capacity, which in turn were caused by Parkinson disease. Sonja did not just accept the diagnosis of major depression and close off her observational skills and clinical reasoning. She observed cues and questioned their meaning and their relation to one another and the diagnosis. She maintained an open mind and a sense of inquiry.

Pattern recognition and interactive reasoning

Studies of pattern recognition by professionals usually focus on identification of concrete cues, such as physical characteristics, and on the procedural aspect of the professional endeavor. However, that is not the only type of pattern recognition. Therapists develop pattern recognition skills related to their interaction with patients. For example, therapists usually recognize behavior patterns that indicate a patient is depressed or excited or lethargic. Therapists also learn specific behavior or body language patterns of their particular patients. They learn to recognize cues within the first few seconds of seeing a patient they have known for a while, and they often assess the situation and make inferences, often accurate ones, about how the subsequent session will go.

Below is an example that is more than, but includes, pattern recognition on the part of a therapist, Kathy, who has been in practice on a spinal cord injury unit for about 2 years. Her story is about John, who did not fit the pattern of the usual spinal cord–injured patient. Actually, this is a story about how they both developed pattern recognition and mutual trust.

CASE STUDY

Using Pattern Recognition in the Interactive Mode

Before admitting a new patient to our unit, all disciplines receive a two-sided face sheet that provides the patient's age, date and mechanism of injury, level of injury, and other important medical information. It was late March of 1989 when I found a new sheet on my desk, indicating I was to pick up "the new patient." Although the face sheet gives limited, objective information, it was easy to read between the lines (or at least try to) to get some idea of who this person was.

From the information given, I learned that John (my new patient) had sustained T12 and L1 fractures as the result of a motor vehicle accident 3 weeks earlier. He was 40 years old, lived in Vermont with his girlfriend, and owned his own

business. John was described as a "big man" under the nutrition section of the face sheet. He had several medical complications before his transfer to us, including a deep vein thrombosis (DVT) for which an intravenous catheter (IVC) filter was placed.

Before I had even cast an eye on John, I began formulating an image of what this man looked like and what kind of person he was. I pictured a gruff, back woods, overweight person who was into fast living and drinking. Simply because of the fact that he was from Vermont, I imagined he was a construction worker or builder with a high school education at most. I wondered how he would fit in with all the other patients, most of whom were from the Boston area. I also wondered what we could possibly have in common to make conversation during the upcoming treatment sessions.

When John arrived from the trauma center in Western Massachusetts, I went to his room to introduce myself and begin my evaluation. I soon discovered that "big man" referred to his build. He was obviously active and well-muscled. He resembled Kenny Rogers, with gray hair and a trimmed beard. He appeared to be in a lot of pain, which he stated was due to the multiple rib fractures that he sustained as a result of the accident. I asked John if he recalled his accident at all, something we typically do to assess for possible head injury. John told me he had been driving home from work late at night after working several 18-hour days. He owned a large excavation company where he worked side-by-side with his employees and typically put in incredibly long days. Exhausted, he had fallen asleep at the wheel, lost control of his truck, and hit a neighbor's tree. Although he could only remember part of what happened after that point, he remembered the volunteer fire department's arriving at the scene. Ironically, John was also on the squad and recognized his rescuers. He remembers many of them being in a state of shock as they tried to remove their friend from his vehicle. Many of the men were crying and could not believe what had happened. As John told me this story, the big man who always was in control began to cry. From that moment on, I realized the man I had imagined was nothing like the man I was to work with for the next few months.

For John, his injury was absolutely devastating. There were many times when I would go into his room in the morning to work with him and find him crying behind his closed curtains. These moments were difficult for me, too, and I had no idea what I could possibly say to comfort him. Sometimes I would ask him if he wanted me to come back in a few minutes since he appeared embarrassed by his display of grief. As I got to know him better, I would sit with him as he tried to pull himself back together. John had every reason to feel the way he did and certainly did not need permission to express his feelings.

Here we see that Kathy knew what sort of functional problems a person with this level of injury would have. She also had an image of a personality pattern that she expected this person to have. Kathy's expectations were based on her prior experience with typical spinal cord unit patients. Such images and "typifications" are useful and often based on real probabilities (Schutz, 1975). For example, most spinal cord injuries appear to be lifestyle-related. Substance abuse and fast driving account for many such injuries. However, this was not the case with John.

Kathy quickly changed her image of the "patient" as she got to know "John," the person. John, in turn, learned to give up part of his image of himself as a person who could tough it out and was able to mourn the losses he experienced and recognize the physical pain he felt. Kathy, as well as his fellow firemen, recognized his loss and helped him to do so as well. John and Kathy developed a pattern of recognition for each other's moods. They also developed a behavioral pattern of creating time and a way for John to mourn the loss and be angry at the pain, which Kathy implied he had every right to do.

Pattern recognition using nonverbal interactions

Much interaction is verbal interaction. As was seen in Langthaler's work, however, much interaction is nonverbal. Therapists learn to give support, encouragement, and other emotional cues using nonverbal behaviors such as facial expressions and body posture. Therapists also learn to "read" the cues and behavior patterns of their patients. This ability to recognize and interpret the patient's interactive cues and patterns is a function of the therapist's interpersonal skills and clinical experience.

Procedural reasoning

Procedural reasoning and focus on the clinical problem

Therapists use procedural reasoning when thinking about the disease or disability and deciding which treatment activities (procedures) they might employ to remediate the person's functional performance problems (Fleming, 1989). Procedural reasoning is a type of hypothetical reasoning aimed at applying specific professional knowledge to the analysis and resolution of a particular clinical problem. Therapists search for both a definition of the problem and the best treatment method. In situations in which problem identification and treatment selection are the central tasks, the reasoning strategies of occupational therapists are similar to those identified by some researchers interested in medical problem solving. The typical medical problem solving sequence of diagnosis, prognosis, and prescription is commonly used; however, the words occupational therapists use to describe this sequence are problem identification, goal setting, and treatment. Below is a case study in which a therapist, Marie, goes quickly through that sequence to guide her procedural reasoning in a difficult situation. The therapist is with a young woman, Ann, who is a patient in a psychiatric hospital. Ann has become upset about a situation of her own and is at the same time concerned about another patient, Rosa, who has become out of control and may need to be restrained. The therapist is concerned about both patients but decides to focus her attention on Ann.

CASE STUDY

Using a Procedural Reasoning Sequence

After getting the go-ahead from Ann's doctor to schedule a meeting with the chaplain, I decided to take a minute to run into Ann's room to make the arrangements. This sounded pretty straightforward. What could be easier than scheduling a meeting between two consenting adults? Timing, I soon found out, is everything.

I walked into Ann's dimly lit room right after she had come from group therapy. She sat on her bed, wiping tears from her eyes, stating that the group was "tough, but good." Knowing that I needed to meet with my student in 15 minutes, I wasn't sure how much I should process the difficult group with Ann. Fortunately, as I was contemplating the pros and cons in my head, Ann's affect brightened. She stood up with an air of accomplishment and tossed her tissue decisively into the trash basket. I took this to mean that Ann had achieved a sense of resolution about what had occurred in group therapy and was ready for the next point of business.

As we began to discuss the planned meeting with the chaplain, noise on the unit began to escalate. I recognized the shrill voice of a Portuguese-speaking patient who had had a number of hysterical crying and screaming episodes on the unit over the past couple of days. The episodes were labeled "behavioral," and the treatment plan involved initial room-restriction followed by placement in the quiet room if the behavior persisted. As Ann and I talked, the screaming on the unit got louder, and Ann grew more tense. She clutched her pillow in her arm and wondered out loud if maybe Rosa was upset because no one could understand her in group therapy (because of the language barrier). The screaming went on for several minutes, which seemed like hours. My conversation with Ann alternated between superficial chit-chat to help distract her from the noise and the deeper discussion of how the screaming made her feel.

Ann stated nervously that the screaming reminded her of when she was in the abortion clinic at age 14. At this point, I was bewildered about what I should do next. Leaving the unit altogether to go to a scheduled meeting with my student was certainly the most appealing option at this time. This, however, was totally out of the question. I thought I might be needed to help escort Rosa to the quiet room. The third choice was to stay with Ann.

I knew from past experiences that restraints cause sexual abuse victims to regress and, in many instances, perform self-destructive acts. I was afraid that if I left Ann to help with the restraint, she would have a flashback or find something with which to cut, scratch, or mutilate herself. I also wondered what Ann was thinking. I'm sure she wondered about Rosa's safety as well as her own, and about how I would react. Would I help with the restraint? Would I abandon Ann? I decided to tell Ann that I needed to leave briefly to see if I was needed for the restraint, but that I would be back. She appeared to be all right with this decision. Going out onto the unit, I was struck by the number of staff that were congregated around Rosa to escort her to the quiet room. It was obvious that additional staff were not needed, so I returned to Ann's room. Before me sat Ann looking totally panic-stricken, and I struggled to figure out what to do next. What was it I remembered about the management of flashbacks? Keep the patient talking. Keep it here and now. Provide reassurance of safety. I wasn't 100% certain that I believed that flashbacks actually occur but decided that now was not the time for skepticism.

Step one. Keep the patient talking. This was easy. At this point, Ann was chattering incessantly about the weather, recent books she read, and anything else that popped into her mind. The pressure of her speech waxed and waned depending on the intensity of the screaming on the unit. During the less pressured moments, I asked Ann to tell me about the things she normally does to cope with stress. What sort of things did she do for fun? What did she do to relax? This appeared to be a good occupational therapy angle on the situation. Ann proceeded to tell a number of stories of her own.

Gardening was one of her interests. She grew copious amounts of flowers and vegetables. At home, she had routinely grown and dried flowers to make floral designs and potpourri. She recently planted a tomato garden and was wondering how to can tomatoes. We looked through an old cookbook she had on her shelf for a while but couldn't find canning techniques. I related the story to her desire to nurture. Ann smiled with recognition, and I could tell that this concept was not a new one for her.

In this story, we see an experienced therapist in a confusing situation. There are many things going on in the scene Marie describes. Although there were several distractions, Marie quickly focused on her most pressing responsibility. She noted that the patient was starting to exhibit a pattern of behaviors that she felt indicated increased anxiety; in other words, Marie *recognized a pattern*. Then she recalled that other patients whose past included sexual abuse "regress and in many instances perform self-destructive acts." Thus, she *identified a potential problem*. Then, seeking to avert the problem, Marie *set a treatment goal*. Then Marie *recalled* the protocol for the treatment of the problem. Then, talking to Ann, she *executed the treatment procedure*. In this case, it was not a specific occupational therapy treatment procedure that the therapist used; rather, it was a protocol given to many health care professionals working in psychiatry. In any case, she recalled it and executed it well. This example provides a useful illustration of the sequence of problem identification, goal setting, and treatment. We also see two additional reasoning features: pattern recognition and recalling a treatment protocol.

Procedural reasoning and the phenomenologic approach

The following case study also illustrates the usual procedural reasoning sequence of problem identification, goal setting, and treatment. In addition, the therapist takes the phenomenologic approach to identifying and resolving the patient's problem. The therapist, Maureen, has no trouble identifying the clinical pattern or the problem. The patient, Sue, had a cerebrovascular accident (CVA) and has the usual pattern of muscle weakness and incoordination on one side of her body. Maureen, an experienced therapist, knows this condition and its usual treatment well. She has a thorough working knowledge of the appropriate treatment procedures. She has a good understanding of the usual sequence and degree of recovery. But this patient is not the typical CVA patient. She is not an elderly person but rather a young mother.

Maureen needs to adjust her procedural work and reasoning slightly to take into account that this young woman is probably stronger than the typical patient with a CVA. More important, Maureen takes the phenomenologic approach. She tries to understand what is important to Sue. Maureen and Sue work together to decide what is the most important problem to work on and what treatment procedures to use. They work together to identify the real problem and to identify the treatment goals. The therapist selects conventional occupational therapy treatment procedures but soon creates her own treatment activities based on the problem, as the patient defines it. Together they find a way to help Sue reach her most valued goal: to be able to hold and care for her baby.

CASE STUDY

Using Procedural Reasoning and the Phenomenologic Approach to the Problem

Sue was a 26-year-old woman who had given birth and subsequently had a stroke. She was admitted to a rehabilitation hospital with right hemiparesis. When I first met Sue, she was depressed about being separated from her new baby, and her main fear was that she would not be able to adequately care for the baby on her own. Adding to this fear was the knowledge that her insurance would not cover any home services. Her husband was her only family. He worked in construction every day, and they lived in a trailer park. To go home with the baby, she would need to be independent.

The initial therapy sessions were centered around tone normalization, with an emphasis on mat activities, along with traditional ADL training in the mornings. Sue's husband visited daily and usually brought the baby with him. At first, this was extremely frustrating to Sue since she could not hold the baby unless she was sitting with pillows to support her right arm. She continued to voice her anxiety around the issue of going home and being able to care for the baby. Her husband was also worried about how this transformation would take place—from Sue as a patient to Sue as wife and mother. I spent a lot of time talking to Sue and her husband about the necessity of normalizing the tone and improving the movement of the upper extremity as a sort of foundation to the more complex functional skills Sue was so anxious to relearn.

Eventually, it was time to spend most of the treatment time on functional skills. The two areas we focused on were homemaking and child care. The homemaking sessions were fairly routine and traditional in nature, but it proved to be a bit more difficult to simulate some of the child-care activities.

Our first step was to find something that would be like a baby. We settled on borrowing a resuscitation baby doll from the nursing education department. We used this doll for the beginning skills, such as feeding and diaper changing. Sue had progressed to a point at which she had slight weakness and incoordination in the right arm, and she was walking with a straight cane. The next step was to tackle walking with the baby. We practiced with a baby carrier. We also had to prepare for the event of carrying without the carrier. I wrapped weights around the doll to equal the weight of the now 3-month-old infant at home. Sue walked down the hall carrying the doll, and I followed behind jostling the doll to simulate squirming (we became the talk of the hospital on our daily walks). Sue was becoming more and more comfortable and confident with these activities, so it was time to make arrangements to have the real baby spend his days on the rehabilitation unit with his mother. This was not as easy as it might seem. The administration was not used to such requests. But, with the right cajoling in the right places, this was eventually approved. The real baby now replaced the doll on our daily walks and in the clinic.

In this part of this story, Maureen moves quickly away from seeing the CVA as the "real" problem and understands Sue's perception of the problem. Yes, the stroke was a terrible accident and has caused this young mother difficult functional problems. These serious losses affect her ability to conduct everyday activities that were meaningful to her. These losses affect her sense of herself and her sense of her own competence as a mother. She will not be able to care for her new baby, something she very much wants to do. So Maureen continues to treat the physical limitations imposed by the stroke with appropriate procedures, but also focuses on the problem as Sue sees it. Maureen takes the phenomenologic point of view to examine and solve the problem. Thus, together, Maureen and Sue *identify the problem*. Next, they *set goals:* to be able to carry the baby. Then Maureen devises and executes a *treatment*. Here, Maureen cannot rely on recalling a protocol for the treatment of relearning how to hold a newborn baby after a stroke. Instead, she devises her own plan using the borrowed resuscitation doll as a treatment tool. Ultimately, Sue returned home and was able to care for her baby during much of the day. A neighbor helped late in the day, and Sue's husband helped at night.

Four features of clinical problem solving

Procedural reasoning usually begins with problem identification. Much of the research that has been conducted regarding problem solving in medicine has focused primarily on the diagnostic, or problem identification, phase of problem solving. Elstein, Shulman, and Sprafka (1978) identified four important features of the problem identification process among medical students and physicians: "cue identification, hypothesis generation, cue interpretation, and hypothesis evaluation" (p. 277). Occupational therapists also use this four-phase strategy. This process moves beyond simple pattern recognition or matching to a more analytic level through the inclusion of hypothesis testing and evaluation. Here, the practitioner gathers cues, mentally arranges them into potential patterns, and then advances two or more hypotheses about what the problem might be.

For example, a therapist might ask a child to color a picture and observes that the child does not take the offered crayon and simply looks down, possibly at the paper. Given these two cues, the therapist might advance the following hypotheses or questions:

Is the child shy? afraid? embarrassed?
Does she understand the task? know how to color?
Does she hate coloring?
Is she deaf?

Since none of these questions or tentative hypotheses can be tested without further inquiry, the therapist takes additional action to elicit more cues. The therapist might try asking the child to take the crayon again, or might offer a different activity, or change her proximity to the child. Each of these variations in the

therapist's behavior would be chosen to elicit some behavior on the part of the child. Observations and interpretations of this behavior would be used to support or reject one or more of the above-mentioned hypotheses, or in some cases, to construct new ones.

When the therapist feels she has sufficient cues to support a particular hypothesis, she holds that as a working hypothesis and then interprets the cues again in light of that hypothesis (cue interpretation). The next step is to reconsider the degree of match between the hypothesis and the interpreted cues (hypothesis evaluation). In this manner, therapists check and recheck the cues and patterns they think they have observed. This checking, or cue interpretation, serves to strengthen or weaken the hypothesis regarding the possible relationship of these cues to a possible cause of the behavior or condition. Hypotheses are then reevaluated and interpreted. The most likely hypothesis then becomes a basis for the therapist's thinking about the problem and potential treatment.

Nature of hypothetical reasoning

Perhaps the most important thing to remember about hypotheses is that they are just that—hypotheses. Hypotheses are propositions that are "tentatively accepted to explain certain facts or to provide a basis for further investigation" (Guralnik, 1970, p. 692). They are useful structures to guide thinking and an efficient way of managing a focus on a stream of thought, but they are not facts or answers. The best hypothetical thinkers generate several hypotheses that range from the usual or obvious to the obscure and unique. They subject those hypotheses to rigorous examination and comparison to both the cues in a particular case and the likelihood of the particular hypothesis being correct given those cues in similar situations (Elstein et. al., 1978) Another quality of effective hypothetical thinkers is that they never settle on a hypothesis too early (Johnson et. al., 1981). They are willing to keep looking, and they are willing to explore many avenues of inquiry. They have a respect for the hypothesis but not a rigid devotion to it. Good hypothetical thinkers are often playful and imaginative and are interested in possibilities, not just in being right.

One observation that we made over and over again was that experienced therapists revised their hypotheses numerous times. This revision usually did not involve the "big" hypotheses, such as the diagnosis or the general functional level the person was likely to attain. Rather, therapists generated myriad "little" hypotheses about the array of small factors and details that they needed to attend to in order to make the fine-tuned adjustments or unique adaptations to individualize therapy. This is especially true in situations in which the person or the condition is unique or in which the outcome possibilities are unknown or unpredictable.

Possible problems with hypothesis generation

Occupational therapy educators and clinical supervisors have observed that when they or their students have difficulty solving a particular problem with a patient, it is often the case that they have failed to generate enough hypotheses to help lead them toward a useful identification of the problem (Cohn & Czycholl, 1990). This observation is also made in the medical problem-solving literature, where various researchers have observed that failure to identify the correct diagnosis is often attributable to "generation of too few hypotheses" (Coughlin & Patel, 1987) or settling too early on a particular hypothesis (Elstein et al., 1978). Therapists should be sensitive to the fact that they need to generate and test several hypotheses about a problem before attempting to solve it.

One great deterrent to useful **hypothesis generation** is false or misleading cues. Some cues can be so large or impressive that they can dominate the therapist's thinking in ways that the therapist is led through the cue identification and hypothesis generation phases quickly, thus settling too early on an hypothesis without proceeding to the cue interpretation and hypothesis generation phases. One way this can happen is when a patient bears a strong resemblance to a prior patient (or a friend or relative), especially if it is a person whom the therapist remembers well, either positively or negatively.

Integrating the procedural and interactive modes

Integrating two perspectives

Procedural reasoning and interactive reasoning are different forms of reasoning. Each has a particular structure and purpose. Each takes a different perspective on knowledge, clinical conditions, patients, and professional practice. They are such different forms of reasoning that they often lead to disparate views about the therapeutic endeavor and process. This sometimes leads to conflicts and frustrations for therapists because it is often difficult to integrate these two perspectives and reasoning strategies. But when therapists are able to achieve this often tricky integration, both the therapist and the patient are more satisfied with the result. This integration of the two forms of reasoning and the two points of view may make the difference between what is simply treatment and what is truly therapy. Below is a therapist's story that illustrates this integration and the therapeutic results.

CASE STUDY

Integrating Both the Procedural and the Interactive Modes of Reasoning

When I first saw Harold, he was lying in his hospital bed looking like almost any other patient admitted to the stroke unit where I worked. I remember the day clearly because that was the day that Hurricane Gloria hit New England.

Harold was a 50-year-old Jamaican who had come to the United States in his late teens to go to school, marry, and raise a family. He began his own electronics installation business and also taught engineering at a university. The more I got to know him, the more I realized that he was not like any other patient with whom I had worked.

Harold had had a stroke that affected his right side, and, as a result, his right upper extremity was low-toned and non-functional. His right leg was extremely weak but did have some movement. Fortunately, his sensations and language were unaffected. As a teen-ager working on the docks in Jamaica, Harold had been in an accident that caused a brachial plexus injury in his left upper extremity, resulting in a nonfunctional left upper extremity. So, as a result of his re-

cent CVA, Harold was unable to use his only remaining functional arm.

Our initial sessions were spent evaluating him and properly positioning his right upper extremity, and, because of Harold's friendly and talkative nature, we became fast friends. However, he did know when it was time to "work" and began referring to me as the "drill sergeant."

Harold's leg improved at a fast pace, but his arm didn't improve quite as quickly. Harold was able to walk around the unit freely but was unable to do any ADL due to lack of upper extremity use. This was frustrating for him, and we discussed this frequently. However, his frame of mind was positive, and he maintained a great level of determination.

Harold continued to slowly develop tone and some active motion in his arm, so we decided to try using a suspension sling on his wheelchair to see if he could use the motion he did have to feed himself. The first few tries were difficult and awkward, but after a few days, Harold was calling all the staff on the unit into the dining room to watch him eat.

As his upper extremity improved and tone normalized, Harold's ADL skills improved. Soon, he learned to dress, bathe, and toilet himself using his remaining strength and coordination. He often improvised and even used his teeth on occasion. His wife, Helen, who had been helping him with ADL, was able to help less as he could do more. As is usually the case, fine motor coordination continued to come slowly. Harold used the button hook and built-up handles until he no longer needed them.

Eventually Harold was ready for discharge. On the last day of his inpatient stay, we were still giving him devices like key-holders and built-up door knobs for home use.

Harold returned to work and teaching, and he comes back and visits often. Each time he comes in, he sings the praises of the hospital and how much it did for him. He never resists saying "Sue, let me squeeze your hand," so he can show me how much strength he has in his right hand.

Putting it all together: Treating the whole person

Therapists often use two phrases to describe their treatment: "putting it all together" and "treating the whole patient." Treating the whole person does not mean that occupational therapists are in charge of the patient's whole medical and psychological treatment. The phrase is intended to convey the sense that occupational therapists concern themselves with the patient as a person, a person with many facets, interests, and concerns.

The phrase "putting it all together" means that while therapists often do think only about the disability at a given moment, they are concerned that they treat the patient as a whole person: person, illness, and condition. Although they use several types of reasoning and address several different types of concerns, therapists always want their reasoning to result in discovering a way to help a person learn or do something that would result in making a better life. Their ultimate goal is to use as many strategies as necessary to improve the individual functional performance of the person.

Since functional performance requires intention, physical action, and social meaning, it is not surprising that people who concern themselves with enabling function have to address problems of the person's sense of self, sense of future, physical body, meanings, and the social and cultural contexts in which actions are taken and meanings are made. Since these areas of inquiry are typically guided by different types of thinking, it is necessary that therapists become facile in thinking about different aspects of humans, using various styles of reasoning. Thus, putting it all together for the whole person to function as a new self in the future is guided by complex and multiple forms of clinical reasoning.

Summary

Several concepts regarding clinical reasoning, especially in occupational therapy, were discussed. Clinical reasoning is not a single form of reasoning. Occupational therapists use several forms of reasoning to guide their practice. Reasoning includes, but is not limited to, hypothetical reasoning, pattern recognition, intuitive reasoning, ethical reasoning, interactive reasoning, and procedural reasoning. Therapists use particular forms of reasoning to interpret and analyze various aspects of the whole problem complex.

The philosophy of the profession strongly influences which aspects of the problem the therapist thinks about and how a thinking process is employed. The profession's unique approach to treating patients, which therapists call *individualizing,* causes therapists to take the phenomenologic perspective toward the patient, the clinical condition, and the patient's family and social context.

Clinical reasoning in occupational therapy is a complex, multifaceted process that is just beginning to be understood. Continued research on the part of many individuals and groups will likely continue to improve our understanding of this fascinating aspect of our professional endeavor.

References

Belenky, M. F., Clinchy, B. M., Goldberger, N. R., & Tarule, J. M. (1986). *Women's ways of knowing.* New York: Basic Books.

Bing, R. K. (1986). Perspectives on values underlying occupational therapy practice. Occupational therapy education: Target 2000. In *Proceedings of forum on promoting excellence in education* (pp. 21–24). Rockville, MD: American Occupational Therapy Association.

Breines, E. (1986). *Origins and adaptations: A philosophy of practice.* Lebanon, NJ: Geri-Rehab, Inc.

Bunge, M. (1967). *Scientific research I: The search system.* New York: Springer-Verlag.

Cohn, E. S. (1989). Fieldwork education: Shaping a foundation for clinical reasoning. *American Journal of Occupational Therapy, 43*(4), 240–244.

Cohn, E. S., & Czycholl, C. (1991). Facilitating a foundation for clinical reasoning. In *Self paced instruction for clinical education and supervision: An instructional guide* (pp. 161–182). Rockville, MD: American Occupational Therapy Association.

Constitution of the National Society for the Promotion of Occupational Therapy (1917). Baltimore: Shippard Hospital Press.

Coughlin, L., & Patel, V. (1987). Processing of critical information by physicians and medical students. *Journal of Medical Education, 62,* 818–828.

Crepeau, E. B. (1991). Achieving intersubjective understanding: Examples from an occupational therapy treatment session. *American Journal of Occupational Therapy, 45,* 1016–1025.

Cutter, P. (1979). *Problem solving in clinical medicine: From data to diagnosis.* Baltimore: Williams & Wilkins.

Dewey, J. (1915). The logic of judgements of practice. *Journal of Philosophy, 12,* 505.

Dunton, W. R. Jr. (1919). Credo. In *Reconstruction therapy.* Philadelphia: W. B. Saunders.

Elstein, A. L., Shulman, L. S., & Sprafka, S. A. (1978). *Medical problem solving: An analysis of clinical reasoning.* Cambridge, MA: Harvard University Press.

Engelhardt, H. T. (1986). The importance of values in shaping professional direction and behavior. Occupational therapy education: Target 2000. In *Proceedings of forum on promoting excellence in education* (pp. 39–44). Rockville, MD: American Occupational Therapy Association.

Feinstein, A. R. (1967). *Clinical judgement.* Baltimore: Williams and Wilkins.

Fidler, G., & Fidler, J. (1963). *Occupational therapy: A communication process in psychiatry.* New York: Macmillan.

Fleming, M. H. (1989). The therapist with the three track mind. In *The AOTA Practice Symposium Program Guide* (pp. 70–75). Rockville, MD: American Occupational Therapy Association.

Fleming, M. H. (1991a). Clinical reasoning in medicine compared to clinical reasoning in occupational therapy. *American Journal of Occupational Therapy, 45*(11), 988–997.

Fleming, M. H. (1991b). The therapist with the three track mind. *American Journal of Occupational Therapy, 45*(11), 1007–1015.

Fondiller, E. D., Rosage, L. J., & Neuhaus, B. E. (1990). Values influencing clinical reasoning in occupational therapy. *Occupational Therapy Journal of Research. 10*(1), 41–55.

Foucault, M. (1973). *The birth of the clinic: An archeology of medical perception.* New York: Vintage Books.

Gardner, H. (1985). *Frames of mind: The theory of multiple intelligences.* New York: Basic Books.

Gillette, N., & Mattingly, C. (1987). Clinical reasoning in occupational therapy. *American Journal of Occupational Therapy, 41*(6), 399–400.

Goldberg, L. R. (1968). Simple models or simple procedures? Some research on clinical judgements. *American Psychologist, 23,* 483–496.

Goldberg, L. R. (1970). Man vs model of man: A rationale, plus some evidence for a method of improving on clinical inferences. *Psychological Bulletin, 73,* 422–432.

Guralnik, D. B. (Editor-in-Chief.) (1970). *Webster's new world dictionary of the American language* (2nd college ed.). New York: The World Publishing Company.

Hammond, K. R. (1988). Judgement and decision making in dynamic tasks. *Information and Decision Making Technologies, 14,* 3–14.

Johnson, J. A. (1981). Old values—new directions: Competence adaptation, integration. *American Journal of Occupational Therapy, 35,* 590–598.

Johnson, P. E., Durán, A. S., Hassebrock, F., Moller, J., Prietula, M. (1981). Expertise and error in diagnostic reasoning. *Cognitive Science, 5,* 235–283.

Karlsson, G. (1988). A phenomenological study of decisions and choice. *Acta Psychologia, 68,* 7–25.

Kassirer, J. P. (1989). Diagnostic reasoning. *Annals of Internal Medicine, 110*(11), 893–900.

Kestenbaum, V. (1982). *The humanity of the ill: Phenomenological perspectives.* Knoxville: University of Tennessee Press.

Kleinman, A. (1980). *Patients and healers in the context of culture.* Los Angeles: University of California Press.

Kockelmans, J. J. (1967). *Phenomenology: The philosophy of Edmund Husserl and it's interpretations.* Garden City, NJ: Anchor Books Doubleday.

Koestler, A. (1967). *The ghost in the machine*. Chicago: Henry Regnery Company.

Langthaler, M. (1990). *The components of therapeutic relationship in occupational therapy*. Unpublished master's thesis, Tufts University, Medford, MA.

Mattingly, C. (1989). *Thinking with stories: Story and experience in a clinical practice*. Unpublished doctoral dissertation, Cambridge, MA: Massachusetts Institute of Technology.

Mattingly, C. (1991a). What is clinical reasoning? *American Journal of Occupational Therapy, 45*(1) 979–986.

Mattingly, C. (1991b). The narrative of clinical reasoning. *American Journal of Occupational Therapy, 45*(1) 998–1005.

Mattingly, C., & Fleming, M. F. (1992). Clinical reasoning: Forms of inquiry in therapeutic practice. Philadelphia: F. A. Davis.

Mattingly, C., & Gillette, N. (1991). Anthropology, occupational therapy, and action research. *American Journal of Occupational Therapy, 45*, 972–978.

Meehl, P. E. (1954). *Clinical versus statistical prediction*. Minneapolis: University of Minnesota Press.

Meyer, A. (1977). The philosophy of occupational therapy. *American Journal of Occupational Therapy, 31*, 639–642.

Mosey, A. C. (1970). *Three frames of reference for mental health*. Thorofare, NJ: Slack.

Neuhaus, B. E. (1988). Ethical considerations in clinical reasoning: The impact of technology and cost containment. *American Journal of Occupational Therapy, 42*, 288–294.

Newell, A., & Simon, H. (1972). *Human problem solving*. Englewood Cliffs, NJ: Prentice Hall.

Paget, M. A. (1988). *The unity of mistakes*. Philadelphia: Temple University Press.

Papa, F. J., Shores, J. H., & Mayer, S. (1990). Effects of pattern matching, pattern discrimination and experience in the development of diagnostic expertise. *Academic Medicine, 65*(9), s21–s22.

Parham, D. (1987). Nationally speaking—Toward professionalism: The reflective therapist. *American Journal of Occupational Therapy, 41*, 555–561.

Pauker, S. G., Gorry, G. A., Kassirer, J. P., & Schwartz, W. B. (1976). Towards the simulation of clinical cognition. Taking a present illness by computer. *American Journal of Medicine, 60*, 981–996.

Polanyi, M. (1967). *The tacit dimension*. New York: Doubleday.

Rogers, C. (1961). *On becoming a person*. Boston: Houghton Mifflin.

Rogers, J. C. (1983). Eleanor Clarke Slagle lectureship—Clinical reasoning: The ethics, science, and art. *American Journal of Occupational Therapy, 37*(9), 601–616.

Sacks, O. (1983). *Awakenings*. New York: E. P. Dutton.

Schon, D. A. (1983). *The reflective practitioner: How professionals think in action*. New York: Basic Books.

Schutz, A. (1975). *On phenomenology and social relations*. London & Chicago: University of Chicago Press.

Serrett, K. D. (1985). *Philosophical and historical roots of occupational therapy*. NY: The Harworth Press.

Siegler, C. C. (1987). *Functions of humor in occupational therapy*. Unpublished master's thesis, Tufts University, Medford, MA.

Sinnett, M. W. (1988). *Clinical specialization in occupational therapy: A pluralistic view of practice*. Unpublished doctoral dissertation, University of Maryland, College Park.

Yerxa, E. (1979). The philosophical base of occupational therapy. In *Occupational therapy 2001 A.D.* Rockville, MD: Occupational Therapy Association.

Occupational therapy code of ethics*

The American Occupational Therapy Association and its component members are committed to furthering people's ability to function fully within their total environment. To this end the occupational therapist renders service to clients in all stages of health and illness, to institutions, to other professionals and colleagues, to students, and to the general public.

In furthering this commitment, the American Occupational Therapy Association has established the Occupational Therapy Code of Ethics. This code is intended to be used as a guide to promoting and maintaining the highest standards of ethical behavior.

This Code of Ethics shall apply to all occupational therapy personnel. The term *occupational therapy personnel* shall include individuals who are registered occupational therapists, certified occupational therapy assistants, and occupational therapy students. The roles of practitioner, educator, manager, researcher, and consultant are assumed.

Principle 1 (beneficence/autonomy)

Occupational therapy personnel shall demonstrate a concern for the welfare and dignity of the recipient of their services.

A. The individual is responsible for providing services without regard to race, creed, national origin, sex, age, handicap, disease entity, social status, financial status, or religious affiliation.
B. The individual shall inform those people served of the nature and potential outcomes of treatment and shall respect the right of potential recipients of service to refuse treatment.
C. The individual shall inform subjects involved in education or research activities of the potential outcome of those activities.
D. The individual shall include those people served in the treatment planning process.
E. The individual shall maintain goal-directed and objective relationships with all people served.
F. The individual shall protect the confidential nature of information gained from educational, practice, and investigational activities unless sharing such information could be deemed necessary to protect the well-being of a third party.
G. The individual shall take all reasonable precautions to avoid

harm to the recipient of services or detriment to the recipient's property.
H. The individual shall establish fees, based on cost analysis, that are commensurate with services rendered.

Principle 2 (competence)

Occupational therapy personnel shall actively maintain high standards of professional competence.

A. The individual shall hold the appropriate credential for providing service.
B. The individual shall recognize the need for competence and shall participate in continuing professional development.
C. The individual shall function within the parameters of his or her competence and the standards of the profession.
D. The individual shall refer clients to other service providers or consult with other service providers when additional knowledge and expertise is required.

Principle 3 (compliance with laws and regulations)

Occupational therapy personnel shall comply with laws and Association policies guiding the profession of occupational therapy.

A. The individual shall be acquainted with applicable local, state, federal, and institutional rules and Association policies and shall function accordingly.
B. The individual shall inform employers, employees, and colleagues about those laws and policies that apply to the profession of occupational therapy.
C. The individual shall require those whom they supervise to adhere to the Code of Ethics.
D. The individual shall accurately record and report information.

Principle 4 (public information)

Occupational therapy personnel shall provide accurate information concerning occupational therapy services.

A. The individual shall accurately represent his or her competence and training.
B. The individual shall not use or participate in the use of any form of communication that contains a false, fraudulent, deceptive, or unfair statement or claim.

Principle 5 (professional relationships)

Occupational therapy personnel shall function with discretion and integrity in relations with colleagues and other professionals, and shall be concerned with the quality of their services.

A. The individual shall report illegal, incompetent, and/or unethical practice to the appropriate authority.
B. The individual shall not disclose privileged information

* This document was approved by the Representative Assembly in April 1988; it replaces the 1977/1979 *Principles of Occupational Therapy Ethics.*

Reprinted with permission from *The American Journal of Occupational Therapy*, December 1988, Volume 42, Number 12.

when participating in reviews of peers, programs, or systems.

C. The individual who employs or supervises colleagues shall provide appropriate supervision, as defined in AOTA guidelines or state laws, regulations, and institutional policies.

D. The individual shall recognize the contributions of colleagues when disseminating professional information.

Principle 6 (professional conduct)

Occupational therapy personnel shall not engage in any form of conduct that constitutes a conflict of interest or that adversely reflects on the profession.

APPENDIX B

Revision: Standards of practice for occupational therapy*

These standards are intended as recommended guidelines to assist occupational therapy practitioners in the provision of occupational therapy services. These standards serve as a minimum standard for occupational therapy practice and are applicable to all individual populations and the programs in which these individuals are served.

These standards apply to those registered occupational therapists and certified occupational therapy assistants who are in compliance with regulation where it exists. The term *occupational therapy practitioner* refers to the registered occupational therapist and to the certified occupational therapy assistant, both of whom are in compliance with regulation where it exists.

The minimum educational requirements for the registered occupational therapist are described in the current *Essentials and Guidelines of an Accredited Educational Program for the Occupational Therapist* (American Occupational Therapy Association [AOTA], 1991a). The minimum educational requirements for the certified occupational therapy assistant are described in the current *Essentials and Guidelines of an Accredited Educa-*

* Developed by the AOTA Commission on Practice, Jim Hinojosa, PhD, OTR, FAOTA, Chair.

Approved by the AOTA Representative Assembly, April 1992.

This document replaces the 1983 Standards of Practice for Occupational Therapy (*American Journal of Occupational Therapy*, 37, 802–804). Reprinted with permission.

tional Program for the Occupational Therapy Assistant (AOTA, 1991b).

Standard I: Professional standing

1. An occupational therapy practitioner shall maintain a current license, registration, or certification as required by law.

2. An occupational therapy practitioner shall practice and manage occupational therapy programs in accordance with applicable federal and state laws and regulations.

3. An occupational therapy practitioner shall be familiar with and abide by AOTA's (1988) Occupational Therapy Code of Ethics.

4. An occupational therapy practitioner shall maintain and update professional knowledge, skills, and abilities through appropriate continuing education or in-service training or higher education. The nature and minimum amount of continuing education must be consistent with state law and regulation.

5. A certified occupational therapy assistant must receive supervision from a registered occupational therapist as defined by the current Supervision Guidelines for Certified Occupational Therapy Assistants (AOTA, 1990) and by official AOTA documents. The nature and amount of supervision must be provided in accordance with state law and regulation.

6. An occupational therapy practitioner shall provide direct and indirect services in accordance with AOTA's standards and policies. The nature and scope of occupational therapy services provided must be in accordance with state law and regulation.

7. An occupational therapy practitioner shall maintain current knowledge of the legislative, political, social, and cultural issues that affect the profession.

Standard II: Referral

1. A registered occupational therapist shall accept referrals in accordance with AOTA's Statement of Occupational Therapy Referral (AOTA, 1989) and in compliance with appropriate laws.

2. A registered occupational therapist may accept referrals for assessment or assessment with intervention in occupational performance areas or occupational performance components when individuals have or appear to have dysfunctions or potential for dysfunctions.

3. A registered occupational therapist, responding to requests for service, may accept cases within the parameters of the law.

4. A registered occupational therapist shall assume responsibility for determining the appropriateness of the scope, frequency, and duration of services within the parameters of the law.

5. A registered occupational therapist shall refer individuals to other appropriate resources when the therapist determines that the knowledge and expertise of other professionals is indicated.

6. An occupational therapy practitioner shall educate current and potential referral sources about the process of initiating occupational therapy referrals.

Standard III: Screening

1. A registered occupational therapist, in accordance with state and federal guidelines, shall conduct screening to determine whether intervention or further assessment is necessary and to identify dysfunctions in occupational performance areas.
2. A registered occupational therapist shall screen independently or as a member of an interdisciplinary team. A certified occupational therapy assistant may contribute to the screening process under the supervision of a registered occupational therapist.
3. A registered occupational therapist shall select screening methods that are appropriate to the individual's age and developmental level; gender; education; cultural background; and socioeconomic, medical, and functional status. Screening methods may include, but are not limited to, interviews, structured observations, informal testing, and record reviews.
4. A registered occupational therapist shall communicate screening results and recommendations to appropriate individuals.

Standard IV: Assessment

1. A registered occupational therapist shall assess an individual's occupational performance components and occupational performance areas. A registered occupational therapist conducts assessments individually or as part of a team of professionals, as appropriate to the practice settings and the purposes of the assessments. A certified occupational therapy assistant may contribute to the assessment process under the supervision of a registered occupational therapist.
2. An occupational therapy practitioner shall educate the individual, or the individual's family or legal guardian, as appropriate, about the purposes and procedures of the occupational therapy assessment.
3. A registered occupational therapist shall select assessments to determine the individual's functional abilities and problems as related to occupational performance areas; occupational performance components; physical, social, and cultural environments; performance safety; and prevention of dysfunction.
4. Occupational therapy assessment methods shall be appropriate to the individual's age and developmental level; gender; education; socioeconomic, cultural, and ethnic background; medical status; and functional abilities. The assessment methods may include some combination of skilled observation, interview, record review, or the use of standardized or criterion-referenced tests. A certified occupational therapy assistant may contribute to the assessment process under the supervision of a registered occupational therapist.
5. An occupational therapy practitioner shall follow accepted protocols when standardized tests are used. Standardized tests are tests whose scores are based on accompanying normative data that may reflect age ranges, gender, ethnic groups, geographic regions, and socioeconomic status. If standardized tests are not available or appropriate, the re-

sults shall be expressed in descriptive reports, and standardized scales shall not be used.
6. A registered occupational therapist shall analyze and summarize collected evaluation data to indicate the individual's current functional status.
7. A registered occupational therapist shall document assessment results in the individual's records, noting the specific evaluation methods and tools used.
8. A registered occupational therapist shall complete and document results of occupational therapy assessments within the time frames established by practice settings, government agencies, accreditation programs, and third-party payers.
9. An occupational therapy practitioner shall communicate assessment results, within the boundaries of client confidentiality, to the appropriate persons.
10. A registered occupational therapist shall refer the individual to the appropriate services or request additional consultations if the results of the assessments indicate areas that require intervention by other professionals.

Standard V: Intervention plan

1. A registered occupational therapist shall develop and document an intervention plan based on analysis of the occupational therapy assessment data and the individual's expected outcome after the intervention. A certified occupational therapy assistant may contribute to the intervention plan under the supervision of a registered occupational therapist.
2. The occupational therapy intervention plan shall be stated in goals that are clear, measurable, behavioral, functional, and appropriate to the individual's needs, personal goals, and expected outcome after intervention.
3. The occupational therapy intervention plan shall reflect the philosophical base of occupational therapy (AOTA, 1979) and be consistent with its established principles and concepts of theory and practice. The intervention planning processes shall include:
   a. Formulating a list of strengths and weaknesses.
   b. Estimating rehabilitation potential.
   c. Identifying measurable short-term and long-term goals.
   d. Collaborating with the individual, family members, other caregivers, professionals, and community resources.
   e. Selecting the media, methods, environment, and personnel needed to accomplish the intervention goals.
   f. Determining the frequency and duration of occupational therapy services.
   g. Identifying a plan for reevaluation.
   h. Discharge planning.
4. A registered occupational therapist shall prepare and document the intervention plan within the time frames and according to the standards established by the employing practice settings, government agencies, accreditation programs, and third-party payers. The certified occupational therapy assistant may contribute to the formation of the intervention plan under the supervision of the registered occupational therapist.

Standard VI: Intervention

1. An occupational therapy practitioner shall implement a program according to the developed intervention plan. The plan shall be appropriate to the individual's age and developmental level, gender, education, cultural and ethnic background, health status, functional ability, interests and personal goals, and service provision setting. The certified occupational therapy assistant shall implement the intervention under the supervision of a registered occupational therapist.
2. An occupational therapy practitioner shall implement the intervention plan through the use of specified purposeful activities or therapeutic methods to enhance occupational performance and achieve stated goals.
3. An occupational therapy practitioner shall be knowledgeable about relevant research in the practitioner's areas of practice. A registered occupational therapist shall interpret research findings as appropriate for application to the intervention process.
4. An occupational therapy practitioner shall educate the individual, the individual's family or legal guardian, and nonoccupational therapy staff, as appropriate, in activities that support the established intervention plan. An occupational therapy practitioner shall communicate the risk and benefit of the intervention.
5. An occupational therapy practitioner shall maintain current information on community resources relevant to the practice area of the practitioner.
6. A registered occupational therapist shall periodically reassess and document the individual's levels of functioning and changes in levels of functioning in the occupational performance areas and occupational performance components. A certified occupational therapy assistant may contribute to the reassessment process under the supervision of a registered occupational therapist.
7. A registered occupational therapist shall formulate and implement program modifications consistent with changes in the individual's response to the intervention. A certified occupational therapy assistant may contribute to program modifications under the supervision of a registered occupational therapist.
8. An occupational therapy practitioner shall document the occupational therapy services provided, including the frequency and duration of the services within the time frames and according to the standards established by the employing facility, government agencies accreditation programs, and third-party payers.

Standard VII: Discontinuation

1. A registered occupational therapist shall discontinue service when the individual has achieved predetermined goals or has achieved maximum benefit from occupational therapy services.
2. A registered occupational therapist, with input from a certified occupational therapy assistant where applicable, shall prepare and implement a discharge plan that is consistent with occupational therapy goals, individual goals, inter-disciplinary team goals, family goals, and expected outcomes. The discharge plan shall address appropriate community resources for referral for psychosocial, cultural, and socioeconomic barriers and limitations that may need modification.
3. A registered occupational therapist shall document the changes between the initial and current states of functional ability and deficit in occupational performance areas and occupational performance components. A certified occupational therapy assistant may contribute to the process under the supervision of a registered occupational therapist.
4. An occupational therapy practitioner shall allow sufficient time for the coordination and effective implementation of the discharge plan.
5. A registered occupational therapist shall document recommendations for follow-up or reevaluation when applicable.

Standard VIII: Quality assurance

1. An occupational therapy practitioner shall monitor and document the continuous quality improvement of practice, which may include outcomes of services, using predetermined practice criteria reflecting professional consensus, recent developments in research, and specific employing facility standards.
2. An occupational therapy practitioner shall monitor all aspects of individual occupational therapy services for effectiveness and timeliness. If actual care does not meet the prescribed standard, it must be justified by peer review or other appropriate means within the practice setting. Occupational therapy services shall be discontinued when no longer necessary.
3. A registered occupational therapist shall systematically assess the review process of patient care to determine the success or appropriateness of interventions. Certified occupational therapy assistants may contribute to the process in collaboration with the registered occupational therapist.

Standard IX: Management

1. A registered occupational therapist shall provide the management necessary for efficient organization and provision of occupational therapy services.
2. A certified occupational therapy assistant, under the supervision of a registered occupational therapist, may perform the following management functions:
    a. Education of members of other related professions and physicians about occupational therapy.
    b. Participation in (1) orientation, supervision, training, and evaluation of the performance of volunteers and other noncertified occupational therapy personnel, and (2) developing plans to remediate areas of skill deficit in the performance of job duties by volunteers and other noncertified occupational therapy personnel.
    c. Design and periodic review of all aspects of the occupational therapy program to determine its effectiveness, efficiency, and future directions.
    d. Systematic review of the quality of service provided, using criteria established by professional consensus

and current research as well as established standards for state regulation; accreditation; American Occupational Therapy Certification Board (AOTCB) certification; and related laws, policies, guidelines, and regulations.

e. Incorporation of a fair and equitable system of admission, discharge, and charges for occupational therapy services.

f. Participation in cross-disciplinary activities to ensure that the total needs of the individual are met.

g. Provision of support (*i.e.*, space, time, money as feasible) for clinical research or collaborative research when such projects have the approval of the appropriate governing bodies (*e.g.*, institutional review board), and the results of which are deemed potentially beneficial to individuals of occupational therapy services now or in the future.

References

American Occupational Therapy Association. (1979). The philosophical base of occupational therapy. *American Journal of Occupational Therapy, 33,* 785.

American Occupational Therapy Association. (1988). Occupational therapy code of ethics. *American Journal of Occupational Therapy, 42,* 795–796.

American Occupational Therapy Association. (1989). Statement of occupational therapy referral. In *Reference manual of the official documents of The American Occupational Therapy Association, Inc.* (AOTA) (p. VIII.1). Rockville, MD: Author (original work published 1969, revised 1980).

American Occupational Therapy Association. (1990). Supervision guidelines for certified occupational therapy assistants. *American Journal of Occupational Therapy, 44,* 1089–1090.

American Occupational Therapy Association. (1991a). Essentials and guidelines of an accredited educational program for the occupational therapist. Rockville, MD: Author.

American Occupational Therapy Association. (1991b). Essentials and guidelines of an accredited educational program for the occupational therapy assistant. Rockville, MD: Author.

Standards of practice for occupational therapy in schools†

These guidelines are to assist AOTA members and school administrators in the management of occupational therapy in the school systems. These standards by themselves cannot be interpreted to constitute a standard of care in any particular locality.

The occupational therapist shall manage the therapy program in accordance with all available Standards of Practice, as defined by the American Occupational Therapy Association, Inc.

The purpose of the Occupational Therapy program in the school system is to enable the student to gain optimum benefit from the educational program.

Direct services

Direct services include screening, referral systems, evaluations, program planning, program implementation, re-evaluation and termination of services.

† Adopted April 1980 by the Representative Assembly, AOTA

Standard I: Screening

The occupational therapist should be involved in the screening process

1. The screening process should allow the therapist to identify those students who need further educational and/or related service evaluation.
2. All screening methods shall be appropriate to the chronological, educational and/or functional level of the student, and shall not be racially or culturally discriminatory.
3. The occupational therapist should refer the results and recommendations to the appropriate school educational planning committee.

Standard II: Referral

A referral for occupational therapy must comply with the AOTA statement on referral.

1. A student should be referred to the occupational therapist for evaluation when the student has or appears to have a dysfunction in any of the following areas:
   a. occupational performance (activities of daily living); self-care activities; home–school–work activities; play/leisure activities; and/or prevocational/vocational activities/skills.
   b. performance components: neuromuscular development; sensory–integrative development; psychological development; social development; and/or cognitive development.
2. A referral may originate through the individual education plan or educational planning committee (including teachers, other student services staff, parents, physicians, etc.).
3. When a referral is received, the therapist shall document:
   a. the date of receipt and referral source; and
   b. services requested in the referral.
4. If in the therapist's judgment there is the need for medical management of the student, the therapist shall immediately apprise the student's parent/guardian or appropriate person and recommend physician involvement, or the therapist shall, after parental/guardian written permission or release has been obtained, contact the physician.

Standard III: Evaluation

The occupational therapist shall evaluate the student's performance.

1. The initial occupational therapy evaluation shall be completed and results documented according to the time frames established by federal and/or state rules and regulations.
2. The occupational therapy evaluation shall include assessment of the developmental level as well as the functional abilities/capacities and deficits/limitations as related to the student's educational level and needs in the following areas:
   a. occupational performance: self-care activities; home–school–work activities; pre-vocational/vocational activities/skills; and/or play/leisure activities.
   b. performance components: neuromuscular development; sensory–integrative development; psychological development; social development and/or cognitive development.

3. If the results of the above evaluation indicate possible deficits in psychological/social, cognitive, physical/medical, speech/language areas, the therapist should refer the student to the appropriate service and/or request consultation if necessary.

4. All evaluation methods shall be appropriate to the chronological age and/or functional level of the student and identify baseline behaviors. The methods may include, but need not be limited to observation of activity performance, interview, record review, testing and individual/group screening.

5. If standardized evaluative measurements are used, the tests should have normative data for the age range of the student. If normative data are not available for the age range of the student, the results should be expressed in a descriptive report and standardized scales are not used.

6. Tests and other evaluation material used in placing handicapped students will be prepared and administered in such a way as not to be racially or culturally discriminatory, and they will be presented in the child's native tongue.

7. As part of the evaluation process, the therapist may make clinical judgments based on observations and recorded progress during intervention programs.

8. The therapist shall document evaluation results in the student's record, indicating evaluation instruments and procedures and also communicate these findings via written reports, oral conferences, and staffings to the appropriate persons and/or community resources.

Standard IV: Program planning and/or individual education plan

The therapist shall prepare and document a program plan based upon an analysis of the data from the occupational therapy and other education planner's evaluation results.

1. The initial program plan shall be prepared and documented according to the time frames established by federal and/or state rules and regulations.

2. The therapist shall utilize the results of the evaluation process to prepare an occupational therapy program that is:
   a. stated in practical outcomes applicable to the student's needs and educational goals,
   b. consistent with principles and concepts of growth and development; and
   c. consistent with expected behavior/progress for the student's defined educational/health problems and needs.

3. The planning process shall include:
   a. Identifying short term and long term (annual) goals;
   b. collaborating with child/family/staff to establish appropriate goals to enhance education;
   c. participation in staffings to coordinate the occupational therapy program with the other programs within the educational setting;
   d. documenting of practical outcomes to be achieved;
   e. selecting the media, methods, environment and personnel to accomplish goals; and
   f. monitoring and modifying the program to meet the established goals.

4. The documented educational program plan shall consist of a statement of when these services will be provided and how long they will last.

5. When the occupational therapy program goal is to prevent or diminish dysfunction in occupational performance and learning or to enhance occupational performance, the program plan shall include the use of one or more of the following types of activities:
   a. self-care activities; may also include instruction in the use of adapted methods and/or equipment, energy conservation, joint protection techniques.
   b. home–work–school activities; may also include instruction in the use of adapted methods and/or equipment.
   c. prevocational/vocational activities/skills may also include improvement of standing or sitting tolerance, general endurance, or awareness and utilization of community resources; and
   d. developmental play/leisure activities; may also include instruction of family in activities appropriate for student's developmental level; instruction in the use of adapted methods and/or equipment.

6. When the goal is to prevent or diminish neuromuscular dysfunction or enhance neuromuscular development and learning, the program plan shall include, but need not be limited to, the use of one or more of the following types of activities:
   a. activities which maintain or increase range of motion and/or muscle strength;
   b. activities which facilitate integration of developmentally appropriate reflex/reaction behavior;
   c. activities which provide appropriate sensory stimulation;
   d. activities which promote the development of normal postural tone, movement patterns and motor control;
   e. instruction in the use of proper positioning and handling techniques;
   f. provision of and instruction in the use of adaptive equipment; and/or
   g. fabrication/recommendation of splints or orthotic devices/equipment.

7. When the goal is to prevent or diminish sensory–integrative dysfunction or to enhance sensory integrative development, the program plan shall include, but need not be limited to, the appropriate use of:
   a. sensory facilitation and/or inhibition techniques for vestibular, tactile, proprioceptive/kinesthetic, visual, auditory, gustatory and olfactory stimulation; and/or
   b. activities to promote adaptive sensorimotor response.

8. When the interdisciplinary educational evaluation results indicate goals to prevent or diminish psychological or social dysfunction, or enhance psychological or social development, the occupational therapy program shall include, but need not be limited to, the appropriate use of activities which assist the student in learning to:
   a. experience and cope with competition, frustration, success and failure;
   b. identify and respond appropriately to feelings;
   c. develop or refine self-esteem or self-identity;
   d. imitate and develop appropriate social behaviors;
   e. listen and communicate; and
   f. develop sensitivity to other persons' feelings and behaviors (interpersonal relationships).

9. When the interdisciplinary education team evaluation results indicate goals to prevent or diminish cognitive dys-

function or to enhance development in the cognitive areas, the occupational therapy program shall include, but need not be limited to, the appropriate use of activities which assist the student in developing:

a. concentration/attention span;
b. memory/recall;
c. decision making and/or problem solving.

The purposes of the occupational therapy program in the above stated areas, (#8 and #9), are not intended to replace academic or other programming. The purposes are to assist the child to receive maximum benefit from educational programming.

Standard V: Program implementation

The therapist shall implement the program according to the program plan.

1. The therapist shall periodically and on an ongoing basis document the occupational therapy services provided (including techniques utilized and the results) and the frequency of the services.
2. The therapist shall periodically re-evaluate and document the changes in the student's occupational performance and performance components.
3. The therapist shall formulate, document and implement program changes consistent with changes in the student's occupational performance and performance components.

Standard VI: Re-evaluation

The therapist shall re-evaluate the student receiving occupational therapy on a yearly basis.

1. The re-evaluation results shall be documented.
2. If the client needs further service, the therapist shall make appropriate recommendations.
3. A re-evaluation does not necessarily constitute a referral for services.

Standard VII: Termination of services

The therapist shall prepare and document the occupational therapy discharge plan.

1. The discharge plan shall be consistent with the student's goals, functional abilities and deficits, expected prognosis and the goals of the educational planners. Consideration should be given to appropriate community resources for referral and environmental factors/barriers that may need modification.
2. The discharge plan shall be consistent with the discharge plan of the other educational planners and appropriately documented through the individual educational planning process.
3. The therapist shall document the comparison of the initial state of functional abilities and deficits in occupational performance and performance components and the current state of these abilities and deficits at the time of discharge.
4. The therapist shall terminate occupational therapy services when the student has achieved the goals, or has achieved maximum benefits from occupational therapy.

5. Recommendations for follow-up or re-evaluation, if appropriate, shall be documented.

Indirect services

With the provision of indirect services, the occupational therapist in a school-based program performs supervision, consultation and administration/management roles.

Standard VIII: Administration/management

The occupational therapist shall provide appropriate management and administrative services.

The management and administrative functions for the school-based therapist shall include:

1. Supervision of other personnel as assigned.
   a. informal and formal training of personnel and volunteers assigned to occupational therapy.
   b. reviewing performances (self and others) and providing evaluations.
2. Design of the occupational therapy program with periodic reviews of all aspects of the total occupational therapy program to determine its effectiveness and efficiency.
3. Occupational therapists shall systematically review the quality, including outcomes, of services delivered, using predetermined criteria reflecting professional consensus and recent developments in research and theory:
   a. to determine if actual service may be justified by peer review.
   b. if justification by peer review fails, a program to improve services shall be planned and implemented.
   c. review will be repeated to assess the success of the corrective action.
4. Maintaining current certification as required by state regulations and AOTA.
5. Maintaining current records and files to meet school requirements and professional standards.
6. Participating in budget planning and is responsible for budget implementation.
7. Responsibility for knowledge, including use of, and utilizing community resources.
8. The therapist shall maintain and update professional knowledge and skills and seek consultation/supervision from others when necessary to assure continued competency.

Standard IX: Consultation

The therapist shall provide consultation services when appropriate.

In the consultation role, the therapist is one member of an interdisciplinary educational team collaborating with a variety of professional personnel to assist students with special needs. The practice of consultation shall include when appropriate:

1. Developing and coordinating occupational therapy programs with the total educational curriculum.
2. Provide consultation for classroom environmental adaptation to enhance the learning potential of students.
3. Provide consultation to teachers and staff regarding the identified special needs of students.
4. Collaborate with the educational team regarding the stu-

dent's program including the IEP (Individualized Education Program).

5. Provide in-service education.
6. Provide consultation for appropriate programs outside the school program.
7. Provide consultation and education to parents to help them understand the special needs of their child.
8. Provide consultation for home environmental adaptation to enhance independent functioning.
9. Provide consultation to school administrators and staff regarding preventive health education and activities to enhance the educational environment and learning potential of students.

Standard X: Legal/ethical components

The occupational therapist shall provide all aspects of direct and indirect services according to legal regulations and ethical standards.

1. The occupational therapist shall practive and manage occupational therapy programs as defined by federal and state laws or legal principles as they apply to issues or situations when relevant to students or themselves in school systems.
2. The therapist shall observe the ethical practices as defined by the American Occupational Therapy Association Standards and Ethics Commission.
3. The therapist should be familiar with and abide by the ethical practices of the specific school district or system in which the therapist serves.

APPENDIX C

*Uniform terminology for occupational therapy— second edition**

Uniform Terminology for Occupational Therapy—Second Edition delineates and defines **OCCUPATIONAL PERFORMANCE AREAS** and **OCCUPATIONAL PERFORMANCE COMPONENTS** that are addressed in occupational therapy direct service. These definitions are provided to facilitate the uniform use of terminol-

* Prepared by the Uniform Terminology Task Force (Linda Kohlman McGourty, MOT, OTR, Chair, and Mary Foto, OTR, Jane K. Marvin, MA, OTR, CIRS, Nancy Mahon Smith, MBA, OTR, and Roger O. Smith, MOT, OTR, task force members) and members of the Commission on Practice, with contributions from Susan Kronsnoble, OTR, for the Commission on Practice (L. Randy Strickland, EdD, OTR, FAOTA, Chair).

Approved by the Representative Assembly, April 1989. Reprinted with permission.

ogy and definitions throughout the profession. The original document, *Occupational Therapy Product Output Reporting System and Uniform Terminology for Reporting Occupational Therapy Services*, which was published in 1979, helped create a base of consistent terminology that was used in many of the official documents of The American Occupational Therapy Association, Inc. (AOTA), in occupational therapy education curricula, and in a variety of occupational therapy practice settings. In order to remain current with practice, the first document was revised over a period of several years with extensive feedback from the profession. The revisions were completed in 1988. It is recognized and recommended that a document of this nature be updated periodically so that occupational therapy is defined in accordance with current theory and practice.

Guidelines for use

Uniform Terminology—Second Edition may be used in a variety of ways. It defines occupational therapy practice, which includes **OCCUPATIONAL PERFORMANCE AREAS** and **OCCUPATIONAL PERFORMANCE COMPONENTS.** In addition, it will be useful to occupational therapists for (a) documentation, (b) charge systems, (c) education, (d) program development, (e) marketing, and (f) research. Examples of how **OCCUPATIONAL PERFORMANCE AREAS** and **OCCUPATIONAL PERFORMANCE COMPONENTS** translate into practice are provided below. It is not the intent of this document to define specific occupational therapy programs nor specific occupational therapy interventions. Some examples of the differences between **OCCUPATIONAL PERFORMANCE AREAS** and **OCCUPATIONAL PERFORMANCE COMPONENTS** and programs and interventions are

1. An individual who is injured on the job may be able to return to work, which is an **OCCUPATIONAL PERFORMANCE AREA.** In order to achieve the outcome of returning to work, the individual may need to address specific **PERFORMANCE COMPONENTS** such as strength, endurance, and time management. The occupational therapist, in cooperation with the vocational team, utilizes planned interventions to achieve the desired outcome. These interventions may include activities such as an exercise program, body mechanics instruction, and job modification, and may be provided in a work-hardening program.
2. An individual with severe physical limitations may need and desire the opportunity to live within a community-integrated setting, which represents the **OCCUPATIONAL PERFORMANCE AREAS** of activities of daily living and work. In order to achieve the outcome of community living, the individual may need to address specific **PERFORMANCE COMPONENTS,** such as normalizing muscle tone, gross motor coordination, postural control, and self-management. The occupational therapist, in cooperation with the team, utilizes planned interventions to achieve the desired outcome. Interventions may include neuromuscular facilitation, object manipulation, instruction in use of adaptive equipment, use of environmental control systems, and functional positioning for eating. These interventions may be provided in a community-based independent living program.

3. A child with learning disabilities may need to perform educational activities within a public school setting. Since learning is a student's work, this educational activity would be considered the **OCCUPATIONAL PERFORMANCE AREA** for this individual. In order to achieve the educational outcome of efficient and effective completion of written classroom work, the child may need to address specific **OCCUPATIONAL PERFORMANCE COMPONENTS,** including sensory processing, perceptual skills, postural control, and motor skills. The occupational therapist, in cooperation with the team, utilizes planned interventions to achieve the desired outcome. Interventions may include activities such as adapting the student's seating to improve postural control and stability and practicing motor control and coordination. This program could be provided by school district personnel or through contracted services.

4. An infant with cerebral palsy may need to participate in developmental activities to engage in the **OCCUPATIONAL PERFORMANCE AREAS** of activities of daily living and play. The developmental outcomes may be achieved by addressing specific **PERFORMANCE COMPONENTS** such as sensory awareness and neuromuscular control. The occupational therapist, in cooperation with the team, utilizes planned interventions to achieve the desired outcomes. Interventions may include activities such as seating and positioning for play, neuromuscular facilitation techniques to enable eating, and parent training. These interventions may be provided in a home-based occupational therapy program.

5. An adult with schizophrenia may need and desire to live independently in the community, which represents the **OCCUPATIONAL PERFORMANCE AREAS** of activities of daily living, work activities, and play or leisure activities. The specific **OCCUPATIONAL PERFORMANCE AREAS** may be medication routine, functional mobility, home management, vocational exploration, play or leisure performance, and social skills. In order to achieve the outcome of living alone, the individual may need to address specific **PERFORMANCE COMPONENTS** such as topographical orientation, memory, categorization, problem solving, interests, social conduct, and time management. The occupational therapist, in cooperation with the team, utilizes planned interventions to achieve the desired outcome. Interventions may include activities such as training in the use of public transportation, instruction in budgeting skills, selection of and participation in social activities, and instruction in social conduct. These interventions may be provided in a community-based mental health program.

6. An individual who abuses substances may need to reestablish family roles and responsibilities, which represents the **OCCUPATIONAL PERFORMANCE AREAS** of activities of daily living and work. In order to achieve the outcome of family participation, the individual may need to address the **PERFORMANCE COMPONENTS** of roles, values, social conduct, self-expression, coping skills, and self-control. The occupational therapist, in cooperation with the team, utilizes planned intervention to achieve the desired outcomes. Interventions may include role and value clarification exercises, role-playing, instruction in stress management techniques, and parenting skills. These interventions may be provided in an inpatient acute care unit.

Because of the extensive use of the original document (*Uniform Terminology for Reporting Occupational Therapy Services,* 1979) in official documents, this revision is a second edition and does not completely replace the 1979 version. This follows the practice that other professions, such as medicine, pursue with their documents. Examples are the *Physician's Current Procedural Terminology First–Fourth Editions (CPT 1–4)* and the *Diagnostic and Statistical Manual First–Third Editions (DSM-I-III-R).* Therefore, this document is presented as *Uniform Terminology for Occupational Therapy—Second Edition.*

Background

Task force charge

In 1983, the Representative Assembly of the American Occupational Therapy Association charged the Commission on Practice to form a task force to revise the *Occupational Therapy Product Output Reporting System and Uniform Terminology for Reporting Occupational Therapy Services.* The document had been approved by the Representative Assembly in 1979 and needed to be updated to reflect current practice.

Background information

The *Occupational Therapy Product Output Reporting System and Uniform Terminology for Reporting Occupational Therapy Services* (hereafter to be referred to as *Product Output Reporting System or Uniform Terminology*) document was originally developed in response to the Medicare–Medicaid Anti-Fraud and Abuse Amendments of 1977 (Public Law 95-142), which required the Secretary of the Department of Health and Human Services to establish regulations for uniform reporting systems for all departments in hospitals. The AOTA developed the documents to create a uniform reporting system for occupational therapy departments. Although the Department of Health and Human Services never adopted the system because of antitrust concerns relating to price fixing, occupational therapists have used the documents extensively in the profession.

Three states, Maryland, California, and Washington, have used the *Product Output Reporting System* as a basis for statewide reporting systems. AOTA's official documents have relied on the definitions to create uniformity. Many occupational therapy schools and departments have used the definitions to guide education and documentation. Although the initial need was for reimbursement reporting systems, the profession has used the documents primarily to facilitate uniformity in definitions.

See Appendix D in the 7th edition of this text for the original *Uniform Terminolgy for Reporting Occupational Therapy Services* (1979).

Development of the uniform terminology—second edition

The task force met in 1986 and 1987 to develop drafts of the revisions. A draft from the task force was submitted to the Commission on Practice in May of 1987. Listed below are several decisions that were made in the revision process by the task force and the Commission on Practice.

1. To not replace the original document (*Uniform Terminology for Reporting Occupational Therapy Services,* 1979) because of the number of official documents based on it and the need to retain a *Product Output Reporting System* as an official document of the AOTA.

2. To limit the revised document to defining **OCCUPATIONAL PERFORMANCE AREAS** and **OCCUPATIONAL PERFORMANCE COMPONENTS** for occupational therapy intervention (i.e., indirect services were deleted and the *Product Output Reporting System* was not revised) to make the project manageable.

3. To coordinate the revision process with other current AOTA projects such as the Professional and Technical Role Analysis (PATRA) and the Occupational Therapy Comprehensive Functional Assessment of the American Occupational Therapy Foundation (AOTF).

4. To develop a document that reflects current areas of practice and facilitates uniformity of definitions in the profession.

5. To recommend that the AOTA develop a companion document to define techniques, modalities, and activities used in occupational therapy intervention and a document to define specific programs that are offered by occupational therapy departments. The Commission on Practice subsequently developed educational materials to assist in the application of uniform terminology to practice.

Several drafts of the revised *Uniform Terminology—Second Edition* document were reviewed by appropriate AOTA commissions and committees and by a selected review network based on geographical representation, professional expertise, and demonstrated leadership in the field. Excellent responses were received, and the feedback was incorporated into the final document by the Commission on Practice.

Outline

OCCUPATIONAL THERAPY ASSESSMENT
OCCUPATIONAL THERAPY INTERVENTION
I. **OCCUPATIONAL THERAPY PERFORMANCE AREAS**
   A. Activities of Daily Living
      1. Grooming
      2. Oral Hygiene
      3. Bathing
      4. Toilet Hygiene
      5. Dressing
      6. Feeding and Eating
      7. Medication Routine
      8. Socialization
      9. Functional Communication
      10. Functional Mobility
      11. Sexual Expression
   B. Work Activities
      1. Home Management
         a. Clothing Care
         b. Cleaning
         c. Meal Preparation and Cleanup
         d. Shopping
         e. Money Management
         f. Household Maintenance
         g. Safety Procedures
      2. Care of Others
      3. Educational Activities
      4. Vocational Activities
         a. Vocational Exploration
         b. Job Acquisition
         c. Work or Job Performance
         d. Retirement Planning
   C. Play or Leisure Activities
      1. Play or Leisure Exploration
      2. Play or Leisure Performance
II. **PERFORMANCE COMPONENTS**
   A. Sensory Motor Component
      1. Sensory Integration
         a. Sensory Awareness
         b. Sensory Processing
            (1) Tactile
            (2) Proprioceptive
            (3) Vestibular
            (4) Visual
            (5) Auditory
            (6) Gustatory
            (7) Olfactory
         c. Perceptual Skills
            (1) Stereognosis
            (2) Kinesthesia
            (3) Body Scheme
            (4) Right-Left Discrimination
            (5) Form Constancy
            (6) Position in Space
            (7) Visual Closure
            (8) Figure-Ground
            (9) Depth Perception
            (10) Topographical Orientation
      2. Neuromuscular
         a. Reflex
         b. Range of Motion
         c. Muscle Tone
         d. Strength
         e. Endurance
         f. Postural Control
         g. Soft Tissue Integrity
      3. Motor
         a. Activity Tolerance
         b. Gross Motor Coordination
         c. Crossing the Midline
         d. Laterality
         e. Bilateral Integration
         f. Praxis
         g. Fine Motor Coordination/Dexterity
         h. Visual-Motor Integration
         i. Oral-Motor Control
   B. Cognitive Integration and Cognitive Components
      1. Level of Arousal
      2. Orientation
      3. Recognition
      4. Attention Span
      5. Memory
         a. Short-Term
         b. Long-Term

    c. Remote
    d. Recent
  6. Sequencing
  7. Categorization
  8. Concept Formation
  9. Intellectual Operations in Space
  10. Problem Solving
  11. Generalization of Learning
  12. Integration of Learning
  13. Synthesis of Learning
C. Psychosocial Skills and Psychological Components
  1. Psychological
    a. Roles
    b. Values
    c. Interests
    d. Initiation of Activity
    e. Termination of Activity
    f. Self-Concept
  2. Social
    a. Social Conduct
    b. Conversation
    c. Self-Expression
  3. Self-Management
    a. Coping Skills
    b. Time Management
    c. Self-Control

Occupational therapy assessment

Assessment is the planned process of obtaining, interpreting, and documenting the functional status of the individual. The purpose of the assessment is to identify the individual's abilities and limitations, including deficits, delays, or maladaptive behavior that can be addressed in occupational therapy intervention. Data can be gathered through a review of records, observation, interview, and the administration of test procedures. Such procedures include, but are not limited to, the use of standardized tests, questionnaires, performance checklists, activities, and tasks designed to evaluate specific performance abilities.

Occupational therapy intervention

Occupational therapy addresses function and uses specific procedures and activities to (a) develop, maintain, improve, and/or restore the performance of necessary functions; (b) compensate for dysfunction; (c) minimize or prevent debilitation; and/or (d) promote health and wellness. Categories of function are defined as **OCCUPATIONAL PERFORMANCE AREAS** and **PERFORMANCE COMPONENTS. OCCUPATIONAL PERFORMANCE AREAS** include activities of daily living, work activities, and play/leisure activities. Performance components refer to the functional abilities required for occupational performance, including sensory motor, cognitive, and psychological components. Deficits of delays in these **OCCUPATIONAL PERFORMANCE AREAS** may be addressed by occupational therapy intervention.

I. Occupational Performance Areas
  A. Activities of Daily Living
    1. *Grooming*—Obtain and use supplies to shave; apply and remove cosmetics; wash, comb, style, and brush hair; care for nails; care for skin; and apply deodorant.
    2. *Oral Hygiene*—Obtain and use supplies; clean mouth and teeth; remove, clean, and reinsert dentures.
    3. *Bathing*—Obtain and use supplies; soap, rinse, and dry all body parts; maintain bathing position; transfer to and from bathing position.
    4. *Toilet Hygiene*—Obtain and use supplies; clean self; transfer to and from, and maintain toileting position on, bedpan, toilet, or commode.
    5. *Dressing*—Select appropriate clothing; obtain clothing from storage area; dress and undress in a sequential fashion; and fasten and adjust clothing and shoes. Don and doff assistive or adaptive equipment, prostheses, or orthoses.
    6. *Feeding and Eating*—Set up food; use appropriate utensils and tableware; bring food or drink to mouth; suck, masticate, cough, and swallow.
    7. *Medication Routine*—Obtain medication; open and close containers; and take prescribed quantities as scheduled.
    8. *Socialization*—Interact in appropriate contextual and cultural ways.
    9. *Functional Communication*—Use equipment or systems to enhance or provide communication, such as writing equipment, telephones, typewriters, communication boards, call lights, emergency systems, braille writers, augmentative communication systems, and computers.
    10. *Functional Mobility*—Move from one position or place to another, such as in bed mobility, wheelchair mobility, transfers (bed, car, tub, toilet, chair), and functional ambulation, with or without adaptive aids, driving, and use of public transportation.
    11. *Sexual Expression*—Recognize, communicate, and perform desired sexual activities.
  B. Work Activities
    1. *Home Management*
      a. *Clothing Care*—Obtain and use supplies, launder, iron, store, and mend.
      b. *Cleaning*—Obtain and use supplies, pick up, vacuum, sweep, dust, scrub, mop, make bed, and remove trash.
      c. *Meal Preparation and Cleanup*—Plan nutritious meals and prepare food; open and close containers, cabinets, and drawers; use kitchen utensils and appliances; and clean up and store food.
      d. *Shopping*—Select and purchase items and perform money transactions.
      e. *Money Management*—Budget, pay bills, and use bank systems.
      f. *Household Maintenance*—Maintain home, yard, garden appliances, and household items, and/or obtain appropriate assistance.
      g. *Safety Procedures*—Know and perform prevention and emergency procedures to maintain a safe environment and prevent injuries.
    2. *Care of Others*—Provide for children, spouse,

parents, or others, such as the physical care, nurturance, communication, and use of age-appropriate activities.

3. *Educational Activities*—Participate in a school environment and school-sponsored activities (such as field trips, work-study, and extracurricular activities).

4. *Vocational Activities*
   a. *Vocational Exploration*—Determine aptitudes, interests, skills, and appropriate vocational pursuits.
   b. *Job Acquisition*—Identify and select work opportunities and complete application and interview processes.
   c. *Work or Job Performance*—Perform job tasks in a timely and effective manner, incorporating necessary work behaviors such as grooming, interpersonal skills, punctuality, and adherence to safety procedures.
   d. *Retirement Planning*—Determine aptitudes, interests, skills, and identify appropriate avocational pursuits.

C. Play or Leisure Activities
   1. *Play or Leisure Exploration*—Identify interests, skills, opportunities, and appropriate play or leisure activities.
   2. *Play or Leisure Performance*—Participate in play or leisure activities, using physical and psychosocial skills.
      a. Maintain a balance of play or leisure activities with work and activities of daily living.
      b. Obtain, utilize, and maintain equipment and supplies.

II. Performance Components
   A. Sensory Motor Component
      1. *Sensory Integration*
         a. *Sensory Awareness*—Receive and differentiate sensory stimuli.
         b. *Sensory Processing*—Interpret sensory stimuli.
            (1) *Tactile*—Interpret light touch, pressure, temperature, pain, vibration, and two-point stimuli through skin contact/receptors.
            (2) *Proprioceptive*—Interpret stimuli originating in muscles, joints, and other internal tissues to give information about the position of one body part in relationship to another.
            (3) *Vestibular*—Interpret stimuli from the inner ear receptors regarding head position and movement.
            (4) *Visual*—Interpret stimuli through the eyes, including peripheral vision and acuity, awareness of color, depth, and figure-ground.
            (5) *Auditory*—Interpret sounds, localize sounds, and discriminate background sounds.
            (6) *Gustatory*—Interpret tastes.
            (7) *Olfactory*—Interpret odors.

         c. *Perceptual Skills*
            (1) *Stereognosis*—Identify objects through the sense of touch.
            (2) *Kinesthesia*—Identify the excursion and direction of joint movement.
            (3) *Body Scheme*—Acquire an internal awareness of the body and the relationship of body parts to each other.
            (4) *Right-Left Discrimination*—Differentiate one side of the body from the other.
            (5) *Form Constancy*—Recognize forms and objects as the same in various environments, positions, and sizes.
            (6) *Position in Space*—Determine the spatial relationship of figures and objects to self or other forms and objects.
            (7) *Visual Closure*—Identify forms or objects from incomplete presentations.
            (8) *Figure-Ground*—Differentiate between foreground and background forms and objects.
            (9) *Depth Perception*—Determine the relative distance between objects, figures, or landmarks and the observer.
            (10) *Topographical Orientation*—Determine the location of objects and settings and the route to the location.

      2. *Neuromuscular*
         a. *Reflex*—Present an involuntary muscle response elicited by sensory input.
         b. *Range of Motion*—Move body parts through an arc.
         c. *Muscle Tone*—Demonstrate a degree of tension or resistance in a muscle.
         d. *Strength*—Demonstrate a degree of muscle power when movement is resisted as with weight or gravity.
         e. *Endurance*—Sustain cardiac, pulmonary, and musculoskeletal exertion over time.
         f. *Postural Control*—Position and maintain head, neck, trunk, and limb alignment with appropriate weight shifting, midline orientation, and righting reactions for function.
         g. *Soft Tissue Integrity*—Maintain anatomical and physiological condition of interstitial tissue and skin.

      3. *Motor*
         a. *Activity Tolerance*—Sustain a purposeful activity over time.
         b. *Gross Motor Coordination*—Use large muscle groups for controlled movements.
         c. *Crossing the Midline*—Move limbs and eyes across the sagittal plane of the body.
         d. *Laterality*—Use a preferred unilateral body part for activities requiring a high level of skill.
         e. *Bilateral Integration*—Interact with both body sides in a coordinated manner during activity.

f. *Praxis*—Conceive and plan a new motor act in response to an environmental demand.

g. *Fine Motor Coordination/Dexterity*—Use small muscle groups for controlled movements, particularly in object manipulation.

h. *Visual-Motor Integration*—Coordinate the interaction of visual information with body movement during activity.

i. *Oral-Motor Control*—Coordinate oropharyngeal musculature for controlled movements.

B. Cognitive Integration and Cognitive Components

1. *Level of Arousal*—Demonstrate alertness and responsiveness to environmental stimuli.

2. *Orientation*—Identify person, place, time, and situation.

3. *Recognition*—Identify familiar faces, objects, and other previously presented materials.

4. *Attention Span*—Focus on a task over time.

5. *Memory*
   a. *Short-Term*—Recall information for brief periods of time.
   b. *Long-Term*—Recall information for long periods of time.
   c. *Remote*—Recall events from distant past.
   d. *Recent*—Recall events from immediate past.

6. *Sequencing*—Place information, concepts, and actions in order.

7. *Categorization*—Identify similarities of and differences between environmental information.

8. *Concept Formation*—Organize a variety of information to form thoughts and ideas.

9. *Intellectual Operations in Space*—Mentally manipulate spatial relationships.

10. *Problem Solving*—Recognize a problem, define a problem, identify alternative plans, select a plan, organize steps in a plan, implement a plan, and evaluate the outcome.

11. *Generalization of Learning*—Apply previously learned concepts and behaviors to similar situations.

12. *Integration of Learning*—Incorporate previously acquired concepts and behavior into a variety of new situations.

13. *Synthesis of Learning*—Restructure previously learned concepts and behaviors into new patterns.

C. Psychosocial Skills and Psychological Components

1. *Psychological*
   a. *Roles*—Identify functions one assumes or acquires in society (e.g., worker, student, parent, church member).
   b. *Values*—Identify ideas or beliefs that are intrinsically important.
   c. *Interests*—Identify mental or physical activities that create pleasure and maintain attention.
   d. *Initiation of Activity*—Engage in a physical or mental activity.
   e. *Termination of Activity*—Stop an activity at an appropriate time.
   f. *Self-Concept*—Develop value of physical and emotional self.

2. *Social*
   a. *Social Conduct*—Interact using manners, personal space, eye contact, gestures, active listening, and self-expression appropriate to one's environment.
   b. *Conversation*—Use verbal and non-verbal communication to interact in a variety of settings.
   c. *Self-Expression*—Use a variety of styles and skills to express thoughts, feelings, and needs.

3. *Self-Management*
   a. *Coping Skills*—Identify and manage stress and related reactors.
   b. *Time Management*—Plan and participate in a balance of self-care, work, leisure, and rest activities to promote satisfaction and health.
   c. *Self-Control*—Modulate and modify one's own behavior in response to environmental needs, demands, and constraints.

References

American Medical Association. (1966–1988). *Physicians' current procedural terminology first–fourth editions (CPT 1–4)*. Chicago: Author.

American Occupational Therapy Association. (1979). *Occupational therapy output reporting system and uniform terminology for reporting occupational therapy services*. Rockville, MD: Author.

American Psychiatric Association. (1952–1987). *Diagnostic and statistical manual of mental disorders first–third editions (DSM-I–III-R)*. Washington, DC: Author.

Medicare-Medicaid Anti-Fraud and Abuse Amendments (Public Law 95–142). (1977). 42 U. S. C. §1305.

APPENDIX D

*Application of uniform terminology to practice**

Winnie Dunn and Linda McGourty

This document was developed to help occupational therapists apply *Uniform Terminology—Second Edition* to practice. A grid format (Dunn,1988) allows a therapist to systematically identify

*Reprinted with permission from Dunn, W., & McGourty, L. (1989). Application of uniform terminology to practice. *American Journal of Occupational Therapy, 43*(12), 817–821.

an individual's deficit and strength areas and to select appropriate activities to address these areas in occupational therapy intervention.

On the grid (see Uniform Terminology Grid), the horizontal axis is composed of the Performance Areas of activities of daily living, work activities, and play or leisure activities. These Performance Areas are the functional outcomes occupational therapy addresses. The Performance Components include sensorimotor components, cognitive integration and cognitive components, and psychosocial skills and pscyhological components and are listed along the vertical axis of the grid. The Performance Components are the skills and abilities that an individual uses to engage in the Performance Areas. During an occupational therapy assessment, the occupational therapist determines an individual's abilities and limitations in the Performance Components and how they affect the individual's functional outcomes in the Performance Areas.

Because occupational therapy is concerned with the outcomes of activities of daily living, work, and play or leisure, any activity chosen for occupational therapy intervention must fit in a cell on this grid. Therefore, if an individual has a Performance Component program but no corresponding Performance Area deficit, occupational therapy intervention would not be indicated. Activities that are therapeutic but that do not relate to both a Performance Area and one or more Performance Components are not considered to be occupational therapy (Dunn & Campbell, in press).

How to use the grid

Initially, an individual is referred for occupational therapy. The referral process will vary according to the practice setting. After the referral is received, the occupational therapist completes an assessment to determine the individual's abilities and limitations. During this process, it is determined which limitations in the Performance Components are effecting function in the Performance Areas. For example, an individual may have limitations in tactile sensory processing, body scheme, range of motion, short-term memory, and self-concept (Performance Components) that affect the individual's ability to dress and groom independently (Performance Areas). This information is used to develop short- and long-term goals; then the intervention or treatment plan is created. In the intervention or treatment planning process, appropriate occupational theapy activities, modalities, and techniques are selected to address the Performance Components and Performance Areas.

The *Uniform Terminology* provides a framework for the program planning process. Strengths and limitations in Performance Components and their effect on functional outcomes in the Performance Areas are identified through the assessment process. Specific limitations are located on the vertical and horizontal axes of the grid; the intersections of the Performance Components and the Performance Areas (called the *cells* of the grid) represent occupational therapy interventions (activities, modalities, or techniques) that are used to address the limitations, and therefore improve functional outcome.

For example, an infant with severe handicaps who needs to learn to play (Performance Area) must first become aware of differentiating sensory stimuli (Performance Components) as persons and objects enter the environment. The therapist de-

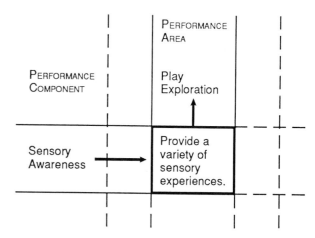

FIGURE 1. *The cell that represents the occupational therapy interventions for an infant with severe handicaps who has poor sensory awareness that limits the outcome of play exploration.*

cides to provide a variety of sensory experiences to develop sensory awareness and, thus, reach the goal of play exploration. This fits on the grid as pictured in Figure 1.

Performance Areas and Performance Components are based on the individual's needs. Therefore, not every box or cell on the grid will be used in one horizontal row or in one vertical column for the individual's intervention or treatment plan.

For example, when the therapist identifies dressing as a Performance Area that an adult cerebrovascular accident patient is unable to complete independently, not all of the Performance Components in the dressing column on the grid would be used for this individual's intervention or treatment plan. Perhaps the assessment revealed the patient had sensory processing, perceptual, and neuromuscular deficits or limitations; the treatment plan would focus on the top half of the grid for dressing with this patient. It would probably not be appropriate to incorporate role, value, and interest components into these early stages of dressing intervention. Table 1 outlines the cells that will be the focus of intervention for this individual.

Treatment planning and intervention are ongoing processes and typically have different areas of focus for each person. During these processes, therapists frequently will develop and use

TABLE 1. *Targets of Intervention for a CVA Patient Who Needs to Improve the Functional Outcome of Dressing*

Performance Components	Performance Area		
	Toilet Hygiene	Dressing	Feeding/ Eating
Sensorimotor components			
Sensory processing		•	
Perceptual skills		•	
Neuromuscular components		•	
Cognitive components			
Psychosocial components			

In this example, sensory processing, perceptual skills, and neuromuscular components are interfering with this outcome. CVA = cerebrovascular accident.

TABLE 2. *Performance Areas That May Be Affected by Poor Oral Motor Control*

| Performance Component | Performance Areas | | | | |
	Oral Hygiene	Bathing	Toilet Hygiene	Feeding/ Eating	Functional Communication
Oral motor control	●			●	●

more than one activity, modality, or technique within a cell on the grid to reach the desired Performance Area outcome.

Conversely, an individual may have a limitation or deficit in a Performance Component that does not affect all of the Performance Areas. For example, a problem with oral motor control may affect oral hygiene, feeding and eating, and functional communication, but may have little or no impact on bathing and toileting. Table 2 summarizes this pattern.

It is important to include the Performance Components' strengths and abilities in the intervention or treatment planning process. This provides a stable base upon which to facilitate success and motivation with difficult tasks (Dunn, in press).

For example, a child with learning disabilities is referred for occupational therapy assessment by the educational team because of difficulty in producing written schoolwork. An occupational therapy assessment reveals that the child is not processing tactile and proprioceptive input from his hands and has poor fine motor skills and poor postural control. He has good auditory processing and visual perceptual skills. The grid helps the therapist consider the impact of this pattern of strengths and limitations on the educational outcome of producing written work. Table 3 illustrates this pattern of strengths and limitations.

A number of intervention strategies would fit into these cells on the grid, including

- Construct art projects (e.g., with glue, clay).
- Plan hand digging and exploration activities.

- Instruct parents in home follow-up.
- Give child responsibility for carrying objects in classroom.
- Adjust seating.
- Supervise manipulation tasks carried out by teacher's aide.
- Allow child to watch others during construction tasks.
- Instruct teacher in auditory cuing strategies.

The Case Example further illustrates the use of the Uniform Terminology Grid (Dunn, 1988) for intervention or treatment planning. The six cases include brief explanations of the individual's problems, followed by two copies of the grid. The first grid (A) displays the performance component limitations and the performance area concerns from the referral, showing how these would intersect on the grid. The second grid (B) displays examples of intervention activities that might be designed for the individual.

References

Dunn, W. (1988). *Uniform Terminology Grid: A framework for applying uniform terminology to occupational therapy practice.* Unpublished grid.

Dunn, W. (Ed.). (in press). *Pediatric occupational therapy: Facilitating effective service provision.* Thorofare, NJ: Slack.

Dunn, W., & Campbell, P. (in press). Designing pediatric service provision. In W. Dunn (Ed.), *Pediatric occupational therapy: Facilitating effective service provision.* Thorofare, NJ: Slack.

TABLE 3. *Strengths and Limitations in Performance Components That Affect Educational Outcomes for a Child With Learning Disabilities*

Performance Components	Performance Area Educational Activities
Sensorimotor components	
Sensory processing	
Tactile	Limitation/deficit
Proprioceptive	Limitation/deficit
Visual	Ability/strength
Auditory	Ability/strength
Neuromuscular components	
Postural control	Limitation/deficit
Motor components	
Praxis	Limitation/deficit
Fine motor coordination/ dexterity	Limitation/deficit

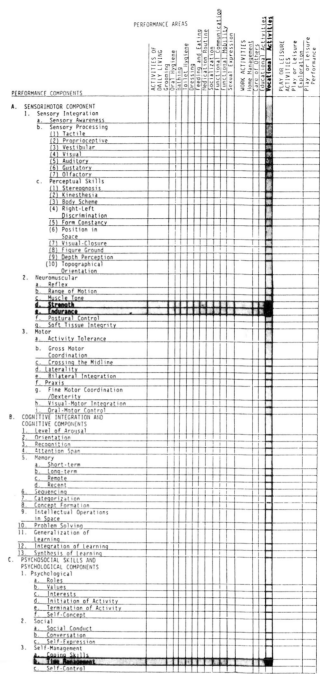

UNIFORM TERMINOLOGY GRID. *Copyright 1988 by Winnie Dunn. Reprinted with permission.*

A

FIGURE 2A. *Illustration of performance area needs in relation to desired performance outcome on the Uniform Terminology Grid. Copyright 1988 by Winnie Dunn. Reprinted with permission.*

Case example

An individual who is injured on the job may be unable to work (Occupational Performance Area on the horizontal axis of the grid). To achieve the outcome of returning to work, the individual may need to address specific Performance Components (on the vertical axis of the grid) such as strength, endurance, and time management. Figure 2A displays the relationship between the Performance Area of work and the Performance Components of strength, endurance, and time management. The black cells represent the focus of program planning and intervention. In this example, the occupational therapist, in cooperation with the vocational team, uses planned interventions to achieve the desired outcome of work. Figure 2B displays examples of activities that might be designed for this individual; other activities might include an exercise program, body mechanics instruction, and job modification. These services might be provided in a work-hardening program.

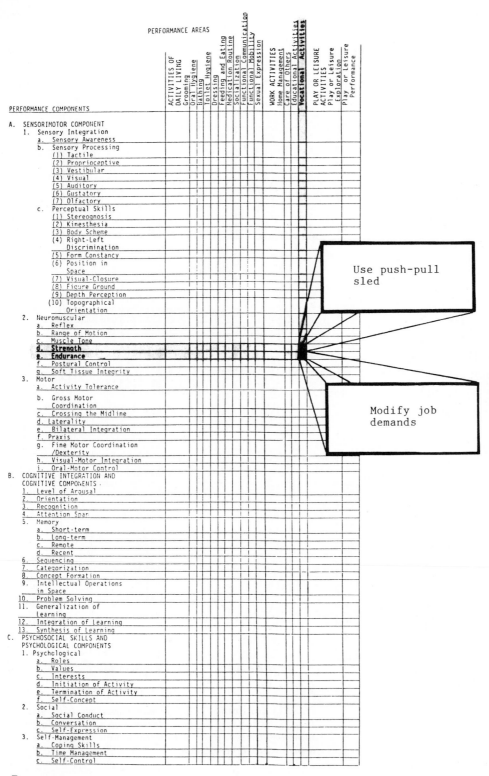

FIGURE 2B. *Sample interventions that fit into the cells on the Uniform Terminology Grid. Copyright 1988 by Winnie Dunn. Reprinted with permission.*

B

APPENDIX E

*Guidelines for occupational therapy documentation**

These guidelines are provided to assist members of the American Occupational Therapy Association (AOTA) in documenting occupational therapy services. Occupational therapy personnel shall document the type and frequency of services provided within the time frames established by facilities, government agencies, and accreditation organizations.

The purpose of documentation is to do the following:

1. Provide a serial and legal record of the patient's condition and the course of therapeutic intervention from admission to discharge.
2. Serve as an information source for patient care.
3. Facilitate communication among health care professionals who contribute to the patient's care.
4. Furnish data for use in treatment, education, research, and reimbursement.

Types of documentation

The various types of documentation are

1. initial note
2. assessment notes and reports
3. treatment plans and goals
4. progress notes
5. treatment records
6. discharge summaries
7. consultation reports
8. special reports (*e.g.,* referrals to other programs and agencies, summary reports for legal reasons, home programs, and correspondence)
9. critical incidents reports or notes

Protocol for documentation

Each patient referred to occupational therapy must have a case record maintained as a permanent file. The record should be:

1. organized
2. legible
3. concise

* Prepared by the Documentation Task Force (Linda Kohlman McGourty, MOT, OTR, Chair; Mary Foto, OTR; Susan Kronsnoble, OTR; Carole Lossing, OTR; Sharon Rask, OTR; and Christine de Renne Stephan, OTR) for the Commission on Practice (Esther Bell, MA, OTR, FAOTA, Chair).

Approved by the Representative Assembly, April 1986.

4. clear
5. accurate
6. complete
7. current
8. objective (clear distinction made between facts and opinions)
9. correct in grammar and spelling

Fundamental elements of documentation

The following ten elements should be present:

1. patient's full name and case number on each page of documentation;
2. date stated as month, day, and year for each entry;
3. identification of type of documentation and department name;
4. signature with a minimum of first name, last name, and professional designation;
5. signature of the recorder directly at the end of the note without space left between the body of the note and the signature;
6. countersignature by a registered occupational therapist (OTR) on documentation written by students and certified occupational therapy assistants (COTA) if required by law or the facility;
7. compliance with confidentiality standards;
8. acceptable terminology as defined by the facility;
9. facility approved abbreviations;
10. errors corrected by drawing a single line through an error, and the correction initialed (liquid correction fluid and erasures are not acceptable), or facility requirements followed.

Content of documentation

The following components should be included in the total occupational therapy or facility record for each patient (see Table 1). Each occupational therapy department must determine the type and frequency of documentation and must abide by the written policies and procedures of the individual facility.

Reference

American Occupational Therapy Association. (1979). *Uniform terminology for reporting occupational services.* Rockville, MD: AOTA. Reprinted with permission.

TABLE 1.   *Components of Total Occupational Therapy or Facility Record for Each Patient*

Content	Clarifications
A. Identification and Background Information	
1. Name, age, sex, date of admission, treatment diagnosis, and date of onset of current diagnosis	Name may be omitted depending on the facility and department policies and procedures
2. Referral source, services requested, and date of referral to occupational therapy	Include who requested occupational therapy services, what specific services were requested, and the date.
3. Pertinent history that indicates prior levels of function and support systems	Include applicable developmental, educational, vocational, socioeconomic, and medical history (may be brief).
4. Secondary problems or preexisting conditions	Include any additional problems or conditions that may affect patient function or treatment outcomes.
5. Precautions and contraindications	May be identified by referral source or occupational therapy staff.
B. Assessment and Reassessment	
Refer to the Uniform Occupational Therapy Checklist (AOTA, 1979) for specific skills and performance.	Independent living/daily living skills and performance components
	Sensorimotor skills and performance components
	Cognitive skills and performance components
	Psychosocial skills and performance components
	Therapeutic adaptations and prevention
1. Tests and evaluations administered and the results	State name and type of evaluation, date administered, and results and whether assessment or reassessment.
2. Summary and analysis of assessment findings	State facts in an objective manner. Analysis of objective findings should include measurable data to define the patient's assets and deficits.
3. References to other pertinent reports and information	Include any additional sources of data or evaluation results that help formulate the total assessment of the patient.
4. Occupational therapy problem list	This list should be compatible with a master problem list developed by the health care team or other health care professionals (when available).
5. Recommendations for occupational therapy services	State whether occupational therapy services are recommended or not.
C. Treatment Planning	
1. Short- and long-term goals	Define clearly the goals established by the patient, family, and therapist. These goals should be measurable and related to the occupational therapy problem list.
2. Activities and/or treatment procedures	State clearly the specific methods to be used in the intervention and relate the methods to the problems identified on the occupational therapy problem list.
3. Type, amount, and frequency of treatment	State skill and performance areas to be addressed and estimate the number, duration, and frequency of treatment sessions to accomplish goals.
4. Anticipated time to achieve goals	State the anticipated number of therapy sessions or days of therapy to reach the desired outcome. This information may be an overall statement not necessarily written for each goal.
5. Statement of potential functional outcome	State the anticipated outcome and clearly relate it to the long-term goals.
D. Treatment Implementation	
1. Activities, procedures, and modalities used	State the specific media and methods used.
2. Patient's response to treatment and the progress toward goal attainment as related to problem list	State the patient's physical and behavioral response to therapy and whether the goals are being achieved.
3. Goal modification when indicated by the response to treatment	If the goals have been modified in the treatment process, state the new goals and rationale for changes.
4. Change in anticipated time to achieve goals	If for any reason the treatment time frame is altered, include the reason for the change and the new anticipated time frame.
5. Attendance and participation with treatment plan (attendance could be a check format)	State if the patient is following through with treatment plan.

(continued)

TABLE 1.   *Components of Total Occupational Therapy or Facility Record for Each Patient (continued)*

Content	Clarifications
D. Treatment Implementation	
6. Statement of reason for patient missing treatment	Write the reasons for treatment not occurring as scheduled.
7. Assistive/adaptive equipment, orthotics, and prosthetics if issued or fabricated, and specific instructions for the application and/or use of the item	State the device, note whether it was fabricated, sold, rented, or loaned, and state the effectiveness of the device.
8. Patient-related conferences and communication	If occupational therapy personnel participated in a conference or made a pertinent contact with a family member, agency, or health care professional, state this information with a brief summary of the conference or communication.
9. Home programs	Include a copy of the home program as established with the patient in the patient record.
E. Discontinuation of Services	
1. Summary of assessment and treatment implementation	State clearly and concisely a summary of the total occupational therapy intervention process, the number of sessions, the goals achieved, and the functional outcome. Compare the initial and discharge status.
2. Home programs	Include the actual written home program that is to be followed after discharge.
3. Follow-up plans	State the schedule and specific plans.
4. Recommendations	State any recommendations pertaining to the patient's future needs.
5. Referral(s) to other health care providers and community agencies	Make referral(s) or recommendations for referral(s) when additional or new services are needed.

APPENDIX F

Entry-level role delineation for registered occupational therapists (OTRs) and certified occupational therapy assistants (COTAs)*

Preamble

The American Occupational Therapy Association, Inc. (AOTA), has the responsibility to define entry-level practice as it projects and represents ideal service provision.

This document describes ideal entry-level practice, unlike a role-analysis, which describes current practice. An entry-level role delineation should be used as a guideline for typical entry-level practice and should not be considered a scope of practice statement. By definition, entry-level is less than 1 year of practice.

Any health care profession must periodically examine the way it describes entry-level practice. The last role delineation was adopted by the Representative Assembly in March 1981. Rapidly changing health care environments, *Essentials* (AOTA, 1983/1989c, 1983/1989d) revisions, and changes in health care provision resulted in the decision to review, revise, and update the 1981 document.

This document reflects the increasing importance of values, attitudes, research, and ethics as important practice components. The increase in specificity of tasks between this document and the 1981 document is a response to multiple requests for a more graphic picture of the expectations of entry-level OTRs and COTAs. As assessment tools, therapeutic intervention techniques and work settings change rapidly, tasks are stated generically and are meant to apply to all areas of clinical practice.

Although successful completion of the American Occupational Therapy Certification Board's Certification Exam permits the new OTR access to independent practice (with regulation, as required), guidelines are given on entry-level OTR supervision and service competency as necessary. It is considered the professional responsibility and therefore a component of practice of the OTR to seek this supervision according to principles of ethics

* Prepared by the Entry-Level Role Delineation Task Force (Linda DiJoseph, MS, OTR, FAOTA, Chair, Winnie Dunn, PhD, OTR, FAOTA, Patricia Lowenstein, OTR, Marie Rabin, MBA, COTA, L. Randy Strickland, EDD, OTR, FAOTA) for The Intercommission Council (Carolyn Van Schroeder, OTR, FAOTA, Chair).

Approved by the AOTA Representative Assembly, April 1990. Reprinted with permission.

This document replaces the 1981 *Entry-Level Role Delineation for OTRs and COTAs.*

and clinical judgment. Supervision of the COTA by an OTR is required professionally and legally. Although the level of this supervision may vary in individual cases and settings, guidelines are also given for COTA supervision and service competency. These guidelines were established to provide support for individuals requesting supervision, for individuals providing supervision, and as guidance to employers regarding staffing patterns.

This description of entry-level COTA and OTR practice can be used by regulatory boards, employers, educators, and practitioners. It is the intent that this document be used to develop job descriptions, guide curriculum development and revision, develop fieldwork objectives, and as a self-assessment tool for individuals entering or returning to practice.

As demands of the health care system continue to change, so will expectations of entry-level practitioners. Periodic reviews and updates of this entry-level role delineation are essential and will occur on a regular basis.

I. Purpose

This document provides a description of **ENTRY-LEVEL PRAC-TICE.** The contents of this document are not to be construed as entirely original, but represent a compilation of resource materials and professional judgment. Application is intended as a foundation for practice and education environments. **REGULATORY AND REIMBURSEMENT SOURCES MUST BE TAKEN INTO CONSIDERATION WHEN USING THIS DOCUMENT.**

II. Introduction

A. Definition of occupational therapy

Occupational therapy is the use of purposeful activity with individuals who are limited by physical injury or illness, psychosocial dysfunction, developmental or learning disabilities, poverty and cultural differences, or the aging process, in order to maximize independence, prevent disability, and maintain health. The practice encompasses evaluation, treatment, and consultation. Specific occupational therapy services include teaching daily living skills; developing perceptual motor skills and sensory integrative functioning; developing play skills and prevocational and leisure capacities; designing, fabricating, or applying selected orthotic and prosthetic devices or selective adaptive equipment; using specifically designed crafts and exercises to enhance functional performance; administering and interpreting tests such as manual muscle testing and range of motion; and adapting environments for persons with handicaps. These services are provided individually, in groups, or through social systems (AOTA, 1989a).

B. Definition of entry-level practice

Entry-level OTRs and COTAs are persons with less than 1 year of experience (AOTA, 1989b).

C. Levels of practice

The OTR and COTA have important but distinct roles in the practice setting. In addition to responsibility to the consumer, both have a responsibility to each other as the service provision process is carried out. The OTR is responsible for all facets of the occupational therapy process and, therefore, professionally supervises the COTA's activity. Both the OTR and the COTA are responsible for performing work within their established levels of competence. Through the communication process, they share mutual responsibility for clarifying competencies and responsibilities (AOTA, 1987).

It is highly recommended that the entry-level OTR practice in a setting in which supervision is provided by an experienced OTR. In this situation, the OTR is able to obtain consultation and guidance as experience is gained. In certain situations, the OTR may be required to establish service competency in more complex aspects of the service provision process. Depending on prior preparation and experience, these may include assessment and treatment interventions related to such areas as prosthetics, sensory integration, augmented communication devices, or management and supervisory functions. It is the OTR's responsibility to practice in an environment in which she or he is competent or has immediate access to and guidance from an experienced OTR.

It is also highly recommended that entry-level COTAs practice in a setting in which they may obtain close supervision as they gain experience in testing and treatment and demonstrate service competency in more complex areas. Initially, the COTA may contribute to the occupational therapy process and, after establishing service competency, may take full responsibility for some components of the service provision process. It is preferable that the entry-level COTA be supervised by an experienced OTR or, if pertinent regulations permit, by an experienced COTA under the direction of the OTR. If an entry-level or experienced COTA practices in a setting in which supervision is provided by an entry-level OTR, this OTR must use sound professional judgment in obtaining consultation on delegation of responsibility, establishment of service competency, or provision of supervision as dictated by the setting, specific treatment situation, or COTA's experience level.

III. Supervision

Supervision is a process in which two or more people participate in a joint effort to promote, establish, maintain, or elevate a level of performance and service. The supervisor is responsible for setting, encouraging, and evaluating the standard of work performed by the supervisee (AOTA, 1987).

Quality supervision is a mutual undertaking between the supervisor and the supervisee that fosters growth and development; ensures the appropriate use of training and potential; encourages creativity and innovation; and provides guidance, support, encouragement, and respect, thereby promoting the goals of the individual and the facility.

In a setting in which both a COTA and an OTR are employed, the OTR and the COTA must cooperate in order to provide the best service. Administrative and service supervision of the OTR and COTA may differ, depending on the employment pattern used. When an agency is contracting services, it is usually responsible for supervising the personnel providing therapy services. Supervision procedures should be carefully coordinated between the agency contracting for therapy services and the agency providing the personnel.

When OTRs and COTAs are employed directly by the agency,

supervision is determined by the administrative structure of the agency. In this situation, supervision falls into two categories: administrative supervision and service supervision.

Department managers, agency administrators, or other supervisory personnel can perform administrative supervision of the OTR and the COTA. The OTR and the COTA are accountable to these persons for such things as work assignment, work schedule, payroll, sick leave and vacation, and permission to attend in-service meetings and conferences. These persons are also responsible for the OTR's and COTA's annual performance evaluations. The OTR contributes to the evaluation of the COTA by sharing with the administrator specific information regarding the COTA's overall job performance and effectiveness in carrying out therapy goals.

An OTR carries out service supervision. An experienced OTR should supervise an entry-level OTR, which is the preferable situation for the beginning therapist. Although a COTA is typically supervised by an OTR, if regulations permit, an experienced COTA may supervise an entry-level COTA. This occurs under the direction of an OTR after the supervising OTR has ensured service and job competencies. The OTR, however, has ultimate overall responsibility for service performance. The supervising OTR determines levels of supervision based on service needs. The supervising OTR should consider the following when identifying supervision levels:

1. Current occupational therapy practice standards and guidelines.
2. Therapy needs within appropriate life environments.
3. Complexity of evaluation and intervention methods used.
4. Proficiencies of the supervisee.
5. Regulations, policies, and procedures of the department or the agency.
6. State laws and regulations.
7. Reimbursement requirements.

Methods of service supervision should be determined before the supervisor and supervisee enter into such a relationship and should be periodically reevaluated for effectiveness.

Two levels of service supervision are identified. Both levels may apply to supervision of the COTA (or the OTR if that situation exists) when that person is providing therapy services. Close supervision requires daily, direct, on-premises contact. Preferably, as part of the process, any notes that the COTA enters into permanent records should be co-signed by the OTR. This promotes the acquisition of knowledge and skills specific to job requirements.

Close, general, or no supervision of the OTR is determined by service competency. The experienced OTR and the entry-level OTR together establish levels of supervision. When an entry-level OTR practices independently in an unsupervised setting, it is that therapist's professional and ethical responsibility to seek consultation as needed.

General supervision of the COTA is used only after service competencies have been determined by the supervising occupational therapist. Contact by the supervising therapist may be less than daily, but should be a minimum of 3 to 5 direct contact hours per week for the full-time COTA; time would be prorated for the part-time COTA. When licensing laws, state regulations, treatment settings, or agencies require more stringent standards for supervision, they must be followed. This supervision may be a combination of record reviews, observations of interventions, informal or formal meetings, or shared assessments and interventions.

In some circumstances, a COTA may receive both types of supervision based on the level of service competency. In the supervisory process, the OTR must be reachable by telephone. It is recommended that the OTR be in the same geographical area and that there be no more than 1½ hours of travel time between the OTR and the COTA. If there are more than 1½ hours of travel time between them, a contingency plan for handling emergencies shall be established. These guidelines reinforce the fact that the OTR is ultimately responsible for the health and safety of each individual in the provision of occupational therapy services.

In extenuating circumstances, when the OTR is absent from the job, the COTA may continue carrying out established programs for up to 30 calendar days under agency supervision while appropriate occupational therapy supervision is sought, except where regulatory or established guidelines supersede this guideline. For an entry-level COTA, it is understood that programs to be continued include routine activities where service competency has been established. Intervention that requires ongoing interpretation is discontinued. Prior to the absence of the OTR, all documentation should be up to date and all intervention plans should be in order.

The supervisor and supervisee have a mutual responsibility to understand each other's educational backgrounds and role competencies and responsibilities in order to work effectively as a team. This understanding will help define a base to establish acceptable service competency. Once service competency has been established, the COTA may be able to work under general supervision rather than close supervision (AOTA, 1987).

IV. Service competency

Service competency is the determination, made by various methods, that two people performing the same or equivalent procedures will obtain the same or equivalent results. In test development, this concept is known as interrater reliability. The same concept can be applied to professionals working together in the service provision process. It stems from the assumption that the OTR employs currently acceptable practices.

When an OTR delegates an assessment or intervention task to a COTA, there must be a high degree of confidence that the COTA will obtain the same information or results as the OTR. Service competency is critical in the working relationship between the OTR and the COTA because the OTR is ultimately responsible for the outcomes of all tasks performed in the occupational therapy service provision process. If a high degree of confidence cannot be assured, the OTR must question the appropriateness of delegating that task.

In a setting in which an entry-level OTR is supervised by an experienced OTR, service competency may be established in the same manner for more difficult procedures or procedures in which the entry-level OTR has no experience. If an entry-level OTR is working independently without supervision, it is highly recommended that an experienced OTR be hired on a part-time consultancy basis or that the entry-level OTR establish a mentor relationship with an experienced OTR.

Standards and methods for establishing service competency vary depending on the task. It is more difficult to obtain clinical competency in observations and other techniques that require a variety of parameters to be rated simultaneously. Service competency can be obtained in many ways that are compatible with the service provision process.

Examples of service competency

For standardized or criterion-referenced tests that do not require special training courses, both the OTR and the COTA can learn the procedures outlined in the manuals. By observation, it can be determined whether the test procedure is being completed in a standardized manner.

For standardized or criterion-referenced tests or for observational recordings, the OTR can administer the test while both the OTR and the COTA independently score the performance to establish that the scoring results are the same.

Videotaping is another useful tool for establishing service competency. Two OTRs or an OTR and a COTA can watch the same performance, rate the performance independently, and compare findings for agreement. This is a time-effective tool, because videotapes that the experienced practitioner has already prepared and scored can be used to check the skills of the entry-level practitioner; each therapist can schedule the check when it is convenient.

When scoring occurs after the testing (e.g., for the Beery Developmental Test of Visual–Motor Integration [Beery, 1967]), a folder containing test protocols and score sheets can be set up. Each person can score the test protocol independently. Results can then be compared and agreement tabulated.

When service competency must be established for intervention procedures, a co-treatment situation is preferable. The experienced practitioner can observe the entry-level practitioner's performance and the decisions that are made as the treatment session progresses to determine whether the same process would have occurred if the experienced practitioner had been providing the intervention. This does not preclude style differences, but it does address the need to ensure that the same outcomes would be produced by both persons.

Periodic videotaping of intervention sessions provided by the entry-level practitioner is another acceptable method for establishing and maintaining service competency for these procedures.

The task of ensuring service competency between the OTR and the COTA should be part of ongoing training and supervision activities. OTRs who regularly spend time with COTAs will find that service competency is easily established for frequently used procedures. Procedures that are used infrequently may require closer supervision.

It is recommended that the acceptable standard percentage of agreement set by the OTR be met on three consecutive occasions before it is recorded that service competency has been established. This standard will ensure that the provision of occupational therapy service is stable among different therapists (AOTA, 1987).

V. Attitudes and values

An attitude is defined as the disposition to respond positively or negatively toward an object, person, concept, or situation. Values are beliefs or ideals to which a person is committed. Actions reflect values and attitudes.

In professional situations, all occupational therapy practitioners must demonstrate actions that reflect nonjudgmental attitudes and values. The following statements provide examples of appropriate professional beliefs and values for OTRs and COTAs:

1. All individuals have the same rights, privileges, and status.
2. All individuals have the right to expect the freedom to exercise choice in their lives.
3. The professional adheres to moral and legal principles, including standards of accuracy, objectivity, honesty, and integrity.
4. The professional exercises self-discipline and sound judgment in actions.
5. The professional is dedicated and responsive to the welfare of others and advocates for creative, adaptable options that produce satisfaction for the consumer (AOTA, 1988b).

VI. Service provision process

A. Assessment

The multifaceted occupational therapy assessment process includes determining the need for intervention, identifying the type and length of intervention, coordinating findings with other professionals and family members, and documenting the assessment process itself. Assessment includes screening, evaluation, and reassessment.

As a general guideline, the OTR is responsible for the assessment process and takes primary responsibility for the initial evaluation. The COTA may contribute to the completion of the assessment process under the OTR's supervision.

Specific guidelines will be outlined under the various types of assessment: screening, evaluation, and reassessment (AOTA, 1987).

1. Screening

Screening is a process by which occupational therapy personnel determine the need for comprehensive evaluation and intervention. Screening is an investigative tool; it is not a substitute for a comprehensive evaluation.

Screening	OTR	COTA
Establishes service competency with COTA for all screening tasks delegated	///////// /////////	
Supervises COTA's activities for tasks that have been delegated after establishing service competency	///////// ///////// /////////	
Determines information to be collected	/////////	
Collects screening data	/////////	::::::::
Reports factual data orally, in writing, or both	/////////	/////////
Analyzes screening information	/////////	
Interprets screening information	/////////	
Summarizes screening information orally, in writing, or both	///////// /////////	
Communicates screening information orally, in writing, or both	///////// /////////	:::::::: ::::::::

Example—screening

Ms. Jones has been admitted to the psychiatric unit with a diagnosis of schizophrenia. The OTR determines that a record review, structured interview, and observation during task performance would provide adequate screening data to determine whether occupational therapy is indicated. Because the observation is a structured format in this facility and the COTA has established service competency with the OTR, the COTA performs this component of screening and reports the findings to the OTR. The OTR combines this data with other screening data to formulate a recommendation that is reported to the team.

2. Evaluation

Evaluation is the process of gathering a database and interpreting findings for the development of an occupational therapy intervention plan. The OTR has the primary role in all evaluation processes that require ongoing interpretation of performance.

The OTR may supervise the COTA in evaluations that are focused primarily on outcome data, such as a standard score. This would be possible only on evaluation tasks for which the OTR has established acceptable service competency with the COTA. In these cases, the COTA may complete the standardized procedure and report the findings to the OTR (AOTA, 1987).

Able to perform the task.	Able to perform the task only after demonstrating service competency.	Contributes to the process but does not complete the task independently.	Does not perform the task.

Evaluation

Evaluation	OTR	COTA
Establishes service competency with COTA for all evaluation tasks delegated	///////// /////////	
Supervises COTA's activities for tasks that have been delegated after establishing service competency	///////// ///////// /////////	
Determines information to be collected	/////////	
Determines evaluation methodology	/////////	
Chooses appropriate evaluation instruments	/////////	
Completes data collection procedures such as record reviews, interviews, general observations, and behavioral checklists	///////// ///////// /////////	:::::::: :::::::: ::::::::
Administers standardized tests	/////////	::::::::
Administers criterion-referenced tests	/////////	::::::::
Administers skilled observations and unstructured tests	///////// /////////	
Scores test protocols	/////////	::::::::
Reports factual data orally, in writing, or both	/////////	/////////
Analyzes evaluation data	/////////	
Interprets evaluation data	/////////	
Summarizes evaluation data orally, in writing, or both	///////// /////////	
Communicates evaluation information orally, in writing, or both	///////// /////////	######## ########

Example—evaluation

Richard is a first grader with mild cerebral palsy. The educational team has determined that occupational therapy may be an appropriate related service to enhance his educational program. The OTR determines the need to gather data in the following areas: sensory processing, perceptual skills, and neuromuscular development.

Because evaluation of sensory processing and neuromuscular development require ongoing judgment of Richard's ability to interact with the environment using stability–mobility patterns, reach–grasp patterns, joint integrity, and sensory input and feedback, the OTR performs these components of the evaluation. Because the COTA will be providing intervention if indicated, he or she observes evaluation procedures, assists in positioning, and records data as specified by the OTR.

To assess Richard's perceptual skills, the OTR decides to include a standardized test in the evaluation protocol. The OTR

assigns the administration and scoring of the Test of Visual–Perceptual Skills (Non-Motor) (TVPS) (Gardner, 1982) to the COTA because they have established service competency for this test. The COTA scores and reports these test results to the OTR. The OTR interprets these data and combines them with other evaluation data to formulate a recommendation and report it to the team.

3. Reassessment

Reassessment is the process of gathering current data and interpreting them to continue intervention, revise the intervention plan, or discontinue intervention. All tasks and criteria related to screening and evaluation apply to reassessment.

Reassessment

Reassessment	OTR	COTA
Tracks the need for reassessment	/////////	/////////
Reports changes in status that might warrant reassessment or referral	///////// /////////	///////// /////////
Performs reassessment as required	/////////	########

B. Program planning

The occupational therapy program planning process contributes to the development of team consensus goals and objectives as well as to the preparation of the occupational therapy intervention plan. The OTR is responsible for accomplishing both of these planning functions and is ultimately responsible for the outcome of the occupational therapy intervention. The COTA contributes to program planning, as directed by the supervising OTR. The OTR contributes to the team's information on the basis of the evaluation results regarding strengths, weaknesses, functional performance, and anticipated changes resulting from therapeutic interventions.

///// Able to perform the task.	:::::: Able to perform the task only after demonstrating service competency.	###### Contributes to the process but does not complete the task independently.		Does not perform the task.

Program Planning

	OTR	COTA
Establishes service competency with COTA for all program planning tasks delegated	///////// /////////	
Supervises COTA's activities for tasks that have been delegated after establishing service competency (supervision may be close or general)	///////// ///////// ///////// /////////	
Reports factual data at meetings	/////////	/////////
Interprets occupational therapy assessment data in relation to overall team goals	///////// /////////	
Develops team goals and objectives based on assessment data	///////// /////////	
Develops occupational therapy goals and objectives based on assessment data	///////// /////////	######### #########
Makes referrals to other occupational therapists for specialty needs	///////// /////////	
Makes referrals to other disciplines or agencies	///////// /////////	######### #########
Develops occupational therapy intervention plan	///////// /////////	######### #########
Documents intervention plan	/////////	#########

Intervention

	OTR	COTA
Establishes service competency with COTA for all intervention tasks delegated	///////// /////////	
Supervises COTA's activities for tasks that have been delegated after establishing service competency (supervision may be close or general)	///////// ///////// ///////// /////////	
Engages client in purposeful activities related to occupational performance areas	///////// /////////	///////// /////////
Provides direct service related to performance components that follows a generally accepted routine	///////// ///////// /////////	///////// ///////// /////////
Provides direct service related to performance components requiring ongoing interpretation	///////// ///////// /////////	:::::::::: :::::::::: ::::::::::
Monitors non-occupational therapy personnel in the implementation of tasks designed to enhance intervention	///////// ///////// /////////	######### ######### #########
Provides case and colleague consultation	/////////	#########
Reports changes in client or environment status that may affect intervention plan	///////// /////////	///////// /////////
Alters intervention plan as indicated	/////////	#########

C. Intervention

Occupational therapy intervention is the implementation of both the documented team goals and objectives and the related occupational therapy intervention plan developed from the evaluation process. The OTR is responsible for the outcome of the intervention plan and for assigning appropriate intervention components to the COTA if available. The COTA's level of competence is determined by the demonstration of skills and the establishment of service competency with the OTR (AOTA, 1987).

Consultation is an intervention option. There are three types of consultation: case, colleague, and system. Case and colleague consultation address individual needs within particular environments. At the entry level, the OTR provides case and colleague consultation regarding routine situations. Practice experience enables the OTR to address more complex situations. At the entry level, the COTA is not prepared to provide case and colleague consultation but contributes to the process as service competency is established.

System consultation addresses the needs of the environments or cultures within which persons function (e.g., a community agency). At the entry level, neither the OTR nor the COTA is prepared to provide system consultation.

Example—intervention

Harriet is a 65-year-old woman who has had a right cerebrovascular accident. Assessment data reveal that Harriet would benefit from occupational therapy intervention to improve motor competency and accomplish independent eating, dressing, and personal hygiene.

The COTA performs the daily dressing and personal hygiene routines with Harriet and constructs a static splint designed by the OTR. The OTR performs the neuromuscular facilitation and inhibition techniques that enable Harriet to move her trunk and limbs in functional patterns for participation in daily life tasks.

As the COTA is performing dressing tasks with Harriet, it becomes apparent that Harriet is experiencing shoulder pain. The COTA reports this finding to the OTR, who alters the intervention plan to incorporate this new information.

Unit staff have reported to the OTR that Harriet is having difficulty at mealtime. After observation, the OTR determines that shoulder pain is affecting Harriet's ability to eat independently. The OTR designs a mealtime routine to be performed by unit personnel. The COTA checks with unit personnel twice a week to determine if the mealtime routine is successful and reports findings to the OTR.

 Able to perform the task.   Able to perform the task only after demonstrating service competency.   ###### Contributes to the process but does not complete the task independently.   Does not perform the task.

D. Documentation

Documentation is the recording of the occupational therapy process. All criteria from other sections regarding documentation apply.

Documentation	OTR	COTA
Countersigns all documentation written by COTA that will become part of the permanent record, if required by relevant regulations	/////////	
Ensures that all official documentation for the permanent record is countersigned by the OTR, if required by relevant regulations		/////////

E. Discontinuation of intervention

Occupational therapy services are provided within diverse agencies. Programs within these agencies have a specific focus. When a person achieves the occupational therapy goals within an agency, occupational therapy services are discontinued. The person may continue services in other disciplines, be referred to another agency if indicated, or be discharged to the community, with or without a recommendation for support services. When persons do not achieve established occupational therapy goals within agency parameters, the same options as previously stated may apply.

Discontinuation of Intervention	OTR	COTA
Recognizes the factors that warrant discontinuation of intervention	/////////	/////////
Reports the factors that warrant discontinuation of intervention orally and in writing	/////////	::::::::
Interprets occupational therapy data in relation to overall goals at time of discharge orally and in writing	/////////	
Formulates the occupational therapy discharge and follow-up plan	/////////	########
Formulates, in collaboration with client, family members, significant others, and staff, discontinuation and follow-up plan	/////////	########
Discontinues occupational therapy services	/////////	
Reports factual data at time of discharge orally and in writing	/////////	/////////
Makes referrals to other OTRs	/////////	
Makes referrals to other disciplines or agencies	/////////	

VII. Service management

Service management refers to those tasks that support the functions of the occupational therapy department or agency service provision.

Service Management	OTR	COTA
Plans daily schedule according to assigned work load	/////////	/////////
Determines space, equipment, and supply needs	/////////	/////////
Manages supplies and equipment according to established procedures	/////////	/////////
Manages records and budget as assigned	/////////	::::::::
Ensures safety of program areas and equipment	/////////	/////////
Summarizes occupational therapy departmental data as required to support departmental function and growth	/////////	/////////
Adheres to all department, agency, regulatory, and government policies and procedures	/////////	/////////
Participates in work-related meetings, as required	/////////	/////////
Provides in-service training	/////////	/////////
Obtains supervision from immediate supervisor to enhance own performance	/////////	/////////
Provides supervision to supervisees, as assigned	/////////	/////////
Manages department personnel, as assigned	/////////	/////////
Implements program evaluation	/////////	::::::::
Participates in accrediting reviews	/////////	/////////
Supervises fieldwork students and non-occupational therapy students, as assigned and according to pertinent regulations	/////////	/////////

VIII. Research

Research provides the basis and validation for both present and future practice. Participation in the research process, as either a consumer or an active researcher, is the responsibility of each OTR in the profession. Following establishment of service competency, COTAs may also participate in the research process through data collection.

////// Able to perform the task.	:::::: Able to perform the task only after demonstrating service competency.	##### Contributes to the process but does not complete the task independently.	Does not perform the task.

Research	OTR	COTA
Understands the importance of research	/////////	/////////
Understands research data	/////////	
Critiques research data	/////////	
Applies research to practice	/////////	
Incorporates research data into service provision process	/////////	
Identifies the need for research	/////////	
Designs research project	#########	
Collects research data	/////////	::::::::
Analyzes research data	::::::::	
Evaluates research results	::::::::	
Reports research results	::::::::	

Promotion of the Profession	OTR	COTA
Explains the purpose and value of the profession	/////////	/////////
Identifies the opportunities to explain the purpose and value of the profession	/////////	/////////
Participates in opportunities to explain the purpose of the profession	/////////	/////////
Serves as a representative of the profession to consumers, associates, and community groups	/////////	/////////
Participates in professional organizations	/////////	/////////

XI. Ethics

Ethical behavior through adherence to the "Occupational Therapy Code of Ethics" (AOTA, 1988a) is assumed. In certain states, adherence to a state code of ethics may be mandated by law. In those instances in which the practitioner does not possess adequate knowledge and skills for a given practice situation, ethical behavior mandates that appropriate consultation be obtained.

IX. Professional competence

Professional competence is attained through the process of self-directed learning and contributes to the development of clinical reasoning. It is the professional and ethical responsibility of each practitioner to continue one's professional growth through varied learning opportunities. Such opportunities may include formal continuing education programs, published materials, and collegial consultation. Consultation or a formal mentoring arrangement with content specialists may provide the entry-level practitioner with a more in-depth learning strategy.

Professional Competence	OTR	COTA
Identifies needs	/////////	/////////
Identifies resources	/////////	/////////
Selects appropriate options	/////////	/////////
Implements professional competence plan	/////////	/////////

X. Promotion of the profession

Promotion of the profession includes such activities as recruitment, public relations, marketing, advocacy, and participation in professional organizations at the local, state, or national level.

References

American Occupational Therapy Association. (1987). Roles of occupational therapists and occupational therapy assistants in schools. *American Journal of Occupational Therapy, 41,* 798–803.

American Occupational Therapy Association. (1988a). Occupational therapy code of ethics. *American Journal of Occupational Therapy, 42,* 795–796.

American Occupational Therapy Association. (1988b). *PATRA: The Professional and Technical Role Analysis Project—Final Report.* Rockville, MD: Author.

American Occupational Therapy Association. (1989a). Definition of occupational therapy for licensure. In *Policy manual of The American Occupational Therapy Association, Inc.* (Policy Number 5.3.1). Rockville, MD: Author. (Original work published 1981)

American Occupational Therapy Association. (1989b). Entry-level role delineation for OTRs and COTAs. In *Reference manual of the official documents of The American Occupational Therapy Association, Inc.* (pp. VI.1–VI.10). Rockville, MD: Author. (Original work published 1981)

American Occupational Therapy Association. (1989c). Essentials and guidelines of an accredited educational program for the occupational therapist. In *Reference manual of the official documents of The American Occupational Therapy Association, Inc.* (pp. II.1–II.5). Rockville, MD: Author. (Original work published 1983)

American Occupational Therapy Association. (1989d). Essentials and guidelines of an approved educational program for the occupational therapy assistant. In *Reference manual of the official documents of The American Occupational Therapy Association, Inc.* (pp. II.7–II.11). Rockville, MD: Author. (Original work published 1983)

| ///// | Able to perform the task. | ::::::: | Able to perform the task only after demonstrating service competency. | ###### | Contributes to the process but does not complete the task independently. | | Does not perform the task. |

Beery, K. (1967). *Beery Developmental Test of Visual–Motor Integration.* Chicago: Follett Educational Corporation.

Gardner, M. F. (1982). *Test of Visual–Perceptual Skills (Non-Motor) (TVPS).* (Available from Special Child Publications, J. B. Preston, Editor & Publisher, PO Box 33548, Seattle, WA 98133)

Related Readings

American Occupational Therapy Association. (1987). *Guidelines for occupational therapy services in school systems.* Rockville, MD: Author.

American Occupational Therapy Association. (1989). Guide for supervision of occupational therapy personnel. In *Reference manual of the official documents of The American Occupational Therapy Association, Inc.* (pp. VII.1–VII.2). Rockville, MD: Author. (Original work published 1981)

American Occupational Therapy Association. (1989). Occupational therapy product output reporting system and uniform terminology for reporting occupational therapy services. In *Reference manual of the official documents of The American Occupational Therapy Association, Inc.* (pp. VII.19–VII.29). Rockville, MD: Author. (Original work published 1978)

American Occupational Therapy Association. (1989). The philosophical base of occupational therapy. In *Policy manual of The American Occupational Therapy Association, Inc.* (Policy Number 1.11). Rockville, MD: Author. (Original work published 1979)

American Occupational Therapy Association. (1989). Standards of practice for occupational therapy [generic]. In *Reference manual of the official documents of The American Occupational Therapy Association, Inc.* (pp. IV.1–IV.3). Rockville, MD: Author. (Original work published 1983)

American Occupational Therapy Association. (1989). Statement of occupational therapy referral. In *Reference manual of the official documents of The American Occupational Therapy Association, Inc.* (p. VIII.1). Rockville, MD: Author. (Original work published 1980)

American Occupational Therapy Association. (1989). Uniform terminology for occupational therapy—second edition. *American Journal of Occupational Therapy, 43,* 808–815.

American Occupational Therapy Association. (1990). Supervision guidelines for certified occupational therapy assistants. *American Journal of Occupational Therapy, 44,* 1089–1090.

Definitions†

Independent living/daily living skills refer to the skill and performance of physical and psychological/emotional self-care, work, and play/leisure activities to a level of independence appropriate to age, life-space, and disability. Life-space refers to an individual's cultural background, value orientation, and physical and social environment.

Physical daily living skills refer to the skill and performance of daily personal care, with or without adaptive equipment. It includes but is not limited to:

Grooming and hygiene refer to the skill and performance of personal health needs, such as bathing, toileting, hair care, shaving, applying make-up.

Feeding/eating refers to the skill and performance of sequentially feeding oneself, including sucking, chewing, swallowing, and using appropriate utensils.

Dressing refers to the skill and performance of choosing appropriate clothing, dressing oneself in a sequential fashion, including fastening and adjusting clothing.

Functional mobility refers to the skill and performance in moving oneself from one position or place to another. It includes skills necessary for activities such as bed mobility, wheelchair mobility, transfers (bed, car, tub, toilet, chair), and functional ambulation, with or without adaptive aids. It also includes use of public and private travel systems, such as driving own automobile and using public transportation.

Functional communication refers to the skill and performance in using equipment or systems to enhance or provide communication, such as writing equipment, typewriters, letterboards, telephone, braille writers, artificial vocalization systems and computers.

Object manipulation refers to the skill and performance in handling large and small common objects, such as calculators, keys, money, light switches, doorknobs, and packages.

Psychological/emotional daily living skills refer to the skill and performance in developing one's self-concept/self-identity, coping with life situations, and participating in one's organizational and community environment. It includes but is not limited to:

Self-concept/self-identity refers to the cognitive image of one's functional self. This includes but is not limited to:

- clearly perceiving others' needs, feelings, conflicts, values, beliefs, expectations, sexuality, and power
- realistically perceiving others' needs, feelings, conflicts, values, beliefs, expectations, sexuality, and power
- knowing one's performance strengths and limitations
- sensing one's competence, achievement, self-esteem, and self-respect
- integrating new experiences with established self-concept/self-identity
- having a sense of psychological safety and security
- perceiving one's goals and directions.

Situational coping refers to skill and performance in handling stress and dealing with problems and changes in a manner that is functional for self and others. This includes but is not limited to:

- setting goals, selecting, harmonizing, and managing activities of daily living to promote optimal performance
- testing goals and perceptions against reality
- perceiving changes and need for changes in self and environment
- directing and redirecting energy to overcome problems
- initiating, implementing, and following through on decisions
- assuming responsibility for self and consequences of actions
- interacting with others, dyadic and group.

Community involvement refers to skill and performance in interacting within one's social system. This includes but is not limited to:

- understanding social norms and their impact on society
- planning, organizing, and executing daily life activities in relationship to society, including such activities as budgeting, time management, social role management and using community resources

---

† Approved by the AOTA Representative Assembly, March 1981.

- recognizing and responding to needs of families and groups
- understanding and responding to organizational/community role expectations as both recipient and contributor.

Work refers to skill and performance in participating in socially purposeful and productive activities. These activities may take place in the home, employment setting, school, or community. They include but are not limited to:

Homemaking refers to skill and performance in homemaking and home management tasks, such as meal planning, meal preparation and clean-up, laundry, cleaning, minor household repairs, shopping, and use of household safety principles.

Child care/parenting refers to skill and performance in child care activities and management. This includes but is not limited to physical care of children, and use of age-appropriate activities, communication, and behavior to facilitate child development.

Employment preparation refers to skill and performance in precursory job activities including prevocational activities. This includes but is not limited to:

- job acquisition skills and performance
- organizational and team participatory skills and performance
- work process skills and performance
- work product quality.

Play/leisure refers to skill and performance in choosing, performing, and engaging in activities for amusement, relaxation, spontaneous enjoyment, and/or self-expression. This includes but is not limited to:

- Recognizing one's specific needs, interests, and adaptations necessary for performance
- Identifying characteristics of activities and social situations that make them play for the individual
- Identifying activities that contain those characteristics
- Choosing play activities for participation, such as sports, games, hobbies, music, drama, and other activities
- Testing out and adapting activities to enable participation
- Identifying and using community resources.

Sensorimotor components refer to the skill and performance of patterns of sensory and motor behavior that are prerequisites to self-care, work, and play/leisure performance. The components in this section include neuromuscular and sensory integrative skills, including perceptual motor skills.

Neuromuscular refers to the skill and performance of motor aspects of behavior. This includes but is not limited to:

Reflex integration refers to skill and performance in enhancing and supporting functional neuromuscular development through eliciting and/or inhibiting stereotyped, patterned, and/or involuntary responses coordinated at subcortical and cortical levels.

Range of motion refers to skill and performance in using maximum span of joint movement in activities with and without assistance to enhance functional performance. The standard levels of performance include:

- active range of motion: movement by patient, unassisted through a complete range of motion
- passive range of motion: movement performed by someone other than patient or by a mechanical device, requiring no muscle contraction on the part of the patient
- active-assistive range of motion: movement performed by the patient to the limit of his/her ability, and then completed with assistance.

Gross and fine coordination refers to skill and performance in muscle control, coordination, and dexterity while participating in activities

- muscle control: skill and performance in directing muscle movement
- coordination: skill and performance in gross motor activities using several muscle groups
- dexterity: skill and performance in tasks using small muscle groups.

Strength and endurance refers to skill and performance in using muscular force within time periods necessary for purposeful task performance. This involves but is not limited to progressively building strength and cardiac and pulmonary reserve, increasing the length of work periods, and decreasing fatigue and strain.

Sensory integration refers to skill and performance in development and coordination of sensory input, motor output, and sensory feedback. This includes but is not limited to:

Sensory awareness refers to skill and performance in perceiving and differentiating external and internal stimuli, such as:

- tactile awareness: the perception and interpretation of stimuli through skin contact
- stereognosis: the identification of forms and nature of objects through the sense of touch
- kinesthesia: the conscious perception of muscular motion, weight, and position
- proprioceptive awareness: the identification of the positions of body parts in space
- ocular control: the localization and visual tracking of stimuli
- vestibular awareness: the detection of motion and gravitational pull as related to one's performance in functional activities, ambulation, and balance
- auditory awareness: the differentiation and identification of sounds
- gustatory awareness: the differentiation and identification of tastes
- olfactory awareness: the differentiation and identification of smells.

Visual-spatial awareness refers to skill and performance in perceiving distances between and relationships among objects, including self. This includes but is not limited to:

- figure-ground: recognition of forms and objects when presented in a configuration with competing stimuli
- form constancy: recognition of forms and objects as the same when presented in different contexts
- position in space: knowledge of one's position in space relative to other objects

Body integration refers to skill and performance in perceiving and regulating the position of various muscles and body parts in relationship to each other during static and movement states. This includes but is not limited to:

- body schema: the perception of one's physical self through proprioceptive and interoceptive sensations
- postural balance: skill and performance in developing and maintaining body posture while sitting, standing, or engaging in activity
- bilateral motor coordination: skill and performance in purposeful movement that requires interaction between both sides of the body in a smooth, refined manner
- right-left discrimination: skill and performance in differentiating right from left and vice versa
- visual-motor integration: skill and performance in combining visual input with purposeful voluntary movement of the hand and other body parts involved in an activity. Visual-motor integration includes eye-hand coordination
- crossing the midline: refers to skill and performance in crossing the vertical midline of the body
- praxis: refers to skill and performance of purposeful movement that involves motor planning.

Cognitive components refer to skill and performance of the mental processes necessary to know or apprehend by understanding. This includes but is not limited to:

Orientation refers to skill and performance in comprehending, defining, and adjusting oneself in an environment with regard to time, place, and person.

Conceptualization/comprehension refers to skill and performance in conceiving and understanding concepts or tasks such as color identification, word recognition, sign concepts, sequencing, matching, association, classification, and abstracting. This includes but is not limited to:

Concentration refers to skill and performance in focusing on a designated task or concept.

Attention span refers to skill and performance in focusing on a task or concept for a particular length of time.

Memory refers to skill and performance in retaining and recalling tasks or concepts from the past.

Cognitive integration refers to skill and performance in applying diverse knowledge to environmental situations. This involves but is not limited to:

Generalization refers to skill and performance in applying specific concepts to a variety of related situations.

Problem solving refers to skill and performance in identifying and organizing solutions to difficulties. It includes but is not limited to:

- defining or evaluating the problem
- organizing a plan
- making decisions/judgments
- implementing plan, including following through in logical sequence
- evaluating decision/judgment and plan.

Psychosocial components refer to skill and performances in self-management, dyadic and group interaction.

Self-management refers to skill and performance in expressing and controlling oneself in functional and creative activities.

Self-expression refers to skill and performance in perceiving one's feelings and interpreting and using a variety of communication signs and symbols. This includes but is not limited to:

- experiencing and recognizing a range of emotions
- having an adequate vocabulary
- having writing and speaking skills
- interpreting and using correctly an adequate range of nonverbal signs and symbols.

Self-control refers to skill and performance in modulating and modifying present behaviors, and in initiating new behaviors in accordance with situational demands. It includes but is not limited to:

- observing own and others' behavior
- conceptualizing problems in terms of needed behavioral changes or action
- imitating new behaviors
- directing and redirecting energies into stress-reducing activities and behaviors

Dyadic interaction refers to skill and performance in relating to another person. This includes but is not limited to:

- understanding social/culture norms of communication and interaction in various activity and social situations
- setting limits on self and others
- compromising and negotiating
- handling competition, frustration, anxiety, success, and failure
- cooperating and competing with others
- responsibly relying on self and others.

Group interaction refers to skill and performance in relating to groups of three to six persons, or larger. This includes but is not limited to:

- knowing and performing a variety of task and social/emotional role behaviors
- understanding common stages of group process
- participating in a group in a manner that is mutually beneficial to self and others.

Therapeutic adaptations refer to the design and/or restructuring of the physical environment to assist self-care, work, and play/leisure performance. This includes selecting, obtaining, fitting, and fabricating equipment, and instructing the client, family, and/or staff in proper use and care of equipment. It also includes minor repair and modification for correct fit, position or use. Categories of therapeutic adaptations consist of:

Orthotics refer to the provision of dynamic and static splints, braces, and slings, for the purpose of relieving pain, maintaining joint alignment, protecting joint integrity, improving function, and/or decreasing deformity.

Prosthetics refer to the training in use of artificial substitutes of missing body parts, which augment performance of function.

Assistive/adaptive equipment refers to the provision of special devices that assist in performance, and/or structural or positional changes such as the installation of ramps, bars, changes in furniture heights, adjustments of traffic patterns, and modifications of wheelchairs.

Prevention refers to skill and performance in minimizing debilitation. It may include programs for persons where predisposition to disability exists, as well as for those who have already incurred a disability. This includes but is not limited to:

Energy conservation refers to skill and performance in applying energy-saving procedures, activity restriction, work simplification, time management, and/or organization of the environment to minimize energy output.

Joint protection/body mechanics refers to skill and performance in applying principles or procedures to minimize stress on joints. Procedures may include the use of proper body mechanics, avoidance of static or deforming postures, and/or avoidance of excessive weight bearing.

Positioning refers to skill and performance in the placement of a body part in alignment to promote optimal functioning.

Coordination of daily living activities refers to skill and performance in selecting and coordinating activities of self-care, work, play/leisure, and rest to promote optimal performance of daily life tasks.

Reassessment refers to the process of obtaining and interpreting data necessary for updating treatment plans and goals. This frequently involves administering only portions of the initial evaluation, documenting results, and/or revising treatment.

Development of standards of quality treatment service refers to the development, implementation, evaluation, and documentation of departmental policy and procedures for the purpose of assuring standardized and quality treatment. This policy includes but is not limited to those procedures governing standards of occupational therapy practice, health, and safety, infection control, and ethical behavior.

Chart audit refers to the evaluation of documentation based on criteria developed within the facility, the profession, Health Systems Agency (Health Planning Act), and/or Professional Standards Review Organizations for a specified geographical area.

Occupational therapy care review refers to the ongoing evaluation and documentation of the quality of care given. Three review programs may be included in the care review process: preadmission screening, concurrent review, and retrospective studies.

Inservice education refers to the participation of regularly employed occupational therapy personnel (e.g., OTR, COTA, OT Aide, or OT orderly) in regularly scheduled classes, in-house seminars, and special training sessions, either in or outside the facility.

Accrediting reviews refer to those activities that are necessary to routinely document the meeting of the standards of a recognized accrediting body such as State Department of Health, Joint Commission on the Accreditation of Hospitals, Commission on Accreditation of Rehabilitation Facilities; or other accreditation procedures, voluntary or mandated by state or local law, and/or by the administration of a particular institution.

Role delineation glossary

1. *structured assessment:* an assessment instrument or form that is constructed and organized to provide guidelines for the content and process of the assessment: e.g., Interest Inventory.
2. *standardized assessment:* an assessment that provides for measurement against a criterion or norm. The assessment must be done according to the testing protocol; e.g., ROM assessment; Southern California Sensory Integration Tests.
3. *non-standardized assessment:* an assessment that provides information but with no precise comparison to a norm; e.g., Social History.
4. *therapeutic activities in occupational therapy:* self-care, work, home management, child care, educational, play/leisure, and cultural activities that have been selected and adapted to meet specific occupational therapy goals.
5. *significant others:* refers to persons, excluding the individual's family and health professionals, who have an important relationship to the individual.
6. *OT program:* refers to the delivery of occupational therapy services to a client.
7. *OT service:* refers to the organizational structure and system within which occupational therapy programs are provided.
8. *level I fieldwork:* is that which occurs as an integral part of didactic course work.

APPENDIX G

Hierarchy of competencies relating to the use of standardized instruments and evaluation techniques by occupational therapists[*]

This hierarchy of competencies has been developed by the AOTA/AOTF Committee on Standardized Assessments/Evaluations in an effort to establish the range of knowledge and skills required of occupational therapists. The hierarchy is intended to provide guidance for educators in the preparation of scholarly practitioners at several levels of practice.

Responding to a charge from the Representative Assembly to design a plan for the development of standardized evaluations for use by occupational therapists, the committee recognized as a first step the need for some agreement across the profession as to the scope and nature of the competencies required in assessment and evaluation. This proposed hierarchy represents the committee's efforts to obtain agreement regarding this aspect of practice.

By definition, items at the beginning (or lower level) of a hierarchy are implied as necessary for later (or higher) level

* Rescinded by the AOTA Representative Assembly in March 1992. Included here for educational purposes only.

functions. Thus, all members of a profession must demonstrate each Basic Competency, in each aspect of practice.

Entry-level competencies of the COTA may be presumed as competencies of the entry-level OTR, and so forth. Higher-level competencies are built on and incorporate the lower-level competencies which precede them. Higher-level competencies may be acquired through practice and experience, or through advanced education. Some competencies at Level IV, and all at Level V, would require advanced education.

Terminology for assessment competencies

Assessment: refers to the process of determining the need for, nature of, and estimated time of treatment, as well as determining the needed coordination with other persons involved (AOTA, 1979).

Clinical reasoning: the process of systematic decision-making based on an identifiable professional frame of reference and utilizing both subjective and objective data accrued through appropriate assessment/evaluation processes.

Entry-level competencies: minimal competence acceptable upon completion of technical or professional education program.

Evaluation: refers to the process of obtaining and interpreting data necessary for treatment. This includes planning for and documenting the evaluation process and results. These data may be gathered through record review, observations, questioning, and testing. Such procedures include but are not limited to the use of standardized tests, performance checklists, interviews, and activities, and tasks designed to evaluate specific performance abilities. Categories of occupational therapy evaluation include independent daily living skills and performance, and their components (AOTA, 1979).

Hierarchy: the basic hierarchical scheme used in this document is the level of professional competence required by the COTA and the OTR.

Instrument: a device for recording or measuring; especially such a device functioning as a control system.

Norms: a standard, a model, or pattern for a specific group; an expected type of performance or behavior for a particular reference group of persons.

Objective: facts or findings which are clearly observable to and verifiable by others, as reflecting reality.

Reliable: the degree to which a test's results may be expected to be consistent.

Standardized: made standard or uniform; to be used without variation; suggests an invariable way in which a test is to be used, as well as denoting the extent to which the results of the test may be considered to be both valid and reliable.

Subjective: an observation not rigidly reflecting measurable reality; may imply observer bias; may not be verifiable by others in the same situation.

Valid: the degree to which a test's results are actually measures of the characteristics it claims to measure.

I. Basic competencies in assessment

A. recognizes the importance of using standardized, reliable, and valid instruments whenever such are appropriate.

B. distinguishes between subjective and objective data, and uses each accordingly.

C. distinguishes the critical differences between standardized and nonstandardized instruments.

D. recognizes the need to use standardized instruments according to the instructions given in the test administration manual.

E. recognizes that using standardized instruments in an unstandardized (or adapted) manner may result in an invalid assessment.

F. recognizes that specialized training may be necessary to administer certain instruments correctly and to interpret the data appropriately.

G. uses assessment data to document work with client so as to provide a logical, continuous record of performance, therapeutic goals and media, and outcomes.

H. follows ethical practices in the use of assessments: recognition of copyright, protection of the security of tests, protection of the confidentiality of test results, use of assessments for which one's education and experience is sufficient.

II. Entry-level competencies, technical education

A. uses a structured interview format as directed by the OTR to elicit background information on family history, self-care function, and leisure interests and experiences.

B. administers other structured instruments as supervised by the OTR.

C. combines information collected through assessment procedures with standards of customary practice and collaborates with the OTR to develop a treatment plan for the client.

D. informs OTR supervisor when client performance seems to indicate need for reassessment or evaluation.

III. Entry-level competencies, professional education

A. identifies available instruments in one's area of practice.

B. identifies behavioral dimension measured by specific instruments.

C. interprets information on reliability, validity, and norms of instruments used.

D. selects instruments based on a clinical/theoretical rationale for their use.

E. identifies areas of practice where instrument development is needed.

F. administers and interprets standardized and other instruments which assess the client's occupational performance and performance components with relation to the given environment.

G. identifies need for further specific assessment of function.

H. integrates data from assessments to formulate a treatment plan using principles derived from theory to show coherence between findings and treatment goals and media.

I. recognizes the need for reassessment or evaluation of client performance.

J. supervises assessments and evaluations done by a COTA in conformance with state and federal laws and regulations.

IV. Advanced-level competencies

A. critiques existing instruments on the basis of reliability, validity, norms, and relationship to theory in occupational therapy.

B. contributes to the development, field testing, and dissemination of instruments clearly linked to theory in occupational therapy.

C. obtains specialized training to use instruments critical to one's area of practice.

V. Scholarly research competencies

A. designs new instruments in accordance with principles of instrument development, and plans research to field tests and standardize the instrument.

B. obtains funding for the development of a new instrument.

C. articulates the need for such an instrument and the rationale for its design so as to increase proper use of it within the profession.

D. designs research linking assessments/evaluations to theory development in occupational therapy.

References

American heritage dictionary of the English language, new college edition (1976). Boston: Houghton Mifflin.

American Occupational Therapy Association (1979). *Uniform terminology for reporting occupational therapy services.* Rockville, MD: Author. Approved by the AOTA Representative Assembly, March 1979

INDEX

Page numbers followed by *f* indicate figures; those followed by *t* indicate tabular material.